MASTERING MEDICINE
MRCP
MADE EASY

Mastering Medicine
MRCP
Made Easy

Archith Boloor MD
Associate Professor
Department of Medicine
Kasturba Medical College, Mangaluru
Manipal Academy of Higher Education
Karnataka, India
(archithb@gmail.com)

Foreword
Gurpreet S Wander MD DM
Professor and Head
Department of Cardiology
Hero DMC Heart Institute
Dayanand Medical College and Hospital
Ludhiana, Punjab, India

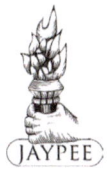

JAYPEE BROTHERS MEDICAL PUBLISHERS
The Health Sciences Publisher
New Delhi | London

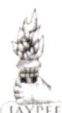 **Jaypee Brothers Medical Publishers (P) Ltd**

Headquarters

Jaypee Brothers Medical Publishers (P) Ltd
4838/24, Ansari Road, Daryaganj
New Delhi 110 002, India
Phone: +91-11-43574357
Fax: +91-11-43574314
Email: jaypee@jaypeebrothers.com

Overseas Office

J.P. Medical Ltd
83 Victoria Street, London
SW1H 0HW (UK)
Phone: +44 20 3170 8910
Fax: +44 (0)20 3008 6180
Email: info@jpmedpub.com

Website: www.jaypeebrothers.com
Website: www.jaypeedigital.com

© 2021, Jaypee Brothers Medical Publishers

The views and opinions expressed in this book are solely those of the original contributor(s)/author(s) and do not necessarily represent those of editor(s) of the book.

All rights reserved. No part of this publication may be reproduced, stored or transmitted in any form or by any means, electronic, mechanical, photocopying, recording or otherwise, without the prior permission in writing of the publishers.

All brand names and product names used in this book are trade names, service marks, trademarks or registered trademarks of their respective owners. The publisher is not associated with any product or vendor mentioned in this book.

Medical knowledge and practice change constantly. This book is designed to provide accurate, authoritative information about the subject matter in question. However, readers are advised to check the most current information available on procedures included and check information from the manufacturer of each product to be administered, to verify the recommended dose, formula, method and duration of administration, adverse effects and contraindications. It is the responsibility of the practitioner to take all appropriate safety precautions. Neither the publisher nor the author(s)/editor(s) assume any liability for any injury and/or damage to persons or property arising from or related to use of material in this book.

This book is sold on the understanding that the publisher is not engaged in providing professional medical services. If such advice or services are required, the services of a competent medical professional should be sought.

Every effort has been made where necessary to contact holders of copyright to obtain permission to reproduce copyright material. If any have been inadvertently overlooked, the publisher will be pleased to make the necessary arrangements at the first opportunity. The **CD/DVD-ROM** (if any) provided in the sealed envelope with this book is complimentary and free of cost. **Not meant for sale.**

Inquiries for bulk sales may be solicited at: jaypee@jaypeebrothers.com

Mastering Medicine: MRCP Made Easy

First Edition: **2021,** Reprint: 2024

ISBN: 978-93-90020-74-4

Printed at Repro India Limited

Dedication

Dedicated to all of my professors, my students and my patients who taught me that the real learning, in both medicine and life, exists beyond books.

CONTRIBUTORS

Sheetal Raj M MD
Associate Professor
Department of Internal Medicine and
Programme Director – Geriatric Medicine
Fellowship
Kasturba Medical College, Mangaluru
Manipal Academy of Higher Education
Mangaluru, Karnataka, India

Madhav H Hande MD
Senior Resident
Department of Internal Medicine
Kasturba Medical College, Manipal
Manipal Academy of Higher Education
Manipal, Karnataka, India

Anudeep Padakanti MD
Department of Internal Medicine
Kasturba Medical College, Mangaluru
Manipal Academy of Higher Education
Mangaluru, Karnataka, India

Ashwini MV
Resident, Department of Internal Medicine
Kasturba Medical College, Mangaluru
Manipal Academy of Higher Education
Mangaluru, Karnataka, India

Mohammed Shaheen
Department of Internal Medicine
Kasturba Medical College, Mangaluru
Manipal Academy of Higher Education
Mangaluru, Karnataka, India

Aditya S Narayan
Department of Internal Medicine
Kasturba Medical College, Mangaluru
Manipal Academy of Higher Education
Mangaluru, Karnataka, India

Nikhil Kenny Thomas MD
Senior Resident
Department of Gastroenterology
PSG Institute of Medical Sciences
and Research
Coimbatore, Tamil Nadu, India

Abu Thajudeen MD
Department of Internal Medicine
Kasturba Medical College, Mangaluru
Manipal Academy of Higher Education
Mangaluru, Karnataka, India

Vivek K Koushik MD
Senior Resident
Department of Internal Medicine
ESIC Medical College and PGIMSR
Chennai, Tamil Nadu, India

Ishika Mahajan
Department of Internal Medicine
Kasturba Medical College, Mangaluru
Manipal Academy of Higher Education
Mangaluru, Karnataka, India

Mohamed Faizan Thouseef
Resident
Department of Internal Medicine
JN Medical College
KLE Academy of Higher Education
and Research
Belgaum, Karnataka, India

FOREWORD

*"Learning gives creativity,
Creativity leads to thinking,
Thinking leads to knowledge,
Knowledge makes you great."*

—APJ Abdul Kalam

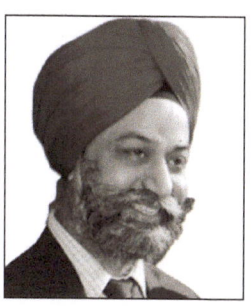

We are happy to bring you the course manual for cracking the MRCP examination. The manual has been titled appropriately as *"Mastering Medicine: MRCP Made Easy"*. This more than 600 pages manual has been written by the author Archith Boloor keeping the pattern of MRCP course in mind. The 30 chapters chosen by the author cover the entire course of medicine with emphasis on the aspects which will help in solving the MCQs for this examination. Each chapter has a text section which covers the topic in an abbreviated manner. The text is in the form of points. He has avoided long sentences and descriptions so as to make it, easy to read. There are some cases also which have been created for better understanding and developing case oriented learning.

The salient features of this book are multiple graphs, tables, algorithms and figures. There are many comparative tables which will help you understand the subject and then remember it. By going through this manual you will develop a wide knowledge of the various subspecialties of medicine. The author has covered all the topics with emphasis on basic understanding. I would recommend you to first read the text of each chapter and only then solve the questions. Each chapter has many best of five type questions with one correct answer. It is in the same pattern as the MRCP examination. Take it as an exercise and solve the questions on your own, without looking at the answers. See how many you have answered correctly and then spend time on the ones which were answered incorrect. The answers to all the questions are available in the preceding text and the tables. This book will not only help you to crack the examination but will also help subsequently in the practice of medicine. As in the MRCP examination, some of the questions are information based and others are to judge your ability to solve clinical challenges. The MRCP examination and the British system follow the NICE guidelines which you should look at, besides this detailed and extensive manual. I am sure you will enjoy reading it, since the language is simple and understandable. I congratulate Dr Archith Boloor for this mammoth effort and for bringing all this information in a comprehensive manner. The Jaypee Brothers Medical Publishers (P) Ltd., has done a great job by making the text readable. The vision of Mr Jitendar P Vij to bring the best information for the medical fraternity is unique and remarkable. He is aided by a very efficient staff including Dr Richa Saxena who has worked hard for putting this project in place. The graphs and tables have been produced very nicely. I wish all the readers a very good luck for the examination and congratulate the author and the publisher for this manual, a first of its kind.

Gurpreet S Wander

PREFACE

As a clinician, an academician and a doctor, a large part of my life revolves around questions. I get concerned questions from my patients. I get plenty of questions from their relatives, some irritating as well (even though I probably should not admit that). I get questions from my family, my neighbours, the mailman and even his wife. And lest I forget, my students: They challenge me, provoke me, prick me and prod me until I finally have questions of my own. Your clinical acumen, your compassion and your worth as a doctor are amplified a thousand-fold by the clarity with which you answer what is asked. When I sat down to write this book, I was faced with the difficult task of compiling years of medical training and experience into a capsule that can help you do the one thing that none of my early training taught me—the ability to understand, analyse and answer a question. *Mastering Medicine: MRCP Made Easy* is your handy, concise and comprehensive cheatbook to developing a skill that would otherwise take years to hone.

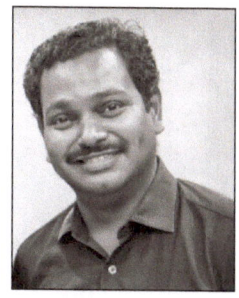

The Membership of the Royal College of Physicians (MRCP) exam is known to be a gruelling war between the internal medicine aspirant and two, huge chunks of paper carrying 100 multiple choice questions (MCQs) each. I would go one step further and claim that it is a bit more challenging for a South Asian doctor to understand the proclivities of infections, autoimmune conditions and other cases. What is common for us is not what is commonly asked. What is commonly asked may not be what is commonly encountered. In every aspect possible, our demographic and our perception of this demographic are different. With this book, I have made a humble effort to bridge that difference with the universal language of medical science. The one thing that does not change, no matter what corner of the world you wish to practice medicine in, is your understanding of it.

Mastering Medicine: MRCP Made Easy covers all known facets of medicine in exquisite detail. Subspecialties, superspecialties and important parts of allied specialties have all made their way into this book. A lot of my colleagues, peers and even students have very graciously contributed their own 'trade secrets' for me to add on in so many sections. As a student, I was and always will be a very visual-tactile learner. So it is only natural that as an author, that too has crept into this book in the form of lists and tables and high-yield concepts and treatment protocols. The way I see it, *Mastering Medicine: MRCP Made Easy* is a book that can fully stand the test of time, holding your hand while you walk into the exam hall, helping you during those 6 hours and continuing to do so long after you have cleared the exam with flying colours.

Every suggestion, recommendation and criticism are welcome. Always: because ultimately, this is a book that caters to you, the reader and the many, many questions that you may have asked while learning medicine. One of them being—'How can I crack the MRCP?'

After years of experience, after understanding and analysing that question: This book is my answer.

Archith Boloor

ACKNOWLEDGEMENTS

Writing a book is much harder than what I thought and much more rewarding than I could have ever imagined. None of this would have been possible without the help of my family, my mentors and my friends.

I thank Dr Sheetal Raj, Dr Anudeep Padakanti, Dr Nikhil Kenny Thomas, Dr Vivek K Koushik and Dr Abu Thajudeen for their constant encouragement and support.

I convey my sincere thanks to Mr Jitendar P Vij (Group Chairman) for offering me this project.

I also thank Dr Richa Saxena (Associate Director – Professional Publishing), Dr Kanav Midha, Dr Nidhi Sood and Prerna Bajaj of M/s Jaypee Brothers Medical Publishers (P) Ltd., New Delhi, India, for their help in formatting and well-received technical assistance. They are responsible for this book to get its form.

To everyone at Jaypee who encouraged me to write, I am honoured to be a part of your team and thank you for helping doctors and authors like me turn their ideas into books.

Special thanks to Dr Ashwini MV, Dr Madhav H Hande, Dr Aditya S Narayan, Dr Mohammed Shaheen, Dr Mohamed Faizan Thouseef and Dr Ishika Mahajan for contributing sections and helping in proofreading and editing.

I am grateful to my department, my college Kasturba Medical College, Mangaluru, and my university, Manipal Academy of Higher Education (MAHE), Manipal, Karnataka, India, for making me what I am today.

Last but not the least, I would also like to express my sincere gratitude to Dr Gurpreet S Wander for sparing time from his busy schedule and contributing his valuable feedback for the book in form of Foreword.

I am thankful to my family—my mom and my sisters—for always being the persons who sustained me in ways that I never knew that I needed and to my niece Ananya and nephew Aaryan—thank you for all the love. I am equally thankful to my great friends and students who have made my existence meaningful. I am very grateful to have you all in my life.

A very special gratitude goes out to all my Teachers, who are solely responsible for what I am today and for having ignited the passion of teaching in me.

Lastly, I thank to Mother Goddess for guiding me through my life and helping me understand the purpose of my existence. I pray to her for a better and a safer tomorrow for the generations to come.

Archith Boloor

CONTENTS

1. **Common Symptoms and Presentations** — 1
   Aditya S Narayan
2. **Emergencies in Medical Practice** — 9
   Madhav H Hande
3. **Cardiology** — 34
   Archith Boloor
4. **Diseases of the Gastrointestinal System** — 77
   Nikhil Kenny Thomas
5. **Hepatobiliary Disorders** — 102
   Nikhil Kenny Thomas
6. **Pancreatic Disorders** — 163
   Nikhil Kenny Thomas
7. **Endocrinology** — 171
   Mohamed Faizan Thouseef
8. **Diabetes Mellitus** — 187
   Mohamed Faizan Thouseef
9. **Rheumatology and Connective Tissue Disorder Diseases** — 208
   Archith Boloor
10. **Nephrology** — 226
    Madhav H Hande
11. **Haematology** — 248
    Archith Boloor
12. **Pulmonology** — 321
    Ashwini MV
13. **Infectious Diseases** — 371
    Abu Thajudeen
14. **HIV Infection and AIDS** — 398
    Abu Thajudeen
15. **Sexually Transmitted Diseases** — 422
    Abu Thajudeen

16.	Diseases of the Nervous System *Vivek K Koushik*	433
17.	Nutrition and Metabolism *Ashwini MV*	470
18.	Psychiatry *Vivek K Koushik*	481
19.	Fluid, Electrolytes and Acid-base Disorders *Madhav H Hande*	498
20.	Dermatology *Archith Boloor*	510
21.	Immunological Factors in Disease *Anudeep Padakanti*	529
22.	Maternal Medicine *Mohammed Shaheen*	542
23.	Environmental Medicine *Mohammed Shaheen*	551
24.	Toxicology *Mohammed Shaheen*	558
25.	Oncology *Anudeep Padakanti*	568
26.	Geriatric Medicine *Sheetal Raj M*	581
27.	Medical Genetics *Ishika Mahajan*	591
28.	Epidemiology *Ishika Mahajan*	602
29.	Clinical Pharmacology *Ishika Mahajan*	610
30.	ECG Interpretation *Archith Boloor*	617
	Index	643

PLATE 1

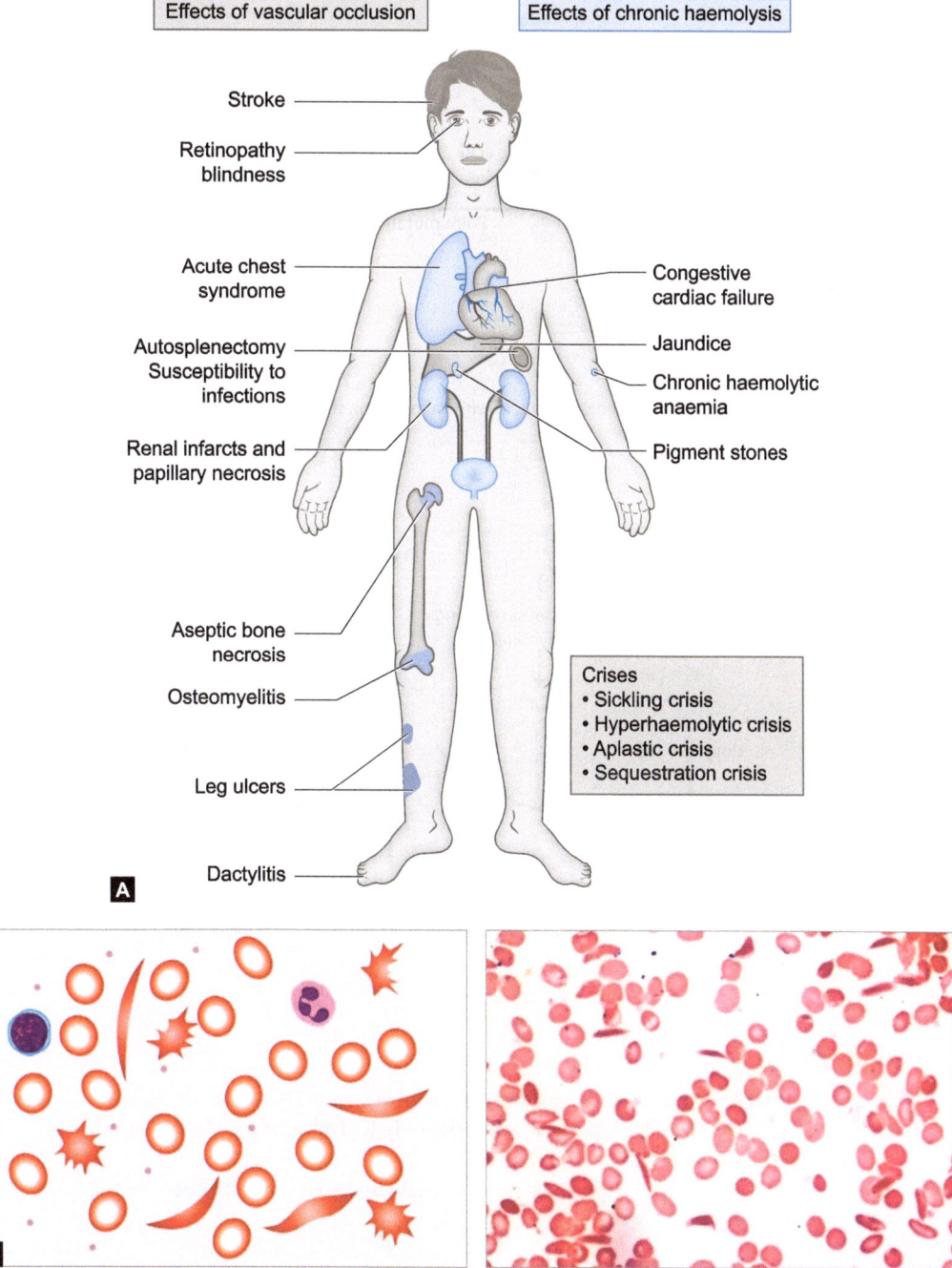

Fig. 11.2A to C:

Continued

PLATE 2

Continued

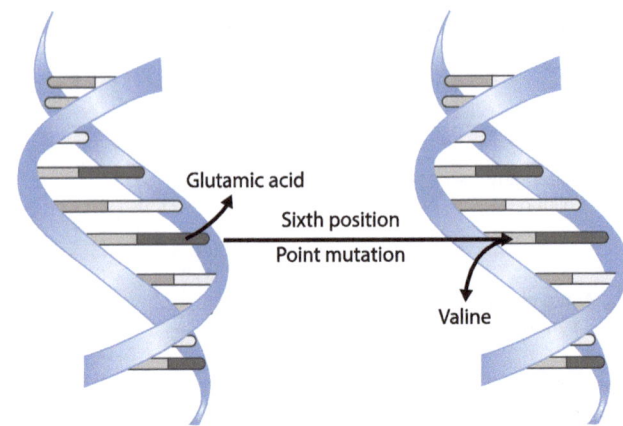

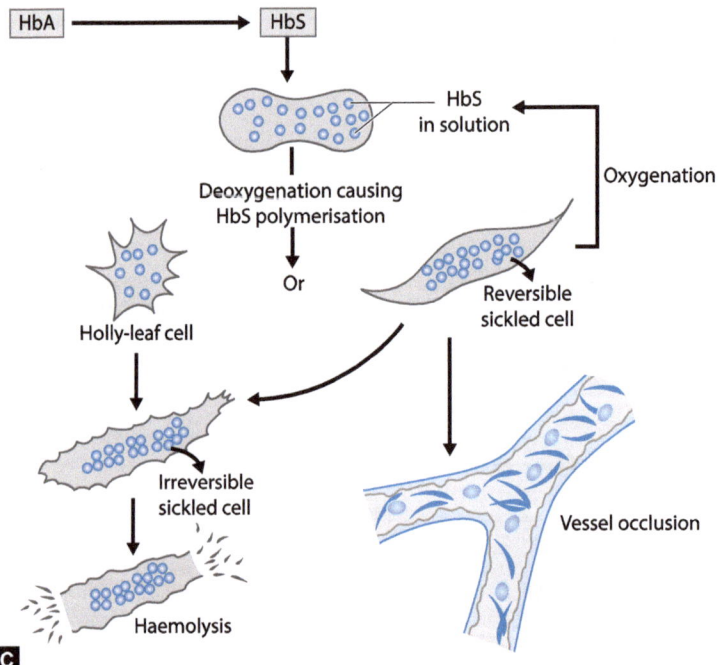

Fig. 11.2A to C: (A) Various effects of vascular occlusion and haemolysis in sickle-cell anaemia; (B) Peripheral smear with sickle cells; (C) Pathogenesis of sickle-cell anaemia. *(Chapter 11)*

Courtesy: Exam Preparatory Manual for Undergradates—Medicine/Archith Boloor and Ramadas Nayak, 2nd edition.

PLATE 3

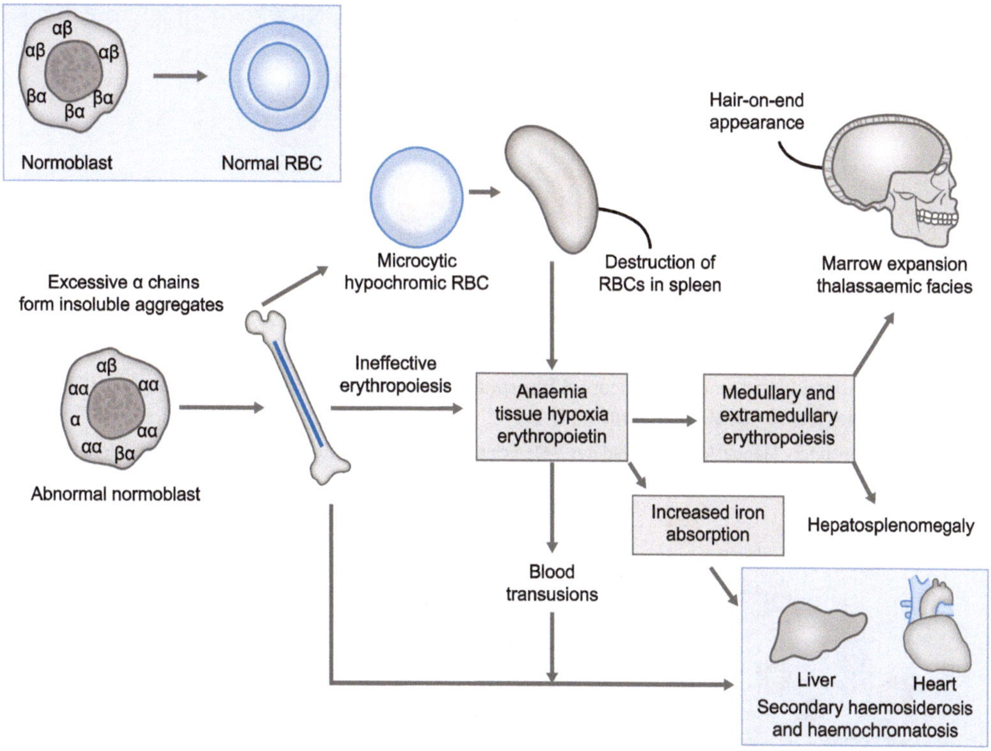

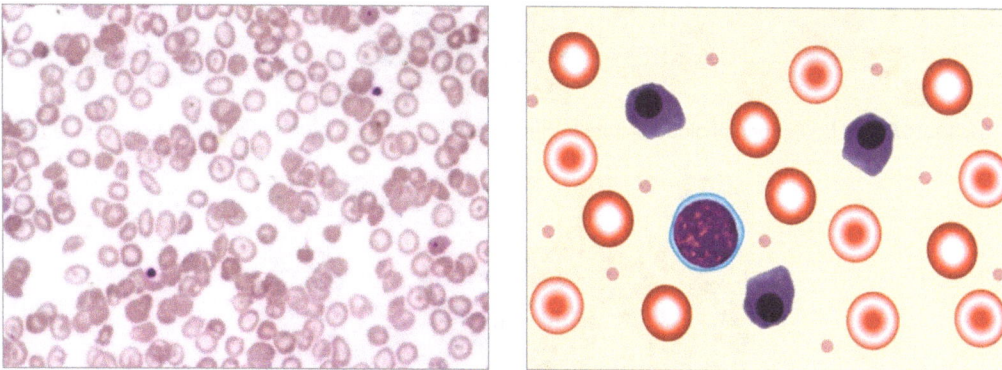

Peripheral blood smear in β-thalassaemia showing target cells and nucleated red cells.

(RBC: red blood cells)

Fig. 11.3: Pathogenesis of β-thalassaemia major and its consequences as well as peripheral blood smear in β-thalassaemia showing target cells and nucleated red cells. *(Chapter 11)*
Courtesy: Exam Preparatory Manual for Undergradates—Medicine/Archith Boloor and Ramadas Nayak, 2nd edition.

PLATE 4

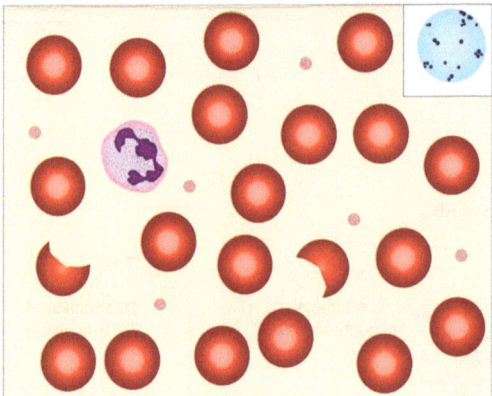

Fig. 11.4: Peripheral blood smear in glucose-6-phosphate dehydrogenase (G6PD) deficiency with "bite cells". Inset: Heinz bodies (supravital stain). *(Chapter 11)*

Courtesy: Exam Preparatory Manual for Undergradates—Medicine/Archith Boloor and Ramadas Nayak, 2nd edition.

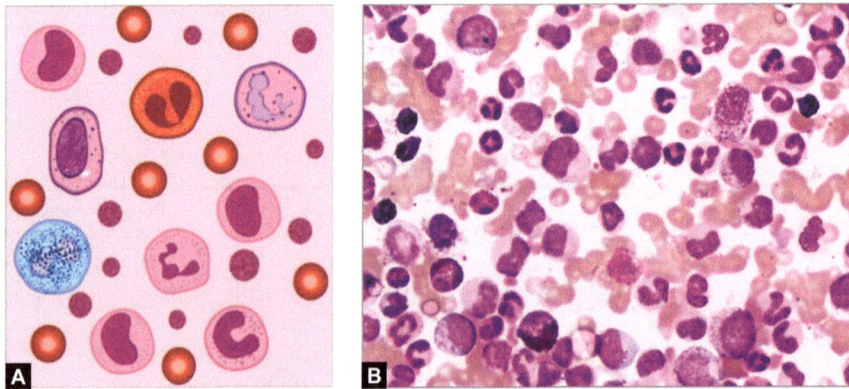

Figs. 11.10A and B: Peripheral blood picture in chronic stable phase of chronic myeloid leukaemia. *(Chapter 11)*

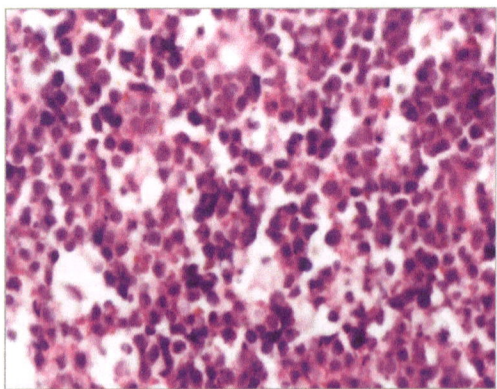

Fig. 11.12: Burkitt lymphoma composed of medium-sized lymphoid cells admixed with benign macrophages giving a "starry sky" appearance. *(Chapter 11)*

Courtesy: Exam Preparatory Manual for Undergradates—Medicine/Archith Boloor and Ramadas Nayak, 2nd edition.

PLATE 5

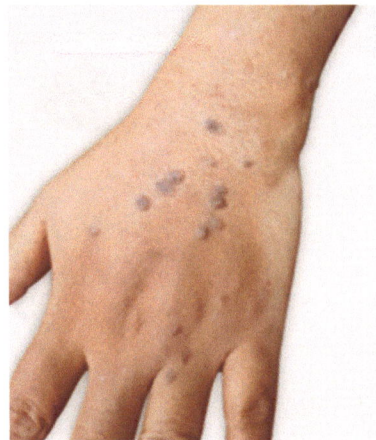

(Chapter 20, Best of Fives, Q.5)

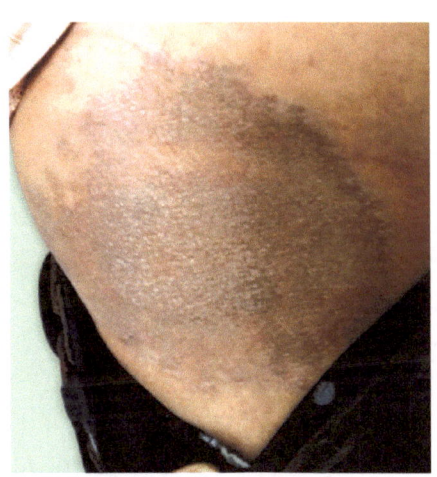 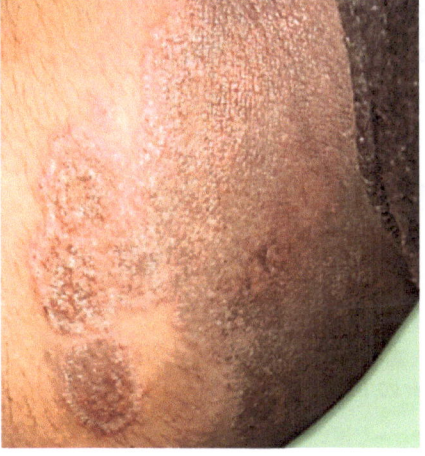

(Chapter 20, Best of Fives, Q.6)

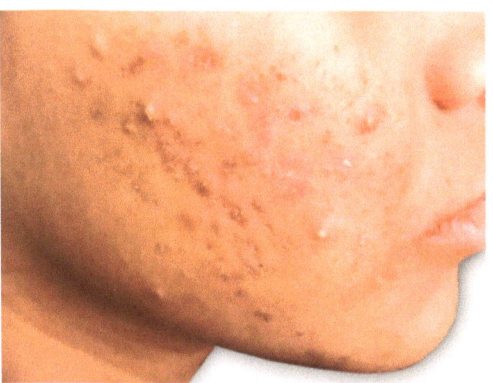

(Chapter 20, Best of Fives, Q.7)

PLATE 6

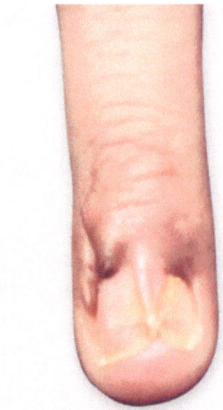

(Chapter 20, Best of Fives, Q.8)

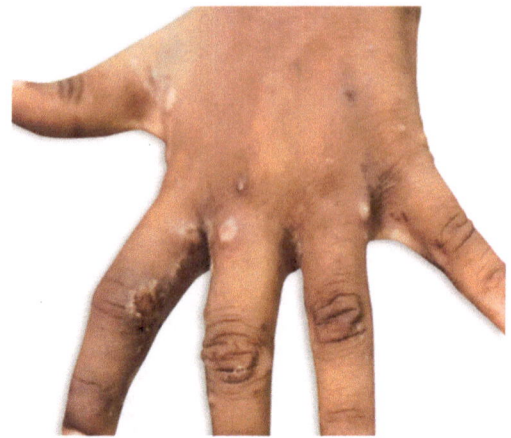

(Chapter 20, Best of Fives, Q.13)

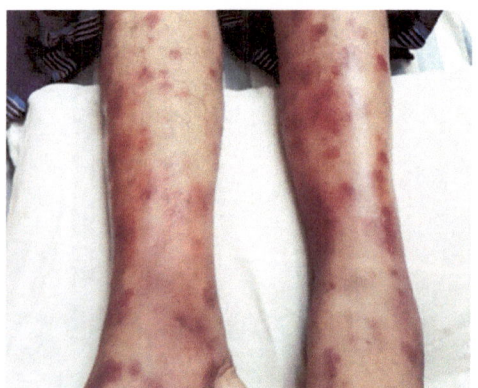

(Chapter 20, Best of Fives, Q.11)

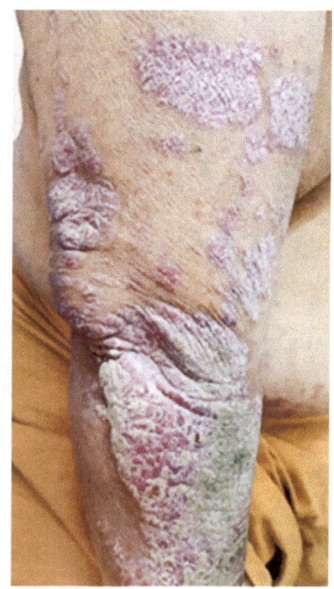

(Chapter 20, Best of Fives, Q.14)

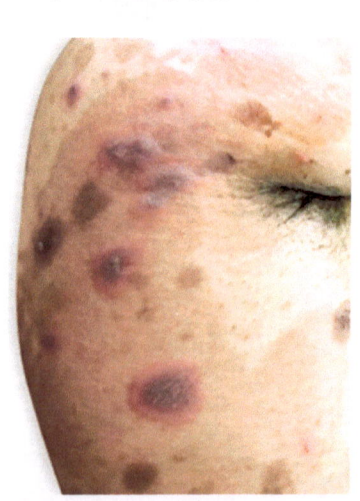

(Chapter 20, Best of Fives, Q.12)

CHAPTER 1

Common Symptoms and Presentations

Aditya Narayan

Symptoms	Causes

Abdominal pain	- Surgical causes: Acute appendicitis, intestinal obstruction, acute cholecystitis, mesenteric ischaemia
	- Non-surgical
	  ○ Gastrointestinal tract (GIT): Acute gastroenteritis, acute hepatitis
	  ○ Renal: Renal colic, ureteric colic
	  ○ Systemic diabetic ketoacidosis (DKA), acute intermittent porphyria

Acute back pain	- Local causes: Spondylolisthesis, spondylitis, muscle spasm - Referred pain: Renal colic, aortic dissection - Systemic causes: Vertebral metastasis as in breast, prostate, myeloma
Blackout/Collapse	- Syncope - Ischaemic: Transient ischaemic attack (TIA), stroke - Central nervous system (CNS): Seizure (Atonic) - Cardiovascular system (CVS): Stokes–Adams attack - Ear, nose and throat (ENT): Drop attacks in Ménière's disease

Breathlessness	- Acute
	  ○ Respiratory: Acute severe asthma, acute exacerbation of chronic obstructive pulmonary disease (COPD), pulmonary embolism, pulmonary infarct, pneumonia, acute respiratory distress syndrome (ARDS)
	  ○ Cardiac: Acute coronary syndrome
	  ○ Psychiatric: Panic attacks
	- Chronic
	  ○ Respiratory: COPD, interstitial lung disease (ILD), bronchogenic carcinoma, pleural effusion, empyema
	  ○ Cardiac: Cor pulmonale, left heart failure

Chest pain	- Cardiac: Acute coronary syndrome (ACS), myocarditis, pericarditis, aortic dissection - Musculoskeletal: Rib fracture, Tietze syndrome - Respiratory: Pleuritic chest pain - GIT: Gastroesophageal reflux disease (GERD), oesophageal motility disorders
Confusion/Delirium	- Metabolic: Electrolyte imbalance, uraemia, hepatic encephalopathy - Toxin: Alcohol, cannabis - Head injury - Substance withdrawal - Infections: Septic encephalopathy

Continued

Continued

Symptoms	Causes

Cough	- Respiratory:
	  - Parenchyma: Pneumonia, ARDS, emphysema, chronic bronchitis, lung abscess
	  - Interstitial: Pneumoconiosis, ILD
	  - Airways: Chronic bronchitis, asthma, bronchiectasis, foreign body
	- Cardiac: Left heart failure causing pulmonary oedema
	- GIT: GERD

Diarrhoea	- Osmotic diarrhoea - Secretory diarrhoea - Infective diarrhoea
Falls	- Vestibular: Labyrinthitis, vestibular neuronitis, Ménière's disease - Cerebellar: Ataxia - Cortical blindness: Anton syndrome - Elderly
Fever	- Infective: Abscess, pneumonia, meningitis, gastroenteritis - Malignancy: Leukaemia, lymphoma - Autoimmune: Systemic lupus erythematosus (SLE), Still's disease, vasculitis - Head injury: Hypothalamic dysfunction - Malignant hyperthermia
Fits/Seizures	- Metabolic: Hyponatraemia, uraemia, hepatic encephalopathy - CNS: Seizure disorders, meningitis, encephalitis, intracranial space occupying lesion (ICSOL) - Substance withdrawal: Alcohol (delirium tremens) - Septic encephalopathy, febrile seizures
Haematemesis/ Melaena	- Oesophagus: Carcinoma, ulcers secondary to caustic injury, varices - Stomach: Peptic ulcer disease, gastric cancer, gastric antral vascular ectasia, Dieulafoy's lesion
Headache	- Primary headaches: Tension, migraine, trigeminal autonomic cephalgias—cluster headache, SUNCT - Secondary headache: Systemic infections, head injury, vascular disorders, haemorrhage, brain tumours
Jaundice	- Prehepatic: Haemolytic anaemia, Crigler–Najjar, Gilbert - Hepatic: Viral hepatitis, alcoholic hepatitis, primary sclerosing cholangitis (PSC), Rotor syndrome, Dubin–Johnson syndrome - Post-hepatic: Choledocholithiasis, oriental cholangiopathies, periampullary carcinoma
Limb pain/Swelling	- Traumatic: Fractures, compartment syndrome - Infective: Cellulitis, necrotising fasciitis, lymphangitis, filariasis
Palpitations	- Arrhythmias: Ectopics, atrial fibrillations, atrial flutter, paroxysmal supraventricular tachycardia (PSVT), ventricular tachycardia (VT) - Endocrine: Hyperthyroidism, phaeochromocytoma - Psychiatric: Generalised anxiety disorder, panic attack - Substance withdrawal

Continued

Continued

Symptoms	Causes
Poisons	- Corrosive poisons: Hydrochloric (HCl), Alkalis - Non-metallic poisons: Phosphorus, iodide - Metallic poisons: Mercury, lead, arsenic - Agricultural poisons: Organophosphate (OP) poisoning, insecticide - Somniferous poisons: Opium, heroin, cocaine - Cardiac poisons
Rash	Based on morphology - Macular - Papular - Plaque Based on aetiology - Infective: Measles, varicella, rubella - Autoimmune: SLE, rheumatoid arthritis (RA) - Malignancy
Vomiting	- GIT: Gastroenteritis, GERD - CNS: Meningitis, encephalitis, raised intracranial pressure (ICP) - Rating disorders: Anorexia nervosa - Substance abuse

Weakness/Paralysis	- Upper motor neuron (UMN) paralysis: Stroke, cerebral palsy, ICSOL
	- Lower motor neuron (LMN) paralysis:
	  ○ Anterior horn cell disorder
	  ○ Nerve: Polio botulism
	  ○ Muscle: Myasthaenia, muscular dystrophies

Hepatosplenomegaly	- Infective: Malaria, kala azar, hydatid cyst, amoebic liver abscess - Congestive: Heart failure, cardiomyopathy - Malignancy: Leukaemia, lymphoma, multiple myeloma - Anaemia: Immune haemolytic anaemias, hereditary spherocytosis, thalassaemia - Storage disorders: Niemann–Pick, Gaucher, mucopolysaccharidosis (MPS)

Constipation	- Organic
	  ○ GIT: Diverticulitis, intestinal obstruction
	  ○ Neurological: Spinal cord disease, autonomic dysfunction
	  ○ Endocrine: Hypothyroidism
	  ○ Metabolic causes: Uraemia, hyponatraemia, hypokalaemia
	- Functional: Low fibre diet, slow peristalsis
	- Drug induced: Anticholinergic, opioids, antibiotics, antipsychiatry

Paraesthesia (Numbness)	- Anatomic: Nerve entrapment, sciatica - Metabolic: Diabetes, thyroid disease, chronic liver disease (CLD), chronic kidney disease (CKD) - Toxic: Heavy metal poisoning - Vitamin deficiencies: B12, thiamine, pyridoxine - Drugs: Amiodarone, isoniazid, digoxin

Continued

Continued

Symptoms	Causes
Spontaneous bleeding	• Thrombocytopaenia 　◦ Infection: Dengue, malaria 　◦ Autoimmune: Immune thrombocytopaenic purpura (ITP) 　◦ Microangiopathic haemolytic anaemia (MAHA): Haemolytic uraemic syndrome (HUS), thrombotic thrombocytopaenic purpura (TTP) 　◦ Malignancies: Leukaemias, myelodysplastic syndrome (MDS) 　◦ Hypersplenism • Drugs: Warfarin, aspirin, clopidogrel • Genetic: Haemophilias
Dyspepsia	• GERD • *Helicobacter pylori* causing peptic ulcer disease • Gastric cancer and other tumours • Cholelithiasis • Malabsorption: Coeliac disease • Medications such as non-steroidal anti-inflammatory drug (NSAID) • Gastroparesis
Dysuria	• Infectious—Cystitis, urethritis, pyelonephritis 　◦ Male: Prostatitis, epididymo-orchitis 　◦ Females: Cervicitis, vaginitis • Dermatologic: Psoriasis, lichen sclerosis • Anatomic: Stricture, benign prostatic hyperplasia (BPH) • Endocrine: Atrophic vaginitis • Neoplastic: Bladder carcinoma
Genital discharge and ulceration	• Discharge 　◦ Gonorrhoea 　◦ Chlamydia 　◦ Non-gonococcal urethritis 　◦ *Trichomonas vaginalis* 　◦ Candidiasis • Ulcer 　◦ Chancroid (painful) 　◦ Genital herpes (painful) 　◦ Syphilis (painless) 　◦ Granuloma inguinale (painless) 　◦ Lymphogranuloma venereum (LGV) (painless)
Haematuria	• Kidney 　◦ Glomerular: Glomerulonephritis, immunoglobulin A (IgA) nephropathy, thin basement membrane disease 　◦ Extraglomerular: Renal cell carcinoma (RCC), polycystic kidney disease (PCKD), renal papillary necrosis, trauma • Ureter: Tumours, stones infection, chronic irritation • Urinary bladder: Tumours, stones, infections, chronic irritation • Prostate: BPH prostate cancer

Continued

Continued

Symptoms	Causes
Haemoptysis	- Infections: Lung abscess, bronchiectasis, tuberculosis (TB), fungal infections - Lung malignancies: Primary, metastasis, bronchial adenoma - Vascular: Arteriovenous (AV) malformations - Autoimmune: Goodpasture disease, SLE
Hoarseness	- Inflammatory or irritant: Allergic, direct trauma as during intubation, infection causing laryngitis [upper respiratory tract infection (URTI)], GERD, vocal abuse - Neoplastic: Benign vocal cord lesions, laryngeal papillomatosis, glottic carcinoma [squamous cell carcinoma (SCC)]
Joint swelling	- Infection: Septic arthritis, gonococcal arthritis - Crystal deposition: Gout, calcium pyrophosphate deposition (CPPD) - Degenerative: Osteoarthritis - Neoplastic: Osteoma, osteosarcoma, osteoclastoma - Autoimmune: RA, psoriatic arthritis
Lymphadenopathy (Generalised)	- Infections: TB, toxoplasmosis, cat scratch disease, psittacosis - Autoimmune: SLE, RA, Sjögren's - Drug hypersensitivity: Phenytoin, carbamazepine - Lymphoproliferative disorders: Non-Hodgkin's lymphoma, Hodgkin's lymphoma, leukaemias
Progressive memory loss	- Degenerative: Alzheimer's, Lewy body dementia, frontotemporal dementia, Huntington's - Vascular: Vascular dementia, CADASIL - Mass lesions - Toxins: Cannabis, alcohol
Neck pain	- Infections: Retropharyngeal abscess, paravertebral abscess - Degenerative arthritis: Cervical spondylosis - Referred pain: Head and neck malignancies, acute coronary syndrome - Spondylolisthesis: Disc protrusion - Trauma: Whiplash injury
Polydipsia	- Psychogenic polydipsia - Endocrine: Central diabetes insipidus, diabetes mellitus types 1 and 2 - Head injuries - Infections: Tubercular meningitis - Multiple sclerosis - Schizophrenia

Polyuria	- Increased fluid intake
	- Increased urinary solute excretion
	  ○ Osmotic diuresis: Diabetes mellitus, Drug—mannitol
	  ○ Salt loss: Adrenal insufficiency, cerebral salt wasting, diuretics
	- Impaired urinary concentration: Diabetes insipidus, renal tubular disorders such as Renal tubular acidosis, Barter's, Gitelman

Continued

Continued

Symptoms	Causes
Pruritus	• Dermatological: Atopic dermatitis, psoriasis, urticaria, prurigo, lichen simplex chronicus • Liver disease: Obstructive jaundice • Drug abuse: Cocaine • Psychological • Metabolic: Uraemia, CLD
Skin and mouth ulcers	• Aphthous ulcer • Dermatological: Pemphigus vulgaris • Autoimmune: Behcet's disease, small vessel vasculitis • Infections: *Candida*, streptococcal

Speech disturbance	• Vocal cord: Inflammatory, neoplastic, traumatic
	• Neurological
	   ○ Aphasia
	   ○ Dysarthria
	• Genetic: Cleft lip, cleft palate

Difficulty swallowing	• Oral causes: Stomatitis, Tonsillitis, oral malignancy, candidiasis, pharyngitis, aphthous ulcer • Obstruction oesophagus: Cancer of oesophagus, pharyngeal pouch, oesophageal web (Plummer–Vinson) • External compression to oesophagus: Lymph nodes, enlarged left atrium in mitral stenosis, dysphagia lusoria • Neuromuscular disorders: Myasthenia gravis, achalasia, oesophageal spasm • MISC: Foreign body, stricture, CREST (calcinosis, Raynaud's phenomenon, esophageal dysmotility, sclerodactyly, and telangiectasia) syndrome
Vertigo	• Peripheral causes: Physiological [motion sickness, benign paroxysmal positional vertigo (BPPV), vestibular neuronitis, labyrinthitis, Ménière's disease, perilymph fistula] • Central causes: Brainstem TIA/Infarct, posterior fossa tumours, temporal lobe epilepsy, basilar migraine
Diplopia	• Supranuclear: Multiple sclerosis [internuclear ophthalmoplegia (INO)] • Nuclear: Mid-brain stroke syndromes • Infranuclear • Myopathic myasthenia gravis • Restrictive: Proptosis, enophthalmos, thyroid ophthalmopathy • Orbital: Trauma, tumours, orbital apex syndrome
Weight loss	• Chronic infectious disease: TB, HIV • Malnutrition • Malignancy: Cachexia • Psychological: Anorexia nervosa

BEST OF FIVES

1. 'Pastia's sign' is seen in:
   A. Kawasaki disease
   B. Scarlet fever
   C. Staphylococcal toxic shock syndrome
   D. Syphilis
   E. Herpes simplex

2. Which of the following scales is used for assessing the severity of the organophosphorus poisoning?
   A. Peradeniya scale
   B. Canadian scale
   C. Hoffman scale
   D. All of the above
   E. Werding scale

3. Which of the following is NOT a component of 'coma cocktail'?
   A. Dextrose
   B. Atropine
   C. Flumazenil
   D. Naloxone
   E. Thiamine

4. Which of the following is not a sign of splenic rupture?
   A. Kehr's sign
   B. Balance's sign
   C. Saegesser's splenic point tenderness
   D. Boas's sign
   E. Loculated hemoperitoneum

5. Worldwide, the major route of transmission of HIV (human immunodeficiency virus) is:
   A. Heterosexual
   B. Homosexual
   C. Parenteral
   D. Vertical
   E. Feco-oral

6. Which of the following is not a component of the classical triad of Reiter's disease?
   A. Non-specific urethritis
   B. Conjunctivitis
   C. Reactive arthritis
   D. Circinate balanitis
   E. None of the above

7. Which of the following is used in post-herpetic neuralgia?
   A. Amitriptyline
   B. Gabapentin
   C. Capsaicin cream
   D. All of the above
   E. None of the above

8. Diffuse soft goitre with bruit is the feature of:
   A. Graves' disease
   B. Hashimoto's thyroiditis
   C. Subacute thyroiditis
   D. Secondary hypothyroidism
   E. Primary Hyperparathyroidism

9. Libman–Sacks endocarditis usually occurs in a lady suffering from:
   A. Systemic lupus erythematosus (SLE)
   B. Rheumatoid arthritis
   C. Immunoglobulin A (IgA) nephropathy
   D. Cervical carcinoma
   E. IV drug abuse

10. Eschar is characteristic of which of the following diseases?
    A. Endemic typhus
    B. Scrub typhus
    C. Epidemic typhus
    D. Leptospirosis
    E. Typhoid

11. Favism is a feature of:
    A. Glucose-6-phosphate dehydrogenase (G6PD) deficiency
    B. Pyruvate kinase deficiency
    C. Pyrimidine 5' nucleotidase deficiency
    D. Galactokinase deficiency
    E. Fructokinase deficiency

12. Kawasaki disease predominantly affects:
    A. Large-sized arteries
    B. Medium-sized arteries
    C. Small-sized arteries
    D. Capillaries
    E. Venules

13. The curative treatment for patients under 30 years of age with severe idiopathic aplastic anaemia is:
    A. Autologous blood transfusion
    B. Autologous bone marrow transplantation
    C. Allogeneic blood transfusion
    D. Allogeneic bone marrow transplantation
    E. Chemoradiation

14. In which of the following diseases is thalidomide used as first-line treatment?
    A. Primary idiopathic acquired aplastic anaemia.
    B. Secondary aplastic anaemia

C. Multiple myeloma
D. Waldenstörm's macroglobulinaemia
E. Immune trhombocytopaenia

15. Which of the following subtypes of myelodysplastic syndrome (MDS) most rapidly progresses to acute myeloid leukaemia (AML)?
    A. Refractory anaemia (RA)
    B. Refractory anaemia with excess blasts (RAEB).
    C. Myelodysplastic syndrome with 5q–
    D. Refractory cytopaenia with multilineage dysplasia (RCMD)
    E. Hypereosinophilic leukaemia

16. Which of the following is the best first-line therapy for remission induction in chronic myeloid leukaemia (CML)?
    A. Imatinib
    B. Dasatinib
    C. Nilotinib
    D. Daunorubicin
    E. Busufan

17. Frontal lobe pathways' disease usually causes:
    A. Spasticity
    B. Rigidity
    C. Paratonia
    D. Cogwheel rigidity
    E. Anosmia

18. Dysexecutive syndrome is usually caused by:
    A. Mesial frontal lesions
    B. Dorsolateral prefrontal cortex lesions
    C. Orbitofrontal lesions of frontal lobes
    D. Temporal lobe lesions
    E. Hippocampus

19. 'Holmes' tremor is a violent, large-amplitude intention tremor that occurs with lesions in:
    A. Superior cerebellar peduncle
    B. Middle cerebellar peduncle
    C. Inferior cerebellar peduncle
    D. Dentate nucleus of cerebellum
    E. Corpus callosum

20. Which of the following is a disorder of pyrimidine metabolism?
    A. Gout
    B. Lesch–Nyhan syndrome
    C. Von Gierke disease
    D. Orotic aciduria
    E. Angelman syndrome

Answers

1-B, 2-A, 3-B, 4-D, 5-A, 6-D, 7-D, 8-A, 9-A, 10-B, 11-A, 12-B, 13-B, 14-C, 15-B, 16-A, 17-C, 18-B, 19-A, 20-D

■ **SUGGESTED READING**

1. Kitabchi AE, Umpierrez GE, Miles JM, Fisher JN. Hyperglycemic crises in adult patients with diabetes. Diabetes Care. 2009;32(7):1335-43.
2. Brophy GM, Bell R, Claassen J, Alldredge B, Bleck TP, Glauser T, et al. Guidelines for the evaluation and management of status epilepticus. Neurocrit Care. 2012; 17(1):3-23.
3. Trinka E, Cock H, Hesdorffer D, Rossetti AO, Scheffer IE, Shinnar S, et al. A definition and classification of status epilepticus--Report of the ILAE Task Force on Classification of Status Epilepticus. Epilepsia. 2015;56(10):1515-23.
4. Pumphrey RS. Lessons for management of anaphylaxis from a study of fatal reactions. Clin Exp Allergy. 2000;30(8): 1144-50.
5. Kearon C, Akl EA, Comerota AJ, Prandoni P, Bounameaux H, Goldhaber SZ, et al. Antithrombotic therapy for VTE disease: Antithrombotic Therapy and Prevention of Thrombosis, 9th ed: American College of Chest Physicians Evidence-Based Clinical Practice Guidelines. Chest. 2012;141(Suppl2):e419S-96S.
6. Siemieniuk RAC, Chu DK, Kim LH, Güell-Rous MR, Alhazzani W, Soccal PM, et al. Oxygen therapy for acutely ill medical patients: a clinical practice guideline. BMJ. 2018;363:k4169.
7. Nieminen MS, Böhm M, Cowie MR, Drexler H, Filippatos GS, Jondeau G, et al. Executive summary of the guidelines on the diagnosis and treatment of acute heart failure: the Task Force on Acute Heart Failure of the European Society of Cardiology. Eur Heart J. 2005;26(4):384-416.
8. Gheorghiade M, Zannad F, Sopko G, Klein L, Piña IL, Konstam MA, et al. Acute heart failure syndromes: current state and framework for future research. Circulation. 2005;112(25):3958-68.
9. Al-Khatib SM, Stevenson WG, Ackerman MJ, Bryant WB, Callans DJ, Curtis AB, et al. 2017 AHA/ACC/HRS Guideline for Management of Patients With Ventricular Arrhythmias and the Prevention of Sudden Cardiac Death: A Report of the American College of Cardiology/American Heart Association Task Force on Clinical Practice Guidelines and the Heart Rhythm Society. J Am Coll Cardiol. 2018;72(14):e91-220.
10. Global Initiative for Asthma (GINA). Global Strategy for Asthma Management and Prevention. [online] Available from: www.ginasthma.org. [Last accessed June, 2020).

CHAPTER 2

Emergencies in Medical Practice

■ MANAGEMENT OF SEVERE HYPERKALAEMIA

Case Scenario

An 80-year-old male was found collapsed at home, with incontinence of urine and faeces. He is a known case of hypertension (HTN) and congestive cardiac failure (CCF). He is on enalapril for HTN and spironolactone and metoprolol for CCF.

On examination: Patient is confused and combative with Glasgow Coma Scale (GCS) of 13.

Blood pressure (BP): 78/60 mmHg   Pulse rate (PR): 74 bpm

Respiratory rate (RR): 32/min   SpO$_2$: 91%

Laboratory data (Fig. 2.1): Arterial blood gas (ABG): pH 7.23; K$^+$: 7.0; Blood glucose: 189 mg/dL

- **Immediate antagonism of cardiac effects of hyperkalaemia:** Membrane stabilisation
  - Calcium gluconate 10 mL 10% slow intravenous (IV) over 10 minutes
  - Calcium chloride 3–4 mL

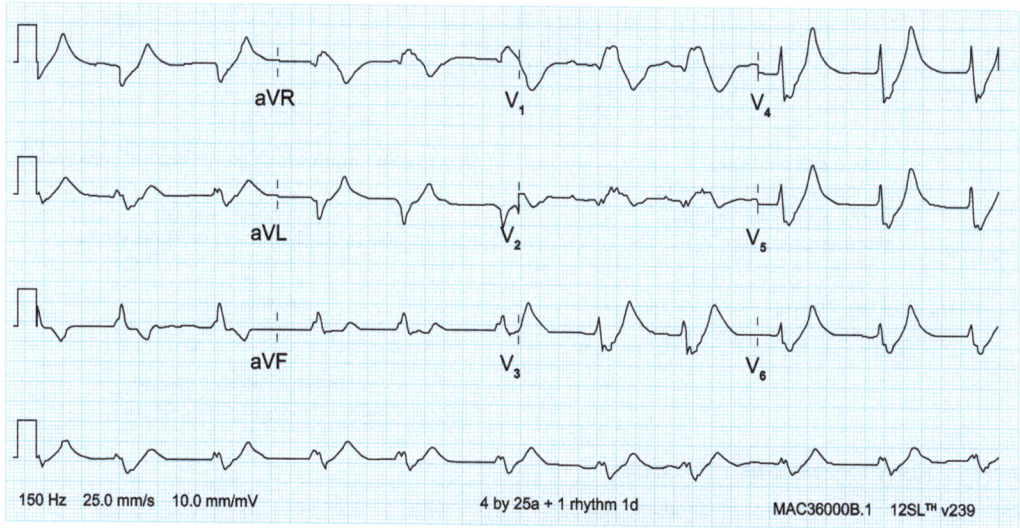

Fig. 2.1: ECG shows tall tented T waves with wide QRS complexes and absent P waves.

- **Rapid reduction in plasma K⁺ by redistribution into the cells:**
    - IV 50 mL of 50% dextrose + 10 units of regular insulin
    - 10–20 mg of nebulised albuterol in 4 mL normal saline (NS) inhaled over 10 minutes
- **Removal of K⁺ from the body:**
    - Ion exchange resin: Sodium polystyrene sulphonate 15–30 g powder
        - Given in a premade suspension with 33% sorbitol
    - IV furosemide and NS
    - Haemodialysis

■ METABOLIC ACIDOSIS

> **Case Scenario**
> A 56-year-old man with a history of alcohol use presents with a 4-day history of severe abdominal pain, nausea and vomiting.
> **On examination,** his blood pressure is 80/50 mmHg and he has tenderness in his epigastrium. His initial laboratory studies reveal:
>
> | Na: 132 | Cl: 92 | HCO$_3$: 16 |
> |---|---|---|
> | Creatinine: 1.5 | Amylase: 400 | Lipase: 250 |
>
> ABG revealed
>
> | pH: 7.28 | PCO$_2$: 34 mmHg | PO$_2$: 88 mmHg |
> |---|---|---|
>
> HCO$_3$: 16.3 mEq/dL

- Identify and treat the underlying cause.
- Determine ΔAG
- Dialysis may be necessary in renal failure with metabolic acidosis.

Management of metabolic acidosis has been shown in **Flowchart 2.1**.

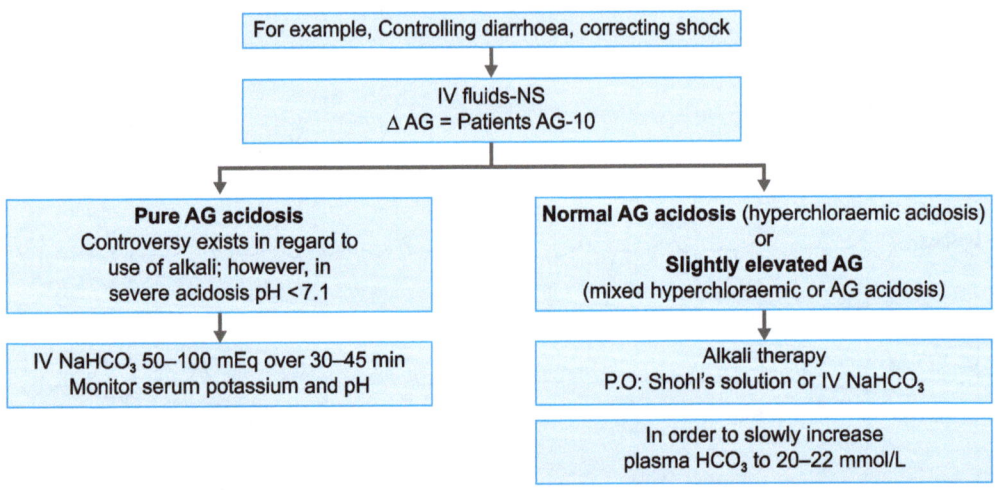

(AG: anion gap; IV: intravenous; NS: normal saline)

Flowchart 2.1: Management of metabolic acidosis.

HYPOGLYCAEMIA

Case Scenario

A 32-year-old patient presented with altered level of consciousness.
Medical history: Diabetes mellitus on Insulin
On examination:

Pulse rate: 72 bpm	BP: 100/56 mmHg
SpO_2: 98%	GCS: 11 (3, 3, 5)
Blood sugar: 32 mg/dL	

MILD: If detected early and patient is able to take orally
↓
Oral carbohydrates in an easily absorbable form

SEVERE:
- Dextrose 75 mL of 20% dextrose IV oral carbohydrate to be given as soon as the patient is able to eat.
- Glucagon 0.5–1 mg SC/IM
- Octreotide
- Identify and treat the cause.
  - For example, adjusting the dose of oral hypoglycaemic agent (OHA) and insulin.
  - Changing the timing of insulin injection.

MANAGEMENT OF ACUTE PULMONARY OEDEMA

Case Scenario

A 62-year-old elderly male patient came with complaint of sudden severe shortness of breath.
Past history (P/H): Myocardial infarction (MI)—6 months back
On examination: Patient is sitting leaning forward.
Appearance: Pale, distressed and sweaty. Productive pink-tinged frothy sputum.

PR: 140 bpm	BP: 200/110 mmHg
RR: 38/min	SpO_2: 78% at room air

Ankle oedema is present bilaterally.
Systemic examination S/E: Cardiovascular system (CVS): Gallop rhythm
Respiratory sound (RS): Basal crepitations are present bilaterally.

- Monitor vitals.
- Oxygen: Non-invasive positive pressure ventilation or intubation and mechanical ventilation
- Furosemide 0.5–1 mg/kg IV bolus
- Morphine 2–4 mg IV
- Management of acute pulmonary oedema has been shown in **Flowchart 2.2**.

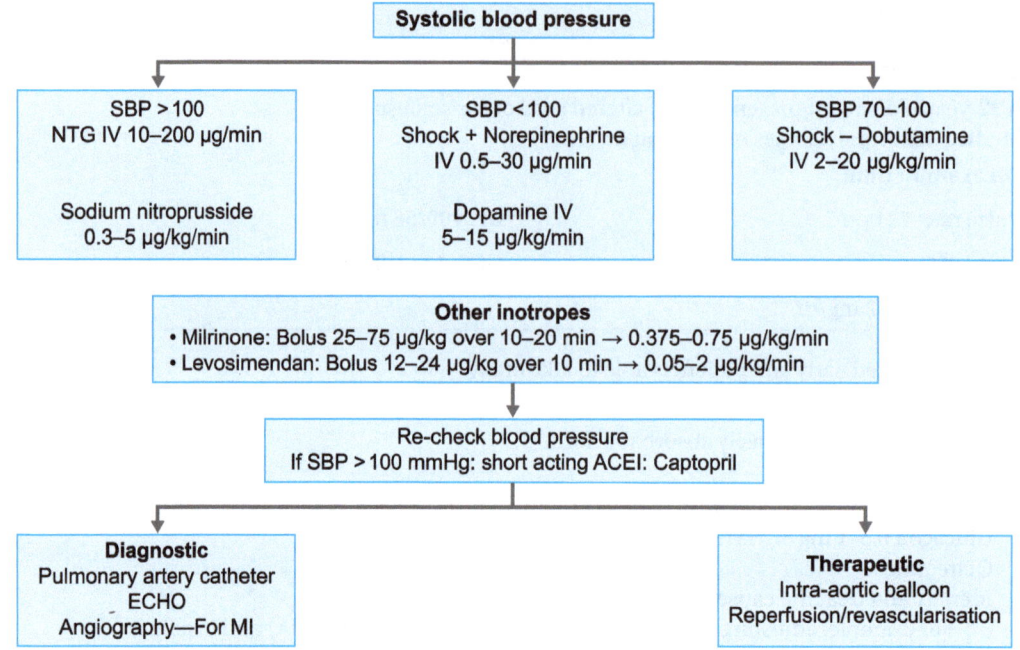

(ACE: angiotensin-converting enzyme; ECHO: echocardiography; MI: myocardial infarction; NTG: nitroglycerin)

Flowchart 2.2: Management of acute pulmonary oedema.

■ MANAGEMENT OF SEVERE HYPERCALCAEMIA

Case Scenario

An 80-year-old woman presented with vomiting, diarrhoea, fatigue, malaise, generalised abdominal pain and weight loss.

P/H: Known case of Metastatic breast cancer

On examination:

PR: 98 bpm   BP: 90/70 mmHg   RR: 14/min

S/E: PA—Generalised abdominal tenderness present
Laboratory data: Serum calcium > 11.0 mg/dL

- **IV normal saline**
  - 4–6 L may be required over first 24 hours.
- **Bisphosphonates:** Inhibit bone resorption
  - Zoledronic acid 4 mg IV over 30 minutes
  - Pamidronate 60–90 mg IV over 2–4 hours
  - Ibandronate 2 mg IV over 2 hours
- **Calcitonin:** Increases calcium excretion
  - 100 U; 3 times/day; IM/SC for first 24–48 hours

- **Gallium nitrate**
  - 200 mg/m² IV daily for 5 days
  - Alternative to bisphosphonates
  - Nephrotoxic
- **Dialysis**

TENSION PNEUMOTHORAX

Case Scenario

A 23-year-old man presents with a single gunshot wound to the right side of his chest.

On examination: Conscious palpable pulse

BP: 100/60 mmHg   RR: 30/min

- Trachea deviated to the left
- Jugular veins are distended
- No breath sounds on the right side of the chest
- Palpable crepitus
- Percussion—hyper-resonance on the right side (**Fig. 2.2**)

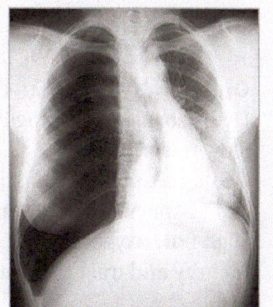

Insertion of wide-bore needle into pleural space through the anterior 2nd ICS. Needle is left in place till a thoracostomy tube is inserted
or
Insertion of a wide-bore plastic cannula, attached to a long rubber tubing, the end of which is placed underwater

↓

Definitive management
Insertion of intercostal drainage tube in 4th/5th/6th ICS in mid-axillary line connected to an underwater seal or one-way Heimlich valve

(ICS: intercostal space)

Fig. 2.2: Management of tension pneumothorax.

MYXOEDEMA COMA

Case Scenario

A 47-year-old female patient, who is a known case of hypothyroidism, presented to office with complaints of falls, leg oedema and pain, drowsiness, headaches and shortness of breath.

On examination:

PR: 50 bpm   BP: 90/70 mmHg   RR: 20/min

Periorbital oedema is present. Non-pitting tibial oedema is present.

S/E: Central nervous system (CNS): Delayed tendon reflexes

Free T3: 0.05 ng/dL (0.93–1.7)   Thyroid stimulating hormone (TSH): 30.12 µIU/mL (0.27–5.0)
Na: 121 mEq/L   K: 4.2 mEq/L   Cl: 87 mEq/L

Treatment must be initiated even before biochemical confirmation of diagnosis.
- Monitor vitals—temperature
- Sepsis screen
- **Investigations:** T4, TSH, creatine phosphokinase (CPK), ABG, random blood sugar (RBS) and electrolytes
- **Levothyroxine**-500 µg IV bolus
  OR
  Triiodothyronine 10–25 µg every 8–12 hourly IV
  ↓
  Followed by

  Oral levothyroxine 50–100 µg daily
- Hydrocortisone 100 mg IV TID
- Slow rewarming
- Cautious use of IV fluids: Hypotonic fluids to be avoided because they increase water retention
- Broad-spectrum antibiotics
- High flow oxygen
- Identify and treat the cause

■ THYROTOXIC CRISIS/THYROID STORM

> **Case Scenario**
>
> A 39-year-old woman presented with a 3-month history of increased sweating and palpitations with weight loss of 7 kg. She had family history of thyroid disease.
>
> **On examination:**
>
> PR: 122 bpm   130/80 mmHg   RR: 20/min
>
> She has warm and moist skin. Her thyroid gland is enlarged bilaterally. Bilateral exophthalmos is present.
>
> **S/E:** CVS: Tachycardia present; PA: Generalised abdominal tenderness
>
> T4: 12.00 ng/dL (0.73–1.84)   T3: 1173.00 ng/dL (123–211 ng/dL)   TSH: < 0.018 µIU/mL

- **Investigations:** T3, T4, TSH, sepsis screen, liver function test (LFT), electrocardiogram (ECG)
- Rehydrate
- **Propranolol**
  - Per oral: 60–80 mg four times a day
  - IV: 1–5 mg four times a day
- **Propylthiouracil (PTU)**
  - 500–1,000 mg loading dose → 250 mg 4th hourly oral or via nasogastric (NG) tube
- **Carbimazole**
  - 15–30 mg STAT → 15 mg TID
- **Lugol's iodine**
  - 10 drops TID—1 hour after PTU/carbimazole
- **Sodium ipodate**
  - 500 mg/day orally
- **Hydrocortisone**
  - 200 mg IV bolus → 100 mg every 8th hourly
- Oxygen, IV fluids and external cooling
- Identify and treat the cause.
- Antibiotics, if infection is present

ACUTE ADRENAL INSUFFICIENCY

> **Case Scenario**
> A 38-year-old female is admitted for complaints of progressive fatigue for 2 weeks. She also complains of nausea and vomiting. She has lost 8 kg in the past 2 weeks. She has history of recent onset of breathlessness.
>
> **On examination:**
>
> PR: 134 bpm   BP: 80/40 mmHg
>
> RR: 18/min   Temperature: 99°F
>
> She appears pale, dehydrated and malnourished.
>
> **S/E:** Unremarkable
>
> Na: 120 mmol/L   K: 5.9 mmol/L
>
> Hb: 12.4 g/dL   White blood cell (WBC): 11,600 and she had a mild oeosinophilia

- **Investigations:** Electrolytes, RBS, complete blood count (CBC), Plasma cortisol
- Monitor vitals
- **Rehydration**
  - Normal saline IV infusion: 1 L/h with continuous cardiac monitoring
- **Hydrocortisone**
  - 100 mg IV bolus

    100 mg 6th hourly for first 24 hours

    Continue parenteral hydrocortisone till patient can take orally
- Treat hypoglycaemia and hyperkalaemia
- Treat the precipitating cause.

MANAGEMENT OF STATUS EPILEPTICUS

- Ensure airway patency—give oxygen.
- Monitor vitals, SpO_2.
- Secure IV access.
- **Investigations:** RBS, electrolytes, antiepileptic drug (AED) levels, LFT, renal function test (RFT), CBC

Early: 5–30 minutes

IV benzodiazepine (BZP)
Lorazepam 0.1 mg/kg
OR
Midazolam 0.2 mg/kg — Repeat only after 15 minutes
OR
Diazepam 10 mg rectally if no IV access

Established and early refractory: 30–40 minutes
- IV ANTIEPILEPTICS with cardiac monitoring
- Phenytoin 15–20 mg/kg or 50 mg/min; OR
- Fosphenytoin 15 mg/kg at 50–100 mg/min; OR
- Phenobarbitone 10 mg/kg at 100 mg/min; OR
- Valproic acid 20–30 mg/kg
- Levetiracetam 20–30 mg/kg

Late refractory: > 48 hours
- IV Midazolam 0.2 mg/kg → 0.2–0.6 mg/kg/h
  and/or
- Propofol 2 mg/kg → 2–10 mg/kg/h
- Consider intubation and mechanical ventilation—general anaesthesia (GA) using propofol or thiopental.
- Consider electroencephalogram (EEG) monitoring—AIM for EEG burst suppression pattern.
- Thiopental 5 mg/kg → 1–5 mg/kg/h
- Once controlled—long-term anticonvulsants

MANAGEMENT OF COMA
- **Investigations:** CBC, RBS, electrolytes LFT, RFT, ABG, blood culture, chest X-ray (CXR), ECG, computed tomography (CT) scan and drug screen, if indicated.
- **General measures:**
  - Monitor vitals
  - Protect the airway: Oropharyngeal airway/intubation, if needed.
  - Avoid secondary insults to the brain such as hypoxia, hypoglycaemia and hypotension.
  - Secure IV access: Hypotonic IV fluids with close monitoring.
- **Specific treatment:**
  - Hypoglycaemic coma: Thiamine followed by dextrose.
  - Fever and meningismus indicate urgent need for cerebrospinal fluid (CSF) analysis followed by IV antibiotics.
- **Long-term management:**
  - Frequent change of position every 2–3 hourly to avoid bedsores
  - Lid taping
  - Catheterisation
  - Prevent aspiration by positioning the patient left lateral.

MANAGEMENT OF SNAKEBITE
- Reassure the patient.
- Immobilise the bitten limb.
- **Investigations:** CBC, coagulation screen, RFT, electrolytes, CPK, ECG, urine routine, fibrinogen degradation product (FDP) and fibrinogen level
- Monitor vitals.
- Intake/output (I/O) charting
- Secure IV access.
- Anti snake venom (ASV) if indicated:
  - Mild cases: 5 vials
  - Moderate cases: 5–10 vials
  - Severe cases: 10–20 vials
  - Given as IV infusion in 5–10 mL/kg of NS and given over 1 hour
- **Never give locally at the site of snakebite.**
- Keep adrenaline ready in case of anaphylaxis.
- For **coagulopathy**: Fresh frozen plasma (FFP)/cryoprecipitate/platelet concentrate
- In case of **neurotoxic snakebite**: If there is respiratory failure or bulbar paralysis (**Flowchart 2.3**)
- Antibiotic prophylaxis
- Antitetanus prophylaxis
- Renal failure managed with haemodialysis

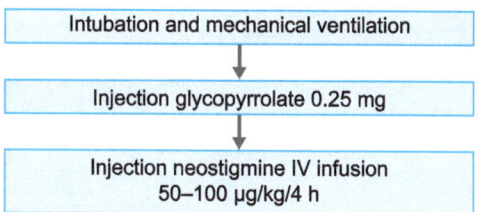

Flowchart 2.3: Dosage of medication for neurotoxic snake bite.

MANAGEMENT OF HYPOVOLAEMIA

- **Investigations:** Haematocrit, blood urea nitrogen (BUN), creatinine, electrolytes, ABG and urinary sodium
- Monitor vitals
- Secure IV line
- Strict input/output charting
- Mild hypovolaemia can be treated with oral hydration.
- Severe hypovolaemia requires IV hydration.
  $$\downarrow$$
  Isotonic NS – 0.9% NaCl, 154 mM Na$^+$
- Calculation of free water deficit

$$\textbf{Free water deficit} = \text{Total body water} \times \frac{(\text{Plasma sodium} - 1)}{140}$$

Total 50% of this calculated deficit is given over the first 24 hours and the remaining over the next 24 hours.
- Patients with bicarbonate loss and metabolic acidosis may need IV bicarbonate.
- Patients with severe haemorrhage should receive red cell transfusion without increasing haematocrit > 35%.
- Identify and treat the cause of hypovolaemia.

MANAGEMENT OF SHOCK

Case Scenario

A 25-year-old male patient is admitted to intensive care unit (ICU) with 3 days' old perforation. History of chills and fever is present.

On examination: Mental status is altered, restless.

Skin warmed and flushed

| PR: 130 bpm | BP: 80/60 mmHg | RR: 40/min |

- **Investigations:** Haemoglobin, haematocrit, sepsis screen, LFT, RFT, electrolytes and ABG.
- Secure IV access
- Assess GCS
- Oxygen/intubation and mechanical ventilation if needed, e.g., GCS < 8.
- Monitor vitals, I/O charting and peripheral perfusion.

Management of shock has been shown in **Flowcharts 2.4** and **2.5**.
- Optimise Hb: Transfuse red cells

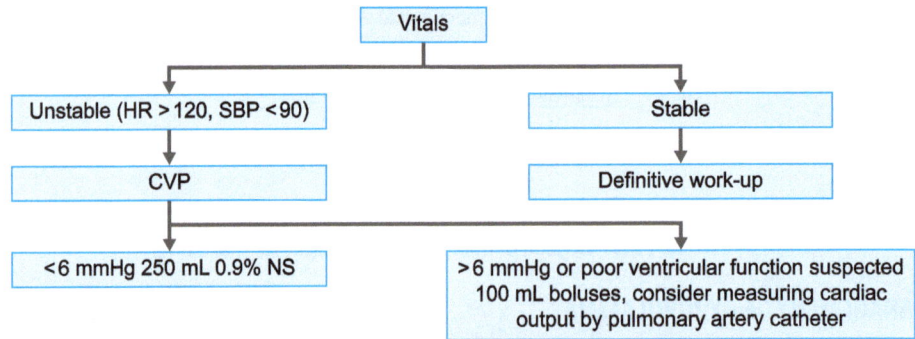

(CVP: central venous pressure; HR: heart rate; NS: nasal saline; SBP: systolic blood pressure)

Flowchart 2.4: Management of shock.

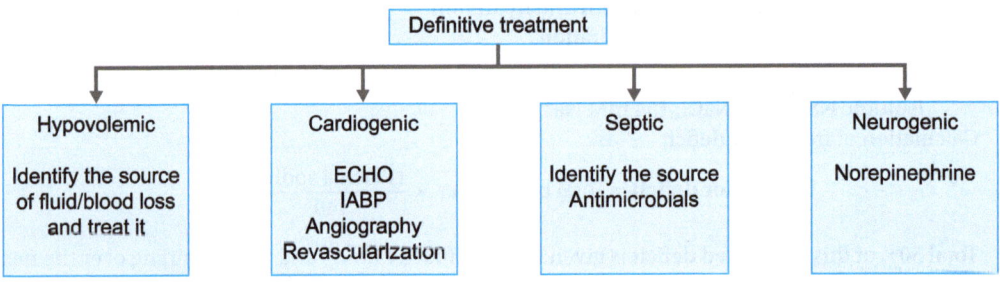

(ECHO: echocardiography; IABP: intra-aortic balloon pump)

Flowchart 2.5: Treatment of shock.

- Achieve target BP: Inotropes once the hypovolaemia is corrected
  - Dobutamine: 2–8 µg/kg/min
  - Adrenaline: 1–8 µg/kg/min

ISCHAEMIC STROKE

> **Case Scenario**
>
> A 41-year-old male patient, alcoholic, K/C/O hypertension presents to casualty with chief complaint of right-sided weakness, slurred speech and loss of balance. Symptoms began 90 minutes prior to arrival.
>
> **On examination:**
>
> PR: 88 bpm and irregular   BP: 177/90 mmHg   RR: 18/min
>
> S/E: CNS: GCS—11/15
>
> Right side facial weakness. Power is reduced on the right side. No sensory deficit on the right side. Plantar extensor on the right side.
>
> Computed tomography (CT) findings are shown in **Figure 2.3**.

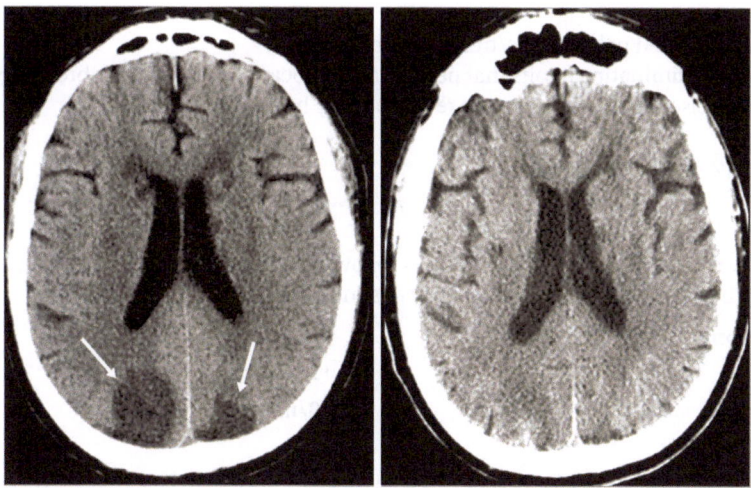

Fig. 2.3: CT brain showing peripheral hypo-dense areas suggestive of ischemic changes.

- **Investigations:** Plain CT Brain, RBS, electrolytes, ECG, suspected atrial fibrillation (AF) → Thyroid function tests, echocardiography (ECHO)
- **General measures:**
  - Airway: Ensure airway patency
  - Breathing: O_2 if SpO_2 is < 95%
  - Circulation: Check PR, BP. Secure IV access-Treat with IV fluids/anti-arrhythmias/inotropes.
- Look for hypoglycaemia and treat accordingly.
- **IV thrombolytics:**
  - IV recombinant tissue plasminogen activator (rtPA) within 3 hours of onset of ischaemic stroke
  - Dose: 0.9 mg/kg → 10% of total dose as IV bolus, remaining as IV infusion over 60 minutes
- **Endovascular mechanical thrombectomy:**
  - If IV thrombolysis is contraindicated or has failed
- **Antiplatelets:**
  - Aspirin 75–150 mg OD
- **Statins:**
  - Atorvastatin, rosuvastatin 10–20 mg OD
- **Medical support:**
  - Catheterisation
  - Ryles tube (RT) feeding
  - Treat fever with antipyretics, surface cooling.
  - Pneumatic compression stockings
  - Prevent bedsores and contractures.
  - Initiate secondary preventive measures.
- **Rehabilitation:**
  - Early physiotherapy, occupational/speech therapy

HYPERVENTILATION

- Identify and treat the initiating factor.
- Reassurance

- Rebreathing into a closed bag
- If there are associated palpitations/tremors: β-blockers.
- Identifying and eliminating habits that perpetuate hypocapnia such as sigh breathing
- Breathing exercises and diaphragmatic retaining may be helpful.

ACUTE PULMONARY EMBOLISM

Case Scenario
A 71-year-old woman bedridden for last 4 days following fall and trauma to right hip is brought to emergency with complaints of sudden onset of dyspnoea and dizziness.

On examination:

PR: 124 bpm   BP: 118/89 mmHg
SpO_2: 84%   RR: 28/min

Diaphoresis is present.
Right lower limb oedema is present extending from mid-thigh to foot. Calf muscle tenderness is present.

- **Investigations:** ECG, CXR, D-dimer and pulmonary angiography
- **Supportive measures:** Oxygen and IV fluids
- **Anticoagulation:**
    - Unfractionated heparin: 80 U/kg bolus → 18 U/kg/h with activated partial thromboplastin time (aPTT) monitoring
    (*Note*: Platelet count to be monitored at least every 3rd day)
    - Low-molecular-weight heparin (LMWH): Subcutaneously
        - LMWH should not be discontinued until international normalised ratio (INR) is ≥ 2 for at least 24 hours
    - Warfarin: 5 mg/day—started on day 1 with INR monitoring
    - Fondaparinux
    - Others: Rivaroxaban, apixaban, argatroban and ximelagatran
    (*Note*: Anticoagulation to be continued for at least 6 months)
- **Thrombolysis:**
    - Indication: Acute massive pulmonary embolism with cardiogenic shock. 100 mg rtPA IV infusion over 2 hours
- **Surgical therapy:**
    - Surgical embolectomy
    - Caval filter

MANAGEMENT OF HAEMOPTYSIS

Case Scenario
A 40-year-old male chronic smoker, with past history of tuberculosis, presents with history of haemoptysis three episodes since day 1.

On examination: He has clubbing, BP: 100/60 mmHg, PR: 100 bpm, and coarse crepitations in the right infraclavicular area.

- **Investigations:** Blood grouping, cross matching, CBC, PT-INR, CXR
- Measure vitals
- Patient should be positioned upright or bleeding side down.

- Secure airway:
  - Intubation with double lumen ET tube is preferable
- Secure IV access: Large bore IV cannula.
- Administer IV fluids or blood transfusion, if needed.
- Vasopressin 0.2–0.4 U/min IV.

↓

Bronchoscopy
- Topical thrombin
- Laser photocoagulation
- Balloon catheter can be inflated proximally in the bleeding bronchus → Endovascular embolisation
- Emergency surgery

■ HYPERTENSIVE EMERGENCY/CRISIS

> **Case Scenario**
> A 69-year-old male patient presented with complaints of chest tightness and shortness of breath. He has been a known case of DM since 10 years and is a chronic smoker. He has a history of hypertension and is not on treatment.
>
> **On examination:**
> HR: 110 bpm   BP: 230/120 mmHg
> S/E: CVS: S3 gallop, No murmur
> RS: Bi-basal fine inspiratory crackles

- **Investigations:** RFT, fundoscopy, ECG and echocardiography
- Reduce the mean arterial pressure (MAP) by no more than 25% within minutes to 2 hours
- Continuous monitoring of BP
- **Labetalol:**
  - 2 mg/min IV; maximum of 300 mg
  - In acute renal failure, subarachnoid haemorrhage (SAH), intracranial (IC) bleed and acute aortic dissection
- **Nitroglycerin (NTG):**
  - 0.6–1.2 mg/h IV
  - In acute pulmonary oedema, acute coronary syndrome and IC bleed
- **Sodium nitroprusside:**
  - 0.3–1 µg/kg/min IV
  - Drug of choice for hypertensive encephalopathy
- **Nicardipine:**
  - 5 mg/h IV titrate by 2.5 mg/h at 5–15 minute intervals → maximum 15 mg/h
- **Esmolol:**
  - 80–500 µg/kg over 1 min → 50–300 µg/kg/min IV
- **Hydralazine:**
  - 10–50 mg at 30 minute intervals

■ SEVERE DEHYDRATION

- **Investigations:** Electrolytes, urea, creatinine and RBS
- **SIGNS:** Sunken eyes, dry tongue, skin pinch going back slowly—two or more positive—SEVERE DEHYDRATION

- Secure IV access
- Monitor vitals
- I/O chartings
- IV fluids started immediately (**Table 2.1**)
  - RL + 5% dextrose
    OR
    Normal saline
- **Oral rehydration solution (ORS)** can be given as soon as the patient is able to take orally (5 mL/kg/h)
- Reclassify dehydration and treat accordingly
  - For example, Some dehydration → discontinue IV fluids and continue ORS
- **Daily fluid requirement:**
  - Up to 10 kg: 100 mL/kg
  - 10–20 kg: 50 mL/kg
  - More than 20 kg: 20 mL/kg

TABLE 2.1: Fluid replacement in dehydration.

Age	30 mL/kg	70 mL/kg
< 12 months	1 h	5 h
> 12 months	30 min	2.5 h

MANAGEMENT OF CARDIAC ARREST

Immediate identification of cardiac arrest and activation of emergency response system (ERS)
↓
Early cardiopulmonary resuscitation (CPR) (30:2)

Basic life support (BLS): Circulation – Chest compression → PUSH HARD – PUSH FAST
- Continue for 2 minutes before re-assessment of rhythm

Management of cardiac arrest has been shown in **Flowcharts 2.6** and **2.7**.

Breathing: Mouth to mouth

Advanced life support (ALS): Airway: Face mask, Ambu bag, Oropharyngeal airway, laryngeal mask airway (LMA) and endotracheal (ET) tube.

Breathing: Supplement oxygen.

Circulation: IV access, attaching a cardiac monitor, assess the rhythm, defibrillation

MANAGEMENT OF VENTRICULAR FIBRILLATION

Management of ventricular fibrillation has been shown in **Flowchart 2.8**.

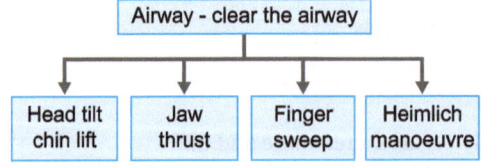

Flowchart 2.6: Management of cardiac arrest.

Emergencies in Medical Practice

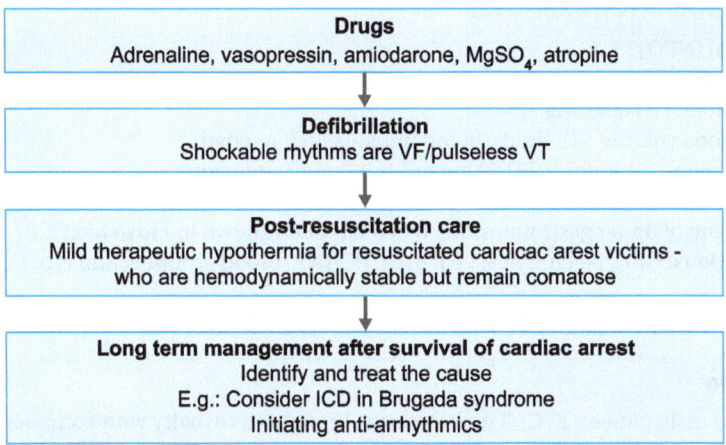

Drugs
Adrenaline, vasopressin, amiodarone, MgSO$_4$, atropine

↓

Defibrillation
Shockable rhythms are VF/pulseless VT

↓

Post-resuscitation care
Mild therapeutic hypothermia for resuscitated cardiac arrest victims - who are hemodynamically stable but remain comatose

↓

Long term management after survival of cardiac arrest
Identify and treat the cause
E.g.: Consider ICD in Brugada syndrome
Initiating anti-arrhythmics

(ICD: implantable cardioverter-defibrillator; VF: ventricular fibrillation; VT: ventricular tachycardia)

Flowchart 2.7: Management of cardiac arrest.

Immediate defibrillation: 150 to 360 J

↓

CPR for 2 min

↓

Repeat shock - 2nd shock repeat the sequence

↓ Circulation fails to return

Continue CPR, intubate, IV access

↓

Epinephrine 1 mg IV every 4 min (alternating cycles)
or
Vasopressin 40 units IV

↓

Repeat shock - 3rd shock

↓ Circulation fails to return

- Epinephrine high dose
- Anti-arrhythmics
  Amiodarone: 150 mg over 10 min
  Lidocaine 1.5 mg/kg
  MgSO$_4$ 1–2 g IV bolus
  Procainamide

↓ Circulation fails to return

Defibrillation, CPR:
Drug-shock-drug-shock

(CPR: cardiopulmonary resuscitation; IV: intravenous)

Flowchart 2.8: Management of ventricular fibrillation.

UPPER GASTROINTESTINAL BLEED

- Nil per oral (NPO)
- Secure IV access
- Monitor vitals, I/O charting
- Restore blood volume—IV fluids/blood transfusion if needed
- IV proton pump inhibitor (PPI) 80 mg bolus → 8 mg/h infusion
- Suspected variceal bleed
- Management of upper gastrointestinal bleed has been shown in **Flowchart 2.9**.
- **Investigations:** CBC, electrolytes, LFT, urea, PT/INR, blood grouping and cross matching

EMERGENCY MANAGEMENT OF ACUTE MYOCARDIAL INFARCTION

> **Case Scenario**
>
> A 60-year-old male patient, K/C/O diabetes, was brought to casualty with complaints of single episode of sudden, rapid onset, severe chest pain, lasting more than 30 minutes, radiating to the medial aspect of his left arm associated with breathlessness, nausea, heavy perspiration, lightheadedness, fever and cold clammy skin.
>
> **On examination:**
>
> PR: 112 bpm   BP: 160/110 mmHg
>
> RR: 20/min   Jugular venous pressure (JVP): Normal
>
> S/E: CVS: S1–S2 + tachycardia
>
> ECG showing acute antero-lateral STEMI in **Figure 2.4**.

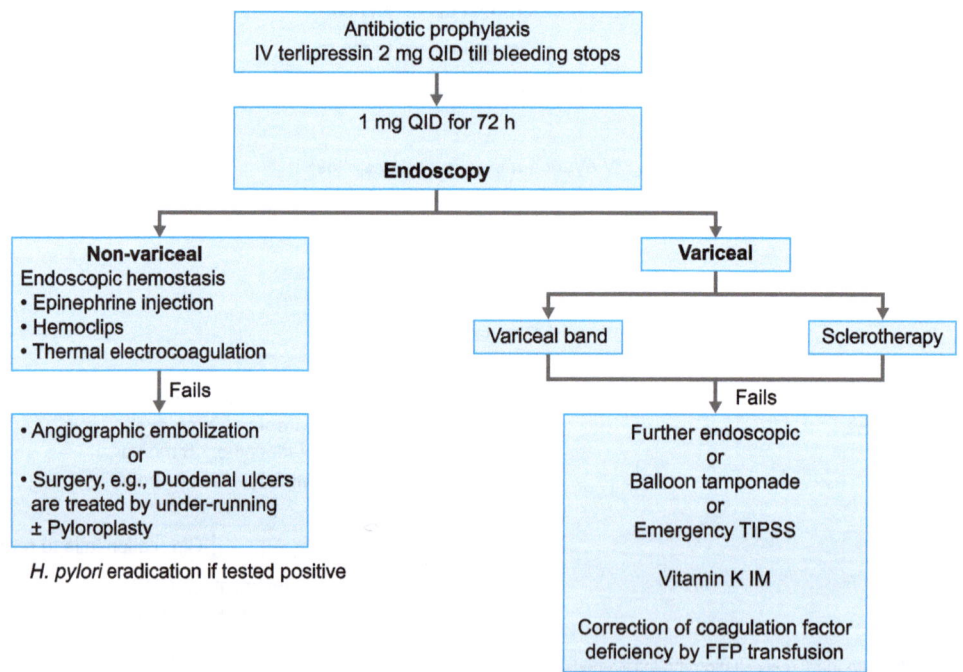

(IM: intramuscular; IV: intravenous; FFP: fresh frozen plasma; TIPSS: transjugular intrahepatic portosystemic shunt)

Flowchart 2.9: Management of upper gastrointestinal bleed.

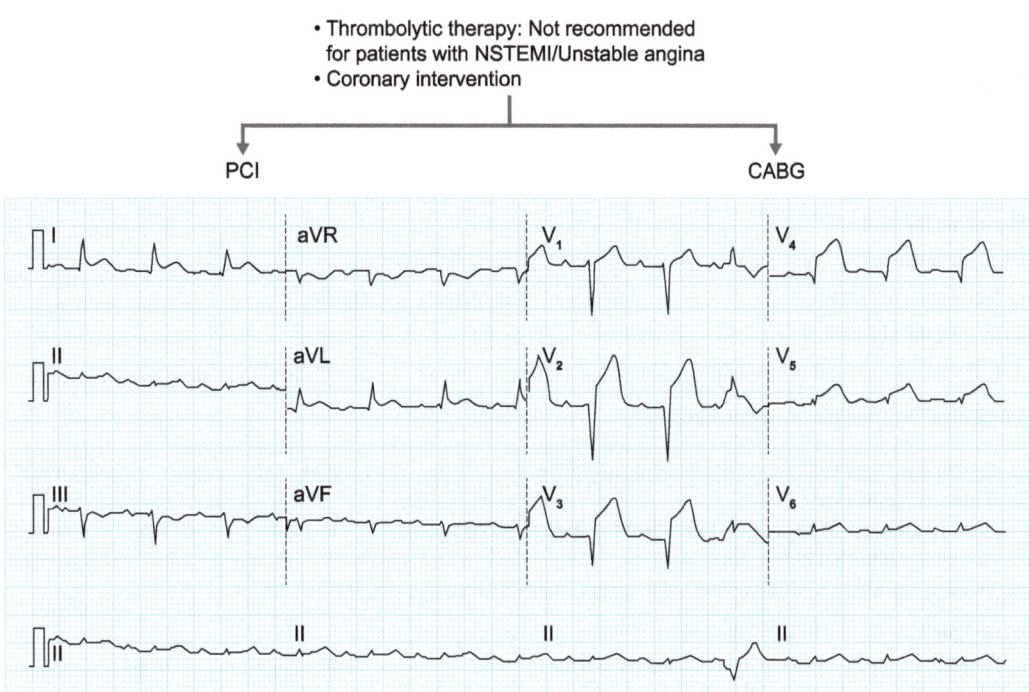

Fig. 2.4: ECG showing acute antero-lateral STEMI.

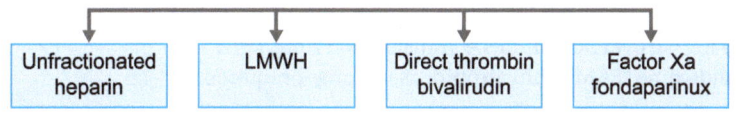

(LMWH: low-molecular-weight heparin)

Flowchart 2.10: Anticoagulants.

Investigations: 12-lead ECG, Cardiac biomarkers: Troponin I, T, creatine kinase-MB (CKMB)
- Monitor vitals
- Oxygen
- Nitrates glyceryl trinitrate 300–500 µg sublingually
  ↓
  If pain persists after three doses given 5 minutes apart
  IV NTG 5–10 µg/min [Maintain systolic blood pressure (SBP) > 40 mmHg]
- *Morphine*: 2–5 mg IV-Analgesia
- Antiplatelets:
  o Aspirin: 325 mg nonenteric formulations → 75–100 mg/day
  o Clopidogrel: 300 mg orally → 75 mg/day
  o Others: Oral—prasugrel, ticagrelor
  o IV—Abciximab, Eptifibatide, Tirofiban
- Anticoagulants (**Flowchart 2.10**)
- Beta-blockers unless contraindicated, angiotensin-converting enzyme (ACE) inhibitors, high-dose statins
- Specific treatment

ORGANOPHOSPHATE POISONING

> **Case Scenario**
> A 27-year-old male was brought to casualty at 1:00 AM with history of sudden loss of consciousness in his room after having a family quarrel. He has history of four episodes of vomiting and incontinence of urine and faeces.
>
> **On examination:**
> PR: 100 bpm   BP: 90/70 mmHg
> RR: 28/min, shallow   Temperature: 102°F
> GCS – E1V2 M4 = 7/15
>
> **S/E:** CNS: Pupils – B/L pinpoint, nonreacting; Tone: Increased; Power: Grade I; Plantar: Non-elicitable
>
> **PA:** Bowel sounds are exaggerated.

- Prevent further exposure: Remove contaminate clothing, wash the skin thoroughly with soap and water, irrigate eyes.
- Airway cleared of excessive secretions → high flow oxygen
- IV access → 0.9% NS infusion
- Monitor vitals, SpO_2, auscultate the lungs. Ventilatory support, if needed.

Investigations: LFT, ABG, ECG, electrolytes, glucose, amylase

- Gastric lavage with activated charcoal if the patient presents within 1 hour of ingestion Management of organophosphate poisoning.

Atropine
Dosage given in **Table 2.2**.

Pralidoxime
- Bolus: 30–45 mg/kg over 30 minutes → Infusion: 8–12 mg/kg/h
  - Give pralidoxime (PAM) until atropine is no longer required.

Benzodiazepine
- Reduces agitation, seizures, fasciculations
- Sedation during ventilation
- **Intensive cardiorespiratory monitoring and support**
- **Others**: $MgSO_4$, $NaHCO_3$, clonidine, haemodialysis

TABLE 2.2: Atropine dosage for treatment of organophosphate poisoning.

Atropine bolus	Atropine infusion
1.8–3 mg IV bolus ↓	Start infusion at 20% of total dose of atropine required for atropinisation
Aim for heart rate (HR) > 80 bpm SBP > 80 mmHg Clear chest ↓If not	Bronchorrhoea is the most important sign for titrating the dose
Double the dose every 5 min ↓Satisfactory improvement	
Start atropine infusion	

Emergencies in Medical Practice

■ MANAGEMENT OF ANAPHYLAXIS

> **Case Scenario**
> A 12-year-old boy is brought to the emergency department after being stung by a bee. He initially complained of localised pain and swelling, but 15 minutes later he began to complain of shortness of breath, weakness and dizziness.
>
> **On examination:**
> PR: 120 bpm   BP: 69/45 mmHg   RR: 39/min
> He has generalised urticaria.
>
> S/E: RS: Mild wheeze bilaterally; CVS: Tachycardia present; PA: No abnormality detected (NAD)

- Prevent further contact with the antigen.
- Ensure airway patency.
- Supportive measures:
  - Oxygen
  - IV fluids
  - β2 agonist

  Drugs that are used in the management of anaphylaxis are given in **Flowchart 2.11**.

■ MANAGEMENT OF ANGINA

> **Case Scenario**
> A 58-year-old male patient who is a non-smoker, diabetic and hypertensive with dyslipidaemia presented with severe shortness of breath and chest tightness since 1 month. Pain is localised to the breast bone and does not radiate. It is aggravated while playing golf and subsides on rest.
>
> **On examination:**
> PR: 88 bpm   BP: 162/80 mmHg
> RR: 24/min   Temperature: Afebrile
> S/E: CVS, RS, PA: NAD

- **Lifestyle modification:**
  - Limit salt intake to < 5 g/day
  - Increase polyunsaturated fatty acid (PUFA) consumption
  - Smoking cessation
  - Limit alcohol intake.
  - Avoid simple carbohydrate.
  - Saturated fatty acids should be < 10% of the total intake.

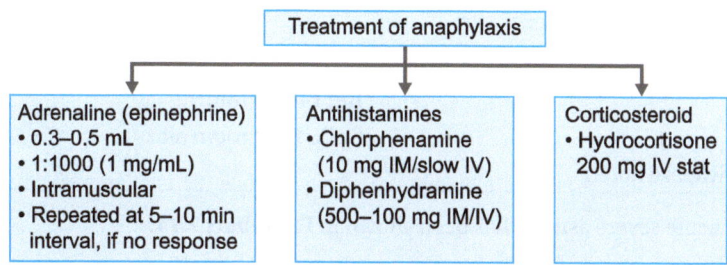

Flowchart 2.11: Drugs used in the management of anaphylaxis.

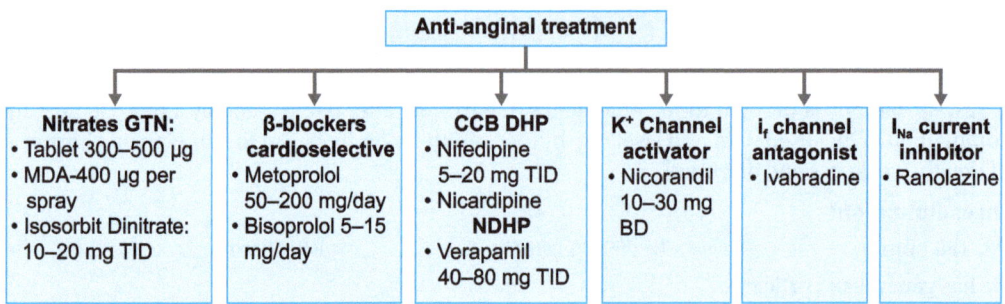

(CCB: calcium channel blocker; DHP: dihydropyridine; GTN: glyceryl trinitrate; MDA: 3,4-methylenedioxyamphetamine; NDHP: nondihydropyridine; I_f: funny current; I_{na}: persistent/late inward sodium current)

Flowchart 2.12: Drugs used in the treatment of angina.

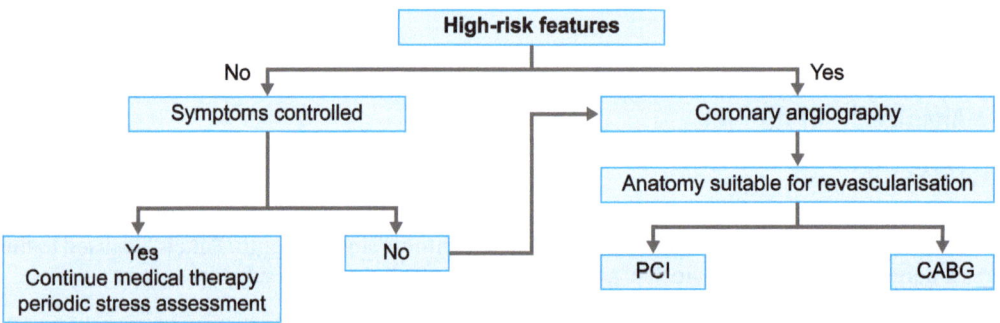

(CABG: coronary artery bypass graft; PCI: percutaneous coronary intervention)

Flowchart 2.13: Management of patients with high-risk features.

- **Aspirin** 75–150 mg daily OR clopidogrel 75 mg daily
- Drugs that are used in the treatment of angina are given in **Flowchart 2.12**.
- Management of patients with high-risk features is given in **Flowchart 2.13**.

■ MANAGEMENT OF ACUTE SEVERE ASTHMA

Case Scenario

A 16-year-old female patient complains of difficulty in breathing. Symptoms increase on exposure to cold. She has positive family history.

On examination:

PR: 126 bpm	BP: 148/86 mmHg
RR: 54/min	SpO_2: 88 at room air
RS: Expiratory wheeze noted	

Management of acute severe asthma has been shown in **Flowchart 2.14**.

Emergencies in Medical Practice

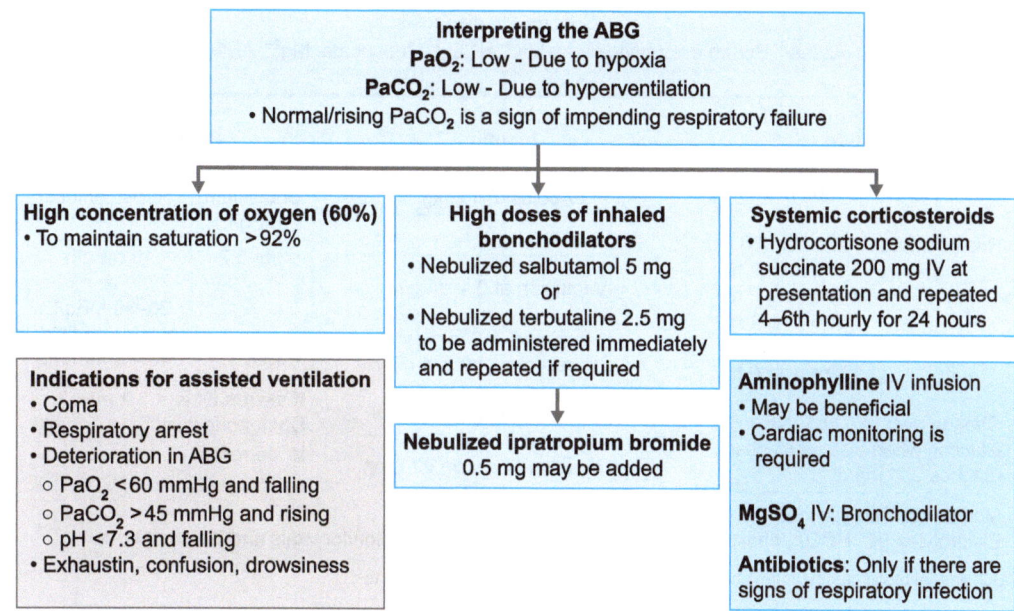

(ABG: arterial blood gas; IV: intravenous)

Flowchart 2.14: Management of acute severe asthma.

MANAGEMENT OF DIABETIC KETOACIDOSIS

Case Scenario

A 32-year-old male patient k/c/o type 1 diabetes mellitus was taken to casualty with complaints of drowsiness, fever, cough, diffuse abdominal pain and vomiting.

On examination: Patient appears confused.

Temperature: 39°C	PR: 104 bpm
BP: 100/70 mmHg	RR: 24/min

Dry mucous membranes, poor skin turgor and rales in right lower chest

pH: 7.12	pCO_2: 17 mmHg
HCO_3: 5.6 mEq/L	

Urinalysis revealed 4+ glucose and 3+ ketones.
Chemistry panel revealed a glucose of 420 mg/dL, BUN of 16 mg/dL, creatinine of 1.1 mg/dL.

Na: 139 mEq/dL	Cl: 112 mEq/dL
HCO_2: 11.2 mEq/L	K: 5.0 mEq/dL

- Confirm the diagnosis
- Assess: Serum electrolytes—Na^+, K^+, HCO_3^-, phosphate, Mg^{2+}
- Management of diabetic ketoacidosis has been shown in **Flowchart 2.15**.

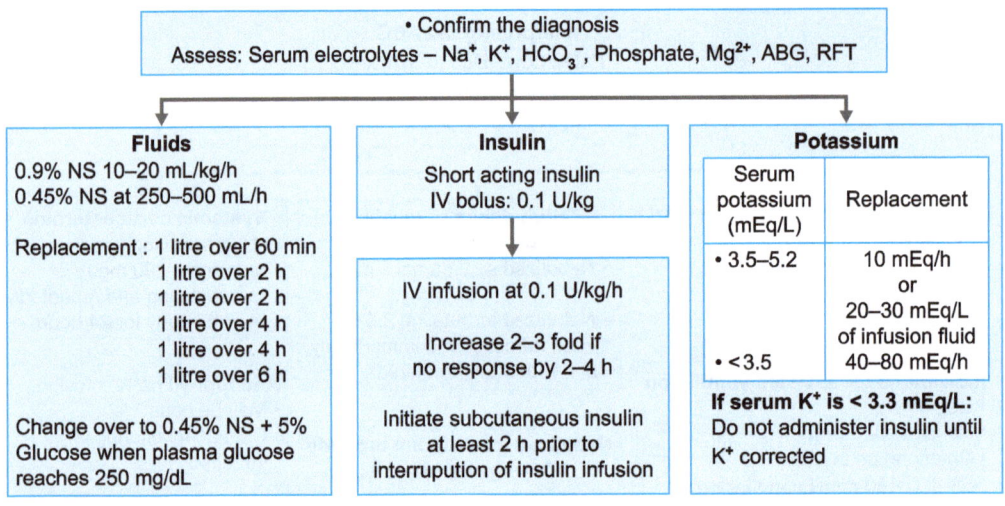

Flowchart 2.15: Management of diabetic ketoacidosis.

BEST OF FIVES

1. A 45-year-old man with no past medical history attends the emergency department with an episode of acute-onset breathlessness and chest pain. He has recently returned from a business trip and had been complaining of a painful, swollen left leg. Which is the next appropriate step?
   A. Focused assessment with sonography for trauma (FAST) scan
   B. Intra-arterial thrombolysis
   C. Intravenous thrombolysis followed by cardiopulmonary resuscitation (CPR) for 90 minutes
   D. Intravenous thrombolysis followed by CPR for 30 minutes
   E. Transthoracic echocardiography to image the right ventricle

2. A 20-year-old female has been found unconscious on her bed in the psychiatry ward. It is suspected that she has consumed lofepramine. Which drug should you ensure is available in the emergency trolley?
   A. Bicarbonate
   B. Calcium chloride
   C. Glucagon
   D. Lidocaine
   E. Verapamil

3. A 73-year-old man is brought to the emergency department in cardiac arrest. He was found unconscious on the floor by his carer. Electrocardiogram (ECG) reveals polymorphic ventricular tachycardia (VT). Which is the next most appropriate management option?
   A. Increase dose of adrenaline.
   B. Increase shock energy.
   C. Administer lidocaine IV.
   D. Administer magnesium sulphate IV.
   E. Repeat dose of amiodarone, at increased dose.

4. A 55-year-old man with a history of depression overdoses on his antihypertensive medication (beta-blocker). His blood pressure is recorded as 96/60 mmHg and his pulse is 45 bpm. A 12-lead electrocardiogram (ECG) reveals a regular rhythm with normal QRS morphology. The PR interval is prolonged but there are no non-conducted P waves. From the given

options, which is the first step in this patient's management?
A. Activated charcoal
B. Atropine
C. Glucagon
D. Observation
E. Temporal transvenous cardiac pacing

5. A 76-year-old man with a history of left ventricular dysfunction secondary to ischaemic heart disease had developed sudden-onset rapid, irregular palpitations and felt breathlessness, so he called the emergency services. He has a heart rate of around 156 bpm and the blood pressure is 60 mmHg systolic. The 12-lead electrocardiogram (ECG) showed a fast, irregular narrow complex tachycardia with absent P waves. From the given options, which is the treatment of choice for this patient?
A. Adenosine
B. Atenolol intravenously
C. Amiodarone intravenously
D. Digoxin intravenously
E. Direct current cardioversion (DCCV)

6. A 25-year-old man with paranoid schizophrenia started depot haloperidol. However, he was admitted by his GP following a 3-day history of confusion and increasing drowsiness. On examination, he was agitated, with a temperature of 38.5°C and blood pressure of 190/110 mmHg. His cardiovascular and chest examination were normal and no enlarged liver, spleen or kidneys were noted. He had bilateral severe rigidity but no tremor. What is the most likely diagnosis?
A. Herpes simplex encephalopathy
B. Hysteria
C. Meningitis
D. Neuroleptic malignant syndrome
E. Non-convulsive status epilepticus

7. A 60-year-old man with chronic alcohol abuse presented in the emergency department with confusion, agitation and ataxia. On examination, he was disoriented in time and place with a mini-mental score of 16/30. He was apyrexial with a blood pressure of 138/90 mmHg. He had bilateral sixth nerve palsies, gaze-evoked nystagmus and gait ataxia. What treatment should this patient receive?

A. Diazepam
B. Immunoglobulins
C. Penicillin
D. Steroids
E. Thiamine

8. A 26-year-old man is admitted to the emergency department after a motor vehicle accident. You are asked to review the patient. He is fully oriented to time, place and person. On questioning, the patient cannot provide any information about the accident; the last he remembers was getting into the car in order to attend a meeting. What course of management would you advise?
A. Admit the patient for observation and consciousness charting
B. Computed tomography (CT) scan of head
C. Discharge home with advice to return if any deterioration
D. Magnetic resonance imaging (MRI) of head
E. Plain X-ray of skull and C-spine

9. A 45-year-old man with a past medical history of multiple sclerosis was admitted to the hospital following an overdose of baclofen. On examination, he was drowsy with a respiratory rate of 5/min. He had a Glasgow coma scale (GCS) of 8/15 and generalised hyporeflexia. The pulse rate was 60/min and blood pressure was 95 mmHg systolic and 60 mmHg diastolic. Examination of respiratory, cardiovascular and abdominal system was unremarkable. What would be your next step in the management of this patient?
A. Increase concentration of inspired oxygen
B. Intravenous doxapram infusion
C. Intubation and mechanical ventilation
D. Non-invasive positive-pressure ventilation (NIPPV)
E. Reduce concentration of inspired oxygen

10. An 18-year-old female presents acutely unwell. Six weeks earlier, she had been diagnosed with hypothyroidism by her general practitioner. On examination, she appears unwell and mildly dehydrated. She has a temperature of 37.5°C and a body mass index (BMI) of 21.3 kg/m^2. Her blood pressure is 72/44 mmHg, with a pulse of 100 bpm.

In the meantime, what is the most appropriate immediate management of this patient?
A. Intravenous cefotaxime
B. Intravenous glucose
C. Intravenous fluids and hydrocortisone
D. Intravenous thyroxine (T4)
E. Intravenous thyronine (T3)

11. A 55-year-old male previously diagnosed with alcoholic liver disease was commenced on the rapid detoxification programme consisting of diazepam 20 mg at a minimum interval of 2-hourly (maximum dose 200 mg on 24 hours, standard regime). The following day, he was found collapsed in the bathroom in the ward. Which of the following agents administered is most likely to lead to an improvement in his conscious level?
A. Cefotaxime
B. Flumazenil
C. Naloxone
D. Thiamine
E. Vitamin K

12. A 24-year-old woman presented at 34 weeks of pregnancy with profuse vaginal bleeding. She had suffered two previous miscarriages. She had a pulse of 95 bpm and blood pressure of 110/84 mmHg and no foetal heart sounds were audible.
Investigations revealed:

Haemoglobin	9.8 g/dL	(11.5–16.5)
Platelets	66 ×10^9/L	(150–400)
Prothrombin time	21 s	(11.5–15.5)
APTT	52 s	(30–40)
Fibrinogen	0.5 g/L	(2–4)

What is the next most appropriate step in management?
A. Antithrombin III infusion
B. Fibrinogen replacement infusion (cryoprecipitate)
C. Intravenous heparin
D. Platelet transfusion
E. Transfusion of two units of group O, rhesus D negative blood

13. The following arterial blood gases (ABGs) were taken from an unconscious 60-year-old man in the emergency department:

pH	7.36	(7.36–7.44)
pO$_2$	13.0 kPa	(11.3–12.6)
pCO$_2$	3.7 kPa	(4.7–6.0)
HCO$_3$	15 mmol/L	(20–28)

Which is the correct interpretation of the ABG result?
A. Compensated metabolic acidosis
B. Compensated metabolic alkalosis
C. Compensated respiratory acidosis
D. Compensated respiratory alkalosis
E. Delayed analysis of ABG sample

14. A 70-year-old lady had a gastrointestinal (GI) bleed 10 months ago related to non-steroidal anti-inflammatory drug (NSAID) use for osteoarthritis. At that time, an endoscopy showed a duodenal ulcer which was treated. She now represents with an acute haematemesis. Her haemoglobin (Hb) on admission is 5.6 g/dL. Oesophago-gastroduodenoscopy (OGD) is performed, showing a single bleeding vessel on the posterior wall of the duodenum. Injection sclerotherapy is attempted but fails to stop the bleeding. What is the next step in her management?
A. Glypressin
B. IV omeprazole
C. Octreotide
D. Repeat attempt at sclerotherapy the following day
E. Urgent referral to on-call surgeons

15. A school girl is brought to the emergency department by her parents. She took a number of paracetamol tablets, but did not intend to kill herself. Which of the following is the best indicator of the degree of hepatocellular damage?
A. Aspartate transaminase level
B. Bilirubin level
C. International normalised ratio (INR)
D. Paracetamol level
E. Quantity of paracetamol ingested

Answers
1-C, 2-A, 3-D, 4-B, 5-E, 6-D, 7-E, 8-B, 9-C, 10-C, 11-B, 12-B, 13-A, 14-E, 15-C

SUGGESTED READING

1. Kitabchi AE, Umpierrez GE, Miles JM, Fisher JN. Hyperglycemic crises in adult patients with diabetes. Diabetes Care. 2009;32(7):1335-43.
2. Brophy GM, Bell R, Claassen J, Alldredge B, Bleck TP, Glauser T, et al. Guidelines for the evaluation and management of status epilepticus. Neurocrit Care. 2012; 17(1):3-23.
3. Trinka E, Cock H, Hesdorffer D, Rossetti AO, Scheffer IE, Shinnar S, et al. A definition and classification of status epilepticus--Report of the ILAE Task Force on Classification of Status Epilepticus. Epilepsia. 2015;56(10):1515-23.
4. Pumphrey RS. Lessons for management of anaphylaxis from a study of fatal reactions. Clin Exp Allergy. 2000;30(8):1144-50.
5. Kearon C, Akl EA, Comerota AJ, Prandoni P, Bounameaux H, Goldhaber SZ, et al. Antithrombotic therapy for VTE disease: Antithrombotic Therapy and Prevention of Thrombosis, 9th ed: American College of Chest Physicians Evidence-Based Clinical Practice Guidelines. Chest. 2012;141(2 Suppl):e419S-96S.
6. Siemieniuk RAC, Chu DK, Kim LH, Güell-Rous MR, Alhazzani W, Soccal PM, et al. Oxygen therapy for acutely ill medical patients: a clinical practice guideline. BMJ. 2018;363:k4169.
7. Nieminen MS, Böhm M, Cowie MR, Drexler H, Filippatos GS, Jondeau G, et al. Executive summary of the guidelines on the diagnosis and treatment of acute heart failure: the Task Force on Acute Heart Failure of the European Society of Cardiology. Eur Heart J. 2005;26(4):384-416.
8. Gheorghiade M, Zannad F, Sopko G, Klein L, Piña IL, Konstam MA, et al. Acute heart failure syndromes: current state and framework for future research. Circulation. 2005;112(25):3958-68.
9. Al-Khatib SM, Stevenson WG, Ackerman MJ, Bryant WB, Callans DJ, Curtis AB, et al. 2017 AHA/ACC/HRS Guideline for Management of Patients With Ventricular Arrhythmias and the Prevention of Sudden Cardiac Death: A Report of the American College of Cardiology/American Heart Association Task Force on Clinical Practice Guidelines and the Heart Rhythm Society. J Am Coll Cardiol. 2018;72(14):e91-220.
10. Global Initiative for Asthma (GINA). Global Strategy for Asthma Management and Prevention. [online] Available from: www.ginasthma.org. [Last accessed June, 2020).

Chapter 3

Cardiology

■ CHEST PAIN
Chest pain is described in **Box 3.1**.

■ PALPITATIONS
Described as an uncomfortable awareness of one's own heartbeat.

Causes of Palpitations
Causes of palpitations are given in **Box 3.2**.

■ SYNCOPE
Comprises generalised weakness of muscles, loss of postural tone, inability to stand upright and momentary loss of consciousness.

Types
Types of syncope are given in **Box 3.3**.

■ CYANOSIS
Bluish discolouration of the skin and mucous membranes, due to an increased amount of reduced haemoglobin (> 5 g/dL).

Box 3.1: Chest pain.

Heart	Intra-abdominal conditions
• Angina pectoris	• Cholecystitis
• Myocardial infarction	• Pancreatitis
• Mitral valve prolapsed	**Aortic**
• Pericarditis	• Dissecting aneurysm
Musculoskeletal	**Oesophageal**
• Rib fracture	• Reflux oesophagitis
• Costochondritis-Tietze syndrome	• Diffuse oesophageal spasm
Lung and pleura	**Truncal neuropathy**
• Pleurisy	**Anxiety state**
• Pneumonia	
• Pneumothorax	
• Pulmonary embolism	

Box 3.2: Causes of palpitations.

Cardiac arrhythmias	Cardiac abnormalities
• Atrial flutter/fibrillation	• Congenital heart disease (atrial septal defect, patent ductus arteriosus, ventricular septal defect)
• Paroxysmal atrial tachycardia	
• Premature atrial contractions	
• Sick sinus syndrome	• Mitral valve prolapsed
• Sinus tachycardia	• Pacemaker (function or failure)
• Premature ventricular contractions	• Prosthetic heart valves
• Ventricular tachycardia	• Aortic or mitral regurgitation
Drug induces	**Metabolic**
• Alcohol	• Hyperthyroidism
• Amphetamines	• Hypoglycaemia
• Anticholinergic agents	• Phaeochromocytoma
• Caffeine, nicotine	**Psychiatric causes**
• Cardiac glycosides	• Generalised anxiety
• Cocaine	• Hypochondriasis
• Epinephrine	• Major depression
• Nitrates	• Panic disorder
High cardiac output states	**Miscellaneous**
• Anaemia	• Emotional stress
• Arteriovenous fistula	• Hyperventilation
• Beriberi	
• Fever	
• Paget's disease	
• Pregnancy	
• Thyrotoxicosis	

Box 3.3: Types of syncope.

Vasovagal syncope
- Causes include emotional stress, warm overcrowded room, sudden pain, mild blood loss, anaemia, fever and fasting

Cardiac syncope
- Due to sudden reduction in cardiac output
    - Acute massive myocardial infarction
    - Aortic stenosis
    - Complete heart block
    - Paroxysmal tachycardias
    - Sick sinus syndrome

Orthostatic syncope (postural syncope)
- When the person suddenly gets up from a lying-down position or stands still for a long time
    - Physiological
    - Antihypertensive drugs
    - Diabetic neuropathy

Neurogenic syncope
- Due to carotid/vertebral occlusion. Physical activity can further reduce the blood flow (which is already compromised) to the brainstem resulting in loss of consciousness

Drug-induced syncope
- Angiotensin-converting enzyme inhibitors, β-blockers, calcium channel blockers, diuretics

Carotid sinus syncope
- Due to compression on the carotid sinus as in turning the head, tight collar or shaving over the region of carotid sinus

Others
- Micturition syncope
- Cough syncope

TABLE 3.1: Cyanosis and its features.

Feature	Central cyanosis	Peripheral cyanosis
Site	Mucous membranes and skin are both involved	Mucous membranes of the oral cavity or those beneath the tongue spared
Tongue	Affected	Unaffected
Temperature of limb	Warm	Cold
Clubbing	Present	Absent
Polycythaemia	Present	Absent
Local warming	Cyanosis remains	Cyanosis disappears
Breathing pure oxygen for 10 min	Cyanosis may disappear	Cyanosis remains
Arterial blood gas studies	Abnormal	Normal
Causes	<ul><li>Cardiac causes<ul><li>Fallot's tetralogy</li><li>Eisenmenger's syndrome</li><li>Congestive cardiac failure</li></ul></li><li>Pulmonary causes<ul><li>Chronic bronchitis</li><li>Interstitial lung disease</li></ul></li><li>High altitude</li></ul>	<ul><li>Congestive cardiac failure</li><li>Shock</li></ul> Due to local vasoconstriction <ul><li>Cold exposure</li><li>Raynaud's disease</li><li>Peripheral vascular disease</li></ul>

Types of Cyanosis and their features are given in **Table 3.1**.

CLINICAL EXAMINATION OF PULSE

Clinical examination of pulse is given in **Box 3.4**.

Rhythm

Types of rhythm are given in **Box 3.5**.

The features of hypokinetic and hyperkinetic pulse are given in **Box 3.6**.

Box 3.4: Clinical examination of pulse.

Bradycardia (< 60 beats/min)
- Athletes
- Hypothyroidism
- Vasovagal syncope
- Drug-β-blockers
- Heart block
- Sick sinus syndrome
- Hypothermia

Tachycardia (> 100 beats/min)
- Anxiety
- Fever
- Pregnancy
- Hyperthyroidism
- Cardiac failure
- Tachyarrhythmias
- Drugs: Salbutamol, terbutaline

Box 3.5: Types of rhythm.

Completely irregular (irregularly irregular)
- Atrial fibrillation
- Frequent extrasystoles

Otherwise regular with occasional irregularity
- Extrasystoles

Irregular with a recurring pattern (regularly irregular)
- Sinus arrhythmia
- Pulsus bigeminus
- Pulsus trigeminus
- Partial atrioventricular blocks

Box 3.6: Features of hypokinetic and hyperkinetic pulse.

Hypokinetic pulse
- Hypovolaemia
- Shock
- Congestive cardiac failure
- Constrictive pericarditis
- Mitral stenosis
- Aortic stenosis

Hyperkinetic pulse
- Hyperkinetic circulation (anaemia, fever, thyrotoxicosis, exercise)
- Mitral regurgitation
- Aortic regurgitation
- Patent ductus arteriosus
- Ventricular septal defect

Character or Quality

The character or quality of pulse is given in **Box 3.7**.

■ JUGULAR VENOUS PULSE/PRESSURE

The causes of raised jugular venous pressure are given in **Box 3.8**.

Abnormalities in Wave Form

Abnormalities in wave form and their conditions are given in **Table 3.2**.

Kussmaul's Sign

- Increase in the height of jugular venous pulsations and hence a rise in jugular venous pressure (JVP) during inspiration
- Is seen in the following conditions:
  - Constrictive pericarditis
  - Restrictive cardiomyopathy

■ APICAL IMPULSE

- Apex beat is the lowermost and outermost point of definite cardiac pulsation.
- Also known as 'point of maximum impulse'

Normal Apex Beat

- With the patient in supine or sitting posture, it is located 1 cm medial to the midclavicular line or 9–10 cm from the midsternal line, in the left fifth intercostals space.
- It is detectable in only one intercostal space and is < 3 cm in diameter.

Abnormalities in Character

- **Hyperdynamic apex**
  - Aortic regurgitation (AR)
  - Mitral regurgitation (MR)
  - Ventricular septal defect

Cardiology

Box 3.7: Character or quality of pulse.

Pulsus parvus: Congestive heart failure or a decrease in systemic arterial pressure
Pulsus tardus: Aortic stenosis
Pulsus parvus et tardus: Aortic stenosis
Anacrotic pulse: Severe aortic stenosis
Collapsing (Water-hammer) pulse
- Patent ductus arteriosus
- Aortic regurgitation
- Hyperkinetic circulatory states (anaemia, fever, thyrotoxicosis, exercise, pregnancy, Paget's diseases, beriberi)

Bisferiens pulse
- Combination of aortic stenosis and aortic regurgitation
- Severe aortic regurgitation
- Hypertrophic cardiomyopathy

Dicrotic pulse
- Dilated (congestive) cardiomyopathy
- Typhoid
- Advanced cardiac failure

Pulsus alternans: Seen in acute left ventricular failure
Pulsus bigeminus: An ectopic beat following each regular beat (digoxin)
Pulsus paradoxus
- Constrictive pericarditis
- Cardiac tamponade
- Chronic obstructive airway disease (severe)
- Severe bronchial asthma
- Tension pneumothorax

Radiofemoral delay
- Occurs in coarctation of aorta

Box 3.8: Causes of raised jugular venous pressure.

- Right heart failure (commonest)
- Tricuspid regurgitation
- Tricuspid stenosis
- Constrictive pericarditis
- Cardiac tamponade
- Superior vena cava obstruction (non-pulsatile)

- **Heaving apex**
   - Aortic stenosis
   - Systemic hypertension
   - Coarctation of aorta (COA)
   - Hypertrophic cardiomyopathy (HCM)
- **Tapping apex:** Occurs in mitral stenosis
- **Hypokinetic apex**
   - Obesity
   - Pericardial effusion

TABLE 3.2: Abnormalities in wave form and their conditions.

Abnormalities	Conditions
• Abnormalities of the *a* wave	
○ Large *a* waves	• Tricuspid stenosis, pulmonary hypertension, pulmonary stenosis, right ventricular hypertrophy
○ Regular 'cannon' *a* waves	• Junctional rhythm
○ Irregular 'cannon' *a* waves	• Complete heart block, multiple ectopics
○ Absent *a* waves	• Atrial fibrillation
• Abnormalities of the *v* wave	
○ Large *v* waves	• Tricuspid regurgitation, right ventricular failure
• Abnormalities of the *x* descent	
○ Increased prominence	• Cardiac tamponade, constrictive pericarditis, atrial septal defect
○ Decreased prominence	• Tricuspid regurgitation (replaced by *c–v* wave), right ventricular failure, atrial fibrillation
• Abnormalities of the *y* descent	
○ Rapid *y* descent	• Tricuspid regurgitation, restrictive heart disease including constrictive pericarditis, severe right heart failure
○ Slow *y* descent	• Tricuspid stenosis, cardiac tamponade

- Shock
- Emphysema
- Constrictive pericarditis
- Myxoedema
- **Double apex:** Hypertrophic cardiomyopathy

FIRST HEART SOUND

First heart sound (S1) and its features are given in **Box 3.9**.

Box 3.9: First heart sound S1 and its features

Loud S1
- Mitral stenosis
- Short PR interval
- Hyperdynamic circulatory states

Soft S1
- Mitral regurgitation
- Calcified mitral valve
- Long PR interval

Varying intensity of S1
- Atrial fibrillation

SECOND HEART SOUND

Types and components of pathological S2 and their causes are described in **Box 3.10**.

THIRD HEART SOUND

Low-pitched sound heard at the end of rapid filling phase (early diastole). Third heart sound (S3) is best heard with the bell of a stethoscope.

Types of S3 and their various causes are listed in **Box 3.11**.

FOURTH HEART SOUND

- It occurs as a result of forceful atrial contraction ('atrial kick').
- It is a low-pitched sound heard in presystole. Types of fourth heart sound (S4) are given in **Box 3.12**.

EJECTION CLICK

- Ejection click is a sharp, high-frequency sound audible immediately after S1.

Box 3.10: Second heart sound S2 and its features.

Aortic component (A_2)
- Increased intensity
  - Essential hypertension
  - Syphilitic aortic regurgitation
- Decreased intensity
  - Aortic stenosis
  - Aortic regurgitation

Wide fixed splitting
- Atrial septal defect

Pulmonary component (P_2)
- Increased intensity
  - Pulmonary hypertension
  - Pulmonary artery dilatation
- Decreased intensity
  - Pulmonary stenosis
  - Tetralogy of Fallot
  - Pulmonary atresia

Reversed (paradoxical) splitting
- Delayed electrical activation of the left ventricle:
  - Left bundle branch block
- Prolonged left ventricular systole
  - Hypertension
  - Severe aortic stenosis

Wide mobile split
- Delayed electrical activation of the right ventricle
  - Right bundle branch block
  - Ectopic from left ventricle
- Prolonged right ventricular systole
  - Pulmonary stenosis
  - Pulmonary hypertension
- Early aortic closure
  - Mitral regurgitation

Single S2
- Severe aortic stenosis (absent A_2)
- Severe pulmonary stenosis (absent P_2)
- Tetralogy of Fallot

Box 3.11: Third heart sound S3 and its types.

Physiological S3
- Children
- Under 40 years
- Athletes
- Pregnancy

Pathological left-sided S3
- Left ventricular failure
- Aortic regurgitation
- Mitral regurgitation

Pathological right-sided S3
- Right ventricular failure

Box 3.12: Fourth heart sound S4 and its types.

Left-sided S4
- Systemic hypertension
- Hypertrophic cardiomyopathy

Right-sided S4
- Pulmonary hypertension
- Pulmonary stenosis

- It can occur with aortic valve stenosis and pulmonary valve stenosis as well as in dilation of ascending aorta and pulmonary artery.

NON-EJECTION CLICK

- Associated with Mitral Valve Prolapse (MVP)
- A mid-systolic click arises from sudden tension on the chordae tendineae or from sudden halt of prolapsing mitral valve leaflet during ventricular systole.

MURMURS

Various systolic murmurs and their causes are given in **Box 3.13**.

Various diastolic murmurs and their causes are given in **Box 3.14**.

Causes of continuous murmurs are given in **Box 3.15**.

Box 3.13: Various systolic murmurs and their causes.

Early systolic murmurs
- VSD (small muscular VSD/large VSD with pulmonary hypertension)
- Acute severe MR
- Acute severe TR

Mid-systolic/ejection systolic murmurs
- Aortic stenosis
- Pulmonary stenosis
- Hypertrophic obstructive cardiomyopathy (HOCM)

Late systolic murmurs
- Mitral valve prolapse
- Tricuspid valve prolapse
- Papillary muscle dysfunction

Pansystolic murmurs
- Mitral regurgitation
- Tricuspid regurgitation
- Ventricular septal defect
- Rare: Early PDA/PDA with Eisenmenger

(MR: mitral regurgitation; PDA: patent ductus arteriosus; TR: tricuspid regurgitation; VSD: ventricular septal defect)

Box 3.14: Various diastolic murmurs and their causes.

Early diastolic murmur
- Aortic regurgitation
- Pulmonary regurgitation

Mid-diastolic murmur (MDM)
- Mitral stenosis
- Tricuspid stenosis
- Carey Coombs murmur of acute rheumatic fever
- Austin Flint murmur of chronic aortic regurgitation
- Flow MDM
  - Across mitral valve: MR, AR, VSD, PDA
  - Across tricuspid valve: ASD, TR, TAPVC (total anomalous pulmonary venous connection)
- Atrial myxoma
- Ball-valve thrombus
- Cor triatriatum
- Rytand's murmur of complete heart block

Late diastolic murmurs/presystolic murmur
- Mitral stenosis
- Tricuspid stenosis
- Myxoma

(AR: aortic regurgitation; ASD: atrial septal defect; MR: mitral regurgitation; PDA: patent ductus arteriosus; TR: tricuspid regurgitation; VSD: ventricular septal defect)

> **Box 3.15: Causes of continuous murmurs.**
>
> - **Systemic to pulmonary communication**
>   - Patent ductus arteriosus
>   - Aortopulmonary window
>   - Anomalous origin of left coronary artery from pulmonary artery (ALCAPA)
>   - Tricuspid atresia
>   - Truncus arteriosus
>   - Shunts for TOF surgery: Waterson, Potts, or Blalock–Taussig shunt
> - **Systemic to right heart connection**
>   - Coronary arteriovenous fistula
>   - Rupture sinus of Valsalva
> - **Left atrium to right atrium connection**
>   - Lutembacher syndrome
> - **Arteriovenous fistula**
>   - Systemic
>   - Pulmonary
> - **Normal flow through constricted arteries**
>   - Coarctation of aorta
>   - Peripheral pulmonary stenosis
>   - Renal artery stenosis
> - **Increased flow through normal vessels**
>   - **Venous:** Cervical venous hum, Cruveilhier–Baumgarten murmur
>   - **Arterial:** Mammary souffle, uterine souffle, thyrotoxicosis, tumours (e.g. hepatocellular carcinoma, renal cell carcinoma)
>
> (TOF: tetralogy of Fallot)

> **Box 3.16: Cardiac arrhythmia and its classification.**
>
> **Disturbances of impulse formation**
> - **Disturbances of sinus mechanism**
>   - Sinus tachycardia
>   - Sinus bradycardia
>   - Sinus arrhythmia
> - **Disturbance of atria**
>   - Atrial premature contraction
>   - Atrial fibrillation
>   - Atrial flutter
>   - Paroxysmal supraventricular tachycardia (PSVT)
> - **Disturbance of atrioventricular node**
>   - Junctional ectopics
>   - Junctional tachycardia
> - **Disturbance of ventricles**
>   - Ventricular ectopics
>   - Ventricular tachycardia
>   - Ventricular fibrillation (VF)
>
> **Disturbances of impulse conduction**
> - **Sinoatrial blocks**
> - **AV nodal blocks**
>   - First-degree block
>   - Second-degree block
>   - Wenckebach (Mobitz type 1) block
>   - Mobitz type II block
>   - Complete or third-degree block
> - **Bundle blocks**
>   - Right bundle branch block
>   - Left bundle branch block
>   - Left anterior hemiblock
>   - Left posterior hemiblock

CARDIAC ARRHYTHMIAS

Classification

Cardiac arrhythmias and their classification is given in **Box 3.16**.

Wide-complex Tachycardias

- Ventricular tachycardia
- Toxicity of certain medications (e.g. tricyclic antidepressants, diphenhydramine, cocaine)
- Hyperkalaemia (usually produces wide complexes with bradycardia)
- Supraventricular and nodal tachycardias may produce widened QRS complexes due to: Antegrade conduction from the atria to the ventricles via an accessory pathway (bundle of Kent and others).
- Underlying pre-existing bundle branch block

VENTRICULAR TACHYCARDIA

Electrocardiogram (ECG) criteria that suggest a ventricular tachycardia—**broad QRS tachycardia with Box 3.17.**

> **Box 3.17: ECG criteria for ventricular tachycardia.**
> - Presence of fusion beats
> - Presence of atrioventricular dissociation
> - Presence of capture beats
> - QRS width > 0.14 s if RBBB is present or > 0.16 s if LBBB is present
> - QRS axis < –90° to +180°
> - Precordial concordance
>
> **RBBB pattern with**
> - RSR or RS pattern in lead V_1
> - R/S < 1 or Qs pattern in V_6
>
> **LBBB pattern with**
> - Q in V_6
> - Notched downstroke S wave in V_1
> - R > 0.03 s in V_1

- The patient may be asymptomatic or may present with palpitations or haemodynamic collapse.
- If the patient is haemodynamically unstable in the form of hypotension, angina, heart failure or altered sensorium, immediate cardioversion in a synchronised mode is required.
- If the patient is stable, **amiodarone** and **lidocaine** are the drugs of choice.
- Amiodarone 150 mg intravenously over 10 minutes, then 1 mg/min for 6 hours and then 0.5 mg/min for the next 18 hours.
- Lidocaine 1–1.5 mg/kg intravenous (IV) over 1 minute followed by infusion at 10–40 µg/kg/min

■ TORSADES DE POINTES

- Type of ventricular tachycardia characterised by gradual changing of QRS axis so that it appears around the isoelectric line
- Usually due to prolonged QT interval
- It can result from ingestion of certain drugs such as quinidine, procainamide, antidepressants and phenothiazines, and the electrolyte imbalances such as hypokalaemia and hypocalcaemia.
- **Magnesium in** a dose of 2–4 kg IV over a period of 30 minutes is quite effective in terminating an episode and preventing its recurrence.

■ ATRIAL FIBRILLATION

- Disorganised and multiple atrial foci fire impulses at a rate of 350–600/min. The ventricles respond at irregular intervals, usually at a rate of 100–140/min.

- Atrial fibrillation can be
  - Paroxysmal atrial fibrillation means that episodes terminate without intervention in lesser than 7 days.
  - Persistent atrial fibrillation means that episodes lasting longer than 7 days or more, usually requiring an intervention.
  - Permanent atrial fibrillation means that the arrhythmia is continuous, and interventions to restore sinus rhythm have either failed or not been attempted.

Aetiology
Aetiology of atrial fibrillation is given in **Box 3.18**.

Symptoms
- Usual symptoms include palpitations, fatigue, syncope and angina.

Signs
- Irregularly irregular pulse
- Varying volumes of pulse
- Pulse deficit (apex pulse deficit) > 10
- Varying intensity of the S1
- Absence of waves on JVP

Electrocardiogram
- An irregularly irregular rhythm of QRS complexes
- Absent P waves
- Small, irregular waves (fibrillary waves)

> **Box 3.18: Aetiology of atrial fibrillation.**
> - Rheumatic heart disease (especially mitral valvular disease)
> - Ischaemic heart disease (especially acute myocardial infarction)
> - Hypertension
> - Thyrotoxicosis
> - Congenital heart diseases (especially atrial septal defect)
> - Cardiomyopathy
> - Pericardial diseases
> - Other rare causes: Alcohol, pulmonary embolism, exercise, chronic lung diseases
> - Lone atrial fibrillation: Elderly patients without underlying heart disease

Complications
- Syncope
- Thromboembolism
  - Risk of stroke in atrial fibrillation
    - A risk index (**CHA$_2$DS$_2$-VASc Score**) has been developed to determine the risk of stroke due to thromboembolism in patients with atrial fibrillation.
  - Warfarin is recommended if score > 2.
- Precipitation/worsening of cardiac failure
- Angina
- Hypotension

Treatment
- If the patient's clinical status is severely compromised, a synchronised direct current (DC) cardioversion is the treatment of choice.
- If the patient's clinical status is not severely compromised, treatment is in two steps (rate and rhythm control):
  - Slowing the ventricular rate with verapamil, diltiazem, propranolol, esmolol or digoxin (rate control)
  - Converting rhythm to normal sinus rhythm (rhythm control)
- Pharmacological cardioversion to sinus rhythm with quinidine, ibutilide, flecainide, propafenone or amiodarone
- Chronic anticoagulation includes warfarin and dabigatran.

■ ATRIAL FLUTTER
- A regular, rapid atrial rate of 250–350/min, where ventricles responded to every second, third or fourth beat [2:1, 3:1 or 4:1 atrioventricular block].
- **Electrocardiographic feature**
  - Characteristic flutter waves are seen as regular saw-toothed waves ('F' waves).
- Management
  - Same as atrial fibrillation

■ PAROXYSMAL SUPRAVENTRICULAR TACHYCARDIA
- It is usually paroxysmal and recurrent and has a rate of 140–220 beats/min with 1:1 conduction.
- It usually results from re-entry of an atrial ectopic in the AV node [AV nodal reentrant tachycardia (AVNRT) or AV reentrant tachycardia (AVRT)].

Causes
- Idiopathic in healthy individuals
- Excessive coffee, tea, alcohol or tobacco
- Anxiety
- Hyperthyroidism
- Organic heart disease (ischaemic, valvular or congenital)

Clinical features
- The onset and termination of the arrhythmia are sudden.
- Patients most commonly complain of palpitations, an odd feeling in the chest and, on occasion, lightheadedness or pain.
- Some patients have polyuria and experience diuresis during or after paroxysmal supraventricular tachycardia (PSVT).

Electrocardiogram
- The P wave is usually buried in the QRS complex or occurs slightly before or after the QRS complex.

■ TREATMENT
- Vagal manoeuvres such as carotid sinus massage, Valsalva manoeuvre and gag reflex
- **Adenosine** is administered as in initial bolus of 6 mg rapidly over 1–3 seconds followed immediately by 20 mL of saline.
- Propranolol, esmolol, verapamil, diltiazem and adenosine
- **Synchronised cardioversion** is performed if the patient is haemodynamically compromised.
- Long-term control can be achieved by **radiofrequency ablation** of the re-entrant pathway.

■ WOLFF–PARKINSON–WHITE SYNDROME
- **Cause:** Presence of an abnormal band of atrial tissue (bundle of Kent) connecting the atria and ventricles and bypassing the AV node
- **ECG:** Short PR interval (< 0.12 s), a delta wave in the beginning of ORS and prolonged QRS complex (> 0.12 s)
- Act as a re-entry pathway and the patient may develop supraventricular tachycardia

- **Treatment:**
  - Disopyramide, quinidine, flecainide and amiodarone to increase the refractory period and reduce the conducting rate through the bypass tract
  - Radiofrequency ablation of the bypass tract can be done.

SICK SINUS SYNDROME

- It includes sinus bradycardia, sinus arrest, combinations of sinoatrial and AV blocks, and supraventricular tachycardias.
- The abnormalities are usually due to ischaemia, fibrosis, drug induced or autonomic dysfunction.
- Clinical features:
  - Many patients are asymptomatic.
- Treatment of recurrent symptomatic bradycardia or prolonged pauses requires implantation of a permanent pacemaker.

BRUGADA SYNDROME

- ST segment elevation (> 2 mm) in right precordial leads (V_1 to V_3), incomplete or complete right bundle branch block
- Susceptibility to ventricular tachyarrhythmia (particularly polymorphic ventricular tachycardia) and sudden cardiac death (SCD)
- Treatment involves implantable cardioverter-defibrillator (ICD).

SUDDEN CARDIAC DEATH

- An unexpected, non-traumatic death due to cardiac causes occurring in a short time period in a person with known or unknown cardiac disease in whom no previously diagnosed fatal condition is apparent.

Causes
Causes of SCD are given in **Box 3.19**.

CARDIAC ARREST

- Cardiac arrest is defined as an abrupt loss of cardiac pump function which may be reversible by a prompt intervention but will lead to death in its absence.
- Cardiac arrest may result from one of the following four mechanisms:
  1. Ventricular fibrillation (VF);
  2. Pulseless ventricular tachycardia;
  3. Asystole;
  4. Pulseless electrical activity (PEA).

Causes of Cardiac Arrest
Causes of cardiac arrest are given in **Box 3.20**.

Management
Cardiopulmonary resuscitation (CPR).

ATRIOVENTRICULAR BLOCKS

First-degree Block
- In the ECG, the PR interval is prolonged to > 0.20 seconds. All the P waves are conducted and the QRS is normal as the delay is most often in the AV mode.

Box 3.19: Causes of sudden cardiac death.
- Coronary artery disease
- Ischaemic cardiomyopathy
- Non-ischaemic cardiomyopathy
- Hypertrophic cardiomyopathy
- Valvular heart disease
- Congenital heart disease
- Brugada syndrome
- Wolff–Parkinson–White syndrome
- Electrolyte abnormalities
- Cocaine
- Myocarditis
- Long QT syndrome

Box 3.20: Causes of cardiac arrest.

Six Hs
1. Hypoxia
2. Hypovolaemia
3. Hypothermia
4. Hydrogen ions (acidosis)
5. Hypokalaemia/hyperkalaemia
6. Hypoglycaemia

Six Ts
1. Tamponade, cardiac
2. Tension pneumothorax
3. Toxins/tablets
4. Thrombosis, coronary (myocardial infarction)
5. Thrombosis, pulmonary embolism
6. Trauma

Second-degree Block
- It can be subdivided into Mobitz type I and Mobitz type II blocks:
  - **Mobitz type I (Wenckebach)** second-degree AV block.
    - The ECG typically shows progressive prolongation of successive PR intervals until one P wave is not conducted. The QRS is usually normal
  - **Mobitz type II** second-degree AV block
    - The block is characterised by a constant PR interval with intermittent failure of atrial impulses to conduct to the ventricles.
    - Patients generally require a pacemaker.

Third-degree or Complete Atrioventricular Block
- Regular and slow pulse (30–40/min)
- High-volume pulse
- Irregular cannon waves on JVP
- Varying intensity of S1
- Stokes–Adams attacks
- The ECG shows constant PP and RR intervals but with complete AV dissociation, i.e. the atria and ventricles beat independently and there is no relation between the P waves and the QRS complexes.

Management
Implantation of a permanent pacemaker.

■ ADAMS–STOKES ATTACKS (STOKES –ADAMS–MORGAGNI ATTACKS)
- An episode of syncope caused by bradycardia related to AV block is called Stokes–Adams–Morgagni syndrome.
- This commonly occurs due to an underlying Mobitz type II block or complete heart block in the distal conduction system.
- Even though ventricular tachycardia can also produce loss of consciousness, it is not typically included under Adams–Stokes attack.
- **Clinical features:**
  - Some patients describe a prodrome preceding the attack.
  - Rapid loss of consciousness and the patient may fall, followed by rapid recovery.
  - Convulsions and later death may result if the asystole or severe bradycardia is prolonged to > 10 seconds.

■ ACUTE CIRCULATORY FAILURE/SHOCK
- Persistent hypotension (systolic blood pressure < 90 mmHg or mean arterial pressure 30 mmHg lower than baseline) with severe reduction in cardiac index (< 1.8/min/m^2 without support or < 2.0–2.2 L/min/m^2 with support), and adequate or elevated filling pressure (e.g. left ventricular end-diastolic pressure > 18 mmHg, right ventricular end-diastolic pressure > 10–15 mmHg)

Classification and Causes
Classification and causes of acute circulatory failure/shock are given in **Table 3.3**.

Cardinal Features of Shock
- Hypotension with a systolic blood pressure < 90 mmHg
- Tachycardia (> 100/min) with a thready pulse
- Cold, clammy skin
- Tachypnoea, Cheyne–Stokes breathing
- Urine output < 30 mL/h

Management of Shock
Patient Monitoring
- Pulse, blood pressure and respiration
- Electrocardiography
- Arterial blood gases
- Central venous pressure monitoring
- Urinary catheterisation to monitor hourly urinary output

General Measures
- Patient should be put in a horizontal position with legs slightly elevated
- Correction of hypovolaemia:
  - Correction is based on the amount and nature of fluid lost, clinical state of the patient and central venous pressure or pulmonary artery wedge pressure.

TABLE 3.3: Classification and causes of acute circulatory failure/shock.

Type of shock	Causes
Hypovolaemic shock	Haemorrhage, severe vomiting and diarrhoea, plasma loss in burns and acute pancreatitis, diabetic ketoacidosis
Cardiogenic shock	Acute myocardial infarction, acute aortic regurgitation, acute mitral regurgitation, right ventricular infarction, acute massive pulmonary embolism, cardiac arrhythmias, dilated cardiomyopathy, pericardial tamponade
Septic shock	Gram-positive and gram-negative bacterial infections, other organisms
Anaphylactic shock	Drugs, insect stings
Neurogenic shock	High cervical cord injury, severe head injury

- ○ Hypovolaemia is corrected by blood, Ringer's lactate solution, isotonic saline solution, dextran, albumin or plasma, depending on the situation.
- Correction of hypoxia with oxygen by face masks or nasal prongs and, if necessary, by intubation and mechanical ventilation.
- Correction of acidosis with IV sodium bicarbonate (if acidosis is severe).
- Treatment of cardiac arrhythmias with drugs, electrical cardioversion or pacing.
- Treatment of sepsis (especially in septic shock) with antibiotics and drainage of any abscesses.
- Low-dose corticosteroids are recommended in early stages of septic shock.

Vasopressors and Inotropic Agents

Sympathomimetic Amines
- Dobutamine
- Dopamine
- Noradrenaline
- Adrenaline
- Isoproterenol
- Phenylephrine
- Vasopressin

Treatment of Cardiogenic Shock

- Early **reperfusion therapy** (prehospital) for myocardial infarction (MI)
- Antithrombotic therapy with aspirin and heparin should be given.
- **Circulatory assist devices**
  - ○ Intra-aortic balloon counterpulsation
  - ○ Partial cardiac bypass (left ventricle assist devices)
  - ○ Extracorporeal membrane oxygenator (ECMO)

Box 3.21: Types of pulmonary oedema.

Cardiogenic pulmonary oedema (primary abnormality is elevated pulmonary capillary pressure)
- Myocardial infarction
- Hypertensive heart disease (including accelerated hypertension)
- Mitral stenosis, mitral regurgitation
- Aortic stenosis, aortic regurgitation
- Congenital heart diseases
- Myocarditis

Non-cardiogenic pulmonary oedema (primary abnormality is not elevated pulmonary capillary pressure)
Disruption of alveolar-capillary membranes, e.g. acute respiratory distress syndrome (ARDS)

■ PULMONARY OEDEMA

- Pulmonary edema is a condition characterised by accumulation of excess fluid in interstitium and alveoli of the lung as a result of an alteration in one or more of starling forces.
- Pulmonary oedema and its types are given in **Box 3.21**.

Clinical Features of Acute Pulmonary Oedema

- Severe dyspnoea and orthopnoea
- Cough that is initially dry, but later with copious, pinkish, frothy expectoration
- Tachycardia, tachypnoea
- Cold, bluish extremities
- Bilateral scattered rhonchi
- Bilateral crepitations, predominantly basal

Investigations
- Arterial blood gas studies show hypoxia.
- Radiological features of acute pulmonary oedema—prominence of the upper lobe veins, Kerley A lines, Kerley B, 'bat's wing' appearance

Treatment of Acute Cardiogenic Pulmonary Oedema
- Propped-up position or sitting position with legs hanging down along the side of the bed to reduce venous return
- 100% oxygen, preferably under positive pressure
- Non-invasive ventilation (NIV)
- Morphine
- IV furosemide
- Vasodilators:
  - Nitrates sublingually (5–10 mg of isosorbide dinitrate) or nitroglycerine intravenously (5–100 µg/min as infusion)
  - IV sodium nitroprusside
  - Nesiritide
- Inotropic agents: IV dopamine or dobutamine or Norepinephrine/Milrinone/Levosimendan
- Correction of precipitating causes such as infection or arrhythmias

■ HEART FAILURE

Types of Heart Failure

Acute and Chronic Heart Failure

Low-output and high-output heart failure
- Low output heart failure is associated with ischaemic heart disease (IHD), hypertension, cardiomyopathy, valvular diseases and pericardial disease.
- High output cardiac failure is associated with hyperthyroidism, anaemia, pregnancy, arteriovenous fistulae, beriberi and Paget's disease.

Left-sided, right-sided and biventricular heart failure
- Systolic and diastolic heart failure
  - **Systolic heart failure** is characterised by an abnormality of ventricular contraction. The ejection fraction is usually below 40%.
  - **Diastolic heart failure:**
    - Diastolic HF is characterised by an impaired ventricular relaxation and increased ventricular stiffness resulting in reduced filling (diastolic dysfunction)

Common Causes of Heart Failure
Common causes of heart failure are given in **Box 3.22**.

Clinical Manifestations of Heart Failure
- Dyspnoea
- Orthopnoea
- Paroxysmal nocturnal dyspnoea (PND)
- Cardiac asthma
- Cough with copious, pinkish frothy expectoration
- Cheyne–Stokes respiration
- Nocturia
- Cerebral symptoms: Confusion, difficulty in concentration, memory impairment, headache, insomnia.
- Non-specific symptoms: Fatigue and weakness from reduced perfusion of skeletal muscles

---

Box 3.22: Common causes of heart failure.
- Ischaemic heart disease
- Systemic hypertension
- Pulmonary hypertension
- Aortic stenosis
- Pulmonary stenosis
- Mitral stenosis
- Tricuspid stenosis
- Endomyocardial fibrosis
- Mitral regurgitation
- Aortic regurgitation
- Ventricular septal defect
- Patent ductus arteriosus
- Atrial septal defect
- Diffuse myocardial disease
- Myocarditis
- Cardiomyopathy
- Segmental myocardial disease
- Myocardial infarction

Signs
Signs of heart failure are given in **Box 3.23**.

Common Diagnostic Studies
- Chest radiograph may show features of pulmonary oedema.
- Electrocardiography (may show presence of ventricular hypertrophy, atria abnormality, arrhythmias, conduction abnormalities, previous MI and active ischaemia)
- Echocardiography
- Brain natriuretic peptide (BNP)

Management of Heart Failure
- Absolute bed rest is only rarely required.
- Correction of obesity by restriction of caloric intake
- Salt-restricted diet and avoidance of salt-retaining medicines
- Angiotensin-converting enzyme (ACE) inhibitors
- β-blockers
- Diuretics
- Digoxin
- Aldosterone receptor blockade with spironolactone
- Vasodilators

- Sympathomimetic amines—if 'shock'
- Vasopressin antagonists: Tolvaptan
- Miscellaneous:
  - Anticoagulation therapy
  - Biventricular pacing and ICD in select group of patients
  - Cardiac resynchronisation therapy (biventricular pacing)

■ RHEUMATIC FEVER
- Rheumatic fever follows an antecedent pharyngeal infection with group A β-haemolytic streptococcus. The latent period ranges from 1 to 5 weeks.
- M-type 5 commonly causes rheumatic fever. The other rheumatogenic serotypes include 1, 3, 5, 14, 18, 19 and 24.
- The peak incidence is between 5 and 15 years.

Clinical Manifestations
- **Sore throat:** Only two-thirds of patients remember having any upper respiratory symptom in the past 1–5 weeks.
- **Polyarthritis:** It is present in nearly 75% of cases.
  - Acute migratory polyarthritis of large joints of the extremities
  - Over a period of time, involved joints heal without any residual deformity.
- **Carditis:**
  - Rheumatic fever may involve endocardium, myocardium and pericardium resulting in pancarditis.

Cardiac involvement in acute rheumatic fever described in **Box 3.24**.

- **Subcutaneous nodules:**
  - Small, pea-sized, painless nodules over bony prominences
  - Common sites: Extensor tendons of hands and feet, elbows, margins of patellae, scalp, occiput, over scapulae and over spinous processes of vertebrae
- **Erythema marginatum:**
  - Erythematous pink rashes with a clear centre and round or serpiginous margins
- **Chorea (Sydenham's chorea: Chorea minor; Saint Vitus' dance):**
  - Long latent period (up to 6 months) after the initial streptococcal infection

---

Box 3.23: Signs of heart failure.

Left ventricular failure
- Dyspnoea, orthopnoea
- Paroxysmal nocturnal dyspnoea (PND)
- Nocturia
- Acute pulmonary oedema
- Tachypnoea, pallor, sweating
- Pulsus alternans
- Narrow pulse pressure
- Third heart sound (S3) gallop of left ventricular origin
- Fourth heart sound (S4) gallop
- Basal crepitations

Right ventricular failure
- Anorexia, nausea, vomiting
- Right hypochondrial pain
- Peripheral oedema and cyanosis
- Raised jugular venous pressure, hepatojugular reflux
- Enlarged tender liver
- Ascites and pleural effusion

> **Box 3.24: Cardiac involvement in acute rheumatic fever.**
>
> **Myocarditis**
> - Tachycardia disproportionate to fever and persisting in sleep
> - Third heart sound, fourth heart sound or a summation gallop
> - Features of congestive heart failure
>
> **Endocarditis**
> - Apical systolic murmur of mitral regurgitation
> - Apical mid-diastolic murmur (Carey-Coombs murmur) due to nodules on the mitral valve leaflets
> - Basal early diastolic murmur of aortic regurgitation
>
> **Pericarditis**
> - Pericardial pain
> - Pericardial friction rub
> - Pericardial effusion

> **Box 3.25: Revised Jones criteria.**
>
> **Major manifestations**
> - Carditis
> - Polyarthritis
> - Chorea
> - Erythema marginatum
> - Subcutaneous nodules
>
> **Minor manifestations**
> - Fever
> - Arthralgia
> - Previous rheumatic fever or rheumatic heart disease
> - Raised ESR
> - Positive CRP
> - Prolonged PR interval
>
> Two major manifestations or one major and two minor manifestations indicate a high probability, with one supporting evidence of preceding streptococcal infection, e.g.:
> - Recent scarlet fever
> - Positive throat culture for group A *Streptococcus*
> - Increased streptococcal antibodies
>
> (CRP: C-reactive protein; ESR: erythrocyte sedimentation rate)

  o Chorea is characterised by sudden, aimless, irregular movements associated with muscle weakness, emotional instability, obsessions and compulsions, tics and psychotic features.

Laboratory Features

- **Isolation of group A streptococci:**
    o Group A streptococci may be isolated by throat culture only in a minority of cases. Hence, serologic tests are preferred.
- **Streptococcal antibody tests (serologic tests):**
    o Common serologic tests done are:
      - Anti-streptolysin O test (ASO)
      - Anti-DNase B
      - Anti-hyaluronidase (AH)
      - Anti-streptozyme test (ASTZ)
- **Electrocardiogram:**
    o Prolongation of the PR interval
- **Chest radiography**
- **Echocardiography**
- **Diagnosis of acute rheumatic fever**
- **Revised Jones Criteria:**
    o Revised Jones Criteria are given in **Box 3.25**.

Management of Acute Rheumatic Fever

- **Bed rest**
- **Antistreptococcal therapy:**
    o Single injection of benzathine penicillin 1.2 million units intramuscularly
    o Daily injection of procaine penicillin 6,00,000 units intramuscularly for 10 days
    o Oral erythromycin 20–40 mg/kg/day in three divided doses, in patients who are sensitive to penicillin or azithromycin in a dose of 500 mg once a day for 5 days
- **Salicylates:**
    o Aspirin is started at doses of 60 mg/kg day in six divided doses.
- **Corticosteroids:**
    o 60–120 mg/day in four divided doses until the erythrocyte sedimentation rate (ESR) is normal.
    o It is then gradually tailed off over a period of 2 weeks.

- **Supportive therapy:**
  - Includes treatment of congestive heart failure, valvular lesions, heart blocks and chorea.

Prevention of Rheumatic Fever

- **Secondary prevention (rheumatic fever prophylaxis):**
  - Intramuscular injection of 1.2 million units of benzathine penicillin G every 3 weeks
  - Oral penicillin V 500 mg twice a day
  - Erythromycin 250 mg twice a day orally or azithromycin 500 mg once a day (in those allergic to penicillins and sulpha)

■ MITRAL STENOSIS

Aetiology of Mitral Stenosis

Aetiology of mitral stenosis is given in **Box 3.26**.

Clinical Features

- Low-volume pulse in severe mitral stenosis, Irregularly irregular rhythm and varying volume in atrial fibrillation.
- Apex beat is tapping in character due to the loud palpable S1.
- Loud S1
- Mitral opening snap—early diastole. It is best heard during expiration, at or just medial to the cardiac apex (sometimes, it is widely heard).
- Mid-diastolic murmur is well localised to the mitral area. It is low pitched, rough and rumbling in character, best heard at the apex with the bell of the stethoscope, with the patient in left lateral position and during expiration. Murmur is accentuated by exercise carried out just before auscultation.

Complications of Mitral Stenosis

Complications of mitral stenosis are given in **Box 3.27**.

Management of Mitral Stenosis

Medical Management

- Treatment of atrial fibrillation with anticoagulants, digoxin, verapamil, diltiazem, β-blockers and cardioversion
- Treatment of right ventricular failure with salt restriction, diuretics, digoxin, etc.
- Infective endocarditis prophylaxis is not recommended in patients with mitral stenosis unless mitral valve replacement (MVR) or mitral valve repair using prosthetic material has been done or patient had previous endocarditis.
- Rheumatic fever prophylaxis

Surgical Management

- Balloon mitral valvotomy (BMV) also known as percutaneous balloon valvuloplasty (PBV)
- Closed surgical mitral commissurotomy/closed mitral valvotomy
- Open mitral commissurotomy (open mitral valvotomy)
- Mitral valve replacement

■ MITRAL REGURGITATION

Aetiology

Aetiology of MR is given in **Box 3.28**.

Box 3.26: Aetiology of mitral stenosis.

- Rheumatic fever
- Congenital mitral stenosis
- Coxsackie B virus carditis
- Systemic lupus erythematosus
- Atrial myxoma
- Methysergide treatment
- Malignant carcinoid
- Gout
- Mitral annular calcification
- Mucopolysaccharidosis
- Infective endocarditis (extremely rare)
- Rheumatoid arthritis (extremely rare)

Box 3.27: Complications of mitral stenosis.

- Atrial fibrillation
- Pulmonary hypertension
- Right ventricular failure
- Systemic thromboembolism
- Haemoptysis
- Winter bronchitis
- Dysphagia due to oesophageal compression by the left atrium
- Ortner's syndrome
- Infective endocarditis (very rare)

> **Box 3.28: Aetiology of mitral regurgitation.**
>
> **Chronic mitral regurgitation**
> - Rheumatic heart disease
> - Rupture of chordae tendineae
> - Mitral valve prolapse
> - Systemic lupus erythematosus, rheumatoid arthritis, ankylosing spondylitis
> - Marfan syndrome
>
> **Acute mitral regurgitation**
> - Infective endocarditis
> - Acute myocardial infarction with rupture of a papillary or one of its heads
> - Chest trauma
> - Cardiac surgery
> - Acute rheumatic fever with carditis

Clinical Features

- **Pulse:** High volume that in severe MR may become collapsing. Irregular rhythm and varying volume in atrial fibrillation
- Wide pulse pressure in severe MR
- Apex beat is shifted downwards and laterally and is hyperdynamic in character.
- First heart sound is usually soft.
- The typical murmur of chronic MR is high pitched, blowing and usually pansystolic best heard at the apex, commonly radiating to the axilla and left interscapular area.

Management

Medical Management

- Infective endocarditis prophylaxis is not indicated in patients with MR. However, it is mandatory for patients after mitral valve repair or after MVR.
- Rheumatic fever prophylaxis
- Treatment of heart failure with salt restriction, digoxin, diuretics, ACE inhibitors and vasodilators
- Treatment of atrial fibrillation with digoxin, verapamil, anticoagulation and cardioversion

Surgical Management

- Reconstruction of mitral valve apparatus by mitral valvuloplasty or mitral annuloplasty Preferred to MVR whenever feasible
- MVR with a prosthesis

MITRAL VALVE PROLAPSE OR BARLOW'S SYNDROME

- More common in females between 15 and 30 years
- Commonly associated with Marfan syndrome and cystic medical necrosis

Symptoms

- Asymptomatic
- Atypical chest pain (precordial stabbing)
- Palpitation (due to ventricular ectopics, supraventricular tachycardia, ventricular tachycardia)
- Syncope or presyncope (light headedness, dizziness)

Signs

- Mid or late systolic click(s)—occur ≥ 0.14 seconds after S1
- Midsystolic or late systolic apical murmur (rarely 'whooping' or 'honking')

Investigations

Echocardiography can confirm the diagnosis.

Complications

- Arrhythmias
- Infective endocarditis
- Transient cerebral ischaemic attacks and embolic episodes (rare)

Management

- Reassurance of asymptomatic patients
- Infective endocarditis prophylaxis is not recommended.
- β-blockers in atypical chest pain
- Antiarrhythmic drugs in arrhythmias
- Aspirin, dipyridamole or anticoagulants in transient ischaemic attacks
- Mitral valve repair or replacement in severe MR

AORTIC STENOSIS

Aetiology of Aortic Stenosis

Aetiology of aortic stenosis (AS) is given in **Box 3.29**.

> **Box 3.29: Aetiology of aortic stenosis.**
>
> **Valvular aortic stenosis**
> - Acquired
>   - Rheumatic heart disease
>   - Fibrocalcific deformity of a bicuspid valve
>   - Aortic sclerosis
>   - Systemic lupus erythematosus (SLE)
>
> **Subvalvular aortic stenosis**
> - Hypertrophic cardiomyopathy
>
> **Supravalvular aortic stenosis**
> - Williams syndrome

Signs

- Pulsus tardus, anacrotic pulse is seen in severe AS.
- Low systolic blood pressure (< 100 mmHg)
- Systolic thrill in carotids
- Heaving apical impulse
- The murmur of AS is an ejection systolic murmur (ESM) best heard at the aortic area, conducted to carotids. It is best heard with the patient sitting up, leaning forwards and breath held in expiration.
  - In calcific AS, the murmur is loud and harsh in the aortic area, but it has a musical quality along the left sternal border and at apes. This difference in the quality of the same murmur at two different sites is referred to as 'Gallavardin phenomenon'.

Treatment

- Infective endocarditis prophylaxis
- Rheumatic fever prophylaxis in aortic stenosis of rheumatic aetiology
- Treatment of angina, atrial fibrillation and left ventricular failure
- Surgery
  - Open commissurotomy or valvuloplasty for non-calcific stenosis
  - Aortic valve replacement for calcific aortic stenosis

■ AORTIC REGURGITATION

Aetiology

Aetiology of AR is given in **Box 3.30**.

> **Box 3.30: Aetiology of aortic regurgitation.**
>
> **Acute aortic regurgitation**
> - Trauma
> - Rheumatic fever
> - Infective endocarditis
> - Dissecting aneurysm
>
> **Chronic aortic regurgitation**
> - Rheumatic (two third of cases)
> - Syphilis
> - Bicuspid aortic valve
> - Atherosclerotic aortic valve
> - Infective endocarditis
> - Marfan syndrome
> - Rheumatoid arthritis
> - Ehlers–Danlos syndrome
> - Systemic lupus erythematosus
> - Ankylosing spondylitis

> **Box 3.31: Peripheral signs of aortic regurgitation.**
>
> - Collapsing pulse (water-hammer pulse)
> - Corrigan's pulse
> - Pulsus bisferiens
> - Wide pulse pressure
> - Corrigan's neck sign
> - de Musset's sign
> - Landolfi's sign
> - Müller's sign
> - Lighthouse sign
> - Quincke's sign
> - Rosenbach's sign
> - Gerhardt's sign
> - Pistol-shot femorals
> - Traube's sign
> - Duroziez's sign

Signs

Peripheral signs of AR are given in **Box 3.31**.
- Prominent neck pulsations
- Hyperdynamic apex that is shifted down and out
- First heart sound may be soft.
- A_2 component of S2 is soft in rheumatic AR, but loud and 'tambour' like in syphilitic AR.
- Third heart sound in patients with left ventricular failure
- Fourth heart sound in prominent left ventricular hypertrophy
- Early diastolic murmur (EDM) of AR: A high-pitched, early diastolic, decrescendo murmur best heard at Erb's area (left third intercostal space near sternum) in rheumatic AR and at aortic area in syphilitic AR. The murmur is best heard with the diaphragm of the stethoscope, with the patient sitting up, learning

forwards, breath held in deep expiration and hands clenched.
- Mid-diastolic murmur (Austin Flint murmur): A mid-diastolic rumbling murmur is heard at the apex in severe AR. It is a functional murmur and does not represent mitral stenosis.

Treatment
- Treatment of the underlying cause
- Infective endocarditis prophylaxis is not indicated.
- Rheumatic fever prophylaxis
- Medical treatment of cardiac failure with digoxin, diuretics, salt restriction and fluid restriction
- Surgical therapy is required in symptomatic patients or in those with left ventricular ejection fraction < 55% or end-systolic left ventricular diameter > 55 mm (even if asymptomatic). It involves aortic valve replacement.

■ INFECTIVE ENDOCARDITIS
Types of Infective Endocarditis
Subacute Endocarditis
- Caused by organisms of relatively low virulence
- Occurs on the damaged valves themselves or at sites where the endothelium is damaged by a high-pressure jet of blood [ventricular septal defect (VSD), patent ductus arteriosus (PDA), MR, aortic stenosis, AR]

Acute Endocarditis
- Caused by highly virulent and invasive organisms
- Can affect damaged valves as well as normal hearts
- Has a fulminant course

Post-operative Endocarditis or Prosthetic Valve Endocarditis
- Follows cardiac surgery using prosthetic valves and other prosthetic materials
- *Staphylococcus aureus* predominates followed by coagulase-negative staphylococci and fungi.
- After 2 months, additional organisms include viridans streptococci and enterococci.

Right-sided Endocarditis
- Occurs in IV drug users
- Caused predominantly by organisms found on the skin (e.g. *S. aureus*, *Candida*).
- Affects right-sided valves, particularly tricuspid valve

Common Organisms
Common organisms of infective endocarditis are given in **Box 3.32**.

Clinical Features of Subacute Endocarditis
- Vague symptoms such as ill-health, fatigue, lassitude, loss of appetite, loss of weight
- Low-grade or high-grade, intermittent or continuous fever with chills and rigors
- Clubbing in fingers
- Splenomegaly
- Features of new murmurs, particularly a diastolic murmur
- Change in the character of an existing murmur

Features of Embolism
- **Cutaneous embolism**—Janeway lesions on palms and soles

Box 3.32: Common organisms of infective endocarditis.

Subacute endocarditis
- Viridans streptococci:
  - *Streptococcus sanguis*
  - *Streptococcus mitis*
- *Streptococcus milleri*
- *Streptococcus bovis*
- *Enterococcus faecalis*
- *Staphylococcus aureus*
- HACEK Group

Acute endocarditis
- *Staphylococcus aureus*
- *Pseudomonas*
- *Candida*
- *Streptococcus pneumonia*
- *Neisseria gonorrhoeae*

Post-operative endocarditis
- *Staphylococcus albus*
- *Candida*
- *Aspergillus*

(HACEK: *Haemophilus* species, *Aggregatibacter* species, *Cardiobacterium hominis*, *Eikenella corrodens* and *Kingella* species)

- **Nails**—splinter haemorrhages
- **Spleen**—painful splenomegaly
- **Peripheral arteries**—claudication, absence of peripheral pulses and gangrene
- **Central nervous system**—convulsions, hemiplegia, aphasia, loss of vision and cerebellar disturbances
- **Kidneys**—loin pain, haematuria and renal failure
- **Lungs**—pulmonary infarction, pleurisy and pleural effusion (right-sided endocarditis)

Features of Immunological Disturbances

- Osler's nodes: Painful tender swollen nodules in pulps of fingers
- Roth's spots: Circular retinal haemorrhages with white central spots
- Glomerulonephritis, haematuria

Clinical Features of Acute Endocarditis

- Severe, abrupt onset of febrile illness
- Prominent and changing heart murmurs
- Embolic episodes more common
- Rapid development of renal and cardiac failure

Investigations

- Normocytic normochromic anaemia
- Leucocytosis
- Microscopic haematuria and albuminuria
- Raised ESR and C-reactive protein (CRP)
- **Blood culture:** Three specimens of 10 mL blood each are taken at intervals of 1 hour. Both aerobic and anaerobic cultures are done; rarely fungal culture also.
- **Echocardiography** can detect the vegetations and identify the valve lesion, chamber dilatation and new prosthetic dehiscence. Transthoracic echocardiography has a sensitivity of about 75% for the diagnosis of vegetations. Transoesophageal echocardiography is mandatory in cases of doubtful transthoracic examination, in prosthetic and pacemaker endocarditis or when an abscess is suspected.

Modified Duke Criteria for Infective Endocarditis

Major Criteria

- **Blood cultures positive**
  - Typical microorganisms consistent with infective endocarditis from blood cultures
- **Evidence of endocardial involvement**
  - Echocardiogram positive for infective endocarditis
  - Oscillating intracardiac mass without alternative explanation, or
  - Abscess, or
  - New partial dehiscence of prosthetic valve, or
  - New valvular regurgitation (worsening or changing of pre-existing murmur not sufficient)

Minor Criteria

- **Predisposition to infective endocarditis:** Predisposing heart condition, injection drug use, previous infective endocarditis, or prosthetic valve or material
- **Fever**, temperature 38°C
- **Vascular phenomena:** Major arterial emboli, septic pulmonary infarcts, mycotic aneurysm, intracranial haemorrhages, subconjunctival petechiae, Janeway lesions
- **Immunologic phenomena:** Glomerulonephritis, Osler's nodes, Roth's spots, positive rheumatoid factor.
- **Microbiological evidence:** Positive blood culture but does not meet a major criterion or serological evidence of active infection with organisms consistent with infective endocarditis

Pathological Criteria

- Positive microbiology or histology of pathologic tissue material attained at surgery or autopsy (vegetations, valve tissue, embolic fragments or tissue/pus from intracardiac abscesses)

Diagnosis of infective endocarditis is definite in the presence of:
- Pathological criteria; or
- Two major criteria; or
- One major and two minor criteria; or
- Five minor criteria

Medical Treatment

Treatment of organisms that cause infective endocarditis are given in **Table 3.4**.

TABLE 3.4: Treatment of organisms that cause infective endocarditis.

Organism	Treatment
Infective endocarditis awaiting culture report	• Benzylpenicillin plus gentamicin at the dose given below OR • Amoxicillin/clavulanate
Suspected staphylococcal endocarditis	• Vancomycin • Rifampicin
Streptococci highly sensitive to penicillin	• Benzylpenicillin • Ceftriaxone
Anaerobic streptococci	• Benzylpenicillin, metronidazole
Staphylococcal endocarditis (methicillin-sensitive)	• Cloxacillin OR Cefazolin PLUS gentamicin
Enterococcal endocarditis	• Ampicillin
Candida	• Amphotericin

Surgical Treatment: Indications
- Progressive cardiac failure from valve damage
- Endocarditis of prosthetic valve
- Large vegetation (10 mm) on a left-sided valve with an episode of embolisation, or very large (15 mm) and mobile vegetation (high risk of embolism).
- Abscess formation, paravalvular involvement and fungal endocarditis are also considered indications for early surgery.

Infective endocarditis prophylaxis for oral procedures

Particular patient groups and their treatment regimen are given in **Table 3.5**.

■ ISCHAEMIC HEART DISEASE
- Ischaemic heart disease (IHD) is a condition in which there is an imbalance between myocardial blood supply and its oxygen demand.

Aetiology
- Most coronary artery diseases are due to **atheromas and their complications**.
- **Uncommon causes include:**
  ○ Severe aortic stenosis
  ○ Congenital abnormalities of coronary arteries
  ○ Arteritis due to connective tissue disorders

■ ATHEROSCLEROSIS: PATHOLOGY TO BE DISCUSSED IN PATHOLOGY

Risk Factors
Risk factors of atherosclerosis are given in **Box 3.33**.

TABLE 3.5: Particular patient groups and their infectious endocarditis treatment regimen.

Patient group	Antibiotic	Dose (single 30–60 min before procedures)
Able to take oral medicine	Amoxicillin	2 g
Unable to take oral medicine	• Ampicillin OR • Cefazolin OR • Ceftriaxone	2 g IM/IV 1 g IM/IV 1 g IM/IV
Allergic to penicillins or ampicillin and able to take oral medication	• Cephalexin OR • Clindamycin OR • Azithromycin/clarithromycin	2 g 600 mg 500 mg
Allergic to penicillins or ampicillin and unable to take oral medication	• Cefazolin OR • Ceftriaxone OR • Clindamycin	1 g 1 g 600 mg

Cardiology

Box 3.33: Risk factors of atherosclerosis.

Modifiable
- Smoking
- Hypercholesterolaemia
- Arterial hypertension
- Diabetes mellitus
- Physical inactivity
- Dietary factors: Deficient in polyunsaturated fatty acids (PUFA)
- Coagulation factors: Fibrinogen and factor VII
- Obesity
- Stress factors

Non-modifiable
- Geographical influences
- Family history of premature coronary artery disease
- Age
    - Men ≥ 45 years
    - Females ≥ 55 years (post-menopausal)
- Genetic factors

Angina Pectoris
- A clinical syndrome causing discomfort due to transient myocardial ischaemia
    - Pain is usually retrosternal in location and brought on by exertion. It is relieved by rest and sublingual nitrates.
    - Pain seldom lasts > 20 minutes.
    - Character of the pain is squeezing, tightening, heaviness or aching.
    - Pain commonly radiates to left arm or less commonly to right arm, throat, back, chin and epigastrium.
- **Nocturnal angina** is an unusual form of angina occurring in AR.
- **Prinzmetal's angina** or variant angina or vasospastic angina is pain that comes capriciously due to coronary arterial spasm and is accompanied by **transient ST segment elevation** on ECG.
- **'Microvascular' angina** indicates angina-such as pain, normal coronary angiograms and positive exercise tests and occurs in patients with metabolic syndrome.
- **Angina equivalents**
    - These include dyspnoea, faintness, fatigue and eructations precipitated by exertion and relieved with rest.

Investigations
- **Electrocardiography:** ECG is normal in most patents at rest and in between attacks.
- **Stress myocardial perfusion scanning** using radioactive thallium (^{201}thallium) or technetium (^{99m}Tc—sestamibi).
- **Echocardiography**
- **Coronary arteriography** provides detailed information about the extent and site of coronary artery stenosis.

Management
Investigation and management of stable angina are shown in **Flowchart 3.1**.

Drug Treatment
- The following group of drugs is used in the management of angina pectoris:
    - Nitrates
    - β-adreno-receptor antagonists (β-blockers)
    - Calcium antagonists
    - Platelet inhibitors: Aspirin, clopidogrel
    - Miscellaneous (ranolazine, trimetazidine, nicorandil, ivabradine)

Intervention
- Percutaneous coronary interventions (PCI)
- Coronary artery bypass grafting (CABG)

■ ACUTE CORONARY SYNDROME
- It includes the following conditions:
    - ST elevation myocardial infarction (**STEMI**)
    - **NSTEMI** (NQMI, previously called subendocardial infarction)
    - Unstable angina (**UA**)

A new classification scheme of acute coronary syndrome is shown in **Flowchart 3.2**.

■ ACUTE MYOCARDIAL INFARCTION

Clinical Features

Symptoms
- Cardinal symptom is chest pain.
- Pain is at the same site as for angina but is more severe and prolonged.
- Other symptoms:

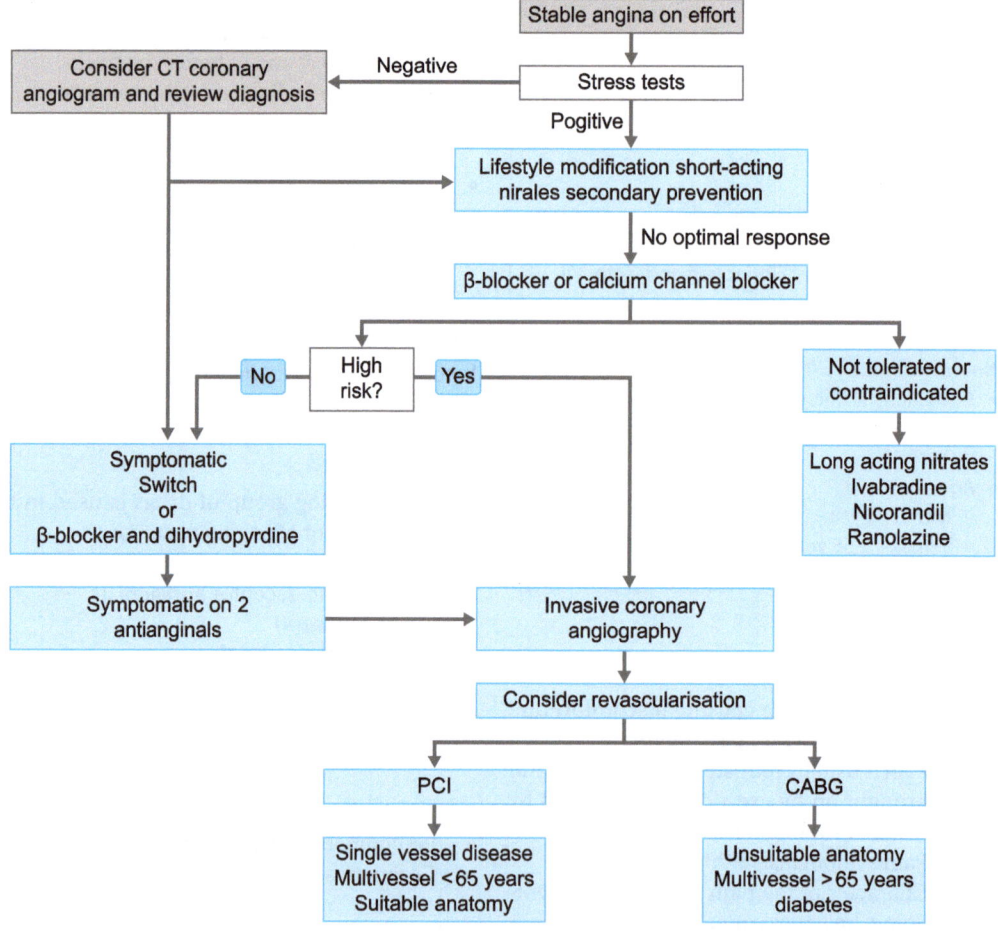

(CABG: coronary artery bypass grafting; PCI: percutaneous coronary intervention)

Flowchart 3.1: Scheme for the investigation and management of stable angina.

- o Breathlessness
- o Syncope
- o Vomiting

Signs
- Mild fever
- Pallor, sweating
- Tachycardia or bradycardia
- Arrhythmias
- Narrow pulse pressure
- Raised JVP
- Diffuse apical impulse
- Soft S1
- Third heart sound
- Pericardial friction rub
- Systolic murmur due to MR or uncommonly due to VSD
- Basal crepitations

Complications
- Arrhythmias
- Cardiogenic shock
- Other complications
  - o Cardiac failure, most commonly manifesting as pulmonary oedema
  - o Infarction of the mitral papillary muscle leading to MR and pulmonary oedema

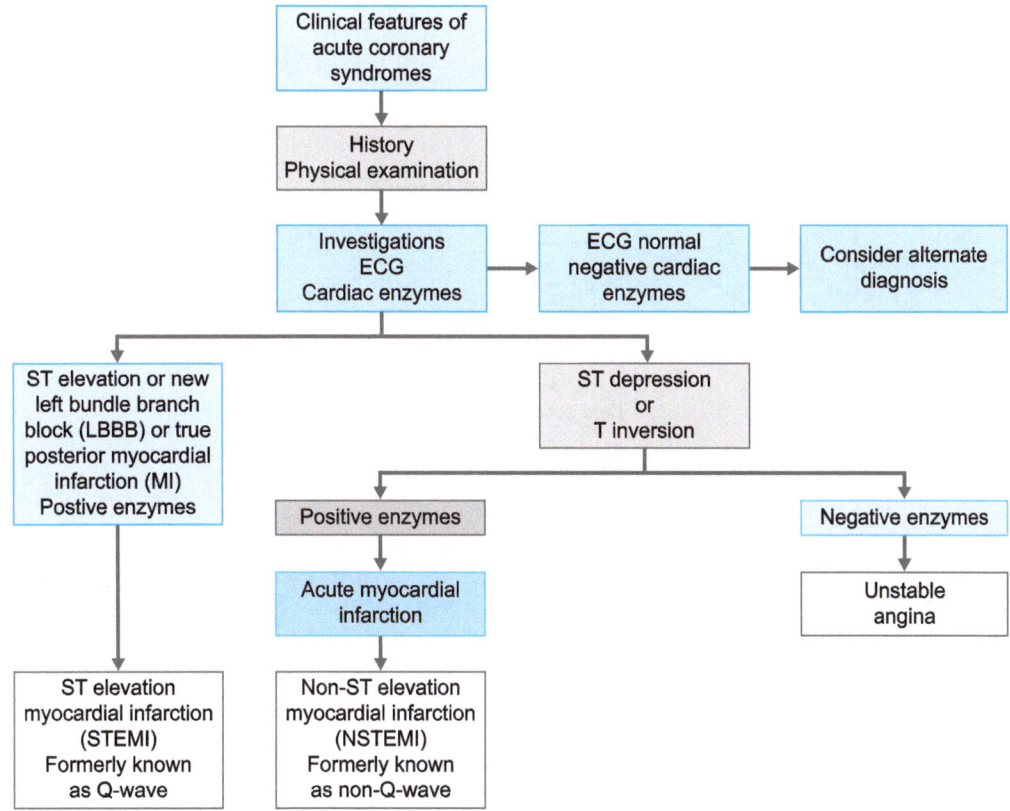

Flowchart 3.2: New classification scheme of acute coronary syndrome.

- Rupture of interventricular septum leading to a murmur of VSD and severe hypotension
- Cardiac tamponade due to rupture of ventricle into pericardial sac
- Cerebral and peripheral embolism resulting from the detachment of a ventricular mural thrombus
- Deep vein thrombosis and pulmonary embolism in patients on prolonged bed rest
- Ventricular aneurysm and dyskinetic or akinetic segments
- Dressler's syndrome—pericarditis

Investigations

- **Electrocardiogram**
  - ST segment elevation (with reciprocal depression in the opposite leads) ≥2 mm in leads V_1–V_3 or ≥1 mm in other leads
  - Appearance of pathologic Q-waves, i.e. initial negative deflections of 0.04 seconds or more in leads other than aVR and V_1
- **Plasma enzymes (cardiac injury enzymes)**
  - Creatine kinase (CK)
  - Aspartate aminotransferase (AST)
  - Lactate dehydrogenase (LDH)
  - Myoglobin
  - Troponins (troponin I and troponin T)

Various enzyme levels following acute myocardial infarction are shown in **Figure 3.1**.

Characteristics of plasma biomarkers for acute myocardial infarction are given in **Table 3.6**.

- **Chest radiography**
- **Radionuclide scanning** shows the site of necrosis and the extent of impairment of ventricular function.
- **Echocardiography** for regional wall motion abnormality and ejection fraction

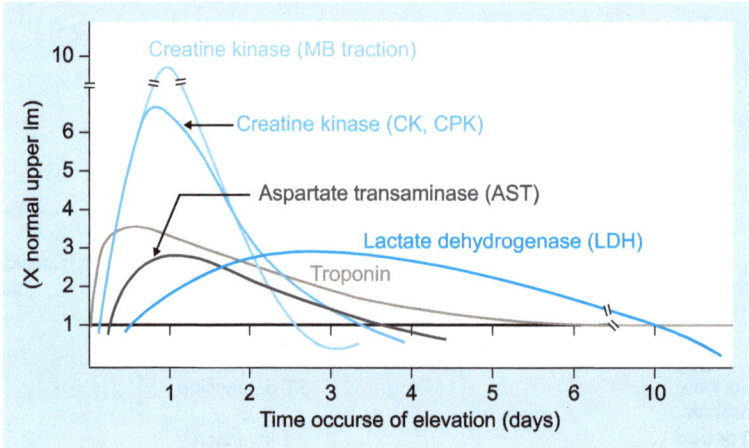

Fig. 3.1: Various enzyme levels following acute myocardial infarction.

TABLE 3.6: Characteristics of plasma biomarkers for acute myocardial infarction (AMI).

Marker protein	Elevation in plasma after AMI (h)	Peak plasma concentration (h)	Normalisation of plasma level (Days)
Myoglobin	2–3	6–12	1–2
Cardiac troponin I	3–8	12–24	7–10
Cardiac troponin T	3–8	12–24	7–10
Creatine kinase myocardial band	2–6	12–24	2–3

Management of Acute Myocardial Infarction

Initial Treatment

- Attach a cardiac monitor.
- Secure an IV line.
- Administer oxygen.
- Administer sublingual nitrate (if not taken by the patient and pain is present).
- If no relief, give IV morphine 3–5 mg along with an antiemetic. May repeat it 5 minutes after the first dose.
- Give aspirin 150 mg to be chewed.
- Give clopidogrel 300 mg orally (unless coronary artery bypass surgery is contemplated).

Specific Therapy

- Thrombolysis or PCI
- β-blockers unless contraindicated
- Treat complications (arrhythmias, congestive failure and shock).

Thrombolytic (or Fibrinolytic) Therapy

- **Thrombolytic agents:** These include:
  - Streptokinase (STK)
  - Urokinase (UK)
  - Recombinant plasminogen activator (rtPA-alteplase, reteplase, tenecteplase)
  - Single-chain UK plasminogen activator (scu-PA)

Indications for Thrombolysis in Acute Myocardial Infarction

- ST segment elevation of greater than 0.1 mV in two or more contiguous leads, with time to therapy 12 hours or less.
- Bundle-branch block (obscuring ST segment analysis) and history suggestive of acute MI for < 12 hours.

Thrombolysis not Indicated/may be Harmful

- ST segment depression only
- Time to therapy > 24 hours

Contraindications to Thrombolytic Therapy

Major Contraindications
- Active bleeding (except menses)
- Severe uncontrolled hypertension
- History of haemorrhagic stroke
- Ischaemic stroke within 3 months (except for acute ischaemic stroke within 3–4.5 h)
- Suspected aortic dissection
- Known intracranial aneurysm or arteriovenous malformation
- Known intracranial neoplasm (primary or metastatic)
- Intracranial/spinal surgery within the last 3 months
- Significant cranial/spinal trauma in the last 3 months

Antithrombin Therapy
- Unfractionated heparin
- Low-molecular-weight heparin (LMWH)
- Direct thrombin inhibitors (hirudin and bivalirudin)

Percutaneous Coronary Interventions
- These interventions include angioplasty [percutaneous transluminal coronary angioplasty (PTCA)] or stent placement in the coronary artery.
- Stents may be bare metallic or drug eluting, the latter containing sirolimus or paclitaxel. Management of acute coronary syndrome is shown in **Flowchart 3.3**.

■ UNSTABLE ANGINA AND NSTEMI

Non-ST Elevation MI
- It is often characterised by ST depression and T inversion along with elevation in cardiac enzymes.
- The myocardial function as shown by ejection fraction is less deranged as compared to STEMI.
- However, **early as well as late reinfarction rates are higher** in the NSTEMI as compared to STEMI.

Unstable Angina
- Unstable angina (UA) includes:
  - Exertional angina of recent onset (within 6 weeks)
  - Angina at rest or minimal exertion
  - Angina of worsening severity
- The ECG and cardiac enzymes are usually normal.
- Patients with UA are at a high risk of developing MI or sudden death as compared to patients with stable angina and therefore require aggressive treatment.

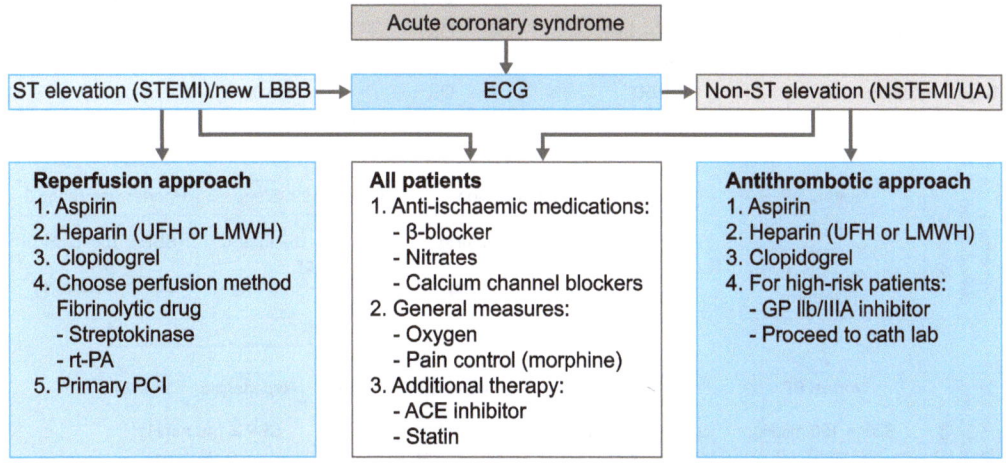

(ACE: angiotensin-converting enzyme; ECG: electrocardiogram; GP: glycoprotein; LMWH: low-molecular-weight heparin; PCI: percutaneous coronary intervention; NSTEMI: non-ST elevation myocardial infarction; rtPA: recombinant tissue plasminogen activator; STEMI: ST elevation myocardial infarction; UFH: unfractionated heparin)

Flowchart 3.3: Management of acute coronary syndrome.

Management

Management of both NSTEMI And UA is similar.

■ HYPERTENSION

Classification

- **Primary or essential hypertension**
  - Accounts for 85% of the cases
  - Not possible to define a specific underlying cause
- **Secondary hypertension**
  - Accounts for 15% of the cases
  - Consequence of a specific disease or abnormality

Hypertension and its classification are given in **Box 3.34** and 2017 updated classification of high blood pressure in adults is shown in **Flowchart 3.4**.

Causes

Causes of hypertension are given in **Box 3.35**.

Clinical Features due to Hypertension Per Se

- Long-standing hypertension leads to left ventricular hypertrophy and heaving apical impulse.

> **Box 3.35: Causes of secondary hypertension.**
> - Coarctation of aorta
> - Renal causes
>   - Glomerulonephritis
>   - Chronic pyelonephritis
>   - Collagen vascular diseases
>   - Polycystic kidney disease
>   - Renal artery stenosis
> - Alcohol and drugs
>   - Oral contraceptives
>   - Anabolic steroids
>   - Corticosteroids
>   - NSAIDs
>   - COX-2 inhibitors
> - Endocrine causes
>   - Phaeochromocytoma
>   - Cushing's syndrome
>   - Conn's syndrome
>   - Hyperparathyroidism
>   - Acromegaly
>   - Primary hypothyroidism
>   - Hyperthyroidism
> - Pre-eclamptic toxaemia
> - Miscellaneous—obstructive sleep apnoea
>
> (NSAIDS: nonsteroidal anti-inflammatory drugs)

Box 3.34: Hypertension and its classification.

Classification	Systolic BP (mmHg)		Diastolic BP (mmHg)
Normal	< 120	AND	< 80
Prehypertension	120–139	OR	80–89
Stage 1 hypertension	140–159	OR	90–99
Stage 2 hypertension	≥ 160	OR	≥ 100

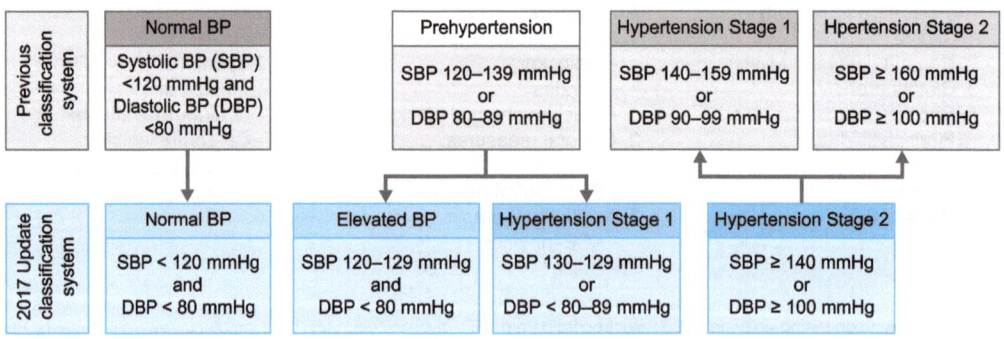

Flowchart 3.4: Updated classification of high blood pressure in adults.

- Left atrial hypertrophy and S4
- Aortic component (A_2) of the S2 is accentuated.
- Very short EDM
- Fundal changes

Complications of Hypertension

Central Nervous System Complications
- Transient ischaemic attacks
- Cerebrovascular accidents (strokes) due to cerebral thrombosis or haemorrhage
- Subarachnoid haemorrhage
- Hypertensive encephalopathy

Ophthalmic Complications
- **Hypertensive retinopathy** is characterised by thickening of the walls of the retinal arterioles.
- Arteriovenous nipping
- Retinal haemorrhages
- Soft and hard exudates and papilloedema
- Severe retinopathy can cause visual field defects and blindness.

Cardiovascular Complications
- Coronary artery disease (angina, MI)
- Left ventricular failure
- Aortic aneurysm
- Aortic dissection

Renal Complications
- Proteinuria
- Progressive renal failure

Malignant Hypertension
It is clinical syndrome of:
- Markedly high blood pressure with retinal haemorrhages and exudates.
- Confusion, headache, vomiting, visual disturbances and deterioration in renal functions.

Investigations

Basic Studies
- Urine analysis for protein, blood and glucose
- Blood urea and creatinine (to assess renal function)
- Serum electrolytes (for hypokalaemia and alkalosis in hyperaldosteronism)
- Fasting and post-prandial blood glucose (for hyperglycaemia)
- Serum cholesterol and triglycerides
- Serum calcium and uric acid
- ECG (for left ventricular hypertrophy)
- Chest radiograph (for cardiac size, evidence of cardiac failure and aortic dilatation)

Various secondary hypertension and their findings and specific investigations are given in **Table 3.7**.

Treatment
- Target for treating hypertension is **< 140/90 mmHg**.
- In patients with hypertension and diabetes or renal disease, the goal is **< 130/80 mmHg**.

General Measures
- Control of obesity
- Low sodium diet (< 100 mEq sodium or < 6 g salt)
- Smoking to be abandoned
- Alcohol consumption to be moderated (males- no more than two alcoholic drinks per day and females- no more than one per day)
- Diuretics
- β adrenoreceptor antagonists (β-blockers)
- ACE inhibitors
- Angiotensin receptor blockers
- Calcium channel blockers (calcium antagonists)
- Centrally acting drugs (**Box 3.36; Fig. 3.2**)
    - Reserpine
    - α-methyldopa
    - Clonidine

Hypertensive Encephalopathy
- Hypertensive encephalopathy is characterised by a very high blood pressure and neurological disturbances, seizures, loss of consciousness and papilloedema.

Treatment
- A controlled reduction of blood pressure over a period of 30–60 minutes to a level of 150/90 mmHg is adequate.
- IV sodium nitroprusside (0.3–1.0 μg/kg/min) is the most effective drug.
- Alternatively, parenteral labetalol may be used.

TABLE 3.7: Findings and specific investigations in various secondary hypertension.

Findings	Disease suspected	Specific investigation
Paroxysmal hypertension, palpitations, headache, diaphoresis	Phaeochromocytoma	Urine vanillylmandelic acid (VMA), metanephrine, plasma metanephrine
Fatigue, weight gain, menstrual irregularities, diastolic hypertension	Hypothyroidism	Serum thyroid stimulating hormone (TSH)
Weight loss, tachycardia, tremors, heat intolerance, systolic hypertension	Hyperthyroidism	Serum TSH
Depression, muscle weakness, kidney stones, osteoporosis	Hyperparathyroidism	Serum calcium, parathormone (PTH)
Headaches, fatigue, visual disturbances, enlarged tongue, enlarged extremities	Acromegaly	Growth hormone (GH)
Weight gain, muscle weakness, striae, obesity, amenorrhoea, moon facies	Cushing's syndrome	Serum cortisol
Obesity, snoring, daytime somnolence	Obstructive sleep apnoea (OSA)	Polysomnography
Enlarged palpable kidneys, family history positive	Autosomal dominant polycystic kidney disease (ADPKD)	Ultrasound abdomen
Proteinuria, elevated serum creatinine, oedema, anaemia	Chronic kidney disease (CKD)	Ultrasound
Abdominal/renal bruit	Renovascular case	MR angiogram
Fatigue, hypokalaemia, hypernatraemia	Aldosteronism	Plasma renin to aldosterone ratio, MRI of abdomen

Hypertensive Emergencies

- A hypertensive emergency involves an elevated blood pressure (usually > 280 mmHg systolic) in association with signs and/or symptoms of acute target organ damage (**Table 3.8**).
- The resultant vascular compromise of the affected organ may include:
    o Hypertensive encephalopathy
    o Acute heart failure with pulmonary oedema
    o Dissecting aortic aneurysm
    o Acute renal failure
    o UA or MI
    o Intracranial bleed, acute ischaemic stroke or subarachnoid haemorrhage

■ PULMONARY HYPERTENSION

Pulmonary hypertension is defined as an increase in blood pressure in pulmonary circulation (either in the arteries, or both in arteries and veins). Normal pressure as measured at right heart catheterisation is 14–18 mmHg at rest and 20–25 mmHg on exercise. Hemodynamically it is defined as an increase in mean pulmonary arterial pressure to 25 mmHg at rest. Definition may be refined by giving consideration of the pulmonary wedge pressure (PWP); the cardiac output and the transpulmonary pressure gradient [mean pulmonary artery pressure (PAP) – mean PWP].

Aetiology and Classification

Aetiology and classification of pulmonary hypertension are given in **Box 3.37**.

Clinical Features

- Fatigue, dyspnoea, syncope and angina due to reduced cardiac output
- Haemoptysis
- Peripheral oedema, tender hepatomegaly and raised JVP due to right ventricular failure

Signs of Pulmonary Hypertension

Jugular Veins
- Prominent *a* waves
- JVP is elevated with right ventricular failure.

Box 3.36: Various antihypertensive drugs (dose).

Diuretics
- **Thiazide diuretics**
  - Chlorothalidone/hydrochlorothiazide (12.5–25 mg once daily)
  - Chlorothiazide (125–500 mg once daily)
  - Indapamide (1.25–2.5 mg once daily)
  - Metolazone (2.5–5.0 mg once daily)
- **Loop diuretics**
  - Furosemide (10–40 mg twice daily)
  - Bumetanide (0.5–1.0 mg twice daily)
  - Torsemide (2.5–10 mg once daily)
- **Potassium-sparing diuretics**
  - Amiloride (5–10 mg once daily)
  - Triamterene (25–100 mg once daily)
- **Aldosterone-receptor blockers**
  - Spironolactone (25–100 mg once daily)
  - Eplerenone (50–100 mg once daily)

β-blockers
- Propranolol (20–80 mg twice or thrice daily)
- Metoprolol (25–100 mg twice daily)
- Atenolol (25–100 mg once daily)
- Bisoprolol (2.5–10 mg once daily)
- Nebivolol (5–10 mg once daily)

Combined α- and β-blockers
- Carvedilol (6.25–25 mg twice daily)
- Labetalol (100–900 mg twice daily)

Angiotensin-converting enzyme (ACE) inhibitors
- Enalapril (2.5–20 mg once daily or twice daily)
- Captopril (12.5–50 mg thrice daily)
- Lisinopril (2.5–40 mg once daily)
- Ramipril (2.5–20 mg once daily)
- Perindopril (2–8 mg once daily)
- Quinapril (10–80 mg once daily)

Angiotensin II receptor antagonists
- Losartan (25–50 mg twice daily)
- Candesartan (8–32 mg once daily)
- Irbesartan (75–300 mg once daily)
- Valsartan (80–320 mg once daily)
- Telmisartan (20–80 mg once daily)
- Olmesartan, Azilsartan (20–40 mg once daily)

Direct renin inhibitors
- Aliskiren (75–300 mg once daily)

Calcium channel blockers
- Nifedipine (SR) (30–60 mg once daily)
- Verapamil and diltiazem (40–160 mg twice daily)
- Diltiazem (SR) (90–360 mg once daily)
- Amlodipine and felodipine (2.5–20 mg once daily)
- Nicardipine (SR) (60–120 mg twice daily)

α-blockers
- Prazosin (1–4 mg once daily and twice daily)
- Terazosin (1–20 mg once daily)
- Doxazosin (1–16 mg once daily)

Direct vasodilators
- Hydralazine (12.5–50 mg twice daily)
- Minaxidil (1.25–40 mg twice daily)

Central α₂-blockers and other centrally acting drugs
- Clonidine (0.05–0.3 mg twice daily)
- Alpha-methyldopa (250–1,000 mg four times/day)
- Reserpine (0.05–0.25 mg once daily)
- Moxonidine (0.2–0.3 mg once daily or twice daily)

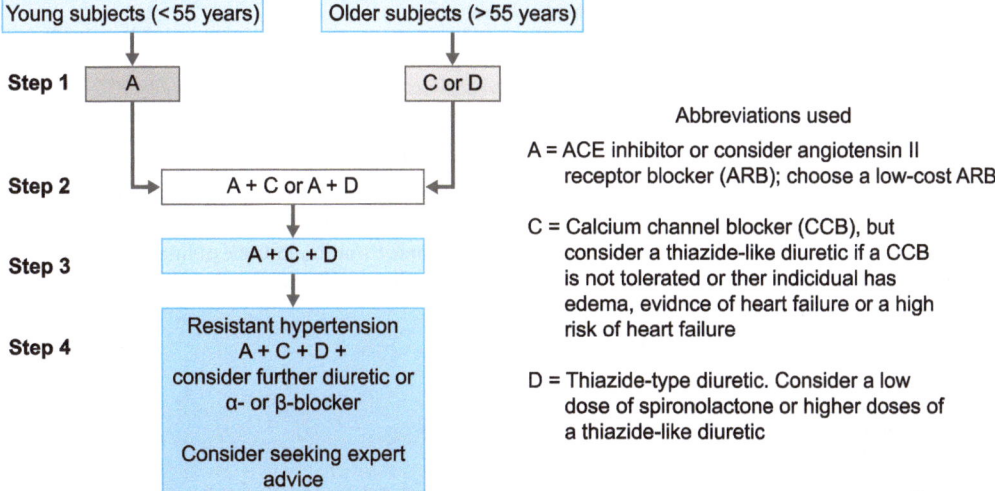

Fig. 3.2: Choosing antihypertensive drug and its combinations for patients newly diagnosed with hypertension.

TABLE 3.8: Various hypertensive emergencies and their treatment.

Diagnosis	Suggested drugs	Targets	Remarks
Acute aortic dissection	Esmolol/labetalol + nitroprusside would be a better combination	Reduce SBP as rapidly as possible down to 100–110 mmHg, simultaneously control tachycardia due to the sympathetic activation	• Avoid volume depletion • Use β-blockers before vasodilators • Hydralazine is contraindicated
Acute pulmonary oedema	• Nitroglycerine infusion, IV enalaprilat • Nitroprusside infusion, IV furosemide	Reduce blood pressure by 20–30%	Hypotension may develop with enalaprilat
Acute coronary syndrome	• Nitroglycerine infusion • β-blockers (metoprolol or labetalol)	Reduce blood pressure by not > 20–30%	• Beware of hypotension in right ventricular infarction • Avoid hypotension
Acute renal failure	Labetalol IV, nicardipine infusion, dialysis	Reduce blood pressure not > 20–30%	Avoid nitroprusside and ACE inhibitors
Subarachnoid haemorrhage	• Labetalol bolus and infusion • Esmolol bolus and infusion • Nicardipine infusion	Systolic pressure < 160 mmHg or mean arterial pressure < 130 mmHg (to reduce recurrence)	Control of pain will help in BP control
Intracranial bleed	• Labetalol and infusion • Nitroglycerine infusion • Nimodipine, a dihydropyridine calcium blocker is effective	To prevent rebleeding and reduce oedema formation May benefit from gradual 20–25% reduction in BP	Avoid lowering blood pressure by > 10–15% in 24 h
Hypertensive encephalopathy	IV sodium nitroprusside is the drug of choice, rapid onset of action. IV labetalol, nicardipine, hydralazine	Mean BP should be reduced by 20% within first hour	–

(ACE: angiotensin-converting enzyme; SBP: systolic blood pressure)

Box 3.37: Aetiology and classification of pulmonary hypertension.

- **Pulmonary arterial hypertension (PAH)**
  - Idiopathic PAH
  - Drug and toxin
  - Connective tissue diseases (e.g. CREST syndrome)
  - HIV infection
  - Congenital heart diseases
- **Pulmonary hypertension owing to left heart disease**
  - Systolic dysfunction
  - Diastolic dysfunction
  - Valvular disease
- **Pulmonary hypertension owing to lung diseases and/or hypoxia**
  - Chronic obstructive pulmonary disease
  - Interstitial lung disease
- **Chronic thromboembolic pulmonary hypertension (CTEPH)**

(CREST: calcinosis, Raynaud phenomenon, esophageal dysmotility, sclerodactyly, and telangiectasia)

Inspection and Palpation
- Apical impulse may be shifted indicating right ventricular hypertrophy and dilatation.
- Visible and palpable left parasternal heave and epigastric pulsations indicating right ventricular hypertrophy
- Visible and palpable pulsations in the second left intercostal space form an underlying dilated pulmonary artery.
- Palpable pulmonary component (P2) of S2 in the pulmonary area

Auscultatory Signs in Pulmonary Hypertension
- Pulmonary ejection sound (ES)
- Right atrial S4
- Right ventricular S3
- Pulmonary ESM
- Pulmonary EDM
- Tricuspid pansystolic murmur (PSM)

Investigations
- **Electrocardiogram**
  - Right axis deviation
  - Right atrial enlargement
  - Right ventricular hypertrophy
- **Chest radiography**
  - Enlargement of the pulmonary trunk and its main branches
  - Peripheral 'pruning' of vascular shadows
  - Enlarged right atrium
  - Enlarged right ventricle
- **Echocardiography** is the most useful modality for detecting pulmonary hypertension and excluding underlying cardiac disease.
- **Autoantibodies** if a collagen vascular disease is suspected.
  - Human immunodeficiency virus (HIV) enzyme-linked immunosorbent assay (ELISA) if the patient has risk factors
  - **Arterial blood gas** to exclude hypoxia and acidosis as contributors to pulmonary hypertension
  - **Sleep studies** if sleep apnoea suspected
  - **Pulmonary function tests** to establish airflow obstruction or restrictive lung disease
  - **High-resolution computed tomography** of chest to exclude occult interstitial lung disease
  - **Ventilation–perfusion (V/Q) scanning**

Treatment
- Pulmonary endarterectomy
- Drugs for treatment include:
  - Prostanoids (epoprostenol, iloprost, treprostinil)
  - Endothelin receptor antagonists (bosentan)
  - Phosphodiesterase-5 inhibitors (sildenafil, tadalafil)
- Lung transplantation

■ DEEP VENOUS THROMBOSIS (DVT)

Common Sites of Venous Thrombosis
- Deep venous system of lower extremities (95% of pulmonary emboli arise from here)
- Other systemic veins, especially pelvic veins
- Right atrium, especially in patients with atrial fibrillation and cardiac failure
- Right ventricle

The risk factors for venous thrombosis and embolism are given in **Box 3.38**.

Clinical Features of Deep Venous Thrombosis
- Clinical detection is difficult as DVT is silent in 50% of cases.

Box 3.38: Risk factors (predisposing factors) for venous thrombosis and embolism.

Primary (genetic)
- **Deficiency of antithrombotic (anticoagulant) factors:** Antithrombin deficiency, protein C and S deficiency
- **Increased prothrombotic factors:** Activated protein C (APC) resistance (factor V mutation/factor Va/factor V Leiden).

Secondary (acquired)
- **Surgery:** Major abdominal/pelvic, hip/knee surgery, post-operative intensive care
- **Obstetrics:** Pregnancy, post-partum
- **Cardiorespiratory disease:** COPD, congestive cardiac failure
- **Lower limb conditions:** Fracture, varicose veins
- **Malignancy:** Abdominal/pelvic, advanced/disseminated cancers, concurrent chemotherapy
- **Antiphospholipid antibody syndrome**
- **Miscellaneous:** Increasing age, prolonged bed rest, prolonged immobilisation, trauma

(COPD: chronic obstructive pulmonary disease)

- Low-grade fever
- Pain, tenderness, warmth and swelling of calf muscles
- 'Homan's sign is pain in the calf on forceful dorsiflexion of foot.
- Later, there is cyanosis, oedema and venous gangrene of the affected limb.

Wells Probability Score

Quantifies pretest probability of DVT

Investigations

- **D-Dimer** is elevated (> 500 ng/mL) in most patients but is not specific.
- **Doppler (duplex) ultrasonography** is useful, but highly operator dependent.

Treatment of Deep Venous Thrombosis

- Bed rest with legs elevated to 15°
- Physiotherapy to legs
- Graduated elastic stockings (compression stockings) should be used routinely to prevent post-thrombotic syndrome.
- Start treatment with heparin (as in pulmonary embolism) as well as warfarin and continue with warfarin.
- Anticoagulation with warfarin should be maintained for 3–6 months.
- Low molecular weight heparins.

■ PULMONARY EMBOLISM

Types

- **Acute massive pulmonary embolism** where the embolus lodges in the main pulmonary artery (may result in death)
- **Pulmonary infarction** from embolism to smaller pulmonary artery
- **Recurrent silent pulmonary embolism** resulting in chronic pulmonary hypertension and chronic right heart failure

Causes and Risk Factors

- Pulmonary embolism usually results from dislodgement of venous thrombi of the deep veins of the lower limb and pelvis.
- Causes of pulmonary embolism are the same as those for venous thrombosis.
- 'Economy class syndrome' (or traveller's thrombosis) is a rare condition.
- The incidence through various studies appears to be in the range of 0.25/1,00,000 passengers in flights longer than 8 hours.

Clinical Features of Pulmonary Embolism and Pulmonary Infarction

- Sudden onset of unexplained breathlessness is the most common symptom.
- Retrosternal discomfort from right ventricular ischaemia
- Syncope
- Pleuritic chest pain and haemoptysis in pulmonary infarction
- Supraventricular tachyarrhythmias
- Sudden onset or worsening of congestive heart failure
- Sudden deterioration in a patient with chronic obstructive lung disease

Physical Findings

- A low-grade fever may occur with infarction.
- Central cyanosis in massive pulmonary infarction
- Pleural friction rub and a small pleural effusion
- Tachycardia is the most consistent and most important physical sign.
- Clinical evidence of DVT may be present (refer venous thrombosis).

Wells Scoring System

To determine probability of pulmonary embolism, Wells scoring system is used.

Diagnosis

- **Electrocardiogram** may show tachycardia, changes of acute pulmonary hypertension and right ventricular enlargement with strain.
  - Other abnormalities include atrial fibrillation or flutter, an S wave in lead I, a Q in Lead III and an inverted T in lead III (S1 Q_3 T_3 pattern).
- **Arterial blood gas studies may** reveal hypoxaemia, hypocapnia and respiratory alkalosis.
- The best screening test is a measurement of the **D-dimer** levels in the blood, **spiral CT pulmonary angiography (CTPA), perfusion scanning of the lungs and pulmonary angiography.**
- A **V/Q scan** uses less radiation and contrast.

Management
Anticoagulation
- Unfractionated heparin is given at an initial dose of 5,000–10,000 units intravenously, followed by maintenance.
- Along with heparin, oral warfarin should be started with the intention of keeping the international normalised ratio (INR) at 2.5–3.0. This may take 4–5 days after which heparin is stopped.
- Anticoagulation is maintained for at least 6 months.

Thrombolytic Therapy
- It is used in patients with major embolism with hypotension.
- Agents currently used for thrombolysis are:
  - Streptokinase
  - Urokinase
  - Tissue plasminogen activator (tPA)

Surgical Therapy
- Inferior vena cava filters to prevent recurrent emboli
- Pulmonary embolectomy

ACUTE MYOCARDITIS
Aetiology
Aetiology of acute myocarditis is given in **Box 3.39** in severe cases and restriction of physical activities
- Treatment of congestive heart failure (using ACE inhibitors, β-blockers, diuretics) and arrhythmias (using amiodarone and β-blockers)
- Aldosterone antagonists (eplerenone or spironolactone)
- Anticoagulation in the setting of concomitant atrial fibrillation or arterial or venous thromboembolism
- Immunosuppressives (including steroids and azathioprine)

CARDIOMYOPATHY
Dilated Cardiomyopathy (Congestive Cardiomyopathy)
Common Causes
The common causes of dilated cardiomyopathy are given in **Box 3.40**.

Box 3.39: Aetiology of acute myocarditis.

Infection
- Viral (Coxsackie A and B, influenza, HIV, dengue virus)
- Bacterial (diphtheria, *Staphylococcus aureus*, *Mycoplasma pneumoniae*),
- Protozoal (trypanosomiasis, toxoplasmosis)
- Spirochaetes (Lyme disease)
- Fungal

Collagen vascular disease
- Scleroderma
- Systemic lupus erythematosus
- Polyarteritis nodosa

Miscellaneous
- Hypersensitivity reactions to drugs: Azithromycin, benzodiazepines, clozapine
- Bee venom, wasp venom, scorpion venom, snake venom
- Acute rheumatic fever, toxins (cocaine, alcohol,

Box 3.40: Common causes of dilated cardiomyopathy.

Inflammatory	Infiltrative
• Post-infective	• Haemochromatosis
• Autoimmune diseases (systemic lupus erythematosus, systemic sclerosis, dermatomyositis)	**Nutritional**
	• Thiamine deficiency
	• Selenium deficiency
	Endocrine
	• Diabetes mellitus
Toxic	• Thyrotoxicosis
• Alcohol	• Hypothyroidism
• Cocaine	**Neuromuscular**
• Adriamycin	• Muscular dystrophies
• Trastuzumab	• Friedreich's ataxia
• Cyclophosphamide	• Myotonic dystrophy
Haematological	**Metabolic**
• Sickle cell anaemia	• Glycogen storage disease
Peripartum	
	Idiopathic

Hypertrophic Cardiomyopathy
Clinical Features
- Many patients are asymptomatic.
- Family history may be positive.
- Dyspnoea, fatigue, angina, syncope or near syncope
- Sudden death during or after physical exertion
- Arrhythmias are common.

- Rapidly rising carotid pulse 'jerky'
- Bisferiens pulse (two systolic peaks)
- Double apical impulse
- Harsh ESM best heard at the lower left sternal border as well as the apex due to left ventricular outflow tract obstruction

Treatment
- β-blockers in angina and syncope
- Amiodarone for controlling arrhythmias
- Disopyramide along with β-blockers to reduce outflow tract obstruction
- Surgical myotomy or myectomy of the hypertrophied septum
- ICD in high-risk patients
- Septal alcohol ablation is increasingly used

■ ACUTE PERICARDITIS

Aetiology
- Tuberculosis
- Viral—Coxsackie B virus, mumps, varicella, rubella
- Post-myocardial infarction syndrome
- Connective tissue disease—systemic lupus erythematosus (SLE), rheumatoid arthritis, systemic sclerosis
- Acute MI
- Rheumatic fever
- Uraemia
- Malignant disease
- Hypothyroidism

Clinical Features
- Pericardial pain
- Pericardial friction rub and pericardial effusion with or without cardiac tamponade and pulsus paradoxus (paradoxical pulse) are the cardinal clinical manifestations of acute pericarditis.
- Non-specific prodrome of fever, malaise and chest pain occurs in viral or idiopathic pericarditis.

■ PERICARDIAL EFFUSION

Clinical Signs
- Apical impulse may not be palpable.
- Increase in cardiac dullness on percussion
- Heart sounds are faint or muffled.
- In a large effusion, there may be an area of dullness and tubular breathing at the angle of left scapula, resulting from compression of lung (Ewart's sign).

Treatment
- Therapeutic paracentesis with aspiration of effusion in selected cases.
- Anti-inflammatory drugs such as aspirin or indomethacin.
- Treatment of underlying cause.
- In neoplastic conditions causing recurrent effusion, intrapericardial instillation of chemotherapeutic agents may be done.

■ CARDIAC TAMPONADE
- Cardiac tamponade results from the accumulation of fluid in the pericardium in an amount sufficient to cause compression of the heart and impairment of diastolic filling.
- Tachycardia
- Pulsus paradoxus or paradoxical pulse is the hallmark of tamponade.
- Hypotension
- Raised JVP with prominent x descent but absence or attenuation of y descent.
- Increase in cardiac dullness to percussion
- Normal respiratory sounds
- Faint heart sounds; pericardial rub uncommon
- Tender hepatomegaly
- Raised JVP, hypotension and muffled heart sounds constitute Beck's triad.

Management
- Emergency pericardiocentesis
- In hypertensive patients, volume expansion with saline, blood, plasma and dextran can be used as a temporary measure.
- Positive pressure mechanical ventilation should be avoided in acute tamponade because it further reduces cardiac filling.
- Treatment of underlying cause

■ CHRONIC CONSTRICTIVE PERICARDITIS

Aetiology
- Tuberculosis (commonest)
- Haemopericardium and cardiac surgery

- Mediastinal irradiation
- Rheumatoid arthritis and SLE
- Uraemia
- Asbestosis

Clinical Features

- Pulse is of low volume and rarely pulsus paradoxus may be present.
- Neck veins are distended (engorged) with a sharp y descent, a deep y trough and rapid ascent to baseline.
- 'Kussmaul's sign' may be positive. This is an increase in the height of jugular venous pulsations (and hence a rise in JVP) during inspiration- venous paradox.
- Heart sounds may be muffled.
- An early diastolic sound; pericardial knock' may be audible (occurs 0.09–0.12 s after A_2).

Treatment

Pericardiectomy (resection of the pericardium) is the only definitive treatment.

CONGENITAL HEART DISEASE

Classification of congenital heart disease is given in **Table 3.9**.

ATRIAL SEPTAL DEFECT

- **Ostium secundum defects** [75–85% of atrial septal defects (ASDs)] are located in the region of the mid-septum (fossa ovalis).
- **Ostium primum** (atrioventricular septal) defects (10–15%) are located in the lower portion of the atrial septum.

TABLE 3.9: Classification of congenital heart disease.

Acyanotic	Cyanotic
With (left-to-right) shunts	With (right-to-left) shunts
• Ventricular septal defect	• Tetralogy of Fallot
• Atrial septal defect	• Tricuspid atresia
• Patent ductus arteriosus	• Ebstein's anomaly
	• Transposition of great vessels
	• Truncus arteriosus
Without shunts (obstructive lesions)	Without shunts (obstructive lesions)
• Aortic stenosis	• Pulmonary stenosis
• Coarctation of aorta	

- **Sinus venosus defects:**
  - **Superior sinus venosus type defect** (5–10%): Defects are located in the superior part of the septum near the orifice of the superior vena cava.
  - **Inferior sinus venosus (IVC) type defect** (1%): Defects are located on the inferior part of the septum near the inferior vena cava entry point.
- **Coronary sinus (1%) septal defect** (in which a defect between the coronary sinus and the left atrium allows a left-to-right shunt to occur through an 'unroofed' coronary sinus)

Signs

- Second heart sound - wide fixed split: Wide, fixed splitting of the S2
- A systolic flow murmur over the pulmonary valve not due to ASD
- Diastolic flow murmur over the tricuspid valve may be heard in children with a large shunt.

VENTRICULAR SEPTAL DEFECT

- Most common congenital heart disease (2 per 1,000 live births).
- Congenital VSDs are due to incomplete septation of the ventricles. Most are perimembranous- at the junction of the membranous and muscular portions. It may be isolated or may be associated with other congenital heart disease.
- Acquired VSDs can be due to—ventricular septal rupture from acute MI, infective endocarditis or rarely from trauma/cardiac catheterisation.
- Pansystolic murmur in the left lower sternal border is pathognomonic.
- Complications include congestive heart failure, pulmonary hypertension, Eisenmenger's syndrome, right ventricular outflow tract obstruction and infective endocarditis.

PERSISTENT DUCTUS ARTERIOSUS (PATENT DUCTUS ARTERIOSUS)

Congenital anomaly in which the **ductus arteriosus remains open after birth producing** a persistent communication between the proximal left pulmonary artery and the descending aorta. This produces a continuous arteriovenous left to right shunt, the volume of which depends on the size of the ductus.

About 50% of the left ventricular output is recirculated through the lungs, with a consequent increase in the work of the heart. PDAs may occur as an isolated anomaly (about 90%) or associated with other abnormalities such as VSD, coarctation of the aorta, or pulmonary or aortic valve stenosis.

- PDA produces a characteristic continuous harsh murmur known as 'machinery-like'/ Gibson's murmur.

■ COARCTATION OF AORTA

It can occur anywhere from the distal part of arch of aorta to bifurcation of the abdominal aorta.

- Major symptoms are the symptoms related to four major complications:
  i. Congestive heart failure
  ii. Infective endocarditis
  iii. Cerebral haemorrhage due to rupture of Berry aneurysm
  iv. Rupture or dissection of aorta
- Hypertension in the upper limbs with low or normal pressure in lower limbs (difference > 20 mmHg)
- Weak and delayed femoral pulses (radiofemoral delay)
- 'Suzman's sign': Dilated, tortuous, pulsatile arteries seen around the scapulae and intercostal regions in the back. It is better seen with the patient bent forwards and hands hanging down.
- 'Cork-screw'-shaped retinal arteries

■ TETRALOGY OF FALLOT

It is the most common congenital cyanotic heart disease in adults (75%).

- **VSD** usually large and similar in aperture to the aortic orifice
- **Pulmonary stenosis:** Right ventricular outflow tract obstruction mostly subvalvular (infundibular) but may be valvular, supravalvular or a combination of these.
- **Overriding of dextroposed aorta**
- **Right ventricular hypertrophy**

Presence of ASD along with tetralogy of Fallot (TOF) is known as pentalogy of Fallot. Trilogy of Fallot is a combination of three congenital heart defects: Pulmonary stenosis, right ventricular hypertrophy, and an atrial septal defect.

■ EISENMENGER'S SYNDROME

- Eisenmenger's syndrome is the consequence of the reversal of a left-to-right shunt to a right-to-left shunt.
- It occurs in patients with congenital heart disease, especially PDA, VSD and ASD.

Clinical Features

- Dyspnoea, cyanosis, fatigue, dizziness and syncope
- Central cyanosis and clubbing occur from mixing of deoxygenated blood with oxygenated blood. It is generalised to ASD and VSD reversal, while it is differential (only lower limbs) in PDA with reversal.
- S2 is loud with palpable P_2.
- S2 is fixed but narrowly split in ASD with reversal.
- S2 is single in VSD with reversal.
- S2 is mobile but narrowly split in PDA with reversal.
- Eventually, patient dies of right heart failure.

Treatment

- Vasodilator therapy using calcium channel blockers may be detrimental as systemic vasodilatation may further increase right-to-left shunt.
- Long-term oxygen inhalation may improve symptoms.
- Phlebotomy in patients with hyperviscosity syndrome due to erythrocytosis.
- The only curative treatment is **heart-lung transplantation**.
- Prostanoids (epoprostenol, iloprost, treprostinil), endothelin receptor antagonists (bosentan) and phosphodiesterase-5 inhibitors (sildenafil, tadalafil) may improve symptoms.

BEST OF FIVES

1. A 54-year-old Asian woman with a recent history of tuberculosis presents with breathlessness. The jugular venous pressure (JVP) shows prominent *x* and *y* descents. The most likely cause is:
   A. Constrictive pericarditis
   B. Dilated cardiomyopathy
   C. Pericardial effusion
   D. Restrictive cardiomyopathy
   E. Severe mitral regurgitation

2. A 40-year-old man undergoes exercise testing 8 weeks following a myocardial infarction. He is currently on aspirin, rosuvastatin, lisinopril and atenolol. Resting heart rate is 70 bpm and blood pressure is 128/70 mmHg. He achieves 4 minutes, stopping secondary to chest pain and associated ST-segment depression in the inferolateral leads. What would be the next stage in his management?
   A. Add diltiazem and review in clinic.
   B. Arrange an echocardiogram.
   C. Increase atenolol 50 mg OD and repeat the exercise test.
   D. Refer for coronary angiography.
   E. Refer for a myocardial perfusion scan.

3. A 60-year-old woman is admitted to a hospital with a swollen left leg 4 weeks after undergoing an elective total hip replacement. An above-knee deep vein thrombosis (DVT) is diagnosed by ultrasound. She is in sinus rhythm at 60 bpm and her blood pressure is 160/80 mmHg. She is commenced on the appropriate dose of low-molecular-weight heparin and warfarin loading. The following day, she becomes acutely short of breath. Examination reveals a resting tachycardia (110 bpm) with a blood pressure of 100/60 mmHg. Her jugular venous pressure (JVP) is elevated at 7 cm above the sternal notch. Arterial blood gas measurement reveals her to be hypoxaemic with a PaO_2 of 7 mmHg. What would be the first-line therapy after administering high-flow oxygen?
   A. Aspirin
   B. Intravenous heparin
   C. Surgical embolectomy
   D. Thrombolysis with reteplase
   E. Vena cava filter

4. A 67-year-old diabetic is admitted with chest pain radiating to his left shoulder and jaw. He is a moderate smoker. Serum cholesterol and low-density lipoprotein (LDL) levels are raised and the electrocardiogram (ECG) shows ST depression in the inferolateral leads. What would be your line of management?
   A. Transfer the following day for coronary angiography followed by angioplasty
   B. Thrombolysis with streptokinase, clopidogrel and aspirin
   C. Oral aspirin, clopidogrel and atenolol
   D. Glyceryl trinitrate, heparin, aspirin, clopidogrel and atorvastatin
   E. Tissue-type plasminogen activator, aspirin, warfarin and simvastatin

5. A 60-year-old man with unstable angina on long-term digoxin was being monitored on the ward with telemetry when the monitor displayed a tachycardia of 180 bpm. The printout showed discrete P waves before each QRS complex and there was an acceleration in the rate after initiation of the arrhythmia. The QRS width was 0.12 second. Which of the following is the most likely arrhythmia?
   A. Automatic supraventricular tachyarrhythmias
   B. Atrioventricular nodal reentrant tachycardia
   C. Bypass tract-mediated macroentrant tachycardia
   D. Intra-atrial re-entry
   E. Ventricular tachycardia

6. A 75-year-old man with congestive cardiac failure presents with atrial fibrillation. He is haemodynamically stable with a ventricular rate of 72 bpm. Which drug option would be most beneficial for this patient?
   A. Aspirin
   B. Digoxin
   C. Frusemide
   D. Lidocaine
   E. Warfarin

7. A 41-year-old man with a family history of sudden death presents to casualty with a second episode of collapse. On this occasion, he is referred to the Cardiology Department for review. Echocardiography reveals asymmetrical septal hypertrophy, abnormal systolic

motion of the anterior mitral valve leaflet and narrowing of the left ventricular outflow tract. The 24-hour electrocardiogram (ECG) monitoring as an outpatient reveals several periods of non-sustained ventricular tachycardia. Which of the following would be most appropriate for the management of his arrhythmia?
A. Oral flecainide 100 mg daily
B. Oral amiodarone 200 mg tds
C. Oral amiodarone 200 mg daily
D. Implantable cardioverter defibrillator
E. Phenytoin 100 mg po daily

8. A 65-year-old man presents to casualty with severe chest pain. The electrocardiogram (ECG) shows anterior ST-segment elevation and he receives prompt thrombolysis with reteplase with good resolution of changes. He is commenced on aspirin, a beta-blocker, an angiotensin-converting enzyme (ACE) inhibitor and a statin. His initial progress is complicated by further pain, worse with inspiration and movement and relieved by non-steroidal drugs. You are called to see him on day 5 post-infarct when he complains of shortness of breath on walking to the bathroom. He looks unwell with a cool periphery and resting tachycardia. Blood pressure is reduced at 90/50 mmHg. Jugular venous pressure is elevated to around 8 cm and rises with inspiration. His ECG shows preserved anterior R waves and anterolateral T-wave inversion together with sinus tachycardia. Chest X-ray shows an increase in the cardiothoracic ratio but clear lung fields. What is the most likely complication to have developed to account for this deterioration?
A. Cardiogenic shock
B. Mitral regurgitation
C. Pericardial tamponade
D. Pulmonary embolism
E. Ventricular septal defect

9. You are called urgently to review a 54-year-old man who has developed acute-onset pulmonary oedema some 36 hours after his myocardial infarction. On arrival, you note that his blood pressure is 95/50 mmHg with a pulse of 100/min regular and a pansystolic murmur is noted. There are crackles on auscultation of the chest consistent with heart failure. Which of the following represents the next investigation of choice in this man?
A. Troponin I
B. Troponin T
C. Urgent chest X-ray
D. Referral for angiography
E. Urgent echocardiogram

10. A 54-year-old man presents with an irregular tachycardia of around 130 bpm. He played in a cricket match the previous day and consumed 28 units of alcohol on the evening of the match. On examination, his blood pressure is 95/50 mmHg. What is the most likely diagnosis?
A. Ventricular tachycardia
B. Sick sinus syndrome
C. Paroxysmal atrial fibrillation
D. Atrial flutter
E. Sinus tachycardia

11. A 16-year-old girl presents to the emergency department with a collapse and palpitations after attending her end-of-term school disco. Only medication history of note includes a recent antibiotic prescription for an infected toe. Past medical history includes allergy to penicillin. Family history reveals that her mother died suddenly at the age of 34 years when the daughter was 3 years old. One aunt and one uncle have also passed away suddenly. Electrocardiogram (ECG) reveals sinus rhythm in the emergency department but the QT interval is prolonged at 550 ms (corrected). Which of the following conditions is most likely to be related to her collapse?
A. Wolff–Parkinson–White type A
B. Wolff–Parkinson–White type B
C. Congenital long QT syndrome
D. Lown–Ganong–Levine syndrome
E. Ebstein's anomaly

12. A 47-year-old man with chest pain of 1-hour duration is diagnosed as having acute myocardial infarction. Which of the following features, if present, would most contraindicate thrombolytic therapy?
A. Blood pressure 160/110 mmHg
B. History of likely ischaemic stroke within the past month
C. ST-segment elevation in electrocardiogram (ECG)

D. Previous aspirin therapy
   E. Elevated serum cholesterol

13. A 57-year-old man with ischaemic heart disease, and a recent transient ischaemic attack, is prescribed clopidogrel. How would the mechanism of action of this drug be best described?
    A. Blocks glycoprotein IIb/IIIa receptors
    B. Blocks thrombin receptors
    C. Blocks thromboxane production
    D. Blocks platelet adenosine diphosphate (ADP) receptors
    E. Potentiates antithrombin-III action

14. A 54-year-old man is referred with increased swelling of his ankles and abdomen, and a degree of shortness of breath on exertion. His jugular venous pressure is elevated with prominent *x* and *y* descents. Echo reveals preserved left ventricular systolic function with biatrial enlargement and an estimated pulmonary artery systolic pressure of around 60 mmHg. Chest X-ray shows atrial enlargement but no other abnormalities. What is the most likely cardiac diagnosis?
    A. Chronic pulmonary emboli
    B. Dilated cardiomyopathy
    C. Restrictive cardiomyopathy
    D. Secundum atrial septal defect (ASD)
    E. Tricuspid regurgitation

15. A 30-year-old-man presents to the outpatient clinic with a 2-month history of progressive effort intolerance. Some 3 weeks ago, he experienced an episode of shortness of breath at rest, suggestive of paroxysmal nocturnal dyspnoea. Examination reveals a jugular venous pressure (JVP) raised up to his earlobes, a soft tender hepatomegaly and a bilateral pitting oedema up to his knees. Chest examination reveals bibasal crepitations and an audible S3 on auscultation of the heart. The chest X-ray shows cardiomegaly with interstitial infiltrates. Echocardiography shows global left ventricular hypokinesia with an ejection fraction of 25–30%.
    Which of the following is the LEAST likely aetiological factor?
    A. Alcohol abuse
    B. Genetic factor
    C. Adenovirus
    D. Eosinophilic states
    E. Human immunodeficiency virus (HIV) infection

16. Which of the following statements is true regarding pulsus alternans?
    A. It is found in beriberi heart disease.
    B. The pulse is irregular.
    C. It is diagnosed electrocardiographically.
    D. It is found in association with a third heart sound.
    E. It is found in patients with pericardial effusion.

17. A 56-year-old lady has a known ventricular septal defect. Which of the following clinical signs would most indicate the presence of established pulmonary hypertension?
    A. Loud systolic murmur
    B. Raised jugular venous pressure (JVP)
    C. Single loud second heart sound
    D. Systolic thrill
    E. Displaced apex beat

18. A 24-year-old woman complains of recurrent syncope. Each attack has occurred after attending an aerobics class. On examination, a systolic murmur is heard which worsens with the Valsalva manoeuvre and improves on squatting. What could be the diagnosis?
    A. Epilepsy
    B. Hypertrophic obstructive cardiomyopathy
    C. Atrial fibrillation
    D. Aortic stenosis
    E. Vasovagal attack

19. A 68-year-old man is admitted with syncope. He is known to have ischaemic cardiomyopathy. His medications include aspirin 75 mg od, frusemide 80 mg bd and lisinopril 10 mg od. An initial electrocardiogram (ECG) shows sinus bradycardia (50 bpm) and right-bundle branch block (RBBB). Results of blood tests are as follows: Sodium, 134 mmol/L; potassium, 3.5 mmol/L; creatinine 124 mmol/L. He has recurrent syncopal episodes in the cardiac care unit (CCU), where monitoring shows episodes of non-sustained torsades de pointes (polymorphic VT).
    Which of the following would be your initial line of treatment?
    A. Direct current (DC) cardioversion
    B. Intravenous amiodarone

C. Intravenous magnesium
D. Oral metoprolol
E. Temporary pacing

20. A 67-year-old man is admitted with chronic congestive heart failure. Based on this history, what is the most important factor to be kept in mind when prescribing drugs for this patient?
    A. Loop diuretic administration would result in a decrease in mortality.
    B. Digoxin is more effective than angiotensin-converting enzyme (ACE) inhibitors in providing symptomatic relief.
    C. Administration of a beta-blocker reduces the time spent in hospital.
    D. Administration of spironolactone has no effect on the incidence of sudden cardiac death.
    E. Angiotensin II-receptor antagonists have a better response rate than ACE inhibitors.

21. A 36-year-old old woman presents with a cerebral infarct following treatment for a deep vein thrombosis. Cardiovascular examination is entirely normal. The most likely underlying cardiac abnormality is:
    A. Partial anomalous pulmonary venous drainage
    B. Ostium primum atrial septal defect (ASD)
    C. Ostium secundum ASD
    D. Common atrium
    E. Patent foramen ovale

22. A 67-year-old lady during pre-operative assessment is found to have a small pericardial effusion located posteriorly on routine echocardiography. Electrocardiogram (ECG) is entirely normal. What is the next most appropriate step in her management?
    A. Cardiac catheterisation
    B. Reassure
    C. Pericardiocentesis
    D. Diuretics
    E. Computed tomography (CT) of the heart

23. A 35-year-old woman presented with a history of intermittent light-headedness. Clinical examination and 12-lead electrocardiogram (ECG) were normal. Which of the following, if present on a 24-hour Holter ECG tracing, would be the most clinically important?
    A. Atrial premature beats
    B. Profound sleep-associated bradycardia
    C. Supraventricular tachycardia
    D. Transient Mobitz type-1 atrioventricular block
    E. Ventricular premature beats

24. The first-line treatment for a 50-year-old man with known poor left ventricular function who presents with a broad complex tachycardia at a rate of 150 beats/min (bpm) and a blood pressure of 120/70 mmHg is:
    A. Amiodarone
    B. Beta-blockers
    C. Flecainide
    D. Lidocaine
    E. Verapamil

25. A 60-year-old man presents to the casualty department with worsening dyspnoea and ankle swelling due to end-stage heart failure. His ejection fraction is 26%. His renal functions are within normal limits and his potassium is 4.4 mmol/L. Which of the following combinations of drugs is best suited for him in terms of mortality benefit?
    A. Ramipril, amiloride and bendrofluazide
    B. Ramipril, amiloride, bendrofluazide and atenolol
    C. Ramipril, frusemide and bendrofluazide
    D. Ramipril, frusemide, bendrofluazide and atenolol
    E. Ramipril, frusemide, bendrofluazide, bisoprolol and spironolactone

26. An obese 45-year-old woman suddenly develops dyspnoea and hypotension 2 days after undergoing a cholecystectomy. There is mild jugular venous distension with prominent *a* waves. The lung fields are clear. The electrocardiogram (ECG) shows sinus tachycardia with a right bundle branch block and minor ST-segment changes. What is the most likely diagnosis?
    A. Acute myocardial infarction
    B. Pulmonary embolism
    C. Aspiration pneumonia
    D. Aortic dissection
    E. Pneumothorax

27. A 74-year-old woman recently diagnosed with multiple myeloma complains of progressively increasing breathlessness and ankle swelling. On examination, there is bilateral pitting leg oedema, ascites and raised jugular venous

pressure (JVP). An electrocardiogram (ECG) shows diffusely diminished voltage. The echocardiogram shows small thick ventricles and dilated atria with a thickened interatrial septum. The ventricular myocardium has a granular sparkling texture on echo, and minimal fluid in the pericardial space is noted. What is the most likely diagnosis?
A. Chronic pericardial effusion with tamponade
B. Chronic pericardial effusion without tamponade
C. Constrictive pericarditis
D. Restrictive cardiomyopathy
E. Congestive heart failure

28. A 65-year-old man is admitted with a broad complex tachycardia. Which of the following features would suggest a diagnosis of supraventricular tachycardia with aberrancy rather than ventricular tachycardia?
A. Capture beats on the electrocardiogram (ECG)
B. Past history of ischaemic heart disease
C. Cannon *a* waves on jugular venous pressure (JVP)
D. Temporary alleviation by carotid sinus massage
E. Variable intensity of the first heart sound

29. An 18-year-old student is admitted from a night club in a state of collapse. Electrocardiogram (ECG) reveals a tachycardia, which is terminated with adenosine. ECG after termination of the tachycardia reveals a PR interval of approximately 100 ms, and a slurred QRS complex with delta wave. What diagnosis fits best with this clinical picture?
A. Amphetamine overdose
B. Cocaine overdose
C. Hypokalaemia-induced arrhythmia
D. Wolff–Parkinson–White syndrome (WPW)
E. Lown–Ganong–Levine syndrome

30. A 72-year-old female has intermittent exertional chest pains and dyspnoea on exertion as well. Her physical examination reveals a III/VI late-peaking crescendo-decrescendo murmur at the right upper sternal border and a III/VI holosystolic murmur at the apex. Her second heart sound is very soft and her carotid upstroke is weak and delayed. Which of the following is most likely causing her symptoms?
A. Aortic valve regurgitation
B. Aortic valve stenosis
C. Mitral valve regurgitation
D. Mitral valve stenosis
E. Mitral valve prolapse

Answers

1-A, 2-D, 3-D, 4-D, 5-A, 6-E, 7-D, 8-C, 9-E, 10-C, 11-C, 12-B, 13-D, 14-C, 15-D, 16-D, 17-C, 18-B, 19-C, 20-C, 21-E, 22-E, 23-C, 24-A, 25-E, 26-B, 27-D, 28-D, 29-D, 30-B

■ SUGGESTED READING

1. Perk J, De Backer G, Gohlke H, Graham I, Reiner Z, Verschuren M, et al. European Guidelines on cardiovascular disease prevention in clinical practice (version 2012). The Fifth Joint Task Force of the European Society of Cardiology and Other Societies on Cardiovascular Disease Prevention in Clinical Practice (constituted by representatives of nine societies and by invited experts). Eur Heart J. 2012;33(13): 1635-701.
2. Body R, Carley S, Wibberley C, McDowell G, Ferguson J, Mackway-Jones K, et al. The value of symptoms and signs in the emergent diagnosis of acute coronary syndromes. Resuscitation. 2010;81(3):281-6.
3. Goodacre S, Locker T, Morris F, Campbell S. How useful are clinical features in the diagnosis of acute, undifferentiated chest pain? Acad Emerg Med. 2002;9(3):203-8.
4. Thrift AG, McNeil JJ, Forbes A, Donnan GA. Risk factors for cerebral hemorrhage in the era of well-controlled hypertension. Melbourne Risk Factor Study (MERFS) Group. Stroke. 1996;27(11):2020-5.
5. Lip GYH, Collet JP, de Caterina R, Fauchier L, Lane DA, Larsen TB, et al. Antithrombotic Therapy in Atrial Fibrillation Associated With Valvular Heart Disease: A Joint Consensus Document From the European Heart Rhythm Association (EHRA) and European Society of Cardiology Working Group on Thrombosis, Endorsed by the ESC Working Group on Valvular Heart Disease, Cardiac Arrhythmia Society of Southern Africa (CASSA), Heart Rhythm Society (HRS), Asia Pacific Heart Rhythm Society (APHRS), South African Heart (SA Heart) Association and Sociedad Latinoamericana De Estimulación Cardíaca Y Electrofisiología (SOLEACE). Europace. 2017;19(11):1757-8.
6. Manuel J Antunes 1, Rodríguez-Palomares J, Prendergast B, Bonis MD, Rosenhek R, Al-Attar N, et al. Management of tricuspid valve regurgitation: Position statement of the European Society of Cardiology Working Groups of Cardiovascular Surgery and Valvular Heart Disease. Eur J Cardiothorac Surg. 2017;52(6):1022-30.

7. January CT, Wann LS, Alpert JS, Calkins H, Cigarroa JE, Cleveland JC, et al. 2014 AHA/ACC/HRS guideline for the management of patients with atrial fibrillation: executive summary: a report of the American College of Cardiology/American Heart Association Task Force on practice guidelines and the Heart Rhythm Society. Circulation. 2014;130(23):2071-104.
8. Kirchhof P, Benussi S, Kotecha D, Ahlsson A, Atar D, Casadei B, et al. 2016 ESC Guidelines for the management of atrial fibrillation developed in collaboration with EACTS. Eur Heart J. 2016;37(38):2893-962.
9. Baumgartner H, Falk V, Bax JJ, Bonis MD, Hamm C, Holm PJ, et al. ESC/European Association for Cardio-Thoracic Surgery (EACTS): Guidelines for the management of valvular heart disease. Eur Heart J. 2017;38(36):2739-791.
10. Chiabrando JG, Bonaventura A, Vecchié A, Wohlford GF, Mauro AG, Jordan JH, et al. Management of Acute and Recurrent Pericarditis: JACC State-of-the-Art Review. J Am Coll Cardiol. 2020;75(1):76-92.
11. Imazio M, Cecchi E, Demichelis B, Chinaglia A, Ierna S, Demarie D, et al. Myopericarditis versus viral or idiopathic acute pericarditis. Heart. 2008;94(4):498-501.
12. Imazio M, Gaita F, LeWinter M. Evaluation and treatment of pericarditis: A systematic review. JAMA. 2015;314(14):1498-506.
13. van Riel AC, Schuuring MJ, van Hessen ID, Zwinderman AH, Cozijnsen L, Reichert CLA, et al. Contemporary prevalence of pulmonary arterial hypertension in adult congenital heart disease following the updated clinical classification. Int J Cardiol. 2014;174(2):299-305.
14. Marelli AJ, Mackie AS, Ionescu-Ittu R, Rahme E, Pilote L, et al. Congenital heart disease in the general population: changing prevalence and age distribution. Circulation. 2007;115(2):163-72.
15. Simonneau G, Montani D, Celermajer DS, Denton CP, Gatzoulis MA, Krowka M, et al. Haemodynamic definitions and updated clinical classification of pulmonary hypertension. Eur Respir J. 2019;53(1): 1801913.

CHAPTER 4

Diseases of the Gastrointestinal System

PERSISTENT VOMITING

- Acute abdominal emergencies or surgical abdomen: Acute appendicitis, acute pancreatitis, acute cholecystitis, intestinal obstruction and acute peritonitis.
- Gastroesophageal reflux and gastroparesis.
- Acute systemic infections with fever: Hepatitis, viral, bacterial and parasitic infestations of intestine.
- Central nervous system disorders: Raised intracranial tension, cerebral tumours, meningitis and encephalitis.
- Disorders of labyrinth or its connections: Acute migraine, acute labyrinthitis and Ménière's disease.
- Endocrine disorders: Diabetic ketoacidosis, adrenal crisis and morning sickness of early pregnancy.
- Congestive cardiac failure and acute myocardial infarction.
- Psychogenic vomiting.

CONSTIPATION

Bowel movements less than three times a week. If stool is hard and difficult to pass, patient is constipated whatever be the frequency.

Causes

Acute
- Dehydration
- Acute intestinal obstruction
- Acute appendicitis

Chronic
- *Functional*:
  o Rectal stasis:
     - Faulty habits
     - Impaired consciousness
     - Painful anal area (anal fissure)
  o Colonic stasis:
     - Decreased food intake
     - Decreased fibre residue
     - Endocrine dysfunction
  o Irritable bowel syndrome (IBS)
- *Organic*:
  o Endocrine and metabolic diseases:
     - Myxoedema
     - Diabetes mellitus
     - Hypercalcaemia
     - Hyperparathyroidism
  o Myopathic diseases:
     - Amyloidosis
     - Systemic sclerosis
     - Myotonic dystrophy
  o Neurological disease:
     - Autonomic neuropathy
     - Cerebrovascular disease
     - Hirschsprung's disease
     - Multiple sclerosis
     - Parkinson's disease
     - Spinal cord diseases
  o Structural disease:
     - Anal fissure
     - Haemorrhoids
     - Megacolon
     - Diverticulitis

- Psychological conditions:
  - Depression
- Medications (antacids, anticholinergics, antidepressants, antihistamines, calcium, calcium channel blockers, clonidine, diuretics, iron opioids).
- Others:
  - Pressure on rectum from tumours or gravid uterus.

Investigations

- Complete blood count, serum glucose, thyroid stimulating hormone, calcium and creatinine levels.
- Stool examination.
- Sigmoidoscopy or colonoscopy to exclude colon cancer.
- Others: Colonic transit time, anorectal manometry and balloon expulsion test.

Treatment

Laxatives

- Bulk laxatives:
  - Contain soluble (ispaghula or psyllium, pectin or guar) or insoluble (cellulose) products.
- Emollient laxatives (stool softeners):
  - Include docusate sodium and docusate calcium.
- Osmotic laxatives:
  - Magnesium hydroxide (milk of magnesia), magnesium citrate and sodium biphosphate, sorbitol and lactulose.
- Stimulant laxatives:
  - Include senna, castor oil and bisacodyl.
  - Increase intestinal motility and secretion of water into the bowel.
- Prokinetic agents:
  - Cisapride, prucalopride and lubiprostone.
  - Lubiprostone in constipation—predominant IBS.

■ DIARRHOEA

Causes of acute diaarhoea (**Box 4.1**).

Chronic Diarrhoea

- Chronic enteric infections:
  - *Salmonella*
  - *Streptococcus*

Box 4.1: Causes of acute diarrhoea.
- Toxin-induced gastroenteritis:
  - Performed toxins
    - *Staphylococcus aureus*
    - *Bacillus cereus*
  - Enterotoxins produced in the intestine
    - *Vibrio cholerae*
    - *Escherichia coli* (enterotoxigenic)
    - *Clostridium perfringens*
    - *Clostridium difficile*
- Gastroenteritis due to changes in mucosa:
  - Mucosal alteration without invasion
    - Rotavirus
    - Norwalk
  - Invasion of mucosa with destruction
    - Shigella
    - *E. coli* (enteroinvasive)
    - Campylobacter
    - *Yersinia enterocolitica*
    - Salmonella
    - *Entamoeba histolytica*
- Other causes:
  - Heavy metals (arsenic)
  - Monosodium glutamate
  - Mushrooms
  - Fungi
  - Viruses
- Parasitic causes:
  - Amoebic colitis
  - Giardiasis
  - *Leishmania donovani*
  - *Strongyloides stercoralis*
  - Trichuriasis
  - *Cryptosporidium*
  - *Microsporidium* [common in patients with acquired immunodeficiency syndrome (AIDS)]
  - *Isospora*
- Malabsorption syndrome
- Post-operative enterocolostomy
- Intestinal, biliary and gastric fistulae
- Pellagra
- Inflammatory bowel diseases:
  - Ulcerative colitis
  - Crohn's disease
- Intestinal tuberculosis
- Diverticulitis and neoplasm
- Colitis due to drugs: Mercury and arsenic

- Laxative abuse
- Miscellaneous: Hyperthyroidism, radiation injury, carcinoid and vipoma.

FOOD POISONING

- A food-borne disease outbreak where a cluster of two or more individuals develop similar symptoms following the ingestion of a common food.
- The commonest type of food poisoning is gastroenteritis.
- Ingestion of contaminated food causes nausea and vomiting which start within 6 hours due to performance of toxins. Diarrhoea is a main feature which is resultant of food poisoning occurring due to toxin production in the gut. It represents within 6–72 hours of exposure.

Examination

Pulse rate (PR), blood pressure (BP) (including postural change) to be monitored. Look for skin turgor, dryness of mucous membranes, mental status and any acidotic breathing.

Severity of Dehydration

Severity of dehydration has been listed in **Table 4.1**.

Laboratory Investigations

- Leucocyte count
- Renal function tests, electrolytes and acid-base status
- Blood cultures
- Stool routine and microscopy
- Stool culture

Management

Most cases are self-limiting and require fluid therapy only.

Rehydration

- Oral rehydration solution (ORS).
- Intravenous fluids:
  - For moderate-to-severe dehydration.
  - Ringer's lactate is usually administered.

Antimotility Drugs

- Opiates (e.g. morphine and codeine)
- Diphenoxylate/atropine combination
- Loperamide
- Bismuth subsalicylate

Antisecretory Agents

- Racecadotril

Antibiotics

- Quinolones: Norfloxacin, ciprofloxacin and levofloxacin.
- In patients with suspected cholera—doxycycline.

HAEMATEMESIS

- It indicates bleeding proximal to the duodenojejunal junction (ligament of Treitz).
- It presents with haematemesis, melaena or both.

TABLE 4.1: Severity of dehydration.

Features	Mild dehydration	Moderate dehydration	Severe dehydration
Urine output	Normal	Reduced	Markedly reduced
Level of consciousness	Normal	Normal	Depressed
Oral mucosa	Dry	Markedly dry	Parched
Skin	Normal	Cool	Cool, mottled
Skin turgor	Normal	Reduced	Markedly reduced
Eyes	Normal	Sunken	Markedly sunken
Pulse rate	Normal or mild increase	Tachycardia	Marked tachycardia
Blood pressure	Normal	Postural drop or reduced	Shock
Respiration	Normal	Normal	Acidotic
Mental status	Normal or irritable	Lethargic	Comatose
Urine specific gravity	< 1.020	> 1.020	> 1.035
Blood urea	Normal	Normal to raised	High

Aetiology
The aetiology of haematemesis has been given in **Table 4.2**.

Clinical Features
- Haematemesis and/or melaena.
- Colour of the vomitus—right red blood suggests a rapid and sizeable haemorrhage while 'coffee ground' colour is consistent with a small bleed.
- Melaena occurs when > 60 mL blood is lost into the upper gastrointestinal tract (GIT).
- Haematochezia in massive bleed.
- Occasionally, presentation with symptoms of blood loss only. These include dizziness, extreme pallor and shock.

Management Strategies
Management strategies of haematemesis have been shown in **Table 4.3**.

■ DYSPHAGIA
- *Congenital*:
  - Congenital stenosis of oesophagus
  - Tracheo-oesophageal fistula
  - Congenital web
- *Acquired*:
  - Oesophageal
  - **Table 4.4** shows the causes of acquired dysphagia.
  - Painful diseases of mouth and pharynx include:
    - Stomatitis
    - Tonsillitis
    - Pharyngitis
    - Retropharyngeal abscess
  - Neuromuscular disorders:
    - Bulbar paralysis
    - Myasthenia gravis
    - Polymyositis
  - Miscellaneous:
    - Sjögren's syndrome
    - Rabies
    - Tetanus

■ GASTROESOPHAGEAL REFLUX DISEASE (REFLUX OESOPHAGITIS)

Causes
- Sliding hiatus hernia.
- Reduction in efficiency of lower oesophageal sphincter (LES) due to cardiomyotomy and vagotomy.

TABLE 4.2: Aetiology of haematemesis.

Oesophageal causes	Gastroduodenal causes	Miscellaneous causes
• Oesophageal varices • Oesophagitis • Oesophageal carcinoma • Mallory–Weiss syndrome	• Erosive gastritis or duodenitis • Stress ulcers • Peptic ulcer (gastric and duodenal) • Gastric carcinoma	• Rupture of aortic aneurysm • Coagulation defects • Angiodysplasia or vascular malformations • Erosive gastritis

TABLE 4.3: Management strategies of haematemesis.

Proton-pump inhibitors: • Omeprazole • Pantoprazole	Balloon tamponade, vasopressin, octreotide	Thermal measures: Lasers, argon plasma coagulation, electrocoagulation and heater probe thermocoagulation
Non-thermal measures: • Endoscopic band ligation • Endoscopic sclerotherapy (EST) • Injection of dilute adrenaline (1:10,000) • Injection of combination of adrenaline and fibrin glue	Embolisation of the bleeding arteries	Surgical measures: • Shunt surgery or transaction-devascularisation of oesophageal varices • In bleeding ulcer, surgery is contemplated • In gastric erosions, total gastrectomy or vagotomy with drainage is required, if medical measures fail

Diseases of the Gastrointestinal System

TABLE 4.4: Causes of acquired dysphagia.

Causes within the oesophageal lumen	Causes in the oesophageal wall	Causes outside the oesophageal wall
• Foreign body	• Strictures • Carcinoma oesophagus • Diverticulum • Reflux oesophagitis • Achalasia cardia • Plummer–Vinson syndrome • Oesophagitis • Diffuse oesophageal spasm • Chagas disease	• Thyroid swelling • Secondaries in the neck • Mediastinal nodes • Mediastinal abscess • Aortic aneurysm

- Rise in the intra-abdominal pressure caused by pregnancy, obesity, ascites, weight lifting or any other act of straining.
- Smoking cigarettes and intake of alcohol, fatty foods or caffeine reduction in the tone of the oesophageal sphincter.
- Systemic sclerosis.
- Certain drugs such as aminophylline, β-agonists, nitrates and calcium channel blockers which decrease the tone of LES.
- *Helicobacter pylori*.

Clinical Features

- Heart burn
- Acid eructation or regurgitation of the gastric contents back in the mouth.
- Tracheal aspiration with coughing or laryngismus or aspiration pneumonia.
- Odynophagia: Painful swallowing.
- Transient dysphagia to solids due to oesophageal spasm.
- Persistent dysphagia to solids due to strictures
- Blood loss causing iron deficiency anaemia
- Extraoesophageal symptoms include hoarseness, sore throat, sinusitis, otitis media, chronic cough, laryngitis, non-atopic asthma, recurrent aspiration and pulmonary fibrosis.

Complications

- Oesophagitis
- Oesophageal ulcers
- Barrett's oesophagus
- Carcinoma of oesophagus
- Strictures
- Aspiration pneumonia
- Iron deficiency anaemia

Investigations

- Endoscopy
- Barium swallow and meal.
- Ambulatory oesophageal pH metry
- Resting ECG (electrocardiogram) and stress ECG to rule out ischaemic heart disease.
- Oesophageal motility studies.

Treatment

- General measures:
  - Weight reduction and cessation of smoking.
  - Small volume and frequent feeds.
  - Avoid alcohol, fatty food, caffeine, mint, orange juice and some medications. Avoid late night meals.
  - Avoid weight lifting, stooping and bending at waist. Head end of the bed should be elevated to 15°.

Medical Treatment

- Liquid antacid
- H2-receptor antagonists such as cimetidine or ranitidine
- Proton pump inhibitors (PPIs); these include omeprazole, pantoprazole, lansoprazole, etc.
- Metoclopramide or domperidone increase the LES tone and promote gastric emptying.
- Therapy for *H. pylori*.
- Oesophageal stricture is treated by repeated dilatations.
- Oral iron or blood transfusion for anaemia.

Surgical Treatment
- Surgical resection of strictures.
- Fundoplication for sliding hiatus hernia.
- Asymptomatic hiatus hernias do not require any treatment.
- If gastroesophageal reflux is present, surgical repair of hernia is done in selected cases—fundoplication combined with an antireflux procedure.

PEPTIC ULCER DISEASE
- Ulcer in the lower oesophagus, stomach or duodenum, in the jejunum after surgical anastomosis to stomach, and in the ileum adjacent to a Meckel's diverticulum.
- Rate of incidence is 10% of all adult males.

Aetiopathogenesis
- **Heredity:**
  - Strong family history with gastric ulcers, but less strong family history with duodenal ulcers.
- **Acid-pepsin versus mucosal resistance:**
  - Digestion of the mucosa with acid and pepsin of gastric juice.
  - **Gastric hypersecretion**
  - Severe ulceration occurs in Zollinger–Ellison syndrome
  - **Mucosal resistance**
  - Prostaglandins regulate the release of mucosal bicarbonate and mucus, inhibit the parietal cell secretion and maintain the mucosal blood flow. This explains the ulcerogenic properties of nonsteroidal anti-inflammatory drugs (NSAIDs).
  - Factors which reduce the resistance of the mucosa.
  - Various drugs, especially those used in rheumatoid arthritis.
  - Aspirin damages the membrane and tight junctions. It inhibits the production of prostaglandin, thereby reducing the secretion of bicarbonate.

Helicobacter pylori
- Majority of gastric and duodenal ulcers can be attributed to NSAIDs and *H. pylori*.
- *H. pylori* also plays a role in the development of gastritis, mucosa-associated lymphoid tissue (MALT) lymphoma, gastric adenocarcinoma, gastroesophageal reflux disease (GERD) and dyspepsia.
- *H. pylori* is a Gram-negative bacillus that produces mucosal damage.
- Transmission occurs following oral–oral or faeco-oral route. **Figure 4.1** describes the natural history and disease spectrum caused by *H. pylori*.

Aetiology of Acute and Stress Ulcers
- Use of aspirin.
- Head injury, burns, severe sepsis, surgery and trauma lead to peptic ulceration known as stress ulcers.
  - Head injury causes ulcers by gastric hypersecretion (Cushing's ulcer).
  - Burns and shock produce ulcers by reflux of duodenal contents and mucosal ischaemia.

Clinical Features
- Peptic ulcer is a chronic condition with spontaneous relapses and remissions lasting.
- Epigastric pain, burning type
- Hunger pain: Pain occurring when the stomach is empty and is relieved by eating food or consumption of antacids.
- Night pain: Pain which causes the patient to be awake from sleep and is relieved by eating food or consumption of antacids.
- Pain relief: Pain is relieved by food, milk, antacids, belching or vomiting.
- Episodic pain:
  - Pain which comes and goes in episodes, lasting 1–3 weeks, 3–4 times a year.
  - Patients are mostly symptomatic during winter and spring.
  - Smokers exhibit more chances of relapse as compared to nonsmokers.
- Other symptoms may include:
  - Water-brash or also called excessive salivation, heartburns, loss of appetite and vomiting.
  - Anorexia, nausea, fullness, bloating and dyspepsia.
  - Anaemia due to chronic blood loss, haematemesis, acute perforation or gastric outlet obstruction may also be present.

Diseases of the Gastrointestinal System

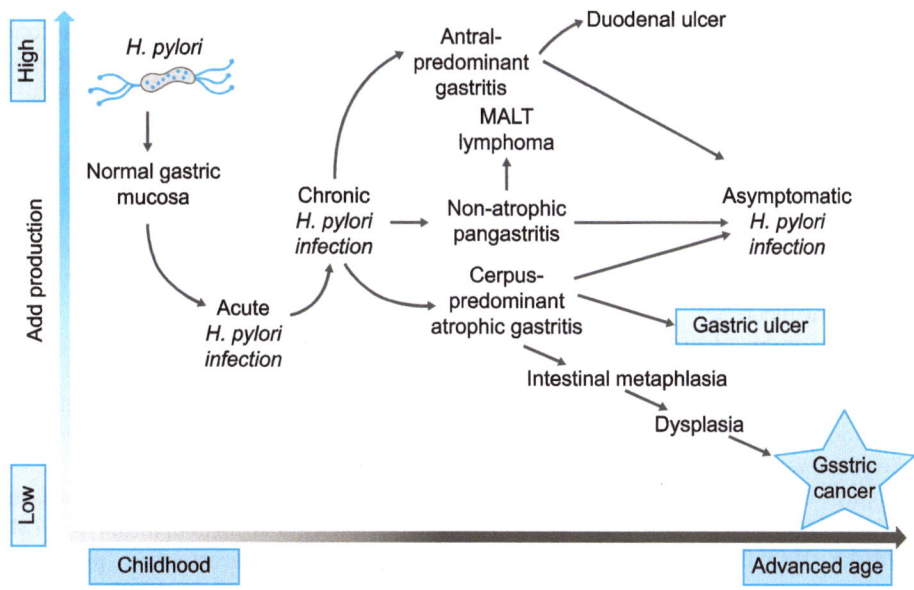

(MALT: mucosa-associated lymphoid tissue)

Fig. 4.1: Natural history of *Helicobacter pylori* (*H. pylori*) infection.

Complications
- Upper gastrointestinal bleed
- Perforation
- Gastric outlet obstruction (with fluid and electrolyte imbalance)
- Gastric malignancy
- Pancreatitis (due to posterior penetration of ulcer)

Investigations
- Double contrast barium meal
- Endoscopy with biopsy
- Tests for *H. pylori*
- Serum gastrin and gastric acid analysis in patients suspected to have Zollinger–Ellison syndrome.

Tests for *H. Pylori*
Table 4.5 shows the tests for *H. pylori*.

Treatment
Short-term management
- **General measures:**
  - Smoking cessation
  - Avoiding use of aspirin and NSAIDs

TABLE 4.5: Tests for *Helicobacter pylori*.

Invasive	Noninvasive
• On endoscopic biopsy material • Rapid urease test • Histology • Culture	• Serology for immunoglobulin G (IgG) • Urea breath test • *H. pylori* stool antigen test

  - Moderation in the consumption of alcohol
  - No special dietary advice
- **Antacids:**
  - A combination of aluminium and magnesium compounds, sodium bicarbonate and calcium carbonate as antacids can be used.
- **Histamine-2 receptor antagonists (H2RA):**
  - Such as cimetidine, ranitidine, famotidine and nizatidine
- **Proton pump inhibitors (PPIs):**
  - Such as omeprazole, lansoprazole, pantoprazole, esomeprazole and rabeprazole
- **Prostaglandin analogues:**
  - Misoprostol

- **Colloidal bismuth compounds:**
  - Bismuth subsalicylate and colloidal bismuth subcitrate
- **Sucralphate (sucralfate):**
  - Forms a protective coating over the ulcers
- **Treatment for *H. pylori* (Tables 4.6 and 4.7)**

Surgical Treatment

- Partial gastrectomy with a Billroth I anastomosis is the primary choice of procedure in case of gastric ulcer.
- For the treatment of duodenal ulcer, the following are recommended:
  - Truncal vagotomy plus pyloroplasty or gastroenterostomy.
  - Selective vagotomy with pyloroplasty.
  - Highly selective vagotomy.

ZOLLINGER–ELLISON SYNDROME

- It defines severe peptic ulcer disease secondary to unregulated gastrin release from a non-β cell endocrine tumour (gastrinoma).
  - More than 80% of gastrinomas are localised in the triangle of the gastrinomas—the convergence of cystic duct and common bile duct, the junction of the second and third portion of duodenum and the function of head and body of pancreas.
- **Clinical features:**
  - Most commonly presents between 30 and 50 years of age.
  - Manifestations of peptic ulcerations but of shorter duration. Ulcers are severe, multiple and occur at unusual sites such as jejunum or oesophagus.
  - Bleeding and perforation
  - Diarrhoea
  - Triad of abdominal pain, weight loss and diarrhoea in the presence of ulcer disease suggests gastrinoma.
  - About one-third of the patients have multiple endocrine neoplasia type I (MEN-I) involving parathyroid, pituitary and pancreas.

Investigations

- Endoscopy
- Fasting gastrin level

TABLE 4.6: First-line treatment of *Helicobacter pylori* infection.

Treatment regimen	Duration	Eradication rate
PPI (omeprazole/lansoprazole/pantoprazole/rabeprazole/esomeprazole), clarithromycin 500 mg, amoxicillin 1,000 mg (each twice daily)	10–14 days	70–85%
PPI, clarithromycin 500 mg, metronidazole 500 mg (each twice daily)	10–14 days	70–85%
Sequential therapy PPI, amoxicillin 1,000 mg (each twice daily) for 5 days **followed by** PPI, clarithromycin 500 mg, tinidazole 500 mg (each twice daily) for next 5 days	10 days	90%
Bismuth subsalicylate 525 mg, metronidazole 500 mg, tetracycline 500 mg (each four time daily) **plus** PPI or H2RA (Ranitidine twice daily)	10–14 days	75–90%

(PPI: proton pump inhibitor; H2RA: histamine-2 receptor antagonists)

TABLE 4.7: Rescue treatment for persistent *Helicobacter pylori* infection.

Regimen	Duration	Eradication rate
Quadruple therapy: Bismuth subsalicylate 525 mg, metronidazole 500 mg, tetracycline 500 mg (each four time daily) **plus** PPI or H2RA (twice daily)	14 days	70%
PPI, amoxicillin 1,000 mg, levofloxacin 250 mg (each twice daily)	10–14 days	57–91%
PPI, amoxicillin 1,000 mg, rifabutin 150 mg (each twice daily)	14 days	60–80%

(PPI: proton pump inhibitor; H2RA: histamine-2 receptor antagonists)

- Tumour localisation by ultrasound, endoscopic ultrasound, CT (computed tomography) of abdomen, somatostatin receptor scintigraphy using Indium-111-pentetreotide with single photon emission computed tomography (SPECT) scanning (octreoscan).

Treatment
- Surgical removal of the tumour
- Omeprazole and other PPIs
- Somatostatin and its analogues (octreotide and lanreotide)
- Total gastrectomy

DYSPEPSIA
- Dyspepsia is a term used for a variety of gastrointestinal symptoms.
- Ulcer dyspepsia: Dyspepsia associated with peptic ulcer.
- Nonulcer dyspepsia (functional dyspepsia) is dyspepsia for which no cause can be found.
- Flatulent dyspepsia is a functional disorder, where dyspeptic symptoms such as early satiety, flatulence, bloating and belching predominate.

Causes
- Functional dyspepsia
- Dyspepsia associated with organic diseases of upper GIT:
  - Peptic ulcer
  - Peptic oesophagitis and GERD
  - Gastric carcinoma
  - Lactose intolerance
- Dyspepsia associated with other conditions:
  - Pancreatic diseases
  - Crohn's disease
  - Colon malignancy
  - Cardiac, renal, hepatic failure
  - Carcinoma of lung
  - Drugs
  - Alcohol
  - Pregnancy
  - Depression
  - Anxiety neurosis

Common Drugs Causing Dyspepsia
- Acarbose
- Bisphosphonates (e.g. alendronate)
- Antibiotics (e.g. erythromycin)
- Codeine
- Corticosteroids
- Iron
- Metformin
- Miglitol
- NSAIDs
- Orlistat
- Theophylline

NONULCER DYSPEPSIA (FUNCTIONAL DYSPEPSIA, NERVOUS DYSPEPSIA; NONORGANIC DYSPEPSIA)

Clinical Features
- Young females (< 40 years of age).
- All the dyspeptic symptoms are present in varying degrees.
- Abdominal pain, nausea and bloating after meals.
- Pain and nausea on walking in the morning are characteristic.
- Symptoms of IBS.
- History of stress factors such as worries, concern about finance, employment and family affairs.
- Examination reveals inappropriate abdominal tenderness.

Investigations
- Blood count, erythrocyte sedimentation rate (ESR) and stool occult blood.
- Liver function tests
- Pregnancy test
- Barium meal
- Endoscopy. Required before a trial of H2-blockers or PPIs in presence of any of the following:
  - Age > 55 years
  - Dysphagia
  - Protracted vomiting
  - Anorexia or unexplained weight loss
  - Melaena
  - Anaemia
  - Palpable mass
  - Previous peptic ulcer disease
  - Jaundice
  - Family history of gastric malignancy
- Non-invasive tests for *H. pylori*, if above-mentioned risk factors are absent.

Management

- Proper explanation and reassurance.
- Stress factors tackled by counselling.
- Avoid cigarette smoking and alcohol abuse.
- If endoscopy is noncontributory, initiate empirical treatment.
    - Metoclopramide or domperidone for nausea, vomiting and bloating.
    - Mosapride or itopride.
    - H2-receptor antagonists or PPIs if pain is predominant symptom
    - *H. pylori* eradication if test is positive
    - Selective serotonin reuptake inhibitors may be effective in some patients.

Table 4.8 shows the distinguishing features of non-ulcer dyspepsia and ulcer dyspepsia.

■ MALABSORPTION SYNDROME

Malabsorption is defined as defective absorption of nutrients from GIT.

Classification and Aetiology

Table 4.9 shows the classification and aetiology of malabsorption syndrome.

Drugs Causing Malabsorption

Drug
- Colchicine
- Neomycin
- Methotrexate
- Cholestyramine
- Laxatives

Systemic Diseases Associated with Malabsorption

- Addison's disease
- Thyrotoxicosis
- Hypothyroidism
- Diabetes mellitus
- Collagen vascular diseases

Clinical Features

- Insidious onset and gradual progression.
- **General features:**
    - Include diarrhoea, abdominal pain, distension, loss of weight, anaemia and vague ill health.
- **Specific features:**
    - Due to defective absorption of different constituents.
    - **Protein:** Progressive emaciation and pitting pedal oedema.
    - **Fat:** Loss of weight, diarrhoea and steatorrhoea.
    - **Carbohydrate:** Abdominal distension, belching, bloating feeling in abdomen.
    - **Vitamins:**
        - Vitamin A: Follicular keratosis, night blindness, xerophthalmia and keratomalacia.
        - Vitamin D: Muscular irritability, tetany and features of osteomalacia.
        - Vitamin K: Haemorrhagic tendencies.
        - Vitamins B_1 and B_2: Angular stomatitis, cheilosis, glossitis and neuropathy.
        - Folic acid: Macrocytic anaemia and glossitis.

TABLE 4.8: Distinguishing features of nonulcer dyspepsia and ulcer dyspepsia.

Characteristics	Nonulcer dyspepsia	Ulcer dyspepsia
Nature of pain	Not episodic	Episodic (periodicity)
Duration of pain	Throughout the day	Occurs only on empty stomach
Relief of pain	Not affected by antacids	Relieved by antacids
Relation of pain with vomiting	Pain is not relieved by vomiting and patient cannot eat afterwards	Pain relieved by vomiting and patient can eat immediately
Relation of pain to food	Pain provoked by food	Pain relieved by food
Location of abdominal pain	Diffuse referred to more than one side	Localised referred to epigastrium
Relation of pain to sleep	Pain at night, waking the patient from sleep is rare	Pain at night, waking the patient from sleep is common

TABLE 4.9: Classification and aetiology of malabsorption syndrome.

Disorders of intraluminal digestion	
• Defect in substrate hydrolysis	• Chronic pancreatitis
	• Cystic fibrosis
	• Pancreatic carcinoma
	• Zollinger–Ellison syndrome
	• Gastroenterostomy
	• Partial gastrectomy
• Defect in fat solublisation	• Parenchymal liver diseases
	• Cholestatic jaundice
	• Zollinger–Ellison syndrome
	• Stagnant loop syndrome or blind loop syndrome
	• Terminal ileal disease (e.g., Crohn's disease and tuberculosis)
• Defect in luminal availability of factors	• Pernicious anaemia
	• Stagnant loop or blind loop syndrome
Disorders of transport in the intestinal mucosal cell	• Lactase deficiency
	• Coeliac disease
	• Tropical sprue
	• Lymphoma
	• Whipple's disease
	• Giardiasis
	• Radiation enteritis
	• Acquired immunodeficiency syndrome (AIDS)
Disorders of transport from mucosal cell	• Abdominal lymphoma
	• Tuberculosis
	• Lymphangiectasia
	• Abetalipoproteinaemia

- **Minerals and electrolytes:**
  - Sodium: Muscle cramps, weakness and hypotension.
  - Potassium: Weakness, areflexia, intestinal distension and cardiac arrhythmias.
  - Calcium: Muscular irritability, tetany, features of rickets and features of osteomalacia.
  - Magnesium: Weakness, tingling sensation and tetany.
  - Zinc: Anorexia, weakness, tingling and impaired taste.
  - Iron: Hypochromic microcytic anaemia, glossitis and koilonychia.
- Water: Dehydration and low blood volume.

Table 4.10 shows the clinical features of specific malabsorption disorders.

Treatment

- Gluten-free diet in coeliac disease.
- Pancreatic supplements in pancreatic insufficiency.
- Low-fat diet and cholestyramine for bile acid deficiency.
- Replacement therapy for anaemia, bone disease and coagulation defects.
- Vitamin D and calcium supplements.
- Vitamin B complex.
- Cholestyramine (bile acid binder) for bile acid malabsorption.
- Treat dehydration and electrolyte deficiency by intravenous infusion.

■ COELIAC DISEASE (NONTROPICAL SPRUE; GLUTEN-INDUCED ENTEROPATHY)

- Chronic disease producing malabsorption and caused by intolerance to gluten.
- Characterised by immune-mediated enteropathy (villous flattening) resulting in maldigestion and malabsorption.
- Immunological damage of the mucosa due to gluten protein of wheat. Gluten is also present

TABLE 4.10: Clinical features of specific malabsorption disorders.

Disorder	Cardinal clinical features
Adrenal insufficiency	Skin darkening, hyponatraemia, hyperkalaemia
Amyloidosis	Renal disease, nephrotic syndrome, cardiomyopathy, neuropathy, carpal tunnel syndrome, macroglossia, hepatosplenomegaly
Carcinoid syndrome	Flushing, cardiac murmur
Coeliac disease	Variable symptoms: Dermatitis herpetiformis, alopecia, aphthous mouth ulcers, arthropathy, neurologic symptoms, (life-threatening) malnutrition, abnormal liver function test result, mid iron deficiency
Crohn's disease	Arthritis, aphthous mouth ulcers, episcleritis uveitis, pyoderma gangrenosum, erythema nodosum, abdominal mass, fistulas, primary sclerosing cholangitis (PSC), laboratory signs of inflammation
Cystic fibrosis	Chronic sinopulmonary disease, meconium ileus, distal intestinal obstruction syndrome (DIOS), elevated sweet chloride
Diabetes mellitus	Long history of diabetes and diabetic complications
Glucagonoma	Migratory necrolytic erythema
Hyperthyroidism, hypothyroidism	Symptoms and signs of thyroid disease
Lymphoma	Enlarged mesenteric or retroperitoneal lymph nodes, abdominal mass, abdominal pain, fever
Pancreatic insufficiency	History of pancreatitis, abdominal pain; or alcoholism; large-volume fatty, oily stools
Parasitic infection	History of travel to endemic areas
Primary biliary cirrhosis	Jaundice, itching
Scleroderma	Dysphagia, Raynaud's phenomenon, skin tightening
Tropical sprue	History of travel to endemic area
Tuberculosis	Specific history of exposure, living in or travel to endemic area, immunosuppression, abdominal mass or intestinal obstruction, ascites
Whipple's disease	Lymphadenopathy, fever, arthritis, cerebral symptoms, heart murmur
Zollinger–Ellison syndrome	Peptic ulcers, diarrhoea

in barley, rye and oats. The toxic component in gluten is gliadin.
- High association with human leucocyte antigen (HLA) DQ2 and DQ8.

Clinical Features

- Diagnosis is made in early childhood around the age of 2 years. A second peak is found around the age of 40 years.
- Features in adults:
    - Range from mild anaemia to florid malabsorptive state.
    - The commonest cause of anaemia is iron deficiency, less commonly, it is due to folate and/or vitamin B12 deficiency.
    - Diarrhoea and weight loss.
    - Peripheral neuropathy (B1 and B2 deficiency); hypoproteinaemia, oedema, bone pain and tetany.
    - Vitamin deficiency features.
    - Clubbing (20%), glossitis, angular stomatitis and skin pigmentation.
    - Amenorrhoea and infertility.
    - Finger prints show epidermal ridge atrophy in 90%.
    - Other autoimmune syndromes have been associated with coeliac disease—type 1 diabetes mellitus, autoimmune thyroid disease, rheumatoid arthritis, systemic lupus erythematosus (SLE), Addison's disease and others.

Complications
- Dermatitis herpetiformis
- Intestinal lymphoma mainly involving jejunum
- Gastrointestinal malignancies
- Pneumococcal infections
- Peripheral neuropathy, epilepsy and ataxia
- Osteomalacia
- Amyloidosis
- Microscopic colitis

Investigations
- Serologic tests:
  - IgA antiendomysial antibodies (85–100% sensitive and 95–100% specific)
  - IgG and IgA antigliadin antibodies
  - Antitransglutaminase antibodies
- Abnormal jejunal biopsy.
- Tests indicating malabsorption of proteins, carbohydrate, fat and vitamins.
- Serologic tests for coeliac disease.

Treatment
- Strict gluten-free diet.
- Rice, corn, soybean, potato, nuts and beans, meat and fruits are safe.
- Corticosteroids are required rarely.
- Vitamin and mineral supplementation including iron administration.
- Dairy products are avoided in beginning as secondary lactase deficiency is often associated with coeliac disease.

■ TROPICAL SPRUE (IDIOPATHIC TROPICAL MALABSORPTION SYNDROME)

Definition
- Malabsorption in patients of tropics in the absence of other intestinal diseases or parasites

Aetiology
- Idiopathic, but some infective organism is suspected as antibiotics are useful in the treatment.
- Some of the implicated bacteria include *Escherichia coli*, *Klebsiella* and *Enterobacter*.
- Folic acid deficiency is another postulation.

Pathology
- Jejunal biopsy shows partial villous atrophy.
- A normal jejunal biopsy rules out tropical sprue, but an abnormal biopsy does not diagnose.

Clinical Features
- Three phases:
  - Initial phase of active diarrhoea
  - Intermediate phase
  - Last phase (Frank malabsorption)
- Spontaneous remissions and relapses may occur.
- Diarrhoea, abdominal distension, anorexia, weight loss and fatigue.
- Megaloblastic anaemia, oedema, glossitis and stomatitis

Investigations
- Stool examination to exclude pathogens
- Megaloblastic anaemia
- Hypoalbuminaemia
- Abnormal tests for fat absorption
- D-xylose test abnormal
- Vitamin B12 malabsorption
- Partial villous atrophy on jejunal biopsy

Treatment
- Tetracycline or oxytetracycline.
- Folic acid 5 mg daily (along with tetracycline)
- Correction of deficiencies of fluids, electrolytes, vitamins and iron.
- Symptomatic treatment for diarrhoea.

■ LACTOSE INTOLERANCE
- Primary lactase deficiency is inherited and characterised by normal intestinal biopsy.
- Secondary lactase deficiency is often associated with abnormal intestinal biopsy. It is seen in coeliac disease, tropical sprue, Crohn's disease, giardiasis and viral gastroenteritis.

Clinical Features
- Abdominal colic, abdominal distension, increased flatus and diarrhoea after ingesting milk or milk products.
- Improvement of symptoms on withdrawal of milk or milk products.

Investigations
- Hydrogen breath test.
- Measurement of lactase activity in a jejunal biopsy specimen.

Treatment
- Avoid milk and milk products.
- Exogenous β-galactosidase
- Use of yogurt and probiotics as a source of β-galactosidase.

■ WHIPPLE'S DISEASE
- It is a chronic multisystem disease associated with malabsorption.
- It is caused by *Tropheryma whipplei*.
- There are characteristic Periodic acid–Schiff (PAS)-positive macrophages in the small intestine and other involved organs. These macrophages cause lymphatic blockade in the lamina propria of small intestine causing malabsorption.

Clinical Features
- M:F = > 8:1
- Diarrhoea, chronic, migratory, non-destructive polyarthritis, weight loss and abdominal pain. Steatorrhoea is uncommon.
- Other features include migratory arthralgias, fever, ophthalmologic features and neurologic features (dementia, nystagmus, myoclonus and ophthalmoplegia in late stages).
- Signs include generalised lymphadenopathy, arthropathy, skin pigmentation, abdominal distension and tenderness.
- Cardiac involvement leads to mitral and aortic regurgitation.

Investigations
Jejunal biopsy and biopsy of other involved tissues show plenty of PAS-positive macrophages that contain small bacilli.

Treatment
Co-trimoxazole

■ GIARDIASIS
Aetiology
Caused by *Giardia lamblia*

Clinical Features
- Incubation period is 1–3 weeks (median 7–10 days).
- It starts as diarrhoea, nausea, vomiting, anorexia, weakness and abdominal pain. Fever and blood in stool are rare.
- Symptoms may persist from a few days to weeks or months to years.
- Chronic giardiasis: Diarrhoea may not be a prominent symptom. They may have increased flatus, loose stools, malabsorption, weight loss and growth retardation.

Treatment
Tinidazole or metronidazole

■ TRAVELLER'S DIARRHOEA
It is caused by ingestion of food and water contaminated with faecal matter.

Aetiology
- *E. coli* (toxigenic and enteroaggregative)
- *Vibrio parahaemolyticus*
- *Vibrio cholerae*—EI Tor biotype
- *Shigella*
- *Salmonella* (non-typhoid)
- *Campylobacter*
- *G. lamblia*
- *Entamoeba histolytica*
- Rotavirus
- Norwalk virus

Clinical Features
- Usually affects inter-continental travellers.
- Abrupt onset, watery diarrhoea, lasting 2–5 days.
- Abdominal cramps, nausea, vomiting, anorexia and fever.
- Diffuse tenderness over abdomen.

Treatment
- Usually self-limited and no treatment is required.
- ORS
- If fever or bloody diarrhoea is present—norfloxacin or ciprofloxacin.
- Rifaximin is highly effective against noninvasive bacterial pathogens.

Prevention
- Doxycycline
- Bismuth subsalicylate
- Norfloxacin or ciprofloxacin or rifaximin

■ CARCINOID TUMOURS AND CARCINOID SYNDROME

Carcinoid tumours are neoplasms of neuroendocrine cells (e.g. enterochromaffin cells). These are now categorised as neuroendocrine tumours (NET).
- Common sites of NET in the GIT are ileum, appendix and rectum.
- Intestinal carcinoids show a high tendency for hepatic metastases.

Secretory products: Serotonin, histamine, motilin, bradykinins, etc.

Clinical Features
- Cutaneous flushing involving head and neck (blush area) associated with lacrimation, periorbital oedema, tachycardia and hypotension.
- Diarrhoea with borborygmic cramps and malabsorption.
- Facial telangiectasia over malar area.
- Right heart valve lesions, especially tricuspid regurgitation (TR) and pulmonary stenosis (PS).
- Wheeze due to bronchoconstriction.
- Pellagra-like lesions due to conversion of tryptophan to serotonin (normally, niacin is produced from tryptophan).
- General features include hepatomegaly due to hepatic intestinal obstruction and bleeding and a tumour-associated myasthenia.

Diagnosis
- Urine: High 5-hydroxyindoleacetic acid (5-HIAA)
- Plasma: High chromogranin A
- High serotonin and platelet levels
- CT, MRI (magnetic resonance imaging), somatostatin receptor scintigraphy, PET (positron emission tomography) with radiolabelled 5-hydroxytryptophan, and occasionally laparotomy for localisation.
- Measurement of increased concentration of serotonin in tumour tissue.

Treatment
- Niacin supplementation
- Bronchodilators for wheeze
- Loperamide for diarrhoea
- Serotonin-receptor antagonists (cyproheptadine, methysergide and ondansetron) to control diarrhoea.
- Analogues of somatostatin (e.g. octreotide, lanreotide) to control flushing.
- Surgical resection of the tumour.
- Excision of hepatic metastases or hepatic artery embolisation with or without chemotherapy.

■ ISCHAEMIC COLITIS

Aetiology
- Systemic hypoperfusion
- Occlusion of the inferior mesenteric artery leading to ischaemia at left colon.
- Occasionally, it can develop due to vasculitis or ingestion of oral contraceptives.
- Drugs (e.g. alosetron, antihypertensive drugs, digoxin and cocaine)

Clinical Features
- Age > 60 years
- Colicky lower abdominal pain, nausea and vomiting.
- Diarrhoea with blood and mucus.
- Tenderness and guarding over left lower abdomen, especially left iliac fossa.
- Persistent bleeding and pain suggest stricture formation.
- It may progress to shock with generalised abdominal pain, indicating peritonitis secondary to gangrene.

Investigation
- Leucocytosis
- Plain radiograph of abdomen—**thumb printing** at splenic flexure and descending colon.
- Double-contrast barium enema
- CT of abdomen
- Sigmoidoscopy
- Arteriography

Treatment
- Conservative management with IV (intravenous) fluids, discontinuation or avoidance

of vasoconstrictive agents, bowel rest and empiric antibiotics.
- Surgical treatment for peritonitis and strictures.

CAUSES OF LOWER GASTROINTESTINAL BLEEDING

Lower GIT extends from below the ligament of Treitz (**Box 4.2**).

PSEUDOMEMBRANOUS COLITIS (ANTIBIOTIC-ASSOCIATED COLITIS)

Aetiology
- Diarrhoea due to a toxin produced by *Clostridium difficile* when the normal bacterial flora is altered or suppressed by antibiotics
- Commonly implicated antibiotics are as follows:
  - Tetracycline
  - Ampicillin
  - Lincomycin
  - Clindamycin

Clinical Features
- It usually occurs in adults.
- Patient is usually on antibiotics or would have received antibiotics within last 8 weeks.
- Profuse watery diarrhoea with abdominal cramps.
- Blood in the stools may occur.
- Complications: Dehydration, electrolyte disturbances, hypoalbuminaemia, toxic megacolon, bowel perforation, hypotension, renal failure, sepsis and death

---

Box 4.2: Causes of lower gastrointestinal bleeding.
- Haemorrhoids and polyps
- Carcinoma colon and rectum
- Diverticular disease
- Angiodysplasia
- Ulcerative colitis
- Ischaemic colitis
- Arteriovenous (AV) malformations
- Meckel's diverticulum

Investigations
- Sigmoidoscopy shows pseudomembrane
- Rectal biopsy
- Stool contains toxin produced by *C. difficile.*
- Stool culture

Treatment
- Withdraw the offending drug
- Oral or IV rehydration
- Oral metronidazole
- Oral vancomycin
- Oral vancomycin plus IV metronidazole in refractory cases
- Oral probiotic therapy
- Faecal transplantation
- Colectomy in severely ill, refractory patients

IRRITABLE BOWEL SYNDROME

Irritable bowel syndrome is characterised by chronic disorder of altered bowel habits with pain in the abdominal region.

Aetiology
- No organic cause.
- Alteration in the mobility of the GIT in the form of exaggerated gastrocolic reflex, altered emptying, increased small bowel contractions and increased small intestinal transit.
- Neurotransmitters such as serotonin may also play a role in causing IBS.
- Various psychological factors such as depression, anxiety, tension and excessive worry are all aetiologically significant.

Clinical Features
- Three clinical variants:
  - Those with spastic colitis, having primarily chronic abdominal pain and constipation (IBS with constipation or constipation predominant IBS).
  - Those with chronic intermittent painless watery diarrhoea (IBS with diarrhoea or diarrhoea predominant IBS).
  - Those with features of alternating diarrhoea and constipation (mixed IBS).
- Mostly occurs in females of the age group 20–40 years.

Diseases of the Gastrointestinal System

Rome III criteria

Recurrent abdominal pain or discomfort at least 3 days per month in the last 3 months (with symptom onset at least 6 months prior to diagnosis) associated with two or more of the following:
- Improvement with defaecation.
- Onset associated with a change in frequency of stool.
- Onset associated with a change in appearance of stool.

Other symptoms that are not essential but support the diagnosis of IBS:
- Abnormal stool frequency (3 bowel movements/day or < 3 bowel movements/week).
- Abnormal stools passage (straining urgency or feeling of incomplete bowel movement).
- Passage of mucus.
- Bloating or feeling of abdominal distension.

Investigations
- Prime aim of investigations is to exclude organic bowel diseases
  - Stool examination for leucocytes, parasites, oval, occult blood.
  - Sigmoidoscopy
  - Barium enema
  - Exclude lactase deficiency, hyperthyroidism and alcohol abuse.
  - Diagnostic criteria

Treatment
- Reassurance
- Treatment (**Table 4.11**)

■ ULCERS IN INTESTINE

Box 4.3 lists the causes of intestinal ulcers.

■ INFLAMMATORY BOWEL DISEASE

- Inflammatory bowel diseases encompass various conditions. The most common ones are discussed in the following text:
  - Ulcerative colitis
  - Crohn's disease

ULCERATIVE COLITIS

- Ulcerative colitis is an inflammatory disease affecting the large intestine, characterised by

TABLE 4.11: Treatment of irritable bowel syndrome (IBS).

Constipation-predominant IBS	Diarrhoea-predominant IBS
• Increase roughage content of the diet • Bulk laxative • Tegaserod, a 5-HT4 agonist • Osmotic agents such as lactulose • If abdominal pain—anticholinergic (dicyclomine) or an antispasmodic (mebeverine) • Psychotropic agents such as amitriptyline	• Loperamide • Cholestyramine • 5-HT3 receptor antagonists—ondansetron, granisetron, alosetron and cilansetron • Anticholinergics for pain control

Box 4.3: Ulcers in the intestine.
- Enteric fever
- Tuberculosis
- Amoebiasis
- Ulcerative colitis
- Crohn's disease
- Zollinger–Ellison syndrome
- Malignant ulcers
- Mesenteric artery occlusion
- Ischaemic colitis

recurrent attacks of bloody diarrhoea and diffuse inflammation of colonic mucosa.
- The extent of the diseases is divided into distal and more extensive disease.
  - Distal disease refers to colitis confined to the rectum (proctitis) or rectum and sigmoid colon (proctosigmoiditis).
  - More extensive disease includes 'left-sided colitis' (up to the splenic flexure), 'extensive colitis' (up to the hepatic flexure) and pancolitis (affecting the whole colon).

Aetiology
- Familial or genetic
- *Infectious*:
  - *Mycobacterium* (*M. avium* paratuberculosis)

- o Measles virus
- o *Listeria monocytogenes*
- o Yeast
- o Endogenous bacteria:
  - Bacteroides
  - *E. coli*
- Dietary factors:
  - o Deficiency or excess of certain nutrients (butyric acid, sulphides, L-arginine, glutamine)
- Smoking:
  - o Smokers are more likely to suffer with Crohn's disease as smoking has been known to aggravate it
  - o There is an increased risk of ulcerative colitis in nonsmokers.
- Psychological:
  - o Psychological stresses and personality of the individual play a vital role in the flare-ups and precipitation of symptoms.
- Ineffective or inefficient regulation of the immune system.

Pathology

- Primarily involves the colonic mucosa
- Mucosal involvement is uniform.
- Rectum is involved in 95% of cases (proctitis).
- Back wash ileitis is involvement of a few centimetres of ileum when the entire colon is involved.
- Macroscopically, the mucosa appears hyperaemic, haemorrhagic or ulcerated. Ulcers do not extend deeper beyond the submucosa.
- 'Pseudopolyps' are regenerating islands of mucosa surrounded by areas of ulceration and denuded mucosa.

Clinical Features

- **General:**
  - o Bloody diarrhoea with pus and mucus.
  - o Pain occurring especially in the lower abdominal region
  - o Fever
  - o Weight loss
  - o Loss of appetite
  - o Signs and symptoms of dehydration and anaemia
  - o Extraintestinal manifestations
  - o Tenderness on palpation over the colon, especially in the left iliac fossa.
  - o Incidence of carcinoma of colon is high, especially in cases of total colitis.
- **Acute variety:**
  - o Entire colon is involved in the disease.
  - o Severe systemic symptoms such as fever, weight loss and loss of appetite.
  - o Diarrhoea and dehydration.
  - o Tachycardia and postural hypotension.
  - o Tenesmus, lower abdominal pain and iliac fossa tenderness due to serosal involvement.
  - o Toxic megacolon and rupture may occur.
- **Chronic variety:**
  - o Bowel is permanently damaged by fibrosis. Colon acts as a rigid tube, losing the capacity to absorbing fluids, acting like a faecal reservoir.
  - o No systemic manifestations or toxaemia.
  - o Patient lives in chronic ill-health with chronic diarrhoea.

Investigations

- Anaemia, raised ESR and leucocytosis
- Electrolyte abnormalities
- Hypoproteinaemia
- Abnormal liver function tests
- Blood culture in septicaemia
- Stool examination and culture to exclude infective pathology.
- Sigmoidoscopy
- Colonoscopy:
  - o Colonoscopy is the choice in case of mild-to-moderate disease in comparison to flexible sigmoidoscopy because the extent of disease can be assessed. In moderate-to-severe disease, there is a higher risk of bowel perforation and flexible sigmoidoscopy is a safer option.
- Rectal biopsy shows mucosal inflammation.
- Serologic markers:
  - o Perinuclear antineutrophil cytoplasmic antibody (pANCA) is positive in 60–70% of patients with ulcerative colitis (seen in only 5–10% of patients with Crohn's disease).
  - o Anti-saccharomyces cerevisiae antibodies (ASCA) in only 10–15% cases (positive in 60–70% case of Crohn's disease).
  - o Anti-goblet cell autoantibodies in 30–40% cases of ulcerative colitis and Crohn's disease.

Treatment

Corticosteroids

- For inducing remission in moderate-to-severe cases
- No role in maintaining remissions
- Local treatment:
  - Hydrocortisone or prednisolone enemas, suppositories or foam.
  - Topical steroids are less effective than topical 5-aminosalicylic acid (5-ASA).
- Systemic treatment:
  - Prednisolone
  - IV hydrocortisone
  - IM or SC long-acting corticotrophin is used in the treatment of relapses.
  - Steroids once started are gradually tapered and withdrawn.

Aminosalicylates

- It is beneficial in the case of acute exacerbation as well and in order to prevent relapses. The risk of colorectal cancer is likely to be reduced by up to 75% on maintenance therapy.
- 5-ASA or mesalazine alone, or combination of 5-ASA with a carrier which releases 5-ASA after splitting by bacteria in colon (sulphasalazine, olsalazine and balsalazide).

Immunosuppressive agents

- Both azathioprine and 6-mercaptopurine are useful in inducing and maintaining remission and have steroid-sparing properties.
- Methotrexate is useful in patients who do not respond to azathioprine.
- Mycophenolate mofetil
- Tacrolimus
- In cases resistant to immunosuppressives, infliximab [antitumour necrosis factor (TNF)-α antibody] has been shown to be effective.

Surgical Management

- Colectomy with ileostomy is carried out as an emergency surgical procedure whereas the rectum and distal colon are removed at a later stage.
- Elective surgical procedure is total proctocolectomy with ileostomy or ileorectal anastomosis or ileoanal anastomosis.

Indications of Emergency Surgery

- Presentation of disease in severe forms
- Toxic dilatation of colon
- Perforation
- Severe haemorrhage

Crohn's Disease

Definition

- It is characterised by patchy, transmural inflammation, which may affect any part of the GIT.
- It may be defined by location (terminal ileal, colonic, ileocolic and upper gastrointestinal) or by pattern of disease (inflammatory, fistulating or structuring).

Pathology

- It affects small and large bowels, but is more common in the small bowel. It can affect any part of the GIT from mouth to anus.
- Commonly involved sites in the order of frequency are:
  - Terminal ileum and right side of colon
  - Colon alone
  - Terminal ileum alone
  - Ileum and jejunum
- Inflammation extends through all the layers of the intestinal wall.
- Bowel wall is thickened and leathery with the lumen narrowed (stenosis).
- Mucosa has a nodular cobble-stoned look.
- Mucosal involvement is characteristically patchy, interrupted by islands of normal mucosa. A small lesion separated from a major area of involvement is known as a 'skip lesion'.
- Fistulae develop between adjacent loops of intestine affected segments of intestine and the bladder, uterus, vaginal or perineum.
- The intestinal ulcers may penetrate to form intra-abdominal abscesses.
- Mesentery and regional lymph nodes are involved.
- Microscopically, the characteristic feature is noncaseating granuloma formation.

Clinical features of Crohn's disease of small intestine/ileum/right colon (ileocolitis) are as follows:
- Chronic disease with exacerbations and remissions.
- Young adults with history of fatigue, weight loss, diarrhoea, fever and pallor.
- Abdominal pain due to peritoneal involvement or intestinal obstruction.
- Right lower quadrant pain, tenderness, guarding and mass.
- Mass palpable per abdomen and rectally suggests adherent loops of intestine and abscess.
- Recurrent episodes of colicky abdominal pain with nausea, vomiting and excessive borborygmi suggest subacute intestinal obstruction.
- Stool usually does not contain Frank blood, mucus or pus unless the colon is involved.
- Anal lesions such as oedematous skin tags, fistulae, fissures, perianal and perirectal abscesses are characteristic.
- Features of malabsorption such as weight loss and anaemia (iron, folic acid and B12 malabsorption).
- Sodium, potassium, water, magnesium and zinc deficiency due to chronic diarrhoea

Intra-abdominal Complications
- Intestinal obstruction
- Fistula formation
  - Ileovesical fistula leads to recurrent urinary infection, cystitis and pneumaturia
  - Fistulae between contiguous segments of intestines
  - Cutaneous fistulae
- Abscesses
- Free perforation
- Rectal fissures
- High incidence of carcinoma of intestine
- Gastric outlet obstruction or duodenal obstruction
- Gall stones and urinary oxalate stones
- Secondary amyloidosis in long-standing cases (hepatosplenomegaly with proteinuria)

Investigations
- Normochromic normocytic or macrocytic or hypochromic anaemia.
- Raised ESR and leucocytosis
- Abnormal liver function tests
- Hypoproteinaemia
- Stool culture and routine examination to exclude infectious causes of diarrhoea.
- Schilling test for malabsorption of vitamin B12
- Sigmoidoscopy and colonoscopy.
- Biopsy of colonic mucosa, ileal mucosa, anal skin tags and perianal inflammatory lesions.
- High-resolution ultrasound and spiral CT scan.
- Radionuclide scan using gallium-labelled polymorphs or indium-labelled leucocytes to identify intestinal and colonic disease and localise extraintestinal abscesses.
- Serologic markers:
  - Antigoblet cell autoantibodies in 30–40% cases of Crohn's disease.
  - Antiglycan antibodies in about 40–50% cases (e.g. antilaminaribioside, antimannobioside antibodies).

Treatment
- 5-ASA as maintenance in mild-to-moderate ileocolonic disease.
- Prednisolone
- Immunosuppressive agents: Azathioprine, 6-mercaptopurine and cyclosporine and newer agents (mycophenolate mofetil, tacrolimus and infliximab). Another TNF-α blocker, adalimumab
- Budesonide
- Metronidazole

Surgical Treatment
- Indicated in repeated episodes of subacute obstruction, abscess, perforation, extensive and severe involvement of colon.
- Minimal resections for strictures and fistulae.

Complications of Inflammatory Bowel Disease
- Complications of inflammatory bowel disease are classified as local and systemic (extraintestinal) (**Box 4.4**).

The differences between ulcerative colitis and Crohn's disease of the colon have been shown in **Table 4.12**.

Box 4.4: Complications of inflammatory bowel disease.

- Local complications:
  - Fistulae, abscess and strictures
  - Perforation
  - Toxic dilatation (toxic megacolon)
  - Carcinoma
- Hepatobiliary:
  - Fatty liver
  - Gallstones
  - Pericholangitis
  - Sclerosing cholangitis
  - Bile duct carcinoma
  - Chronic hepatitis
  - Cirrhosis
- Haematological:
  - Venous thrombosis and thromboembolism
  - Autoimmune haemolytic anaemia
- Nutritional and metabolic:
  - Weight loss and anaemia
  - Electrolyte imbalance
  - Hypoalbuminaemia
- Musculoskeletal:
  - Ankylosing spondylitis
  - Seronegative arthritis
  - Sacroiliitis
- Renal:
  - Acalculous disease
  - Amyloidosis
  - Pyelonephritis
- Eyes:
  - Iritis and uveitis
  - Episcleritis and conjunctivitis
- Skin and mucous membranes
  - Erythema nodosum
  - Pyoderma gangrenosum
  - Aphthous stomatitis
  - Finger clubbing

TABLE 4.12: Differences between ulcerative colitis and Crohn's disease of the colon.

Characteristics	Ulcerative colitis	Crohn's disease
Pathological features		
<ul><li>Involvement of bowel</li><li>Inflammation</li><li>Noncaseating granulomas</li><li>Crypt abscess</li><li>Goblet cell depletion</li><li>Strictures, fissures and fistulae</li><li>Mesenteric and lymph nodal involvement</li></ul>	<ul><li>Continuous involvement</li><li>Restricted to mucosa and submucosa</li><li>Absent</li><li>Common</li><li>Seen</li><li>Uncommon</li><li>Absent</li></ul>	<ul><li>Segmental involvement (skip lesions)</li><li>Transmural</li><li>Common</li><li>Uncommon</li><li>Absent</li><li>Common</li><li>Common</li></ul>
Clinical features		
<ul><li>Rectal bleeding</li><li>Abdominal pain</li><li>Abdominal masses</li><li>Fistulae, fissures and perianal skin tags</li><li>Small bowel involvement</li><li>Rectal and colonic involvement</li><li>Recurrence after surgery</li><li>Toxic dilatation</li></ul>	<ul><li>Common</li><li>Less common</li><li>May be palpable</li><li>Uncommon</li><li>Uncommon</li><li>Common</li><li>Not common</li><li>Relatively common</li></ul>	<ul><li>Uncommon</li><li>More common</li><li>Not usually palpable</li><li>Common and characteristic</li><li>Common</li><li>Rare</li><li>Common</li><li>Uncommon</li></ul>

BEST OF FIVES

1. Which of the following has a well-established association with gastroesophageal reflux?
   A. Chronic sinusitis
   B. Dental erosion
   C. Pulmonary fibrosis
   D. Recurrent aspiration pneumonia
   E. Sleep apnoea

2. A 36-year-old woman complains of 6 months of epigastric pain that is worst between meals. She also reports symptoms of heartburn. The pain is typically relieved by over-the-counter antacid medications. She comes to the clinic after noting her stools' darkening. Her stools for heme is positive. She undergoes esophagogastroduodenoscopy (EGD), which demonstrates a well-circumscribed, 2-cm duodenal ulcer that is positive for *Helicobacter pylori*. Given these findings, which of the following is the recommended initial therapy?
   A. Lansoprazole plus clarithromycin plus amoxicillin for 14 days
   B. Pantoprazole plus amoxicillin for 21 days
   C. Pantoprazole plus clarithromycin for 14 days
   D. Omeprazole plus bismuth plus tetracycline plus metronidazole for 14 days
   E. Omeprazole plus metronidazole plus clarithromycin for 7 days

3. All of the following are direct complications of short bowel syndrome except:
   A. Cholesterol gallstones
   B. Coronary artery disease
   C. Gastric acid hypersecretion
   D. Renal calcium oxalate calculi
   E. Steatorrhoea

4. A 45-year-old male presents with 1 month of diarrhoea. He states that he has 8–10 loose bowel movements a day. He has lost 4 kg during this time. Vital signs and physical examination are normal. Serum laboratory studies are normal. A 24-hour stool collection reveals 500 g of stool with a measured stool osmolality of 200 mOsmol/L and a calculated stool osmolality of 210 mOsmol/L. Based on these findings, what is the most likely cause of this patient's diarrhoea?
   A. Coeliac sprue
   B. Chronic pancreatitis
   C. Lactase deficiency
   D. Vasoactive intestinal peptide tumour
   E. Whipple disease

5. Cobalamin malabsorption may occur in all of the following diseases except:
   A. Bacterial overgrowth syndrome
   B. Chronic pancreatitis
   C. Crohn's disease
   D. Pernicious anaemia
   E. Ulcerative colitis

6. A 36-year-old man with ulcerative colitis has been treated for the past 5 years with infliximab with excellent resolution of his bowel symptoms and endoscopic evidence of normal colonic mucosa. He is otherwise healthy. He is evaluated by a dermatologist for a lesion that initially was a pustule over his right lower extremity but has since progressed in size with ulceration. The ulcer is moderately painful. He does not recall any trauma to the area. On examination, the ulcer measures 15 cm by 7 cm and central necrosis is present. The edges of the ulcer are violaceous. No other lesions are identified. Which of the following is the most likely diagnosis?
   A. Erythema nodosum
   B. Metastatic Crohn's disease
   C. Psoriasis
   D. Pyoderma gangrenosum
   E. Pyoderma vegete

7. Your 43-year-old patient with Crohn's disease (CD) has had a disappointing disease response to glucocorticoids and 5-aminosalicylic acid (ASA) agents. He is interested in steroid-sparing agents. He has no liver or renal disease. You prescribe once-weekly methotrexate injections. In addition to monitoring hepatic function and complete blood count, what other complication of methotrexate therapy do you aware the patient of?
   A. Disseminated histoplasmosis
   B. Lymphoma
   C. Pancreatitis
   D. Pneumonitis
   E. Primary sclerosing cholangitis

8. After a careful history, physical examination and a cost-effective workup, you have diagnosed a 22-year-old female patient with irritable bowel syndrome. What other condition

would you reasonably expect to find in this patient?
A. Abnormal brain anatomy
B. Autoimmune disease
C. History of sexually transmitted diseases
D. Psychiatric diagnosis
E. Sensory hypersensitivity to peripheral stimuli

9. Which of the following statements regarding anorectal abscess is true?
A. Anorectal abscess is more common in diabetic patients
B. Anorectal abscess is more common in women
C. Difficulty voiding is uncommon and should prompt further evaluation of anorectal abscess
D. Examination in the operating room under anaesthesia is required for adequate exploration in most cases
E. The peak incidence is the seventh decade of life

10. All of the following are potential causes of appendix obstruction and appendicitis except:
A. Ascaris infection
B. Carcinoid tumour
C. Cholelithiasis
D. Fecalith
E. Measles infection

11. Which of the following organisms is most likely to be causative in acute appendicitis?
A. *Clostridium* species
B. *Escherichia coli*
C. *Mycobacterium tuberculosis*
D. *Staphylococcus aureus*
E. *Yersinia enterocolitica*

12. Enteric pathogens can produce diarrhoeal illness through a variety of mechanisms that lead to specific clinical characteristics. All of the following are characteristics of diarrhoea caused by *Vibrio cholerae* except:
A. Disease localised to the proximal small intestine
B. Faecal leucocytes
C. Faecal lactoferrin
D. Toxin production
E. Watery diarrhoea

13. Two hours after attending a company picnic, many individuals who attended the picnic developed an acute gastrointestinal illness. Food poisoning caused by *Staphylococcus aureus* is suspected. All of the following characteristics would be a common feature of food poisoning due to this organism except:
A. Abdominal cramping
B. Diarrhoea
C. Fever
D. Vomiting
E. Toxin mediated

14. Which of the following is a common manifestation of *Clostridium difficile* infection?
A. Fever
B. Nonbloody diarrhoea
C. Adynamic ileus
D. Recurrence after therapy
E. All of the above

15. Which of the following antibiotics has the weakest association with the development of *Clostridium difficile*-associated disease?
A. Ceftriaxone
B. Ciprofloxacin
C. Clindamycin
D. Moxifloxacin
E. Piperacillin/tazobactam

16. *Helicobacter pylori* colonisation increases the odds ratio of developing all of the following conditions except:
A. Duodenal ulcer disease
B. Oesophageal adenocarcinoma
C. Gastric adenocarcinoma
D. Gastric mucosa-associated lymphoid tissue (MALT) lymphoma
E. Peptic ulcer disease

17. All of the following statements regarding Norwalk virus gastroenteritis are true except:
A. Fever is common
B. Incubation period is typically 5–7 days
C. Infection is common worldwide
D. It is a major cause of non-bacterial diarrhoea outbreaks in the United States
E. Transmission is typically faecal–oral

18. All of the following statements regarding rotavirus gastroenteritis are true except:
A. Fever occurs in > 25% of cases

B. Inflammatory diarrhoea distinguishes rotaviral illness from Norwalk gastroenteritis
C. It is a major cause of diarrhoeal death among children in the developing world
D. Nausea is common
E. Vaccination is recommended for all children in the United States

19. A 22-year-old college student presents to the emergency department with crampy abdominal pain and watery diarrhoea that have worsened over 3 days. He recently returned from a volunteer trip to Mexico. He has no past medical history and felt well throughout the trip. Stool examination shows small cysts containing four nuclei, and stool antigen immunoassay is positive for *Giardia* species. Which of the following is a recommended treatment regimen for this patient?
    A. Albendazole
    B. Clindamycin
    C. Giardiasis is self-limited and requires no antibiotic therapy
    D. Paromomycin
    E. Tinidazole

20. All of the following are clinical manifestations of *Ascaris lumbricoides* infection except:
    A. Asymptomatic carriage
    B. Fever, headache, photophobia, nuchal rigidity and eosinophilia
    C. Nonproductive cough and pleurisy with eosinophilia
    D. Right upper quadrant pain and fever
    E. Small bowel obstruction

21. Which is the most common site for chronic gastric ulcer?
    A. Lesser curvature at incisura
    B. High on lesser curvature
    C. Greater curvature
    D. Prepyloric region
    E. Fundus

22. Rockall scoring system is used in the prognosis of patients with
    A. Upper gastrointestinal (GI) bleeding
    B. Lower GI bleeding
    C. Hepatic encephalopathy
    D. Inflammatory bowel disease (IBD)
    E. Pancreatitis

23. Diffuse oesophageal spasm can be treated with:
    A. Pneumatic dilation
    B. Oxybutynin
    C. Nitrates
    D. Atropine
    E. Proton-pump inhibitor (PPI)

24. The most common site for iatrogenic rupture of oesophagus is:
    A. Cervical oesophagus
    B. Thoracic below aortic arch
    C. Thoracic above aortic arch
    D. Abdominal
    E. Gastroesophageal (GE) junction

25. Heller's operation is done for:
    A. Achalasia cardia
    B. Diffuse oesophageal spasm
    C. Peptic ulcer disease
    D. Cancer of the oesophagus
    E. Gastroesophageal reflux disease (GERD)

26. Schatzki's ring is:
    A. Mucosal ring at squamous columnar junction
    B. Muscular ring
    C. Dysphagia is presenting symptom
    D. Inflammatory stricture
    E. Seen in iron deficiency

27. Bleeding from lesser curvature in gastric ulcer is from:
    A. Right gastroepiploic artery
    B. Right omentoduodenal artery
    C. Pancreaticoduodenal artery
    D. Left gastric artery
    E. Left gastroepiploic artery

28. All the following statements are true about dumping syndrome except:
    A. It is caused by early emptying of stomach
    B. It can be medically managed
    C. It can be controlled by small diets
    D. It needs re-surgery
    E. It can cause hypoglycaemia

29. The best screening test for Crohn's disease is:
    A. Anti-Saccharomyces cerevisiae antibody (ASCA)
    B. Perinuclear antineutrophil cytoplasmic antibodies (p-ANCA)
    C. Faecal alpha-1 anti-trypsin

D. Faecal calprotectin
E. ANA

30. The most common manifestation of Whipple disease is:
A. Ataxia
B. Ophthalmoplegia
C. Seizure
D. Dementia
E. Fever

Answers

1-B, 2-A, 3-B, 4-D, 5-E, 6-D, 7-D, 8-D, 9-A, 10-C, 11-E, 12-B, 13-C, 14-E, 15-E, 16-B, 17-B, 18-B, 19-E, 20-B, 21-A, 22-A, 23-C, 24-A, 25-A, 26-A, 27-D, 28-D, 29-A, 30-D

SUGGESTED READING

1. Malfertheiner P, Megraud F, O'Morain CA, Atherton J, Axon ATR, Bazzoli F, et al. Management of Helicobacter pylori infection--the Maastricht IV/Florence Consensus Report. Gut. 2012;61(5):646-64.
2. ASGE Standards of Practice Committee, Banerjee S, Cash BD, Dominitz JA, Baron TH, Anderson MA, et al. The role of endoscopy in the management of patients with peptic ulcer disease. Gastrointest Endosc. 2010;71(4):663-8.
3. Hosokawa O, Watanabe K, Hatorri M, Douden K, Hayashi H, Kaizaki Y. Detection of gastric cancer by repeat endoscopy within a short time after negative examination. Endoscopy. 2001;33(4):301-5.
4. Gomollón F, Dignass A, Annese S, Dias FJM, Rogler G, Lakatos PL, et al. 3rd European Evidence-based Consensus on the Diagnosis and Management of Crohn's Disease 2016: Part 1: Diagnosis and Medical Management. J Crohns Colitis. 2017;11(2):135-49.
5. Lichtenstein GR, Loftus EV, Isaacs KL, Regueiro MD, Gerson LB, Sands BE. ACG clinical guideline: Management of Crohn's disease in adults. Am J Gastroenterol. 2018;113(4):481-517.
6. Lamb CA, Kennedy NA, Raine T, Hendy PA, Smith PJ, Limdi JK, et al. British Society of Gastroenterology consensus guidelines on the management of inflammatory bowel disease in adults. Gut. 2019;68(Suppl 3):s1-106.
7. Schiller LR. Evaluation of chronic diarrhea and irritable bowel syndrome with diarrhea in adults in the era of precision medicine. Am J Gastroenterol. 2018;113(5):660-669.
8. Hogenauer C, Hammer HF. Maldigestion and malabsorption. In: Feldman M, Friedman LS, Brandt LJ (Eds). Sleisenger and Fordtran's Gastrointestinal and Liver Disease, 10th edition, Philadelphia: Saunders; 2016. p.1788.
9. Barkun AN, Almadi M, Kuipers EJ, Laine L, Sung J, Tse F, et al. Management of nonvariceal upper gastrointestinal bleeding: Guideline Recommendations From the International Consensus Group. Ann Intern Med. 2019;171(11):805-22.
10. Hwang JH, Fisher DA, Ben-Menachem T, Chandrasekhara V, Chathadi K, Decker GA, et al. The role of endoscopy in the management of acute non-variceal upper GI bleeding. Gastrointest Endosc. 2012;75(6):1132-8.
11. Laine L, Jensen DM. Management of patients with ulcer bleeding. Am J Gastroenterol 2012;107(3):345-60.
12. Malagelada JR, Bazzoli F, Boeckxstaens G, Looze DD, Fried M, Kahrilas P, et al. World gastroenterology organisation global guidelines: dysphagia--global guidelines and cascades update September 2014. J Clin Gastroenterol. 2015;49(5):370-8.
13. Tack J, Talley NJ, Camilleri M, Holtmann G, Hu P, Malagelada JR, et al. Functional gastroduodenal disorders. Gastroenterology. 2006;130(5):1466-79.

CHAPTER 5

Hepatobiliary Disorders

■ LIVER FUNCTION TESTS

Liver Biochemistry

Serum Bilirubin
- Normal level: 1.0–1.5 mg/dL (almost all unconjugated)
- Hyperbilirubinaemia—conjugated or unconjugated type (**Table 5.1**)
- **Conjunctival icterus:** Total serum bilirubin level less than at least 3.0 mg/dL does not differentiate between conjugated and unconjugated hyperbilirubinaemia. Tea- or cola-coloured urine may indicate the presence of bilirubinuria and thus conjugated hyperbilirubinaemia.
- **Fluctuating hyperbilirubinaemia:**
    - Gall stones
    - Carcinoma of ampulla of Vater
    - Chronic hepatitis
    - Haemolytic anaemias
    - Gilbert's syndrome

Serum Enzymes (Tables 5.2 and 5.3)
- **Aminotransferases (transaminases):** Aspartate aminotransferase (AST, SGOT), Alanine aminotransferase (ALT, SGPT).
    - Present in hepatocytes and leak into the blood with liver cell damage
    - Normal value: 10–40 U/L.
    - Poor correlation between the degree of liver cell damage and level of aminotransferases.
    - **AST:** Mitochondrial and cytoplasmic isoenzymes. High concentration also in heart, muscle, kidney and brain. Raised in hepatic necrosis, myocardial infarction, muscle injury and congestive cardiac failure.
    - **ALT:** Cytosolic enzyme; more specific for liver injury.
    - **AST:ALT ratio:**
        - AST:ALT > 1: Chronic viral hepatitis and non-alcoholic fatty liver disease.
        - AST:ALT ratio > 2:1 is suggestive, while a ratio > 3:1 is highly suggestive of alcoholic liver disease. A low level of ALT in the serum in alcoholic patients is due to an alcohol-induced deficiency of pyridoxal phosphate.

TABLE 5.1: Types of hyperbilirubinaemia.

Type	Bilirubin level	Causes	Bilirubinuria, liver function test (LFT)
Unconjugated hyperbilirubinaemia	< 6 mg/dL	• Haemolytic anaemia • Ineffective erythropoiesis • Gilbert's syndrome	• Absent • LFT otherwise normal
Conjugated hyperbilirubinaemia	Higher levels	• Parenchymal liver diseases • Biliary tract obstructions	• Present • LFT deranged

TABLE 5.2: Chronic mild elevations (< 150 U/L).

ALT > AST		AST > ALT	
Hepatic	**Non-hepatic**	**Hepatic**	**Non-hepatic**
Alpha-1 antitrypsin deficiency	Celiac disease	Alcohol-related liver injury	Hypothyroidism
Autoimmune hepatitis	Hyperthyroidism	Cirrhosis	Macro-AST
Chronic viral hepatitis (B,C,D)			Myopathy
Haemochromatosis			Strenuous exercise
Medications and toxins			
Wilson's disease			
Steatosis and steatohepatitis			

(ALT: alanine aminotransferase; AST: aspartate aminotransferase)

TABLE 5.3: Acute severe elevations (> 1,000 U/L).

ALT > AST		AST > ALT	
Hepatic	**Non-hepatic**	**Hepatic**	**Non-hepatic**
Acute bile duct obstruction	None	Medications or toxins in a patient with underlying alcoholic liver injury	Acute rhabdomyolysis
Acute Budd–Chiari syndrome			
Acute viral hepatitis			
Autoimmune hepatitis			
Hepatic artery ligation			
Ischaemic hepatitis			
Medications/toxins			
Wilson's disease			

(ALT: alanine aminotransferase; AST: aspartate aminotransferase)

Causes of Elevated Serum Aminotransferases

- **Enzymes that reflect cholestasis:**
  - **Alkaline phosphatase (ALP):**
    - Many distinct isoenzymes: Liver, bone, kidney, placenta, small intestine and their origin can be determined by electrophoretic separation.
    - Normal serum level: 3–13 KA units (80–240 IU/L).
    - Raised levels of liver-derived ALP are not totally specific for cholestasis.
    - **Low levels:** Wilson's disease, with fulminant hepatitis and haemolysis, possibly because of reduced activity of the enzyme owing to displacement of the cofactor zinc by copper.
  - **Raised serum ALP levels:**
    - **Less than 2.5 times:** Hepatocellular jaundice
      ◊ More than 4 times:
      ◊ Obstructive jaundice (intrahepatic or extrahepatic obstruction)
      ◊ Infiltrative liver diseases, e.g. cancer, metastases, amyloidosis
      ◊ Bone lesions with rapid bone turnover, e.g. Paget's disease
      ◊ Primary biliary cirrhosis
- **Gamma glutamyl transpeptidase (GGTP):**
  - Microsomal enzyme present in liver, renal tubules, pancreas and intestine.

- Identify source of isolated elevation in serum ALP (GGTP is normal in bone disease)
- Screening test for alcoholism: If ALP is normal, raised serum GGTP is a good guide to alcohol intake of > 60 g/day.
- **Elevated GGTP levels:**
  - Biliary obstruction
  - Alcoholism
  - Liver parenchymal damage
  - Non-alcoholic fatty liver
  - Other causes: Chronic obstructive lung disease, diabetes mellitus, hyperthyroidism, obesity and renal failure
  - Patients taking phenytoin, barbiturates and antiretroviral therapy—non-nucleoside reverse transcriptase inhibitors and abacavir
- **5'-nucleotidase (5'-NT):**
  - Microsomal enzyme similar significance to that of GGTP
  - 5'-NT levels not increased in bone disease, increased in hepatobiliary disease
- **Lactic dehydrogenase (LDH):**
  - Not useful in diagnosis of liver diseases.
  - Moderate elevations: Ischaemic hepatitis and hepatic metastasis.
  - ALT/LDH ratio > 1.5 suggests ischaemic hepatitis while ratio < 1.5 is seen with paracetamol toxicity.

Biosynthetic Function of the Liver

Plasma proteins:
- **Serum albumin:**
  - Synthesised exclusively in liver and marker of synthetic function
  - Normal serum albumin level: 4–5.5 g/100 mL.
  - Hypoalbuminaemia: Chronic liver diseases: Cirrhosis, chronic hepatitis; reflects severe liver damage and decreased albumin synthesis. Bad prognostic sign
- **Serum globulins (Table 5.4):**
  - Made of gamma globulins, synthesized by b-lymphocytes and α and β globulins synthesised primarily by hepatocytes
  - Normal serum globulin level: 1.5–3.5 g/100 mL
  - Increased in chronic liver disease (e.g. chronic hepatitis and cirrhosis).

TABLE 5.4: Specific types of elevated immunoglobulin and its associated conditions.

Specific types of immunoglobulin	Condition in which it is raised
IgG	Chronic hepatitis and cryptogenic cirrhosis
IgA	Alcoholic liver disease
IgM	Primary biliary cirrhosis

Coagulation factors:
- Liver produces all the coagulation factors except factor VIII.
- Vitamin K: Activation of coagulation factors II, VII, IX and X.
- Factors have short half-life time, best measure of current hepatic synthetic function for diagnosis and prognosis of acute parenchymal liver disease.
- Prothrombin time (PT):
  - Normal: 11–12.5 seconds.
  - PT collectively measures factors II, V, VII and X.
  - Prolonged:
    - Severe liver damage: Acute hepatitis (e.g. viral hepatitis) and cirrhosis
    - Vitamin K deficiency: Obstructive jaundice, fat malabsorption, poor intake and antibiotic therapy
    - Disseminated intravascular coagulation
  - Marked prolongation of the PT (> 5 s) above control, if not corrected by parenteral administration of vitamin K, is a poor prognostic sign in acute viral hepatitis and other acute and chronic liver diseases.

Ceruloplasmin:
- Acute phase reactant synthesised by the liver
- Major carrier for copper by binding to it in plasma
- Normal plasma level: 20–60 mg/dL
- **Elevated levels:** Infections, liver diseases, obstructive jaundice, rheumatoid arthritis and pregnancy.
- **Decreased levels:** Wilson's disease (due to decreased rate of synthesis), neonates, Menkes disease, kwashiorkor, marasmus, protein-losing enteropathy and copper deficiency.

Other tests above Brompsulpthalein (BSP) test
- **Bromosulphthalein (BSP) clearance:** Delayed in Dubin–Johnson syndrome
- **Urine tests:**
  o **Bilirubin:**
    - Normally, cannot be detected in urine
    - In unconjugated hyperbilirubinaemia, urine does not contain bilirubin (acholuric jaundice).
    - In conjugated hyperbilirubinaemia, urine contains bilirubin.
    - Detected by Fouchet's test
  o **Urine urobilinogen:**
    - Normally present in urine in trace amount (1–2 mg/dL), insufficient for significant positive reaction.
    - **Increased urobilinogen:**
      ▪ Haemolytic anaemias (without bilirubin in urine): Thalassaemia, sickle cell anaemia and hereditary spherocytosis
      ▪ Liver diseases (bilirubinuria present): Preicteric phase of infective hepatitis, drugs or toxic hepatitis, cirrhosis
    - **Cause of absent urobilinogen:** Obstructive jaundice (bilirubinuria present)
    - Detected by Ehrlich's aldehyde test

Summary of main liver function tests (LFT) and their significance is given in **Table 5.5**.
- **Alpha-foetoprotein:**
  o Normally produced by foetal liver, levels fall after birth
  o Reappearance in increasing and high concentrations in the adult is abnormal
  o Causes of **elevated levels of α-foetoprotein are:**
    - Hepatocellular carcinoma (HCC) (hepatoma)
    - Carcinomas of stomach, pancreas, gall bladder, bile ducts and lungs
    - Teratomas
  o Slightly raised with regenerative liver tissue in patients with:
    - Viral hepatitis
    - Chronic hepatitis
    - Cirrhosis
- Increased concentrations in pregnancy: Neural tube defects of the foetus

Liver Biopsy

Indications, contraindications and complications of liver biopsy are given in **Box 5.1**.

Hepatic Elastography

- *Hepatic fibrosis:* Early stage of chronic liver disease and cirrhosis
- Conventional liver tests and imaging studies do not detect hepatic fibrosis.
- Non-invasive method for measurement of hepatic fibrosis.
- **Methods:**
  o **Ultrasound elastography:** Mild-amplitude, low-frequency (50 Hz) vibration transmitted through the liver. The velocity of wave correlates with tissue stiffness; the wave travels faster through denser fibrotic tissue.
  o **Magnetic resonance elastography:** More reliable than ultrasound elastography

Endoscopic Retrograde Cholangiopancreatography

- Endoscopic retrograde cholangiopancreatography (ERCP) is used to outline the biliary and pancreatic ducts.
- **Uses:**
  o **Diagnostic procedure:**
    - Biopsy of ampullary carcinoma
    - Administration of brachytherapy for cholangiocarcinoma
    - Direct visualisation of the ampulla and common bile duct

TABLE 5.5: Summary of main liver function tests (LFT) and their significance.

Tests	Function determined/assessed
Serum bilirubin	Transport
Serum enzymes	
Serum aminotransferases (ALT and AST)	Hepatocellular damage
Serum alkaline phosphatase (ALP)	Biliary tract obstruction
Plasma proteins	Synthesis
Prothrombin time	Synthesis

(ALT: alanine aminotransferase; AST: aspartate aminotransferase)

> **Box 5.1: Indications, contraindications and complications of liver biopsy.**
>
> - **Indications:**
>   - Cirrhosis of liver
>   - Unexplained hepatomegaly, splenomegaly and jaundice
>   - Hepatitis: Chronic or acute
>   - Tumours: Primary or secondary
>   - Granulomatous diseases: Tuberculosis, leprosy and sarcoidosis
>   - Storage and metabolic disorders: Amyloidosis, storage disorders, haemochromatosis and Wilson's disease
>   - After liver transplantation: Assess for rejection and disease recurrence
>   - Brucellosis
>   - Pyrexia of unknown origin (with hepatomegaly)
>   - Malignancy
>   - Miliary tuberculosis
>   - Lymphoma staging
>
> - **Complications of liver biopsy:**
>   - Pleurisy, perihepatitis
>   - Haemorrhage
>   - Intrahepatic haematoma
>   - Biliary peritonitis
>   - Haemobilia
>   - Arteriovenous fistula
>   - Infection
>   - Organ perforation
>   - Carcinoid crisis
>
> - **Contraindications:**
>   - Hepatocellular failure
>   - Congenital coagulation disorders
>   - Hepatobiliary infections
>   - Massive ascites
>   - Obstructive jaundice
>   - Severe jaundice
>   - Prolonged prothrombin time: > 3 seconds over control
>
> - **Relative contradictions:**
>   - Hydatid cyst liver
>   - Haemangioma liver

  - Placement of stents
  - Sphincterotomy
  - **Therapeutic procedure:**
    - Removal of common bile duct stones
    - Sphincterotomy
    - Dilatation of benign strictures
    - Placement of nasobiliary catheters and biliary stents
    - Obtain samples for culture. Cytology
- **Complications:** The complication rate in diagnostic ERCP is 2–3%.
  - Pancreatitis
  - Cholangitis
  - Bleeding
  - Duodenal perforation

Percutaneous Transhepatic Cholangiography

- **Uses:**
  - Identification and localisation of the site of obstruction of the biliary tract
  - Pre-operative planning of surgery
  - Introduction of stent in malignant strictures

- **Complications:**
  - Bleeding
  - Cholangitis
  - Infection with septicaemia
  - Biliary peritonitis

Magnetic Resonance Cholangiopancreatography

- Magnetic resonance cholangiopancreatography (MRCP) is a non-invasive technique largely replacing diagnostic (but not therapeutic) ERCP.
- A heavily T2-weighted sequence enhances visualisation of the water-filled biliary and pancreatic ducts to produce high-quality images of ductal anatomy.
- **Advantages of MRCP over ERCP:**
  - No need for contrast media or ionising radiation
  - Images can be acquired faster.
  - Less operator dependent
  - No risk of pancreatitis

- **Indications:**
  - Diagnosis of bile duct obstruction and pancreatic duct abnormalities
  - Unsuccessful ERCP or a contraindication to ERCP

Endoscopic Ultrasound

- Gradually replacing diagnostic ERCP
- **Advantages:**
  - High-resolution ultrasound imaging
  - Accurate staging of small, potentially operable pancreatic tumours
  - Offers a less invasive method for bile duct imaging
- **Uses:**
  - **Diagnostic:**
    - Imaging pancreatic and biliary diseases, e.g. choledocholithiasis, pancreatic and biliary cancers, and cystic lesions of the pancreas
    - Ampullary carcinoma: To know the local extension, regional nodal metastasis
    - Guided fine-needle aspiration from suspicious lesions
  - **Therapeutic:** Increasingly used for interventions
    - Pain relief in unresectable pancreatic carcinoma, injecting bupivacaine and alcohol into celiac ganglia
    - Endoscopic management of pancreatic pseudocysts
- **Disadvantages:** Cost is high; high degree of training is required.

■ JAUNDICE

- **Yellowish pigmentation** of **skin, mucous membranes and sclera** due to **increased levels of bilirubin** in the blood.
- Scleral involvement—rich elastic tissue that has special affinity for bilirubin
- **Normal serum bilirubin level:** 0.3–1.2 mg/dL.
- Clinically detected when the serum bilirubin 2.0–2.5 mg/dL.
- **Latent jaundice** bilirubin level: 1.2–2.5 mg/dL.
- Carotenaemia—yellowish pigmentation of skin by carotene but not of sclera
- Cassification of jaundice is given in **Tables 5.6** and **5.7**.

Haemolytic Jaundice

- Increased destruction of red blood cells or their precursors produces increased production of bilirubin.
- Unconjugated bilirubin accumulates in the plasma and results in jaundice.
- Usually mild, because normal liver can easily handle the increased bilirubin production.

TABLE 5.6: Classification of jaundice.

Predominantly unconjugated hyperbilirubinaemia	Predominantly conjugated hyperbilirubinaemia
Increased production of bilirubin: • Haemolytic anaemias • Resorption internal haemorrhage [e.g. gastrointestinal (GI) bleeding and haematomas] • Ineffective erythropoiesis	**Decreased hepatocellular excretion:** • Liver damage or toxicity (e.g. hepatitis) • Deficiency of membrane transporters: Dubin–Johnson syndrome, Rotor syndrome
Reduced hepatic uptake: • Drug that interfere with membrane carrier systems • Diffuse liver disease (hepatitis and cirrhosis) • Some cases of Gilbert's syndrome	**Impaired intra-/extrahepatic bile flow:** • Inflammatory destruction of bile ducts (e.g. primary biliary cirrhosis) • Gall stones • Carcinoma: Head of pancreas, peri-ampullary carcinoma and cholangiocarcinoma
Impaired bilirubin conjugation: • Physiologic jaundice of the newborn • Crigler–Najjar syndrome types I and II • Gilbert's syndrome • Diffuse liver disease (hepatitis and cirrhosis)	

TABLE 5.7: Classification of jaundice based on the pathological mechanism.

Haemolytic jaundice	
Intracorpuscular defects	**Extracorpuscular defects**
• Hereditary: Spherocytosis, sickle cell disease, thalassaemia, glucose-6-phosphate dehydrogenase (G6PD) deficiency • Acquired: Vitamin B12 and folate deficiency	• Autoimmune, alloimmune haemolytic anaemias • Fragmentation syndromes: Prosthetic valves • Drugs, e.g. sulphasalazine and dapsone • Infections of RBCs: Malaria

Hepatocellular jaundice	
• Viral, alcoholic hepatitis • Chronic hepatitis • Cirrhosis: Any type • Infiltrations	• Ischaemic liver • Drug-induced hepatitis: Chlorpromazine, imipramine, isoniazid (INH), rifampicin, erythromycin, amitriptyline, halothane and methyldopa

Cholestatic (obstructive) jaundice	
Intrahepatic (small duct obstruction)	**Extrahepatic (large duct obstruction)**

• Primary biliary cirrhosis
• Primary sclerosing cholangitis
• Alcohol and drugs
• Viral hepatitis
• Cirrhosis
• Chronic hepatitis
• Secondaries in liver
• Severe bacterial infections
• Inherited cholestatic liver disease
• Pregnancy
	• Gall stones in the common bile duct (CBD)
	• Parasitic: Helminths in the CBD
	• Carcinoma:
	   o Head of pancreas
	   o Ampulla of Vater
	   o Bile duct (cholangiocarcinoma)
	   o Liver metastases
	• Stricture of bile ducts
	• Sclerosing cholangitis
	• Chronic pancreatitis

- **Clinical features:** Depend on the cause of anaemia:
   o **Pallor**
   o **Mild jaundice** without any signs of liver disease
   o **Hepatosplenomegaly**
   o Gallstones and leg ulcers may be seen depending on the cause of anaemia.
   o **Dark stools** (stercobilinogen)
   o **Urine turns dark yellow** on standing (increased urobilinogen converted to urobilin).
- **Investigations:**
   o **Haemolysis**
   o **Unconjugated hyperbilirubinaemia** (< 6 mg%)
   o **No bilirubin in urine,** unconjugated bilirubin—water insoluble (acholuric jaundice)
   o **Urinary urobilinogen** is increased (> 4 mg/24 h).
   o Other liver function tests (LFTs) are normal.

Hepatocellular Jaundice

- Parenchymal liver disease causing inability of liver to transport bilirubin from hepatocytes into bile.
- Defect in bilirubin transport across the hepatocyte may occur at any point between the uptake of unconjugated bilirubin into the hepatocyte and transport of conjugated bilirubin into biliary canaliculi.
- In hepatocellular jaundice, both unconjugated and conjugated bilirubin levels rise in the blood.
- **Investigations:**
   o Raised AST and ALT.
   o Acute jaundice with AST > 1,000 U/L is highly suggestive of an infectious cause (e.g. hepatitis A, B), drugs (e.g. paracetamol) or hepatic ischaemia.
   o Imaging and liver biopsy

Cholestatic (Obstructive) Jaundice

- Failure of bile flow: Its cause may be anywhere between hepatocyte and duodenum.

- Surgical jaundice—causes require surgical intervention.
- **Types of cholestasis:**
  - **Extrahepatic cholestasis:** Due to large duct (extrahepatic bile ducts) obstruction between the porta hepatis and the ampulla of Vater
  - **Intrahepatic cholestasis:** Due to small duct obstruction—failure of hepatocytes to initiate bile flow or obstruction of bile flow in the bile ducts or portal tracts
- There is retention of bile acids and bilirubin in the liver and blood and deficiency of bile acids in the intestine.

Clinical features and differentiating the types of jaundice given in **Tables 5.8** and **5.9**.

- **Investigations:**
  - **Serum findings:**
    - Marked conjugated hyperbilirubinaemia
    - Serum ALP increased (3-4 times normal)
    - Minimal biochemical changes of liver parenchymal damage
    - Antimitochondrial antibodies (AMA) in primary biliary cirrhosis
  - **Urine findings:** Bilirubin present and urobilinogen absent
  - **Ultrasonography** to detect the underlying cause
  - **ERCP or MRCP**

TABLE 5.8: **Clinical features.**

Symptoms	Signs
Jaundice (gradually progressive/ fluctuating)	Deep jaundice with a greenish hue
Pruritus	Scratch marks
Pale, clay-coloured stools	Xanthelasmas on eyelids
Dark urine (increased conjugated bilirubin)	Xanthomas over tendons
Depending on the cause: • Fever with chills and rigors (cholangitis) • Weight loss (malabsorption) • Bleeding tendency (vitamin K deficiency) • Bone pains (calcium, vitamin D deficiency) • Abdominal pain (gall stones)	**Depending on the cause:** • Palpable gall bladder in carcinoma head of pancreas • Large hard irregular liver (malignancy) • Late features: Secondary biliary cirrhosis and signs of liver cell failure

TABLE 5.9: **Clinical features useful in differentiating different types of jaundice.**

Features	Haemolytic	Hepatocellular	Obstructive
Jaundice			
Colour	Lemon yellow	Orange yellow	Greenish yellow
Depth	Mild	Variable	Deep
Pruritus	–	Variable	+
Bleeding tendency	–	+	+ (late)
Anaemia	+	–	–
Splenomegaly	+	Variable	Absent (may develop later)
Palpable gall bladder	–	–	May be present
Features of liver cell failure	–	+ (early)	+ (late)

- Percutaneous transhepatic cholangiography (PTC)
- Liver biopsy performed if there is evidence of liver cell disease

CONGENITAL NON-HAEMOLYTIC HYPERBILIRUBINAEMIAS

Gilbert's Syndrome

- Relatively **common**, autosomal **recessive, harmless** and inherited disorder
- **Aetiology: Mutations in *UGT1* gene**—inadequate synthesis of UGT1A1 enzyme (about 30% of normal)
- **Clinical features:**
    - More common in males
    - Usually asymptomatic, jaundice is incidentally detected
    - **Mild, chronic unconjugated fluctuating hyperbilirubinaemia**
    - No other functional derangements
    - Depth of jaundice increases with infections, fatigue, exertion and fasting.
    - Physical examination is otherwise normal.
- **Investigations:**
    - Unconjugated hyperbilirubinaemia (< 6 mg%). Raised bilirubin levels during fasting are the most common diagnostic tool.
    - Urine: Increased urobilinogen and absent bilirubinuria
    - Peripheral smear, reticulocyte count and serum haptoglobin: Normal
- **Treatment:** Usually no treatment is required. Glucuronosyltransferase activity may be increased by administering phenobarbital 60 mg bd.

Crigler–Najjar Syndrome Type I

- Rare, **autosomal recessive** disorder. Invariably fatal.
- **Aetiology:** Due to **complete absence of hepatic UGT1A1**
- Chronic, severe, **unconjugated hyperbilirubinaemia** with severe jaundice, icterus and **death** secondary to kernicterus **within 18 months** of birth.
- **Bile** does contain conjugated into bilirubin; hence, it is **colourless**.
- **Treatment: Daily phototherapy** and **liver transplantation**. Phenobarbital has **no effect**.
- Liver is **morphologically normal** by light and electron microscopy.

Crigler–Najjar Syndrome Type II

- Less severe, non-fatal disorder, also known as Arias syndrome
- Autosomal recessive inheritance in most cases
- Partial deficiency of UGT1A1 enzyme (10% of normal)
- Jaundice is milder than type I and does not develop kernicterus.
- **Treatment** includes ultraviolet light therapy and liver transplantation. Phenobarbital treatment can improve bilirubin glucuronidation by inducing hypertrophy of hepatocellular endoplasmic reticulum.

Dubin–Johnson Syndrome

- Benign autosomal recessive disorder
- **Aetiology: Complete absence** of the **multidrug resistance protein 2 (MRP2)** which is required for secretion of conjugated bilirubin from hepatocytes into canaliculi. This leads to defect in hepatocellular excretion of bilirubin glucuronides across biliary canalicular membrane.
- **Clinical features:** Chronic, recurrent conjugated hyperbilirubinaemia, generally after puberty.
- **Investigations:**
    - Conjugated hyperbilirubinaemia (usually 2–5 mg/dL)
    - BSP clearance—impaired with reflux into blood at 90 minutes
    - Bilirubinuria
    - Gall bladder is usually not visualised on oral cholecystography.
    - Liver biopsy—**dark pigment** in centrilobular hepatocytes, **coarse melanin-like pigmented granules** within the enlarged lysosomes, present in the cytoplasm. Pigment composed of polymers of epinephrine metabolites.
- **No treatment** is required in most cases. Have a normal life expectancy.

Rotor Syndrome

- Rare, autosomal recessive, asymptomatic conjugated hyperbilirubinaemia
- Defects in hepatocellular uptake, intracellular binding and excretion of bilirubin pigments
- Clinical presentation—mild jaundice
- *Investigations*:
  - Conjugated hyperbilirubinaemia
  - Bilirubinuria
  - BSP clearance test—impaired without reflux back into blood
  - Gall bladder is visualised on oral cholecystography
- Liver is morphologically normal.

■ CHARCOT'S TRIAD

Consists of following in the presence of stones in bile ducts:
- Pain in the right hypochondrium
- Intermittent or persistent jaundice
- Fever with chills and rigors due to acute cholangitis
- **Reynolds pentad** adds mental status changes and sepsis to the triad.

■ COURVOISIER'S LAW

- In obstruction of common bile duct due to a stone, the gall bladder as a rule is impalpable (no distension) as it is already shrivelled, fibrotic and non-distensible.
- In obstruction from other causes (e.g. carcinoma head of pancreas), distension of the gall bladder is common and hence gall bladder may be palpable.

■ ACUTE VIRAL HEPATITIS

- **Infection of hepatocytes** that produces necrosis and inflammation of the liver (**Table 5.10**).

Hepatitis A

- **Aetiology:** Hepatitis A virus (HAV), non-enveloped, 27 nm, RNA virus, Picornaviridae.
- Most common type and often occurs in epidemics and affects children and young adults.
- **Source of infection:** Acutely infected person
- Replicates in liver, excreted in bile, then excreted in faeces of infected person for 2 weeks before symptoms and for a further 2 weeks or so.
- **Maximally infectious just before the onset of jaundice.**
- **Mode of spread: Faecal–oral route,** ingestion of contaminated water or food. Spreads through water, milk, shellfish. Survives on human hands and fomites. Overcrowding and poor sanitation facilitate spread. Resistant to freezing, detergents and acids, inactivated by formalin and chlorine.
- Viremia—transient. No blood-borne transmission
- **Incubation period:** 15–45 days (mean 4 weeks)
- No carrier state
- **Prevention:** Good hygiene and improving social conditions
- **Prophylaxis:**
  - **Active:** It probably provides life-long immunity. Role of the vaccine in India is

TABLE 5.10: Aetiology of viral hepatitis.

Hepatitis caused by common (hepatotropic) viruses		Other viruses
Type of hepatitis	**Causative agent**	• Cytomegalovirus
Hepatitis A	Hepatitis A virus (HAV)	• Epstein–Barr virus
Hepatitis B	Hepatitis B virus (HBV)	• Herpes simplex virus
Hepatitis C	Hepatitis C virus (HCV)	• Yellow fever virus
Delta hepatitis	Hepatitis D virus (HDV)	• Hepatitis G virus
Hepatitis E	Hepatitis E virus (HEV)	• Dengue virus

not clear as most individuals get infection in early childhood when the disease has a mild course.
- **Passive immunisation:** Normal human immunoglobulin (Ig) [0.02 mL/kg intramuscular (IM)] is used if exposure to HAV is < 2 weeks and protects from infection for 3 months. HAV vaccine should also be administered.

Hepatitis B

- **Aetiology:** Hepatitis B virus (HBV), DNA virus, Hepadnaviridae.
- **Structure:** Complete infective virion is called Dane particle. Spherical, 42 nm particle, double-layered comprising an inner core or nucleocapsid (27 nm) with an outer envelope of surface protein [hepatitis B surface antigen (HBsAg)].
- **Viral genome:** Consists of partially double-stranded circular DNA and has four genes.
    i. **HBsAg (*S* gene):** It is a product of *S* gene which is secreted into the blood in large amounts. HBsAg is immunogenic. It is also called Australia antigen. It is identified by haemagglutination and radioimmunoassay methods.
    ii. **Hepatitis B core antigen [HBcAg (*C* gene)]:** The *C* gene produces two antigenically different products:
        a. **HBcAg:** Intracellular in the hepatocytes and do not circulate in the serum.
        b. **Hepatitis B e antigen (HBeAg):** It is secreted into serum and is a surrogate marker for **high levels of viral replication**. Signifies persistent infection.
    iii. **HBV polymerase (*P* gene):** A polymerase (Pol) is a product of *P* gene and DNA polymerase enzyme is needed for virus replication.
    iv. **HBxAg (*X* gene): HBx protein** is necessary for virus infectivity and has been implicated in the **pathogenesis of liver cancer** in HBV infection.
- **Source: Cases** of hepatitis (acute/chronic) **or carriers** are the only source of infection. 100 times as infectious as human immunodeficiency virus (HIV) and 10 times as infectious as hepatitis C virus (HCV).
- **Mode of transmission:**
    - **Vertical/congenital transmission:** From mother (HBV carrier) to child may occur in utero, during parturition or soon after birth. Not transmitted by breastfeeding.
    - **Horizontal transmission:** Dominant mode of transmission
    - **Parenteral:** Is the major route of transmission but occasionally non-parenteral.
        - **Percutaneous, mucous membrane** exposure to infectious body fluids, through minor cuts/abrasions. HBV can survive for long periods on household articles and may transmit the infection.
        - **Intravenous (IV) route:** Through transfusion of unscreened infected blood or blood products. This mode of spread is rare now, because of routine screening of all blood donors for HBV and HCV. IV drug abuse with sharing of needles and syringes, tattooing and acupuncture are other ways of developing infection.
    - **Close personal contact:** Spread through body fluids such as saliva, urine, semen and vaginal secretions. Requires close personal contact, unprotected heterosexual or homosexual intercourse.
- **Incubation period:** 30–180 days (mean, 8–12 weeks)
- **Chronic carrier state** can develop with HBV infection (1–20%)
- **Prevention:** Avoiding risk factors such as not sharing needles, having safe sex, transfusing safe blood and blood products, and enforcing strict standard safety precautions in laboratories and hospitals to avoid accidental needle punctures and contact with infected body fluids.
- **Prophylaxis:**
    - **Active immunisation:** By using recombinant vaccines (containing HBsAg). Advised in:
        - *Children:* In India, non-percutaneous routes of transmission are quite prevalent.
        - *High-risk groups:* Healthcare personnel, haemodialysis patients, injection drug users, haemophiliacs and sexual contacts of HBsAg carriers

- **Dosage regimen:** Three doses into the deltoid muscle at 0, 1, 6 months; 10 μg (children < 10 years) and 20 μg (children > 10 years). More frequent, larger doses are required in individuals over 50 years of age or clinically ill and/or immunocompromised.
- **Combined prophylaxis:** This consists of vaccination and Ig. Advised in:
  o Accidental needle-stick injury, gross personal contamination with infected blood and exposure to infected blood in the presence of cuts and grazes
  o All newborn babies of HBsAg-positive mothers.
  o Regular sexual partners of HBsAg-positive patients, who are HBV-negative.
  o Dosage: Adults, 500 IU of hepatitis B Ig (HBIg); newborns, 200 IU and the vaccine (IM) at another site.
- **Treatment:** Pegylated interferon alpha, lamivudine, adefovir, entecavir, telbivudine or tenofovir may be used as initial therapy but lamivudine and telbivudine are not preferred because of high rates of resistance.

Hepatitis C

- Previously called blood-borne non-A, non-B hepatitis
- **Aetiology:** Small, **enveloped, single-stranded RNA virus,** Flaviviridae.
- **Unstable genomic and antigenic variability,** leading to emergence of an endogenous, newly mutated strain, making production of an **effective HCV vaccine difficult**
- HCV has six genotypes and in India, the most prevalent is HCV 3.
- **Mode of spread: Parenteral route** (transfusion of blood, blood products and IV drug abusers) as blood-borne infection, sexual contact and perinatal transmission. Not transmitted by breastfeeding
- **Incubation period:** 15–160 days (mean, 7 weeks)
- Nearly 80% develop chronic hepatitis.

■ Hepatitis D (Delta Hepatitis)

- **Aetiology:** Hepatitis D virus (HDV or delta virus), defective/incomplete RNA virus, Deltaviridae. RNA genome is covered by an outer coat/shell of HBsAg.
- No independent existence requires HBV for replication and expression.
- Duration of HDV infection is determined by the duration of HBV infection.
- Causes **delta hepatitis**—two clinical patterns:
  i. **Acute co-infection:** Simultaneous exposure to serum containing both HDV and HBV. The HBV infection first becomes established and the HBsAg is necessary for development of complete HDV virions.
  ii. **Super-infection:** When a chronic carrier of HBV is exposed to a new dose HDV.
- **Mode of spread:** Parenteral route and sexual contact
- Fulminant hepatitis can follow both patterns of infection but is more common after co-infection.

Hepatitis E

- Previously called epidemic or enterically transmitted non-A, non-B hepatitis.
- **Aetiology:** Unenveloped, single-stranded RNA, 32–34 nm, *Hepeviridae* family.
- Occurs primarily in young to middle-aged adults.
- **Source: Zoonotic disease** with animal reservoirs, such as monkeys, cats, pigs, rodents and dogs. Virions are shed in stool during the acute illness.
- **Modes of transmission: Enterically transmitted, water-borne** infection. Common after contamination of water supplies as after monsoon flooding.
- **Incubation period:** 14–60 days (mean, 5–6 weeks).
- **Outcome:** More than 30–60% cases of sporadic acute hepatitis (similar to hepatitis A) in India. Acute self-limiting hepatitis with a high mortality rate (about 20%) among pregnant women. Does not cause chronic liver disease
- **Prevention:** Good sanitation and hygiene. Vaccine has been developed and used successfully in China.

Clinical Features of Viral Hepatitis

Clinical features of viral hepatitis are given in **Box 5.2.**

> **Box 5.2: Clinical features of viral hepatitis.**
>
> **Phase 1: Incubation period**
> - Varies according to the virus
>
> **Phase 2: Symptomatic pre-icteric phase**
> - Lasts for 1–2 weeks before onset of jaundice
> - *Prodromal symptoms*: Systemic and variable
> - *Constitutional symptoms*: Anorexia, nausea, vomiting, poor appetite, fatigue, malaise, headache, etc.
> - *Low-grade fever*: More in hepatitis A and E than in hepatitis B or C.
> - Hepatitis B may present with serum sickness—like immunological syndrome consisting of rashes and small joints polyarthritis
> - Upper vague abdominal pain due to stretching of liver capsule
> - Dark urine and clay-coloured stools
>
> **Phase 3: Symptomatic icteric phase**
> - With the onset of clinical jaundice, the constitutional prodromal symptoms usually diminish
> - Liver becomes enlarged and tender. Pruritus may develop due to bile salt retention
> - Splenomegaly and cervical lymphadenopathy may be observed in about 10–20% of patients
> - Dark urine and pale stool
>
> **Phase 4: Recovery (convalescence) phase**
> - Symptoms disappear, appetite improves, jaundice decreases, stools and urine are normal and liver size decreases
> - Duration is variable, 2–12 weeks. More prolonged in acute hepatitis B and C
> - Complete clinical and biochemical recovery within 1–2 months in A and E and 3–4 months in B and C

- **Fulminant hepatitis:** In hepatitis B, D and E. Uncommon in C and rare in A. With hepatitis E, fulminant hepatitis occurs in nearly 20% cases in pregnant females.

Summary of various hepatotropic viruses is given in **Table 5.11**.

Investigations

Investigations for viral hepatitis are given in **Table 5.12**.

Serological Markers for Viral Hepatitis

Serological markers for viral hepatitis are given in **Table 5.13**.

Summary of serological findings in HBV are given in **Table 5.14**.

Complications and poor prognostic features of acute viral hepatitis are given in **Tables 5.15** and **5.16**, respectively.

Treatment

- General measures:
  - Avoid drugs metabolised in the liver, e.g. sedatives and narcotics.
  - Avoid alcohol during the acute illness.
  - No specific dietary modifications are required.
  - Elective surgery should be avoided, as there is risk of post-operative liver failure.
- Liver transplantation can be performed for complications of cirrhosis due to chronic hepatitis B, C.

Extrahepatic manifestations of HCV infection are given in **Table 5.17**.

Causes for Acute Hepatitis

Causes for acute hepatitis are given in **Box 5.3**.

■ CHRONIC PARENCHYMAL LIVER DISEASE

Chronic Hepatitis

- Chronic persistent hepatitis (CPH)
- Chronic active hepatitis (CAH)
- Chronic lobular hepatitis (CLH)

■ CHRONIC HEPATITIS

- **Symptomatic, biochemical or serologic evidence of hepatic disease for > 6 months.** Microscopically, there should be inflammation and necrosis in the liver.
- **Classification:** To assess response to therapy and prognosis, it is based on:
  - Causes of hepatitis (**Table 5.18**)
  - Histologic activity or grade
  - Degree of progression or stage
  - **Based on the grade of chronic hepatitis:**
    - Histological assessment of inflammation and necrosis observed on liver biopsy. Indicates severity of liver disease.
    - Scoring system: Histologic activity index (HAI) and METAVIR score, can be graded as mild, moderate and severe (**Table 5.19**).

TABLE 5.11: Summary of various hepatotropic viruses.

Feature	HAV	HBV	HCV	HDV	HEV
Incubation period in days (range)	30 (15–45)	90 (30–180)	50 (15–160)	90 (30–180)	40 (14–60)
Onset	Acute	Insidious or acute	Insidious	Insidious or acute	Acute
Age group affected	Children and young adults	Young adults, babies and toddlers	Adults, but any age	Any age (similar to HBV)	Young adults
Mode of transmission	Faecal-oral	Parenteral, sexual contract and perinatal	Parenteral	Parenteral	Faecal-oral
Clinical					
Severity	Mild	Occasionally severe	Moderate	Occasionally severe	Mild
Frequency of chronic liver disease	Never	10%	80%	5% with co-infection; ≤ 70% for super-infection	Never
Carrier state	None	1–30%	1.5–3.2%	Variable	None
Progression to cancer	None	+ (neonatal infection)	+	±	None
Prognosis	Good	Worse	Moderate	Acute, good chronic, poor	Good
Prophylaxis	Immunoglobulin inactivated vaccine	Hepatitis B immunoglobulin, recombinant vaccine	None	HBV vaccine (none for HBV carriers)	Vaccine

(HAV: hepatitis A virus; HBV: hepatitis B virus; HCV: hepatitis C virus; HDV: hepatitis D virus; HEV: hepatitis E virus)

TABLE 5.12: Investigations for viral hepatitis.

Urine	Blood	Biochemistry
Biliruburia (in early stages)	Leucopaenia, relative lymphocytosis	AST, ALT—raised, maximum during the prodromal phase, progressively decline during icteric, recovery phase
Increased urinary urobilinogen	PT is prolonged (best prognostic feature)	Conjugated, unconjugated bilirubin levels raised
Slight microscopic haematuria	ESR is raised	ALP—may be raised
Mild proteinuria		Serum protein—normal
		Blood glucose—may be low

(ALP: alkaline phosphatase; ALT: alanine aminotransferase; AST: aspartate aminotransferase; ESR: erythrocyte sedimentation rate; PT: prothrombin time)

TABLE 5.13: Serological markers for viral hepatitis.

Hepatitis A	
IgM anti-HAV	Appears at the onset of symptoms, reliable marker of acute infection
IgG anti-HAV	Persists for years, provides lifelong immunity against reinfection
Hepatitis B (Table 5.9; Figs. 5.1 and 5.2)	
HBsAg	• First marker to appear in serum before symptoms, undetectable in 3–6 months • Significance: Presence in acute and chronic hepatitis B indicates infectious state • Loss of HBsAg with development of anti-HBs denotes recovery
Anti-HBs	• Antibody to HBsAg, appear after its disappearance. Present on vaccination • Significance: Protective antibody; may persist for life providing protection
IgM anti-HBc	• Appears in serum 1–2 weeks after appearance of HBsAg • Significance: Earliest antibody marker; indicates recent infection (1st 6 months) • High titresin acute hepatitis B and low titres in chronic hepatitis B
IgG anti-HBc	• Significance: Indicates remote infection (beyond 6 months). Indicates previous infection with HBV even when all the other viral markers are not detectable
HBeAg	• Detected transiently, early in the course • Significance: Persistence 6 weeks after the onset indicates infectivity, severe disease progressing to chronic hepatitis. Absence is a favourable serologic finding
Anti-HBe	• Significance: Found in recovery phase. Seroconversion
HBV-DNA, DNA polymerase	• Found in serum and liver soon after HBsAg • Significance: Not helpful in diagnosis of hepatitis B, valuable in assessing prognosis. Indicates active viral replication
Hepatitis C	
Anti-HCV	Appears after infection; disappears after recovery; persists in chronic hepatitis C
HCV-RNA	Appears after exposure
Hepatitis D (delta hepatitis)	
HDV-RNA	It is detectable in the blood and liver before and in the early days of acute disease
Anti-HDV	IgM anti-HDV is the most reliable indicator of recent HDV exposure
Hepatitis E	
HEV-RNA, HEV virions	Before the onset of clinical illness, can be detected in stool and serum
IgM anti-HEV	After the onset of clinical illness, serum aminotransferases rises, and elevated titres also occur simultaneously
IgG anti-HEV	After recovery, the IgM is replaced with a persistent IgG anti-HEV titre

(Anti-HBc: antibodies against hepatitis B core antigen; Anti-HBe: antibodies against hepatitis B e antigen; Anti-HBs: antibodies against hepatitis B surface antigen; Anti-HCV: antibody against hepatitis C virus; Anti-HDV: antibody against hepatitis D virus; DNA: deoxyribonucleic acid; HAV: hepatitis A virus; HBV: hepatitis B virus; HCV: hepatitis C virus; HDV: hepatitis D virus; HEV: hepatitis E virus; HBeAg: hepatitis B e antigen; HBsAg: hepatitis B surface antigen; RNA: ribonucleic acid; Anti-HAV: antibody against hepatitis A virus; Anti-HEV: antibody against hepatitis E virus; Ig: immunoglobulin)

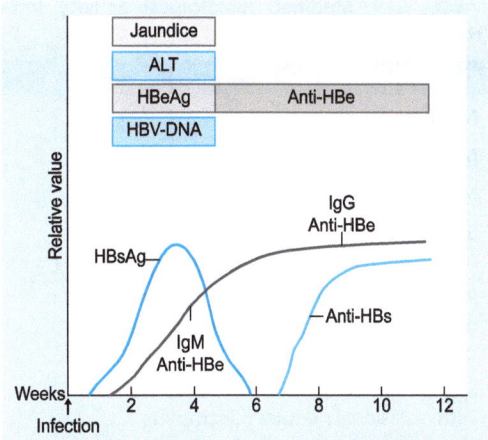

(ALT: alanine aminotransferase; Anti-HBe: antibodies against hepatitis B e antigen; Anti-HBs: antibodies against hepatitis B surface antigen; DNA: deoxyribonucleic acid; HBeAg: hepatitis B e antigen; HBV: hepatitis B virus; HBsAg: hepatitis B surface antigen; Ig: immunoglobulin)

Fig. 5.1: Sequence of serologic markers in acute hepatitis with resolution caused by HBV.

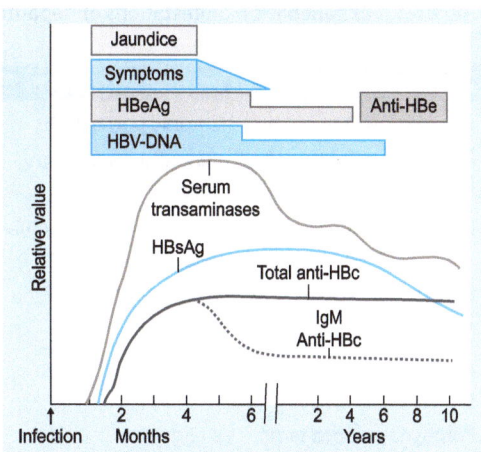

(Anti-HBe: antibodies against hepatitis B e antigen; Anti-HBs: antibodies against hepatitis B surface antigen; DNA: deoxyribonucleic acid; HBeAg: hepatitis B e antigen; HBV: hepatitis B virus; HBsAg: hepatitis B surface antigen; Anti-HBc: antibodies against hepatitis B core antigen)

Fig. 5.2: Sequence of serologic markers in chronic hepatitis caused by HBV.

TABLE 5.14: Summary of serological findings in HBV.

Antigens		Antibodies			Interpretation
HBsAg	HBeAg	Anti-HBc	Anti-HBs	Anti-HBe	
+	+	IgM	–	–	Acute hepatitis B, highly infectious
+	+	IgG	–	–	Chronic infection, carrier, high infectivity
+	–	IgG	–	+/–	Chronic infection, carrier, low infectivity
–	–	–	+	–	Immunity following HBV vaccine
–	–	+	+		Immune due to natural infection

(Anti-HBc: antibody to hepatitis B core antigen; Anti-HBe: antibody to hepatitis e-antigen; Anti-HBs: antibody to hepatitis B surface antigen; HBeAg: hepatitis B e antigen; HBsAg: hepatitis B surface antigen; HBV: hepatitis B virus; Ig: immunoglobulin)

TABLE 5.15: Complications of acute viral hepatitis.

Hepatic complications	Extrahepatic complications
• Fulminant hepatic failure • Cholestatic viral hepatitis • Relapsing hepatitis • Post-hepatitis syndrome • Chronic hepatitis • Cirrhosis • Hepatocellular carcinoma	• Aplastic anaemia • Renal failure • Polyarteritis nodosa • Henoch–Schönlein purpura • Myocarditis • Transverse myelitis • Peripheral neuropathy

TABLE 5.16: Poor prognostic features of viral hepatitis.

Laboratory findings	Other features
Marked increase in AST and ALT levels	Liver not enlarged
Serum bilirubin > 20 mg/dL	Renal failure
Prolongation prothrombin time by > 5 s that control	Recurring attacks of hypoglycaemia
	HBV, HCV or HDV infection

(ALT: alanine aminotransferase; AST: aspartate aminotransferase; HBV: hepatitis B virus; HCV: hepatitis C virus; HDV: hepatitis D virus)

TABLE 5.17: Extrahepatic manifestations of hepatitis C virus (HCV) infection.

Proven associations	Possible associations
Autoimmune thyroiditis	Chronic polyarthritis
B-cell non-Hodgkin's lymphoma	Idiopathic pulmonary fibrosis
Diabetes mellitus	Non-cryoglobulinaemia nephropathies
Lichen planus	Sicca syndrome
Mixed cryoglobulinaemia	Thyroid cancer
Monoclonal gammopathies	Renal cell carcinoma
Porphyria cutanea tarda	Vitiligo

Box 5.3: Causes for acute hepatitis.
- **Infectious:** Viruses (described earlier), bacterial, parasites and fungi
- **Toxin/drugs:** Alcohol (described later)
- **Immunological:** Autoimmune hepatitis, primary sclerosing cholangitis

Metabolic or hereditary:
- Non-alcoholic fatty liver disease (NAFLD)
- Haemochromatosis
- Wilson's disease

Pregnancy-related:
- Pre-eclampsia
- Acute fatty liver of pregnancy
- Haemolysis, elevated liver enzymes, low platelet count (HELLP) syndrome

Ischaemic and vascular:
- Cardiogenic shock
- Hypotension
- Cocaine, methamphetamine and ephedrine
- Acute Budd–Chiari syndrome

TABLE 5.18: Based on the causes of chronic hepatitis.

Chronic viral hepatitis	Chronic hepatitis B ± hepatitis D, chronic hepatitis C
Drug-associated chronic hepatitis	Methyldopa, isoniazid, ketoconazole and nitrofurantoin
Autoimmune hepatitis	
Hereditary	Wilson's disease
Unknown cause	Cryptogenic chronic hepatitis
Others	Ulcerative colitis, rarely alcohol

TABLE 5.19: Modified histological activity index (HAI)—Staging.

Degree of fibrosis	Stage
No fibrosis	0
Mild fibrosis of some portal areas	1
Moderate fibrosis of most portal areas	2
Severe fibrosis of most portal areas with occasional portal–portal (P–P) bridging	3
Fibrous expansion of portal areas with marked bridging of P–P and portal–central (P–C)	4
Marked bridging (P–P and/or P–C) with occasional nodules (incomplete cirrhosis)	5
Cirrhosis	6

- **Interface hepatitis** (piecemeal/periportal necrosis): **Spillover of inflammatory cells** (lymphocytes and plasma cells) from **portal tract into the adjacent** periportal hepatocytes at the limiting plate, with degenerating and apoptosis of periportal hepatocytes.
- **Bridging necrosis:** Confluent necrosis of hepatocytes observed in severe acute hepatitis. Forms bridges from **portal tract to portal tract, central vein to central vein, or portal-to-central** regions of adjacent lobules
- Degree of hepatocyte degeneration and focal intralobular necrosis
- Degree of portal inflammation
- **Fibrosis:** Hallmark of chronic liver damage
  o **Classification based on stage of chronic hepatitis:** Indicates level of progression and based on the degree of hepatic fibrosis.

Autoimmune Chronic and Progressive Hepatitis (Lupoid)

- Chronic and progressive hepatitis (CAH) of unknown cause, characterised by un-resolving inflammation of liver and by presence of interface hepatitis on histology, hypergammaglobulinaemia and autoantibodies.

- **Diagnosis:** No absolute diagnostic features. Recognition of a constellation of compatible features and exclusion of other diseases
- **Clinical features:**
  - Seen in females, peri- and post-menopausal age groups
  - Asymptomatic or present with fatigue, anorexia and jaundice
  - Acute hepatitis: Jaundice, marked rise of serum aminotransferase which do not resolve
  - Other autoimmune symptoms: Fever, polyarthritis, glomerulonephritis, pleurisy, pulmonary infiltration or fibrosing alveolitis
  - Other autoimmune diseases: Hashimoto's thyroiditis, ulcerative colitis, glomerulonephritis, Sjögren's syndrome
  - Jaundice may be mild-to-moderate.
  - Signs of chronic liver disease: Spider telangiectasia and hepatosplenomegaly
- **Investigations:**
  - **Biochemical findings:**
    - Serum aminotransferases: High and > 10 times during relapses
    - Serum bilirubin: Mildly raised usually > 6 mg/dL
    - Serum ALP: Mildly raised
    - Serum γ-globulins: High
    - Serum albumin: Low
    - Serum alpha-1 antitrypsin (A1AT), serum ceruloplasmin, iron and ferritin levels: Normal
  - **Autoantibodies:** Autoimmune hepatitis may be of three types:
    - **Type I:** With antibodies to (1) antinuclear and (2) anti-smooth muscle (anti-actin)
    - **Type II:** With antibodies to anti-liver/kidney microsomal (anti-LKM-1). Seen more in girls and young women
    - **Type III:** With soluble liver antigen (anti-SLP/LP). This behaves as type I.
    - About 13% of patients do not have above autoantibodies.
  - HBsAg: Negative.
  - PT: Prolonged.
  - Liver biopsy: Chronic hepatitis, variable amounts of interface hepatitis, cirrhosis and bridging necrosis.
- **Treatment:**
  - Prednisolone: About 30 mg given orally daily for 2 weeks. Gradually tapering dose as LFT improves. Maintenance dose of 10–15 mg daily for at least 2 years after LFT has become normal
  - Azathioprine: Dose of 1–2 mg/kg daily, added as a steroid-sparing agent and some patients for sole long-term maintenance therapy or if dose of prednisolone is > 10 mg/day.
  - Other immunosuppressive agents: Mycophenolate, ciclosporin and tacrolimus for resistant cases
  - Duration of treatment: Lifelong in most cases
  - Liver transplantation: If treatment fails
- **Course and prognosis:**
  - Exacerbations and remissions are common. Progression, steroid and azathioprine therapy produce remission in over 80% of patients.
  - May progress to hepatic failure and death.
  - Some may develop cirrhosis and its complications
  - HCC is uncommon.

Chronic Hepatitis B

- Follows acute HBV infection (may be subclinical), in about 1–10% of patients.
- HBsAg persists for > 6 months. May progress to cirrhosis and HCC
- Risk of chronic hepatitis: Depends on:
  - Age: More common with neonatal (90%) or childhood (20–50% < 5 years) infection rather than in adults (< 10%).
  - Immune status: In immunocompetent adults, the incidence of acute hepatitis is high while chronic infection is rare (1–2% of cases).
    - **High-risk comorbid states**
      - Down's syndrome
      - Lepromatous leprosy
      - Leukaemias
      - Hodgkin's lymphoma
      - Polyarteritis nodosa

- Patients on chronic haemodialysis
- Needle used by drug addicts—HIV infection
- Phases of infection: Three major phases:
  i. **Immune-tolerant phase:**
     - Asymptomatic, may last for decades
     - Active viral replication in liver but little or no evidence of disease activity
     - Associated with HBsAg and HBeAg positive and very high levels of serum HBV-DNA
     - Liver without inflammation with normal LFTs
  ii. **Immune-active phase (chronic hepatitis):** Progression from immune-tolerant phase. Criteria for chronic HBV hepatitis are:
     - HBsAg positive > 6 months
     - Liver biopsy: Chronic hepatitis with moderate-to-severe necroinflammation
     - Evidence of HBV replication: HBeAg and/or anti-HBe and HBV-DNA (> 20,000 IU/mL) in their serum.
     - Persistent or intermittent elevation of ALT/AST
  iii. **Inactive carrier phase with chronic HBV infection:** Incidence varies. Most patients eventually enter inactive carrier phase as they clear HBeAg and develop anti-HBe. Criteria for inactive carrier state:
     - HBsAg positive in the serum > 6 months
     - HBeAg negative and HBe antibody positive
     - Undetectable or low levels (< 400 IU/L) of HBV-DNA in the serum
     - Normal aminotransferase (ALT) levels
     - Liver biopsy does not show any significant hepatitis.
- Liver abnormalities generally do not progress to more severe disease. Low risk for HCC
- May be reactivated by severe immunosuppression
- Age at which infection occurs:
  o Infected during adults, adolescents—inactive carriers after they clear HBeAg
  o Infection during birth, early childhood—prolonged immune-tolerant phase, disease progresses even after disappearance of HBeAg in some. Therefore, lifelong monitoring is necessary.
- HBV genotype C (prevalent in India)—increased risk of cirrhosis and HCC
- **Clinical features:**
  o Asymptomatic or may develop severe end-stage liver disease
  o Fatigue, malaise, anorexia, persistent or intermittent jaundice
  o In end-stage liver disease: Symptoms due to complications of cirrhosis
  o Extrahepatic manifestations: Arthralgias, arthritis, vasculitis, glomerulonephritis, polyarthritis nodosa
  o Mild hepatomegaly
  o Long-standing cases may develop HCC.
- **Investigations:**
  o Biochemical investigations:
     - ALT, AST elevated. ALT > AST (SGOT). Once cirrhosis develops, AST > ALT.
     - Serum bilirubin: May be normal or raised up to 10 mg/dL
     - Serum proteins: Hypoalbuminaemia in severe cases and hyperglobulinaemia
     - PT: Prolonged
     - Serological markers: Positive HBsAg, positive IgG anti-HBc, negative IgM anti-HBc, positive HBe antigen or rarely, positive anti-HBe and positive HBV-DNA
  o **Indications:**
     - Serum HBV-DNA above 2,000 IU/mL (about > 10,000 copies/mL)
     - Serum ALT level greater than two times normal
     - Moderate-severe active necroinflammation and/or fibrosis in the liver biopsy
- **Treatment (Flowcharts 5.1 and 5.2):**
  o In cirrhosis: Oral antiviral agents are recommended; liver transplantation may be necessary.
  o Immunotolerant patients, usually young with normal ALT and high HBV-DNA levels, without evidence of liver disease do not need therapy but be regularly followed-up
  o Aims of treatment:
     - Seroconversion. When HBeAg disappears, remission may be attained for several years.

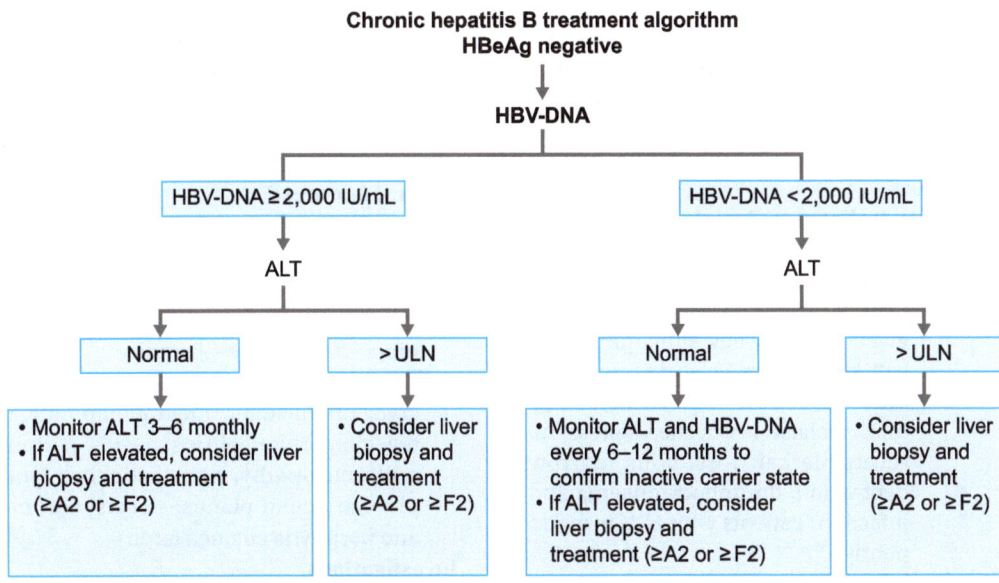

Flowchart 5.1: Chronic hepatitis B treatment algorithm for HBeAg-negative patients.

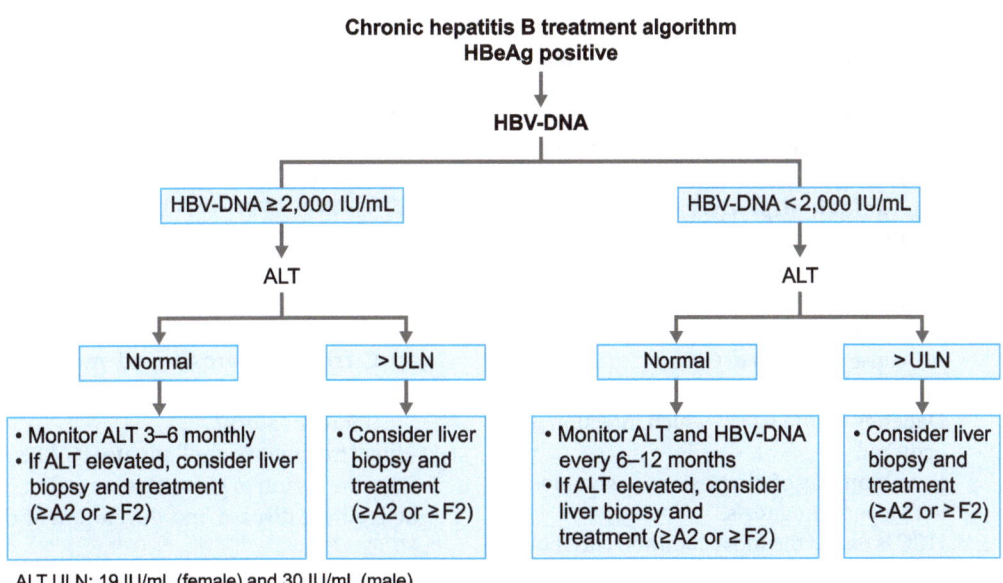

Flowchart 5.2: Chronic hepatitis B treatment algorithm for HBeAg-positive patients.

- Reduction of HBV-DNA < 400 IU/L.
- Achieve normal levels of serum ALT.
- Histological improvement in inflammation and fibrosis in the liver biopsy.
- Patients usually remain HBsAg positive, but loss of serum HBsAg indicates a good response.
  - **Antiviral agents:** Interferon, entecavir, tenofovir—commonly used
    - Pegylated α-2a interferon b: Response occurs in 25–40% of cases. 180 µg given once a week subcutaneously with response in 48 weeks.
    - Side effects: Acute flu-like symptoms, malaise, headache, depression, reversible hair loss, bone marrow depression, thrombocytopaenia and infection. Patients with HIV respond poorly.
  - **Oral therapy:**
    - **Entecavir:** Potent, cyclopentylguanosine analogue, reduces HBV-DNA by 48 weeks
    - **Tenofovir:** Cytosine nucleoside analogue, very effective, used for HIV-HBV infection.
    - **Lamivudine:** Well tolerated, development of resistance (80%) is high and itself may cause hepatitis; monotherapy—no longer recommended. 100 mg/day orally once a day until HBeAg becomes negative
    - **Adefovir dipivoxil:** A nucleotide reverse transcriptase inhibitor. It may be used in patients who develop resistance to lamivudine.
    - **Telbivudine:** L-nucleoside that may cause elevation of CPK.
- **Prognosis:**
  - Depends on the age at which infection is acquired
  - Development of cirrhosis is associated with a poor prognosis.
  - HCC is one of the most common carcinomas in HBV-endemic areas.

Chronic Hepatitis C

- About 70–85% of **individuals infected by HCV**
- **Cirrhosis** develops over 5–20 years in 20–30% of patients, **HCC** develops in several patients, especially with cirrhosis.
- Accelerate progression in alcoholism, HIV or HBV coinfection, and older age at the time of acquiring the infection
- **Clinical features:**
  - Usually asymptomatic. Detected on routine biochemical tests with mild elevations of ALT.
  - Similar to chronic hepatitis B. Most common—fatigue, rare—jaundice
  - **Extrahepatic features:** Essential mixed cryoglobulinaemia, membranoproliferative glomerulonephritis, uveitis, peripheral neuropathy, non-Hodgkin's lymphoma, lichen planus, sicca syndrome and porphyria cutanea tarda.
- **Investigations:**
  - HCV antibody in serum detected—> 95% cases
  - HCV-RNA in all patients
  - Liver biopsy if active treatment is considered. Histological changes—highly variable. Features—chronic hepatitis with lymphoid follicles in portal tracts, fatty change
  - Other features are similar to chronic hepatitis B
- **Treatment:**
  - **Indications:**
    - Chronic hepatitis on histology, HCV-RNA in serum and serum aminotransferases for > 6 months
    - Chronic hepatitis with persistently normal aminotransferases
    - Cirrhosis, fibrosis and moderate inflammation on liver biopsy (biopsy not mandatory)
  - Aim of treatment is to eliminate HCV-RNA from the serum to prevent progression of active liver disease and development of HCC.
  - **Combination therapy:** Pegylated interferon (once a week) and ribavirin
  - **Newer drugs (Box 5.4):**
  - **Liver transplant:** For patients with decompensated cirrhosis

> **Box 5.4: New drugs for hepatitis C.**
>
> **NS3/4A protease inhibitors:**
> - Becoprevir
> - Glecaprevir
> - Grazoprevir
> - Paritaprevir
> - Simeprevir
> - Telaprevir
> - Voxilaprevir
>
> **NS5A inhibitors:**
> - Daclatasvir
> - Elbasvir
> - Ledipasvir
> - Ombitasvir
> - Pibretasvir
> - Velpatasvir
>
> **NS5B polymerase inhibitors:**
> - Dasabuvir
> - Sofosbuvir

Chronic Hepatitis D (Plus Hepatitis B)

- Acute coinfection with hepatitis B or with superinfection in a patient with hepatitis B
- Relatively infrequent chronic hepatitis; spontaneous resolution is rare.
- About 60–70% of patients develop cirrhosis and develop more rapidly than with HBV infection.
- **Investigations:** Anti-delta antibody with chronic liver disease with HBsAg-positive. HDV in liver or HDV-RNA in serum by reverse transcription polymerase chain reaction
- **Treatment:** Usually supportive. Alpha-interferon at a high dose of 10M units three times weekly for 12 months gives a poor response. Lamivudine and adefovir are not useful.

■ FULMINANT HEPATITIS FAILURE (TABLE 5.14)

- Rapid development of hepatocellular dysfunction, specifically coagulopathy and mental status changes (encephalopathy) in a patient without a known prior liver disease
- Severe hepatic failure (insufficiency) in which encephalopathy develops within 4 weeks (8–28 days) from onset of symptoms in a patient with a previously normal liver
- **Subacute/subfulminant hepatic failure (FHF):** If hepatic failure develops at a slower pace (4–12 weeks)
- **Hyperacute hepatic failure:** If encephalopathy develops within 7 days, better prognosis than acute hepatic failure
- **Aetiology:** Rare but often life-threatening (**Table 5.20**)
- **Clinical features:**
    - **General features:** Jaundice, weakness, nausea, vomiting; right hypochondrial pain, small liver, liver dullness absent on percussion, ascites and oedema develop later
    - **Hepatic encephalopathy (HE):**
        - Mental state: Mild drowsiness, confusion and disorientation (grades I and II) to unresponsive coma (grade IV) with convulsions
        - Fetor hepaticus and flapping tremor (asterixis)

TABLE 5.20: Important causes of fulminant hepatic failure (FHF).

Viruses: HAV and HBV. Occasionally, HCV and others

Non-infectious causes

- **Drugs**
    - Analgesics (e.g. paracetamol)
    - Monoamine oxidase inhibitors
    - Anti-tuberculosis (e.g. isoniazid)
    - Anti-epileptic (e.g. valproate)
    - Halogenated anaesthetics
    - Social drugs (e.g. 'Ecstasy')
- **Toxins:** *Amanita phalloides* (mushroom) poisoning
- **Miscellaneous**
    - Wilson's disease
    - HELLP syndrome, eclampsia, Pre-eclampsia, acute fatty liver of pregnancy
    - Reye's syndrome
    - Autoimmune hepatitis
    - Budd–Chiari syndrome
    - Shock, ischaemic hepatitis
- Unknown

(HAV: hepatitis A virus; HBV: hepatitis B virus; HCV: hepatitis C virus; HELLP: haemolysis, elevated liver enzymes, low platelet count)

- Ascites and splenomegaly are rare.
- Fever, vomiting, hypotension and hypoglycaemia
- Spasticity and extension of the arms and legs and plantar responses remain flexor until late.
- **Cerebral oedema:** Develops in ~80% of patients
  - Bradycardia, intracranial hypertension and irregular respiration (Cushing's triad)
  - Pupils: Unequal, abnormally reacting or fixed pupils
  - Hyperventilation and hyperreflexia
  - Death due to intracranial hypertension and brain herniation
- **Investigations:**
  - **Serum findings:**
    - Hyperbilirubinaemia
    - Serum aminotransferases: Raised, but not useful indicators
    - Decreased levels of clotting factors. PT—prolonged.
    - Hypoalbuminaemia
    - Plasma and urine amino acids are increased.
    - Blood ammonia levels: Raised
  - **Urine:** Shows protein, bilirubin and urobilinogen
  - Leucocytosis and thrombocytopaenia
  - **Electroencephalography (EEG):** Grading of encephalopathy
  - **Ultrasound:** To detect liver size and for any evidence of underlying liver pathology
  - Intracranial pressure (ICP) is raised, but CSF is normal.

Box 5.5: Complications of fulminant hepatic failure (FHF).

• Encephalopathy	• Gastrointestinal bleeding and hypotension
• Cerebral oedema	
• Respiratory failure	• Hypoglycaemia, hypokalaemia
• Renal failure	
• Pancreatitis	• Hypothermia
• Hypocalcaemia	• Acid–base imbalance
• Bacterial and fungal infections	• Hypomagnesaemia

Complications of fulminant hepatic failure are given in **Box 5.5**.

Pathogenesis and management of major complications of acute liver failure are given in **Table 5.21**.

- **General measures:**
  - Monitor vital signs, urine output, renal functions, central venous pressure and electrolytes.
  - Maintain fluid–electrolyte balance.
  - Supply of adequate calories: Glucose (300 g/day) orally, nasogastric tube (NGT), infusion.
  - Ventilatory support for respiratory failure
  - Renal failure is treated with dialysis
  - Drugs:
    - Antibiotic prophylaxis—bacterial, fungal infection and infection treatment
    - H_2-receptor antagonists (omeprazole, pantoprazole): Prevent GI bleeding.
  - Fresh frozen plasma: If PT is prolonged > 1.5 times the normal
- **Encephalopathy:** Supportive therapy:
  - Protein-restricted diet (starting with 0.5 g/kg/day), suitable antibiotic therapy (e.g. ampicillin, rifaximin, metronidazole or neomycin), bowel washes, etc.
  - Reduce plasma ammonia level: Lactulose is catabolised by colonic bacterial flora to short-chain fatty acids that reduce pH of colon. Lowered pH favours formation of non-absorbable ammonium ion from ammonia, trapping ammonia in the colon, leading to decreased plasma ammonia.
  - Avoid sedatives. For restlessness and excitement, IV diazepam or midazolam.
- **Cerebral oedema:**
  - Head elevated at 30°, elective ventilation, in patients with grade 3 or 4 encephalopathy.
  - Raised ICP: Mannitol 20% (1 g/kg body weight) given intravenously over half an hour. Dose may need repetition every 6 hours and maintain the serum osmolarity below 310 mOsm/L.
  - Controlled hyperventilation so as to maintain $PaCO_2$ between 30 and 35 mmHg.

TABLE 5.21: Pathogenesis and management of major complications of acute liver failure.

Complication	Pathogenesis	Management
Hypoglycaemia	Reduced synthesis of hepatic glucose	Close monitoring of blood glucose and supplementation of intravenous (IV) glucose/10–20% dextrose
Encephalopathy	Cerebral oedema	• ICP monitoring (in case of 3rd or 4th stage encephalopathy) • In case of advanced encephalopathy computed tomography (CT) scan is suggested • Osmotherapy or treatment with mannitol or barbiturates • Treatment of other factors which are contributing • Elevating the head to > 30° • Antibiotics/antipyretic drugs to alleviate fever • Moderate hypothermia • Use of medication such as benzodiazepines and sedative medications
Coagulopathy	• Decrease in synthesis of the clotting factor • Breakdown of fibrin collagen • Thrombocytopaenia	• Administering vitamin K via parenteral route • Cryoprecipitate for bleeding with hypofibrinogenaemia • Recombinant factor VIIa • Infusion of platelets or plasma for controlling bleeding and prior to any procedures
GI haemorrhage	Stress ulceration	• Placement of nasogastric tube • Administering IV H2 receptor agonist/PPI (proton-pump inhibitor)
Infections	Compromised immunity	• Aseptic medical, nursing care • Routine or daily cultures of sputum, blood and urine • Prone to various fungal as well as bacterial infections • Administration of antibiotic • Prescribing antifungal therapy in case patient worsens
Renal failure	• Hypovolaemia • Hepatorenal syndrome • Acute tubular necrosis	• Central venous pressure monitoring • Repletion of the fluid volume with colloid or blood • Refraining use of agents such as aminoglycosides, contrast dye and non-steroidal anti-inflammatory drugs which are nephrotoxic in nature • Oral N-acetylcysteine prior to IV contrast agent • Haemofiltration, dialysis
Pancreatitis	Questionable hypoxia	• CT of the abdomen to rule out necrotising pancreatitis • Supplementary oxygen administration
Hypotension	• Hypovolaemia • Reduction in the resistance in the vessels	• Central venous pressure monitoring • Repletion of the fluid volume with colloid or blood
Respiratory failure	Acute respiratory distress syndrome)	• Initiating mechanical ventilation of the patient/continuous monitoring of the central venous pressure

- **Other measures:**
   o Coagulopathy—IV vitamin K, platelets, blood or fresh frozen plasma.
   o Steroids, exchange transfusion, haemodialysis using special membranes—not useful.
   o Liver transplantation: It is a major advance in the treatment of FHF.
- **Prognosis:** Mortality ~80% without liver transplantation, ~35% with transplantation.

Reye's Syndrome
- Children and adolescents with history of aspirin intake
- Develops after viral infections such as influenza or chicken pox
- Acute presentation with vomiting, lethargy during the recovery period of a viral illness followed by encephalopathy and cerebral oedema.
- Liver shows severe fatty change. Raised ammonia levels and liver enzymes. Usually no jaundice.

■ FATTY LIVER/STEATOSIS
- Abnormal accumulations of triglycerides within cytosol of the parenchymal cells Causes of fatty liver are given in **Box 5.6**.

Alcoholic Steatosis and Steatohepatitis
- Degree of fatty change is roughly proportional to the duration and amount of alcohol intake.
- **Features: Hepatomegaly** with or without tenderness or discomfort, **icterus** and **nausea**, **cirrhosis** with associated complications
- **Laboratory features:** Raised ALT and AST with AST:ALT > 1.
- **Ultrasound:** Diffuse increase in echogenicity
- **CT scan:** Fatty infiltration produces a low-density liver
- **Treatment:** Complete abstinence of alcohol and nutritional support

---

Box 5.6: Causes of fatty liver.

Alcohol
NAFLD/non-alcoholic steatohepatitis (NASH)
Drugs: Glucocorticoids, amiodarone, tetracycline, aspirin, methotrexate, didanosine, zidovudine, tamoxifen and amiodarone
Nutritional: Protein-calorie malnutrition, total parenteral nutrition and rapid weight loss/obesity
Metabolic: Diabetes, lipodystrophy and acute fatty liver of pregnancy
Miscellaneous: Inflammatory bowel disease, HIV infection, chronic hepatitis C, toxic mushrooms (*Amanita phalloides*), Reye's syndrome, obstructive sleep apnoea and Indian childhood cirrhosis

---

Non-alcoholic Fatty Liver Disease, Non-alcoholic Steatosis, Non-alcoholic Steatohepatitis
- Disease of affluent societies; prevalence increases proportionately with obesity
- Increasingly recognised; most common cause of chronic liver disease after hepatitis B, C and alcohol
- **Classification:**
  o Simple fatty liver disease [non-alcoholic fatty liver (NAFL)] with favourable prognosis
  o Non-alcoholic steatohepatitis (NASH) with fibrosis, progression to cirrhosis, HCC
- **Risk factors:**
  o Metabolic syndrome
  o Obesity, **hypertension**, type 2 diabetes mellitus, hyperlipidaemia and insulin resistance
  o **Rare:** Tamoxifen, amiodarone and exposure to certain petrochemicals
- Induced by two steps: Excess fat accumulation and subsequent necroinflammation in the liver
- **Clinical features:**
  o Mostly asymptomatic, obesity
  o Fatigue, malaise, sensation of fullness in the upper abdomen
  o Hepatomegaly
- **Diagnosis:** Mild moderate elevation of serum transaminases, no history of alcohol abuse, negative chronic liver disease screen
- **Investigations:**
  o Mild elevation of AST, ALT with AST:ALT < 1. Increases as fibrosis advances. May be only isolated elevation of the GGT. Elevated ALP in about 30% of patients
  o Ferritin levels increased in 20–50% of patients.
  o Autoantibodies in about 25% patients with more advanced fibrosis
  o Ultrasound and CT features: Similar to those in alcoholic fatty liver
  o Liver biopsy: Best diagnostic tool for confirmation and staging. Microscopic changes are similar to alcohol-induced

hepatic injury—steatosis, steatohepatitis and fibrosis. Characterised by fat, Mallory bodies, neutrophil infiltration, pericellular fibrosis
- **Management:**
  - Weight loss, control of diabetes, hyperlipidaemia
  - Drugs: Metformin, thiazolidinediones, ursodeoxycholic acid (UDCA), pentoxifylline and atorvastatin have shown some promise.
  - Liver transplantation for end-stage cirrhosis. May recur in graft
  - Regular follow-up, particularly for steatohepatitis

CIRRHOSIS

- **End stage** of any chronic liver disease, **diffuse process** (entire liver is involved) characterised by **fibrosis** and conversion of normal architecture to structurally **abnormal regenerating nodules** of liver cells.
- Main morphologic characteristics—**fibrosis, regenerating nodules, loss of architecture**

- **Pathology and pathogenesis:**
  - Widespread liver cell necrosis
  - Cirrhotic changes affect the whole liver, but not necessarily every lobule
  - Extensive fibrosis causing loss of liver architecture
  - Regenerating nodules due to hyperplasia of surviving liver cells
  - Destruction and distortion of vasculature by fibrosis causing obstruction of blood flow. Vascular reorganisation leads to portal hypertension, gastroesophageal varices and splenomegaly
  - Hepatocellular insufficiency and portal hypertension: Ascites and HE
  - Hepatocellular damage: Jaundice, oedema, coagulopathy, metabolic abnormalities

Alcoholic Cirrhosis

- Safe limits in males: 200 g, females: 140 g/week. About 40–80 g/day for men, 20–40 g/day for women for 10 years
- About 10 g of alcohol = 30 mL whisky, 100 mL wine, 250 mL of beer

TABLE 5.22: Morphological classification of cirrhosis (Fig. 5.3).

Micronodular cirrhosis (Laennec's cirrhosis)	Macronodular cirrhosis
- Regular, small nodules < 3 mm - Uniform thin regular fibrous connective tissue septa - Involvement of every lobule of whole liver - Most common cause: Alcoholic cirrhosis	- Irregular, coarse nodules of variable size, > 3 mm - Fibrous connective tissue septa, broad, vary in thickness; liver surface is grossly distorted - Most common cause: Chronic viral hepatitis - Increased risk of developing carcinoma of liver
Mixed cirrhosis	
Both micronodular and macronodular cirrhosis	

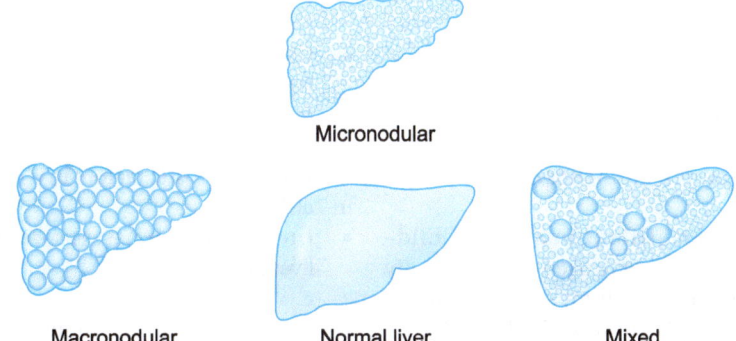

Fig. 5.3: Morphological classification of cirrhosis.

TABLE 5.23: Aetiological classification.

Alcohol	Non-alcoholic fatty liver disease
Chronic viral hepatitis Hepatitis B, hepatitis C, Delta hepatitis (hepatitis D) + hepatitis B	**Intra-/extrahepatic biliary obstruction:** Recurrent biliary obstruction (e.g. gallstones)
Autoimmune hepatitis	**Cryptogenic or idiopathic**
Biliary cirrhosis Primary biliary cirrhosis, secondary biliary cirrhosis, primary sclerosing cholangitis, autoimmune cholangiopathy	**Inherited metabolic liver disease** Haemochromatosis, Wilson's disease, α1-AT deficiency, cystic fibrosis, glycogen storage disease
Drug-induced cirrhosis Methotrexate, methyldopa, isoniazid, phenylbutazone, sulphonamides	**Others** Indian childhood cirrhosis, cardiac cirrhosis, chronic venous outflow obstruction

TABLE 5.24: Clinical features.

Signs	Symptoms

• Jaundice
 • Hepatomegaly/shrunken liver, ascites
 • **Circulatory changes:** Spider naevi, palmar erythema
 • **Endocrine changes:** Loss of libido, diminished body hair and hair loss, gynaecomastia, testicular atrophy, impotence in males, irregular menses, amenorrhoea, breast atrophy in females
 • **Haemorrhagic tendency:** Bruises, purpura, epistaxis
 • **Portal hypertension:** Splenomegaly, portosystemic collateral vessels, variceal bleeding
 • Flapping tremors
 • Pigmentation, clubbing, cyanosis, white nails
 • Dupuytren's contracture, parotid enlargement
	• Asymptomatic, diagnosed at ultrasound
	 • **Non-specific:** Weakness, fatigue, muscle cramps, weight loss, anorexia, nausea, vomiting, upper abdominal discomfort
	 • **Hepatic insufficiency**
	 • **Portal hypertension, sequelae**
	 • **Endocrine changes:**
	   ○ Males: Gynaecomastia, loss of libido, hair loss
	   ○ Females: Irregular menses, amenorrhoea, breast atrophy
	 • **Haemorrhagic tendency:** Easy bruising, purpura, epistaxis, menorrhagia and gastrointestinal bleeding

- About 180 g of alcohol/day for 25 years increases, risk of cirrhosis by 25 times
- Cirrhosis is 6-fold when consumption is double safety limit.
- Hepatitis C infection is an important contributory factor for progression to cirrhosis.
Classification of cirrhosis is given in **Tables 5.22** and **5.23**.
Clinical features of cirrhosis are given in **Table 5.24**.
- **Prognostic classifications:** The Child–Pugh (CP) scoring was used to risk-stratify patients undergoing shunt surgery. Modifications of Child's grading (A, B and C) are useful to classify severity of liver disease and prognosis in patients with established cirrhosis (**Table 5.25**).
  ○ CP class A: Points 5–6; CP class B: 7–9; CP class C: > 9 (range 5–15)
- **Characteristics of end stage of cirrhosis:** Jaundice; progressive, refractory ascites; worsening of signs of portal hypertension; progressive renal dysfunction; HE (**Box 5.7**).
Poor prognostic factors in cirrhosis are given in **Table 5.26**.
- **Investigations:** Assess severity and type of liver disease
  ○ **LFTs:**
    – Hyperbilirubinaemia: Conjugated and unconjugated

TABLE 5.25: Modified Child's–Pugh classification or Child–Turcotte–Pugh score.

Parameter	Score		
	1	2	3
Encephalopathy	None	Mild	Marked
Ascites	None	Mild/diuretic controlled	Moderate/severe
Prothrombin time (seconds over normal)	< 4	4–6	> 6
Serum albumin (g/dL)	> 3.5	2.8–3.5	< 2.8
Serum bilirubin (mg/dL)	< 2	2–3	> 3

Box 5.7: Complications of cirrhosis.
- Portal hypertension and sequelae
- Ascites
- Spontaneous bacterial peritonitis
- Hepatic encephalopathy
- Portal gastropathy
- Hepatorenal syndrome
- Hepatopulmonary syndrome
- Hepatocellular carcinoma
- Bleeding manifestations
- Cirrhotic cardiomyopathy
- Hepatic hydrothorax

TABLE 5.26: Poor prognostic factors in cirrhosis.

Laboratory findings	Clinical findings
• Serum albumin < 2.5 g/dL • Serum sodium < 120 mmol/L • Rising serum creatinine • Prothrombin time > 1.5 times of control (> 6 s above normal)	• Persistent jaundice (bilirubin > 20 mg/dL) • Ascites—poor response to therapy • Encephalopathy • Variceal haemorrhage with poor liver function • Neuropsychiatric complications • Persistent hypotension • Small liver

- Serum proteins: Show reversal of A:G ratio. Hypoalbuminaemia—reduced synthesis, hyperglobulinaemia—stimulation of reticuloendothelial system
- Serum transaminases: AST, ALT—raised, usually < 300 U/dL. AST:ALT ratio is > 2 in alcoholic cirrhosis. AST is disproportionately raised relative to ALT, due to proportionately greater inhibition of ALT synthesis by alcohol. < 2 in cirrhosis complicating viral hepatitis
  - ALP: May be slightly elevated
  - PT: Prolonged due to reduced synthesis of clotting factors
- **Haematological tests:** Peripheral smear shows anaemia, acanthocytosis (spur-like projections on RBC), leucopaenia, thrombocytopaenia (hypersplenism, bone marrow suppression)
- **Serological markers:** For hepatitis B and C
- **Serum electrolytes:** Hyponatraemia—severe disease due to defect in free water clearance or to excess diuretic therapy; hypokalaemia; hypomagnesaemia, hypophosphataemia
- **Blood ammonia estimation:** Reliable when HE is suspected. Caused due to decreased clearance by liver and shunting of portal venous blood to systemic circulation.
- Respiratory alkalosis may develop due to central hyperventilation.
- Glucose intolerance
- **Ultrasound:**
  - Changes in size and shape of the liver; nodularity
  - Fatty change and fibrosis produce a diffuse increased echogenicity.
  - Distortion of the arterial vascular architecture, patency and size of the portal and hepatic veins.
  - Detect HCC.
  - Splenomegaly, ascites

- CT scan: Detects hepatosplenomegaly, dilated collaterals. Phase-contrast-enhanced scans to detect HCC
- Endoscopy: Detecting and treating varices, portal hypertensive gastropathy
- Liver biopsy: Done to confirm diagnosis, assess severity and type of liver disease. Special stains may be necessary for iron and copper. Immunocytochemical stains can identify viruses.
- Special investigations depending on the aetiology:
  - Chemical measurement of iron (serum transferrin saturation level, serum ferritin) and copper (ceruloplasmin) is required to confirm diagnosis of iron overload or Wilson's disease.
  - Serum α-foetoprotein, α-1-antitrypsin, antinuclear antibodies, anti-smooth muscle antibodies, etc., depending on the aetiology
- Ascitic fluid examination

PORTAL HYPERTENSION

- Prolonged elevation of portal venous pressure (> 30 cm saline)
- Elevation of hepatic venous pressure gradient (HVPG) > 7 mmHg. HVPG > 10 mmHg is significant portal hypertension.
- Portal vein is formed by the union of the superior mesenteric and splenic veins. Normal pressure: 5–8 mmHg (or 10–15 cm saline).
- Develops due to combination of two simultaneously occurring haemodynamic processes:
  - Increased intrahepatic resistance to the blood flow through the liver caused by cirrhosis and regenerative nodules
  - Increased splanchnic blood flow secondary to vasodilatation within the splanchnic vascular bed
- **Classification of portal hypertension:** Site of obstruction: **pre-hepatic, intrahepatic, post-hepatic (Fig. 5.4):**

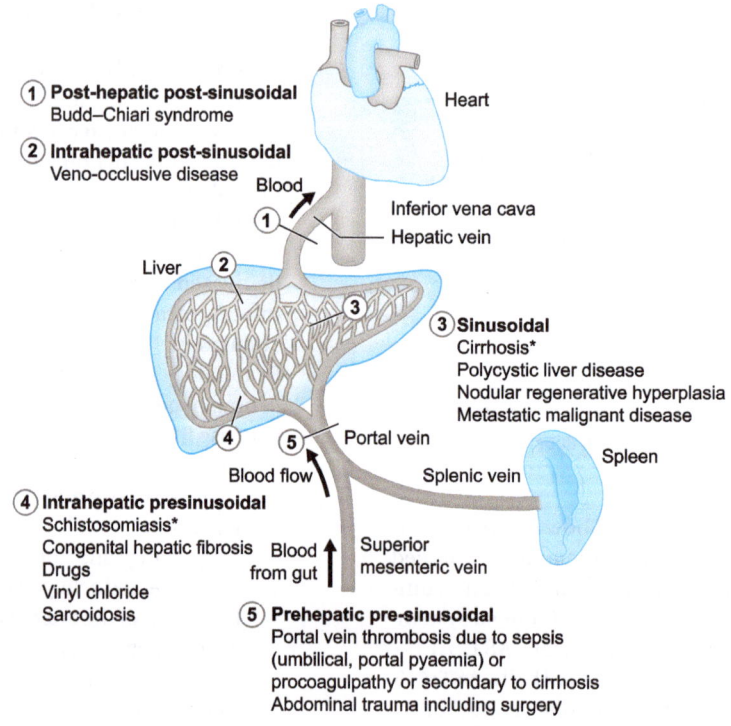

*Most common cause. Note that splenic vein occlusion can also follow pancreatitis leading to gastric varices.

Fig. 5.4: Classification of portal hypertension according to site of vascular obstruction.

- Pre-hepatic causes: Obstruction/blockage of portal vein before it ramifies within the liver—portal vein thrombosis, splenic vein thrombosis, massive splenomegaly (Banti's syndrome)
- Intrahepatic causes: Distortion of architecture and may be further divided into pre-sinusoidal (schistosomiasis), sinusoidal (cirrhosis), post-sinusoidal (veno-occlusive syndrome).
- Post-hepatic causes: Due to venous blockage outside the liver and are rare, e.g. severe right-sided heart failure, Budd–Chiari syndrome, constrictive pericarditis and hepatic vein outflow obstruction

- Clinical features of portal hypertension are given in **Table 5.27** and **Figure 5.5**.
- **Investigations:** Diagnosis can be made on clinical grounds.
  - Barium swallow: Varices as filing defects in lower-third of oesophagus ('bag of worms appearance')
  - **Upper gastrointestinal (GI) scopy:** Most reliable method. Appear as blue rounded projections (red spots and red stripes) under submucosa. 'Cherry red spots' indicate impending rupture of varices.
  - **Ultrasonography:** Detects the size of liver and spleen. Size and patency of portal vein and splenic vein. Presence of collaterals and ascites

Box 5.8: Complications of portal hypertension.
- Variceal bleeding: Oesophageal and gastric
- Hepatic encephalopathy
- Ascites
- Renal failure
- Congestive gastropathy
- Hypersplenism
- Iron deficiency anaemia

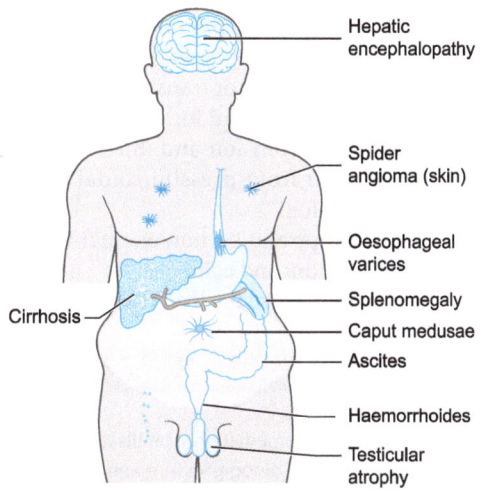

Fig. 5.5: Major clinical consequences of portal hypertension in cirrhosis.

TABLE 5.27: Clinical features of portal hypertension.

Asymptomatic	History: Alcoholism, hepatitis	Caput medusae
Splenomegaly (required for diagnosis)	Features due to liver cell failure, HE	Hypersplenism: Leucopaenia, thrombocytopaenia
Fetor hepaticus: Musty odour of breath due to shunting of blood allowing mercaptans to pass directly to lungs, bypassing liver	• Bleeding—oesophageal varices or portal gastropathy—haematemesis and melaena • Haemorrhoids—dilation of rectal veins due to development of collaterals	• Splanchnic arteriovenous fistula—bruit in left or right upper quadrant • Cruveilhier–Baumgarten hum—epigastric venous hum, collateral flow in the falciform ligament
Enlarged or shrunken liver. Small, contracted, fibrotic liver is found when the portal venous pressure is very high. Soft liver—extrahepatic portal vein obstruction		
Ascites		

> **Box 5.9: Drugs used in the treatment of portal hypertension.**
>
> | Drugs that decrease portal blood flow | Drugs that decrease intrahepatic resistance |
> |---|---|
> | • Non-selective β-adrenergic blocking agents
• Somatostatin and its analogues
• Vasopressin | • α1-adrenergic blocking agents (e.g. prazosin)
• Angiotensin receptor blocking agents
• Nitrates |

- Complications of portal hypertension are given in **Box 5.8**.
- **Treatment:**
  - Treatment of underlying disease (**Box 5.9**).

■ VARICEAL BLEEDING

- About 90% patients with cirrhosis develop gastroesophageal varices, but only one third will bleed.
- The most common site is oesophageal varices within 3–5 cm of the oesophago-gastric junction.
- Factors that predispose to rupture of varices are:
  - Large varices
  - 'Red sign' on endoscopy suggests imminent rupture
  - Associated with severe liver disease
  - High portal venous pressure
  - Salicylates and other non-steroidal anti-inflammatory drugs

- Portal venography rarely done nowadays
- **Measurement of portal venous pressure:** By either wedged hepatic venous pressure (WHVP) or transhepatic venous pressure. It is useful for confirmation of portal hypertension and differentiating sinusoidal from pre-sinusoidal portal hypertension.
- Proctoscopy and barium enema: Varices in the rectum and colon
- LFTs: To confirm the liver diseases

> **Box 5.10: Management of acute variceal bleeding.**
>
> - **General measures**
>   - Resuscitation. Immediate hospitalisation: Intensive-care nursing. Nil by mouth until bleeding stops
>   - Assess pulse and blood pressure and maintain fluid and electrolyte balance
>   - Investigations: Haemoglobin, blood group, urea-creatinine, electrolytes, liver function, cultures
>   - Grade cirrhosis by Child–Pugh score
>   - Blood transfusion avoids saline infusions. Prompt correction of hypovolaemia.
>   - Coagulation factor deficiency correction—fresh frozen plasma
>   - Platelet transfusions and vitamin K I
>   - Prevent stress ulcers give H_2 receptor antagonists or proton-pump inhibitors
> - **Complication prevention**
>   - Prophylactic antibiotics: Reduce infection, mortality—prevent spontaneous bacterial peritonitis (SBP)
>   - Oral and intravenous quinolones are used (e.g. ciprofloxacin 500 mg twice daily)
>   - Prevent hepatic encephalopathy: Precipitated when the amount of bleeding is large because blood contains protein
>   - Treatment of ascites: Ascitic tap (paracentesis), administration of spironolactone or amiloride
>   - Monitor for alcohol withdrawal and give thiamine
> - **Urgent endoscopy**
>   - Confirms diagnosis of oesophageal varices. Excludes bleeding from other sites (e.g. gastric ulceration)
>   - Reduces oesophageal ulceration following therapy, sucralfate—1 g four times daily
> - **Local measures**
>   - Endoscopic procedures—sclerotherapy and variceal banding [endoscopic variceal band ligation (EVBL)]. They arrest bleeding in 80% of cases and reduce early rebleeding
>   - Balloon tamponade
> - **Vasoconstrictor therapy**
>   - Reduce portal pressure for constricting splanchnic vessels and portal inflow of blood
>   - Terlipressin, somatostatin, octreotide and vasopressin

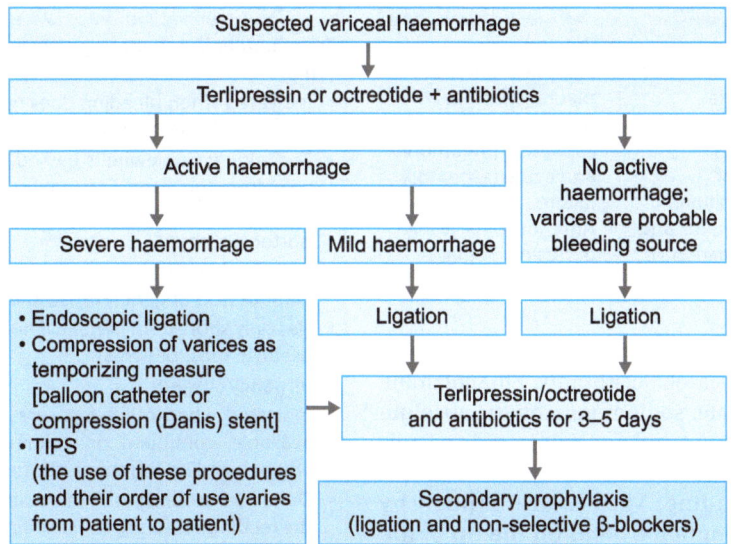

(TIPSS: transjugular intrahepatic portosystemic shunt)

Flowchart 5.3: Treatment of acute variceal haemorrhage.

- **Clinical features:** Painless, mild-massive haematemesis, with or without associated melaena. Depending on the amount of blood loss, they may vary from mild postural tachycardia to shock. Features of liver cell failure, ascites and portal hypertension
- **Diagnosis:**
  - **Fibreoptic endoscopy:** Within 8 hours of bleeding, it reveals bleeding site and the presence of varices.
  - **Ultrasonography:** It is useful to confirm the patency of portal vein.
- **Management:** Management of the active bleeding episode, prevention of rebleeding, prophylactic measures to prevent the first haemorrhage (**Box 5.10, Flowchart 5.3**).
  - **Vasoconstrictor therapy:**
    – Used for emergency control of bleeding before endoscopy and in combination with endoscopic techniques by reducing portal inflow of blood and pressure by constricting splanchnic vessels
    – **Drugs used:**
      ▪ Terlipressin: About 2 mg IV 6-hourly till bleeding stops, 1 mg 4-hourly after 48 hours if prolonged dosage regimen is used. Contraindicated in ischaemic heart disease. Side effects: Abdominal colic, evacuation of bowels, facial pallor due to generalised vasoconstriction.
      ▪ Somatostatin, octreotide stops bleeding > 80% patients, equivalent to vasopressin, endoscopic therapy. Few side effects. Administered as somatostatin infusion of 250–500 µg/h followed by 250 µg/h for 2–5 days; octreotide—50 µg as bolus followed by 50 µg/h for 2–5 days. Given if terlipressin is contraindication.
      ▪ Vasopressin: It was used in the past but is not commonly used now.
    – **Drugs that are used in the reduction of portal venous pressure:** Terlipressin, somatostatin, octreotide, propranolol, nadolol and nitroglycerine
  - **Injection sclerotherapy or variceal banding:**
    – Sclerotherapy: Injection of sclerosing agent into the varices may arrest

> **Box 5.11: Complications of sclerotherapy.**
> - 1% mortality
> - Abdominal pain, fever and dysphagia
> - Oesophageal complications: Recurrence of varices, ulceration, perforation, reflux and stricture formation
> - Pulmonary complications: Pain, pleural effusion, mediastinitis, aspiration pneumonia and acute respiratory failure
> - Anterior spinal artery occlusion: Spinal paralysis

> **Box 5.12: Management of acute rebleed.**
> **Transjugular intrahepatic portosystemic shunt (TIPS)**
> - Indicated when bleeding does not stop after two sessions of endoscopic therapy within 5 days
> - **Technique:** Guidewire is passed from the jugular vein into the liver. Expandable metal shunt is forced over it into the liver substance to form a portocaval shunt
> - Reduces hepatic sinusoidal, portal vein pressure without risks of general anaesthesia or surgery
> - Has only short-term benefit. If no response, TIPS is useful in most patients
>
> **Emergency surgery**
> - Indicated when other measures fail, TIPS is not available, continued or recurrent haemorrhage and or bleeding is from gastric fundal varices
> - Done by oesophageal transection and ligation of the feeding vessels to the bleeding varices
> - Infrequently acute portosystemic shunt surgery and oesophageal staple transaction

bleeding by producing thrombosis of vessel. Sclerosants: Ethanolamine oleate, sodium morrhuate, absolute alcohol and sodium tetradecyl sulphate
  – Banding: Varices are banded by mounting a band on the tip of the endoscope, sucking the varix just into the end of the scope and dislodging the band over the varix.
  – Complications of sclerotherapy are given in **Box 5.11**.
 o **Balloon tamponade:**
  – Indicated in variceal bleeding if endoscopic therapy or vasoconstrictors fails/contraindicated or exsanguinating haemorrhage. Useful in initial hours of bleeding in 90% cases.
  – Sengstaken–Blakemore tube, Minnesota tube: Four-lumen tubes with two balloons— oesophageal and gastric balloons
  – Complications: Aspiration pneumonia, oesophageal rupture, necrosis, ulcerations of oesophageal mucosa and obstruction to pharynx.
- **Management of an acute rebleed:**
 o Post one therapeutic endoscopy, nearly 30% of patients suffer rebleeding.
 o Source: Established by endoscopy. Can be due to ulcer from sclerotherapy; difficult to manage.
 o **Management:** Repeat endoscopic therapy once only to control rebleeding and further sclerotherapy or banding should not be done (**Box 5.12**).
- **Prevention of variceal bleeding: Prophylaxis**
 o Prophylactic measures are given in **Box 5.13**.

HEPATIC (PORTOSYSTEMIC) ENCEPHALOPATHY

- Chronic neuropsychiatric syndrome (alteration in mental status and cognitive function) secondary to chronic liver disease.
- Acute and potentially reversible, or chronic and progressive.
- **Aetiology:** It develops due to spontaneous 'shunting' in chronic liver disease with portal hypertension or following a portosystemic shunt procedure, e.g. TIPS or FHF.
- **Pathogenesis:** Mechanism is unknown, but many factors play a role. Mechanisms proposed:
 o Gut-derived neurotoxins
 o Brain water homeostasis
 o Oxidative/nitrosative stress
 o Astrocyte dysregulation
 o Neurotransmitter dysfunction—decreased glutamine, increased GABA, serotonin
 o Infection and inflammation

Toxic substances involved in hepatic encephalopathy are mentioned in **Box 5.14**.

Precipitating factors for portosystemic encephalopathy are given in **Box 5.15**.

Clinical features of acute and chronic hepatic (portosystemic) encephalopathy are given in **Box 5.16**.

Box 5.13: Prophylactic measures.

Primary prophylactic measures

Useful in patients with cirrhosis and varices, who have not bled

Non-selective β-blockers: Propranolol, nadolol—
- Reduce chances of upper GI bleeding, cost-effectiveness and recurrence
- Efficacy is similar to prophylactic banding
- Act by vasodilatation of splanchnic arterial bed and portal venous system

Nitrates: Nitroglycerine, isosorbide dinitrate—
- Given with β-blockers—reduce risk of variceal bleed

Variceal banding is done if there are contraindications or intolerance to non-selective β-blockers

Recurrent variceal bleeding (secondary prophylaxis)

Bleeding recurs in about 60–80% of patients within 2 years after initial bleed

Long-term measures

Non-selective β-blockers—treatment of choice

Propranolol: About 80–160 mg/day oral, decreases portal pressure, decreases frequency of rebleed (as effective as sclerotherapy or ligation), prevents bleeding from portal hypertensive gastropathy

Endoscopic treatment: Injection sclerotherapy or variceal banding. Repeated courses of banding done every 2 weeks until the varices are obliterated. It is superior to sclerotherapy.

Transjugular portosystemic stent shunts: Reduce rebleeding rates compared to endoscopic techniques but associated with increased rate of encephalopathy. Used if endoscopic or medical therapy fails

Surgical portosystemic shunting

Performed in patients with good liver function (Child–Pugh A, B), when medical therapy, EVBL and sclerotherapy are unsuccessful with very low risk of rebleeding

Types of portal systemic shunts:
- Non-selective shunt with end-to-side portocaval anastomosis decompresses entire portal venous system, produces significant post-operative hepatic encephalopathy
- Selective distal splenorenal (Warren) shunt- decompress only varices while maintaining blood flow to liver via superior mesenteric vein, produces less encephalopathy

Complications of portosystemic shunts:
About 5% mortality, shunt closure, hepatic encephalopathy due to reduction in portal pressure and hepatic blood flow, post-operative jaundice because of deterioration of liver function

Oesophageal transection: Devascularisation procedure that does not produce encephalopathy

Liver transplantation: Treatment of choice when liver function is poor

(EVBL: endoscopic variceal band ligation; GI: gastrointestinal)

Box 5.14: Toxic substances involved in hepatic encephalopathy.

- Ammonia
- Free-fatty acids
- Mercaptans derived from methionine
- Gamma-aminobutyric acid (GABA)
- Aromatic amino acids—tyrosine, phenylalanine
- Reduced branched-chain amino acids
- Phenol, indole
- False neurotransmitters (octopamine)

Box 5.15: Precipitating factors for portosystemic encephalopathy.

- Increased dietary protein
- Gastrointestinal bleeding
- Electrolyte disturbance: Hypokalaemia, hyponatraemia
- Large-volume paracentesis
- Overzealous use of diuretics
- Vomiting and diarrhoea
- Constipation
- Acute infections: Spontaneous bacterial peritonitis
- Drugs, e.g. sedatives
- Viral/alcoholic hepatitis
- Portosystemic shunt operations
- Development of hepatocellular carcinoma
- Uraemia

> **Box 5.16: Clinical features.**
>
> - **Acute hepatic (portosystemic) encephalopathy**
>   - Usually has a precipitating factor, patient becomes drowsy and comatose within weeks to months
>   - Brain oedema may occur with severe encephalopathy and may lead to cerebral herniation
> - **Chronic hepatic (portosystemic) encephalopathy**
>   - Disturbances in consciousness and behaviour: Which may fluctuate
>   - Hypersomnia—earliest feature
>   - Reversal of sleep rhythm
>   - Violent and difficult to manage
>   - Very sleepy and difficult to rouse
>   - Irritable, confused, disoriented and slurred speech
>   - Drowsiness progressing to coma
>   - Change in personality, mood and intellect
>   - General features: Nausea, vomiting and weakness
>   - Signs:
>   - Fetor hepaticus (a sweet smell to the breath)
>   - Asterixis or coarse flapping tremor (outstretched hands, head and trunk). Also seen in uraemia, respiratory failure, severe heart failure
>   - Fluctuating neurological signs: Constructional apraxia with the patient being unable to write or draw, hypertonia, hyperreflexia, decreased mental function

TABLE 5.28: Types of hepatic encephalopathy.

Type A	Associated with acute liver failure
Type B	Associated with portosystemic bypass with no intrinsic liver disease
Type C	Associated with cirrhosis, portal hypertension or portosystemic shunts
• Minimal HE	
• Episodic HE	Persistent, spontaneous, recurrent
• Persistent HE	Mild, severe, treatment dependent

(HE: hepatic encephalopathy)

TABLE 5.29: West Haven criteria.

Grade	Consciousness	Intellect and behaviour	Neurological findings
0	Normal	Normal	Normal examination or impaired psychomotor testing
1	Mild lack of awareness	Shortened attention span; impaired addition or subtraction	Mild asterixis or tremor
2	Lethargic	Disoriented, inappropriate behaviour	Obvious asterixis, slurred speech
3	Somnolent but arousable	Gross disorientation, bizarre behaviour	• Muscular rigidity and clonus • Hyperreflexia
4	Coma	Coma	Decerebrate posturing

Types of hepatic encephalopathy are given in **Table 5.28**.

Classification of encephalopathy according to West Haven criteria is given in **Table 5.29**.

- **Diagnosis:** Based on clinical features:
  - **Reitan's number connection test:** Used for > 50 years to assess mental function.
- **Investigations:**
  - Blood ammonia levels: Raised (upper limit of normal is 0.8–1 µg/mL).

> **Box 5.17: Treatment measures for encephalopathy.**
>
> - **General measures:**
>   - Removal of the precipitating factors. Stop alcohol
>   - Maintain nutrition with glucose 300 g/day. Maintain hydration, correct electrolyte imbalance
>   - No restriction of dietary proteins for > 48 h. Administer 0.8–1.0 g/kg of proteins daily preferably vegetable protein. Restriction is reserved for resistant cases
>   - Zinc supplementation may be helpful
>   - Stop or reduce diuretic therapy
>   - Treat any infection
> - **Bowel evacuation:**
>   - Evacuating, sterilising the bowels of nitrogenous toxins and bacteria
>   - Lactulose: Non-absorbable disaccharide, osmotic purgative; metabolised by colonic bacteria—produces colonic acidification. Promotes 2–3 soft stools per day
>   - Eliminates nitrogenous waste, limits ammonia absorption, favours conversion of ammonia to ammonium (poorly absorbed). Lactitol has a similar action, more palatable and better than lactulose
>   - Dose: 15–30 mL three times orally per day
> - **Poorly absorbed antibiotics:**
>   - Sterilise gut in patients having difficulty with lactulose. Reduce bacterial intestinal ammonia production
>   - Alternating administration of neomycin and metronidazole to reduce the individual side effects
>   - Rifaximin: 550 mg twice daily is very effective and without any side effects of neomycin or metronidazole. It has only 0.4% systemic absorption
> - **Other measures:**
>   - GI bleeding: Ryles tube aspiration, bowel washes to remove the blood and blood products. Reduces the production of nitrogen in the gut
>   - Mannitol, judicious use of IV fluids to reduce spontaneous cerebral oedema in acute liver failure
> - **Other drugs tried:**
>   - Bromocriptine, L-ornithine L-aspartate (LOLA), branched-chain amino acids, probiotics, sodium benzoate, flunarizine
> - **Novel treatment strategies:**
>   - L-carnitine, rivastigmine, endocannabinoids, mGluR1 antagonists
>   - Molecular adsorbent recirculating system (MARS)—purifies the blood by removal of albumin bound as well as water-soluble substrates
> - **Liver transplantation**

- EEG: A decrease in the frequency of the normal α-waves (8–13 Hz) to α-waves of 1.5–3 Hz is seen before coma develops.
- Cerebrospinal fluid—glutamine: Increased; proteins and cell count—normal.
- Visual evoked potential abnormalities may be present during subclinical encephalopathy.
- LFTs confirm presence of liver disease.
- **Treatment:** Multifactorial (**Box 5.17**)

HEPATORENAL SYNDROME

- Form of functional renal failure without renal pathology in patients with advanced cirrhosis or acute liver failure.
- Urine output is low, tubular function is normal, kidneys are histologically normal.
- About 10% of patients with advanced cirrhosis with jaundice and ascites.
- **Pathogenesis**: Severe peripheral vasodilatation leads to severe reduction in effective blood volume and hypotension, activating homeostatic mechanisms, renin–angiotensin–aldosterone system leading to vasoconstriction of the renal vessels. Increased preglomerular vascular resistance directs the flow of blood away from the renal cortex. This leads to a reduced glomerular filtration rate. Eicosanoids are also implicated.

> **Box 5.18: Types of hepatorenal syndrome (HRS).**
>
> **Type 1 hepatorenal syndrome**
> - Progressive oliguria, rapid rise of serum creatinine to > 2.5 mg/dL
> - Very poor prognosis
> - Precipitated by spontaneous bacterial peritonitis
> - Without treatment, median survival is < 1 month, die within 10 weeks after onset of renal failure
>
> **Type 2 hepatorenal syndrome**
> - Reduction in glomerular filtration, moderate, stable increase of serum creatinine (> 1.5 mg/dL)
> - Better prognosis than Type 1 HRS
> - Usually occurs in patients with refractory ascites (resistant to diuretics)
> - Median survival is 3–6 months

- **Precipitating factors:** GI bleeding, aggressive paracentesis, diuretic therapy, sepsis including SBP and diarrhoea.
- **Clinical types:** There are two types (**Box 5.18**).
- **Clinical features:**
    o Develops in advanced cirrhosis, almost always with ascites.
    o Anorexia, weakness, fatigue, oliguria, nausea, vomiting and thirst.
    o Terminally coma deepens and hypotension develops.
- **Investigations:**
    o Urea and creatinine levels: High
    o Serum sodium: Less than 120 mEq/L. Urine sodium excretion: Less than 10 mEq/day
    o Urinalysis: Normal. Urine:Plasma osmolality ratio is > 1.5.
- **Diagnosis:** Usually made in the presence of a large amount of ascites in patients who have a stepwise progressive increase in creatinine.
- **Diagnostic criteria:** All must be present—
    o Cirrhosis with ascites
    o Serum creatinine > 1.5 mg/dL, no improvement (decrease to a level of 1.5 mg/dL or less) after at least 2 days of diuretic withdrawal and volume expansion with albumin (1 g/kg body weight/day up to a maximum of 100 g/day)
    o Absence of shock
    o No current or recent treatment with nephrotoxic drugs
    o Absence of parenchymal kidney disease as indicated by proteinuria > 500 mg/day, microhaematuria (> 50 red blood cells per high power field) and/or abnormal renal ultrasonography
- **Treatment:** Liver transplantation is the treatment of choice.
- **Prevention:**
    o Avoid over-vigorous diuretic therapy, slow treatment of ascites.
    o Early recognition of electrolyte imbalance and haemorrhage. Screen, treat infection (SBP).
    o Correct hypovolaemia by IV plasma protein solution or salt-poor albumin.
    o Albumin infusions with vasopressin analogues are effective short-term medical therapy.
    o Currently, midodrine (α-agonist) along with octreotide is also being used.
    o TIPS if vasoconstrictors fall

ASCITES

- Accumulation of excess fluid within the peritoneal cavity
- **Pathogenesis:** Complex; involving the following mechanisms (**Table 5.30**)
- **Classification of ascitic fluid infection:**
    o Culture-negative neutrocytic ascites
    o Monomicrobial non-neutrocytic bacterascites
    o Polymicrobial bacterascites
    o Secondary bacterial peritonitis
    o SBP
- **Investigations:** 10–20 mL of ascitic fluid
    o **Cell count:** Neutrophil count above 250 cells/mm^3—SBP
    o **Gram stain and culture:** Bacteria and acid-fast bacilli
    o **Protein:** Total ascetic fluid protein > 1.5 g/dL—increased risk of SBP
    o **Serum ascites albumin gradient (SAAG):** Difference between serum albumin and ascitic fluid albumin. Better indicator than simple estimation of protein in the ascetic fluid. A high SAAG of > 1.1 g/dL suggests portal hypertension, and a low gradient < 1.1 g/dL is associated with abnormalities of the peritoneum, e.g. inflammation, infections and neoplasms.

TABLE 5.30: Mechanisms of pathogenesis of ascites.

In cirrhosis	Absence of cirrhosis
Portal hypertension	**Inflammation of peritoneum**
Increase in portal vein hydrostatic pressure, causing extravasation of fluid from plasma into the peritoneal cavity	Peritonitis: From bacteria or mycobacteria causes increased vascular permeability and exudation of fluid into peritoneal cavity
Hypoalbuminaemia	**Venous obstruction**
Decreased synthetic function in cirrhosis reduces plasma oncotic pressure and results in extravasation of fluid (ascites and oedema)	Inferior vena cava obstruction increases the hydrostatic pressure and leads to transudation of fluid into peritoneal cavity
Splanchnic vasodilation	**Lymphatic obstruction**
Reduction of arterial blood pressure activates renin–angiotensin–aldosterone system causing secondary hyperaldosteronism. Liver fails to metabolise aldosterone increased hyperaldosteronism. It causes sodium and fluid retention	Obstruction of lymphatic flow due to involvement of mesenteric lymph nodes, thoracic duct and abdominal lymphatic ducts can cause leakage of chyle into peritoneal cavity and can lead to chylous ascites
Percolation of lymph	**Rupture of a viscus**
In cirrhosis, hepatic lymphatic flow exceeds thoracic duct capacity. Excess lymph oozes freely from the surface of cirrhotic liver into the peritoneal cavity causing ascites	Outpouring of blood, cystic fluid, contaminated material, favouring ascites. Pancreatic ascites results from leakage of pancreatic enzymes into the peritoneum (pancreatitis)
Combination of portal hypertension, splanchnic arterial vasodilation, and sodium and water retention increases the hydrostatic pressure as well as permeability of interstitial capillaries. It causes extravasation of fluid into the peritoneal cavity	**Malignancy**
	Primary peritoneal malignancies (mesothelioma, sarcoma), abdominal malignancies (gastric, colonic adenocarcinoma) or metastatic disease from breast, lung or melanoma

TABLE 5.31: Ascitic fluid changes in cirrhosis.

Features	Findings
Appearance	Clear, straw coloured or light green
Specific gravity	< 1.018
Protein	< 2.5 g/dL
Total cell count	Normal (< 250/µL)
Differential cell count	Mesothelial cells and lymphocytes
Gram's stain	Negative
Culture	Negative
Malignant cells	Absent
Serum ascites albumin gradient	≥ 1.1g/dL

- o **Cytology:** For malignant cells to exclude neoplasms
- o **Amylase:** To exclude pancreatic ascites. It is increased in acute pancreatitis.
- o **Ultrasonography:** Very sensitive, detects small amounts of fluid and identifies the cause also.
- o Paracentesis and evaluation of ascitic fluid (**Tables 5.31** and **5.32**)
- o Laparoscopy and biopsy of peritoneum
- **Nature of ascitic fluid:** The ascitic fluid may be transudate or exudate.
- Various causes of ascites are given in **Box 5.19**.
- Examination of ascetic fluid and its interpretation are given in **Table 5.33**.

TABLE 5.32: Differences between transudate and exudate.

Characteristics	Transudate	Exudate
Cause	Non-inflammatory process	Inflammatory process
Mechanism	• Ultrafiltrate of plasma • Increased hydrostatic pressure	Increased vascular permeability
Appearance	Clear, serous	Turbid, chylous, purulent, haemorrhagic
Colour	Straw yellow	Yellow to red
Specific gravity	< 1.018	> 1.018
Protein	Low, < 2 g/dL, mainly albumin	High, > 2 g/dL
Clot	Absent	Clots spontaneously (high fibrinogen)
Cell count	Low (< 250/µL)	High (> 250/µL)
Type of cells	Few lymphocytes and mesothelial cells	• Acute: Neutrophils • Chronic: Lymphocytes
Bacteria	Absent	Usually present
LDH	Low	High
Oedema	Pitting type	No pitting

(LDH: lactate dehydrogenase)

> **Box 5.19: Various causes of ascites categorised depending on the nature of ascitic fluid.**
>
> **Transudates**
> - Cirrhosis and portal hypertension
> - Nephrotic syndrome
> - Hypoproteinaemia
> - Congestive cardiac failure
> - Constrictive pericarditis
> - Beriberi
> - Inferior vena cava obstruction
>
> **Exudates**
> - Tuberculous, bacterial peritonitis
> - Malignant peritonitis
> - Pancreatic ascites
>
> **Miscellaneous (exudate/transudate)**
> - Meigs's syndrome
> - Chylous ascites
> - Budd–Chiari syndrome

Serum Ascites Albumin Gradient

- Useful for differentiating ascites caused by portal hypertension from other causes.
- Serum albumin concentration:Ascitic albumin concentration (does not change with diuresis)
- **Significance**:
    - **SAAG ≥ 1.1 g/dL:** Portal hypertension, ascites is due to increased pressure in hepatic sinusoids.
    - **SAAG < 1.1 g/dL:** Non-portal hypertensive ascites such as tuberculous peritonitis, peritoneal carcinomatosis or pancreatic ascites.
    - Depending on the total protein level in the ascitic fluid, it is divided into transudate or exudate. However, many patients with SBP have a low rather than high total protein in the ascetic fluid, and many patients with portal hypertension secondary to heart failure have a high protein rather than the expected low total protein level in ascetic fluid. In these situations, SAAG is a highly sensitive method.

Causes of high and low serum ascites albumin gradient are given in **Box 5.20**.

Causes of ascites according to the nature of ascitic fluid are given in **Box 5.21**.

- **Management:** Produce a net reabsorption of fluid from the ascites into the circulating volume by reducing sodium intake and increasing renal excretion of sodium.
    - General measures:
        – Hospitalisation is necessary if there is massive ascites.
        – Check serum electrolytes, renal function tests at the start and twice a week.

TABLE 5.33: Examination of ascetic fluid and its interpretation.

Features	Interpretation
Gross appearance	
Clear, straw-coloured or light green	Cirrhosis, congestive heart failure and nephritic syndrome
Haemorrhagic	Malignancy, tuberculosis, pancreatitis
Cloudy, turbid	Bacterial peritonitis
Milky white (chylous)	Lymphatic obstruction
Biochemistry	
Specific gravity	• Transudates < 1.018 • Exudates > 1.018
Protein	• Transudates < 2.5 g/dL • Exudates > 2.5 g/dL
SAAG	Refer text
Glucose	Low in malignancy, tuberculosis, peritonitis
Amylase activity	> 1,000 U/L in pancreatitis
Microscopy	
Polymorphs	< 250/mm³ in cirrhosis > 250/mm³ in bacterial peritonitis
Lymphocytes	Tuberculosis, malignancy
Cytological examination	Malignancy
Special stains	
Gram's stain	Bacterial peritonitis
Ziehl–Neelsen staining	Tuberculosis
Culture	
Pyogenic bacteria	Bacterial peritonitis
Mycobacteria	Tuberculosis

(SAAG: serum ascites albumin gradient)

Box 5.20: Causes of high and low serum ascites albumin gradient.

High serum ascites albumin gradient (> 1.1 g/dL)	Low serum ascites albumin gradient (< 1.1 g/dL)
• Portal hypertension, e.g. cirrhosis of liver • Hepatic outflow obstruction • Budd–Chiari syndrome • Hepatic veno-occlusive disease • Right-sided heart failure • Constrictive pericarditis	• Peritoneal tuberculosis • Carcinoma involving peritoneal cavity • Pancreatitis • Nephrotic syndrome

---

Box 5.21: Causes of ascites according to the nature of ascitic fluid.

Straw-coloured
- Malignancy (most common cause)
- Cirrhosis
- Infective: Tuberculosis, intra-abdominal perforation
- Chronic pancreatitis
- Heart disorders: Congestive cardiac failure, constrictive pericarditis
- Hepatic vein obstruction: Budd–Chiari syndrome
- Meigs' syndrome (ovarian tumour)
- Hypoproteinaemia (e.g. nephrotic syndrome)

Chylous
- Obstruction of lymphatic duct (e.g. by carcinoma)
- Cirrhosis

Haemorrhagic
- Malignant tumours
- Ruptured ectopic pregnancy
- Trauma to abdomen
- Acute pancreatitis

- Measure abdominal girth and weight daily.
- Strict intake–output recording
- Urinary electrolyte determination
○ Bed rest alone induces diuresis in a small proportion of people because renal blood flow increases in the horizontal position, but in practice is not helpful.
○ Dietary restriction sodium by reducing sodium intake to 40 mmol in 24 hours and maintain an adequate protein and calorie intake with a palatable diet.
○ Fluid restriction to 1,000–1,500 mL/day if serum sodium is under 128 mmol/L (hyponatraemia)
○ Diuretics:
  - Aim at producing a net loss of fluid of about 700 mL/day (0.7 kg weight loss in patients with ascites alone or 1.0 kg if both ascites and peripheral oedema are present). The maximum rate at which ascites can be mobilised is 500–700 mL/day. This is to prevent diuretic-induced renal failure and/or hyponatraemia.
  - **Aldosterone antagonists:** As there is secondary hyperaldosteronism,

diuretics of first choice are aldosterone antagonists (potassium-sparing diuretics), e.g. spironolactone, triamterene and amiloride. Spironolactone—25 mg QID (100 mg daily), and gradually stepped up every week to a maximum of 400 mg/day (provided there is no hyperkalaemia). Chronic administration—gynaecomastia. Eplerenone 25 mg once daily does not produce gynaecomastia.
   - **Loop diuretics:** When a large dose of spironolactone has failed, add a loop diuretic, such as furosemide 20–40 mg or bumetanide 0.5 or 1 mg daily. Usually, spironolactone combines with furosemide. Disadvantages of loop diuretics include development of hyponatraemia, hypokalaemia and volume depletion.
   - Stop all diuretics, if severe hyponatraemia (sodium < 120 mEq/L), progressive renal failure or worsening of HE occurs.
- **Treatment of refractory ascites:**
   o **IV salt-poor albumin:** 25 g in 3 hours
   o **Large-volume paracentesis** is indicated in refractory ascites, to relieve symptomatic tense ascites, e.g. cardiorespiratory distress due to gross ascites and if there is risk of impending rupture of a hernia.
      - Complication: Hypovolaemia and renal dysfunction (post-paracentesis circulatory dysfunction) are more likely with removal of > 5 L and worse liver function.
      - Paracentesis and diuretics usually reduce ascites.
- **Shunts:**
   o Transjugular intrahepatic portosystemic shunt (TIPS): It is used for resistant ascites, if there is no spontaneous portosystemic encephalopathy and no disturbance of renal function.
   o LeVeen shunt: Peritoneovenous shunt that allows peritoneal fluid to drain directly into the internal jugular vein. Its use has been abandoned in most centres due to a high rate of blockage. It may be considered in patients with refractory ascites who cannot undergo paracentesis, or TIPS or liver transplant.
   o Side-to-side portocaval shunt
- **Complications:** Infection, thrombosis of superior vena cava, bleeding from oesophageal varices, pulmonary oedema and disseminated intravascular coagulation.
- Liver transplantation

■ SPONTANEOUS BACTERIAL PERITONITIS

- Common, severe complication of ascites characterised by spontaneous infection of ascetic fluid in the absence of a recognisable intra-abdominal source of peritonitis.
- **Causative agents:** Most commonly due to *Escherichia coli*, *Klebsiella*, enterococci, gut bacteria. Others—streptococci and enterococci.
- **Route of infection:** Infective gut flora traverse the intestine into mesenteric lymph nodes, leading to bacteraemia and seeding of ascitic fluid by haematogenous spread.
- **Clinical features:**
   o Suspected in any patient with ascites who clinically deteriorates
   o Sudden deterioration or HE in a cirrhotic patient with ascites
   o Fever, abdominal pain or discomfort, rebound abdominal tenderness
- **Investigations:**
   o Peripheral blood: Leucocytosis
   o Ascitic fluid:
      - Cloudy fluid
      - Leucocyte count: More than 500/mm^3. Neutrophil count > 250/mm^3 in ascites, alone is sufficient for diagnosis and to start treatment immediately.
      - pH: Less than 7.3
      - Culture: Positive. *E. coli* is the most common organism.
- **Diagnosis:** Diagnostic aspiration should always be performed in patients with high clinical suspicion.
- **Treatment:**
   o **Third-generation cephalosporins:** Cefotaxime, ceftazidime. Modified on the basis of culture results. Dose of Cefotaxime: 2 g IV 8 hourly for 5 days.

- Alternative therapy in patients without shock or HE
    - Amoxicillin/clavulanate (1.2 g IV 8 hourly followed by 625 mg orally)
    - Ciprofloxacin (200 mg IV 12 hourly followed by 500 mg bd orally)
    - Ofloxacin (400 mg twice daily). Quinolones avoided if norfloxacin is used for prophylaxis.
- Antibiotic therapy and albumin (1.5 g/kg body weight within 6 hours, 1 g/kg on day 3 reduces risk of type 1 HRS).
- **Prophylaxis:** Recurrence is common (70% within a year) and prophylaxis is indicated.
    - Acute GI bleed (reduces rate of rebleed): Cefotaxime/norfloxacin (400 mg BID for 7 days)
    - Previous episode of SBP and recovered: Quinolones—norfloxacin (400 mg/day)
    - Low total ascites protein content < 1.5 g/dL: Quinolones—norfloxacin (400 mg/day)
    - Severe liver disease and no prior history of SBP
    - Alternative, less effective drugs: Co-trimoxazole (800 mg sulphamethoxazole + 160 mg trimethoprim od) or ciprofloxacin (750 mg once a week).

DRUG AND LIVER

- Types of drug and toxin-induced hepatitis (**Box 5.22**):
    - **Direct toxic hepatitis:** Characterised by a predictable and dose-related toxicity, short latent period and absence of extrahepatic manifestations.
    - **Idiosyncratic drug reactions**: Characterised by unpredictable, most often dose-independent toxicity with a variable latent period and presence of extrahepatic manifestations (e.g. fever, rashes, arthralgia and eosinophilia). However, for many drugs, idiosyncratic hepatotoxicity can be dose dependent.
- **Severity**: Range from asymptomatic (raised enzymes) to chronic disease to FHF.
- **Treatment:**
    - Withdrawal of the drug/toxin
    - Supportive therapy

Clinicopathologic classification of drug-induced liver disease is given in **Table 5.34**.

Box 5.22: Common hepatotoxic drugs and toxins with associated morphologic changes.

Cholestasis
- Erythromycin estolate
- Methimazole
- Chlorpromazine
- Chlorpropamide
- Methyltestosterone
- Anabolic steroids
- Cyclosporin
- Nimesulide
- Amoxicillin/clavulanate

Toxic (necrosis)
- Paracetamol
- Carbon tetrachloride
- Mushroom (*Amanita phalloides*)
- Yellow phosphorus

Fatty liver
- Zidovudine
- Amiodarone
- Indinavir
- Ritonavir
- Methotrexate
- Tetracyclines
- Valproic acid

Granuloma
- Phenylbutazone
- Sulphonamides
- Carbamazepine
- Allopurinol
- Quinidine

Hepatitis
- Halothane
- Isoniazid
- Rifampicin
- Phenytoin
- Methyldopa
- Ibuprofen
- Ketoconazole
- Zidovudine
- Chlorothiazide

Hepatic fibrosis: Methotrexate

Chronic hepatitis
- Phenytoin
- Isoniazid

TABLE 5.34: Clinicopathologic classification of drug-induced liver disease.

Category	Description	Drugs
Hepatic adaptation	No symptoms; raised serum GGTP and ALP levels (occasionally raised ALT)	Phenytoin, warfarin
	Hyperbilirubinaemia	Rifampicin, flavaspidic acid
Dose-dependent hepatotoxicity	Symptoms of hepatitis; zonal, bridging, and massive necrosis; serum ALT level > 5-fold increased, often > 2,000 U/L	Acetaminophen, nicotinic acid, amodiaquine, hycanthone
Other cytopathic toxicity, acute steatosis	Microvesicular steatosis, diffuse or zonal; partially dose-dependent, severe liver injury, features of mitochondrial toxicity (lactic acidosis)	Valproic acid, didanosine, highly active antiretroviral therapy (HAART) agents, fialuridine, l-asparaginase, some herbal medicines
Acute hepatitis	Symptoms of hepatitis; focal, bridging, and massive necrosis; serum ALT level > 5-fold increased; extrahepatic features of drug allergy in some cases	Isoniazid, dantrolene, nitrofurantoin, halothane, sulphonamides, phenytoin, disulfiram, acebutolol, etretinate, ketoconazole, terbinafine, troglitazone
Chronic hepatitis	Duration > 3 months; interface hepatitis, bridging necrosis, fibrosis, cirrhosis; clinical and laboratory features of chronic liver disease; autoantibodies with some types of reaction	Nitrofurantoin, etretinate, diclofenac, minocycline, nefazodone
Granulomatous hepatitis	Hepatic granulomas with varying hepatitis and cholestasis; raised serum ALT, ALP, GGTP levels	Allopurinol, carbamazepine, hydralazine, quinidine, quinine
Cholestasis without hepatitis	Cholestasis, no inflammation; serum ALP levels > twice normal	Oral contraceptives, androgens
Cholestatic hepatitis	Cholestasis with inflammation; symptoms of hepatitis; raised serum ALT and AP levels	Chlorpromazine, tricyclic antidepressants, erythromycins, amoxicillin-clavulanic acid
Cholestasis with bile duct injury	Bile duct lesions and cholestatic hepatitis; clinical features of cholangitis	Chlorpromazine, flucloxacillin, dextropropoxyphene
Chronic cholestasis	Cholestasis present > 3 months	Chlorpromazine, haloperidol, erythromycin, cimetidine/ranitidine, nitrofurantoin, imipramine, azathioprine
Vanishing bile duct syndrome	Paucity of small bile ducts; resembles primary biliary cirrhosis, but AMA negative	Chlorpromazine, flucloxacillin, trimethoprim-sulphamethoxazole
Sclerosing cholangitis	Strictures of large bile ducts	Intra-arterial floxuridine, intra-lesional scolicidals
Steatohepatitis	Steatosis, focal necrosis, Mallory's hyaline, pericellular fibrosis, cirrhosis; chronic liver disease, portal hypertension	Perhexiline, amiodarone,
Vascular disorders	Sinusoidal obstruction syndrome, nodular regenerative hyperplasia, others	Contraceptive drugs, anabolic steroids, azathioprine
Tumours	Hepatocellular carcinoma, adenoma, angiosarcoma, others	Contraceptive pill, danazol

(AMA: antimitochondrial antibody; ALP: alkaline phosphatise; ALT; alanine transaminase; GGTP: gamma-glutamyl transpeptidase)

VASCULAR LIVER DISEASE

Hepatic Venous Outflow Tract Obstruction

- Obstruction to the hepatic venous outflow tract (HVOT) can occur at different levels. These include:
  - Small central hepatic veins→Veno-occlusive disease
  - Large hepatic veins→Budd-Chiari syndrome
  - Inferior vena cava (IVC)
  - Heart
- **Clinical features:** Depends on cause and on the speed with which obstruction develops. Common features are congestive hepatomegaly and ascites.

Budd–Chiari Syndrome

- Obstruction of HVOT owing to occlusion of the hepatic vein.
- Obstruction may be at any level from small hepatic veins to junction of IVC with the right atrium.
- Classically results from thrombosis of one or more hepatic veins at their openings into the IVC.
- The deleterious physiologic changes of hepatic venous obstruction are transmitted directly to the hepatic sinusoids, resulting in sinusoidal congestion, portal vein hypertension and reduced portal vein blood flow.
- The result is hepatomegaly, pain, ascites and impaired hepatic function. The ascitic fluid typically has a high SAAG.

Box 5.23 mentions various causes of Budd–Chiari syndrome.
- **Pathology:** Initially, liver shows congestion of centrilobular area with haemorrhage and central necrosis of hepatocytes. In later stages, centrilobular fibrosis develops and eventually progresses to cardiac cirrhosis.
- **Clinical features:** Triad of abdominal pain, ascites and hepatomegaly with hepatic histology showing centrilobular sinusoidal distension and pooling.
  - **Acute Budd-Chiari** follows sudden venous occlusion (e.g. by renal cell carcinoma, HCC and polycythaemia). Acute upper abdominal pain, nausea, vomiting, tender hepatomegaly, marked ascites and mild jaundice. With total venous occlusion: Delirium, coma and hepatocellular failure.
  - **Fulminant Budd-Chiari** presents with FHF in the setting of an additional predisposing factor (e.g. factor V Leiden mutation). Occurs particularly in pregnant women.
  - **Chronic Budd-Chiari:** More gradual occlusion presents with pain in the abdomen, tender hepatomegaly and gross ascites. With the enlarged caudate lobe, the liver becomes palpable. There is splenomegaly with portal hypertension; jaundice is mild or absent. Bilateral pedal oedema and distended veins over abdomen, flanks and back, with IVC obstruction, negative hepatojugular reflux, i.e.

Box 5.23: Various causes of Budd–Chiari syndrome.	
Venous thrombosis	**Compression (may also produce thrombosis)**
Hypercoagulability states: • Haematological disorders: Polycythaemia vera, paroxysmal nocturnal haemoglobinuria, antithrombin III, protein C or S deficiencies, antiphospholipid syndrome, sickle cell disease, leukaemia • Pregnancy • Use of oral contraceptive pills	• Hepatic infections • Hydatid cyst • Liver abscess • Obstruction due to tumours • Renal cell carcinoma • Adrenal tumours • Hepatocellular carcinoma • Posterior abdominal wall sarcomas
Radiation injury	**Congenital venous webs**
Trauma to the liver	**Idiopathic (40–50% of cases)**

pressure over the liver fails to fill the jugular veins. Features of cirrhosis and portal hypertension are seen in patients who survive the acute event. HCC may develop.

- **Investigations:**
  - **LFTs:** Mild hyperbilirubinaemia, raised ALP, low albumin, raised AST, ALT.
  - **Ascitic fluid examination:** High protein content (> 2.5 g/dL, i.e. exudate) in the early stages; however, this often falls later in the disease.
  - **Ultrasound:** Enlargement of caudate lobe, intrahepatic collaterals, echogenic areas, ascites. It also may show compression of the IVC, if present.
  - **Pulsed Doppler sonography:** Obliteration of hepatic veins, reversed flow or associated thrombosis in the portal vein with high accuracy. Doppler ultrasonography: Sensitivity and specificity rates > 80% and is the diagnostic procedure of first choice
  - **CT or magnetic resonance imaging (MRI):** Reveals occlusion in hepatic veins, IVC as well as diffuse abnormal parenchyma on contrast enhancement. An enlargement of the caudate lobe with independent supply of blood and venous drainage may also be seen.
  - **Hepatic venography:** It is used to determine the extent of the blockage and to estimate the caval pressures in case if CT and MRI do not demonstrate clear anatomy of the hepatic venous system.
  - **Liver biopsy:** Based on the duration of the disease, a liver biopsy is done to reveal the centrilobular congestion haemorrhage, fibrosis and cirrhosis. Other investigations: To identify a cause (e.g. blood tests and coagulation studies).
- **Differential diagnosis:** Similar clinical picture can be produced due to obstruction of IVC, right-sided cardiac failure or constrictive pericarditis. Relevant investigations should be done.
- **Management:**
  - Prevention and treatment of the predisposing factors.
  - Acute with recent thrombosis: Thrombolytic therapy—intrahepatic vein streptokinase (in very early cases of thrombosis), followed by heparin and oral anticoagulation (warfarin).
  - Short hepatic venous strictures: Treated with angioplasty.
  - Extensive hepatic vein occlusion: Insertion of a covered TIPS followed by anticoagulation may be useful in opening of the hepatic veins.
  - Ascites: Initially treated medically with low-salt diet and diuretics; the underlying cause (e.g. polycythaemia) is treated as well. If not relieved, it may be treated with surgical shunts such as LeVeen shunt and portosystemic shunts.
  - Percutaneous balloon angioplasty for membranous obstruction of the IVC and hepatic vein
  - Congenital web can be treated radiologically or resected surgically
  - Liver transplantation is indicated for chronic Budd–Chiari syndrome and for progressive liver failure, followed by lifelong anticoagulation.
- **Prognosis:** Without transplantation or shunts, acute and fulminant types have poor prognosis.

Veno-occlusive Disease

- Sinusoidal obstruction syndrome is a rare condition characterised by widespread occlusion of the small central hepatic veins.
- **Aetiology:** Develops as a complication of:
  - Total body irradiation/myeloablative regimens used before haematopoietic stem cell transplantation. It carries a high mortality.
  - Antineoplastic drugs have been implicated—gemtuzumab, ozogamicin, actinomycin D, dacarbazine, cytosine arabinoside, mithramycin and 6-thioguanine.
  - Chronic immunosuppression with azathioprine or 6-thioguanine.
  - Herbal teas made with pyrrolizidine alkaloids in Senecio and Heliotropium plants.

- Ingestion of alkaloids in inadequately winnowed wheat or in 'bush tea'.
- Hepatic irradiation.
- **Pathogenesis:**
    - Develops due to injury of the hepatic veins and presents like Budd–Chiari syndrome.
    - Characterised by obliteration and fibrosis of terminal hepatic venules.
    - Associated with circulatory obstruction due to deposition of red cells, hemosiderin-laden macrophages and coagulation factors.
- **Clinical features:** Similar to those of the Budd–Chiari syndrome. Classically, sinusoidal obstruction syndrome manifests with mild hyperbilirubinaemia (bilirubin levels > 2 mg/dL), painful hepatomegaly, weight gain of > 2% and development of ascites.
- **Investigations:**
    - Large hepatic veins appear patent radiologically.
    - Transjugular liver biopsy (with portal pressure measurements) confirms diagnosis.
    - Liver biopsy: Evidence of venous outflow obstruction
- **Treatment:** Supportive and includes control of fluid overload, ascites and hepatocellular failure. Defibrotide-Oligodeoxyribonucleotide with anti-ischaemic, antithrombotic, thrombolytic activity but minimal systemic anti-coagulant effect. Several studies have shown efficacy of defibrotide in the prevention and treatment of sinusoidal obstruction syndrome with no major toxicity.

■ HEPATOCELLULAR CARCINOMA

- Hepatocellular carcinoma is the most common primary malignancy of liver from hepatocytes or their precursors.
- Predominantly in males with a M:F ratio of 2.4:1. The number of men and number of women with HCC in the absence of cirrhosis are almost equal.
- **Aetiology:**
    - Risk factors for hepatocellular carcinoma are given in **Box 5.24**.
- **Clinical features:**
    - Usually develops in patients with underlying cirrhosis
    - **Non-specific symptoms** include ill-defined upper abdominal pain in the right hypochondrium, malaise, weakness, anorexia, fatigue, weight loss and ascites. Rapid development of these symptoms in a patient with cirrhosis is suggestive of HCC.
    - **On examination:** Liver is enlarged, irregular, nodular with pain or tenderness and friction rub or a hepatic bruit over the liver due to vascularity of tumour.
- **Paraneoplastic syndromes** associated with HCC
    - Carcinoid syndrome
    - Hypercalcaemia
    - Hypertrophic osteoarthropathy
    - Hypoglycaemia
    - Neuropathy
    - Osteoporosis
    - Polycythaemia (erythrocytosis)
    - Polymyositis
    - Porphyria
    - Sexual changes—isosexual precocity, gynaecomastia, feminisation

---

Box 5.24: Risk factors for hepatocellular carcinoma (HCC).

Major risk factors:
- Chronic hepatitis B, C
- Viruses
- Alcoholic cirrhosis
- Aflatoxin B1 (fungal toxin)
- Non-alcoholic steatohepatitis (NASH)

Minor risk factors:
- Hereditary haemochromatosis
- Wilson's disease
- Primary biliary cirrhosis
- Tyrosinaemia
- α1-AT deficiency
- Glycogen storage disease
- Hormones: Anabolic steroids, oestrogens and androgens
- Oral contraceptives
- Cigarette smoking
- Betel quid chewing
- Thorotrast and arsenic exposure
- Obesity
- Ataxia telangiectasia
- Hypercitrulinaemia

- Systemic arterial hypertension
- Thyrotoxicosis
- Thrombophlebitis migrans
- Watery diarrhoea syndrome
- **All patterns of HCCs have a strong tendency for invasion of vessels.** The portal vein and its branches are infiltrated by tumour. Occasionally, long, snake-like tumour masses may **invade the portal vein** and occlude portal circulation. Rarely tumour may invade IVC and extend into the right side of the heart through the hepatic veins. It may metastasise to the lungs.
- **Investigations:**
  - **Serum markers:**
    - **Alpha-foetoprotein:** About 50% HCC is associated with high (> 500 μg/L) or rising levels of alpha-foetoprotein. However, levels are raised in other neoplastic and non-neoplastic liver diseases and in some extrahepatic disorders.
    - **α-L-fucosidase:** It is raised in HCC and also in cirrhosis.
    - **Serum des-γ-carboxy prothrombin** is raised in a majority of HCC.
    - Serum ALP: Very high
  - **Ultrasound scans** show filling defects.
  - **CT scan** (triple-phase) or MRI abdomen
  - Blood-tinged **ascites**
  - **Hepatic artery angiography** shows 'tumour blushes.' Liver scintigraphic scans
  - **Liver aspiration or biopsy** particularly under ultrasonic guidance confirms the diagnosis. Microscopy: Consists of cells resembling hepatocytes.
- **Prevention:** Widespread vaccination against HBV.
- **Management:** Treatment is different for patients with cirrhosis and those without. Therapy depends on tumour size, multicentricity, extent of liver disease (Child–Pugh score) and performance status.
  - **Surgical resection:** Indicated when lesions 1–3 in number, < 5 cm in size; without metastasis; with Child score A. Local or segmental resections are preferred to major resections. After successful resection, tumour recurs in the cirrhotic liver in about 70% of patients after 5 years.
  - **Non-surgical therapy:** Majority of patients are diagnosed at an advanced stage of HCC and cannot be treated by surgical resection.
    - **Local ablation strategies:**
      - **Radiofrequency ablation (RFA):** Uses heat to kill tumour cells. A single electrode inserted into the tumour under CT or ultrasound guidance.
      - **Trans arterial embolisation (TAE):** Hepatic artery embolisation with Gelfoam and doxorubicin
      - **Transarterial chemoembolisation (TACE):** With drugs such as doxorubicin but is contraindicated in decompensated cirrhosis and when HCC is multifocal.
    - **Local injection therapy:** Percutaneous ethanol injection (PEI) or percutaneous acetic acid injection (PAI). It not only causes direct destruction of tumour cells, but also destroy normal cells in the vicinity. It usually requires multiple injections (average three) and the maximum size of tumour treated is 3 cm.
    - Conventional chemotherapy and radiotherapy are unsuccessful.
    - Chemotherapy using IV **sorafenib**: This drug is a multikinase inhibitor with activity against Raf, vascular endothelial growth factor (VEGF) and platelet-derived growth factor (PDGF) signalling.
- **Liver transplantation:** Indicated in presence of localised tumour and underlying advanced liver disease. Unfortunately, the underlying liver disease (e.g. hepatitis B and C) may recur in the transplanted liver.
- **Prognosis:** Depends on the size of the tumour, the extent of spread (e.g. presence of vascular invasion) and liver function in those with cirrhosis.

LIVER TRANSPLANTATION

- Useful in treating patient with end-stage liver disease or acute/fulminant liver failure, and 5-year survival rate in good centres is about 75%.

- **Split livers:** In which one liver is used for two recipients. It is helpful in tackling organ shortage and in shortening the time on the waiting list.
- **Orthotopic liver transplantation:** Most common form of liver transplantation. Orthotopic means that the graft is placed in its correct anatomical location. In this technique, the donor organ after removal of the native organ is transplanted in the same anatomic location.
- **Auxiliary orthotopic transplantation (APOLT):** A segment of donor liver is transplanted in a recipient who has undergone hemihepatectomy to make room for the graft.
  - *Advantages:* If the donor's liver fails, the recipient's own organ can function as a backup until a new liver is found. It can be used as a temporary measure in fulminant liver failure, where the recipient's liver has the potential of regeneration and full functional recovery. This avoids life-long immunosuppression and the liver graft can be allowed to undergo atrophy or may be surgically removed.
  - *Disadvantages:* Not appropriate in patients having cirrhosis or where there is a risk of hepatic malignancy (e.g. tyrosinaemia, multicentric HCC).
- **Living donor liver transplantation:** In this technique, a portion of a healthy person's liver is removed and used for transplantation. The donor of the liver segment is a first-degree living relative.
- **Bioartificial liver:** Cultured hepatocytes are used in patients with acute liver failure till the donor liver becomes available.
- **Immunosuppressive treatment:** Corticosteroids along with tacrolimus or cyclosporine are used.

Indications and contraindications of liver transplantation are given in **Boxes 5.25** and **5.26**, respectively.

Complications of liver transplantation are given in **Box 5.27**.

PYOGENIC LIVER ABSCESS (BACTERIAL LIVER ABSCESS)

- Uncommon
- **Aetiology:**
  - Commonly liver abscesses are caused by echinococcal, amoebic infections; less commonly—other protozoans and helminths.
  - Bacterial infections in the liver may be manifest as pyogenic abscess. Develop

---

Box 5.25: Indications of liver transplantation.

Causes of cirrhosis:
- Chronic viral hepatitis C and B
- Alcoholic liver disease
- Non-alcoholic steatohepatitis
- Autoimmune diseases
- Primary biliary cirrhosis

Acute/fulminant liver failure:
- Seronegative hepatitis
- Drug-induced liver injury

In children:
- Biliary atresia
- Inborn errors of metabolism:
- Wilson's disease
  - Glycogen storage diseases
  - Crigler–Najjar syndrome type I
  - Familial hypercholesterolaemia
- α1-AT deficiency

Failure of previous liver transplant

Complications of cirrhosis:
- Ascites
- Portal hypertensive gastropathy, refractory variceal haemorrhage
- Encephalopathy
- Synthetic dysfunction

Hepatocellular carcinoma:
- No single lesion > 5 cm or no more than three lesions with the largest being 3 cm or smaller

Liver-based metabolic conditions:
- Alpha-1-antitrypsin deficiency
- Familial amyloidosis
- Glycogen storage disease
- Primary oxaluria
- Tyrosaemia
- Urea cycle enzyme deficiencies
- Wilson's disease

Hepatopulmonary syndrome

Portopulmonary hypertension

> **Box 5.26: Contraindications of liver transplantation.**
>
> | Absolute | Relative |
> |---|---|
> | *Expected outcome is poor:* | *Co-morbidities with potential to reduce survival:* |
> | • Multi-system organ failure | • Renal insufficiency |
> | • Extrahepatic/extra-biliary malignancy, infection | • Primary hepatobiliary malignancy > 5 cm, haemochromatosis |
> | • Advanced cardiac or pulmonary disease | • Spontaneous bacterial peritonitis |
> | • Human immunodeficiency virus infection | • Age older than 65 years, poor social support |
> | • Active alcohol or illicit substance abuse | • Inability to comply with immunosuppressants |

> **Box 5.27: Complications of liver transplantation.**
>
> **Hepatic complications:**
> - Reperfusion injury—graft failure due to ischaemia
> - Acute graft rejection
> - Surgical complications—failure or obstruction of biliary anastomosis
> - Chronic graft rejection
> - Recurrent disease
> - Infection and drug-induced liver injury
> - Jaundice
>
> **Non-hepatic complications:**
> - Infections/sepsis
> - Fluid overload
> - Renal dysfunction
> - Intraperitoneal bleed

as a complication of a bacterial infection elsewhere. Commonly—*E. coli*. *Streptococcus milleri* and *Bacteroides*. Others—*Enterococcus faecalis*, *Proteus vulgaris*, *Staphylococcus aureus*. Often mixed infection.

- **Route of infection:**
  - **Portal vein:** Intra-abdominal infections (appendicitis, diverticulitis, colitis, perforated bowel)
  - **Arterial blood supply:** During systemic bacteraemia, organism may reach liver via hepatic artery
  - **Ascending infection** in the biliary tract (ascending cholangitis)
  - **Direct invasion of the liver** from a nearby source (e.g. subphrenic abscess, perinephric abscess) or a penetrating injury
- **Clinical features:**
  - Fever, chills, rigors
  - Right upper quadrant pain radiating to the right shoulder
  - Weight loss, anorexia
  - Nausea and vomiting
  - Pleuritic chest pain
  - Tender hepatomegaly
  - Mild jaundice if there is extra hepatic biliary obstruction.
  - Respiratory findings at the base of the right lung -pleural effusion, crepitations or a pleural rub.
- **Investigations:** Patients who are not acutely ill, often diagnosed as pyrexia of unknown origin.
  - **Serum bilirubin:** Raised in 25% of cases
  - **Serum ALP:** Markedly elevated
  - **Blood cultures:** Positive in only 30% of cases
  - **Normochromic normocytic anaemia** with polymorphonuclear leucocytosis
  - **ESR and CRP** are often raised.
  - **Chest radiograph**: Elevation of right dome of diaphragm, and in severe cases right basilar atelectasis and pneumonia or effusion.
  - **Ultrasonography:** Confirms the diagnosis
  - **CT scan of abdomen**: Helpful when ultrasound is normal
  - **Needle aspiration** of pus for culture and sensitivity
- **Management:**
  - **Antibiotics:** Initiate treatment with antibiotics (combination of ampicillin, gentamicin and metronidazole) to cover gram-positive, gram-negative and anaerobic organisms till the causative organism is identified. Later, change the antibiotic according to the culture and sensitivity reports. Duration of treatment is 4–8 weeks.
  - **Ultrasound-guided aspiration of the abscess:** Indications include:
    - Large abscess (> 6 cm)

- Abscess in the left lobe
- Lack of response within 48–72 hours of medical therapy
- Ultrasonography is suggestive of large abscess impending rupture.
  o **Surgical drainage** via a large-bore needle for those who fail to respond
  o Treat the underlying cause.

■ AMOEBIC LIVER ABSCESS

- Most common extraintestinal complication of amoebic dysentery.
- *Entamoeba histolytica*: Carried from the bowel to the liver in the portal venous system with the development of multiple microabscesses and eventually single or multiple large abscesses.
- Amoebic abscess ranges from 8 to 12 cm in diameter, well circumscribed. Cavity contains thick, dark material that has been linked to anchovy sauce.
- **Clinical features:**
  o Symptoms are similar to pyogenic abscesses (such as fever, anorexia, weight loss and malaise).
  o Onset is usually gradual but may be sudden.
  o Past history of dysentery. Jaundice is rare.
  o On examination, patient looks ill, tender hepatomegaly and signs of an effusion or consolidation in the base of the right side of the chest.
  o Rare complications: Intraperitoneal, intrathoracic or pericardial rupture and multiorgan failure.
- **Investigations:** These are same as for pyogenic abscess, plus:
  o **Serological tests** for amoeba [e.g. haemagglutination, amoebic complement fixation test, enzyme-linked immunosorbent assay (ELISA)].
  o **Diagnostic aspiration** of abscess: Anchovy sauce.
- **Treatment:**
  o Metronidazole, 750 mg tid for 7–10 days orally or IV, or tinidazole, 2 g orally for 3 days, followed by iodoquinol, 650 mg orally tid for 20 days; diloxanide furoate, 500 mg orally tid for 10 days; or aminosidine (paromomycin) 25–35 mg/kg/day orally in three divided doses for 7–10 days
  o If an amoebic abscess continues to grow, it may rupture into the peritoneal cavity, where it produces peritonitis, a complication associated with a mortality rate as high as 40%. The amoebae may also invade the blood, in which case abscesses of the brain and lung may ensue.

■ IRON OVERLOAD

Classification of iron overload is given in **Box 5.28**.
- **In secondary** iron overload, iron accumulates in Kupffer cells rather than hepatocytes compared to that of hereditary haemochromatosis.

Hereditary Haemochromatosis

- Inherited disease characterised by abnormal (excessive) accumulation of iron in various parenchymal organs leading to eventual fibrosis and functional organ failure
- In symptomatic patients, total body iron is 20–40 g, compared to 3–4 g in a normal individual.

Box 5.28: Classification of iron overload.

Hereditary
- Mutations of genes encoding HFE, transferrin receptor 2 (TfR2) or hepcidin
- Mutations of genes encoding haemojuvelin (HJV)

Haemosiderosis (secondary haemochromatosis)
- Parenteral iron overload
- Exogenous: Multiple blood transfusions, repeated iron injections, long-term haemodialysis
- Endogenous: Sickle cell disease
- Increased oral intake of iron
- Ineffective erythropoiesis, increased erythroid activity: β-thalassaemia, sideroblastic anaemia, porphyria
- Chronic liver disease: Chronic alcoholic liver disease

- Associated with high incidence of HCC
- **Aetiology:**
  - *HFE* gene (chromosome 6) regulates intestinal absorption of dietary iron. *HFE* gene product along with proteins hemojuvelin (HJV) and transferrin receptor 2 (TfR2) regulate iron metabolism through hepcidin. Hepcidin synthesised in the liver is the central regulator of iron homeostasis. It controls iron absorption and storage. When hepcidin levels rise, iron gets stored within enterocytes forming mucosal ferritin and is shed with the cells.
  - **Mutations in HJV, TfR2** and **HFE** lead to absence of hepcidin, causing absorption of iron even when there is substantial **elevation of body iron stores.** The free iron produces reactive oxygen metabolites which cause cell injury and fibrosis.
  - Most are inherited as autosomal recessive genetic disorders, associated with HLA-B3, B7 and B14 histocompatibility antigens.
  - About 90% patients—males. Unlikely in females due to loss of iron—menstruation and pregnancy.
- **Pathology:** Excess iron is deposited in liver, joint, heart, pancreas, endocrine glands and skin.
- **Clinical features:**
  - Develop due to toxic damage of cells by accumulated iron and consequent fibrosis
  - Muscle aches, weakness, abdominal and/or joint pain
  - **Classic triad:** Bronze skin pigmentation (melanin deposition in exposed parts, axillae, groin, genitalia), hepatomegaly, diabetes mellitus (bronzed diabetes) in patients with gross iron overload.
  - **Late features:** Loss of libido, testicular atrophy, cardiac complaints (heart failure and cardiac arrhythmias), hepatosplenomegaly, spiders, loss of body hair, jaundice and ascites.
  - Cirrhosis (disease and scarring of the liver)
  - **Cardiac manifestations:** Heart failure, arrhythmias are in younger patients. Hypogonadism, related to involvement of pituitary gland and genitalia
- **Complications:** Chondrocalcinosis (asymmetrical deposition of calcium pyrophosphate in both large and small joints and leads to an arthropathy), HCC, multiorgan failure.
- **Investigations:**
  - **Serum iron profile:**
    - **Serum iron** is elevated (> 30 μmol/L).
    - **Total iron binding capacity (TIBC):** Reduced
    - **Transferrin saturation of > 45%:** Highly sensitive for diagnosis
    - **Serum ferritin** is elevated (usually > 500 μg/L or 240 nmol/L): Less sensitive than transferring saturation in screening for haemochromatosis because it is also increased in alcoholic liver disease, hepatitis C infection, NASH
- Acute phase reactant are increased in other inflammatory and neoplastic conditions.
  - **Biochemical tests for liver function are** often normal, even with established cirrhosis.
  - **Genetic testing:** Is performed if iron studies are abnormal.
  - **CT scan:** Shows increased density of liver due to deposits of iron.
  - **MRI:** Sensitive to detect liver iron content
  - **Liver biopsy:** Shows iron deposition and hepatic fibrosis leading on to cirrhosis
- **Screening:** All first-degree family members of hereditary haemochromatosis must be screened to detect early and asymptomatic disease.
- **Diagnosis:** The association of hepatomegaly, skin pigmentation, diabetes mellitus, heart disease, arthritis and hypogonadism suggests the diagnosis. However, significant iron overload may exist without or with only few of these manifestations; a high index of suspicion is necessary for early diagnosis.
- **Management:** Started before permanent organ damage occurs due to iron toxicity. Excess iron should be removed as rapidly as possible and prolongs life and may reverse tissue damage.
  - **Venesection:** Venesection of 500 mL blood (removes 250 mg of iron) is performed twice weekly until the serum iron is normal. Takes 2 years or more.

Thereafter, reaccumulation of iron can be prevented by three or four venesections per year to keep the serum ferritin normal range. Blood removed can be utilised for routine transfusion.
- **Chelation therapy:** Rarely in patients who cannot tolerate venesection because of severe cardiac disease or anaemia, chelation therapy with desferrioxamine (40–80 mg/kg/day subcutaneously) can be used. It removes about 10–20 mg of iron/day.
- Treatment of diabetes, congestive heart failure and cardiac arrhythmias
- Treatment of cirrhosis: There is a risk of malignancy if cirrhosis is present.

WILSON'S DISEASE (HEPATOLENTICULAR DEGENERATION)

- **Normal copper metabolism:** Copper in the diet is absorbed from the stomach and upper small intestine and is transported to the liver, loosely bound to albumin in the blood. In the liver, copper is incorporated into proceruloplasmin and forms ceruloplasmin (a glycoprotein synthesised in the liver) and secreted into the blood. Remaining copper is excreted in the bile and excreted in stool.
- **Wilson's disease** is a very rare inborn error of copper metabolism characterised by increased total body copper.
- Excess copper gets deposited in the liver, basal ganglia of the brain, cornea, kidneys and skeleton.
- It is a potentially treatable condition.
- Excessive accumulation of copper in the body due to failure of incorporation of copper into proceruloplasmin leads to low serum ceruloplasmin and failure of biliary copper excretion, causing its accumulation in the body.
- **Aetiology:** Autosomal recessive disorder due to a molecular defect within a copper-transporting ATPase encoded by a gene (*ATP7B*) located on chromosome 13. More than 300 mutations have been identified. Rare in India and Asia. Consanguinity is risk factor.
- **Pathology:** Microscopic features are non-diagnostic and differ from those of chronic hepatitis to macronodular cirrhosis. Stains for copper are suggestive of periportal distribution of copper.
- **Clinical features:**
  - **Presents** between 5 and 30 years. Children with hepatic problems. Young adults with more neurological problems
  - **Liver involvement:** Varies from acute hepatitis, FHF, chronic hepatitis to cirrhosis.
  - **Brain involvement:** Tremor, dysarthria, involuntary movements (especially resting and intention tremors, wing beating), eventually dementia.
  - **Psychiatric manifestations:** Phobia, depression, compulsive behaviour
  - **Features of eye involvement:** Kayser–Fleischer rings:
    - Characteristic sign due to deposition of copper in Descemet's membrane of cornea.
    - Greenish-brown or golden-brown ring at the corneo-scleral junction, appearing first at the upper periphery, best identified by slit-lamp examination.
    - Absent in young children and disappears with treatment
    - May be associated with 'sunflower cataracts'.
    - Not specific for Wilson's disease; found occasionally with other types of chronic liver disease, with a prominent cholestatic component, such as primary biliary cirrhosis, primary sclerosing cholangitis or familial cholestatic syndromes.
  - **Other manifestations:** Renal tubular damage, osteoporosis, arthropathy.
- **Investigations:**
  - **Slit-lamp examination** of the eyes for Kayser–Fleischer ring
  - **Serum copper:** Reduced but can be normal
  - **Serum ceruloplasmin levels:** Low and < 29 mg/dL.
  - **Urinary copper:** Increased 100–1,000 µg in 24 hours (1.6–16 µmol)
  - **Liver biopsy:** Diagnosis dependent on amount of copper in liver (> 250 µg/g dry weight)
  - **Haemolysis and anaemia** may be found.

- **Treatment and management:** Started early, improvement seen clinically and biochemically.
  - **Chelating drugs:**
    - Penicillamine: Pyridoxine (1–1.5 g daily) should be given lifetime which effectively chelates copper.
    - Asymptomatic cases, maintenance therapy (after maximal improvement with penicillamine): Trientine dihydrochloride—in the dose of 1.2–1.8 g/day. Zinc acetate: Dose 150 mg/day; blocks absorption of copper from intestine. However, it should not be administered with penicillamine or trientine as both chelate zinc.
  - For severe neurologic involvement: Patients who do not improve with penicillamine or trientine may be treated with (1) IM dimercaprol or (2) ammonium tetrathiomolybdate.
  - **Liver transplantation:** In FHF and decompensated/advanced cirrhosis
  - All siblings and children of the patient should be screened for Wilson's disease and treated even if they are asymptomatic and if there is evidence of copper accumulation.

ALPHA-1-ANTITRYPSIN DEFECIENCY

- Alpha-1 antitrypsin—serum acute-phase protein with alpha mobility on electrophoresis.
- Normally synthesised by liver and immediately secreted into the blood. Forms 90% of serum α_1-globulin seen on electrophoresis.
- It is a protease inhibitor (P_i) with antiproteolytic properties that inactivate the proteases (trypsin) released by active neutrophils; prevents breakdown of elastin and collagen by proteases.
- The gene is located on chromosome 14.
- There are three genetic variants of α1-AT characterised by their electrophoretic mobilities as medium (M), slow (S) or very slow (Z).
- Several phenotypes occur in the population: Normal phenotype is MM (PiMM). Heterozygotes are PiMZ and PiSZ. Abnormal phenotype most often causing clinical disease is ZZ (PiZZ), where the glycoprotein is misfolded and cannot be secreted from the liver cells.
- It is associated with cirrhosis and pulmonary emphysema especially in smokers, due to unopposed action of neutrophil enzymes damaging alveolar walls.
- **Clinical features:**
  - In neonates, the deficiency of α1-AT produces cholestatic jaundice.
  - In adults:
    - Liver: Chronic hepatitis, cirrhosis, HCC and cholangiocarcinoma
    - Lung: Emphysema and chronic bronchitis
    - Others: Panniculitis, vasculitis, pancreatitis, glomerulonephritis
- **Investigations:**
  - Serum α1-AT is low (normal above 150 mg/dL).
  - Serum protein electrophoresis shows absence of α-1-globulin peak.
  - Liver biopsy: α1-AT accumulates in periportal hepatocytes and can be seen periodic acid–Schiff (PAS)-positive, diastase-resistant globular inclusions in these hepatocytes. The injury to these hepatocytes results in progressive fibrosis and cirrhosis.
- **Treatment:** No treatment apart from dealing with the complications of liver disease. Stop cigarette smoking and alcohol intake. Liver or lung transplantation.

BILIARY CIRRHOSIS

- Cirrhosis secondary to prolonged obstruction of biliary system (between the small interlobular bile ducts and the papilla of Vater). Obstruction results in progressive destruction of bile ducts.
- Subdivided into **primary biliary cirrhosis** and **secondary biliary cirrhosis.**

Primary Biliary Cirrhosis

- Progressive chronic autoimmune liver disease characterised by non-suppurative, inflammatory destruction of small intrahepatic bile ducts (cholangitis), eventually leading to cirrhosis.

- Early lesions are inflammatory, true cirrhosis develops several years after the onset of disease. Most patients are diagnosed at a pre-cirrhotic stage.
- Destruction of bile ducts leads to impaired secretion of bile, cholestasis and inflammatory reaction in the portal tract. This results in hepatic damage, fibrosis and ends up in cirrhosis and liver failure.
- **Gender:** It usually affects middle-aged women, with a female to male ratio of > 6:1.
- **Aetiology and pathogenesis:**
    - May be **autoimmune**, but exact pathogenesis is unknown. It may be due to an environmental factor acting on a genetically predisposed individual via molecular mimicry to initiate autoimmunity.
    - Many mechanisms have been proposed for destruction of intrahepatic bile ducts.
    - Aberrant expression of major histocompatibility complex (MHC) class II molecules on bile duct epithelial cells, but it is not known whether this expression is the cause or result of the inflammatory response.
    - Impaired cell-mediated immunity: Accumulation of autoreactive cytotoxic $CD4^+$ and $CD8^+$ T lymphocytes around bile ducts and directly produce damage to the biliary epithelium.
- **Autoantibodies:**
    - **Serum AMA:** To hepatocytes—specific to PBC, found in almost all patients. Target E2 component of the pyruvate dehydrogenase complex titres are unrelated to clinical or microscopic appearance and its role in pathogenesis is unclear. Specific T cells are also detected in these patients, supporting immune-mediated pathogenesis.
    - **Antibodies against nuclear antigens:** Anti-glycoprotein-210 is observed in about 50% of patients and correlate with progression towards liver failure.
- **Pathology:** Three distinct stages: **Small-duct** inflammation destroying the interlobular bile ducts, **biliary fibrosis**/scarring and **cirrhosis**. It is a focal and variable disease, showing different degrees of severity in different portions of the liver.
- **Clinical features:** Insidious onset, asymptomatic in some (**Box 5.29**)
- **Investigations:**
    - **AMA:** Characteristic, essential for the diagnosis. Apart from the M2 antibodies which are normally found in 90–95% of patients, other non-specific antibodies—antinuclear factor and smooth muscle may also be present.

Box 5.29: Clinical features of biliary cirrhosis.

General: Pruritus (earliest symptom), fatigue, skin pigmentation (melanin), abdominal discomfort

Liver involvement	Hypercholesterolaemia	Malabsorption
• Intense pruritus (bile salts): Much before jaundice, more at night. Scratch marks	• Xanthelasmas (cholesterol-rich macrophages) around the eyes	• Steatorrhoea, diarrhoea: Fat malabsorption
• Progressive jaundice	• Xanthomas over joints, tendons, hand creases, elbows and knees	• Easy bruising, ecchymosis—vitamin K deficiency
• Patient acquires a 'bottle green colour'		• Night blindness due to vitamin A deficiency
• Clubbing of fingers	• Pain, tingling, numbness over feet and hands—peripheral neuropathy (lipid infiltration of peripheral nerves)	• Dermatitis due to vitamin E deficiency
• Hepatosplenomegaly		• Osteomalacia and/or osteoporosis due to malabsorption of vitamin D
• Hepatic decompensation, portal hypertension, ascites and variceal bleeding develop		

Extrahepatic manifestations: These include autoimmune disorders such as Sjögren syndrome, keratoconjunctivitis sicca (dry eyes and mouth), systemic sclerosis, autoimmune thyroiditis, rheumatoid arthritis, Raynaud phenomenon, membranous glomerulonephritis and celiac disease

- Marked rise of serum 5'-nucleotidase activity. **High serum ALP** (2–5-fold rise) Mild elevation of transaminases
- **Serum cholesterol** is raised. **Hyperlipidaemia** is present.
- **Hyperbilirubinaemia** of the conjugated type occurs in late stage.
- Possible high levels of **serum IgM**
- **Ultrasound:** Shows mild changes in liver architecture.
- **MRCP (or ERCP):** Reveals normal biliary tree
- **Liver biopsy:** Portal tract infiltration by lymphocytes and plasma cells and about 40% have granulomas. Later portal tract fibrosis and eventually progress to cirrhosis.
- **Hepatic granulomas:** Not specific, found in sarcoidosis, tuberculosis, schistosomiasis, drug reactions, brucellosis, parasitic infestation (e.g. strongyloidiasis) and other conditions.
- **Management/treatment:**
  - **Ursodeoxycholic acid (10–15 mg/kg):** Improves levels of bilirubin and aminotransferase alters composition of bile to become less toxic for the injured biliary epithelium, reducing the retention of bile acids in hepatocytes and inhibiting bile-induced apoptosis of hepatocytes. It should be started early in the asymptomatic phase.
  - **Steroids:** Show biochemical and histological improvement of disease but indice risk of osteoporosis
  - **Other therapies:** Azathioprine, colchicine, methotrexate and cyclosporine may be beneficial.
  - **Steatorrhoea:** Reduced fat intake of fat, substitute long-chain with medium-chain triglycerides.
  - Supplementing vitamins A, D and K with monthly injections (calciferol 1 mg/day), bisphosphonates (e.g. alendronate) for osteoporosis, calcium supplementation
  - Pruritus is difficult to control but following can be helpful: Cholestyramine (4 g sachet tid), but is unpalatable, antihistamines, rifampicin, naloxone hydrochloride, ondansetron and opiate antagonists (naloxone and naltrexone).
  - Liver transplantation
- **Complications:** Cirrhosis, osteoporosis and osteomalacia, polyneuropathy, increased risk of HCCs
- **Cause of death:** Liver failure, massive haemorrhage—oesophageal varices and intercurrent infection.

Secondary Biliary Cirrhosis

- Cirrhosis developing secondary to prolonged obstruction of the extrahepatic biliary tree
- **Causes:** Gallstones, bile duct strictures, sclerosing cholangitis, malignant tumours of bile duct or pancreas rarely survive long enough to develop secondary biliary cirrhosis.
- **Clinical features:**
  - **Gall stones:** Recurrent abdominal pain, fluctuating jaundice
  - **Bile duct strictures:** History of previous abdominal surgery
  - **Sclerosing cholangitis:** Chronic cholestasis with episodes of ascending cholangitis, right upper quadrant pain.
  - **Late features:** Cirrhosis, ascites and portal hypertension
- **Investigations:**
  - Serum bilirubin: Conjugated hyperbilirubinaemia
  - Serum ALP: Markedly raised
  - Ultrasound and CT of abdomen
  - ERCP or PTC: Outlines the ducts
  - Liver biopsy
- **Treatment:** Relief of biliary obstruction by ERCP or surgery, antibiotics in sclerosing cholangitis

■ CARDIAC CIRRHOSIS

- **Cause:** Damage primarily due to congestion may develop in all types of right heart failure.
- **Mechanism:**
  - Right heart failure causes retrograde transmission of raised venous pressure via the IVC and hepatic vein into the liver, leading to passive congestion of liver.

- When passive venous congestion becomes chronic/ prolonged, the liver becomes enlarged, tender and shows a 'nutmeg appearance' (alternating red—congested and pale—fibrotic areas).
- Very rarely, prolonged, severe right-sided heart failure and hepatic congestion cause cardiac cirrhosis.
- **Clinical features** are usually dominated by the heart disease, and features of severe right heart failure
- **Diagnosis:**
  - Firm enlarged liver with signs of chronic liver disease in a patient with valvular heart disease, constrictive pericarditis or chronic cor pulmonale
  - Non-pulsatile liver despite the presence of tricuspid regurgitation
  - Liver biopsy confirms the diagnosis (not required in most cases)
- **Treatment** of the underlying cardiovascular disorder

NON-CIRRHOTIC PORTAL FIBROSIS

- Non-cirrhotic portal fibrosis (NCPF) is an idiopathic disease characterised by periportal fibrosis, involving small and medium branches of portal vein.
- Causes development of portal hypertension and splenomegaly without features of liver cell failure
- **Aetiology:** Bacterial infections, exposure to toxins, immunological abnormalities and hypercoagulable states may play role.
- **Clinical features:** Upper GI bleed, massive splenomegaly with anaemia with preserved liver function. Ascites, jaundice and HE are uncommon.
- **Investigations:**
  - **LFTs:** Usually normal.
  - **Peripheral blood:** Pancytopaenia may develop due to hypersplenism.
  - **Doppler ultrasound:** Shows patent splenoportal axis and hepatic veins
  - **Splenoportovenography (SPV):** Reveals massive dilatation of the portal and splenic veins, and the presence of collaterals.
  - **Liver biopsy:** Lobular architecture maintained, portal fibrosis of variable degree, sclerosis and obliteration of small-sized portal vein radicals.
- **Diagnosis:** NCPF is to be considered in patients with no evidence of cirrhosis or extrahepatic portal vein obstruction.
- **Treatment:** Endoscopic sclerotherapy or banding to prevent variceal bleed and shunt surgery

LIVER MISCELLANEOUS

Bilirubin Metabolism

Bilirubin Production

Sources

- **Major** (85%): Catabolism of **haemoglobin** from breakdown of senescent red cells in the Kupffer cells of the liver and in the reticuloendothelial system.
- **Minor:** Degradation of other haeme-containing proteins (cytochromes, myoglobin, catalases) and premature destruction of red cell precursors in bone marrow

Bilirubin Formation

- Haeme liberated is oxidised to **biliverdin** by haeme oxygenase.
- Biliverdin is immediately reduced to **bilirubin** by the enzyme biliverdin reductase. The bilirubin formed is known as unconjugated bilirubin.

Transport of Bilirubin/Bilirubin Binding

- Unconjugated bilirubin formed in the periphery is liberated into the circulation and reversibly binds to serum albumin (albumin–bilirubin complex) in the plasma.
- Unconjugated bilirubin is insoluble in aqueous solutions at physiologic pH.
- The unconjugated bilirubin is **transported to the liver** in plasma.

Hepatic Processing of Bilirubin

Hepatic Uptake from the Circulation

- On reaching the sinusoidal plasma membrane of the hepatocyte, the unconjugated bilirubin (albumin-bilirubin complex) is dissociated and the unconjugated bilirubin enters the hepatocytes.

Binding
- Within the hepatocyte, bilirubin binds to several proteins in the cytosol known collectively as glutathione-S-transferases (formally termed ligandin).

Conjugation with Glucuronic Acid
- In the hepatocyte, **unconjugated bilirubin** (not water-soluble) combines with one or two molecules of glucuronic acid in the presence of uridine diphosphate (UDP)–glucuronyl-transferase (UGT1A1) and forms **water-soluble bilirubin diglucuronide (conjugated bilirubin)**.
- Two-step process: Formation of bilirubin monoglucuronide and then bilirubin diglucuronide.

Biliary Excretion/Secretion
- Conjugated bilirubin is water-soluble and actively secreted into bile canaliculi, is excreted into bile and reaches the small intestine.

Intestinal Phase of Bilirubin Metabolism
- In the intestine, conjugated bilirubin (bilirubin diglucuronide and bilirubin monoglucuronide) as such is not reabsorbed by the intestinal mucosa because of its large molecular size.
- In the terminal ileum, bacterial enzymes (β-glucuronidases) hydrolyse the conjugated bilirubin, releasing free bilirubin, which is then reduced to colourless urobilinogen.
- **Excretion of urobilinogen:** Most (80%) of it is excreted in stools as stercobilinogen (responsible for normal colour of the stool).
- In obstructive jaundice stercobilinogen is absent in the stool, and hence stools are pale, or clay coloured
- **Reabsorption of urobilinogen:** About 20% is absorbed by terminal ileum, passes into liver via enterohepatic circulation and is re-excreted into the bile.
- Small amount of the bound form enters systemic circulation and is excreted in the urine as urobilinogen. In obstructive jaundice, it is absent in urine. In hepatocellular and haemolytic jaundice, it is markedly increased.

Renal Excretion of Bilirubin
- Normal individuals—no urine bilirubin. Unconjugated bilirubin is tightly bound to albumin; cannot be filtered by glomeruli, not excreted in the urine.
- Unconjugated hyperbilirubinaemia—acholuric jaundice.
- About 5% of conjugated bilirubin is less tightly bound to albumin; a smaller fraction unbound, can be filtered by glomeruli and appears in the urine (bilirubinuria). In conjugated hyperbilirubinaemia, bilirubin appears in the urine (obstructive jaundice).

Van Den Bergh Reaction
- Measures the levels of conjugated and unconjugated bilirubin in the blood.
- Unconjugated bilirubin requires the presence of alcohol for the reaction while conjugated bilirubin reacts directly without alcohol.
- Hence conjugated bilirubin—direct bilirubin and unconjugated bilirubin—indirect bilirubin.

■ ALCOHOLIC LIVER DISEASE
- Chronic and excessive consumption of alcohol can produce a wide spectrum of liver disease—fatty liver, alcoholic hepatitis and alcoholic cirrhosis (**Table 5.35**).
- Effects of alcohol are worse in women compared to men. For women, values should be reduced by 50%.

Alcoholic Fatty Liver
- **Clinical features:**
    - Asymptomatic or may present with discomfort in right upper quadrant, nausea and jaundice
    - Hepatomegaly
    - Progression to cirrhosis not common

TABLE 5.35: Amount of alcohol consumption and its associated risk of alcoholic liver disease in male.

Amount of ingestion per day	Degree of risk
160 g ethanol (20 single drinks)	High
80 g ethanol (10 single drinks)	Medium
40 g ethanol (5 single drinks)	Low

- **Investigations:**
  - **Biochemical findings:** Moderate elevations of AST and ALT. GGT level is a sensitive test to determine whether the individual is taking alcohol
  - **Ultrasound or CT:** Demonstrates fatty liver
  - **Liver biopsy:** Shows accumulation of fat in perivenular hepatocytes and later in entire hepatic lobule.
- Cessation of alcohol consumption results in normalisation of biochemical findings and histological changes.

Alcoholic Hepatitis

- **Clinical features:**
  - May be asymptomatic or present with fever, rapid onset of jaundice, abdominal discomfort and proximal muscle wasting
  - Portal hypertension, ascites and bleeding due to oesophageal varices can occur without cirrhosis
  - Hepatomegaly
- **Investigations:**
  - **Biochemical findings:**
    - Serum aminotransferase (AST and ALT) raised to 2–7 times of normal (usually < 400 IU)
    - AST:ALT ratio is > 1 (generally > 2). Mildly elevated serum ALP
    - Raised bilirubin
    - Decreased albumin
  - **Haematological findings:** Prolonged PT and leucocytosis
  - **Liver biopsy:** Ballooning degeneration of hepatocytes with leucocyte infiltration. Mallory bodies often seen.
- **Prognosis:**
  - Variable. Despite abstinence, disease progresses in many. Conversely, a few patients continue to drink heavily without developing cirrhosis.
  - Mortality high in patients with severe alcoholic hepatitis
  - **Poor prognostic factors:**
    - PT > 5 seconds of control
    - Anaemia
    - Albumin < 2.5 g/dL
    - Serum bilirubin > 8 mg/dL
    - Progressive encephalopathy
    - Renal failure
    - Presence of ascites
    - Maddrey discriminant function > 32
- **Treatment:**
  - Advised to stop alcohol consumption for life, because this is a pre-cirrhotic condition
  - Severe hepatitis needs bed rest.
  - Nutrition: Feeding via a fine-bore NGT or sometimes intravenously (> 3,000 kcal/day; multivitamins, mainly vitamins B and C)
  - Treatment for encephalopathy and ascites
  - Corticosteroids: Tried in severe cases (discriminant function > 32) in the absence of any infection.
  - Antibiotics (pentoxyfylline) in severe cases (discriminant function > 32) and antifungal prophylaxis.

Causes of Tender Hepatomegaly

Causes of tender hepatomegaly are given in **Box 5.30**.

Causes of Splenomegaly

Causes of splenomegaly are given in **Table 5.36**.

Box 5.30: Causes of tender hepatomegaly

- Hepatitis: Viral, drug-induced, alcoholic, chronic
- Amoebic liver abscess
- Pyogenic liver abscess
- Malignancies: HCC, secondaries
- Acute Budd–Chiari syndrome
- Congestive cardiac failure

TABLE 5.36: Causes of splenomegaly.

Mild splenomegaly (up to 5 cm)	
Acute infections	Septic shock, infective endocarditis, enteric fever, infectious hepatitis, infectious mononucleosis, brucellosis, cytomegalovirus, toxoplasmosis
Chronic infections	Tuberculosis, syphilis, brucellosis, chronic bacteraemia, HIV
Parasitic infestations	Malaria, kala-azar and schistosomiasis

Continued

Continued

Inflammation	Rheumatoid arthritis, sarcoidosis, SLE
Others	Congestive cardiac failure, thalassaemia minor
Moderate splenomegaly (upto umbilicus) (5–8 cm)	
Neoplastic	Lymphomas, acute leukaemias, chronic lymphocytic leukaemia, chronic myeloid leukaemia
Non-neoplastic	Cirrhosis of liver (with portal hypertension), chronic haemolytic anaemia, malaria, kala-azar, sarcoidosis, infectious mononucleosis, splenic abscess, amyloidosis, haemochromatosis, polycythaemia vera
Massive splenomegaly (below umbilicus) (> 8 cm)	
Common causes	Chronic myeloid leukaemia, myelofibrosis, kala-azar, hairy cell leukaemia, tropical splenomegaly, portal hypertension (extrahepatic portal vein thrombosis), chronic malaria
Uncommon causes	Lymphomas, Gaucher's disease, Niemann–Pick disease, thalassaemia major, Splenic cysts and tumours of spleen, myeloid metaplasia, hairy cell leukaemia, sarcoidosis

BEST OF FIVES

1. Which of the following is the most common symptom or sign of liver disease?
   A. Fatigue
   B. Itching
   C. Jaundice
   D. Nausea
   E. Right upper quadrant pain

2. For females, what is the average amount of reported daily alcohol intake that is associated with the development of chronic liver disease?
   A. 1 drink
   B. 2 drinks
   C. 3 drinks
   D. 6 drinks
   E. 12 drinks

3. Elevations in all of the following laboratory studies would be indicative of liver disease except:
   A. 5'-Nucleotidase
   B. Aspartate aminotransferase
   C. Conjugated bilirubin
   D. Unconjugated bilirubin
   E. Urine bilirubin

4. Which of the following viral causes of acute hepatitis is most likely to cause fulminant hepatitis in a pregnant woman?
   A. Hepatitis A
   B. Hepatitis B
   C. Hepatitis C
   D. Hepatitis D
   E. Hepatitis E

5. A 44-year-old male presents with fatigue and tea-coloured urine for 5 days. Physical examination reveals jaundice and tender hepatomegaly. Laboratories are remarkable for an aspartate aminotransferase (AST) of 2,400 U/L and an alanine aminotransferase (ALT) of 2,640 U/L. Alkaline phosphatase is 210 U/L. Total bilirubin is 8.6 mg/dL. Which of the following diagnoses is least likely to cause this clinical picture and these laboratory abnormalities?
   A. Acute hepatitis A infection
   B. Acute hepatitis B infection
   C. Acute hepatitis C infection
   D. Acetaminophen ingestion
   E. Budd-Chiari syndrome

6. Which of the following drugs has a direct toxic effect on hepatocytes?
   A. Acetaminophen
   B. Chlorpromazine
   C. Halothane
   D. Isoniazid
   E. Rosuvastatin

7. A 29-year-old woman is evaluated for elevated transaminase levels that were identified during routine laboratory testing for life insurance. She has no significant past medical history. She had one uncomplicated pregnancy at the age of 22 years. She recalls an episode of

jaundice that she did not seek evaluation for about 15 years ago. It resolved spontaneously. There are no stigmata of chronic liver disease. Her laboratory studies reveal an aspartate aminotransferase (AST) of 346 U/L, alanine aminotransferase (ALT) of 412 U/L, alkaline phosphatase of 98 U/L and total bilirubin of 1.5 mg/dL. Further workup includes the following viral studies: hepatitis A immunoglobulin G (IgG) +, hepatitis B surface antigen +, hepatitis B e antigen +, anti-hepatitis B virus (HBV) core IgG +, and hepatitis C IgG negative. The HBV DNA (deoxyribonucleic acid) level is 4.8×10^4 IU/mL.
What treatment do you recommend for this patient?
   A. Entecavir
   B. Pegylated interferon
   C. Pegylated interferon plus entecavir
   D. No treatment is necessary
   E. Either A or C

8. In chronic hepatitis B virus (HBV) infection, the presence of hepatitis B e antigen (HBeAg) signifies which of the following?
   A. Development of liver fibrosis leading to cirrhosis
   B. Dominant viral population is less virulent and less transmissible.
   C. Increased likelihood of an acute flare in the next 1–2 weeks
   D. Ongoing viral replication
   E. Resolving infection

9. A 42-year-old man with cirrhosis related to hepatitis C and alcohol abuse has ascites requiring frequent large-volume paracentesis. All of the following therapies would be indicated for this patient except:
   A. Fluid restriction to less than 2 L daily
   B. Furosemide 40 mg daily
   C. Sodium restriction to less than 2 g daily
   D. Spironolactone 100 mg daily
   E. Transjugular intrahepatic portosystemic shunt if medical therapy fails

10. All of the following are associated with an increased risk for cholelithiasis except:
    A. Chronic haemolytic anaemia
    B. Female sex
    C. High-protein diet
    D. Obesity
    E. Pregnancy

11. Cryoglobulinaemia is seen with:
    A. Hepatitis A
    B. Hepatitis C
    C. Leukaemia
    D. Ovarian cancer
    E. Hepatitis B

12. Which of the following serum markers for liver fibrosis can replace the need for liver biopsy?
    A. Serum glutamic-oxaloacetic transaminase (SGOT) and serum glutamic pyruvic transaminase (SGPT)
    B. Serum hyaluronic acid
    C. Gamma-glutamyl transpeptidase (GGT) and fibronectin
    D. Fibronectin and factor V levels
    E. Serum albumin

13. All the following are used for treatment of chronic hepatitis B except:
    A. Entecavir
    B. Telbivudine
    C. Zidovudine
    D. Lamivudine
    E. A and C

14. Reverse transcriptase of hepatitis B virus is coded on the following gene:
    A. *C* gene
    B. *P* gene
    C. *S* gene
    D. *X* gene
    E. *Q* gene

15. De Ritis ratio of aspartate aminotransaminase (AST)/alanine aminotransferase (ALT) of 3:1 is present in:
    A. Non-alcoholic steatohepatitis
    B. Alcoholic hepatitis
    C. Wilson's disease
    D. Paracetamol toxicity
    E. All the above

16. Micronodular cirrhosis is commonly seen in all except:
    A. Chronic hepatitis B
    B. Alcoholic liver disease
    C. Haemochromatosis
    D. Chronic extrahepatic biliary obstruction
    E. Caroli diseases

17. 5'-nucleotidase activity is increased in:
    A. Bone disease
    B. Prostrate cancer
    C. Chronic renal failure

D. Cholestatic disease
E. Haemolysis

18. Raised unconjugated bilirubin is seen in:
    A. Gilbert syndrome
    B. Dubin-Johnson syndrome
    C. Drug-induced haemolysis
    D. Hepatocellular necrosis
    E. Pancreatic cancer

19. Microvascular steatosis is seen in all except:
    A. Haemolysis, elevated liver enzymes, low platelet count (HELLP) syndrome
    B. Acute fatty liver of pregnancy
    C. Methotrexate toxicity
    D. Reye's syndrome
    E. Non-alcoholic steatohepatitis (NASH)

20. In Budd-Chiari syndrome, the site of venous thrombosis is:
    A. Infrahepatic inferior vena cava
    B. Infrarenal inferior vena cava
    C. Hepatic veins
    D. Portal veins
    E. Splenic vein

21. Model for end-stage liver disease (MELD) score includes all except:
    A. Bilirubin
    B. International normalised ratio (INR)
    C. Serum creatinine
    D. Serum albumin
    E. All the above

22. A child has serum ascites albumin gradient (SAAG) < 1.1 g/dL. The probable diagnosis is:
    A. Cirrhosis
    B. Portal hypertension
    C. Congestive cardiac failure
    D. Nephrotic syndrome
    E. Chronic kidney diseases

23. All the following are risk factors for hepatocellular carcinoma except:
    A. Hepatitis C infection
    B. Alcoholism
    C. Aflatoxins
    D. Animal fat in diet
    E. Non-alcoholic steatohepatitis (NASH)

24. Incorrect about Wilson's disease is:
    A. Decreased urine copper
    B. Decrease serum copper
    C. Decrease serum ceruloplasmin
    D. Increase serum copper
    E. Both B and D

25. Factors of importance in predicting the virulence of *Helicobacter pylori* are:
    A. CagA protein
    B. JamA protein
    C. VacA protein
    D. Metronidazole resistance
    E. Both A and C

Answers

1-A, 2-B, 3-D, 4-E, 5-C, 6-A, 7-E, 8-D, 9-A, 10-C, 11-B, 12-B, 13-C, 14-B, 15-B, 16-A, 17-D, 18-A, 19-C, 20-C, 21-D, 22-D, 23-D, 24-A, 25-E

■ SUGGESTED READING

1. Pratt DS, Kaplan MM. Evaluation of abnormal liver-enzyme results in asymptomatic patients. N Engl J Med. 2000;342(17):1266-71.
2. Kwo PY, Cohen SM, Lim JK. ACG Clinical Guideline: Evaluation of Abnormal Liver Chemistries. Am J Gastroenterol. 2017;112(1):18-35.
3. Newsome PN, Cramb R, Davison SM, Dillon JF, Foulerton M, Godfrey EM, et al. Guidelines on the management of abnormal liver blood tests. Gut. 2018;67(1):6-19.
4. Sarin SK, Kumar M, Lau GK, Abbas Z, Chan HLY, Chen CJ, et al. Asian-Pacific clinical practice guidelines on the management of hepatitis B: a 2015 update. Hepatol Int. 2016;10(1):1-98.
5. European Association for the Study of the Liver. EASL 2017 Clinical Practice Guidelines on the management of hepatitis B virus infection. J Hepatol. 2017;67(2):370-98.
6. Terrault NA, Lok ASF, McMahon BJ, Chang KM, Hwang JP, Jonas MM, et al. Update on prevention, diagnosis, and treatment of chronic hepatitis B: AASLD 2018 hepatitis B guidance. Hepatology. 2018;67(4):1560.
7. European Association for the Study of the Liver. EASL Recommendations on Treatment of Hepatitis C 2016. J Hepatol. 2017;66(1):153-94.
8. Rehm J, Samokhvalov AV, Shield KD. Global burden of alcoholic liver diseases. J Hepatol. 2013;59(1):160-8.
9. Blachier M, Leleu H, Peck-Radosavljevic M, Valla DC, Roudot-Thoraval F. The burden of liver disease in Europe: a review of available epidemiological data. J Hepatol. 2013;58(3):593-608.
10. Forner A, Reig M, Bruix J. Hepatocellular carcinoma. Lancet. 2018; 391(10127):1301-14.
11. Yu SJ. A concise review of updated guidelines regarding the management of hepatocellular carcinoma around the world: 2010-2016. Clin Mol Hepatol. 2016;22(1):7-17.
12. Wong RJ, Aguilar M, Cheung R, Perumpail RB, Harrison SA, Younossi ZM, et al. Nonalcoholic steatohepatitis is the second leading etiology of liver disease among adults awaiting liver transplantation in the United States. Gastroenterology. 2015;148(3):547-55.

CHAPTER 6

Pancreatic Disorders

■ ACUTE PANCREATITIS

Aetiology
Causes of acute pancreatitis are given in **Box 6.1**.

Clinical Features
Symptoms
- Abdominal pain
  - Severe intensity
  - Dull, boring and steady
  - Usually located in the epigastric region
  - Radiates to the back.
  - Partial relief if patient sits up and leans forwards
- Nausea and vomiting
- Anorexia

Signs
- Fever (low grade)
- Tachycardia
- Tachypnoea
- Hypotension
- Abdominal tenderness, muscular guarding and distension
- Bowel sounds often hypoactive
- Lungs—cyanosis, basal crepitations, pleural effusion
- Skin
  - Bluish discolouration around the umbilicus 'Cullen's sign'
  - Bluish or green-brown discolouration in the flanks 'Turner's sign' due to haemoperitoneum
- Others
  - Haematemesis or melaena
  - Ischaemic injury to retina is seen on fundus examination (Purtscher retinopathy).

Investigations
- Serum amylase
  - Levels increase for the initial 72 hours and then decline to normal in 1–2 weeks.

Box 6.1: Causes of acute pancreatitis.

Trauma
Accidental: Blunt trauma to the abdomen
Iatrogenic injury: Post-operative, post-endoscopic retrograde cholangiopancreatography, endoscopic sphincterotomy, sphincter of Oddi manometry

Vascular
Ischaemia: Hypoperfusion (e.g. post-cardiac surgery) or atherosclerotic emboli
Vasculitis: Systemic lupus erythematosus, periarteritis nodosa, malignant hypertension

Miscellaneous
Penetrating peptic ulcer
Pregnancy-associated Reye syndrome

Infectious
Viral: **Mumps**, rubella, viral hepatitis, **coxsackievirus B**, echovirus, cytomegalovirus, human immunodeficiency virus
Bacterial: Mycoplasma, Campylobacter jejuni, tuberculosis, *Legionella* species, **Leptospirosis**

Idiopathic
Pancreas divisum

Genetic
Mutations in the pancreatic trypsin inhibitor (*SPINK1*) gene and in the cystic fibrosis transmembrane regulator (CFTR)

- Serum lipase
  - Preferable for diagnosis as its elevation is more specific than that of amylase

Other Blood Investigations
- Blood glucose, total leucocyte count, platelet count, blood urea, serum calcium and other electrolytes, triglycerides
- Blood gas

Plain X-ray of Abdomen and Chest
- To exclude other causes of acute abdominal pain (e.g. perforation)
- If abscess forms in the necrotic pancreas, the X-ray may show multiple extraluminal gas shadows in the pancreatic area.
- Calcification in pancreas in chronic pancreatitis

Ultrasound of Abdomen
- To evaluate gallbladder and biliary tree
- It can detect acute pancreatitis in > 60% of cases. However, pancreatic evaluation may be obscured by bowel gas.

CT Scan/MRI of Abdomen
- May show solid mass of swollen pancreas, pseudocyst or pancreatic abscess

Endoscopic Ultrasound
- Can be used to evaluate common bile duct for the presence of stones

Prognostic Features
Ranson Criteria
Ranson criteria are given in **Box 6.2**.

Complications
Complications of acute pancreatitis are given in **Box 6.3**.

Treatment
- Nil orally initially
- Intravenous fluids to maintain intravascular volume
- Pain control with analgesics
- Nasogastric aspiration if pain continues, if the patient has protracted vomiting or if obstruction is seen on plain X-ray of abdomen.

Box 6.2: Ranson criteria.

At admission	During the initial 48 hours
• Age > 55 years	• Fall in haematocrit > 10% of baseline
• Leucocytosis > 6,000/mm³	• Fluid sequestration > 4,000 mL
• Blood sugar > 200 mg/dL	• Hypocalcaemia < 8 mg/dL
• Serum LDH > 400 IU/L	• Hypoxaemia with PaO$_2$ < 60 mmHg
• Serum AST > 250 IU/L	• Rise in blood urea > 10 mg/dL after IV fluids
	• Hypoalbuminaemia < 3.2 g/dL

0–2 Criteria: Mortality 2%
3–4 Criteria: Mortality 15%
5–6 Criteria: Mortality 40%
More than 6 Criteria: Mortality 100%
(AST: aspartate aminotransferase; LDH: lactate dehydrogenase)

- Monitor pulse, blood pressure, abdominal girth, urine output, blood glucose and calcium, and blood gases. Severe cases should be monitored in intensive care units.
- Antibiotics, carbapenems (imipenem or meropenem) or ceftazidime, in severe cases
- Other drugs include proton-pump inhibitors, glucagon, octreotide and aprotinin (protease inhibitor).
- Surgery is indicated for:
  - Infected pancreatic necrosis
  - Complications
- Endoscopic retrograde cholangiopancreatography (ERCP) within the first 36–48 hours in patients with gallstone pancreatitis who are in a very severe group

■ CHRONIC PANCREATITIS
- Chronic inflammation of pancreas presenting as recurrent pain, endocrine deficiency (diabetes mellitus), exocrine deficiency (malabsorption) or a combination of two of all three features.

Aetiology
- Chronic alcohol ingestion
- Cholelithiasis

> **Box 6.3: Complications of acute pancreatitis.**
>
> **Local**
> - **Pseudocyst**
> - **Necrosis:** Sterile/infected necrosis/walled-off necrosis
> - **Abscess**
> - **Pancreatic ascites**
> - Disruption of main pancreatic duct
> - Leaking pseudocyst
> - Involvement of contiguous organs by necrotising pancreatitis
> - Massive intraperitoneal haemorrhage
> - Thrombosis of blood vessels (splenic vein, portal vein)
> - Bowel infarction
> - Obstructive jaundice
> - Abdominal compartment syndrome
>
> **Systemic**
> - Systemic inflammatory response syndrome (SIRS) due to increased vascular permeability caused by release of cytokine platelet aggregating factor and kinin
> - **Respiratory complications:** Pleural effusion, hypoxia—adult respiratory distress syndrome (ARDS) due to microthrombi in pulmonary vessels, pneumonia
> - **Cardiovascular:** Hypotension and shock, hypovolaemia
> - **Gastrointestinal complications: Upper gastrointestinal bleeding** due to gastric or duodenal erosions and paralytic ileus
> - **Hepatobiliary complications:** Jaundice, common bile duct obstruction (obstructive jaundice), splenic or portal vein thrombosis, variceal haemorrhage
> - **Renal:** Oliguria azotaemia renal artery and/or renal vein thrombosis, acute tubular necrosis
> - **Metabolic:** Hyperglycaemia (due to disruption of islets of Langerhans with altered insulin glucagon release), hypocalcaemia due to sequestration of calcium in fat necrosis
> - **Haematological complications:** Disseminated intravascular coagulation (DIC), Increased factor VII or fibrinogen
> - Fat Necrosis (subcutaneous nodules), polyarthritis
> - **Retinopathy (Purtscher's retinopathy):** Sudden blindness
> - **Central nervous system:** Psychosis, encephalopathy and coma

- Stenosis of sphincter of Oddi
- Associated with autoimmune diseases (Sjögren's syndrome, primary biliary cirrhosis)
- Cystic fibrosis
- Familial

Clinical Features

- Pain, continuous or intermittent. May be referred to chest or back
- Pain is often increased by alcohol or heavy meals.
- Features of malabsorption: Diarrhoea, steatorrhoea, weight loss, features of fat-soluble vitamin deficiency and vitamin B12 deficiency
- Diabetes mellitus
- In late stages, mechanical obstruction of common bile duct can occur.

Investigations

- Serum amylase and lipase are usually normal.
- Plain X-ray of abdomen
  - Calcification in pancreatic area (in 30%)
  - Sensitivity for picking calcification increases when both anteroposterior and oblique views are taken.
- Ultrasound of abdomen and CT scan of abdomen
  - Pancreatic atrophy
  - Calcifications
  - Dilatation of bile duct
  - Stricture of bile duct

- ERCP is the gold standard for diagnosis as it most accurately demonstrates pancreatic ducts.
- Magnetic resonance cholangiopancreatography (MRCP) may replace ERCP.
- Endoscopic ultrasound to evaluate pancreas
- Pancreatic function tests
  - Secretin/cholecystokinin (CCK) stimulation test
  - Faecal chymotrypsin or elastase concentration
  - 24-hour faecal fat
  - Oral glucose tolerance test

Treatment
- Abstinence of alcohol
- Diet rich in medium-chain triglycerides that do not require lipase for digestion
- Pancreatic enzymes, particularly lipase, 20,000–75,000 U before each meal to reduce faecal fat excretion
- Proton-pump inhibitors or H2-blockers
- Treatment of pain by opioids or non-steroidal anti-inflammatory drugs (NSAIDs)
- Treatment of diabetes
- Surgery for unremitting pain; includes pancreatectomy and pancretojejunostomy

■ TROPICAL PANCREATITIS
- It is a juvenile form of chronic calcific pancreatitis that is not related to alcohol intake.
- It is seen almost exclusively in tropical countries.
- In India, it is more common in southern states (Kerala and Tamil Nadu).

Aetiology
- Malnutrition
- Diet rich in cassava that contains cyanogenic glycosides
- Oxidant stress
- Infections (Coxsackie and viral hepatitis)
- Familial

Clinical Features
- Affects young males
- Presents with recurrent abdominal pain, typically in the epigastric area with radiation to back. Pain gets precipitated by heavy meals.
- Associated features include malnutrition, enlarged parotid glands, abdominal distention and a peculiar cyanotic hue of the lips.
- Pancreatic exocrine deficiency presents with steatorrhoea and malabsorption.
- Diabetes mellitus is common.

Investigations
- Plain X-ray and ultrasound of abdomen show multiple, large intraductal calculi.

Treatment
- As with chronic pancreatitis
- High doses of insulin are often required with careful watch over hypoglycaemia.

Autoimmune Pancreatitis/Autoimmune Chronic Pancreatitis
- Association with other autoimmune disease: Autoimmune pancreatitis (AIP) may also develop in association with other autoimmune disorders such as Sjögren's syndrome, primary sclerosing cholangitis (PSC), inflammatory bowel disease and retroperitoneal fibrosis.
- Associated with immunoglobulin G4 (IgG4)-related disorders
- *Treatment:* Glucocorticoids, azathioprine

■ PANCREATIC CANCER
Pancreatic tumours and their types are shown in **Flowchart 6.1**.

Endocrine Tumours of Pancreas (Table 6.1)
- Classified as functioning or non-functioning according to the type and level of their hormonal secretion
- Insulinomas (50%) and gastrinomas (30%) are the most frequent.
- Tumours secreting vasoactive intestinal peptide (VIPomas), glucagon (glucagonomas) and somatostatin (somatostatinomas) are much rarer (5–10%).
- Those secreting growth-hormone-releasing factor (GHRH), adrenocorticotropic hormone (ACTH) or corticotropin-releasing factor (CRF), and parathyroid hormone related peptide (PTHrP) are anecdotal.

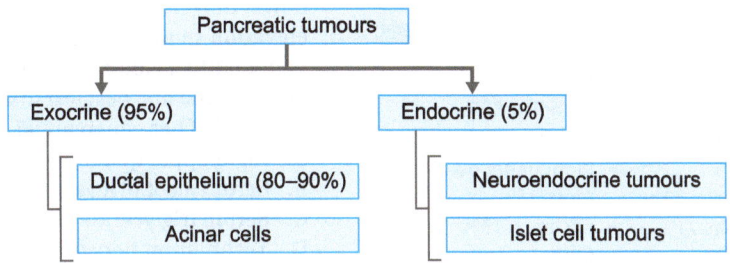

Flowchart 6.1: Pancreatic tumours and their types.

TABLE 6.1: Pancreatic endocrine tumors.

Tumour type	Corresponding syndrome	Localisation	Malignancy rate
Insulinoma	Fasting, hypoglycaemia, overweight	Pancreas	5%
Gastrinoma	Diarrhoea, atypical peptic ulcer disease	Duodenum (pancreas)	40–60%
VIPomas	Watery diarrhoea, muscle weakness	Pancreas (retroperitoneum, duodenum)	60%
Somatostatinoma	Steatorrhoea, weight loss, glucose intolerance, gallbladder disease	Pancreas (duodenum)	50%
Glucagonoma	Skin rash, diabetes, denutrition, thrombophlebitis	Pancreas	80%
Non-functioning (PPomas)	Epigastric pain, dyspepsia, jaundice, abdominal mass	Pancreas	60–80%

- Conversely, at least 15% of endocrine tumors of the pancreas (ETP) are non-functioning or secrete non-clinically active peptides such as human pancreatic polypeptide (PPomas).
- Zollinger–Ellison syndrome is characterised by hyperacidity and non-healing ulcers (gastric, duodenal, jejunal or in atypical locations). Epigastric pain with duodenal ulcer is seen in 90% of cases; one third have diarrhoea, and weight loss is common (40% of cases). Oesophagitis, dysphagia (30%), stricture and perforation may occur.
- VIPoma [Watery diarrhoea, hypokalaemia, achlorhydria (WDHA) syndrome, Verner–Morrison syndrome, pancreatic cholera] characterised by severe secretory diarrhoea secondary to the stimulation of adenylyl cyclase within the enterocyte large-volume diarrhoea (> 3 L/day), hypokalaemia, and hypo- or achlorhydria forms part of the syndrome; hence the term WDHA syndrome.

Ductal Adenocarcinoma of Pancreas

- Ductal adenocarcinoma accounts for 85–90% of pancreatic tumours.
- About 60–70% of these tumours are localised in the head of the gland, 5–10% in the body and 10–15% in the tail.
- Risk factors: Excess intake of alcohol, cigarette smoking, high fat and protein diet, excessive intake of coffee and tea consumption and chronic calcific pancreatitis.
- Genetic predisposition: About 5–10% of patients with pancreatic cancer have a family history of the disease. Familial atypical multiple mole melanoma (FAMMM) syndrome, hereditary non-polyposis colorectal cancer (HNPCC) syndrome, hereditary pancreatitis, multiple endocrine neoplasia (MEN), and Peutz–Jeghers syndrome have an increased risk of pancreatic cancer.
- Symptoms and signs of ductal adenocarcinoma of pancreas are given in **Box 6.4**.

> **Box 6.4: Symptoms and signs of ductal adenocarcinoma of pancreas.**
>
> **Symptoms**
> - Asthenia: 86%
> - Weight loss: 85%
> - Anorexia: 83%
> - Abdominal pain: 79%
> - Epigastric pain: 71%
> - Dark urine: 59%
> - Jaundice: 56%
> - Nausea: 51%
> - Back pain: 49%
> - Diarrhoea: 44%
> - Vomiting: 33%
> - Steatorrhoea: 25%
> - Thrombophlebitis: 3%
>
> **Signs**
> - Jaundice: 55%
> - Hepatomegaly: 39%
> - Right upper quadrant mass: 15%
> - Cachexia: 13%
> - Courvoisier sign (non-tender but palpable distended gallbladder at the right costal margin): 13%
> - Epigastric mass: 9%
> - Ascites: 5%

- Ultrasound, contrast CT and ERCP yield in localisation of tumour, assessing the spread as well as operability; guided biopsy/cytology helps to confirm diagnosis.
- Tumour markers: Carcinoembryonic antigen (CEA) and CA-19-9 [high sensitivity (80%) but a high false-positive rate]
- Treatment
    - Surgical resection: It is the only method of effecting cure. Resectable tumours in the head and periampullary region are removed by Whipple's pancreaticoduodenectomy or its modifications.
    - Chemotherapy: For inoperable cases chemotherapy with gemcitabine, capecitabine, nab-paclitaxel, cisplatin, docetaxel, oxaliplatin, irinotecan, 5- fluorouracil, mitomycin, streptozotocin and high-dose methotrexate, alone or in combination, may be beneficial. Tyrosine kinase inhibitors of EGFR (e.g. erlotinib) and monoclonal antibodies cetuximab are under trials.
    - Radiotherapy may be supportive.

BEST OF FIVES

1. A 24-year-old woman is admitted to the hospital with acute-onset severe right upper quadrant pain that radiates to the back. The pain is constant and not relieved with eating or bowel movements. Her labs show a marked elevation in amylase and lipase, and acute pancreatitis is diagnosed. Which of the following is the first best test to demonstrate the aetiology of her pancreatitis?
    A. Right upper quadrant ultrasound
    B. Serum alcohol level
    C. Serum triglyceride level
    D. Technetium hepatobiliary iminodiacetic acid (HIDA) scan
    E. Urine drug screen

2. A 36-year-old man is admitted to the hospital with acute pancreatitis. In order to determine the severity of disease and risk of mortality, the bedside index of severity in acute pancreatitis (BISAP) is calculated. All of the following variables are used to calculate this score except:
    A. Age > 60 years
    B. Blood urea nitrogen (BUN) > 35
    C. Impaired mental status
    D. Pleural effusion
    E. White blood cell count > 15,000 leucocytes/µL

3. A 25-year-old female with cystic fibrosis is diagnosed with chronic pancreatitis. She is at risk for all of the following complications except:
    A. Vitamin B12 deficiency
    B. Vitamin A deficiency
    C. Pancreatic carcinoma
    D. Niacin deficiency
    E. Steatorrhoea

4. The most common complication of acute pancreatitis is:
    A. Pancreatic abscess
    B. Pseudocyst of pancreas
    C. Phlegmon
    D. Pleural effusion
    E. Pancreatic cancer

5. Pancreatitis can be produced by the following drug:
    A. Ciprofloxacin
    B. Nalidixic acid
    C. Colchicine
    D. L-Asparaginase
    E. Ceftriaxone

6. This is the most diagnostic investigation for acute pancreatitis:
   A. Serum lactate dehydrogenase (LDH)
   B. Serum amylase
   C. Serum lipase
   D. Serum P-isoamylase
   E. Urinary lipase

7. Which of the following are common causes of acute pancreatitis?
   A. Hypertension, gallstones, diabetes mellitus
   B. Chronic obstructive pulmonary disease, hypertriglyceridaemia, medications
   C. Ethanol abuse, gallstones, pregnancy
   D. Hereditary predisposition, obesity, gallstones
   E. Obesity, hypertension, hypertriglyceridaemia

8. Complications of acute pancreatitis may include all of the following except:
   A. Acute respiratory distress syndrome
   B. Acute kidney injury
   C. Abscess formation
   D. Hypertension
   E. Pancreatic infection

9. Which of the following are complications of chronic pancreatitis?
   A. Ascites
   B. Glucose intolerance
   C. Malnutrition
   D. Both B and C
   E. Sepsis

10. Which of the following tests should be reviewed to work up a patient for pancreatitis?
    A. Lipase, amylase, triglycerides
    B. Amylase, serum calcium, haemoglobin
    C. Triglycerides, haemoglobin, serum glucose
    D. Alanine aminotransferase (ALT), lipase, serum magnesium
    E. Serum calcium, lipase, C-reactive protein

11. Which of the following is not an indicator that the patient may require transfer to an intensive care unit (ICU)?
    A. Systolic blood pressure < 80 mmHg
    B. Multiple organ dysfunction
    C. Temperature > 38°C with altered mental status
    D. Respiratory rate > 35 breaths/min
    E. Food intolerance

12. Which of the following are risk factors for chronic pancreatitis?
    A. Obesity and race
    B. Hypertension, enalapril use
    C. Ethanol, tobacco and enalapril use
    D. Aspirin, ibuprofen, ethanol and tobacco use
    E. Gallstones, dyslipidaemia

13. Which of the following bacteria are likely to be implicated in infected pancreatic necrosis?
    A. *Listeria monocytogenes*
    B. *Haemophilus influenzae*
    C. *Klebsiella pneumoniae*
    D. *Streptococcus agalactiae*
    E. *Mycobacterium tuberculosis*

14. Which statement best describes the pathophysiology of chronic pancreatitis?
    A. Pancreatic necrosis secondary to damage to the pancreatic tissue
    B. Autolysis of the pancreas secondary to early activation of pancreatic enzymes
    C. An inflammatory process leading to endocrine and exocrine dysfunction secondary to diffuse scaring and fibrosis
    D. Inflammation of the pancreas secondary to a predominantly neutrophilic inflammatory response
    E. Immune destruction of alpha cells leading to hyperglycaemia

15. Differences between acute pancreatitis and chronic pancreatitis include which of the following?
    A. Serum creatinine is elevated in acute but not chronic pancreatitis.
    B. Serum thromboplastin is elevated in acute but not chronic pancreatitis.
    C. Serum creatine kinase (CK) is elevated in acute but not chronic pancreatitis.
    D. Serum amylase is elevated in acute but not chronic pancreatitis.
    E. Serum potassium is elevated in acute but not chronic pancreatitis.

16. What % of pancreas must be damaged before maldigestion is manifested?
    A. 25%
    B. 50%

C. 90%
D. 100%
E. 60%

17. When does serum amylase rise in acute pancreatitis?
    A. 6 hours
    B. 24 hours
    C. 72 hours
    D. 3–5 days
    E. 48 hours

18. Normal serum amylase in pancreatitis is seen in all except:
    A. Delay of 3 days before blood samples are obtained in acute pancreatitis
    B. Delay of 5 days before blood samples are obtained
    C. Chronic pancreatitis
    D. Hyperglycaemia
    E. Hypertriglyceridaemia

19. Which is not a manifestation of pancreatitis and pancreatic insufficiency?
    A. Hypertriglyceridaemia
    B. Hypocalcaemia
    C. Hypoglycaemia
    D. Normal blood amylase levels
    E. Pleural effusion

Answers

1-A, 2-E, 3-D, 4-B, 5-D, 6-C, 7-D, 8-D, 9-D, 10-A, 11-E, 12-C, 13-C, 14-C, 15-E, 16-C, 17-B, 18-D, 19-C

■ SUGGESTED READING

1. Tenner S, Baillie J, DeWitt J, Santhi Swaroop Vege, American College of Gastroenterology. American College of Gastroenterology guideline: management of acute pancreatitis. Am J Gastroenterol. 2013;108(9):1400-15.
2. Working Group IAP/APA Acute Pancreatitis Guidelines. IAP/APA evidence-based guidelines for the management of acute pancreatitis. Pancreatology. 2013;13(4 Suppl 2): e1-15.
3. Crockett SD, Wani S, Gardner TB, Falck-Ytter Y, Barkun AN, American Gastroenterological Association Institute Clinical Guidelines Committee. American Gastroenterological Association Institute Guideline on initial management of acute pancreatitis. Gastroenterology. 2018;154(4):1096-101.
4. Majumder S, Chari ST. Chronic pancreatitis. Lancet. 2016;387(10031):1957-66.
5. Gardner TB, Adler DG, Forsmark CE, Sauer BG, Taylor JR, Whitcomb DC, et al. ACG clinical guideline: Chronic pancreatitis. Am J Gastroenterol. 2020;115(3):322-39.
6. Whitcomb DC, Frulloni L, Garg P, Greer JB, Schneider A, Yadav D, et al. Chronic pancreatitis: An international draft consensus proposal for a new mechanistic definition. Pancreatology. 2016;16(2):218-24.
7. Allen PJ, Kuk D, Castillo CF, Basturk O, Wolfgang C, Cameron J, et al. Multi-institutional Validation Study of the American Joint Commission on Cancer (8th Edition). Changes for T and N staging in patients with pancreatic adenocarcinoma. Ann Surg. 2017;265(1):185.
8. Dasari A, Shen C, Halperin D, Zhao B, Zhou S, Xu Y, et al. Trends in the incidence, prevalence, and survival outcomes in patients with neuroendocrine tumors in the United States. JAMA Oncol 2017;3(10):1335-42.

CHAPTER 7

Endocrinology

◼ HYPOPITUTARISM

Aetiology
- **Congenital hypothalamic causes**—deficiencies of gonadotropin-releasing hormone (GnRH) (Kallmann syndrome), thyrotropin-releasing hormone (TRH), growth hormone-releasing hormone (GHRH)
- **Acquired hypothalamic causes**—craniopharyngioma, sarcoidosis, tuberculosis, histiocytosis-X, surgery, radiotherapy, tumours, head trauma
- **Pituitary causes**—pituitary adenoma, postpartum necrosis (Sheehan's syndrome), autoimmune (lymphocytic hypophysitis), surgery, radiotherapy, haemorrhage, empty sella syndrome, haemochromatosis

Clinical Features
- Pituitary tumors cause symptoms related to mass effects (e.g. headache, visual impairment, electrolyte alterations)
- Symptoms related to deficiency of hormones

Management
- Replacement of deficient hormone
- Treat underlying cause

◼ ACROMEGALY
- Excess secretion of growth hormone (GH) prior to closure of epiphyseal growth plates in long bone causes **pituitary gigantism**.
- Excess secretion after puberty causes **acromegaly**.

Aetiology
- Pituitary tumour (somatotroph pituitary adenoma) is the most common cause.
- Other tumours: Pancreas, lungs and adrenal glands (they produce GHRH).

Clinical Features
- Local tumour effects—visual-field defects, cranial nerve palsy, headache
- Somatic systems—thickness of soft tissue of hands and feet
- Gigantism, prognathism, jaw malocclusion, widely spaced teeth, arthritis
- Neurological—carpal tunnel syndrome, proximal myopathy
- Skin and integumental—skin tags, acanthosis nigricans, enlargement of lips, nose, increased heel pad thickness
- Gastrointestinal tract (GIT)—macroglossia, colonic polyps, visceromegaly
- Cardiovascular system (CVS)—left ventricular hypertrophy, cardiomyopathy, hypertension, congestive heart failure, coronary artery disease (CAD)
- Respiratory system (RS)—sleep apnoea
- Reproduction—menstrual abnormalities, galactorrhoea, gynaecomastia
- Carbohydrate metabolism—impaired glucose tolerance

Investigations
- Raised GH levels and insulin-like growth factor (IGF) levels
- Imaging—X-ray skull, magnetic resonance imaging (MRI) of brain

Treatment
- Surgical excision of tumour
- Medical therapy
    - Somatostatin receptor ligands (SRL)—octreotide, pasireotide or lanreotide
    - GH receptor antagonist—**pegvisomant**
    - Dopamine receptor agonists—bromocriptine or cabergoline
- Radiotherapy

■ DIABETES INSIPIDUS
Disorder resulting from deficiency of vasopressin/antidiuretic hormone (ADH) or its action.

Types of Diabetes Insipidus
- Primary deficiency [neurogenic, pituitary, hypothalamic, cranial or **central diabetes insipidus (DI)**]: It is due to agenesis or destruction of neurohypophysis.
- Secondary deficiency: It is due to inhibition of ADH secretion (primary polydipsia).
- Deficient action of ADH (**nephrogenic DI**)

Clinical Features
- Polyuria and polydipsia: Urinary frequency (polyuria) 4–18 L/day, nocturia and compensatory excessive thirst (polydipsia)
- Other features: Change in mentation, insomnia, weight loss
- Can lead to hypernatraemia, restlessness, seizures

Investigation
- Measurement of plasma and urine osmolality
- Water deprivation test
- Hypernatraemia
- MRI of pituitary

Treatment
Drugs
- Desmopressin (DDAVP)
- Chlorpropamide
- Carbamazepine
- Clofibrate
- Thiazide diuretics (e.g. bendrofluazide) for nephrogenic DI

■ THYROID DISORDERS
Thyroid Function Tests
Basic evaluation of thyroid is shown in **Figure 7.1**.

■ THYROTOXICOSIS
Thyrotoxicosis and its types are given in **Box 7.1**.

Clinical Features
- Gastrointestinal system—weight loss, increased appetite, vomiting, increased frequency of stool

Basic thyroid evaluation

Free thyroxine (FT4)	Low TSH	Normal TSH	High TSH
High	Primary hyperthyroidism	Non-thyroid illness (NTI) or patient on eltroxin	Secondary hyperthyroidism
Normal	Subclinical hyperthyroidism	Euthyroid	Subclinical hypothyroid
Low	Secondary hypothyroid	NTI	Primary hypothyroid

Fig. 7.1: Basic thyroid evaluation.

Box 7.1: Thyrotoxicosis and its types.

Primary hyperthyroidism
- Graves' disease
- Toxic multinodular goitre
- Toxic adenoma
- Iodine excess (Jod-Basedow)

Thyrotoxicosis without hyperthyroidism
- Subacute thyroiditis, hashitoxicosis
- Amiodarone induced
- Radiation induced
- Thyrotoxicosis factitia
- Struma ovarii

Secondary hyperthyroidism
- TSH-secreting pituitary adenoma
- Human chorionic gonadotropin-mediated hyperthyroidism
- Gestational thyrotoxicosis

(TSH: thyroid-stimulating hormone)

- Cardiovascular system—palpitations, angina, sinus tachycardia, atrial fibrillation, wide pulse pressure, cardiac failure
- Nervous system—nervousness, irritability, fine tremors, hyperreflexia, proximal myopathy
- Skin and integumentary system—increased sweating, pruritus, palmar erythema, spider naevi, onycholysis, pretibial myxoedema (Graves), clubbing (thyroid acropachy)
- Reproductive system—menstrual disturbances (amenorrhoea or oligomenorrhoea), repeated abortions, infertility
- General—heat intolerance, fatigue, gynaecomastia, apathy, thirst
- Eyes—lid lag, exophthalmos, proptosis, extraocular diplopia, exposure keratitis, lagophthalmos (classically seen in Graves' disease)

Investigations

- Thyroid-stimulating hormone (TSH) levels: Very low or undetectable
- Serum T3 and T4 levels: Raised in most cases
- ^{131}I uptake by the thyroid gland: It may be increased
- TSH receptor antibody (TRAb): Present in most cases

Approach to hyperthyroidism discussed in **Flowchart 7.1**.

Management

Medical

Indications: Primary therapy in pregnancy, in children and adolescents and severe Graves' disease with eye changes. The drugs include:
- Thionamides: Propylthiouracil, carbimazole, methimazole
- Potassium perchlorate
- Potassium iodide: Only in (1) preparation for thyroidectomy and (2) thyrotoxic crisis
- Beta-adrenergic blockers: Propranolol
- Lithium

Surgical Treatment

- Subtotal thyroidectomy is the treatment of choice.

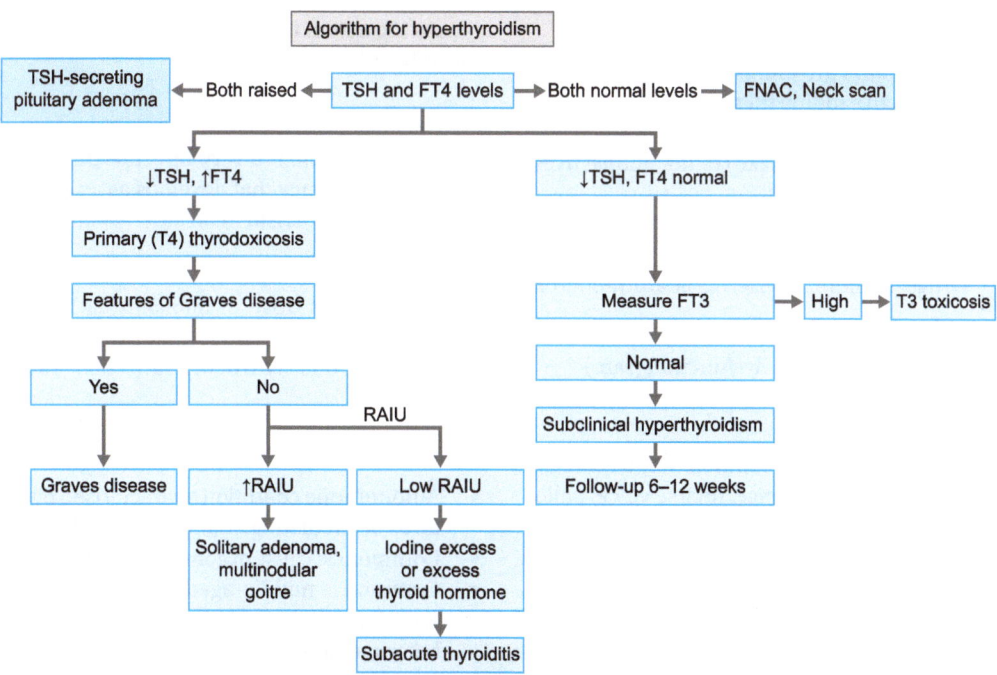

(FT4: free thyroxine; FT3: free triiodothronine; TSH: thyroid-stimulating hormone; RAIU: radioactive iodine uptake)

Flowchart 7.1: Approach to diagnosis in hyperthyroidism.

Radioactive Iodine

[using ^{131}I]

HYPERTHYROID CRISIS/THYROTOXIC CRISIS/THYROID STORM

Treatment

- Rehydration and given antibiotics if there is infection
- Control hyperthermia: By external cooling. DO NOT administer salicylates, as they convert T4 to T3.
- Propranolol: Either orally (80 mg 4 times daily) or intravenously (1–5 mg 4 times daily)
- Propylthiouracil 800–1200 mg orally every 4 hours
- Lugol's iodine: 10 drops tid about 1 hour after propylthiouracil or carbimazole
- Sodium iopodate: 500 mg/day orally
- Benzodiazepines: For agitation
- Corticosteroids: Intravenous (IV) hydrocortisone 100–200 mg every 6 hours
- Bile acid sequestrants, cholestyramine

HYPOTHYROIDISM

Primary:
- Hashimoto's thyroiditis
- Radioactive iodine therapy
- Subtotal thyroidectomy
- Excessive iodide intake (radiocontrast dyes)
- Subacute thyroiditis
- Post-partum thyroiditis
- Iodide deficiency
- Drugs: Lithium, interferon-alfa, amiodarone

Secondary: Hypopituitarism

Tertiary: Hypothalamic dysfunction (rare)

Clinical Features

- General—lethargy, somnolence, weight gain, goitre, cold intolerance, hoarse voice, pallor
- Thyroid—enlargement of the gland
- Gastrointestinal—reduced appetite, constipation, ileus, macroglossia
- Cardiorespiratory—angina, bradycardia, hypertension (diastolic), cardiac failure, pericardial effusion, pleural effusion
- Neuromuscular—delayed relaxation of tendon reflexes (Woltman's sign), carpal tunnel syndrome, depression, cerebellar ataxia, proximal myopathy
- Skin—myxoedema (non-pitting oedema of the skin of hands, feet and eyelids), xanthelasmas, madarosis
- Reproductive—menorrhagia, infertility, galactorrhoea, impotence
- Haematological—macrocytosis, anaemia
- Miscellaneous—obstructive sleep apnoea (OSA), hyponatraemia, weight gain

Investigations

- Serum TSH→High TSH level confirms primary hypothyroidism
- Serum T4 levels: Low
- Thyroid antibodies
- Other abnormalities:
  - Hypercholesterolaemia and hypertriglyceridaemia
  - Hyponatraemia

Treatment

- Replacement therapy with levothyroxine sodium, once-daily dosage (1.6–1.8 µg/kg/day)

An algorithm for hypothyroidism is shown in **Flowchart 7.2**.

Myxoedema Coma

Myxoedema coma is a very rare, life-threatening medical emergency that develops as a complication of hypothyroidism in an elderly patient.

Treatment

- Intravenous dose of 300–500 µg T4; if no response within 48 hours, add T3.
- Intravenous hydrocortisone 200–400 mg daily.

Hashimoto's Thyroiditis

- Autoimmune condition characterised by high titres of circulating antibodies to TPC and Tg
- Commonest cause of goitrous hypothyroidism
- Common in middle-aged females and is often associated with ulcerative colitis or type 1 diabetes mellitus

Investigations

- Thyroid function test (TFT)

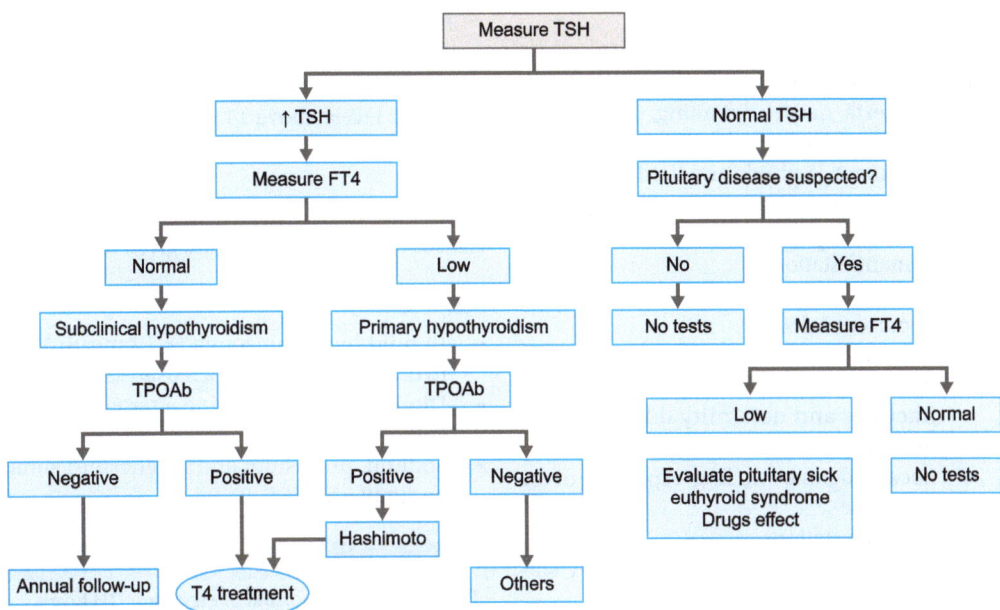

(FT4: free thyroxine; FT3: free triiodothronine; TSH: thyroid-stimulating hormone; TPOAb: thyroid peroxidase antibodies)

Flowchart 7.2: Algorithm for hypothyroidism.

TABLE 7.1: Classification and causes of hyperparathyroidism.

Type	Serum calcium	Serum PTH	Causes
Primary: Autonomous secretion of PTH by parathyroid	Raised	Raised	Single adenoma (90%), multiple adenomata, nodular hyperplasia and carcinoma of parathyroid
Secondary: Parathyroid hyperplasia with increased PTH secretion in an attempt to compensate for prolonged hypocalcaemia	Low	Raised	Chronic renal failure, malabsorption, osteomalacia and rickets
Tertiary: Adenoma formation and autonomous PTH secretion. Occurring cases of secondary hyperparathyroidism	Raised	Raised	• Chronic secondary hyperparathyroidism • Post-renal transplantation

(PTH: parathyroid hormone)

- Anti-thyroid peroxidase (anti-TPO) antibody
- Fine needle aspiration cytology (FNAC) of thyroid

Treatment
- Thyroxine supplements

HYPERPARATHYROIDISM

Classification and Causes

Classification and causes of hyperparathyroidism are shown in **Table 7.1**.

Clinical Features
- Incidental finding of hypercalcaemia
- Non-specific symptoms
  - Anorexia, nausea, vomiting, constipation and weight loss
  - Weakness, lassitude and tiredness
  - Drowsiness, poor concentration, memory loss and depression
- Renal manifestations
  - Polyuria and polydipsia
  - Recurrent calculus
- Skeletal manifestations
  - Bone pain, osteopaenia, osteoporosis, fractures and deformity due to osteitis fibrosa cystic
  - Localised bone swelling, especially of the mandible
- Other manifestations
  - Corneal calcification, best seen by slit-lamp examination
  - Calcification of arterial walls and soft tissues of hand
  - Peptic ulceration
  - Hypertension
  - Myopathy

Investigations
- Serum calcium and parathyroid hormone (PTH)
- Vitamin D
- Serum phosphate
- Serum chloride
- Serum alkaline phosphatase
- Electrocardiogram (ECG)
  - Shortened QT interval
- Radiological abnormalities
  - Demineralisation and subperiosteal erosions of phalanges, most marked on the radial side of the middle phalanx
  - Resorption of the terminal phalanges
  - 'Pepper-pot' appearance of the skull
  - Nephrocalcinosis
- Dual-energy X-ray absorptiometry (DEXA) and CT scan
- Investigations for localisation of the tumour

Treatment
- Treatment of hypercalcaemia
- Adenoma—surgical removal

■ HYPERCALCAEMIA
- Mild if the total serum calcium level is between 10.5 and 12 mg/dL (2.6–3 mmol/L) while levels above 14 mg/dL indicate severe hypercalcaemia.

Causes
Causes of hypercalcaemia are given in **Box 7.2**.

Management
- In mild hypercalcaemia (< 12 mg/dL), oral hydration along with increased salt intake
- Diuretics like furosemide after correction of volume
- Sodium, potassium and magnesium should be supplemented.

Box 7.2: Causes of hypercalcaemia.

PTH related with normal or elevated PTH levels
- Primary hyperparathyroidism (commonest) or tertiary hyperparathyroidism
- Lithium therapy–induced hyperparathyroidism
- Familial hypercalciuric hypercalcaemia

Malignancy related with low PTH levels (second commonest cause)
- Multiple myeloma
- PTH related protein secretion: Tumours of lung and kidney
- Secondary deposits in bone: Breast carcinoma
- Production of osteoclastic factor by tumours

Associated with renal failure
- Secondary hyperparathyroidism
- Aluminium intoxication

Vitamin D related with low PTH levels
- Vitamin D intoxication: Iatrogenic or self-administered excess
- Granulomatous diseases (sarcoidosis, tuberculosis, berylliosis)
- Lymphoma
- Idiopathic hypercalcaemia of infancy

High bone turnover
- Long-term immobilisation
- Hyperthyroidism
- Drugs: For example, thiazide diuretics
- Paget's disease with immobilisation

Excessive calcium intake
Milk-alkali syndrome

(PTH: parathyroid hormone)

- Prednisolone or hydrocortisone
- Oral phosphate
- Mithramycin
- Intravenous bisphosphonates
- Serum calcitonin
- Haemodialysis with a low-calcium bath

■ HYPOPARATHYROIDISM

- The common clinical manifestation is tetany, irrespective of the cause
- Characteristically, serum calcium is low and serum phosphate is high.

Causes

- Post-operative hypoparathyroidism
- Infantile hypoparathyroidism
- Idiopathic hypoparathyroidism
- Pseudohypoparathyroidism (resistance to PTH)

Treatment

- In the acute phase, calcium is given intravenously as for tetany.
- Substitution therapy is provided by 1-α-hydroxycholecalciferol (alphacalcidol) or 1, 25 dihydroxycholecalciferol (calcitriol).

■ TETANY

Causes

Tetany is caused by an increased excitability of peripheral nerves due to hypocalcaemia or alkalosis or hypomagnesaemia (**Box 7.3**).

Box 7.3: Causes of tetany.

Due to hypocalcaemia
Increased phosphate levels
- Chronic renal failure (common)
- Phosphate therapy

Hypoparathyroidism
- Surgical—after neck exploration (thyroidectomy, parathyroidectomy—common)
- Congenital deficiency (DiGeorge syndrome)
- Idiopathic hypoparathyroidism (rare)
- Severe hypomagnesaemia

Resistance to PTH
- Pseudohypoparathyroidism

Vitamin D deficiency
- Osteomalacia/rickets
- Vitamin D resistance

Others
- Acute pancreatitis (quite common)
- Citrated blood in massive transfusion (not uncommon)
- Low plasma albumin, e.g. malnutrition, chronic liver disease
- Malabsorption, e.g. coeliac disease

Drugs
- Calcitonin
- Bisphosphonates

Due to alkalosis
- Repeated vomiting of gastric juice
- Excessive intake of oral alkali
- Hyperventilation, e.g. hysteria
- Primary hyperaldosteronism

Due to hypomagnesaemia

(PTH: parathyroid hormone)

Clinical Features

- In children, the characteristic triad of carpopedal spasm, stridor and convulsions occurs. In '**carpal spasm**', the metacarpophalangeal joints are flexed, the interphalangeal joints are extended and there is opposition of the thumb (main d'accoucheur).
- In adults there is tingling in the hands, feet and around the mouth (circumoral paraesthesia).
- Latent tetany may be present when signs of overt tetany are lacking. It is recognised by eliciting two signs:
  1. **Trousseau's sign**—inflation of sphygmomanometer cuff on the upper arm to more than systolic pressure is followed by the characteristic carpal spasm within 3 minutes.
  2. **Chvostek sign**—tapping over the branches of facial nerve as they emerge from the parotid gland produces twitching of the facial muscles.

Treatment

Control of Tetany

- Slow intravenous injection of calcium gluconate
- Administration of magnesium

Correction of Alkalosis
- Hysterical hyperventilation→re-breathing expired air from a suitable bag or inhalation of 5% carbon dioxide in oxygen.

■ CUSHING'S SYNDROME
Causes
Causes of Cushing's syndrome are given in **Table 7.2**.

Clinical Features
Clinical features of Cushing's syndrome are given in **Table 7.3**.

Investigations
- Plasma cortisol levels
- 24-hour urinary cortisol excretion→raised
- Overnight dexamethasone suppression test
- Low-dose dexamethasone suppression test

TABLE 7.2: Causes of Cushing's syndrome.

ACTH dependent	ACTH independent
• Cushing's disease • Ectopic ACTH syndrome (tumours) • Ectopic corticotropin-releasing hormone syndrome	• Iatrogenic (use of corticosteroids) • Adrenal adenoma • Adrenal carcinoma

(ACTH: adrenocorticotropic hormone)

TABLE 7.3: Clinical features of Cushing's syndrome.

Symptom	Sign
• Weight pain • Hirsutism • Back pain • Muscle weakness • Oligomenorrhoea, amenorrhoea and impotence • Depression, irritability, psychosis	• Central obesity ('lemon on matchstick') • Buffalo hump • Plethoric appearance • Moon face • Bruising • Purplish striae over abdomen, buttocks and thighs • Hypertension • Proximal myopathy • Skin infections

- Blood sugar, cholesterol and low-density lipoproteins (LDL) may be elevated.
- Plain radiograph of the skull
- CT/MRI of head
- Radiograph of chest to detect bronchogenic carcinoma
- CT scan of anterior mediastinum and upper abdomen including pancreas to rule out tumours
- MRI of abdomen

An algorithm of Cushing's syndrome is shown in **Flowchart 7.3**.

Management
Adrenal Tumours
- Metyrapone or aminoglutethimide
- Adrenal carcinomas are resected surgically.

Cushing's Disease
- Metyrapone or ketoconazole
- Trans-sphenoidal surgical removal of the adenoma
- Radiotherapy and radiosurgery for the treatment of recurrent or residual adrenocorticotropic hormone (ACTH)-secreting tumours

■ NELSON'S SYNDROME
- Develops in patients with Cushing's disease (pituitary-dependent bilateral hyperplasia) treated by bilateral adrenalectomy with no definitive treatment for pituitary
- Characterised by an aggressive locally invasive pituitary tumour with very high levels of ACTH in the blood and hyperpigmentation of skin
- Treatment includes surgery and radiotherapy.

■ PRIMARY HYPERALDOSTERONISM
Aetiology
- Adenoma (**Conn's syndrome**)
- Bilateral zona glomerulosa hyperplasia
  - Idiopathic
  - ACTH dependent (glucocorticoid-responsive or dexamethasone-suppressible). In this type of hyperaldosteronism, the secretion of aldosterone is under ACTH control. Therefore, treatment is administering glucocorticoids that suppress ACTH release.

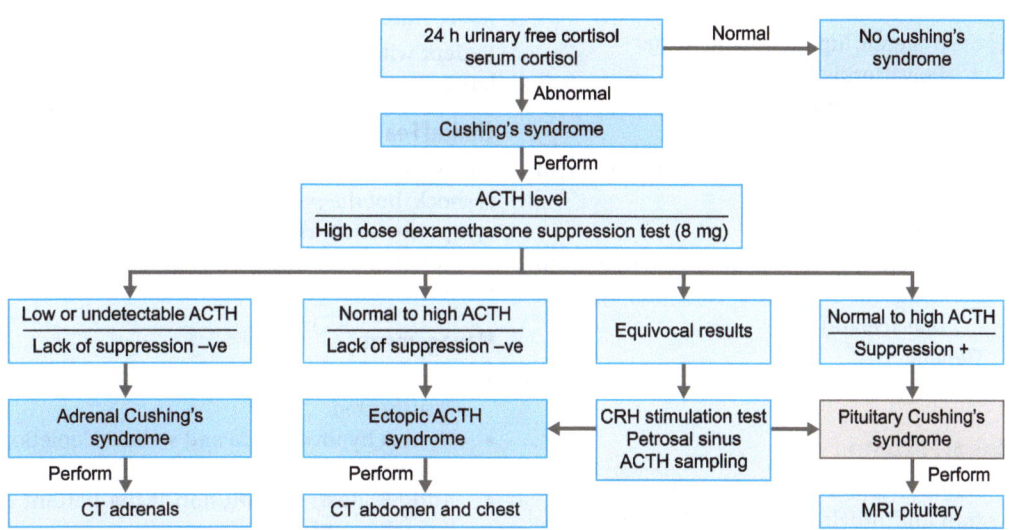

Flowchart 7.3: Algorithm of Cushing's syndrome.

(ACTH: adrenocorticotropic hormone; CRH: corticotropin-releasing hormone; CT: computed tomography; MRI: magnetic resonance imaging)

Pathophysiology
- Excess aldosterone produces sodium retention, potassium loss and metabolic alkalosis.

Clinical Features
- Hypertension and hypokalaemia
- Muscle weakness from hypokalaemia
- Tetany due to metabolic alkalosis

Investigations
Diagnosis
- Hypokalaemia: Elevated urinary potassium
- Plasma aldosterone concentration (PAC) is elevated.
- Plasma renin activity (PRA) is suppressed.
- PAC:PRA ratio is the accepted screening test for primary hyperaldosteronism. A level above 20 is considered abnormal.
- CT/MRI scanning can detect adenoma and hyperplasia.
- Adrenal vein catheterisation
- Measurement of 18-OH-cortisol levels

Management
- Aldosterone antagonists, spironolactone and eplerenone are effective in patients where surgery cannot be done.
- Unilateral adrenalectomy may be done in an adenoma.
- Angiotensin receptor blockers may be given for control of hypertension.

■ SECONDARY HYPERALDOSTERONISM
- Physiological—salt depletion from inadequate intake or excessive loss through kidney or GIT; pregnancy.
- Pathological—excessive diuretic therapy, nephrotic syndrome, cirrhosis with ascites, congestive heart failure, Bartter's syndrome accelerated or malignant phase of hypertension, severe renal artery stenosis.

■ ADDISON'S DISEASE
- Indicates adrenocortical insufficiency due to destruction of the entire adrenal cortex.

Causes
- Autoimmune adrenalitis
- Infectious adrenalitis
  - Tuberculosis
  - Fungal (histoplasmosis)
- Adrenal haemorrhage
  - Waterhouse–Friderichsen syndrome
  - Anticoagulation therapy

- Adrenal infarction (due to thrombosis)
  - Systemic lupus erythematosus
  - Polyarteritis nodosa
  - Antiphospholipid syndrome
- Metastases in the adrenal
  - Lung, breast, stomach carcinomas, lymphoma
- Drug induced
  - Adrenolytic therapy (e.g. mitotane, ketoconazole, etomidate, rifampin, cyproterone acetate)
- Genetic
  - Congenital adrenal hyperplasia

Clinical Features

- Cardinal features—hypotension, pigmentation and previous history of acute adrenal crisis following stress or slow recovery from illness
- **Glucocorticoid deficiency** results in malaise, weakness, weight loss, anorexia, nausea, vomiting, postural hypotension and hypoglycaemia.
- **Mineralocorticoid deficiency** manifests as hypotension. Many patients have salt carving.
- **ACTH excess** results in pigmentation of exposed areas, pressure areas such as elbows, knees and knuckles, palmar creases, mucous membranes, conjunctive and recently acquired scars.

Investigations

- Elevated blood urea, hyponatraemia and hyperkalaemia
- Low blood sugar levels
- Mild anaemia, mild eosinophilia
- Plasma cortisol measured between 8 and 9 am < 3 mg/dL
- ACTH stimulation test

Management

- Patients with Addison's disease require lifelong glucocorticoid and mineralocorticoid replacement therapy—cortisone or prednisolone and fludrocortisones
- Addison's disease due to tuberculous adrenalitis should be treated with antitubercular treatment (ATT)

Acute Adrenal Crisis

Patient with primary adrenal insufficiency who has a serious infection or other acute stress.

Clinical Features

The predominant manifestation of adrenal crisis is shock, but the patients often have non-specific symptoms such as anorexia, nausea, vomiting, abdominal pain, weakness, fatigue, lethargy, confusion or coma.

Management

- Initiate therapy as soon as acute adrenal crisis is suspected.
- Correct hypovolaemia and sodium depletion with normal saline.
- Add 5% dextrose solution if the patient is hypoglycaemic.
- Administer hydrocortisone.

WATERHOUSE–FRIDERICHSEN SYNDROME

- Acute haemorrhagic destruction of both the adrenal glands, usually associated with fulminant meningococcal septicaemia.
- It is characterised by vasomotor collapse and shock.
- Petechiae, purpuric lesion and haemorrhage into the skin occur.

PHAEOCHROMOCYTOMA

- Phaeochromocytoma is a tumour of the chromaffin tissue that secretes catecholamines (adrenaline and noradrenaline).
- About 90% of the tumours arise from the adrenal medulla (phaeochromocytoma), while 10% are paragangliomas.
- About 90% are benign while 10% are malignant.

Clinical Features

- Paroxysmal hypertension associated with episodes of pallor or flushing, palpitations, sweating, headache and anxiety
- Gastrointestinal symptoms such as abdominal pain, vomiting, constipation and weight loss
- Glucose intolerance
- Complications of hypertension such as stroke, myocardial infarction, cardiomyopathy and left ventricular failure

Investigations

- 24-hour urine vanillylmandelic acid (VMA) is raised.
- 24-hour urine metanephrines and normetanephrines are raised.
- 24-hour urine free catecholamines are raised.
- CT scan to localise tumour
- Metaiodobenzylguanidine (MIBG) scintigraphy

Management

- Excision of the tumour if possible
- If excision is not possible, long-term treatment with α- and β-adrenoreceptor-blocking drugs (phenoxybenzamine and propranolol, or labetalol) is advocated. β-blockers should never be given alone.

■ HYPERLIPIDAEMIA

Causes

- Primary hyperlipidaemia (Genetic)
- Secondary hyperlipidaemia (**Table 7.4**)

Management Strategies

- Lipid profile of a person is always interpreted with the risk factors for CAD.
  Risk factors that modify LDL goals are given in **Table 7.5**.

Management

Therapeutic Lifestyle Changes

- Reduced intake of saturated fats and cholesterol
- Increased intake of soluble fibre
- Weight reduction
- Increased physical activity

Pharmacotherapy

- Statins—simvastatin, atorvastatin, lovastatin, pravastatin and rosuvastatin (**Table 7.6**)
- Bile acid sequestrants—cholestyramine and colestipol
- Niacin
- Fibrates—gemfibrozil
- Ezetimibe—inhibits the absorption of cholesterol from the diet
- Omega-3 fatty acid
- Newer agents
  - Torcetrapib is a cholesteryl ester transfer protein (CETP)
  - Proprotein convertase subtilisin/kexin 9 (PCSK9) inhibitors—evolocumab and alirocumab

TABLE 7.5: Risk factors that modify low-density lipoproteins (LDL) goals.

Positive risk factors	Negative risk factors
• Age (males ≥ 45 years; females > 55 years) • Low HDL cholesterol (40 mg/dL) • Smoking • Hypertension (with or without treatment) • Family history of premature CAD (at the age of < 55 years in males and < 65 years in females)	• High HDL cholesterol (> 60 mg/dL)

(CAD: coronary artery disease; DI: diabetes insipidus; HDL: high-density lipoproteins

TABLE 7.4: Cuses of secondary hyperlipidaemia.

Increased LDL cholesterol level	Increased triglyceride level	Decreased HDL cholesterol level

• Diabetes mellitus
• Hypothyroidism
• Nephrotic syndrome
• Obstructive liver disease
• Drugs:
  ○ Anabolic steroids
  ○ Progestins
  ○ Beta-adrenergic blockers (without intrinsic sympathomimetic action)
  ○ Thiazides
	• Alcoholism
	• Diabetes mellitus
	• Hypothyroidism
	• Obesity
	• Renal insufficiency
	• Drugs:
	  ○ Beta-adrenergic blockers (without intrinsic sympathomimetic action)
	  ○ Bile acid binding resins
	  ○ Oestrogens
	  ○ Ticlopidine
		• Cigarette smoking
		• Diabetes mellitus Hypertriglyceridaemia
		• Menopause
		• Obesity
		• Uraemia
		• Anabolic steroids
		• Beta-adrenergic blockers (without intrinsic sympathomimetic action)
		• Progestins

(LDL: low-density lipoprotein; HDL: high-density lipoprotein)

TABLE 7.6: Cardiovascular risk categories and recommendations for LDL-C—2019 ESC/EAS (European Society of Cardiology/European Atherosclerosis Society) Guidelines for the management of dyslipidaemias.

Risk	Description	Recommendation	
		Target	Intervention
Very-high-risk	• Documented ASCVD, either clinical or unequivocal on imaging • Documented ASCVD—includes previous ACS, stable angina, coronary revascularisation, stroke and TIA, and peripheral arterial disease • Unequivocally documented ASCVD on imaging—such as significant plaque on coronary angiography or CT scan or on carotid ultrasound, known to be predictive of clinical events • DM with target organ damage, ≥ 3 major risk factors or early onset of T1DM of long duration (> 20 years) • Severe CKD (eGFR < 30 mL/min/1.73 m²) • Family history with ASCVD or with another major risk factor • Apparently healthy people with calculated SCORE ≥ 10% for 10-year risk of fatal CVD	• An LDL-C reduction of at least 50% from baseline and an LDL-C goal of < 1.4 mmol/L (< 55 mg/dL) are recommended • LDL-C goal of < 1.0 mmol/L (< 40 mg/dL) may be considered for patients with ASCVD who experience a second vascular event within 2 years while taking maximally tolerated statin therapy	Secondary prevention: • Lifestyle interventions recommended and pharmacological intervention considered for all patients with very-high cardiovascular risk • Pharmacological intervention recommended for patients with LDL-C > 55 mg/dL Primary prevention: • Lifestyle interventions recommended and pharmacological intervention considered for patients with LDL levels above target (> 55 mg/dL) • Pharmacological intervention recommended for patients with LDL-C > 70 mg/dL
High-risk	• Markedly elevated single risk factor, in particular TC > 8 mmol/L (> 310 mg/dL), LDL-C > 4.9 mmol/L (> 190 mg/dL) or BP ≥ 180/110 mmHg • Patients with FH without other major risk factors • Patients with DM without target organ damage, with DM duration ≥ 10 years or another additional risk factor • Moderate CKD (eGFR 30–59 mL/min/1.73 m²) • Apparently healthy people with calculated SCORE ≥ 5% and < 10% for 10-year risk of fatal CVD	An LDL-C reduction of at least 50% from baseline and an LDL-C goal of < 1.8 mmol/L (< 70 mg/dL) are recommended	Primary prevention: • Lifestyle interventions recommended and pharmacological intervention considered for patients with LDL levels above target (> 70 mg/dL) • Pharmacological intervention recommended for patients with LDL-C levels > 100 mg/dL

Continued

Continued

Risk	Description	Recommendation	
		Target	Intervention
Moderate-risk	• Young patients (T1DM < 35 years; T2DM < 50 years) with DM duration < 10 years, without other risk factors • Apparently healthy people with calculated SCORE ≥ 1% and < 5% for 10-year risk of fatal CVD	An LDL-C goal of < 2.6 mmol/L (< 100 mg/dL) should be considered	Primary prevention: • Lifestyle interventions recommended and pharmacological intervention considered for patients with LDL levels above target (> 100 mg/dL) • Pharmacological intervention recommended for patients with LDL-C levels ≥ 190 mg/dL
Low-risk	• Apparently healthy people with calculated SCORE < 1% for 10-year risk of fatal CVD	An LDL-C goal < 3.0 mmol/L (< 116 mg/dL) may be considered	Primary prevention: Lifestyle interventions recommended and pharmacological intervention considered for patients with LDL levels above target (> 116 mg/dL) Pharmacological intervention recommended for patients with LDL-C levels ≥ 190 mg/dL

- Pharmacological therapy includes:
  - For patients with no current statin use: Add high-intensity LDL-lowering therapy
  - For patients on LDL-lowering treatment: Increase treatment intensity

(ACS: acute coronary syndrome; ASCVD: atherosclerotic cardiovascular disease; CKD: chronic kidney disease; CVD: cardiovascular disease; DM: diabetes mellitus; eGFR: estimated glomerular filtration rate; FH: familial hypercholesterolaemia; LDL-C: low-density lipoprotein-cholesterol; SCORE: Systematic Coronary Risk Estimation; TC: total cholesterol; TIA: transient ischaemic attack ; CT: computed tomography; T1DM: type 1 diabetes mellitus; T2DM: type 2 diabetes mellitus)

BEST OF FIVES

1. All of the following hormones are produced by the anterior pituitary except:
   A. Adrenocorticotropic hormone
   B. Growth hormone
   C. Oxytocin
   D. Prolactin
   E. Thyroid stimulating hormone (TSH)

2. A 19-year-old woman presents to the clinic complaining of months of weight gain, fatigue, amenorrhoea and worsening acne. She has noted a 12.3-kg weight gain over the past 6 months. She has been amenorrhoeic for several months. On examination, she is noted to have truncal obesity with bilateral purplish striae across both flanks. Which of the following tests should be used to make the diagnosis?
   A. 24-hour urine free cortisol
   B. Basal adrenocorticotropic hormone (ACTH)
   C. Corticotropin-releasing hormone (CRH) level at 8 AM
   D. Inferior petrosal venous sampling
   E. Overnight 1 mg dexamethasone suppression test

3. Which of the following is common in patients with Kallmann syndrome?
   A. Anosmia
   B. White forelock
   C. Precocious (early) puberty in females
   D. Syndactyly in males
   E. Hyperphagia—obesity

4. All of the following are risk factors for the development of osteoporotic fractures except:
   A. African-American race
   B. Current cigarette smoking
   C. Female sex
   D. Low body weight
   E. Physical inactivity

5. All of the following biochemical markers are a measure of bone resorption except:
   A. Serum alkaline phosphatase
   B. Serum cross-linked N-telopeptide
   C. Serum cross-linked C-telopeptide
   D. Urine hydroxyproline
   E. Urine total free deoxypyridinoline

6. A 40-year-old woman presents to your clinic complaining of difficulty in swallowing, sore throat and tender swelling in her neck. She has also noted fevers intermittently over the past week. On physical examination, she is noted to have a small goitre that is painful to the touch. Her oropharynx is clear. Laboratory studies are sent, and they reveal a white blood cell count of 14,100 cells/μL with a normal differential, erythrocyte sedimentation rate (ESR) of 53 mm/h and a thyroid-stimulating hormone (TSH) of 21 μIU/mL. Thyroid antibodies are negative. What is the most likely diagnosis?
   A. Autoimmune hypothyroidism
   B. Cat-scratch fever
   C. Graves' disease
   D. Ludwig's angina
   E. Subacute thyroiditis

7. Differentiating primary dysmenorrhoea from other causes of chronic cyclical pelvic pain is important because there is a specific treatment for primary dysmenorrhoea. What is the pathophysiology/treatment for primary dysmenorrhoea?
   A. Ectopic endometrium/oral contraceptives
   B. History of sexual abuse/counselling
   C. Increased stores of prostaglandin precursors/anti-inflammatory medication
   D. Ruptured Graafian follicle/oral contraceptives
   E. Nutritional intervention/ supplementation of vitamins

8. Post-menopausal oestrogen therapy has been shown to increase a female's risk of all of the following clinical outcomes except:
   A. Breast cancer
   B. Hip fracture
   C. Myocardial infarction
   D. Stroke
   E. Venous thromboembolism

9. Inhibition of renin activity is a contemporary target mechanism for treatment of hypertension. All of the following physiologic alterations will cause an increase in renin secretion except:
   A. Decreased effective circulating blood volume
   B. High-potassium diet
   C. Increased sympathetic activity
   D. Low solute delivery to the distal convoluted tubules
   E. Upright posture

10. Which of the following statements regarding autoimmune hypothyroidism is true?
    A. About 10% of 40–60-year-old adults have subclinical hypothyroidism.
    B. Absence of a goitre makes autoimmune hypothyroidism unlikely.
    C. Family history of autoimmune disorders does not significantly increase risk.
    D. It is more common in the Pacific Rim where diets are lower in iodine.
    E. Viral thyroiditis does not induce subsequent autoimmune thyroiditis.

11. A patient is asked to undergo a testing protocol to assess adrenocortical function. After 5 days of severe sodium restriction (10 mmol/d), blood is drawn for analysis. Which hormone abnormality may be detected using this protocol?
    A. Hypercortisolism
    B. Glucocorticoid deficiency
    C. Mineralocorticoid deficiency

D. Mineralocorticoid excess
E. Vasopressin excess

12. All of the following are direct actions of parathyroid hormone (PTH) except:
    A. Increased calcium resorption from the bone
    B. Increased calcium resorption from the kidney
    C. Increased calcium resorption from the gastrointestinal tract
    D. Increased synthesis of 1,25-dihydroxyvitamin D
    E. Decreased phosphate resorption from the kidney

13. A comprehensive metabolic panel of a 45-year-old male shows a serum calcium level of 11.2 mg/dL. Serum phosphate is 3.0 mg/dL. Serum creatinine is normal. He denies bone pain, lethargy, weakness or weight loss. What is the most common cause of hypercalcaemia in outpatients?
    A. Malignancy
    B. Medications
    C. Milk-alkali syndrome
    D. Primary hyperparathyroidism
    E. Granulomatous disease

14. A patient is seen in the clinic for follow-up of type 2 diabetes mellitus (T2DM). Her glycated haemoglobin (HbA1c) has been poorly controlled at 9.4% recently. The patient can be counselled to expect all of the following improvements with improved glycaemic control except:
    A. Decreased microalbuminuria
    B. Decreased risk of nephropathy
    C. Decreased risk of neuropathy
    D. Decreased risk of peripheral vascular disease
    E. Decreased risk of retinopathy

15. During a routine check-up, a 75-year-old male is found to have a level of serum alkaline phosphatase three times the upper limit of normal. Serum calcium and phosphorus concentrations and liver function test results are normal. He is asymptomatic. The most likely diagnosis is:
    A. Metastatic bone disease
    B. Primary hyperparathyroidism
    C. Occult plasmacytoma
    D. Paget's disease of bone
    E. Osteomalacia

16. Which of the following statements regarding hormone release from the anterior pituitary is true?
    A. All hormones are released in a pulsatile manner.
    B. Follicle-stimulating hormone (FSH) and luteinising hormone (LH) release are suppressed prior to puberty and after menopause.
    C. Somatostatin acts in a feedback loop to inhibit adrenocorticotropin hormone (ACTH) release.
    D. Thyroid-stimulating hormone (TSH) is released primarily at night.
    E. With the exception of prolactin, none of the anterior pituitary hormones are present in a foetus until week 28 of gestation.

17. Which of the following is the most common sign of Cushing's syndrome?
    A. Amenorrhoea
    B. Hirsutism
    C. Obesity
    D. Purple skin striae
    E. Skin hyperpigmentation

18. All of the following are effects of hypercalcaemia except:
    A. Diarrhoea
    B. Confusion
    C. Polyuria
    D. A shortened QT interval
    E. Nephrolithiasis

19. Which of the following statements regarding hypothyroidism is true?
    A. Hashimoto's thyroiditis is the most common cause of hypothyroidism worldwide.
    B. The annual risk of developing overt clinical hypothyroidism from subclinical hypothyroidism in patients with positive thyroid peroxidase (TPO) antibodies is 20%.
    C. Histologically, Hashimoto's thyroiditis is characterised by marked infiltration of the thyroid with activated T cells and B cells.
    D. A low thyroid-stimulating hormone (TSH) level excludes the diagnosis of hypothyroidism.
    E. Thyroid peroxidase antibodies are present in < 50% of patients with autoimmune hypothyroidism.

20. Obesity is associated with an increased incidence of all of the following except:
    A. Diabetes mellitus
    B. Cancer
    C. Hypertension
    D. Biliary disease
    E. Chronic obstructive lung disease

21. All of the following would be expected to increase prolactin levels except:
    A. Chest wall trauma
    B. Hyperthyroidism
    C. Pregnancy
    D. Renal failure
    E. Sexual orgasm

22. The common site for infection of islet cells in islet cell transplantation for diabetes mellitus is:
    A. Around umbilicus
    B. Pancreas
    C. Portal vein
    D. Forearm muscles
    E. Urinary bladder

23. Nelson's syndrome is most likely seen after:
    A. Hypophysectomy
    B. Adrenalectomy
    C. Thyroidectomy
    D. Orchidectomy
    E. Mastectomy

24. Which of the following is produced by argentaffinoma of ileum?
    A. Gamma-aminobutyric acid (GABA)
    B. Serotonin
    C. Epinephrine
    D. Norepinephrine
    E. Histamine

25. The most common presentation of a sick euthyroid state is:
    A. Low T3 and normal T4
    B. Low T3 and low T4
    C. Low T4 and high T3
    D. High T3 and high T4
    E. Normal T3 and normal thyroid-stimulating hormone (TSH)

Answers

1-C, 2-A, 3-A, 4-A, 5-A, 6-E, 7-C, 8-B, 9-B, 10-E, 11-C, 12-C, 13-D, 14-D, 15-D, 16-A, 17-C, 18-A, 19-C, 20-E, 21-B, 22-C, 23-B, 24-B, 25-A

■ SUGGESTED READING

1. Jonklaas J, Bianco AC, Bauer AJ, Burman KD, Cappola AR, Celi FS, et al. Guidelines for the treatment of hypothyroidism: prepared by the American thyroid association task force on thyroid hormone replacement. Thyroid. 2014;24(12):1670-751.
2. Ross DS, Burch HB, Cooper DS, Greenlee MC, Laurberg P, Maia AL, et al. 2016 American Thyroid Association Guidelines for diagnosis and management of hyperthyroidism and other causes of thyrotoxicosis. Thyroid. 2016;26(10):1343-421.
3. Bornstein SR, Allolio B, Arlt W, Barthel A, Don-Wauchope A, Hammer GD, et al. Diagnosis and treatment of primary adrenal insufficiency: An Endocrine Society Clinical Practice Guideline. J Clin Endocrinol Metab. 2016;101(2):364-89.
4. Nieman LK, Biller BM, Findling JW, Murad MH, Newell-Price J, Savage MO, et al. Treatment of Cushing's Syndrome: An Endocrine Society Clinical Practice Guideline. J Clin Endocrinol Metab. 2015;100(8):2807-31.
5. Lenders JW, Duh QY, Eisenhofer G, Gimenez-Roqueplo AP, Grebe SKG, Murad MH, et al. Pheochromocytoma and paraganglioma: An Endocrine Society Clinical Practice Guideline. J Clin Endocrinol Metab. 2014;99(6):1915-42.
6. Fleseriu M, Hashim IA, Karavitaki N, Melmed S, Murad MH, Salvatori R, et al. Hormonal replacement in hypopituitarism in adults: An Endocrine Society Clinical Practice Guideline. J Clin Endocrinol Metab. 2016;101(11):3888-921.
7. Melmed S. Acromegaly pathogenesis and treatment. J Clin Invest. 2009;119(11):3189-202.
8. Katznelson L, Laws ER Jr, Melmed S, Molitch ME, Murad MH, Utz A, et al. Acromegaly: An Endocrine Society Clinical Practice Guideline. J Clin Endocrinol Metab. 2014;99(11):3933-51.
9. Silverberg SJ, Clarke BL, Peacock M, Bandeira F, Boutroy S, Cusano NE, et al. Current issues in the presentation of asymptomatic primary hyperparathyroidism: proceedings of the Fourth International Workshop. J Clin Endocrinol Metab. 2014;99(10):3580-94.
10. Lopes MP, Kliemann BS, Bini IB, Kulchetscki R, Borsani V, Savi L, et al. Hypoparathyroidism and pseudohypoparathyroidism: Etiology, laboratory features and complications. Arch Endocrinol Metab. 2016;60(6):532-36.
11. Di Iorgi N, Napoli F, Allegri AE, Olivieri I, Bertelli E, Gallizia A, et al. Diabetes insipidus--diagnosis and management. Horm Res Paediatr. 2012;77(2):69-84.

CHAPTER 8

Diabetes Mellitus

CLASSIFICATION

Classification of diabetes mellitus is given in **Table 8.1**.

CLINICAL FEATURES

General Characteristics

The general characteristics of diabetes mellitus are given in **Table 8.2**.

Diabetes mellitus and its types are shown in **Flowchart 8.1**.

Symptoms

Diabetes may present with polyuria, polydipsia, polyphagia and significant weight loss despite polyphagia.
- Depressed immune status may result in flare-ups of pulmonary tuberculosis, non-healing

TABLE 8.1: Classification of diabetes mellitus.

Type 1 diabetes mellitus	Type 2 diabetes mellitus
• Type 1-A (immune-mediated)	• Other endocrine diseases (acromegaly, Cushing syndrome, phaeochromocytoma, hyperthyroidism)
• Type 1-B (idiopathic)	• Infections (congenital rubella, cytomegalovirus)
• Monogenic diabetes: Maturity onset diabetes of the young (MODY)	• Drug/toxin-induced (glucocorticoids, T4, β-agonists, thiazides, protease inhibitors)
• Genetic defects in insulin action	• Gestational diabetes mellitus (GDM)
• Pancreatic diseases: Pancreatitis, pancreatectomy, haemochromatosis, fibrocalculus pancreatopathy	• Latent autoimmune diabetes in adults (LADA)
• Insulin receptor defects or insulin receptor antibodies	
• Other genetic syndromes (Down syndrome, Klinefelter syndrome)	

TABLE 8.2: General characteristics of diabetes mellitus.

Feature	Type 1 diabetes mellitus	Type 2 diabetes mellitus
• Age of onset	• < 40 years	• > 40 years
• Duration of symptoms	• Days or weeks	• Months or years
• Body habitus	• Normal to thin	• Obese
• Plasma insulin	• Low to absent	• Normal to high
• Acute complication	• Ketoacidosis	• Hyperosmolar hyperglycaemic state
• Insulin therapy	• Responsive	• Responsive to resistant
• Sulphonylurea therapy	• Unresponsive	• Responsive
• Autoantibodies	• Yes	• No
• Other autoimmune diseases	• Yes	• Absent
• Family history of diabetes	• No	• Present

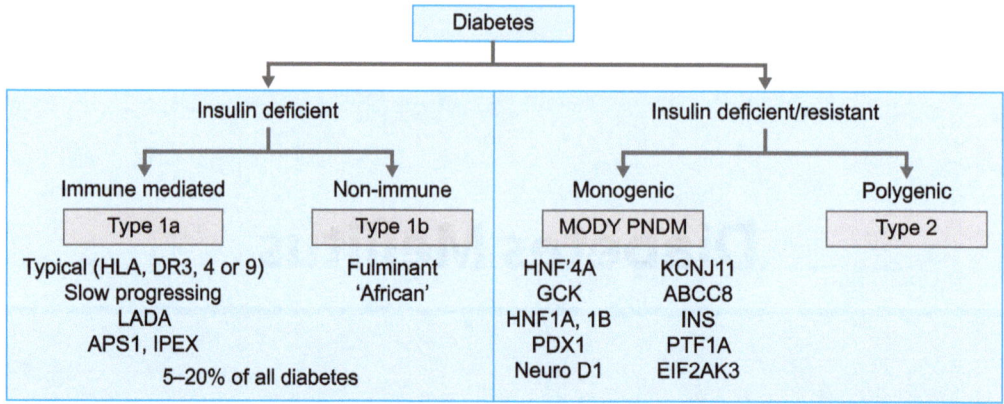

(ABCC8: ATP-binding cassette transporter sub-family C member 8; APS1: autoimmune polyendocrinopathy syndrome type 1; EIF2AK3: eukaryotic translation initiation factor 2-alpha kinase 3; GCK: glucokinase; HNF4: hepatocyte nuclear factor 4; IPEX: immune dysregulation, polyendocrinopathy, enteropathy, X-linked; INS: insulin; KCNJ11: potassium inwardly-rectifying channel, subfamily J, member 11; LADA: latent autoimmune diabetes of adults; MODY: maturity onset diabetes of the young; Neuro D1: neurogenic differentiation 1; PDX1: pancreatic and duodenal homeobox 1; PNDM: permanent neonatal diabetes mellitus; PTF1A: pancreas transcription factor 1 subunit alpha)

Flowchart 8.1: Types of diabetes mellitus.

of wounds, recurrent styes, candidal pruritus vulvae, balanitis and recurrent urinary tract infections.
- Some patients may present with end-organ involvement.

The pathophysiology of type 2 diabetes mellitus (T2DM) is shown in **Figure 8.1**.

■ OTHER TYPES OF DIABETES

Latent Autoimmune Diabetes in Adults (LADA)
- 'Slow-onset type 1' diabetes mellitus (T1DM) and 'type 1.5'.
- *Age*: Usually ≤25 years age.
- *Clinical presentation*: Similar to non-obese T2DM
- Initial control achieved with diet alone or diet plus oral antidiabetic drugs (OADs). Insulin dependency occurs within months (rarely can take years). LADA shares an increased frequency of risk for an HLA-DQB1 genotype than patients with T1DM and for a variant in the transcription factor 7-like 2 (*TCF7L2*) gene with patients with T2DM.
- Other features of T1DM
  o Low fasting and post glucagon stimulated C peptide levels.
  o Islet cell antigen (ICA) and glutamic acid decarboxylase antibodies (GADA) positive

- *Importance of diagnosis*: High risk of progression to insulin dependency
  o Avoid metformin treatment.
  o Early introduction of insulin therapy

Maturity Onset Diabetes of the Young (MODY)
- *Age*: Young onset of diabetes < 25 years of age
- Strong family history of early onset diabetes (2–3 generations affected)
- Evidence of macrovascular complications in earlier generation
- Sulphonylurea sensitivity. Non-insulin dependence (not requiring insulin even after 5 years of diagnosis)
- Absence of insulin resistance phenotype: Normal blood pressure, triglycerides (TGs), high-density lipoproteins (HDL)
- Mutations in several transcription factors or in glucokinase result in insufficient insulin release from pancreatic β-cells, causing MODY. Almost 11 subtypes of MODY are identified based on the mutated gene.
- MODY can occur at any age. About 70% forms of MODY are MODY-3 (hepatic transcription factor-1 gene) and 10% MODY-2 (glucokinase gene).

The differences between T1DM, T2DM and MODY are given in **Table 8.3**.

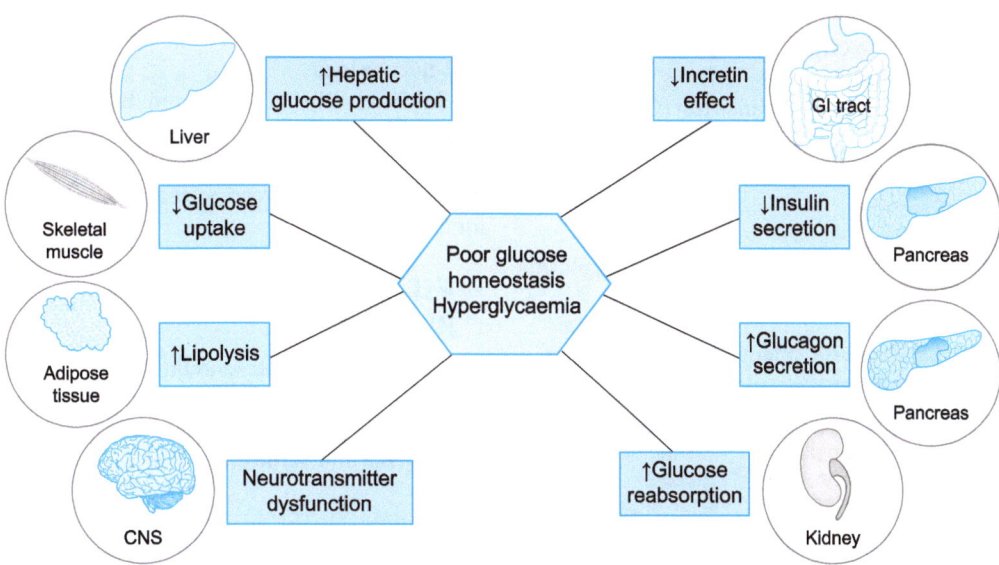

Fig. 8.1: Pathophysiology of type 2 diabetes mellitus—THE OMINOUS OCTET. Multiple drugs in combination may be needed to improve glucose homeostasis. The treatment should target the underlying pathophysiology.

TABLE 8.3: **Differences between T1DM, T2DM and MODY.**

Features	T1DM	T2DM	MODY
Frequency	Common	Increasing	2–5% of T2DM
Genetics	Polygenic	Polygenic	Monogenic autosomal dominant
Family history	< 15%	> 50%	100%
Ethnicity	Different races	Different races	Asians, Polynesians, indigenous Australians
Age of onset	Throughout childhood	Post-puberty	< 25 years
Severity of oneset	Acute and severe	Mild	Mild/asymptomatic
Ketosis/diabetic ketoacidosis	Common	Uncommon	Rare
Obesity association	–	> 90%	+/–
Acanthosis nigricans and metabolic syndrome	Absent	Common	Absent
Autoimmunity	Positive	Negative	Positive
Pathophysiology	β-Cell destruction	Insulin resistance and relative insulinopaenia	β-cell dysfunction

(MODY: maturity onset diabetes of the young; T1DM: type 1 diabetes mellitus; T2DM: type 2 diabetes mellitus)

Diagnostic Criteria

The diagnostic criteria of diabetes mellitus are given in **Table 8.4**.
- The oral glucose tolerance test (OGTT) should be performed with 1.75 g/kg up to 75 g, anhydrous glucose dissolved in water.

Prediabetes

Impaired fasting glucose (IFG)—fasting plasma glucose ≥100 mg/dL but < 125 mg/dL.

TABLE 8.4: Diagnostic criteria of diabetes mellitus.

	Impaired glucose tolerance	Diabetes
Diagnostic criteria	Fasting plasma glucose: 100–125 mg/dL OR 2-hour plasma glucose during OGTT: 140–199 mg/dL OR HbA1c: 5.7–6.4%	Fasting plasma glucose: ≥126 mg/dL OR 2-hour plasma glucose during OGTT: ≥200 mg/dL OR Random plasma glucose: ≥200 mg/dL with symptoms of polyuria and weight loss. OR HbA1c: ≥6.5%

(HbA1c: glycosylated haemoglobin; OGTT: oral glucose tolerance test)

Impaired glucose tolerance (IGT)—plasma glucose between 140 and 200 mg/dL 2 hours after oral glucose load.

Additionally, glycosylated haemoglobin (HbA1c) in the range of 5.7–6.4% is also included in 'prediabetes'. Recently, the term 'prediabetes' has been changed to 'categories of increased risk for diabetes'.

■ MEDICAL NUTRITION THERAPY IN DIABETES

- People with diabetes should receive individualised dietary advice (medical nutrition treatment) as needed to achieve treatment goals (**Fig. 8.2** and **Table 8.5**).

■ PHARMACOLOGICAL TREATMENT OF DIABETES

The agents used for the treatment of T1DM and T2DM are given in **Table 8.6**.

■ GENERAL INDICATIONS FOR INSULIN THERAPY

- T1DM
- Diabetic ketoacidosis (DKA)
- Hyperosmolar hyperglycaemic state (previously called non-ketotic hyperglycaemic coma)

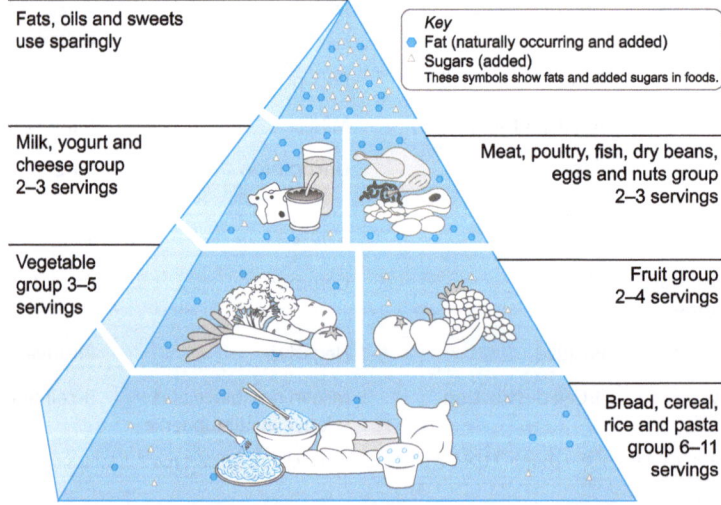

Fig 8.2: Medical nutrition therapy for T2DM.

TABLE 8.5: Recommended dietary goals for patients with diabetes.

Estimation of the total daily caloric requirement of the individual patient	Recommended proportion of calories to be derived from each	Distribution of the calories throughout the day
• Sedentary individuals—30 kcal/kg/day • Moderately active individual—35 kcal/kg/day • Heavily active individuals—40 kcal/kg/day	• Carbohydrate—50 to 65% • Protein—10 to 20% • Total fat—25 to 30% • Saturated fat—≤7% • Polyunsaturated fat—10% • Monounsaturated fat—10 to 15%	• 20% of the total calories—for breakfast • 35% of the total calories—for lunch • 30% of the total calories—for dinner • 15% of the total calories—for late-evening feed

TABLE 8.6: Agents used for treatment of type 1 diabetes mellitus and type 2 diabetes mellitus.

	Mechanism of action	Examples	HbA1c reduction (%)	Specific advantages	Specific disadvantages
Oral					
Biguanides	Hepatic glucose production	Metformin	1–2	Weight neutral/mild weight loss do not cause hypoglycaemia, inexpensive	Diarrhoea, nausea, lactic acidosis, vitamin B12 deficiency (0.5%)
Insulin secretagogues: Sulphonylureas	Insulin secretion	Glibendamide (glyburide), glipizide	1–2	Inexpensive	Hypoglycaemia, weight gain, sulphonamide allergies
Insulin secretagogues: Non-sulphonylureas	Insulin secretion	Repaglinide, nateglinide, nitiglinide	1–2	Short onset of action, lower post-prandial glucose	Hypoglycaemia
Insulin secretagogues: Dipeptidyl peptidase IV inhibitors	Prolong endogenous GLP-1 action	Saxagliptin, sitagliptin, vildaglipion	0.5–0.8	Do not cause hypoglycaemia	Nasopharyngitis Meniscus lesions Headache contact Dermatitis Osteoarthritis tremor
α-Glucosidase inhibitors	↓GI glucose absorption	Acarbose, miglitol	0.5–0.8	Reduce post-prandial glycaemia	GI flatulence, liver function abnormalities Contraindicated in kidney disease, inflammatory bowel disease
Thiazolidinediones Cotraindication: CHF, liver disease	↓Insulin resistance ↑Glucose utilisation	Rosiglitazone, pioglitazone	0.5–1.4	Lower insulin requirements	Peripheral oedema, CHF, weight gain, fractures, macular oedema, rosiglitazone may increase cardiovascular rsik

Continued

Continued

	Mechanism of action	Examples	HbA1c reduction (%)	Specific advantages	Specific disadvantages
Sodium glucose contransporter-2 (SGLT-2) inhibitors	Help eliminate glucose in the urine	Canagliflozin, dapagliflozin, empagliflozin	0.4–1.1	No hypoglycaemia, weight loss	Genital and urinary infections
Bile acid sequestrants					
Bile acid sequestrants Contraindications: Elevated plasma triglycerides	Bind bile acids, mechanism of glucose lowering not known	Colesevelam	0.5		Constipation, dyspepsia, abdominal pain, nausea, triglycerides interfere with absorption of other drugs, intestinal obstruction
Parenteral					
Insulin	↑Glucose utilisation, ↓Hepatic gluocse production, and other anabolic actions	Refer to Table 8.9	Not limited	Know safety profile	Injection, weight gain, hypoglycaemia
GLP-1 receptor agonists Contraindications: Renal disease, agents that also slow GI motility	↑Insulin, ↓Glucagon, slow gastric emptying satiety	Exenatide, liraglutide	0.5–10	Weight loss, do not cause hypoglycaemia	Injection, nausea, risk of hypoglycaemia with insulin secretagogues, pancreatitis, renal failure
Amylin agonists Contraindication: Agents that also GI motility	Slow gastric emptying, ↓Glucagon	Pramlintide	0.25–0.5	Reduce post-prandial glycaemia; weight loss	Injection, nausea, risk of hypoglycaemia with insulin
Medical nutrition therapy and physical activity	↓Insulin resistance, ↑Insulin secretion	Low-calorie, low-fat diet, exercise	1–3	Other health benefits	Compliance difficult, long-term sucess low

CHF: congestive heart failure; GI: gastrointestinal; GLP-1: glucagon-like peptide 1)

- Stress of surgery, infections and trauma
- Diabetes during pregnancy
- Non-obese T2DM unresponsive to oral drugs.
- Post-renal transplantation diabetic patients

Insulin Preparations

Various insulin preparations and their duration of action are given in **Table 8.7**.

Insulin Regimens

Insulin regimens are given in **Box 8.1**.

■ GOALS OF TREATMENT IN DIABETES

The guidelines for glycaemic, blood pressure and lipid control by American Diabetes Association are given in **Table 8.8**.

TABLE 8.7: Duration of action (in hours) of various insulin preparations.

Class	Type	Oneset of effect (hours)	Peak effect (hours)	Effective duration of action (hours)
Rapid-acting	Insulin analogues: lispro, aspart, glulisine	< 0.25	0.5–1.5	2–4
Short-acting	Regular (crystalline, soluble, plain)	0.5–1	2–3	3–6
	Semilente	0.5–1	2–6	10–12
Intermediate	Isophane (NPH)	2–4	4–10	10–16
	Lente (excess zinc ions)*	1–3	6–12	18–24
Long-acting	Protamine zinc (PZI)	2–4	14–24	36
	Ultralente	2–4	18–24	36
	Insulin analogues: glargine, detemir	1–4	None	18–24

*Lente (intermediate acting) insulin is mixture of semilente and ultralente in the ratio of 30:70, respectively.

Box 8.1: Insulin regimens.

Conventional insulin therapy
One or two injections a day of intermediate-acting insulin with or without the addition of small amounts of regular insulin

Multiple subcutaneous injections (MSI)
Intermediate or long-acting insulin in the evening as a single dose together with regular insulin prior to each meal

Continuous subcutaneous insulin infusion (CSII)
Battery-driven pump as a means of mimicking the physiological basal plus prandial pattern of insulin secretion

TABLE 8.8: Guidelines for glycaemic, blood pressure and lipid control by American Diabetes Association.

	American Diabetes Association Goals
HbA1c	< 7.0% (individualisation)
Pre-prandial glucose	70–130 mg/dL (3.9–7.2 mmol/L)
Post-prandial glucose	< 180 mg/dL
Blood pressure	< 130/80 mmHg
Lipids	LDL: < 100 mg/dL (2.59 mmol/L) < 70 mg/dL (1.81 mmol/L) (with overt CVD) HDL: > 40 mg/dL (1.04 mmol/L) > 50 mg/dL (1.30 mmol/L) TG: < 150 mg/dL (1.69 mmol/L)

(HDL: high-density lipoprotein; LDL: low-density lipoprotein; PG: plasma glucose; TG: triglycerides)
Source: American Diabetes Association. Standards of Medical Care in Diabetes. Diabetes Care. 2012; 35:S11-63.

A stepwise approach for the management of T2DM is given in **Flowchart 8.2**.

■ COMPLICATIONS OF DIABETES

Complications of diabetes are given in **Table 8.9**.

■ DIABETIC KETOACIDOSIS

State of hyperglycaemia and acidaemia due to insulin deficiency: Glucose > 250 mg/dL, acidosis (pH < 7.3), ketosis

Causes

Triggers include infection, myocardial ischaemia, medication non-compliance, steroid use, alcohol abuse, pregnancy, stroke, pancreatitis, renal failure.

Signs

Acetone odour on breath, Kussmaul respirations, hypotension, tachycardia, altered mental status, abdominal tenderness

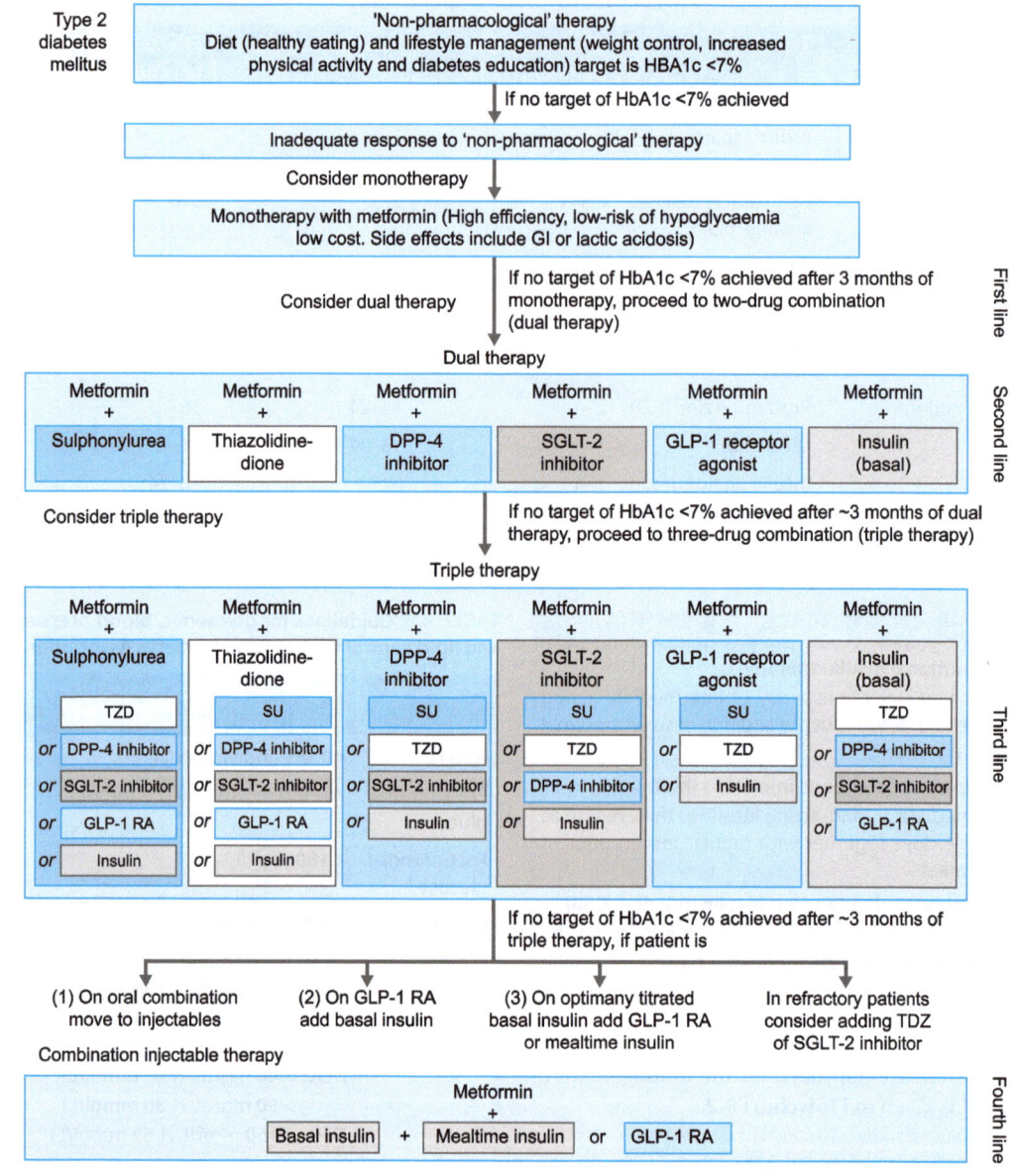

Flowchart 8.2: Stepwise approach to the management of type 2 diabetes mellitus.

(DPP-4: dipeptidyl peptidase 4; GLP-1 RA: glucagon-like peptide-1 receptor agonist; SGLT-2: sodium and glucose transporter-2; SU: sulphonylures; TZD: thiazolidinedione)

Investigations

- Serum glucose (usually > 350 mg/dL).
- Anion gap metabolic acidaemia.
- Electrolytes: Hypokalaemia, hyponatraemia, azotaemia
- Urinalysis: For ketones
- Electrocardiogram (ECG): To rule out infarction
- Septic workup

TABLE 8.9: Complications of diabetes.

Acute metabolic complications	Chronic (long-term) complications	
• Diabetic ketoacidosis (DKA) • Hyperosmolar hyperglycaemic state (hyperosmolar non-ketotic diabetic coma) • Hypoglycaemia • Lactic acidosis	**Microvascular** Diabetic retinopathy (non-proliferative and proliferative) Cataract Glaucoma Neuropathy • Sensory • Motor • Sensory motor • Autonomic Nephropathy • Microalbuminuria • Macroalbuminuria • Chronic kidney disease	**Macrovascular** Coronary artery disease Peripheral vascular disease Cerebrovascular disease • Others • Gastrointestinal (gastroparesis, diarrhoea) • Genitourinary (uropathy/sexual dysfunction) • Dermatologic • Infectious • Cataracts • Glaucoma • Periodontal disease • Hearing loss

---

Box 8.2: Treatment of DKA.

IV fluids:
- Patients often have loss of > 6 L. Start with 10–20 cc/kg in fluid-depleted patients.
- May need to repeat fluid boluses for hydration → consider providing 200 mL/h of IV fluid
- Normal saline (NS) is the typical fluid of choice

Insulin:
- Insulin infusion at 0.1–0.14 units/kg IV per hour is recommended → continue the insulin drip rate the same until serum bicarbonate and anion gap are improving.
- If serum glucose is dropping (or once it drops to < 250–300 mg/dL), begin dextrose 5% 50–200 mL/h.

Hyponatraemia: Corrects with hyperglycaemia treatment. If hyponatraemic after correction, use NS for fluid repletion.

Potassium
- If K > 5.2 mEq/L, no replacement is necessary, and insulin can be started.
- If K is 3.3–5.2 mEq/L, provide PO K (20 mEq) and peripheral IV at 10 mEq/h while starting insulin.
- If K < 3.3 mEq/L, hold insulin until > 3.3. Start PO and IV potassium.

Magnesium is often low due to hypokalaemia. If the patient is hypokalaemia and hypomagnesemia, provide 1–2 g $MgSO_4$ IV.

Phosphorus < 1 requires replacement.

Bicarbonate: Correct bicarbonate for patients with pH < 6.9.

Supportive care
- Intubation, mechanical ventilation
- Antibiotics
- Renal replacement
- Treatment of complications

Management

Start with ABCs (airway, breathing, circulation), bilateral IVs (often require multiple medications), monitor, ECG.

- Search for the underlying aetiology/inciting event (infection).
- **Box 8.2** treatment of DKA

HYPERGLYCAEMIC HYPEROSMOLAR STATE

- Mostly a complication of T2DM.
- This is a syndrome characterised by extreme dehydration resulting from a sustained hyperglycaemia in the absence of significant ketoacidosis.
- Precipitating factors
  - Infections
  - Cerebrovascular accidents
  - Steroids, immunosuppressive agents, phenytoin and diuretics

Clinical Features

- Insidious onset
- Extreme dehydration present
- Central nervous system manifestations → altered level of consciousness and convulsions (transient hemiplegia)

Laboratory Findings

- Plasma glucose is markedly elevated, usually around 1,000 mg/dL (range 600–2,400 mg/dL).
- Serum osmolarity is markedly raised.
- Prerenal azotaemia with elevation of blood urea nitrogen (BUN) and creatinine
- A mild metabolic acidosis is present.

Management

Management of HHS is given in **Box 8.3**.

The differences between DKA and HHS are given in **Table 8.10**.

Box 8.3: Management of hyperglycaemic hyperosmolar state.

- Fluid replacement. The average fluid deficit is about 10 L that should be corrected intravenously. Initially, 2–3 L isotonic (0.9%) saline should be given over 1–2 hours. Subsequently, half-strength (0.45%) saline should be used.
- Insulin. Regular insulin should be given as low-dose intravenous infusion, as for diabetic ketoacidosis (DKA). The goal is to keep the plasma glucose around 200 mg/dL.
- Potassium supplementation is required early, as for DKA.
- Lactic acidosis should be treated with intravenous sodium bicarbonate.
- Infections should be treated with antibiotics.

The pathogenesis of DKA and HHS are given in **Flowchart 8.3**.

HYPOGLYCAEMIA

- Hypoglycaemia commonly complicates therapy with insulin and oral hypoglycaemic drugs.
- Other causes such as pentamidine, didanosine, alcohol intoxication, insulin-secreting tumours, chronic kidney disease, severe infections, malaria

Clinical Features

- Poorly controlled diabetic patients develop symptoms at higher levels (80 mg/dL) while well-controlled diabetic patients develop symptoms at lower levels.
- Symptoms of hypoglycaemia fall into two main categories:
  - Adrenergic symptoms induced by excessive secretion of adrenaline include sweating, tremor, tachycardia, anxiety and hunger.
  - Central nervous system dysfunction causes dizziness, headache, clouding of vision, loss of fine motor skill, confusion, abnormal behaviour, convulsions and loss of consciousness.

Management

- *Oral carbohydrate*: If hypoglycaemia is recognised early, it may be corrected by ingestion of carbohydrate, preferably in an easily absorbable form.
- *Intravenous dextrose*: 50 mL of 50% dextrose should be given initially, followed by infusion of 5–10% dextrose.
- *Glucagon*: Severe hypoglycaemia may be treated with glucagon 1 mg subcutaneously or intramuscularly.

CARDIOVASCULAR COMPLICATIONS OF DIABETES

Cardiovascular risk in patients with type T2DM is shown in **Flowchart 8.4**.

- Intermittent claudication, gangrene and impotence
- Coronary artery disease leading to ischaemic heart disease, especially silent myocardial infarctions

TABLE 8.10: Differences between diabetic ketoacidosis and hyperglycaemic hyperosmolar state.

Features	Diabetic ketoacidosis (DKA)	Hyperglycaemic hyperosmolar state (HHS)
Clinical features		
Type of diabetes	Both type 1 diabetes mellitus and type 2 diabetes mellitus	Type 2 diabetes mellitus
Evolution/onset	Over hours	Over days
Fruity (acetone) odour of breath	Observed	Not present
Kussmaul's respiration	Seen	Not seen
Abdominal pain/tenderness	Present	Absent
Laboratory findings		
Plasma glucose level	> 250 mg/dL	> 600 mg/dL
Serum sodium	Normal or low (< 140 mmol/L)	Usually high (> 155 mmol/L)
Blood/urine ketones	Moderate ketonuria or ketonaemia	Absent/minimal ketonuria and ketonaemia
Arterial pH	< 7.3	> 7.3
Serum bicarbonate	< 15 mEq/L	> 15 mEq/L
Serum osmolality	Variable	> 320 mosm/L
Anion gap	> 12	Variable
Fluid deficit	6 L	> 10 L
Mortality rate	1%	20–30%

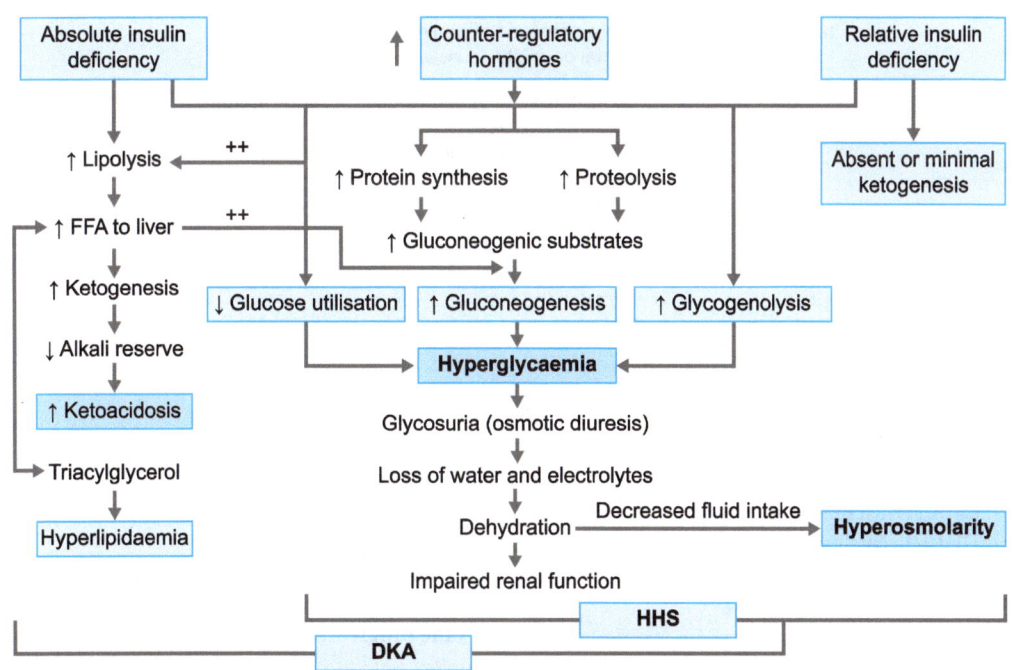

(DKA: diabetic ketoacidosis; FFA: free fatty acid; HHS: hyperglycaemic hyperosmolar state)

Flowchart 8.3: Pathogenesis of DKA and HHS.

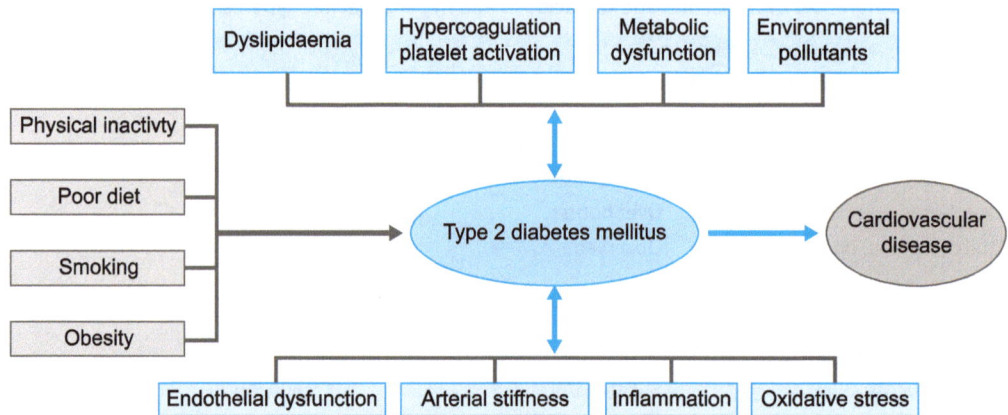

Flowchart 8.4 : Pathways of cardiovascular risk in patients with type 2 diabetes mellitus.

Stage	Features
Hyperfiltration	• Glomerular hyperfiltration and hypertrophy • Normoalbuminuria (<30 mg/g) • GFR increased
Silent	• Mild GBM thickening and focal mesangial sclerosis • Normoalbuminuria (<30 mg/g) • GFR normal
Incipient	• Mild-to-moderate GBM thickening and variable mesangial sclerosis • Moderately increased albuminuria (30–300 mg/g) • GFR normal or mildly decreased
Overt	• Marked GBM thickening and diffuse mesangial sclerosis (with or without nodules) • Severely increased albuminuria (>300 mg/g) • GFR decreased • Hypertension
ESRD	• Diffuse global glomerulosclerosis • Decreasing albuminuria • GFR <15 mL/min • Hypertension

(ESRD: end stage renal disease; GBM: glioblastoma multiforme; GFR: glomerular filtration rate)

Fig. 8.3: Stages of diabetic nephropathy.

- Cerebrovascular accidents
- Diabetic cardiomyopathy

DIABETIC NEPHROPATHY

Management

- **Figure 8.3** describes the stages of diabetic nephrpathy

- Stop smoking and control dyslipidaemia.
- Strict control of diabetes.
- Angiotensin-converting enzyme inhibitors and Angiotensin receptor blockers can retard the progression of nephropathy at this stage.

DIABETIC NEUROPATHY

Box 8.4 classification of diabetic neuropathy.

Box 8.4: Classification of diabetic neuropathy.

Generalised symmetrical polyneuropathies
- Distal sensory or sensorimotor polyneuropathy
- Small-fibre neuropathy
- Autonomic neuropathy
- Large-fibre sensory neuropathy

Focal and asymmetrical neuropathies
- Cranial neuropathy
- Truncal neuropathy
- Limb mononeuropathy
- Proximal motor neuropathy (amyotrophy)

Box 8.5: Clinical features of autonomic neuropathy.

- Cardiovascular—postural hypotension, resting tachycardia, absence of sinus arrhythmia, abnormal Valsalva response, sudden cardiac death
- Gastrointestinal—oesophageal dysmotility, dysphagia, gastroparesis, nocturnal and post-prandial diarrhoea, constipation, anal incontinence
- Genitourinary—vesicopathy, incontinence, impotence, retrograde ejaculation
- Secretomotor—gustatory sweating, nocturnal sweat without hypoglycaemia, anhidrosis
- Vasomotor—dependent pedal oedema
- Papillary—decreased pupil size, resistance to mydriatics

Autonomic Neuropathy

The clinical features of autonomic neuropathy are given in **Box 8.5**.

■ DIABETIC RETINOPATHY

Features of diabetic retinopathy are given in **Table 8.11**.

■ GESTATIONAL DIABETES MELLITUS

Gestational diabetes mellitus (GDM) is defined as any degree of glucose intolerance that begins or is first recognised during pregnancy.

The importance of proper diagnosis can be appreciated as GDM is known to cause increased foetal loss and congenital malformations such as foetal macrosomia. Also, females with GDM are at increased risk of obesity and diabetes.
- The diagnosis of GDM is based on an OGTT done at 24–38 weeks of gestation in women with moderate-to-high risk.

TABLE 8.11: Features of diabetic retinopathy.

Non-proliferative/simple background (NPDR)	Proliferative (PDR)
• Develops late in the first decade or early in the second decade	• New blood vessel formation/neovascularisation
• Increased capillary permeability	• Pre-retinal or subhyaloid haemorrhage
• Marked retinal vascular microaneurysms, capillary closure and dilatation	• Vitreous haemorrhage
• Haemorrhages: Dot (capillary microaneurysms) and blot (leakage of blood into deeper retinal layers)	• More numerous microaneurysms and haemorrhages
• Cotton wool spots/cytoid bodies (caused by microinfarcts within the retina due to occluded vessels)	• Changes in calibre of venous vessel
• Hard exudates (exudation of plasma rich in lipids and protein)	• Retinal fibrosis/scar (retinitis proliferans)
• Atreriovenous shunts and dilated veins	• Traction retinal detachment

TABLE 8.12: Criteria for diagnosis of gestational diabetes mellitus.

Time (hour)	Upper limit of normal values (mg/dL)	
	Whole blood (O'Sullivan)	Plasma (Carpenter and Coustan)
0 (fasting)	85	95
1	160	180
2	140	155
3	125	140

- **Criteria for diagnosis of GDM**
  The criteria for diagnosis of GDM are given in **Table 8.12**.
  100 g OGTT is recommended at present. (Two or more of these values must be abnormal.)
- **Management**—these pregnant diabetic patients should be managed meticulously with insulin. Oral hypoglycaemic agents (OHAs) such as Glyburide and metformin have been safely recommended for use in GDM.

METABOLIC SYNDROME

- Metabolic syndrome (previously known as syndrome X or insulin resistance syndrome) refers to the clustering of cardiovascular risk factors and includes abdominal obesity, hyperglycaemia, dyslipidaemia [high TGs, low high-density lipoprotein (HDL)] and elevated blood pressure. The pathophysiological hallmark is insulin resistance.

Clinical Diagnosis

National Cholesterol Education Program's Adult Treatment Panel III (ATP III)
- Waist circumference of > 102 cm in men and > 88 cm in women;
- Triglyceride levels of at least 150 mg/dL;
- HDL lipoprotein cholesterol levels of < 40 mg/dL in men and < 50 mg/dL in women;
- Blood pressure of at least 130/85 mmHg; and
- Fasting glucose levels of at least 110 mg/dL.

Associated Risks

The risks associated with metabolic syndrome are given in **Box 8.6**.

Treatment

- Components of therapy include:
   - Exercise
   - Hypocaloric diet
   - Weight reduction
   - Diet high in fibres
- Control of diabetes, hypertension and lipid abnormalities by various drugs
- In the absence of diabetes, hypoglycaemic drugs (e.g. metformin, acarbose) are not recommended to control insulin resistance.

Box 8.6: Risks associated with metabolic syndrome.

- Cardiovascular diseases
- Type 2 diabetes mellitus
- Polycystic ovary syndrome
- Sleep-disorder breathing
- Chronic kidney disease
- Non-alcoholic fatty liver disease

BEST OF FIVES

1. A 50-year-old diabetic woman recently sustained a left Colles fracture and you suspect underlying osteoporosis. Current medication includes metformin, pioglitazone, BD mixed insulin, ramipril, indapamide and amlodipine. On examination, her blood pressure is 140/72 mmHg and pulse is 78 bpm and regular. Her body mass index (BMI) is 34 kg/m².

   Which of her medications is most likely to be linked to the risk of osteoporotic fracture?
   A. Indapamide
   B. Insulin
   C. Metformin
   D. Pioglitazone
   E. Ramipril

2. A 62-year-old man presents to the diabetes clinic for review. His current diabetes medication includes metformin and pioglitazone. Past history of note includes transurethral resection of bladder tumours some 3 years earlier. Which of the following is the most appropriate way to manage his diabetes?
   A. Add BD mixed insulin.
   B. Add liraglutide.
   C. Add sitagliptin.
   D. Continue current therapy.
   E. Stop pioglitazone and substitute an alternative.

3. A 22-year-old woman presents to the emergency department with a severe viral upper respiratory tract infection. She has a history of T1DM for which she takes a basal bolus insulin regime and a recent HbA1c was elevated at 8.2%. You diagnose DKA. She is started on an insulin infusion and is rehydrated aggressively; however, she has become unconscious. What is most likely to have occurred?
   A. Cerebral haemorrhage
   B. Cerebral infarct
   C. Cerebral oedema
   D. Worsening sepsis
   E. Worsening tissue acidosis

4. A 45-year-old man is obese and is currently on treatment for hypertension with indapamide

and ramipril. On examination, his blood pressure is 128/72 mmHg, pulse is 70 bpm and regular and BMI is 28 kg/m². There are no other significant findings on clinical examination. Investigations show glucose 6.7 mmol/L (fasting). IGT is confirmed on glucose tolerance testing.

Which of the following has been proven to have a positive impact on cardiovascular risk in patients with this clinical picture?
A. Acarbose
B. Gliclazide
C. Insulin glargine
D. Metformin
E. Pioglitazone

5. A 22-year-old woman who has a history of T1DM comes to the emergency department. She has suffered a viral upper respiratory tract infection which has worsened over the past 3 days. Her glucose has risen to 33 mmol/L on her latest BM estimation. On examination, she is pyrexial at 37.9°C, her blood pressure is 100/60 mmHg and her pulse is 95 bpm. There are signs of pharyngitis and she has a cough. Her respiratory rate is elevated at 30 bpm.

Which of the following is correct when discussing the management of her DKA?
A. Potassium replacement is 40 mmol/L of fluid given and potassium is monitored closely.
B. Ketones < 0.5 mmol/L define resolution of DKA.
C. Prophylaxis against thromboembolism is not required.
D. She can be converted back to subcutaneous insulin when the pH is above 7.2.
E. She should be treated with a sliding scale insulin regime.

6. A 24-year-old woman with a history of T1DM has lost weight and had problems with diarrhoea which is hard to flush away. Her current insulin regime is meal-time Actrapid and Insulatard at night. On examination her blood pressure is 110/72 mmHg, pulse is 65 bpm and regular, and her BMI is 19 kg/m². She looks pale and thin. Investigations show:

| Creatinine | 129 µmol/L | (79–118) |
| HbA1c | 6.0% | (< 7.0) |

Which of the following is likely to be the most effective treatment?
A. Carbimazole
B. Codeine phosphate
C. Erythromycin
D. Gluten-free diet
E. Pancreatic enzyme supplementation

7. A 71-year-old man is managed with a BD mixed insulin and metformin. Previously well controlled, he has lost weight over recent months and now has troublesome hypoglycaemia mid-afternoon. On examination, his BMI is 27 kg/m², blood pressure is 125/72 mmHg and pulse is 75 bpm and regular.

Which of the following is the most appropriate way to manage him?
A. Change his insulin to pioglitazone
B. Change his insulin to sitagliptin
C. Keep his insulin dose the same and transfer him to basal bolus
D. Reduce his insulin dose
E. Stop his metformin

8. A 70-year-old man with a history of T2DM comes to the clinic for review. He is managed with BD mixed insulin and metformin to limit insulin-associated weight gain. The patient has severe painful bilateral symmetrical sensorimotor polyneuropathy.

Which of the following is the most appropriate way to manage his neuropathic pain according to the National Institute for Health and Care Excellence (NICE) guidance?
A. Amitriptyline
B. Duloxetine
C. Gabapentin
D. Pregabalin
E. Topical lidocaine

9. A 22-year-old man presents to the diabetes nurse specialist for review after being diagnosed with new-onset T1DM. He is a second-year medical student and engages in recreational sports with fellow members of his college.

Which of the following is the most appropriate initial insulin regime for him?
A. Meal-time Actrapid and Insulatard at night
B. Meal-time Actrapid and glargine at night

C. Meal-time Actrapid and detemir at night
D. Meal-time Actrapid and BD detemir
E. BD mixed insulin

10. A 16-year-old male comes to the clinic for review. His 13-year-old brother has been recently diagnosed with T1DM. He wants to know about his risk of developing the disorder. Which of the following features is most closely associated with the imminent development of T1DM?
    A. Anti-insulinoma antigen 2 (IA2) antibodies
    B. Anti-insulin antibodies
    C. Anti-zinc transporter 8 (ZnT8) antibodies
    D. Loss of first-phase insulin response
    E. Loss of second-phase insulin response

11. A 50-year-old woman comes to the diabetes nephropathy clinic for review. She is known to have a chronically elevated creatinine and microalbuminuria. Medication includes basal-bolus insulin, ramipril 10 mg, amlodipine 5 mg and bisoprolol 10 mg. Her blood pressure is 154/72 mmHg and pulse is 72 and regular. She has neuropathy and retinopathy. Which of the following is the correct way to manage her blood pressure?
    A. Add diltiazem
    B. Add doxazosin
    C. Add indapamide
    D. Exchange her ramipril for doxazosin
    E. Exchange her ramipril for indapamide

12. A 40-year-old female with a family history of diabetes smokes 10 cigarettes per day and drinks approximately 10 units of alcohol weekly. On examination, her BMI is 31.2 kg/m^2 and she has a blood pressure of 140/84 mmHg. Her investigations reveal:

Fasting plasma glucose	5.5 mmol/L
Total cholesterol	4.5 mmol/L
High-density lipoprotein (HDL)	1.8 mmol/L
Triglycerides	2.1 mmol/L

    Which of the following is the most appropriate description for this patient?
    A. Impaired fasting glucose
    B. Metabolic syndrome
    C. Obesity
    D. Pre-diabetes
    E. T2DM

13. A 72-year-old female presents with a 6-month history of weight gain and nocturia. More recently, she has developed candidal infection of the vulva. Dipstick urine reveals ++ glucose. A diagnosis of diabetes is subsequently confirmed with a fasting plasma glucose of 10.2 mmol/L and her HbA1c is 8.2%. Which of the following is the likely pathological entity that would underlie her diabetes?
    A. Islet amyloid deposition
    B. Islet ferritin deposition
    C. Islet fibrosis
    D. Islet granuloma formation

14. A 55-year-old male presents with a 6-month history of nocturia. He is diagnosed with T2DM mellitus based on a fasting plasma glucose concentration of 10.1 mmol/L. His HbA1c is 7.5% and he has a BMI of 35.2 kg/m^2. Which of the following most adequately describes the likely beta-cell mass found in this patient?
    A. Beta-cell mass is increased by approximately 20%.
    B. Beta-cell mass is increased by approximately 60%.
    C. Beta-cell mass is reduced by approximately 20%.
    D. Beta-cell mass is reduced by approximately 60%.
    E. Beta-cell mass is normal.

15. A 68-year-old male presents with a 6-month history of weight loss and thirst. He has a past history of hypertension for which he takes bendroflumethiazide and ramipril. On examination, his pulse is 80 bpm and regular, blood pressure is 138/84 mmHg and BMI is 23.5 kg/m^2. Dipstick urine analysis reveals ++ glucose. His investigations reveal:

Fasting plasma glucose	13.3 mmol/L (3.5–6)
HbA1c	8.9% (< 6)

Which of the following is the most appropriate investigation in determining the aetiology of this patient's diabetes?
A. Glutamic acid decarboxylase (GAD) antibodies
B. Human leucocyte antigen (HLA) typing
C. Insulin autoantibodies
D. Tryptophan hydroxylase autoantibodies
E. Urine free cortisol measurement

16. A 16-year-old female with T1DM is admitted with dysuria, fever and rigors. She has been using mixed insulin twice daily and her last HbA1c was 7.2% at annual review 3 months ago. On examination, she has a temperature of 39°C, a blood pressure of 112/76 mmHg and a pulse of 110 bpm. The patient is commenced on a fixed rate of insulin infusion IV. Investigations reveal:

pH	7.1 (7.35–7.45)
Standard bicarbonate	9 mmol/L (22–28)

Which of the following is the most appropriate management strategy of her pH status?
A. IV bicarbonate infusion should be administered in a high-dependency unit (HDU).
B. IV bicarbonate should be administered and the patient transferred to a medical ward.
C. IV bicarbonate should be given as an infusion.
D. Oral bicarbonate should be administered.
E. There is no requirement to administer IV bicarbonate.

17. A 32-year-old male with T1DM and on insulin presents to the rheumatology clinic with stiffness and deformity of the small joints of the hands which has developed over the last 12 months. He has retinopathy. Investigations reveal:

HbA1c	7.6% (3.8-6.4)
Sodium	140 mmol/L (137-144)
Potassium	4.0 mmol/L (3.5-4.9)
Urea	7.8 mmol/L (2.5-7.5)
Creatinine	135 μmol/L (60-110)
Liver function tests	Normal -
Haemoglobin	11.0 g/dL (13.0-18.0)
MCV	83.0 fL (80-96)
White cell count	10×10^9/L (4-11)
Platelets	205×10^9/L (150–400)
Total cholesterol	4.9 mmol/L (< 5.2)
HDL cholesterol	1.0 mmol/L (0.8–1.2)
LDL cholesterol	2.5 mmol/L (< 3.5)
Triglycerides	2.2 mmol/L (0.8–1.5)
Estimated glomerular filtration rate	50 mL/min/1.73 m²
Microalbumin screen	45 mg/mmol (< 2.5)

What is the rheumatological diagnosis?
A. Cheiroarthropathy
B. Dupuytren's contracture
C. Reflex sympathetic dystrophy
D. Scleroderma
E. Secondary hyperparathyroidism

18. A 52-year-old male T2DM patient is admitted with ST-elevation myocardial infarction (STEMI). Rescue percutaneous coronary intervention (PCI) is not available and so he receives tenecteplase and his BM glucose concentrations show values between 7 and 12 mmol/L. His plasma glucose concentration obtained from the laboratory is 10.8 mmol/L (3.0–6.0). What is the most appropriate treatment for his glycaemic control?
A. Add gliclazide to metformin.
B. Change metformin to gliclazide.
C. Commence intravenous insulin infusion.
D. Continue the current dose of metformin.
E. Increase metformin.

19. A 48-year-old male diabetic has become increasingly distressed about his impotence. On examination he has a BMI of 29 kg/m², a blood pressure of 132/78 mmHg and a pulse of 90 bpm. His investigations reveal:

HbA1c	7.9% (3.8–6.4)
Serum testosterone	6.5 nmol/L (9–35)
Plasma luteinising hormone	0.5 mU/L (1–10)
Plasma follicle stimulating hormone	0.9 mU/L (1–7)
Plasma prolactin	322 mU/L (< 360)

Which of the following investigations would you request next for this patient?
A. Karyotype
B. MRI of pituitary
C. Short Synacthen test
D. Thyroid function tests
E. Ultrasound testes

20. A 60-year-old male with a history of diabetes mellitus and who was receiving glibenclamide 10 mg daily and metformin 1 g twice daily presents with a 3-month history of lethargy and weight loss. On examination, he was noted to have a BMI of 22.6 kg/m², a pulse of 88 bpm and a blood pressure of 156/90 mmHg. There was evidence of retinopathy and neuropathy. Investigations reveal:

Serum creatinine	220 μmol/L	(60–110)
HbA1c	9.5%	(3.8–6.4)
Urinalysis	Protein++	

Which of the following is the most appropriate therapeutic strategy for this patient?
A. Change glibenclamide to insulin
B. Maximise his current oral hypoglycaemic therapy
C. Pioglitazone
D. Stop metformin
E. Stop metformin and glibenclamide and start insulin

21. A young female presents with recurrent vulval candidiasis. There is a strong family history of coronary artery disease; both her father and paternal uncle died in their fifties of heart disease. Her mother has diabetes and takes thyroxine for a thyroid problem. On examination, she has a BMI of 35.5 kg/m². Her pulse is 82 bpm and regular and her blood pressure is 138/88 mmHg. Investigations reveal:

HbA1c	7.8%	(3.8-6.4)
Fasting plasma glucose	10.3 mmol/l	(3.0-6.0)

Which of the following treatments in addition to lifestyle advice should this patient receive?
A. Gliclazide
B. Insulin
C. Metformin
D. Pioglitazone
E. Sitagliptin

22. A 25-year-old female developed diabetes mellitus at the age of 15 years and is currently treated with human mixed insulin twice daily. Her blood pressure is 116/76 mmHg. Investigations show:

HbA1c	9%	(3.8–6.4)
Fasting plasma glucose	12.1 mmol/L	(3.0–6.0)
Serum creatinine	90 μmol/L	(60–110)
Urinalysis	Glucose +	
24-hour urine protein	220 mg/24 hours	(< 200)

What would be the best therapeutic option to prevent progression of renal disease?
A. Improve glycaemic control with insulin.
B. Prescribe a low-protein diet.
C. Treat with angiotensin-converting enzyme (ACE) inhibitors.
D. Treat with prolonged antibiotics.
E. Treat with steroids.

23. A 66-year-old male with a 12-year history of diabetes mellitus presents for annual review. He is currently receiving gliclazide at a dose of 80 mg twice daily. Examination reveals a pulse of 80 bpm and regular and a blood pressure of 152/90 mmHg. Fundal examination reveals bilateral dot haemorrhages with scattered hard exudates. He has loss of vibration

sensation into the ankles but all pulses are palpable. Investigations reveal:

Serum sodium	139 mmol/L (137–144)
Serum potassium	3.8 mmol/L (3.5–4.9)
Serum urea	10.2 mmol/L (2.5–7.5)
Serum creatinine	160 µmol/L (60–110)
Glucose	12.1 mmol/L (3.0–6.0)
HbA1c	9.5% (3.8–6.4)
Cholesterol	5.5 mmol/L (< 5.2)
Triglycerides	2.8 mmol/L (0.45–1.69)

Which of the following measures would you adopt to improve this patient's prognosis?
A. Angiotensin-converting enzyme (ACE) inhibitor and insulin
B. Beta-blocker
C. Increased dose of gliclazide
D. Insulin
E. Calcium channel blocker

24. A 16-year-old boy has insulin-dependent diabetes mellitus. On examination, he is alert and oriented. His mouth is dry but there is no loss of skin turgor. Examination is otherwise unremarkable. Investigations reveal:

Hb	16.9 g/dL	(13.0–18.0)
WBC	13.1 ×109/L	(4–11)
Platelets	350 ×109/L	(150–400)
Sodium	138 mmol/L	(137–144)
Potassium	4.0 mmol/L	(3.5–4.9)
Urea	10.9 mmol/L	(2.5–7.5)
Creatinine	180 µmol/L	(60–110)
Bicarbonate	12 mmol/L	(20–28)
Glucose	28.4 mmol/L	(3.0–6.0)
Urinalysis protein trace		
Ketones	+++	
Glucose	2%	

He is treated with intravenous fluids and with an intravenous insulin sliding scale and his symptoms improved within 24 hours. After 36 hours, he has good glycaemic control and is able to eat and drink without feeling nauseated. His repeat investigations reveal:

Sodium	110 mmol/L	(137–144)
Potassium	7.2 mmol/L	(3.5–4.9)
Urea	12.4 mmol/L	(2.5–7.5)
Bicarbonate	14 mmol/L	(20–28)

What single test would be best to determine the cause of these biochemical abnormalities?
A. Adrenal autoantibodies
B. HbA1c
C. Paired insulin and C peptide
D. Serum amylase
E. Tetracosactrin (synacthen) test

25. A 55-year-old man is found to have ++ glycosuria and had a maternal history of T2DM. He is a smoker of 20 cigarettes per day. He has a BMI of 30 kg/m². Blood pressure is 132/88 mmHg. Investigations reveal:

Serum creatinine	80 µmol/L	(60110)
Plasma glucose (fasting)	11.3 mmol/L	(3.0–6.0)
Total serum cholesterol	5.5 mmol/L	(< 5.2)
HDL cholesterol	1.4 mmol/L	(> 1.55)

What is most likely to improve his life expectancy?
A. Metformin 500 mg twice daily
B. Ramipril 10 mg daily
C. Simvastatin 10 mg daily
D. Lifestyle modification and stopping smoking
E. Weight loss to achieve a BMI of 25 kg/m²

26. A 50-year-old male with long-standing diabetes presents with severe pain in his left thigh. On examination, there is marked wasting of his quadriceps on the left side and loss of knee reflex. There is no sensory loss. You diagnose the condition as amyotrophy. What is most useful for the management?
A. Weight loss
B. Good glycaemic control
C. Non-steroidal anti-inflammatory drugs (NSAIDs)
D. B12 supplementation
E. Gabapentin

27. A patient who is 16 weeks pregnant and has a BMI of 35 kg/m² is found to have a fasting glucose of 6.0 mmol/L. What is the next course of action?
    A. Nil required as diabetes is excluded
    B. Glucose tolerance test
    C. Dip urine to ensure no ketones
    D. Repeat fasting glucose at 28 weeks
    E. Glucose tolerance test at 28 weeks

28. An 18-year-old girl with T1DM has been unwell for the last couple of days and has not been taking her insulin as she has not been eating. She is alert and is now feeling much better and is managing to eat and drink and is no longer vomiting; however, there are ketones in her urine. Bloods reveal a glucose of 14 mmol/L, a bicarbonate of 13 mmol/L and a pH of 7.25. Which of the following is the most appropriate management option?
    A. Admit—commence IV fluids and IV insulin.
    B. Admit—commence IV fluids and normal subcutaneous insulin dose.
    C. No admission required—monitor for few hours to ensure eating and drinking and give normal insulin dose and then manage as outpatient.
    D. Admit—commence oral fluids and normal subcutaneous insulin dose.
    E. Admit—commence oral fluids and IV insulin.

29. A 20-year-old male has been brought by his family as he has become increasingly drowsy over the last few days. He has T1DM and was commenced on antibiotics a few days ago for a urinary tract infection. He has not been able to eat or drink much. On examination, he is tachycardic and hypotensive and he looks unwell and dry. Bloods reveal a lab glucose of 35 mmol/L, bicarbonate of 17 mmol/L and serum osmolality of 350 mOsmol/kg. His urea is 11.3 mmol/L, creatinine 220, sodium 147 mmol/L and potassium of 5.2 mmol/L.
    A. 1 L of 0.45 NaCl over 30 minutes
    B. 1 L of 0.45% NaCl over 1 hour
    C. 1 L of 0.9% NaCl over 30 minutes
    D. 1 L of 0.9% NaCl over 1 hour
    E. 1 L of 0.9% NaCl over 2 hours

30. A 55-year-old gentleman with T2DM was on the maximum dose of metformin and gliclazide. However, his recent HbA1c was 8.2% and he has been struggling with his blood sugars. What treatment option would be least appropriate in this case?
    A. Sitagliptin
    B. Pioglitazone
    C. Vildagliptin
    D. Exenatide
    E. Insulin

Answers

1-D, 2-E, 3-C, 4-A, 5-A, 6-D, 7-D, 8-D, 9-A, 10-D, 11-C, 12-B, 13-A, 14-D, 15-A, 16-E, 17-A, 18-C, 19-B, 20-E, 21-C, 22-C, 23-A, 24-E, 25-D, 26-B, 27-E, 28-C, 29-D, 30-E

■ SUGGESTED READING

1. Buse JB, Wexler DJ, Tsapas A, Rossing P, Mingrone G, Mathieu C, et al. 2019 Update to: Management of Hyperglycemia in Type 2 Diabetes, 2018. A Consensus Report by the American Diabetes Association (ADA) and the European Association for the Study of Diabetes (EASD). Diabetes Care. 2019; dci190066.
2. Davies MJ, D'Alessio DA, Fradkin J, Kernan WN, Mathieu C, Mingrone G, et al. Management of hyperglycemia in type 2 diabetes, 2018. A Consensus Report by the American Diabetes Association (ADA) and the European Association for the Study of Diabetes (EASD). Diabetes Care. 2018;41(12):2669-701.
3. Cosentino F, Grant PJ, Aboyans V, Bailey CJ, Ceriello A, Delgado V, et al. 2019 ESC Guidelines on diabetes, pre-diabetes, and cardiovascular diseases developed in collaboration with the EASD: The Task Force for diabetes, pre-diabetes, and cardiovascular diseases of the European Society of Cardiology (ESC) and the European Association for the Study of Diabetes (EASD). Eur Heart J. 2020;41(2):255-323.
4. Heinemann L, Fleming GA, Petrie JR, Holl RW, Bergenstal RM, Peters AL. Insulin pump risks and benefits: A clinical appraisal of pump safety standards, adverse event reporting and research needs. A joint statement of the European Association for the Study of Diabetes and the American Diabetes Association Diabetes Technology Working Group. Diabetologia. 2015;58(5):862-70.
5. Sinclair A, Morley JE, Rodriguez-Mañas L, Paolisso G, Bayer T, Zeyfang A, et al. Diabetes Mellitus in Older People: Position Statement on Behalf of the International Association of Gerontology and Geriatrics (IAGG), the European Diabetes Working Party for Older People (EDWPOP), and the International Task Force of Experts in Diabetes. J Am Med Dir Assoc. 2012;13(6):497-502.

6. American Diabetes Association. 2. Classification and Diagnosis of Diabetes: Standards of Medical Care in Diabetes-2020. Diabetes Care. 2020;43:S14-31.
7. American Diabetes Association. 2. Classification and Diagnosis of Diabetes: Standards of Medical Care in Diabetes-2018. Diabetes Care. 2018;41:S13-27.
8. American Diabetes Association. 4. Comprehensive Medical Evaluation and Assessment of Comorbidities: Standards of Medical Care in Diabetes-2020. Diabetes Care. 2020;43:S37-47.
9. American Diabetes Association. 11. Microvascular Complications and Foot Care: Standards of Medical Care in Diabetes-2020. Diabetes Care. 2020;43:S135-51.
10. Davies MJ, D'Alessio DA, Fradkin J, Kernan WN, Mathieu C, Mingrone G, et al. Management of Hyperglycemia in Type 2 Diabetes, 2018. A Consensus Report by the American Diabetes Association (ADA) and the European Association for the Study of Diabetes (EASD). Diabetes Care. 2018;41(12):2669-701.
11. Qaseem A, Wilt TJ, Kansagara D, Horwitch C, Barry MJ, Forciea MA, et al. Hemoglobin A1c targets for glycemic control with pharmacologic therapy for nonpregnant adults with type 2 diabetes mellitus: A Guidance Statement Update From the American College of Physicians. Ann Intern Med. 2018;168(8):569-76.

CHAPTER 9

Rheumatology and Connective Tissue Disorder Diseases

Differences between inflammatory and non-inflammatory arthritis discussed in **Table 9.1**. Causes of acute and chronic arthritis is listed in **Box 9.1**.

TABLE 9.1: Inflammatory versus noninflammatory arthritis.

Features	Inflammatory (rheumatoid arthritis)	Non-inflammatory (osteoarthritis)
Age of onset	Usually 20–40 years but may begin at any age	Most commonly over 50 years of age
Speed of onset	Rapid over weeks to months	Slow; over years
Systemic symptoms	Fatigue, low-grade fever, anorexia Extra-articular manifestations: Rheumatoid nodules, Sjögren's syndrome, Felty syndrome	No systemic symptoms
Joint affection	Symmetrical	Asymmetrical
Joint symptoms	Painful, swollen stiff joints and muscle aches	Joints painful without swelling
Joints involved	Primarily affects small joints [metacarpophalangeal (MCP) and proximal interphalangeal (PIP)]	Affects large weight bearing joints (hip, knee or the spine). Affects PIP and distal interphalangeal (DIP) joints
Stiffness	Morning stiffness for > 1 h. Stiffness occurs after periods of rest/inactivity (the so-called gel phenomenon)	Morning stiffness for < 30 min. Stiffness is generally mild and occurs after periods of activity
Relation of movement with pain	Movement or mild-to-moderate activity decreases pain	Movement increases the pain (worsens with activity) and improves with rest
Examination of joint	Swollen, red, warm, tender and painful	Swollen, cool and hard on palpation. When severely inflamed (as in acute gout or septic arthritis), can have erythema of the overlying skin
Radiological findings	Bony erosion, soft tissue swelling, angular deformities, periarticular osteopaenia	Loss of joints space and articular cartilage, routine wear and tear, osteophytes

Continued

Continued

Features	Inflammatory (rheumatoid arthritis)	Non-inflammatory (osteoarthritis)
Laboratory findings		
Rehumatoid factor (RF), antinuclear antibody	Positive	Negative
Erythrocyte sedimentation rate (ESR) and C-reactive protein (CRP)	Both are often raised	Usually normal but transient elevation of ESR may occur due to synovitis
White blood cell (WBC) count in the synovial fluid	WBC count is > 2,000/mm^3 in septic arthritis and not in rheumatoid arthritis (RA)	< 200/mm^3

Box 9.1: Causes of acute and chronic arthritis.

Actue monoarthritis
- **Inflammatory:** Crystal disease (e.g. gout), infectious disease, spondyloarthropathy, rheumatoid arthritis (RA)
- **Mechanical/inflammatory:** Trauma, avascular necrosis

Acute polyarthritis
- **Infectious:** Bacterial, HIV
- **Non-infectious:** Rheumatoid arthritis, spondyloarthropathy, other connective tissue diseases, crystal (gout), sarcoidosis, malignancy, leukaemia, sickle cell anaemia

Chronic monoarthritis
- **Inflammatory:** Crystal disease, infectious disease (e.g. tuberculosis, fungal), spondyloarthropathy, RA
- **Non-inflammatory:** Osteoarthritis, avascular necrosis, neuropathic arthropathy, villonodular synovitis

Chronic polyarthritis
- **Inflammatory:** Rheumatoid arthritis, spondyloarthropathy, other connective tissue diseases
- **Mechanical:** Osteoarthritis
- **Crystal:** Gout
- **Metabolic:** Infiltrative, metabolic, hypothyroidism
- **Malignancy**

Clinical Features
- Fatigue, anorexia, weakness and vague musculoskeletal symptoms
- Joint involvement is usually **symmetric**.
- The metacarpophalangeal (MCP) and proximal interphalangeal (PIP) joints of the hands, wrists, knees, and the metatarsophalangeal (MTP) and PIP joints of the feet are the most common joints involved.
- '**Morning stiffness**' lasting > 1 hour is a characteristic feature.

Deformities Seen
- 'Spindling' of the fingers
- 'Swan-neck' deformity
- 'Boutonniere' deformity
- 'Z' deformity
- 'Broadening' of the forefoot
- Hallux valgus deformity

Extra-articular Manifestations
- Rheumatoid nodules
- **Rheumatoid vasculitis:** Polyneuropathy and mononeuritis multiplex
- **Pleuropulmonary manifestations:** Effusion, interstitial fibrosis and nodules (Caplan syndrome)
- Premature atherosclerosis
- **Neurological manifestations:** Carpal and tarsal tunnel syndromes, atlanto-axial subluxation
- **Ophthalmological manifestations:** Scleritis, episcleritis and scleromalacia perforans
- **Felty's syndrome:** Splenomegaly and granulocytopenia with rheumatoid arthritis (RA)

■ RHEUMATOID ARTHRITIS
- Females:Males (3:1)
- Fourth and fifth decades of life
- Association with human leucocyte antigen **(HLA)-DR4** in 70% of patients

- Osteoporosis
- **Haematological manifestations:** Anaemia and thrombocytosis

Diagnosis: ACR/EULAR Criteria
- **American College of Rheumatism/European League** Against Rheumatism (ACR/EULAR) criteria are given in **Table 9.2**.

Investigations
- Markers of acute inflammation: Raised Erythrocyte sedimentation rate (ESR), anaemia, thrombocytosis, increased C-reactive protein (CRP)
- Rheumatoid factor (RF)
- Anti-citrullinated peptide antibody (ACPA)

Management
- **Analgesics:**
  Nonsteroidal anti-inflammatory drugs (NSAIDs) are the first-line drugs.
- **Disease-modifying antirheumatic drugs (DMARDs):**
  - Hydroxychloroquine
  - Oral gold (auranofin)
  - Parenteral (intramuscular) gold
  - D-penicillamine
  - Sulphasalazine
  - Methotrexate
  - Leflunomide
- **Biological response modifiers (or biologicals):**
  - Anti-tumour necrosis factor alpha (TNF-α) inhibitors (infliximab, adalimumab, golimumab and certolizumab) and a soluble receptor fusion protein (etanercept)
  - Other biological include:
    - Rituximab (anti-CD20 antibody that blocks CD20 present on B cells)
    - Tocilizumab [a monoclonal antibody that binds to interleukin 6 (IL-6) receptors]
    - Abatacept (T-cell receptor CTLA-4 that downregulates T cells)
    - Anakinra (IL-1 receptor blocker)
- **Corticosteroids**

ADULT-ONSET STILL'S DISEASE
- A triad of:
  - High-spiking fever
  - Characteristic evanescent skin rash
  - Arthritis/arthralgias
- Investigations show anaemia, leucocytosis, thrombocytosis, raised ESR, elevated liver enzymes.
- Ferritin levels usually higher.
- Treatment is with NSAIDs and steroids. Role of DMARDs in not clear.

SJÖGREN'S SYNDROME
- A triad of:
  - Keratoconjunctivitis sicca
  - Xerostomia
  - Mononuclear cell infiltration of salivary gland

Clinical Features
- Dryness of eyes
- Xerostomia
- Enlargement of the parotid occurs with primary Sjögren's syndrome.

TABLE 9.2: ACR/EULAR criteria.

Features	Score
• Joint involvement:	
○ 1 large joint	0
○ 2–10 large joints	1
○ 1–3 small joints	2
○ 4–10 small joints	3
○ > 10 joints	5
• Serology:	
○ Negative rheumatoid factor (RF) and negative anti-citrullinated peptide antibody (ACPA)	0
○ Low-positive RF or low-positive ACPA	2
○ High-positive RF or high-positive ACPA	3
• Acute-phase reactants:	
○ Normal C-reactive protein (CRP) and normal erythrocyte sedimentation rate (ESR)	0
○ Abnormal CRP or abnormal ESR	1
• Duration of symptoms:	
○ Less than 6 weeks	0
○ 6 weeks or more	1

(ACR/EULAR: American College of Rheumatism/European League Against Rheumatism)

- Interstitial nephritis or glomerulonephritis
- Cutaneous and systemic vasculitis
- Polyneuropathies or mononeuritis multiplex

Laboratory Investigations
- Raised ESR, leucopoenia and thrombocytosis.
- Antibodies to Ro/SSA or La/SSB, antinuclear antibody (ANA) or RF are positive

Treatment
- Ocular and mucosal lubricants such as artificial tears, ophthalmologic lubricating ointments and lubricating agents for dryness of mouth
- Cyclosporine emulsion is useful in ocular dryness.
- Pilocarpine and cevimeline
- Hydroxychloroquine

ANKYLOSING SPONDYLITIS/ MARIE-STRUMPELL DISEASE
- Seronegative
- Primarily affects the axial skeleton with a predilection for lumbar spine and sacroiliac joints
- About 90% of the affected people carry the histocompatibility antigen HLA-B27.
- Male-to-female ratio of 4:1

Clinical Features
- Low back pain with nocturnal exacerbations
- Low back morning stiffness that improves with activity
- Schober's test positive
- Figure of four tests (Patrick's test) positive
- Enthesitis
- Diminished chest expansion (< 5 cm) and thoracic kyphosis

Extra-articular Manifestations
- Acute anterior uveitis
- Iritis
- Aortic regurgitation and heart failure
- Apical pulmonary fibrosis and cavitation
- Osteoporosis
- Myelopathy secondary to atlanto-axial subluxation and spinal fracture
- Cauda equina syndrome
- Amyloidosis

Investigations
- ESR is raised. Tests for RF are negative.
- HLA-B27 is present in > 90% cases.
- Magnetic resonance imaging (MRI) and bone scan can pick up early sacroiliitis.

Management
- Indomethacin is the most effective drug.
- Sulphasalazine and methotrexate
- Infliximab, etanercept and adalimumab

REITER'S SYNDROME
- Classical Reiter's syndrome is a triad of:
  i. Non-specific urethritis
  ii. Conjunctivitis
  iii. Arthritis 2–4 weeks following enteric or urogential infections
- Common enteric pathogens triggering the disease are *Shigella, Salmonella, Yersinia* and *Campylobacter* species.
- Enthesitis and dactylitis (inflammation of entire digit) are very common.
- Keratoderma blennorrhagica
- Circinate balanitis

Investigations
- Raised ESR
- Anaemia and polymorphonuclear leucocytosis
- HLA-B27 is positive in > 75% of cases.
- Serum tests for RF and ANAs are negative.

Management
- Rest and NSAIDs
- Intra-articular or local steroid injections
- Non-specific urethritis is treated with a short course of tetracycline or ciprofloxacin.
- Biologicals such as infliximab, etanercept, adalimumab and thalidomide in refractory cases.

PSORIATIC ARTHRITIS

Types
- Symmetric psoriatic arthritis
- Asymmetric psoriatic arthritis
- Arthritis mutilans
- Psoriatic spondylitis
- Predominant distal interphalangeal arthritis

Clinical Features
- Involvement of proximal and distal interphalangeal joints with characteristic 'sausage-shaped' digits
- Distal interphalangeal predominant type of psoriatic arthritis
- Characteristic skin lesion of psoriasis may be present.
- Characteristic nail changes of psoriasis are pitting, onycholysis, subungual hyperkeratosis and horizontal ridging.
- Uveitis, unilateral or bilateral, generally chronic

Diagnosis
- Raised ESR and negative tests for RF and ANAs
- Radiological findings are similar to those of RA.
- Radiographs of distal interphalangeal joints may show pencil-in-cup changes because of marked resorption of bone.

Management
- Majority of the patients respond to NSAIDs.
- Other modalities of treatment include:
  - Sulphasalazine
  - Methotrexate
  - Photochemotherapy
  - Infliximab, etanercept and adalimuimab

■ BEHCET'S DISEASE
Criteria of Behcet's disease are given in **Table 9.3**.

Diagnosis
- Based on clinical features
- Pathergy test

TABLE 9.3: Major and minor criteria of Behcet's disease.

Major criteria	Minor criteria
• Recurrent aphthous stomatitis • Erythema nodosum • Genital ulcerations • Iritis	• Inflammatory arthritis of large joints (non-deforming) • Intestinal ulceration • Meningoencephalitis • Epididymitis • Thrombophlebitis

Treatment
- For mucocutaneous manifestations, local steroids and oral colchicine
- For joint manifestations, NSAIDs are sufficient.
- Aspirin for thrombophlebitis
- Systemic steroids along with cytotoxic drugs (methotrexate, azathioprine, chlorambucil, cyclosporine A or cyclophosphamide) for uveitis

■ HENOCH–SCHÖNLEIN PURPURA/ ANAPHYLACTOID PURPURA
- Small-vessel vasculitis
- The characteristic features are vasculitic purpura, abdominal pain, haematuria and acute arthritis.

Treatment
- Most patients respond to bed rest and NSAIDs.
- Corticosteroids are indicated in severe systemic disease.

■ SYSTEMIC LUPUS ERYTHEMATOSUS
- Second and third decades, with a female/male ratio of 9:1.

Clinical Features
- Fatigue, malaise, fever, anorexia, nausea and weight loss.

Renal Disease
- Characterised by proteinuria (> 0.5 g/24 h) and/or red cell casts (**Box 9.2**)

Musculoskeletal Features
- Arthralgia and myalgia in most patients
- The classical 'Jaccoud's arthropathy' occurs without any erosion.

Box 9.2: Classification of lupus nephritis.
- Class I: Minimal mesangial lupus nephritis
- Class II: Mesangial proliferative lupus nephritis
- Class III: Focal lupus nephritis
- Class IV: Diffuse lupus nephritis
- Class V: Membranous lupus nephritis
- Class VI: Advanced sclerosing lupus nephritis

Mucocutaneous Features
- Malar rash
- Discoid rash
- Photosensitivity
- Alopecia
- Painless mouth ulcers

Haematological Features
- Normocytic normochromic anaemia
- Coombs-positive haemolytic anaemia
- Thrombocytopaenia
- Leucopoenia

Cardiovascular Features
- Myocarditis and pericarditis
- Endocarditis (Libman–Sacks endocarditis)

Pulmonary Features
- Pleurisy
- Pleural effusion
- Pneumonitis
- Vanishing lung syndrome
- Pulmonary haemorrhage

Gastrointestinal Features
- Hepatosplenomegaly
- Mesenteric vasculitis

Investigations

Immunological Abnormalities
Autoantibodies in patients with systemic lupus erythematosus (SLE) are given in **Box 9.3**.

Diagnostic Criteria
ACR criteria: Presence of four or more criteria is diagnostic (**Table 9.4**).

Systemic lupus international collaboration clinics (SLICC) classification 2012 criteria are given in **Table 9.5**.

Box 9.3: Autoantibodies in patients with systemic lupus erythematosus (SLE).
- ANA
- Anti-DNA (anti-dsDNA and anti-ssDNA)
- Anti-Sm (Anti-Smith)
- Anti-RNP
- Anti-Ro (SSA)
- Anti-La (SSB)
- Anti-histone
- Anti-cardiolipin (aCL)
- Anti-erythrocyte
- Anti-platelet
- Anti-lymphocyte
- Anti-neuronal

TABLE 9.4: ACR (American College of Rheumatism) criteria.

Criteria:	
1. Malar rash	
2. Discoid rash	
3. Photosensitivity	
4. Oral ulcers	
5. Arthritis	
6. Serositis	Pleuritis or pleural effusion/pericarditis or pericardial effusion
7. Renal disorder	Persistent proteinuria > 0.5 g/day/cellular casts
8. Neurologic disorder	Seizures/psychosis
9. Haematologic disorder	Haemolytic anaemia/ leucopoenia/ lymphopoenia/ thrombocytopaenia
10. Immunologic disorder	Anti-DNA antibody/anti-Sm antibody
11. Antinuclear antibody	

TABLE 9.5: Systemic lupus international collaborating clinics (SLICC) classification 2012 criteria.

Lupus nephritis proved by biopsy and ANA or anti-DNA or at least four criteria (one needs to be immunological)	
Clinical	Immunological
• Acute cutaneous LE	• ANA
• Chronic cutaneous LE	• Anti-dsDNA
• Oral ulcer	• Anti-Sm
• Alopecia	• aPL antibodies
• Synovitis	• Low complement
• Serositis	• Direct Coombs' test positive
• Renal	
• Neurologic	
• Haemolytic anaemia	
• Leucopoenia/lymphopaenia	
• Thrombocytopenia	

(ANA: antinuclear antibody; Anti-Sm: autoantibodies against Smith antigen; aPL: antiphospholipid; dsDNA: double stranded deoxyribonucleic acid; LE: lupus erythematosus)

Management

- NSAIDs
- Skin lesions and arthritis—hydroxychloroquine
- Photosensitive skin lesions—sun-screen lotions
- Patients with severe symptoms or life-threatening features—corticosteroids
- Acutely ill patients and patients with proliferative glomerulonephritis
    - 'Pulses' of methylprednisolone for 3 days (1 g/day) followed by oral steroids
- Azathioprine, methotrexate, cyclophosphamide and mycophenolate mofetil

Treatment algorithm for SLE is shown in **Flowchart 9.1**.

■ DRUG-INDUCED LUPUS

- Drugs implicated:
    - Antiarrhythmics- procainamide, diltiazem, disopyramide, and propafenone
    - Antihypertensive- hydralazine, methyl dopa, angiotensin-converting enzyme inhibitors, beta-blockers
    - Antithyroid drugs- propyl-thiouracil
    - Antipsychotics- chlorpromazine and lithium
    - Anticonvulsants- carbamazepine and phenytoin)
    - Antibiotics -isoniazid, minocycline
    - Antirheumatic -sulphasalazine
    - Diuretic- hydrochlorothiazide
    - Antihyperlipidemics- lovastatin and simvastatin).
    - Biologic agents- Interferons and TNF inhibitors.
- Less female predilection than SLE
- Kidneys or brain involvement rare, less cutaneous involvement
- ANAs positive; antihistone antibodies positive (95%); autoantibodies to dsDNA absent
- C3 levels normal

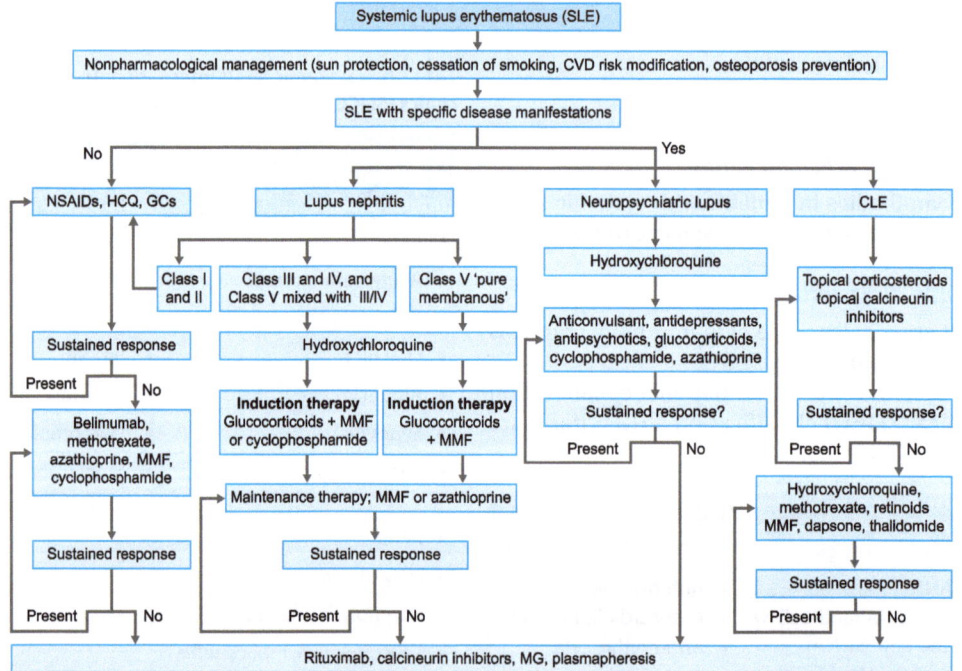

(CLE: cutaneous lupus erythematosus; GCs: glucocorticoids; HCQ: hydroxychloroquine; MMF: mycophenolate mofetil; NSAIDs: non-steroidal anti-inflammatory drugs; CVD: cardiovascular disease)

Flowchart 9.1: Treatment algorithm for systemic lupus erythematous.

ANTIPHOSPHOLIPID ANTIBODY SYNDROME

Clinical Features
Clinical features of antiphospholipid antibody (APLA) syndrome are given in **Table 9.6**.

Diagnosis
- Anticardiolipin (aCL) antibodies
- Lupus anticoagulant (LA) antibodies
- Anti-β2-glycoprotein I (IgG and/or IgM)

Treatment
Treatment of venous thrombosis:
- Anticoagulation with heparin and oral warfarin
- Steroids are often added to this treatment.
- In severe cases of generalised thrombosis, plasmapheresis or intravenous immunoglobulin may be tried.

Prevention of recurrence of arterial thrombosis: Aspirin

SYSTEMIC SCLEROSIS
- Diffuse cutaneous systemic sclerosis/limited cutaneous systemic sclerosis

Clinical Manifestations
- Raynaud phenomenon
- Diffuse cutaneous scleroderma is characterised by symmetrical skin thickening of proximal and distal extremities, face and trunk.
- Kidney and other systemic involvement
- Limited cutaneous scleroderma is associated with:
  o Skin thickening limited to distal extremities and face
  o CREST syndrome (calcinosis, Raynaud phenomenon, oesophageal dysfunction, sclerodactyly and telangiectasia)
  o Muscle weakness
  o Arthralgia
  o Resorption of terminal phalanges
  o Dysphagia, reflux oesophagitis and sliding hiatus hernia
  o Pulmonary fibrosis

Investigations
- Elevated ESR
- Anaemia
- Anti-topoisomerase I (previously called anti-Scl-70) and anti-centromere antibodies

Treatment
- Control of Raynaud phenomenon
- Management of gastroesophageal reflux disease (GERD)
- D-Penicillamine—reduces skin thickening
- Cyclophosphamide—lung disease and severe skin disease
- Methotrexate—scleroderma overlap syndromes

TABLE 9.6: **Clinical features of antiphospholipid antibody (APLA) syndrome.**

Organ/system	Manifestations
Arterial/venous	Thrombosis in any artery or vein
Cardiac	Angina, myocardial infarction, valvular vegetations
Haematologic	Thrombocytopaenia (in 40–50%) haemolytic anaemia, disseminated intravascular coagulation
Neurologic	Transient ischaemic attack, stroke, headache, mononeuritis multiplex
Obstetrical	Pregnancy loss, intrauterine growth retardation
Ophthalmologic	Retinal artery/vein thrombosis
Renal	Thrombosis of renal artery/vein, acute renal failure, haematuria
Gastrointestinal (GI)	Budd–Chiari syndrome, intestinal infarction, splenic infarction, pancreatitis
Cutaneous	Ulcers and infarcts in the skin, gangrene
Pulmonary	Pulmonary embolism and pulmonary hypertension

POLYMYOSITIS AND DERMATOMYOSITIS

- The skeletal muscle is damaged by an inflammatory process dominated by lymphocytic infiltration.
- Polymyositis spares the skin.
- **Dermatomyositis**—associated with a characteristic skin rash.

Clinical Manifestations

- Weakness of the proximal muscles of the lower limbs (hips and thighs)
- Weakness of the proximal muscles of the upper limbs (should girdle muscles)
- The distal muscles are spared.
- Other features are dysphagia, respiratory impairment, myocarditis resulting heart failure and arrhythmias, arthralgia and interstitial lung disease.
- **Characteristic skin changes:**
  - Classic lilac-coloured (heliotrope) rash is seen on the upper eyelids.
  - Gottron's papules
  - Shawl sign or the V sign
  - Mechanic's hand

Diagnosis

- ESR is usually raised.
- ANAs
- Characteristic electromyography (EMG) findings (myopathic pattern) may be present.
- Muscle biopsy shows the typical pathologic changes in myositis.

Management

- Prednisolone
- If no improvement, azathioprine is to be added.

The differences between dermatomyositis, polymyositis and inclusion-body myositis are given in **Table 9.7**.

POLYMYALGIA RHEUMATICA

- Proximal myalgias are characteristic.
- There are chronic, symmetric, proximal muscle aching and stiffness usually involving shoulder, pelvic girdles and neck. Muscles may be tender on palpation.
- Neuropsychiatric manifestations are frequent, particularly depression.
- About 10–30% of these patients have associated temporal arteritis.

Investigations

- Elevated ESR (> 50 mm/h) and CRP, and normocytic normochromic anaemia
- Tests for RF and ANAs may be positive.
- Muscle enzymes are characteristically normal.

Treatment

- Prednisolone

TABLE 9.7: Differences between dermatomyositis, polymyositis and inclusion-body myositis.

Features	Dermatomyositis	Polymyositis	Inclusion-body myositis
Sex	F > M	M = F	M > F
Age of oneset	Any	20 years +	50 years +
Onset	Subacute/acute	Chronic	Chronic
Distribution of weakness	Proximal	Proximal	Proximal + distal + asymmetric (typically quadriceps + finger flexors)
Muscle pain/swelling	In acute cases	No	No
Skin involvement	Often	No	No
Raynaud's arthralgia	Frequent	Infrequent	No
Dysphagia	In severe cases	Infrequent	Occasional
Association with cancer	Up to 20%	Probably no	No
Cardiac involvement	Yes	No	No
Interstitial lung disease	Associated with anti-Jo	Associated with anti-Jo	No

VASCULITIS

Classification of Vasculitis is described in **Figure 9.1**.

TEMPORAL ARTERITIS, CRANIAL ARTERITIS OR GIANT-CELL ARTERITIS

- Exclusively in people over the age of 55 years
- Often occurs in the carotid arteries and their branches.
- The disease is characterised by the classic complex of:
  - Fever
  - Anaemia
  - High ESR
  - Headache (usually temporal) in an elderly patient
- The temporal artery may become tender, thickened and cord-like or nodular.
- Scalp pain, and claudication of tongue and jaw are frequent.
- Visual symptoms including diplopia and even sudden blindness may result from ischaemic optic neuritis.
- This condition is very sensitive to corticosteroid therapy.

POLYARTERITIS NODOSA

- Necrotising vasculitis of small- and medium-sized muscular arteries
- Kidneys, heart, liver and GI tract are involved.
- It does not involve pulmonary arteries.

Clinical Features

- Predominantly affects males
- Common clinical manifestations are:
  - Hypertension
  - Renal failure
  - Polyarthritis
  - Myalgia
  - Peripheral neuropathy
  - Mononeuritis multiplex

Diagnosis

- Anaemia, raised ESR and neutrophilic leucocytosis
- About 30% are positive for hepatitis B surface antigen (HBsAg).

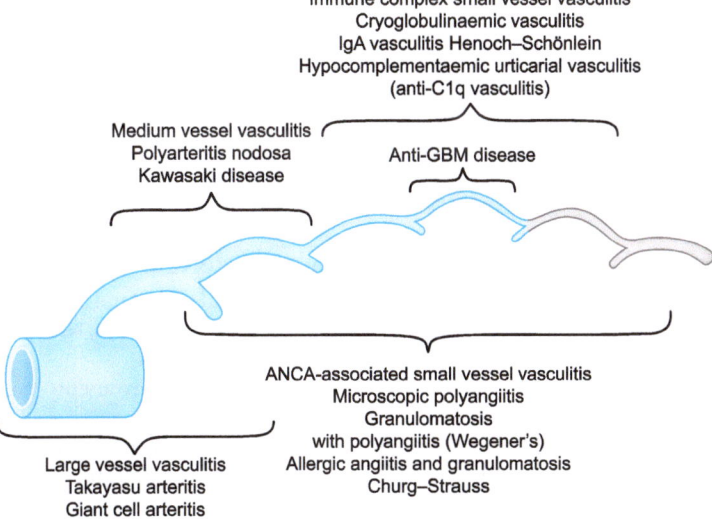

(ANCA: antineutrophil cytoplasmic antibody; GBM: glomerular basement membrane)

Fig. 9.1: Classification of vasculitis.

- Perinuclear anti-neutrophil cytoplasmic antibody (p-ANCA) is present in only about 20% of cases.
- Characteristic findings of vasculitis on biopsy material of involved organ confirm the diagnosis.

Treatment
- Corticosteroids, cyclophosphamide and plasma exchange

■ MICROSCOPIC POLYANGIITIS
- Most common ANCA-associated small-vessel vasculitis
- Characterised by absence of immune deposits in the involved vessels

Clinical Features
- About 40–60 years. More common in males compared to females
- Presentation is by variable combinations or renal involvement.
- Palpable purpura
- Abdominal pain
- Cough and haemoptysis
- Kidney involvement is present in nearly 90% cases.

Diagnosis
- Most patients have positive p-ANCA, although cytoplasmic ANCA (c-ANCA) may also be present in 40% cases.

Treatment
- Combined treatment with cyclophosphamide and corticosteroids has reduced mortality and morbidity significantly.

■ CHURG–STRAUSS SYNDROME
- Allergic granulomatous angiitis affects small- to medium-sized arteries and veins.

Clinical Features
- History of asthma and allergic rhinitis that is followed by small-vessel vasculitis and granulomatous inflammation
- Common features are:
  - Arthralgia and arthritis
  - Purpura
  - Myocarditis, congestive heart failure, pericarditis and myocardial infarction
  - Abdominal pain, diarrhoea and GI bleed
  - Mononeuritis multiplex
  - Stroke
  - Coronary arteritis and myocarditis are the principal causes of morbidity and mortality.

Investigations
- Eosinophils > 10% in peripheral blood
- Elevated ESR and CRP
- Urine showing RBC casts and proteinuria
- Increased IgE levels
- Positive antinuclear cytoplasmic antibodies against myeloperoxidase (p-ANCA) in 15–60% of cases
- Chest X-ray may show infiltrates and pleural effusion.

Treatment
- Most patients respond to high-dose steroids though some cases may require addition of cytotoxic drugs.
- In severe cases, anti-TNF-α agents such as infliximab and etanercept

■ WEGENER'S GRANULOMATOSIS
- Granulomatous vasculitis of upper and lower respiratory tracts together with glomerulonephritis

Clinical Features
- Paranasal sinus pain and discharge, nasal mucosal ulcerations, saddle-nose deformity and hearing loss
- Pulmonary involvement—cough, haemoptysis and dyspnoea
- Renal involvement-glomerulonephritis, resulting in proteinuria, haematuria

Diagnosis
- The ESR is markedly elevated.
- Serum anti-proteinase 3 (c-ANCA) is positive.
- Kidney or lung biopsy

Treatment
Treatment is similar to that for microscopic polyangiitis.

■ GOUT AND HYPERURICAEMIA
Aetiology
Aetiology of gout and hyperuricaemia is given in **Box 9.4**.

Clinical Features
- Asymptomatic hyperuricaemia
- Acute gouty arthritis
- Intercritical period
- Chronic tophaceous gout (tophi and chronic gouty arthritis)
- The MTP joint of the great toe (podagra) in 70% of patients
- Gout can also cause bursitis and tenosynovitis.
- In chronic tophaceous gouty arthritis, crystal deposits appear in cartilage, synovial membranes, tendons and soft tissues. The classic location of a tophus is the helix and antihelix of the ear.

Box 9.4: Aetiology of gout and hyperuricaemia.

Increased purine synthesis de novo:
- Hypoxanthine-guanine-phosphoribosyl transferase (HGPRT) deficiency
- Phosphoribosyl pyrophosphate (PRPP) synthetase overactivity
- Glucose-6 phosphatase deficiency
- Idiopathic

Decreased renal excretion of uric acid:
- Renal failure
- Lead poisoning
- Alcohol
- Drugs: Diuretics, aspirin, pyrazinamide, cyclosporine and levodopa
- Lactic acidosis
- Hyperparathyroidism
- Myxoedema

Increased turnover of purines:
- Myeloproliferative disorders
- Lymphoproliferative disorders
- Cancer chemotherapy
- Haemolysis

- Urate nephropathy
- Obstructive uropathy (nephrolithiasis)

Diagnosis
- Increase in serum uric acid concentration (> 7.0 mg/dL in males and > 6.0 mg/dL in females)
- Aggregated deposits of monosodium urate monohydrate (tophi) in and around the joints
- Synovial fluid examination by compensated polarised microscopy can demonstrate urate crystals. They are seen as slender, needle-shaped, negatively birefringent structures.

Management
Treatment of acute attack:
- NSAIDs are the agents of choice. All NSAIDs are equally effective. Commonly used NSAIDs are indomethacin (50 mg 6 hourly), naproxen and fenoprofen.
- Colchicine is the second choice of drug.
- In patients with polyarticular involvement not responding to NSAIDs or colchicines

Drugs for prophylaxis:
- Allopurinol
- Febuxostat
- Uricosuric agents such as probenecid and sulphinpyrazone

■ PSEUDO-GOUT, CALCIUM PYROPHOSPHATE DIHYDRATE DEPOSITION DISEASE AND PYROPHOSPHATE ARTHROPATHY

- Crystal deposition occurs in fibrous and articular cartilage.
- Release of calcium pyrophosphate dihydrate (CPPD) crystals into the joint space provokes an acute attack of synovitis—'pseudo-gout'.
- Mostly asymptomatic; identified as an incidental finding on radiographs.
- The knee is the most frequently affected joint.
- Acute attacks of pseudo-gout may be precipitated by trauma, joint surgery, sprain or even a long walk.
- Chronic pyrophosphate arthropathy resembles osteoarthritis involving
  - Knees
  - Wrist

- Metacarpophalangeal joints (particularly second and third)
- Shoulders and hips

Diagnosis

- Radiographs of joints may show chondrocalcinosis.
- Ultrasound may be more sensitive than plain radiography.
- CPPD crystals—rod- or rhomboid-shaped weakly positive birefringent crystals

Treatment

- Joint aspiration
- NSAIDs
- Intra-articular corticosteroids and colchicine

BEST OF FIVES

1. A 38-year-old Asian woman presents with polyarthritis. The pain is progressively accompanied by more than an hour of morning stiffness. On physical examination, synovitis of the proximal interphalangeal joints, elbows, left knee and ankles is noted. Which of the following is the most likely diagnosis?
   A. Fibromyalgia
   B. Osteoarthritis
   C. Polymyalgia rheumatica
   D. Rheumatoid arthritis (RA)
   E. Psoriatic arthritis

2. An 18-year-old man is hospitalised for a 1-month history of daily high-spiking fever, arthralgia, myalgia and weight loss. There are enlarged cervical lymph nodes. A salmon-coloured rash is noted on the trunk and proximal extremities. Abdominal examination discloses hepatosplenomegaly. Musculoskeletal examination reveals tenderness of the wrists, knees and ankles. Laboratory studies reveal haemoglobin—10.8 g/dL, leucocyte count—24,000/μL, platelet count—560,000/μL, erythrocyte sedimentation rate (ESR)—102 mm/h and serum ferritin—5,250 ng/mL. Which of the following is the most likely diagnosis?
   A. Adult-onset Still disease
   B. Lymphoma
   C. Parvovirus B19 infection
   D. Systemic lupus erythematosus (SLE)
   E. Acute leukaemia

3. A 30-year-old man is evaluated for a 1-day history of left shoulder pain while throwing a football. The pain is located over the left lateral deltoid muscle. On physical examination, there is pain in the left shoulder with active abduction beginning at approximately 60°, and he has difficulty actively abducting the left arm beyond 60°. Which of the following is the next most appropriate step in management?
   A. Magnetic resonance imaging of the left shoulder
   B. Non-steroidal anti-inflammatory drug therapy
   C. Physical therapy
   D. Subacromial glucocorticoid injection
   E. Surgical correction

4. A 47-year-old woman presents with a 4-week history of fatigue, bilateral hand pain and stiffness, and hand and wrist joint swelling. About a month before presentation, she noticed that her hands were stiffer in the morning but thought that it was due to too much typing. However, the stiffness has worsened and she now needs about an hour each morning to 'loosen up' her hands. Physical examination reveals warm, erythematous wrists and metacarpal joints bilaterally. What is your diagnosis?
   A. Carpel tunnel syndrome
   B. Scaphoid fractures secondary to too much typing
   C. Subdeck's osteodystrophy
   D. Rheumatoid arthritis (RA)
   E. Osteoarthritis

5. A 58-year-old man with a long history of treated essential hypertension and mild renal insufficiency presents to the clinic complaining of pain in the right knee. His primary care provider saw him 1 week ago and added a thiazide diuretic to improve his blood pressure control. Physical examination confirmed the presence of a swollen right knee, which was erythematous and warm. Joint aspiration recovered copious dark yellow, cloudy synovial fluid. Microscopic analysis demonstrated

30,000 leucocytes/L, a negative Gram stain and many needle-like, negatively birefringent crystals.
What is the precipitating factor for this episode?
A. Infection
B. Diet
C. Diuretic
D. Mild renal insufficiency
E. Trauma

6. A 22-year-old African-American woman with a family history of systemic lupus erythematosus (SLE) reports intermittent arthralgias in her knees. She denies any facial rash, photosensitivity, chest pain or shortness of breath. She is convinced that she has lupus and requests confirmatory blood tests. What is the test that you will advice?
A. Anti-neutrophil cytoplasmic antibodies (ANCA)
B. Anti-citrullinated peptide antibody (ACPA)
C. Anti-ds deoxyribonucleic acid (DNA)
D. Rheumatoid factor (RF)
E. Antistreptolysin O (ASO)

7. Which of the following statements is TRUE regarding management of gout?
A. Xanthine oxidase inhibitors are appropriate for treatment of uric acid overproducers, and uricosuric agents for treating uric acid underexcretors.
B. Xanthine oxidase inhibitors are appropriate for treatment of uric acid underexcretors, and uricosuric agents for treating uric acid overproducers.
C. Xanthine oxidase inhibitors and uricosuric agents are appropriate for treating uric acid overproducers.
D. Xanthine oxidase inhibitors and uricosuric agents are appropriate for treatment of uric acid underexcretors.
E. Xanthine oxidase inhibitors and uricosuric agent are appropriate for treatment of uric acid underexcretors and uric acid overproducers.

8. The drug used for the treatment of post-menopausal osteoporosis that reduces the risk of vertebral fractures by 40% and non-vertebral fractures by about 25% is:

A. Alendronate
B. Strontium ranelate
C. Parathyroid hormone
D. Denosumab
E. Vitamin D3

9. Features of simple mechanical low back pain include all EXCEPT:
A. Pain varies with physical activity (improved with rest)
B. Sudden onset, precipitated by lifting or bending
C. Recurrent episodes
D. Clear-cut nerve root distribution
E. Relieved by rest and analgesics

10. Inflammatory enthesitis is characteristically seen in:
A. Polymyositis
B. Systemic lupus erythematosus (SLE)
C. Ankylosing spondylitis
D. Fibromyalgia
E. Rheumatoid arthritis (RA)

11. A 30-year-old female from South Asia presents with claudication in upper limbs, fever, and arthralgia and weight loss. Clinical examination may reveal loss of bilateral radial and brachial pulses, bilateral subclavian bruits and hypertension. Biopsy of the vessels revealed granulomatous inflammation of the vessel wall leading to vessel occlusion. What is your diagnosis?
A. Polyarteritis nodosa
B. Wegener's granulomatosis
C. Takayasu's arteritis
D. Cryoglobulinaemic vasculitis
E. Polymyalgia rheumatica

12. An elderly female came with blindness in one eye. She had a history of headache, localised to the temporal region and jaw claudication. On examination, she had tenderness over the temporal region. On fundoscopy, the optic disc may appear pale and swollen with haemorrhages. Her erythrocyte sedimentation rate (ESR) was 120. What is your diagnosis?
A. Giant cell arteritis
B. Polymyalgia rheumatica
C. Glaucoma
D. Migraine
E. Meningioma

13. Scaly erythematous or violaceous psoriasiform plaques occurring over the extensor surfaces of proximal and distal interphalangeal joints and a heliotrope rash which is a violaceous discoloration of the eyelid in combination with periorbital oedema are characteristically seen in:
    A. Psoriasis
    B. Systemic lupus erythematosus (SLE)
    C. Dermatomyositis
    D. Sjogren's syndrome
    E. Pellagra

14. A 20-year-old female gives birth to a baby with complete heart block who subsequently requires pacemaker insertion. Which of the following antibodies is most likely to be detected in the maternal serum?
    A. Anti-double-stranded deoxyribonucleic acid (dsDNA) antibodies
    B. Anti-endomysial antibodies
    C. Anti-Ro/SSA antibodies
    D. Anti-SCL70 antibodies
    E. Rheumatoid factor (RF)

15. A woman taking hydralazine for hypertension presents with joint pain and chest pain. On examination, the patient has a pericardial rub and bilateral pleural effusion. What is the diagnosis?
    A. Dermatomyositis
    B. Systemic lupus erythematosus (SLE)
    C. Polymyalgia rheumatic
    D. Felty syndrome
    E. Drug-induced lupus

16. A 25-year-old lady with known systemic lupus erythematosus (SLE) presents with the nephrotic syndrome. A renal biopsy is performed and this confirms diffuse proliferative glomerulonephritis (WHO Class IV). Which of the following treatment regimens would you advise?
    A. Azathioprine alone
    B. Prednisolone alone
    C. Azathioprine and prednisolone
    D. Prednisolone and intravenous cyclophosphamide
    E. Prednisolone and methotrexate

17. Allopurinol is used in the management of gout. Which of the following statements is correct?
    A. Allopurinol is effective by increasing glomerular filtration of uric acid.
    B. Allopurinol is effective by reducing the tubular reabsorption of uric acid.
    C. Allopurinol is effective by inhibiting the conversion of xanthine to uric acid.
    D. Allopurinol is indicated in a 37-year-old man with a uric acid concentration of 0.42 mg/L and a history of one attack of gout.
    E. Allopurinol is associated with aplastic anaemia in 1% of cases.

18. A 20-year-old man presents with palpable purpura on the legs and haemoptysis. A radiograph of the chest shows a thin-walled cavity in the bilateral lower zone. Investigations reveal proteinuria and red cell casts in the urine and an elevated serum creatinine level (3.2 mg/dL). What is the most probable diagnosis?
    A. Henoch–Schönlein purpura
    B. Polyarteritis nodosa
    C. Granulomatosis with polyangiitis
    D. Disseminated tuberculosis
    E. Churg–Strauss syndrome

19. A 3-year-old boy presents with fever and conjunctivitis. Physical examination reveals oral erythema and fissuring along with a generalised maculopapular rash and cervical lymphadenopathy. What is the most likely diagnosis?
    A. Henoch–Schönlein purpura
    B. Polyarteritis nodosa
    C. Kawasaki disease
    D. Takayasu's arteritis
    E. Lymphoma

20. A 40-year-old female, with a known case of asthma for the last 4 years, presented with a 2-month history of numbness in the right upper and both lower limbs. Examination revealed asymmetric neuropathy and palpable purpura over the lower limbs. Investigations revealed eosinophilia. What is the likely diagnosis?
    A. Systemic lupus erythematosus (SLE)
    B. Polyarteritis nodosa (PAN)
    C. Giant cell arteritis (GCA)
    D. Churg–Strauss syndrome
    E. Tropical eosinophilia

21. A 40-year-old banker is evaluated for an abnormal serum uric acid level of 7.9 mg/dL (0.47 mmol/L) obtained at a health screening performed at his place of employment. He drinks two alcoholic beverages each weekend and eats meat several times weekly. Medical history is otherwise unremarkable. Family history is notable for his father who has gout. Which of the following is the most appropriate treatment at this time?
    A. Allopurinol
    B. Colchicine
    C. Febuxostat
    D. Probenecid
    E. No treatment is required

22. An 80-year-old woman presents with a 3-year history of progressive pain of the fingers and knees, along with morning stiffness lasting for 10 minutes. Musculoskeletal examination reveals tenderness, erythema and some soft-tissue swelling. She has bilateral knee joint pain, tenderness and crepitus. Blood investigations including erythrocyte sedimentation rate (ESR), C-reactive protein (CRP), rheumatoid factor (RF) and anti-cyclic citrullinated protein (anti-CCP) are negative. X-ray of the hands reveals joint-space narrowing, subchondral sclerosis and linear calcification of the cartilage. Which of the following is the most likely diagnosis?
    A. Calcium pyrophosphate dihydrate deposition disease
    B. Haemochromatosis
    C. Osteoarthritis
    D. Rheumatoid arthritis (RA)
    E. Gout

23. A 40-year-old woman is evaluated for a 6-month history of progressive joint pain of hand, knee and foot associated with 90 minutes of morning stiffness. Musculoskeletal examination reveals tenderness and synovial thickening. Laboratory studies reveal erythrocyte sedimentation rate (ESR) 88 mm/h and rheumatoid factor (RF) 38 U/mL (40 kUI/L). Anti-cyclic citrullinated peptide antibodies are positive. Which of the following is the most appropriate therapy?
    A. Diclofenac
    B. Infliximab
    C. Methotrexate
    D. Sulphasalazine
    E. Cyclophosphamide

24. A 33-year-old female has been diagnosed with rheumatoid arthritis (RA) 6 months ago, and methotrexate was begun at that time. She also takes ibuprofen and acetaminophen. Despite this treatment, she still has 2–3 hours of morning stiffness daily and wakes frequently during the night with pain and stiffness. Laboratory studies show an erythrocyte sedimentation rate (ESR) of 45 mm/h. Radiographs of the hands show periarticular osteopaenia and erosion of the right ulnar styloid. Which of the following is the next most appropriate step in this patient's treatment?
    A. Add etanercept.
    B. Add hydroxychloroquine.
    C. Add cyclophosphamide.
    D. Discontinue methotrexate and begin sulphasalazine.
    E. Add steroids.

25. A 22-year-old woman is evaluated for a 3-month history of fatigue, a photosensitive rash on her face, and hand pain accompanied by morning stiffness. She has a history of two mid-trimester abortions. Anti-nuclear antibody assay results are positive with a titre of 1:160. Which of the following tests is most specific for confirming this patient's diagnosis?
    A. Anti-double-stranded DNA antibodies
    B. Anti-cardiolipin antibody
    C. Anti-U1-ribonucleoprotein antibodies
    D. Antiproteinase-3 antibodies
    E. Anticentromere antibody

26. A 25-year-old woman is evaluated for systemic lupus erythematosus (SLE). Laboratory studies are significant for a serum creatinine level of 1.0 mg/dL (88.4 µmol/L) and a urinalysis showing 2+ protein, 3+ blood, 5–10 leucocytes/high-power field (hpO, 15–20 erythrocytes/hpf, and 1 erythrocyte cast/hpf). Serum complement levels (C3 and C4) are decreased. Which of the following is the next most appropriate step in this patient's treatment?
    A. High-dose prednisone
    B. Ibuprofen
    C. Lisinopril
    D. Low-dose prednisone
    E. Hydroxychloroquine

27. A 20-year-old man is evaluated for a 6-month history of bilateral buttock pain accompanied by prolonged morning stiffness. On physical examination, there is loss of normal lumbar lordosis, and flexion of the lumbar spine is decreased. The low back and pelvis are tender to palpation. Pain increases when the patient crosses his legs. Which of the following studies is most likely to establish the diagnosis in this patient?
    A. Bone scan
    B. Computed tomography (CT) of the sacroiliac joints
    C. Magnetic resonance imaging (MRI) of the lumbar spine
    D. MRI of the sacroiliac joints
    E. Ultrasound of lumbosacral spine

28. A 24-year-old man with Crohn's disease diagnosed 4 years ago complains of low backache. Musculoskeletal examination reveals moderate tenderness to palpation over the low back, with decreased ability to flex at the waist. The remainder of the examination is unremarkable. Laboratory studies include a normal haemoglobin level and leucocyte count and negative rheumatoid factor (RF). Which of the following is the most likely diagnosis?
    A. Enteropathic arthritis
    B. Psoriatic arthritis
    C. Reactive arthritis
    D. Rheumatoid arthritis (RA)
    E. Ankylosing spondylitis

29. A 36-year-old woman is evaluated for pain and colour changes in her fingers and hands. During an episode, her fingers turned white and became very painful, then blue, and over 15–20 minutes became red with eventual resolution of her pain. Her episodes are worsening despite her efforts to avoid cold exposure and minimise stress. Examination of the hands shows sclerodactyly. The radial and ulnar pulses are normal bilaterally. Which of the following is the most appropriate additional treatment for this patient?
    A. Amlodipine
    B. Isosorbide dinitrate
    C. Metoprolol
    D. Prednisone
    E. Methotrexate

30. A 38-year-old woman is evaluated for a gritty, burning sensation in her eyes that worsens over the course of the day and dry mouth with difficulty salivating at times. Laboratory studies are significant for a positive antinuclear antibody (ANA) assay, rheumatoid factor (RF), and anti-Ro/SSA and anti-La/SSB titres. Which of the following is the most likely diagnosis?
    A. Lacrimal gland dysfunction
    B. Primary Sjögren's syndrome
    C. Rheumatoid arthritis (RA)
    D. Systemic lupus erythematosus (SLE)
    E. Sarcoidosis

31. A 70-year-old woman is evaluated for a sudden loss of vision in the left eye that began 30 minutes ago. She has a past history of temporal headache and jaw claudication. On physical examination, the left temporal artery is tender. Funduscopic examination reveals a pale, swollen optic disc. Which of the following is the most appropriate next step in this patient's management?
    A. Magnetic resonance imaging (MRI) of brain
    B. High-dose intravenous methylprednisolone
    C. Low-dose oral prednisone
    D. Temporal artery biopsy
    E. Aspirin and Rosuvastatin

Answers

1-D, 2-A, 3-A, 4-D, 5-C, 6-C, 7-A, 8-A, 9-D, 10-C, 11-C, 12-A, 13-C, 14-C, 15-E, 16-D, 17-C, 18-C, 19-C, 20-D, 21-E, 22-A, 23-C, 24-A, 25-B, 26-A, 27-D, 28-A, 29-A, 30-B, 31-B

■ SUGGESTED READING

1. Singh JA, Furst DE, Bharat A, Jeffrey R Curtis, Arthur F Kavanaugh, Kremer JM, et al. 2012 update of the 2008 American College of Rheumatology recommendations for the use of disease-modifying antirheumatic drugs and biologic agents in the treatment of rheumatoid arthritis. Arthritis Care Res (Hoboken). 2012;64(5):625-39.
2. Smolen JS, Aletaha D, Bijlsma JW, Breedveld FC, Boumpas D, Burmester G, et al. Treating rheumatoid arthritis to target: recommendations of an international task force. Ann Rheum Dis. 2010;69(4):631-7.
3. van Vollenhoven RF, Mosca M, Bertsias G, Isenberg D, Kuhn A, Lerstrøm K, et al. Treat-to-target in systemic lupus

erythematosus: recommendations from an international task force. Ann Rheum Dis. 2014;73(6):958-67.
4. Bertsias G, Ioannidis JP, Boletis J, Bombardieri S, Cervera R, Dostal C, et al. EULAR recommendations for the management of systemic lupus erythematosus. Report of a Task Force of the EULAR Standing Committee for International Clinical Studies Including Therapeutics. Ann Rheum Dis. 2008;67(2):195-205.
5. Drozdinsky G, Hadar E, Shmueli A, Gabbay-Benziv R, Shiber S. Obstetric antiphospholipid syndrome and long-term arterial thrombosis risk. J Thromb Thrombolysis. 2017;44(3):371-5.
6. Terkeltaub R. Update on gout: new therapeutic strategies and options. Nat Rev Rheumatol. 2010;6(1):30-8.
7. Sundy JS. Progress in the pharmacotherapy of gout. Curr Opin Rheumatol. 2010;22(2):188-93.
8. Kontzias A, Efthimiou P. Adult-onset Still's disease: pathogenesis, clinical manifestations and therapeutic advances. Drugs. 2008;68(3):319-37.
9. Henter JI, Samuelsson-Horne A, Aricò M, Egeler RM, Elinder G, Filipovich AH, et al. Treatment of hemophagocytic lymphohistiocytosis with HLH-94 immunochemotherapy and bone marrow transplantation. Blood. 2002;100(7):2367-73.
10. Trottestam H, Horne A, Aricò M, Egeler RM, Filipovich AH, Gadner H, et al. Chemoimmunotherapy for hemophagocytic lymphohistiocytosis: long-term results of the HLH-94 treatment protocol. Blood. 2011;118(17):4577-84.
11. van der Heijde D, Ramiro S, Landewé R, Baraliakos X, van den Bosch P, Sepriano A, et al. 2016 update of the ASAS-EULAR management recommendations for axial spondyloarthritis. Ann Rheum Dis. 2017;76(6):978-91.
12. Ward MM, Deodhar A, Akl EA, Lui A, Ermann J, Gensler LS, et al. American College of Rheumatology/Spondylitis Association of America/Spondyloarthritis Research and Treatment Network 2015 Recommendations for the Treatment of Ankylosing Spondylitis and Nonradiographic Axial Spondyloarthritis. Arthritis Rheumatol. 2016;68(2):282-98.

CHAPTER 10

Nephrology

Definitions
- Azotaemia: Increase in the concentration of urea and creatinine in the blood
- Oliguria: Usually < 400 mL of urine/day
- Anuria refers to complete cessation of urine flow, i.e. daily urinary output < 100 mL.
- Polyuria denotes persistent increase in urine volume of > 3 L/day.

PROTEINURIA
- Normal adults may excrete up to 150 mg of proteins daily.
- Pathological proteinuria may be 'mild' (< 1.0 g/day), 'moderate' (1.0–3.5 g/day) or 'massive' (> 3.5 g/day).
- **Microalbuminuria**. Normal urine contains albumin in a concentration of < 30 mg/L. Elevation of albumin in the urine from > 30 to < 300 mg/day—microalbuminuria.
  - It is known to be an early indicator of diabetic nephropathy and is an established risk for the presence of cardiovascular disease even in normotensive persons.
  - Angiotensin-converting enzyme (ACE) inhibitors or Angiotensin receptor II blockers (ARBs) decrease proteinuria and control of diabetes.

An algorithm approach to proteinuria is shown in **Flowchart 10.1**.

HAEMATURIA
- Haematuria may be macroscopic (visible on gross examination) or microscopic [three or more red blood cells (RBCs) per high-power field].
  - The presence of red-cell casts in the urine is diagnostic of bleeding from the kidney, most often due to glomerulonephritis.
- Kidney: Glomerulonephritis, infective endocarditis, renal tuberculosis, benign familial haematuria, Immunoglobulin A (IgA) nephropathy, severe acute pyelonephritis, papillary necrosis (more common in diabetes mellitus and sickle cell trait or disease), renal cell carcinoma, microscopic polyangiitis, Wegener's granulomatosis
- Ureter: Neoplasms
- Bladder: Neoplasms, trauma, schistosomiasis
- Prostate: Prostatitis, neoplasms
- Urethra: Trauma

CREATINE CLEARANCE
- Renal clearance given as an estimate of the glomerular function of the kidney.
- Formula: 'C = UV/P'
  - C is the renal clearance.
  - U is the urinary concentration of any substance.
  - P is the plasma concentration of the same substance.
  - V is the minute volume of urine.
- Renal clearance of inulin can be used to estimate the glomerular filtration rate (GFR).
- The GFR for an average adult is about 125 mL/min.
- Creatinine clearance (and hence GFR) can also be calculated by using the **Cockcroft–Gault formula** if serum creatinine is stable:

$$Cl_{cr} \text{ (mL/min)} = 140 - \text{age} \times \text{Ideal body weight}/72 \times \text{Serum creatinine (mg/dL)}$$ (for females, the value is multiplied by 0.85).

Nephrology

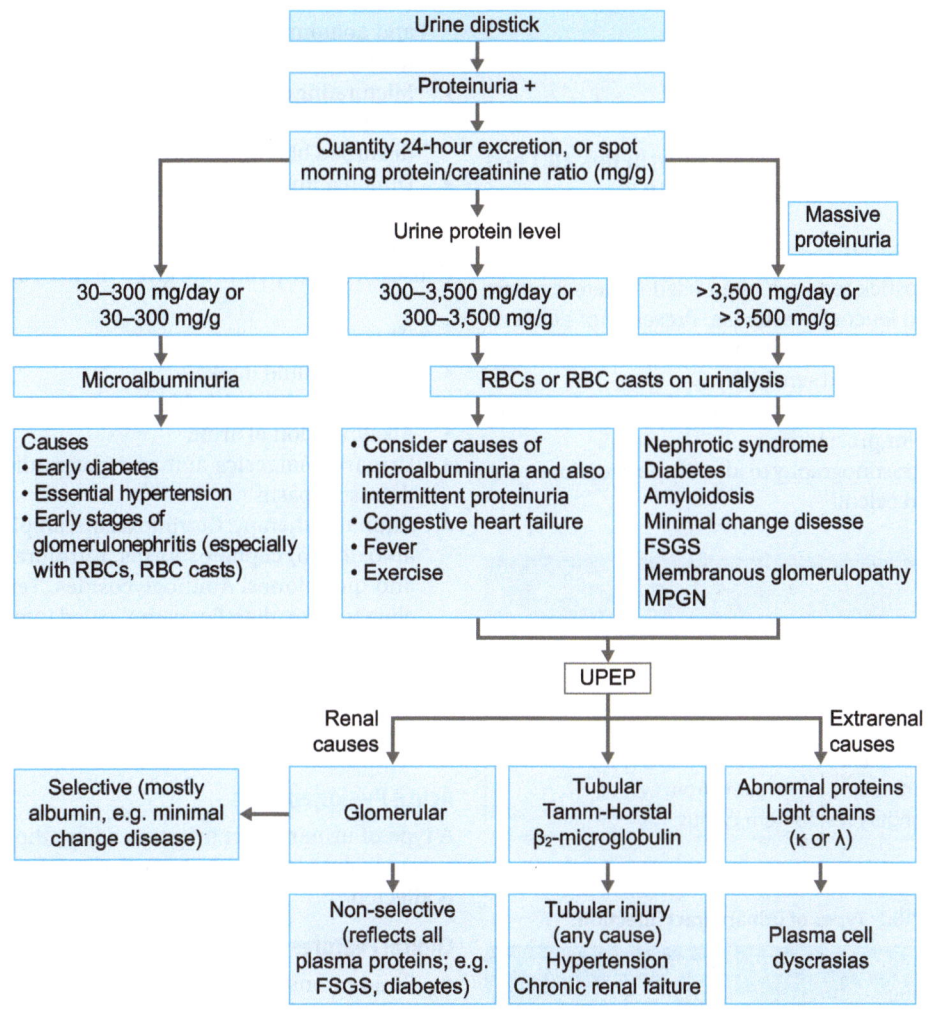

Flowchart 10.1: Algorithm approach to proteinuria.

(FSGS: focal segmental glomerulosclerosis; MPGN: membranoproliferative glomerulonephritis; RBC: red blood cell; UPEP: urine protein electrophoresis)

■ URINARY TRACT INFECTION

Urinary tract infection (UTI) is defined by the presence of > 10^5 organism/mL in the midstream sample of urine, i.e. 'significant bacteriuria'.

Types of bacteriuria are given in **Table 10.1**.

Aetiology

- *Escherichia coli* (80% cases)
- *Proteus, Klebsiella, Enterobacter*

TABLE 10.1: Bacteriuria and its types.

Asymptomatic bacteriuria	Symptomatic bacteriuria
• Presence of bacteriuria (> 10^5/mL on 2 occasions in women and on 1 occasion in men) but without symptoms	• Lower tract infections (urethritis, prostatitis and cystitis) • Upper tract infections (pyelonephritis and perinephric abscess)

- *Pseudomonas, Serratia, Chlamydia trachomatis*
- *Neisseria gonorrhoeae*

Clinical Features

Clinical features of UTI are given in **Box 10.1** and types of UTI are given in **Table 10.2**.

Investigations

- Dipstick tests are often used to detect nitrite and leucocyte esterase. Presence of either of them increases the possibility of UTI.
- Culture and sensitivity
- Prostatic massage followed by urine culture → for prostatitis.
- Ultrasonography to identify obstruction, cysts and calculi
- Intravenous urography (IVU) → physiological and anatomical abnormalities of the urinary tract
- Micturating cystourethrogram (MCU) to identify and quantitate vesicoureteric reflux and disturbed bladder emptying
- Dimercaptosuccinic acid (DMSA) renal scan for pyelonephritis
- Cystoscopy in suspected bladder lesions

Causes of sterile pyuria are given in **Box 10.2**

Treatment

- Adequate fluid intake
- Regular complete bladder emptying
- Alkalinisation of urine
- Urinary analgesics and antispasmodics for detrusor spasm
- Antibiotic therapy: Cotrimoxazole, ampicillin, amoxicillin, cephalosporins, nitrofurantoin and quinolones. Aminoglycosides. Tetracycline (chlamydia). For complicated infection, parenteral antibiotics preferable
- In females, maintenance of adequate perineal hygiene, emptying the bladder before and after intercourse

Acute Pyelonephritis

A type of urinary tract infection where the renal parenchyma along with the upper urinary tract is affected.

Clinical Features

- Sudden onset of pain in one or both loins, radiating to the iliac fossa
- Frequent passage of small amount of scalding Cloudy urine may be a symptom.
- Fever with chills and rigors
- Tenderness and guarding at the renal angle

Box 10.1: Clinical features of urinary tract infection.

- Fever with chills and rigors
- Frequency of micturition
- Dysuria or scalding micturition
- Urgency
- Haematuria
- Suprapubic pain resulting from cystitis
- Strangury results from cystitis

TABLE 10.2: Types of urinary tract infection.

Uncomplicated urinary tract infection	Complicated urinary tract infection
• Includes cystitis or urethritis due to bacterial colonisation of the bladder or urethra • Females are significantly more affected than males • Sequelae rare	• Infection involving renal parenchyma (pyelonephritis) or prostate (prostatitis) • Infection in men often considered complicated • Presence of obstructive lesions or following instrumentations on urinary tract • Sequelae such as sepsis, metastatic abscesses and renal failure are common

---

Box 10.2: Causes of sterile pyuria.

- Partially treated urinary tract infection
- Calculi in urinary tract
- Urinary tuberculosis
- Chlamydia
- Bladder tumours
- Chemical cystitis
- Appendicitis

Investigations

- Peripheral blood leucocytosis
- Microscopic examination of urine shows numerous pus cells and organisms, some red cells and epithelial cells.
- Culture of MSU may grow the organism.
- Ultrasound studies
- Computed tomography (CT)

Management

Intravenous (IV) ampicillin, amoxicillin plus aminoglycosides, such as tobramycin, or cephalosporin, such as cefuroxime, or quinolone for 10–21 days.

Chronic Pyelonephritis (Reflux Nephropathy)

- Chronic interstitial nephritis that occurs as a result of recurrent UTIs, commonly due to severe vesicoureteric reflux in children.

Clinical Features

- Lassitude, vague ill-health, or symptoms of uraemia or hypertension
- Frequency of micturition, dysuria and aching lumbar pain

Investigations

- Culture of the urine
- Ultrasound of kidneys
- DMSA scan
- IV urogram shows contraction of the renal substance associated with clubbing of the adjacent calyces.
- An MCU will disclose vesicoureteric reflux.
- Cystoscopy and urography may help to identify any abnormality causing obstruction to the flow of urine.

Management

- Appropriate antibiotics should be given for 7 days.
- Suppressive therapy may be required with trimethoprim (100 mg at bed time) or nitrofurantoin (50 mg at bed time) for several months.
- 'Double micturition' to be practiced. The patient is advised to empty the bladder and then again attempt to empty a second time, approximately 10–15 minutes later.
- Surgery is indicated if the vesicoureteric reflux persists.

■ NEPHRITIC SYNDROME

Aetiology

Causes of Glomerulonephritis

Causes of glomerulonephritis are given in **Box 10.3**.

Spectrum of glomerular diseases is listed in **Flowchart 10.2** and **Figure 10.1**.

Clinical Features

- Haematuria
- RBC casts
- Oliguria
- Oedema
- Hypertension
- Proteinuria
- Uraemia

■ POST-STREPTOCOCCAL GLOMERULONEPHRITIS

- Post-streptococcal glomerulonephritis (PSGN) occurs after a pharyngeal or cutaneous infection with group A β-haemolytic *Streptococcus*.
- Following pharyngeal infection, the latent period is about 6–10 days. Cutaneous infections are associated with a longer latent period of about 2 weeks.
- Children are commonly affected.

Box 10.3: Causes of glomerulonephritis.

- **Infectious diseases (postinfectious glomerulonephritis):** Poststreptococcal glomerulonephritis (PSGN), infective endocarditis, syphilis, mumps, measles, hepatitis B, infectious mononucleosis, Epstein–Barr virus infection, malaria, HIV-associated nephropathy
- **Multisystem diseases:** Systemic lupus erythematosus, Henoch–Schönlein purpura, microscopic polyangiitis, Wegner's granulomatosis, Goodpasture syndrome
- **Primary glomerular disease:** Diffuse proliferative glomerulonephritis, IgA nephropathy, mesangiocapillary glomerulonephritis, crescentic glomerulonephritis, membranous glomerulonephritis, focal segmental glomerulosclerosis
- **Miscellaneous:** Malignancy, eclampsia, penicillamine

Glomerulonephritis
Non-proliferative
Proliferative
Minimal change glomerulonephritis
Abnormal podocytes seen on electron microscopy
Treat with supportive cane + prednisolone
Most respond well
Membranous Glomerulopathy/ Nephropathy (MGN) Thickened glomerular basement membrane Usually idiopathic 1/3 go chronic MGN 1/3 go into remission 1/3 progress to renal failure
Focal segmental glomerulosclerosis Segments of glomeruli develop sclerosis Presents with nephrotic syndrome Genetic causes identified
Steroids often ineffective 50% progress to renal failure
IgA nephropathy Most common type of GN in adults Macroscopic haematuria Appears 24–48 hours post URTI/GII infection
IgA deposits seen in the matrix
Membranoproliferative glomerulonephritis Primary (immune mediated) Secondary (SLE, hepatitis)
Usually progresses to end-stage renal failure
Rapidly progressive glomerulonephritis (Crescentic)
Vasculitic disorders
Wegener granulomatosis Vasculitis Lung, kidneys, and other organs c-ANCA +ve
Treat with steroids + cyclophosphamide
Microscopic polyangiitis Small vessel vasculitis p-ANCA +ve
Treat with long-term steroids +/– cytotoxic agents
Goodpasture syndrome Autoimmune anti-GBM antibody Glomerulus and lung affected
Haematuria and hemoptysis
Treat with steroids +/– steroid sparing agents
Post-infectious glomerulonephritis Occurs weeks after URTI Usually Streptococcus pyogenes
Supportive treatment
Resolves over 2–4 weeks

(ANCA: antineutrophil cytoplasmic antibodies; GBM: glomerular basement membrane; GN: glomerulonephritis; SLE: systemic lupus erythematosus; URTI: upper respiratory tract infection)

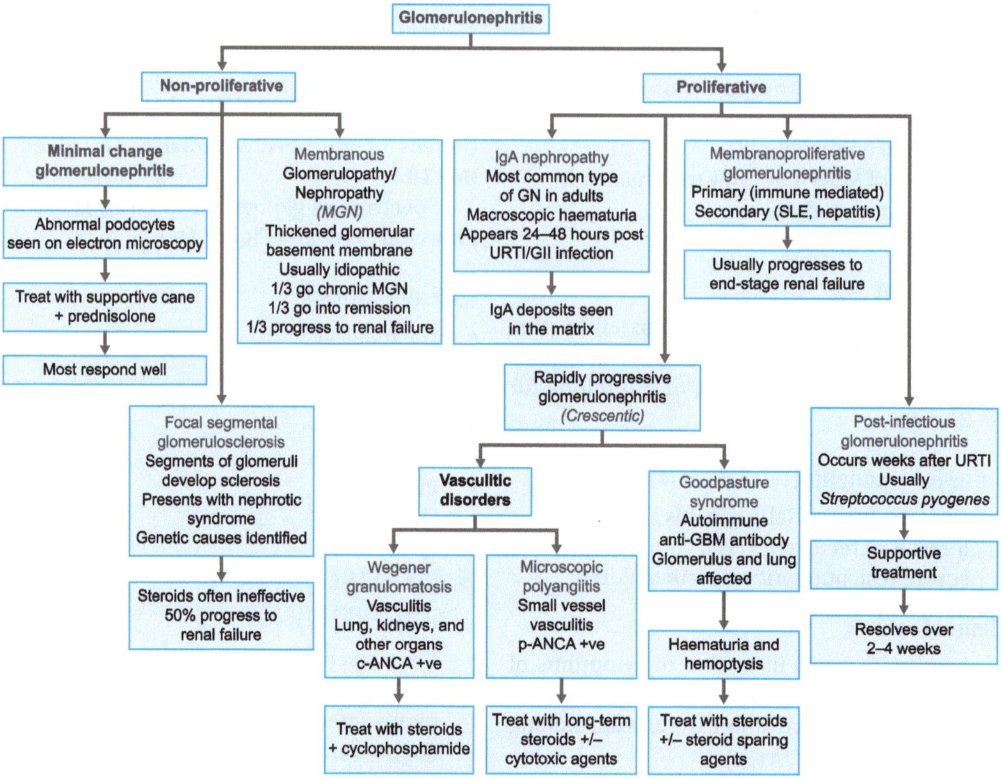

Flowchart 10.2: Spectrum of glomerular diseases.

SLE
IgA nephropathy
Minimal change nephropathy
Anti-GBM disease
FSGS
Diabetic nephropathy
Small vessel vasculitis
MPGN
Membranous nephropathy
Amyloidosis
Post-streptococcal glomerulonephritis
Nephrotic
Mechanism
• Injury to podocytes
• Changed architecture:
– Scarring
– Deposition of matrix or other elements
Nephritic
Mechanism
• Inflammation
• Reactive cell proliferation
• Breaks in GBM
• Crescent formation
Haematuria
Proteinuria

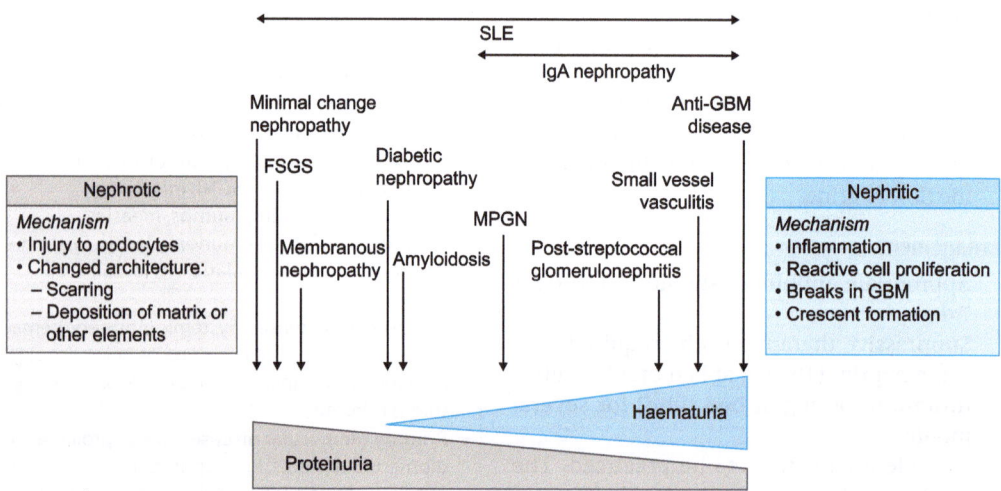

(FSGS: focal segmental glomerulosclerosis; GBM: glomerular basement membrane; IgA: immunoglobulin A; MPGN: membranoproliferative glomerulonephritis; SLE: systemic lupus erythematosus)

Fig. 10.1: Various causes of proliferative and non-proliferative glomerulonephritis.

- The onset is often abrupt with puffiness of face, oliguria, smoky urine or reddish urine, hypertension and oedema and may lead to ascites and/or pleural effusion.

Investigations
- Urine microscopy—red cells (particularly dysmorphic, i.e. distorted and fragmented red cells), red cell casts
- Cultures—throat swab and swab inflamed skin may grow group A β-haemolytic *Streptococci*.
- Antistreptolysin-O (ASO) titre—elevated
- C3 level (complement)—may be reduced
- Urinary protein—increased
- Urea and creatinine—may be elevated
- Renal biopsy—features of glomerulonephritis

Treatment
- Supportive
- The measures include rest, salt restriction, diuretics and antihypertensives.
- Antibodies are given for presumed throat infection as this may result in a milder form of nephritis. Further, treatment of a carrier state may prevent spread to other household members.
- Dialysis is required in severe oliguria, fluid overload and hyperkalaemia.
- Steroids and cytotoxic drugs are of no value.
- Complications include pulmonary oedema, hypertensive encephalopathy and renal failure.

IMMUNOGLOBULIN A NEPHROPATHY BERGER'S DISEASE
- IgA deposition in the glomerular mesangium
- Presents with painless haematuria, generally within 1–2 days of upper respiratory infection
- May be detected on routine urine examination (microscopic haematuria)
- Occasionally presents as acute renal failure (ARF) or nephritic syndrome
- Diagnosis by renal biopsy
- Complete remission uncommon
- No specific therapy is available.
- Therapeutic options include ACE inhibitors if significant proteinuria is present; also for control of hypertension.

RAPIDLY PROGRESSIVE GLOMERULONEPHRITIS/CRESCENTIC GLOMERULONEPHRITIS
- Extensive crescents (usually > 50%) as the principal histologic finding and by a rapid loss of renal function (usually a 50% decline in the GFR within 3 months)
- Rapidly progressive glomerulonephritis (RPGN) is classified pathologically into these categories:
  - Anti-glomerular basement membrane (GBM) antibody disease—linear deposits of antibodies on immunofluorescence
  - Immune-complex disease—granular deposits of immune complexes on immunofluorescence
  - Pauci-immune disease [generally anti-neutrophil cytoplasmic antibody (ANCA) positive]—little or no deposit on immunofluorescence

Causes of Rapidly Progressive Glomerulonephritis
Causes of RPGN are given in **Table 10.3**.

Clinical Features
Presents with moderate proteinuria, haematuria, oliguria and uraemia

TABLE 10.3: Causes of rapidly progressive glomerulonephritis.

Anti-GBM antibody	Pauci-immune	Immune complex
• Goodpasture syndrome	• Granulomatosis with Polyangiitis (Wegener's granulamatosis) • Microscopic polyangiitis • Eosinophilic Granulomatosis with Polyangiitis (Churg–Strauss syndrome)	• Post-streptococcal • IgA nephropathy • Membranoproliferative glomerulonephritis • Henoch–Schönlein purpura • Lupus nephritis • Mixed cryoglobulinaemia

(GBM: glomerular basement membrane; IgA: immunoglobulin A)

Investigations

- Leucocytosis and anaemia
- Blood urea and serum creatinine levels usually elevated
- Urinalysis shows modest proteinuria (1–4 g/day), microscopic haematuria and RBC and white blood cell (WBC) casts
- Complement levels (C3 and C4) may be decreased.
- Anti-GBM antibodies in Goodpasture syndrome
- ANCA in patients with pauci-immune RPGN
- Serum cryoglobulin levels may be elevated in cryoglobulinaemias.
- Abdominal ultrasound shows normal-sized kidneys.
- Chest X-ray in patients with Goodpasture syndrome and vasculitides may show diffuse opacities, if pulmonary haemorrhage occurs.
- Kidney biopsy

Treatment

- Supportive therapy
  - Control of infection
  - Control of volume status
  - Dialysis, if required
- Specific therapy
  - Immunosuppressive therapy (e.g. glucocorticoids, azathioprine, mycophenolate cyclophosphamide,) plasma exchange
  - Infliximab and rituximab

Algorithm of approach to the patient presenting with acute glomerulonephritis/nephritic syndrome is shown in **Flowchart 10.3**.

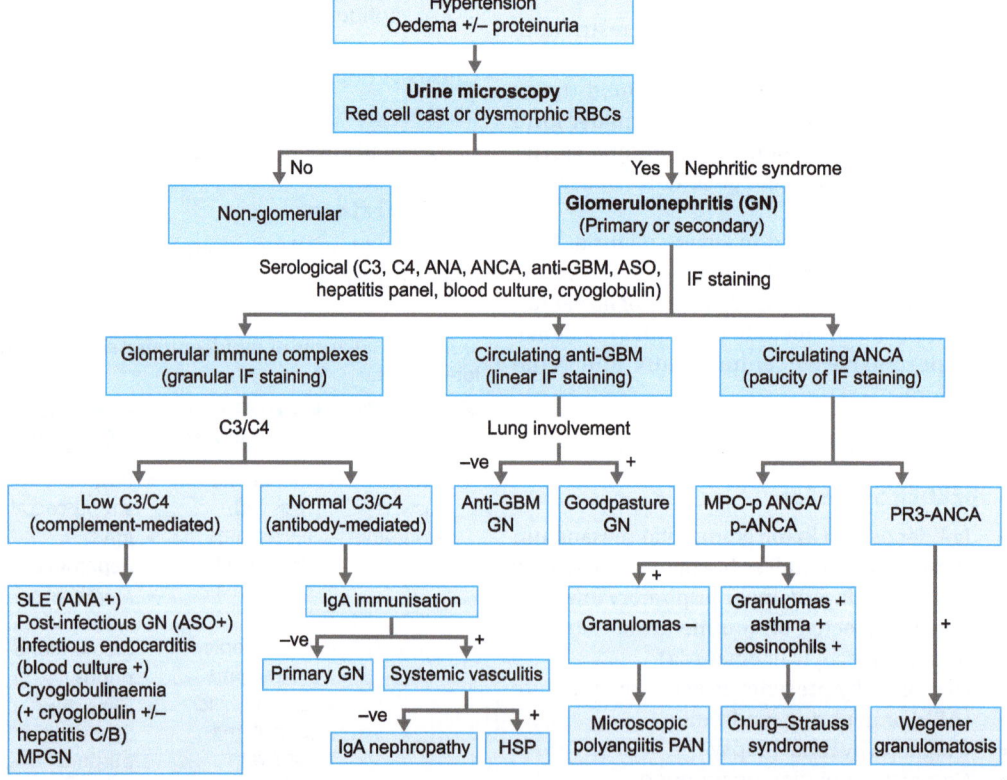

[ANA: antinuclear antibody; ANCA: antineutrophil cytoplasmic antibody; ASO: antistreptolysin O; GBM: glomerular basement membrane; HSP: Henoch–Schonlein purpura; MPGN: membranoproliferative glomerulonephritis; MPO-ANCA: antimyeloperoxidase (perviously called p-ANCA); PR3-ANCA: anti-proteinase-3; PAN, polyarteritis nodosa; IF: immunofluorescence; SLE: systemic lupus erythematosus]

Flowchart 10.3: Algorithm of approach to the patient presenting with acute glomerulonephritis/nephritic syndrome.

NEPHROTIC SYNDROME

Characterised by the following abnormalities:
- Proteinuria (> 3.5 g in 24 h)
- Hypoalbuminaemia
- Generalised oedema
- Hyperlipidaemia

Pathogenesis
- Excessive leakage of plasma proteins into the urine → hypoalbuminaemia → oedema
- Hypovolaemia → renin–angiotensin–aldosterone system activation → oedema
- Stimulate hepatic lipoprotein synthesis → hyperlipidaemia → increases risk of cardiovascular disease

Consequences of Protein Loss
- Oedema
- Increased susceptibility to infections
- Pleural effusion and ascites
- Loss of thyroxine-binding globulin → hypothyroidism
- Deficiency of antithrombin III → hypercoagulable state, deep vein thrombosis (DVT), pulmonary embolism, myocardial infarction and renal vein thrombosis and stroke
- Loss of globulins → spontaneous bacterial peritonitis
- Loss of cholecalciferol-binding protein → vitamin D deficiency
- Loss of transferrin → microcytic hypochromic anaemia
- Loss of binding proteins → deficiency of zinc, copper
- Loss of drug-binding proteins → altered drug pharmacokinetics

Causes
Causes of nephrotic syndrome are given in **Table 10.4**.

Minimal Change Disease
- Most common cause of nephrotic syndrome in children (80%) and 20% of all cases in adults
- Normal-appearing glomeruli on light microscopy and effacement of foot processes of epithelial cells on electron microscopy

TABLE 10.4: Causes of nephrotic syndrome.

Primary (idiopathic)	Secondary
Idiopathic glomerular diseases such as minimal change disease, membranous glomerulonephritis, mesangial proliferative glomerulonephritis, focal and segmental glomerulosclerosis and mesangiocapillary glomerulonephritis	• Infections: Bacterial endocarditis, malaria, syphilis, hepatitis B, leprosy, HIV infection • Connective tissue disease: SLE, rheumatoid arthritis • Neoplasms: Hodgkin's lymphoma, carcinomas, leukaemias • Drugs and toxins: Penicillamine, captopril, gold, mercury, contaminated heroin • Metabolic: Diabetes mellitus, amyloidosis

(HIV: human immunodeficiency virus; SLE: systemic lupus erythematosus)

Membranous Glomerulonephritis
- Most common primary renal cause of nephrotic syndrome in adults

Investigations
- 24-hour urinary protein estimation
- Serum albumin
- Serum cholesterol concentrations
- Urine routine
- Renal biopsy—histological diagnosis
- For suspected secondary causes, appropriate investigations are required.

Management
Measures to Reduce Proteinuria
- ACE inhibitors reduce proteinuria and slow the rate of progression of renal failure by lowering the intraglomerular pressure.
- Steroids and immunosuppressive drugs and treatment of the underlying cause.

Treatment of Complications
- Oedema → salt restriction, rest and use of diuretics. IV salt-poor albumin may be used.
- Dietary proteins should be about 0.8–1.0 g/kg as excessive proteins.
- Vitamin D supplementation

- Hyperlipidaemia → dietary restrictions and lipid-lowering drugs
- Anticoagulants → deep venous thrombosis or arterial thrombosis

Measures to Treat the Underlying Disease
- **Minimal change disease**
  - Corticosteroids in the form of daily prednisolone
  - Frequent relapses or develop unacceptable corticosteroid side effects → cyclophosphamide (2 mg/kg/day) for 6 weeks OR mycophenolate mofetil, cyclosporine and tacrolimus, and rituximab
- **Focal and segmental glomerulosclerosis**
  - Steroids may be beneficial in only 20–30% cases.
  - Cyclophosphamide, tacrolimus and cyclosporine are of little use in steroid-resistant cases.
- **Membranous glomerulonephritis**
  - Spontaneous remission may occur in 40% cases.
  - Another 3–40% cases remit and relapse repeatedly.
  - Rest 10–20% patients develop progressive renal failure. Cyclophosphamide, cyclosporine and chlorambucil in combination with steroids may retard the progression in this subset of patients.

■ CHRONIC KIDNEY DISEASES
- GFR of < 60 mL/min/1.73 m² for 3 months or more, with or without kidney damage.
  OR
- Kidney damage for 3 or more months with or without decreased GFR, as evidenced by any of the following:
  - Microalbuminuria
  - Macroalbuminuria
  - Abnormal renal biopsy
  - Scarring or polycystic kidneys on renal ultrasound

Stages
Stages of chronic kidney disease are given in **Table 10.5**.

A revised classification of chronic kidney disease based upon GFR and albuminuria by Kidney disease: Improving Global Outcomes (KDIGO, 2013) is shown in **Figure 10.2**.

TABLE 10.5: Stages of chronic kidney disease.

Stage	Description	GFR (mL/min/1.73 m²)
1	Slight kidney damage with normal or increased filtration	> 90
2	Mild decrease in kidney function	60–89
3	Moderate decrease in kidney function	30–59
4	Severe decrease in kidney function	15–29
5	Requiring dialysis or transplantation/ESRD	< 15

(ESRD: end-stage renal disease; GFR: glomerular filtration rate)

Causes
Causes of chronic kidney disease are given in **Box 10.4**.

Clinical Features
Various clinical features of chronic kidney disease are shown in **Figure 10.3**.
- Uraemia: All signs and symptoms seen in various systems (**Table 10.6**)

Investigations
- Important urinary abnormalities include a fixed specific gravity around 1.010 (isosthenuria) and broad casts.
- Elevated levels of blood urea and creatinine are observed.
- Hypocalcaemia, hyperphosphataemia, hyperuricaemia and hyperkalaemia. Bicarbonate levels are reduced.
- Renal ultrasound typically shows shrunken kidneys. In diabetic glomerulosclerosis, amyloidosis, polycystic kidney diseases, bilateral hydronephrosis and myeloma kidney, the kidneys may be of normal size.

Management
Some of the reversible factors in chronic renal failure (CRF) which require treatment are given in **Box 10.5**.

				Persistent albuminuria categories, description and range		
				Normal to mildly increased	Moderately increased	Severely increased
				<30 mg/g (<3 mg/mmol)	30–300 mg/g (3–30 mg/mmol)	>300 mg/g (>30 mg/mmol)
GFR categories (mL/min/1.73 m²) stage, description and range	1	Normal or high	≥90			2
	2	Mildly decreased	60–89	1 if CKD	1	2
	3a	Mildly to moderately decreased	45–59	1	2	3
	3b	Moderately to severely decreased	30–44	2	3	3
	4	Severely decreased	15–29	3	3	4⁺
	5	Kidney failure	<15	4⁺	4⁺	4⁺

(CKD: chronic kidney disease; GFR: glomerular filtration rate)

Fig. 10.2: Revised chronic kidney disease classification based upon glomerular filtration rate and albuminuria KDIGO 2013.

Box 10.4: Causes of chronic kidney disease (CKD).
- Primary or secondary glomerulonephritis
- Diabetic nephropathy
- Hypertensive nephrosclerosis
- Polycystic kidney disease
- Chronic pyelonephritis
- Analgesic neuropathy
- Vesicoureteric reflux
- Renal tuberculosis
- Nephrocalcinosis
- Obstruction uropathy
- Family history of CKD
- Infections such as Hepatitis C and HIV
- Autoimmune diseases

(CKD: chronic kidney disease; HIV: human immunodeficiency virus)

Treatment

Treatment of chronic kidney disease is given in **Box 10.6**.
- Kidney transplantation offers the possibility of restoring normal kidney functions.

Indications for Urgent Dialysis
- A—Acidosis
- E—Electrolyte disturbance, usually hyperkalaemia
- I—Intoxications (lithium, ethylene glycol, etc.)
- O—Overload (volume overload)
- U—Uraemia (pericarditis, encephalopathy)

RENAL REPLACEMENT THERAPIES

Types of Renal replacement therapies are given in **Table 10.7**.

Haemodialysis

- Accumulated uraemic toxins diffuse across a semipermeable membrane from the blood, where they are in high concentrations, to the dialysis fluid on the other side of the membrane.
- For long term, an arteriovenous fistula is created, usually in the forearm.
- Indications for haemodialysis listed in **Box 10.7**.

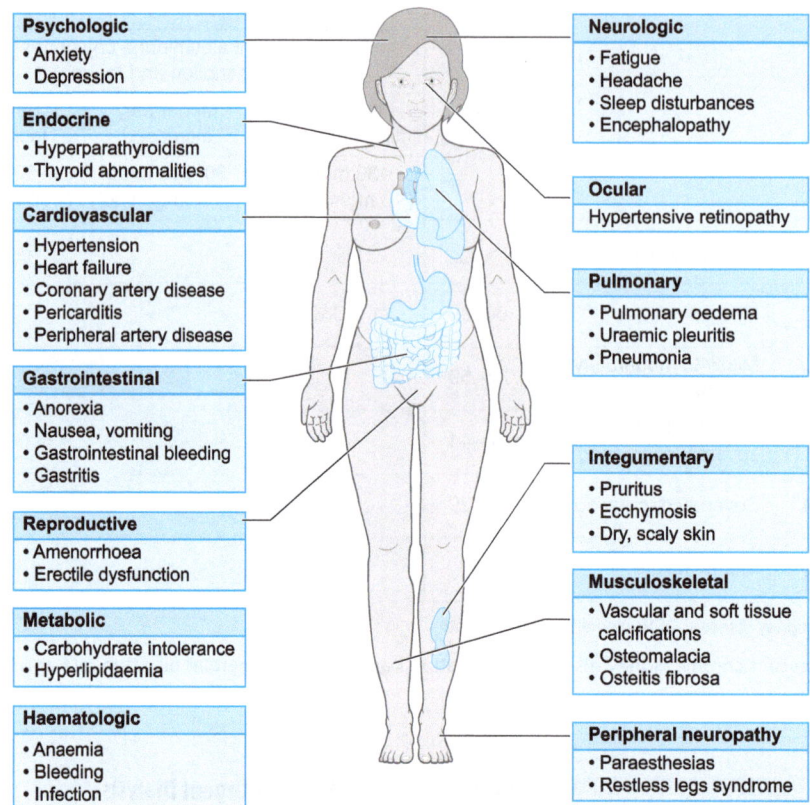

Fig. 10.3: Various clinical manifestations of chronic kidney disease (CKD).

Complications
- Hypotension during dialysis
- Muscle cramps, anaphylaxis, air embolism, infections, haemolysis and pulmonary oedema
- Dialysis disequilibrium
- Dialysis dementia

Peritoneal Dialysis
- In peritoneal dialysis, the peritoneum of the patient acts as a semipermeable membrane across which diffusion of water and solutes takes place.
- The main complication is the occurrence of peritonitis and infections around the catheter site. **Continuous ambulatory peritoneal dialysis (CAPD)**
- Here, the dwelling time of fluid is long so that only three to five cycles are done in a day. The patient infuses 1.5–3 L of dialysate in the peritoneal cavity. The solution is allowed to remain for more than 4 hours during the day and 8–12 hours at night. This technique is useful for maintenance of dialysis in patients with CRF.

Continuous cycling peritoneal dialysis (CCPD)
- Here, the dwelling period is longer than CAPD during the daytime but at night-time an automated cycler performs short exchanges.

■ RENAL TRANSPLANTATION

Contraindications
- Reversible renal involvement
- Un-reconstructable coronary artery disease
- Refractory congestive heart failure
- Disseminated or untreated cancer
- Severe mental retardation
- Active glomerulonephritis
- Severe psychiatric disease
- Persistent substance abuse

TABLE 10.6: Signs and symptoms of uraemia seen in various systems.

Urinary system	Polyuria • Results from inability of kidneys to concentrate urine • Occurs most often at night	As CKD worsens, oliguria, and anuria set
Metabolic disturbances	BUN ↑ and serum creatinine levels ↑	Nausea, vomiting, lethargy, fatigue, delirium, encephalopathy
Electrolyte/acid–base imbalances	• Hyponatraemia • Hyperkalaemia	• Metabolic acidosis • Hypocalcaemia, hyperphosphataemia
Haematologic system	Anaemia: Normocytic normochromic • Decreased erythropoietin • Reduced dietary intake due to anorexia • Impaired intestinal iron absorption • Anaemia of chronic disease • Uraemic toxin depression on marrow • Reduced red cell survival • Poor platelet function and capillary fragility	Bleeding tendencies • Defect in platelet function • Infection • Changes in leucocyte function • Altered immune response and function • Diminished inflammatory response
Cardiovascular system	• Hypertension • Heart failure • Left ventricular hypertrophy	• Dysrhythmias • Uraemic pericarditis • Peripheral oedema
Respiratory system	• Kussmaul's respiration • Dyspnoea • Pulmonary oedema • Uraemic pleuritis	• Pleural effusion • Respiratory infections • Depressed cough reflex • Uraemic lung
Gastrointestinal system	• Mucosal ulcerations • Stomatitis • Uraemic fetor	• Gastrointestinal bleeding • Anorexia • Nausea, Vomiting
Neurologic system	• Seizures and Coma • Dialysis dementia and dialysis disequilibrium • Peripheral neuropathy	• Restless leg syndrome • Muscle twitching • Irritability • Myopathy
Reproductive system	• Infertility • Decreased libido	• Azoospermia • Amenorrhoea
Musculoskeletal system	Renal osteodystrophy	

Integumentary system	• Yellow-grey discolouration of the skin
	  ○ Pruritus
	  ○ Uraemic frost
	  ○ Dry, pale skin
		• Dry, brittle hair
		• Thin nails
		• Petechiae
		• Ecchymoses

(BUN: blood urea nitrogen; CKD: chronic kidney disease)

■ ACUTE KIDNEY INJURY

Definition

Introduction—Defined by a rapid decline in GFR, resulting in disturbance of renal physiological functions

RIFLE criteria are used to classify acute kidney injury (AKI) (**Table 10.8**).
- As per the Acute Kidney Injury Network (AKIN) classification, AKI is classified into three stages:

Box 10.5: Reversible factors in chronic renal failure that require treatment.

- Hypertension
- Urinary tract infection (UTI)
- Urinary tract obstruction
- Haemorrhage
- Septic shock
- Cardiogenic shock
- Infections
- Nephrotoxic drugs

Box 10.6: Treatment of chronic kidney disease.

Nutritional therapy
- Protein restriction
  - 0.6–0.8 g/kg body weight/day
- Water restriction
  - Intake depends on daily urine output
- Sodium restriction
  - Varies from 2 to 4 g
- Potassium restriction
  - 2–4 g
- Phosphate restriction
  - 1,000 mg/day

Control of hypertension: The blood pressure should be reduced to < 130/80 mmHg.
Hypocalcaemia requires treatment with calcitriol or alphacalcidol (1-α-hydroxyvitamin D3) or paricalcitol (19-nor-1,25-dihydroxyvitamin D3) and calcium supplementation.

Phosphate binders:
- Aluminium hydroxide, calcium carbonate and calcium acetate
- Sevelamer carbonate
- Lanthanum carbonate

Treating hyperparathyroidism:
- Use of calcimimetics: Cinacalcet has been approved for use in patients on dialysis.

Metabolic acidosis should be corrected with sodium bicarbonate.
Hyperkalaemia usually responds to dietary restrictions, potassium-exchange resins.
Anaemia
- Erythropoietin: Administered intravenously or subcutaneously
- Addition of iron, folate and vitamin B12

- Stage 1 is the same as Risk category of RIFLE with addition of increase in serum creatinine by 0.3 mg/dL.
- Stages 2 and 3 are same as Injury and Failure categories of RIFLE.

TABLE 10.7: Renal replacement therapies.

Haemodynamically stable	Haemodynamically unstable
• Intermittent haemodialysis	• CRRT: Continuous renal replacement therapy • PD: Peritoneal dialysis • SLED: Slow low-efficiency dialysis

Box 10.7: Indication of dialysis or hemofiltration in acute renal failure (ARF).

- Fluid overload refractory to diuretics and refractory pulmonary oedema*
- Severe metabolic acidosis (pH < 7.1)*
- Resistant hyperkalaemia*
- Complications of uraemia (e.g. pericarditis, encephalopathy, neuropathy)*
- Increased plasma urea (> 180 mg/dL) and creatinine (> 6.8 mg/dL)
- ESRD (end-stage renal disease)
- Severe biochemical derangement in the absence of symptoms (especially in oliguric and hypercatabolic patients)
- Removal of drugs causing the ARF (e.g. gentamicin, lithium, severe aspirin overdose)
- Severe hyperphosphataemia (defined as > 12 mg/dL)
- Tumour lysis syndrome
- Anuria for > 12 hours

* Absolute indications

TABLE 10.8: RIFLE criteria.

Criteria	Definition
• Risk	• Increased creatinine × 1.5 times OR Urine output < 0.5 mL/kg/h × 6 hours
• Injury	• Increased creatinine × 2 times OR Urine output < 0.5 mL/kg/h × 12 hours
• Failure	• Increased creatinine × 3 times or creatinine = 4 mg/dL (acute rise of 0.5 mg/dL) OR Urine output < 0.3 mL/kg/h × 24 hours OR Anuria × 12 hours
• Loss	
• End-stage kidney disease	• Persistent AKI = Complete loss of renal function > 4 weeks End-stage kidney disease (> 3 months)

(AKI: acute kidney injury)

Nephrology

The causes of ARF can therefore be categorised as **Prerenal, Renal** or **Postrenal** (Flowchart 10.4; Table 10.9).

Prerenal—Prerenal azotaemia results from either:

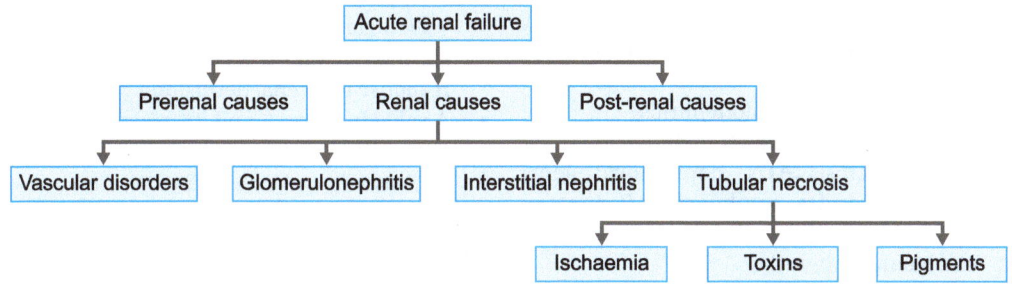

Flowchart 10.4: Causes of acute renal failure.

TABLE 10.9: Clinical features of acute kidney injury.

Type of acute kidney injury	History findings	Physical examination findings
Prerenal	• Volume loss (e.g. history of vomiting, diarrhoea, diuretic overuse, haemorrhage, burns) • Reduced fluid intake • Cardiac disease • Liver disease	• Orthostatic hypotension and tachycardia • Cardiac disease • Poor skin turgor • Dilated neck veins, S3 heart sound, pulmonary rales, peripheral oedema • Ascites, caput medusae, spider angiomas
Intrinsic renal		
Acute tubular necrosis	History of receiving nephrotoxic medications (including over-the-counter, illicit and herbal), hypotension, trauma or myalgias suggesting rhabdomyolysis, recent exposure to radiographic contrast agents	Muscle tenderness, compartment syndrome, assessment of volume status
Glomerular	Lupus, systemic sclerosis, rash, arthritis, uveitis, weight loss, fatigue, hepatitis C virus infection, human immunodeficiency virus infection, haematuria, foamy urine, cough, sinusitis, haemoptysis	Periorbital, sacral and lower-extremity oedema, rash, oral/nasal ulcers, hypertension
Interstitial	Medication use (e.g. antibiotics, proton pump inhibitors), rash, arthralgias, fever, infectious illness	Fever drug-related rash (skin) Eosinophilia
Vascular	Nephrotic syndrome, trauma, flank pain, anticoagulation (atheroembolic disease), vessel catheterisation or vascular surgery	Skin changes, livedo reticularis, fundoscopic examination (showing malignant hypertension), abdominal bruits
Postrenal	Urinary urgency or hesitancy, gross haematuria, polyuria, stones, medications, cancer	Bladder distention, pelvic mass, prostate enlargement

- Volume depletion: Surgery, trauma, gastrointestinal bleeding, vomiting, diarrhoea, diuretics or burns

Intrinsic Renal Disorders
- **Vascular**: Thrombosis (arterial and venous), haemolytic–uraemic syndrome (HUS), malignant hypertension
- **Glomerular**: Glomerulonephritis
- **Tubular and interstitial disease**: Acute tubular necrosis (ATN), nephrotoxic agents (aminoglycosides, amphotericin B, contrast agents, myoglobinuria due to rhabdomyolysis and haemoglobinuria)

Postrenal: Bilateral urinary tract obstruction (posterior urethral valves)

Evaluation and Diagnosis

Serum Creatinine Concentration

Serum blood urea nitrogen (BUN)/creatinine (Cr) ratio: It is normal at 10–15:1 in ATN and may be > 20:1 in prerenal.

Urinalysis: The urinalysis is the most important non-invasive test in the diagnostic evaluation, since characteristic findings on microscopic examination of the urine sediment strongly suggest certain diagnoses (**Flowchart 10.5**).

Fractional excretion of Sodium (FENa)

$$\text{FENa (\%)} = \frac{UNa \times PCr}{PNa \times UCr} \times 100$$

UCr and PCr = urine and serum Cr, respectively; UNa and PNa = urine and serum Na^+, respectively.

The FENa is a screening test that differentiates between prerenal ARF and ATN in children.
- < 1% suggests prerenal disease, where reabsorption of almost all filtered Na^+ represents response to ↓ renal perfusion.
- A value between 1 and 2% may be seen with either disorder.
- > 2% usually indicates ATN.

Urine osmolality: ATN urine osmolality usually being below 350 mOsmol/kg, a urine osmolality > 500 mOsmol/kg is highly suggestive of prerenal disease.

Complete blood count: Severe microangiopathic haemolytic anaemia associated with thrombocytopaenia—HUS.

Urine sodium excretion: Measurement of urine Na^+ concentration is helpful in distinguishing ATN from prerenal ARF due to effective volume depletion. The urine Na^+ concentration is usually > 30–40 mEq/L in ATN and < 10 mEq/L in prerenal ARF (**Flowchart 10.6**).

Other Abnormalities
- Hyperkalaemia
- Hyperphosphataemia
- Hypocalcaemia
- Antinuclear antibody (ANA), ANCA, compliment levels, ASO

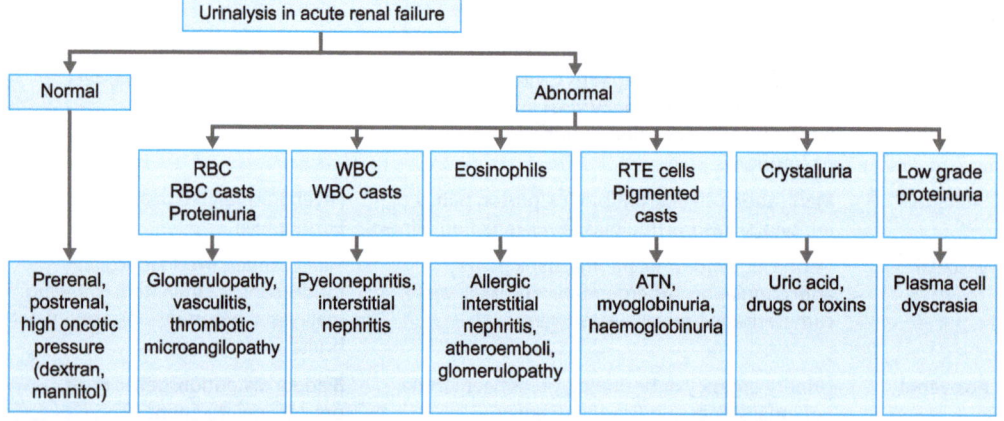

(ATN: acute tubular necrosis; RBC: red blood cell; WBC: white blood cell)

Flowchart 10.5: Urinalysis in acute renal failure.

- Eosinophilia and/or urine eosinophiluria may be present in some cases of interstitial nephritis.

Renal imaging: Diagnosing urinary tract obstruction or occlusion of the major renal vessels.

Renal biopsy: Establish the correct diagnosis.

ARF Management (Flowchart 10.7)
- Maintenance of electrolyte and fluid balance
- Adequate nutritional support
- Avoidance of life-threatening complications
- Treatment of the underlying cause

Hyperkalaemia

- Around 10% Ca gluconate: 0.5–1.0 mL/kg IV over 5–15 minutes
- IV glucose and insulin
- IV sodium bicarbonate
- β-agonists, such as salbutamol via neb
- Kayexalate
- Diuretics can be given to patients with continued urine output.
- Renal replacement

Acidosis
Although the administration of oral or parenteral sodium bicarbonate may provide temporary benefit in children with concurrent hyperkalaemia or maximal respiratory compensation

Intravascular volume: Appropriate immediate fluid management is crucial with ARF.

Hyperphosphataemia and Hypocalcaemia

Oral phosphate binders and dietary restriction of phosphorus are commonly used to decrease intestinal absorption of phosphorus.

Hypertension: Diuretics, calcium channel blocker (CCB)

Renal replacement therapy: Already discussed under CKD section.

RENAL TUBULAR ACIDOSIS

Types of renal tubular acidosis (RTA) are given in **Table 10.10**.

An algorithm approach to RTA is shown in **Flowchart 10.8**.

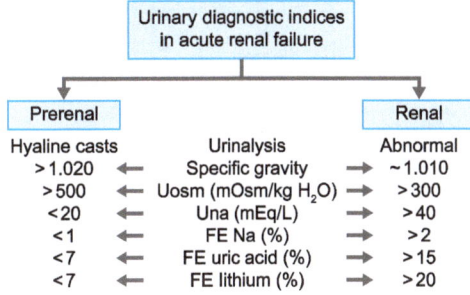

Flowchart 10.6: Urinary diagnostic indices in acute renal failure.

TABLE 10.10: Types of renal tubular acidosis.

Type of RTA	Primary defect	Plasma HCO3 (mEq/L)	Urine pH	Plasma potassium	Causes
RTA type 1	Impaired distal acidification	< 10	> 5.3	Hypokalaemia	• Hereditary • Sjögren's syndrome • Cirrhosis of liver • Nephrocalcinosis
RTA type 2	Reduced proximal HCO3 reabsorption	12–20	< 5.3	Hypokalaemia	• Cystinosis • Galactosaemia • Glycogen storage disease (type I)
RTA type 4	• Decreased aldosterone secretion • Aldosterone resistance	> 17	Variable	Hyperkalaemia	• Primary adrenal insufficiency • Congenital adrenal hyperplasia • Potassium-sparing diuretics

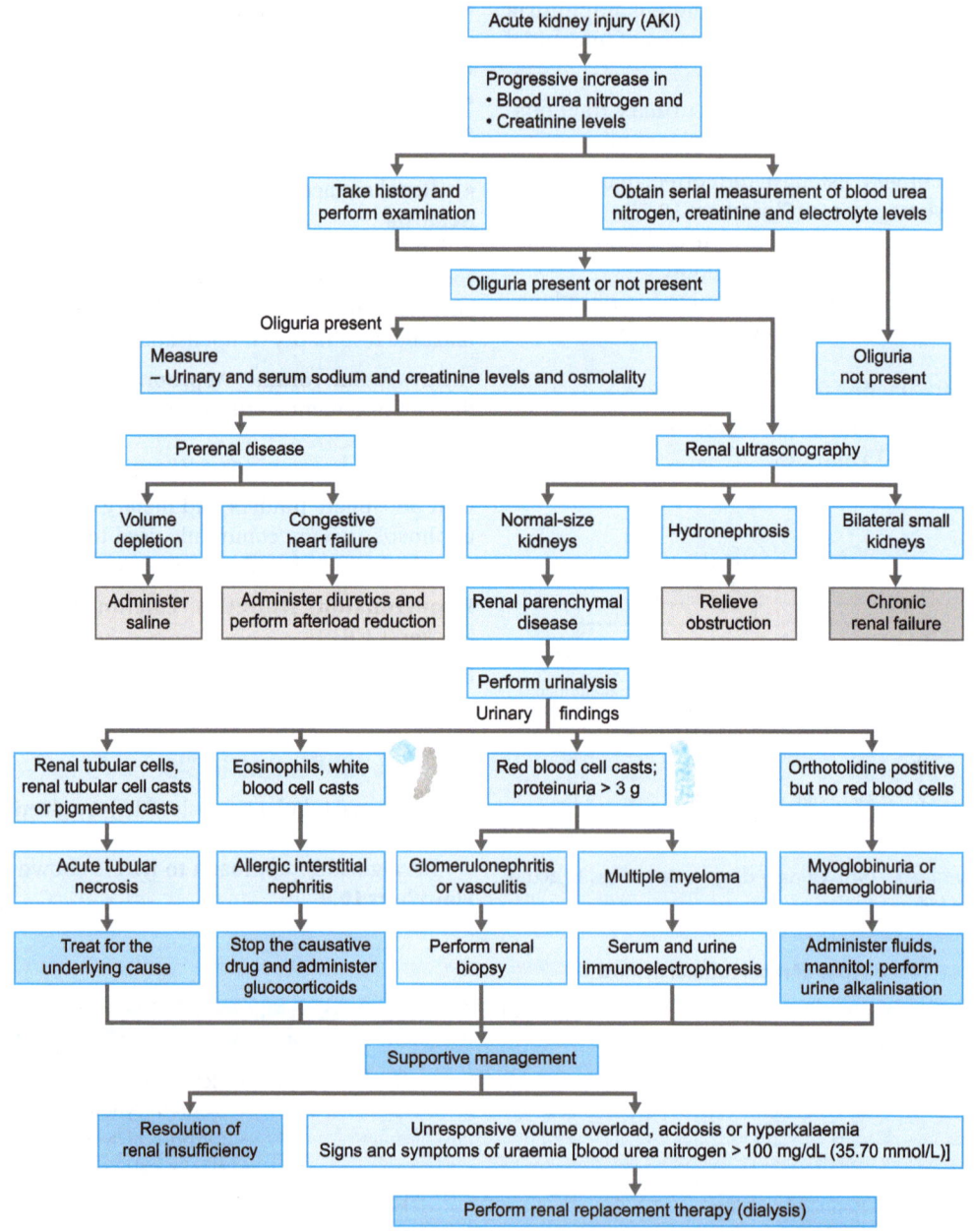

Flowchart 10.7: Approach to acute kidney injury.

POLYCYSTIC KIDNEY DISEASES

- There are two types:
    - Infantile polycystic kidney disease is an autosomal recessive disorder, which is usually fatal.
    - The more common adult polycystic kidney disease is an autosomal dominant polycystic kidney disease (ADPKD). The cortex and medulla of both kidneys are usually filled with thin-walled, spherical

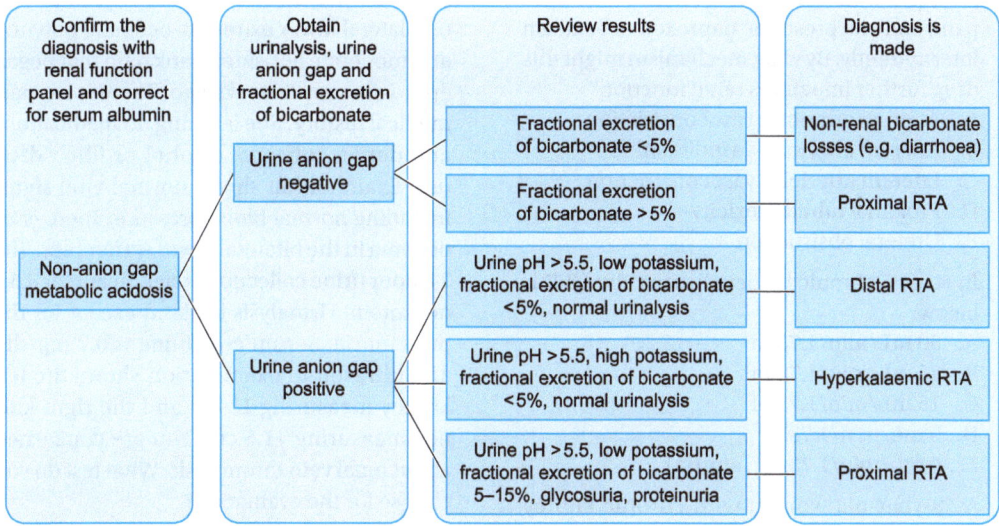

Flowchart 10.8: Algorithm approach to renal tubular acidosis (RTA).

- cysts that enlarge and compress intervening renal tissue → resulting in CKD.
- Associations: Hepatic cysts (75%), 15–30% berry aneurysms, mitral valve prolapse
- Clinical features: Hypertension, acute loin pain and haematuria resulting from haemorrhage into a cyst, symptoms of uraemia and UTI (pyelonephritis and renal cyst infection)
- Physical examination reveals large palpable irregular kidneys.
- Abdominal ultrasound is the investigation of choice. IVU may demonstrate the characteristic 'drooping water lily sign'. MRI is more sensitive than ultrasound to detect small cysts.
- Supportive treatment includes control of hypertension, control of pain, treatment of infection and renal replacement by dialysis or transplantation, if required.
- Tolvaptan has been tried to decrease the size of the cysts.

BEST OF FIVES

1. Which of the following is a potential aetiology for ischaemic ARF?
   A. Apoptosis and necrosis of tubular cells
   B. Decreased glomerular vasodilation in response to nitric oxide
   C. Increased glomerular vasoconstriction in response to elevated endothelin levels
   D. Increased leucocyte adhesion within the glomerulus
   E. All of the above

2. In evaluation for AKI in a patient who has recently undergone cardiopulmonary bypass during mitral valve replacement, which of the following findings on urine microscopy is most suggestive of cholesterol emboli as the source of renal failure?
   A. Calcium oxalate crystals
   B. Eosinophiluria
   C. Granular casts
   D. Normal sediment
   E. WBC casts

3. Which of the following is an extrarenal manifestation of autosomal dominant polycystic kidney disease?
   A. Aortic regurgitation
   B. Aortic root dilation
   C. Colonic diverticulae
   D. Intracranial aneurysm
   E. All of the above

4. It is hospital day 6 for a 50-year-old patient with prerenal azotaemia secondary to dehydration. His creatinine was initially 3.6 mg/dL on admission, but it has improved today to

2.1 mg/dL. He complains of mild lower back pain, and you prescribe naproxen to be taken intermittently. By what mechanism might this drug further impair his renal function?
A. Afferent arteriolar vasoconstriction
B. Afferent arteriolar vasodilatation
C. Efferent arteriolar vasoconstriction
D. Proximal tubular toxicity
E. Ureteral obstruction

5. In stage 5 chronic kidney disease, the GFR is below:
A. 50 mL/min/1.73 m²
B. 25 mL/min/1.73 m²
C. 15 mL/min/1.73 m²
D. 5 mL/min/1.73 m²
E. 0 mL/min/1.73 m² (anuria)

6. A 59-year-old woman with chronic kidney disease is undergoing haemodialysis and is found to be hypotensive during her treatment. Which of the following is a potential mechanism for hypotension during haemodialysis?
A. Antihypertensive agents
B. Excessive ultrafiltration
C. Impaired autonomic responses
D. Osmolar shifts
E. All of the above

7. A 21-year-old male college student is evaluated for profound fatigue that has been present for several years but has recently become debilitating. He also reports several foot spasms and cramps, and occasional sustained muscle contractions that are uncontrollable. He is otherwise healthy, takes no medications and denies tobacco or alcohol use. On examination, he is well developed with normal vital signs including blood pressure. The remainder of the examination is normal. Laboratory evaluation shows a sodium of 138 mEq/L, potassium of 2.8 mEq/L, chloride of 90 mEq/L and bicarbonate of 30 mmol/L. Magnesium level is normal. Urine screen for diuretics is negative, and urine chloride is elevated. Which of the following is the most likely diagnosis?
A. Bulimia nervosa
B. Diuretic abuse
C. Gitelman syndrome
D. Liddle's syndrome
E. Type 1 pseudohypoaldosteronism

8. A 38-year-old female presents with complaints of bilateral lower extremity oedema, polyuria and moderate left-sided flank pain that began approximately 2 weeks ago. There is no past medical history. She is taking no medications and denies tobacco, alcohol or illicit drug use. Examination shows normal vital signs, including normal blood pressure. There is 2+ oedema in the bilateral lower extremities. The 24-hour urine collection is significant for 3.5 g of protein. Urinalysis is bland except for the proteinuria. Serum creatinine is 0.7 mg/dL, and ultrasound examination shows the left kidney measuring 13 cm and the right kidney measuring 11.5 cm. You are concerned about renal vein thrombosis. What test do you choose for the evaluation?
A. Computed tomography of the renal veins
B. Contrast venography
C. Magnetic resonance venography
D. 99Tc-labelled pentetic acid (DPTA) imaging
E. Ultrasound with Doppler evaluation of the renal veins

9. A 48-year-old man with diabetes mellitus and hyperlipidaemia presents to the emergency department for evaluation of right flank pain and groin pain that has been severe and present for approximately 3 hours. He is diagnosed with a kidney stone. Which of the following is most likely to be found as the constituent of his stone?
A. Calcium
B. Cysteine
C. Oxalic acid
D. Struvite
E. Uric acid

10. The pain associated with acute urinary tract obstruction is a result of which of the following?
A. Compensatory natriuresis
B. Decreased medullary blood flow
C. Increased renal blood flow
D. Vasodilatory prostaglandins
E. Uraemia

11. During the first 2 weeks after solid organ transplantation, which family of infection is most common?

A. Cytomegalovirus and Epstein–Barr virus reactivation
B. Humoral immunodeficiency-associated infections (e.g. meningococcaemia, invasive *Streptococcus pneumoniae* infection)
C. Neutropaenia-associated infection (e.g. aspergillosis, candidaemia)
D. T-cell deficiency–associated infections (e.g. *Pneumocystis jiroveci*, nocardiosis, cryptococcosis)
E. Typical hospital-acquired infections (e.g. central line infection, hospital-acquired pneumonia, UTI)

12. The biomarker not involved in AKI is:
    A. NGAL
    B. KIM-1
    C. Micro RNA 122
    D. Cystatin C
    E. AKI protein 1

13. Dialysis disequilibrium occurs due to:
    A. Cerebral oedema
    B. Hypertension
    C. Aluminium toxicity
    D. Beta-2 amyloid deposition
    E. Hyponatraemia

14. The most common ocular infection after renal transplantation is by:
    A. Cytomegalovirus
    B. Toxoplasma
    C. Herpes virus
    D. Epstein–Barr virus
    E. Tuberculosis

15. The most common nephropathy associated with malignancy is:
    A. Membranous nephropathy
    B. Minimal change disease
    C. IgA nephropathy
    D. Focal segmental glomerulonephropathy
    E. Membranoproliferative nephropathy

16. Hypercoagulation in nephrotic syndrome is caused by:
    A. Loss of antithrombin III
    B. Decreased fibrinogen
    C. Decreased metabolism of Vit K
    D. Increase in protein C
    E. Loss of globulin

17. The presence of which of the following in the urine is diagnosis of glomerular injury?
    A. Bright red cells
    B. 20% dysmorphic cells
    C. 100 RBCs per high-power field
    D. Beta-2 microglobulin
    E. Tamm–Horsfall protein

18. All are true with respect to haemolytic uraemic syndrome except:
    A. Uraemia
    B. Hypofibrinogenaemia
    C. Thrombocytopaenia
    D. Coombs positive haemolytic anaemia
    E. Coagulopathy

19. Which of the following is a possible complication of administration of gadolinium to a patient with chronic kidney disease?
    A. ARF
    B. Hyperthyroidism
    C. Hypocalcaemia
    D. Lactic acidosis
    E. Nephrogenic systemic sclerosis

20. A 68-year-old man with chronic renal insufficiency presents with weakness, paraesthesias and progressively worsening shortness of breath. He has been experiencing these symptoms for 4 days. Laboratory findings show a potassium level of 7.2; an electrocardiogram reveals peaked T waves and widening of the QRS complex. Which of the following is NOT indicated in the initial treatment of this patient?
    A. IV calcium
    B. IV glucose and insulin
    C. Dialysis
    D. Sodium polystyrene sulfonate
    E. Beta blockers

21. A 28-year-old man presents to the clinic with a complaint of haematuria of 1 day's duration. He was well until 3 days ago, when he developed a sore throat, low-grade fever and malaise, which lasted for approximately 48 hours. He had a similar episode approximately 1 year ago. He denies having rash, joint pains or dysuria. On examination, he appears well and is afebrile. His blood pressure is 118/62 mmHg. Urine dipstick assay is significant for 2+ blood

and trace protein. Microscopic examination of the urine reveals 10–15 red cells per high-powered field; dysmorphic red cells and occasional red cell casts are noted as well. Further testing reveals a normal antistreptolysin-O (ASO) titre and serum complement level. What is the diagnosis?

A. Acute post-infectious glomerulonephritis
B. Henoch–Schönlein purpura
C. IgA nephropathy
D. Oxalate stones
E. Minimal change disease

22. A 28-year-old woman presents to you after a recent hospital admission for flash pulmonary oedema. She was diagnosed with hypertension several months ago. Her blood pressure remains poorly controlled despite compliance with a regimen of hydrochlorothiazide, amlodipine and metoprolol. She denies having headache and palpitation. Her physical examination is remarkable for a blood pressure of 204/106 mmHg in the left arm and bilateral abdominal bruits. Your diagnosis is:

A. Renal artery stenosis (RAS) secondary to fibromuscular dysplasia (FMD)
B. Coarctation of aorta
C. Pheochromocytoma
D. Carcinoid syndrome
E. Takayasu arteritis

23. Medullary cystic kidney disease type 2 has been associated with mutations in which gene?

A. *LMX1B*
B. *TSC1*
C. *Polycystin*
D. *UMOD*
E. *EPO*

24. A patient with CRF, treated with regular haemodialysis, attends the renal clinic. He has been treated for 6 months with oral ferrous sulphate, 200 mg three times a day. His haemoglobin is 7.6 g/dL. His previous result was 10.6 six months ago. Which of the following is the most appropriate treatment?

A. Blood transfusion
B. Commence subcutaneous (SC) erythropoietin
C. Increase the dose of oral ferrous sulphate
D. IV iron
E. IV iron and subcutaneous erythropoietin

25. A 25-year-old lady with known systemic lupus erythematosus (SLE) presents with the nephrotic syndrome. A renal biopsy is performed and this confirms diffuse proliferative glomerulonephritis (WHO Class IV). Which of the following treatment regimens would you advise?

A. Azathioprine alone
B. Prednisolone alone
C. Azathioprine and prednisolone
D. Prednisolone and IV cyclophosphamide
E. Prednisolone and methotrexate

26. A 22-year-old obese man presents with mild ankle oedema and urinalysis shows protein +++ with no blood. A diagnosis of nephrotic syndrome is made on the basis of a cholesterol of 6.9 mmol/L, an albumin of 30 g/dL and proteinuria of 8 g/24 hours. What is the most likely diagnosis?

A. Amyloid
B. Focal segmental glomerulosclerosis
C. Membranoproliferative glomerulonephritis
D. Membranous nephropathy
E. Minimal change nephropathy

27. A 49-year-old woman has been an inpatient for the past 10 days for treatment of a bronchopneumonia. She has developed the onset of chills, fever and skin rash over the past 2 days. A peripheral blood film reveals eosinophilia. On urinalysis, she has ++ proteinuria. There is no past history of renal disease. Her glycosylated haemoglobin (HbA1c) is normal. These findings would most strongly suggest which of the following diagnoses?

A. Acute serum sickness
B. Acute tubular necrosis
C. Drug-induced interstitial nephritis
D. IgA nephropathy
E. Post-streptococcal glomerulonephritis

28. What is the most likely outcome of minimal change nephropathy at 16 years of age?

A. A tendency to relapse
B. Full renal recovery
C. Permanent renal impairment
D. Persistent hypertension
E. Persistent proteinuria

29. A 50-year-old man presents with a 6-week history of general malaise and a 2-day history of a right foot drop, a left ulnar nerve palsy and a widespread purpuric rash. He complains of arthralgia but has no clinical evidence of inflammatory joint disease. Echocardiogram is normal, blood cultures are negative, erythrocyte sedimentation rate (ESR) 100 mm/h, ANCA negative, ANA negative, rheumatoid factor strongly positive, C3 0.8 g/L (0.75–1.6) and C4 0.02 g/L (0.14–0.5). Dipstick urinalysis shows blood ++ but no protein. What is the most probably diagnosis?
    A. ANA negative SLE
    B. Cryoglobulinaemia
    C. Infective endocarditis
    D. Polyarthritis nordosa
    E. Rheumatoid arthritis

30. Renal papillary necrosis is found in the following condition:
    A. Polycystic disease
    B. Sickle cell disease
    C. Medullary cystic disease
    D. Diabetes insipidus
    E. Renal artery stenosis

31. Oliguria is defined as reduction in urine output:
    A. < 400 mL/24 h
    B. < 300 mL/24 h
    C. < 200 mL/24 h
    D. < 100 mL/24 h
    E. < 50 mL/24 h

Answers

1-E, 2-B, 3-E, 4-A, 5-C, 6-E, 7-C, 8-C, 9-A, 10-C, 11-E, 12-C, 13-A, 14-A, 15-A, 16-A, 17-B, 18-D, 19-E, 20-E, 21-C, 22-A, 23D, 24-E, 25-D, 26-D, 27-C, 28-B, 29-D, 30-B, 31-A

■ SUGGESTED READING

1. Carroll MF, Temte JL. Proteinuria in adults: a diagnostic approach. Am Fam Physician. 2000;62(6):1333-40.
2. KDIGO Clinical Practice Guideline for Acute Kidney Injury. Kidney Disease: Improving Global Outcomes (KDIGO) Acute Kidney Injury Work Group. Kidney Int Suppl. 2012;2(1):1.
3. Balasubramanian G, Al-Aly Z, Moiz A, Rauchman M, Zhang Z, Gopalakrishnan R, et al. Early nephrologist involvement in hospital-acquired acute kidney injury: a pilot study. Am J Kidney Dis. 2011;57(2):228-34.
4. Levey AS, Eckardt KU, Tsukamoto Y, Levin A, Coresh J, Rossert J, et al. Definition and classification of chronic kidney disease: a position statement from Kidney Disease: Improving Global Outcomes (KDIGO). Kidney Int 2005;67(6):2089-100.
5. Levey AS, Stevens LA, Coresh J. Conceptual model of CKD: applications and implications. Am J Kidney Dis. 2009;53(3 Suppl 3):S4-16.
6. Hemodialysis Adequacy 2006 Work Group. Clinical practice guidelines for hemodialysis adequacy, update 2006. Am J Kidney Dis. 2006; 48(Suppl 1):S2-90.
7. Dickinson BL. Unraveling the immunopathogenesis of glomerular disease. Clin Immunol. 2016;169:89-97.
8. George JN, Nester CM. Syndromes of thrombotic microangiopathy. N Engl J Med. 2014;371(7):654-66.
9. Fwu CW, Eggers PW, Kimmel PL, Kusek JW, Kirkali Z. Emergency department visits, use of imaging, and drugs for urolithiasis have increased in the United States. Kidney Int. 2013;83(3):479-86.
10. Singh P, Enders FT, Vaughan LE, Bergstralh EJ, Knoedler JJ, Krambeck AE, et al. Stone Composition Among First-Time Symptomatic Kidney Stone Formers in the Community. Mayo Clin Proc. 2015;90(10):1356-65.
11. Hart A, Smith JM, Skeans MA, Gustafson SK, Stewart DE, Cherikh WS, et al. Kidney. Am J Transplant. 2016;16(Suppl 2):11-6.
12. Gupta K, Hooton TM, Naber KG, Wullt B, Colgan R, Miller LG, et al. International clinical practice guidelines for the treatment of acute uncomplicated cystitis and pyelonephritis in women: A 2010 update by the Infectious Diseases Society of America and the European Society for Microbiology and Infectious Diseases. Clin Infect Dis. 2011;52(5):e103-20.
13. Czaja CA, Scholes D, Hooton TM, Stamm WE. Population-based epidemiologic analysis of acute pyelonephritis. Clin Infect Dis. 2007;45(7):273-80.

CHAPTER 11

Haematology

ANAEMIA

■ INTRODUCTION

Decrease of haemoglobin (Hb) concentration/red blood cells (RBC) count/haematocrit packed-cell volume (PCV) below normal for the patient's age, sex, and altitude of residence.

Normal adult haemoglobin—Males: 13–17 g/dL, Females: 12.0–15.0 g/dL

Classification of anaemia has been explained in **Table 11.1**.

■ CLINICAL FEATURES (FIG. 11.1)

- *Pallor*: Skin, palms, oral mucous membrane, nail beds, and palpebral conjunctiva.
- *Pulse*: Tachycardia, wide pulse pressure.
- *Cardiovascular system*: Cervical venous hum, hyperdynamic precordium, ejection systolic

TABLE 11.1: Classification of anaemia.

Morphological classification		
Normocytic normochromic	Microcytic hypochromic	Macrocytic
Aetiological classification		
BLOOD LOSS		
Acute	Chronic	
• Loss of large volume over short period • **Trauma,** post-partum bleeding	Small volume over long period peptic ulcer, haemorrhoids, carcinoma colon, hookworms, excessive menstrual loss	
IMPAIRED RED CELL PRODUCTION		
Disturbed proliferation and maturation	Marrow replacement	
Defective DNA synthesis	Primary haematopoietic neoplasms:	
• Megaloblastic anaemias: Deficiency or impaired utilisation of vitamin B12 and folic acid • Anaemia of renal failure: Deficiency of erythropoietin (EPO) • Anaemia of chronic disease: Iron sequestration and relative EPO deficiency • Anaemias of endocrine disorders	• Acute leukaemia • Myelodysplastic syndromes	
	Marrow Infiltration (myelophthisic anaemia)	
	Metastatic neoplasms	
	Disturbed proliferation and differentiation of stem cells	
Defective haemoglobin synthesis	• Aplastic anaemia • Pure red-cell aplasia	
• Defective heme-synthesis: Iron deficiency, sideroblastic anaemia • Defective globin synthesis: Thalassaemia		

Continued

Continued

INCREASED RED-CELL DESTRUCTION (HAEMOLYTIC ANAEMIAS)	
Intrinsic (Intracorpuscular)	**Extrinsic (Extracorpuscular)**
Hereditary • Abnormal membrane: Spherocytosis, elliptocytosis • Enzyme deficiencies: Glucose-6-phosphate dehydrogenase, pyruvate kinase • Disorders of haemoglobin synthesis 　○ Deficient globin synthesis: Thalassaemia 　○ Haemoglobinopathies: Sickle-cell anaemia **Acquired** • Membrane defects: Paroxysmal nocturnal haemoglobinuria (PNH)	**Antibody-mediated** • Isohaemagglutinins: Transfusion reactions, Rh disease of the newborn • Autoantibodies: Idiopathic, primary, drug-associated, systemic lupus erythematosus (SLE) **Mechanical trauma to RBCs:** • Microangiopathic haemolytic anaemia: Disseminated intravascular coagulation **Infections:** Malaria

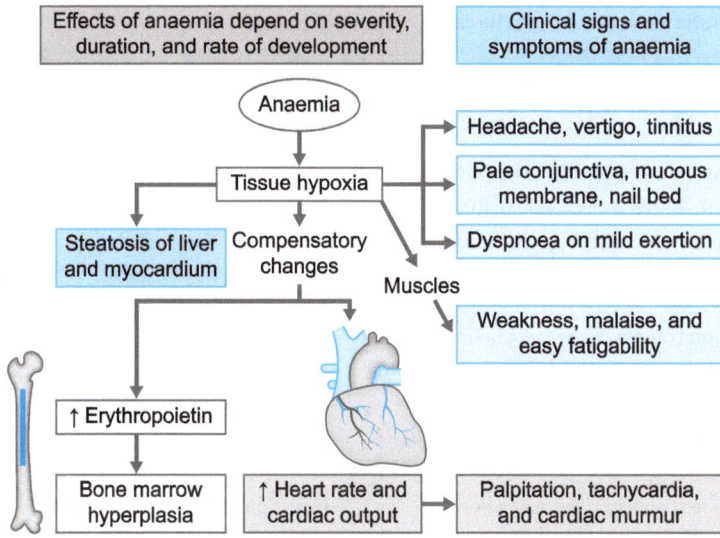

Fig. 11.1: Clinical features of anaemia.

murmur (best heard over the pulmonary area), cardiac dilatation and later signs of cardiac failure.
- *Oedema*

■ IRON-DEFICIENCY ANAEMIA

Causes of iron-deficiency anaemia have been well explained in **Table 11.2**.

Clinical Features

- Usual symptoms and signs of anaemia
- Advanced iron deficiency:
  ○ Cheilosis/angular stomatitis
  ○ Glossitis
  ○ Brittle fingernails, platynychia and **koilonychia** (spooning of the fingernails)
  ○ Blue-tinged sclerae
  ○ **Pica:** Unusual craving for substances with no nutritional value such as clay or chalk. Craving for ice (pagophagia) specific to iron deficiency or for clay (geophagia) or starch (amylophagia).
  ○ **Plummer–Vinson syndrome/Patterson-Kelly-Brown/Sideropenic dysphagia:** Esophageal/post-cricoid webs resulting in dysphagia for solids than liquids.

TABLE 11.2: Causes of iron-deficiency anaemia.

Decreased iron intake
- Milk fed infants
- Elderly with improper diet, poor dentition
- Low socioeconomical sections
- Vegetarians (poorly absorbable inorganic iron)

Decreased absorption of iron
- Total/partial gastrectomy
- Intestinal absorption is impaired in sprue, other causes of intestinal steatorrhoea and chronic diarrhoea
- Specific items in the diet, such as phytates of cereals, tannates, carbonates, oxalates, phosphates, and drugs can impair iron absorption

Increased demand/requirement for iron
- Rapid growth in infancy or adolescents
- Pregnancy and lactation

Increased iron loss
- Chronic blood loss due to bleeding from the gastrointestinal tract [peptic ulcers, gastric or colonic carcinoma, haemorrhoids, hookworm infestation, schistosomiasis, or non-steroidal anti-inflammatory drug (NSAID)]
- Urinary tract (renal or bladder tumours)
- Genital tract (menorrhagia and uterine cancer)

TABLE 11.3: Laboratory investigations: The cause of iron deficiency.

To confirm iron deficiency	Investigation of the cause of iron deficiency
Haemoglobin and haematocrit (PCV): Decreased **Red cell indices:** • MCV: < 80 fL; MCH: < 25 pg; MCHC: < 27 g/dL • RDW: Increased, > 15%. Earliest sign of iron deficiency	Stool: Examine for occult blood and hookworm infestation
• **Peripheral smear:** Microcytic hypochromic RBCs • Severe anaemia: Ring/pessary, pencil/cigar-shaped cells with moderate anisocytosis and poikilocytosis	Endoscopy: This includes upper gastrointestinal endoscopy, sigmoidoscopy, and colonoscopy
Reticulocyte count: Low for degree of anaemia	
Bone marrow: Moderate erythroid hyperplasia and micronormoblastic maturation	Urine: Examine for parasites such as schistosomiasis
Absence of bone marrow iron: "Gold standard" test, demonstrated by negative Prussian blue reaction	
Hepcidin: Decreased. Hepcidin regulates iron concentrations and tissue iron distribution	Investigations for malabsorption

(MCV: mean corpuscular volume; MCH: mean corpuscular haemoglobin; MCHC: mean corpuscular haemoglobin concentration; PCV: packedcell volume; RBC: red blood cells; RDW: red cell distribution width)

Laboratory Investigations

Investigation of the cause of iron deficiency has been mentioned in **Table 11.3**.

Serum iron profile in iron-deficiency anaemia has been elaborated in **Table 11.4**.

Differential diagnosis for microcytic hypochromic anaemia has been discussed in **Table 11.5**.

Management

- Identify and treat the underlying cause for deficiency.
- **Oral iron therapy:** Most patients can be treated with oral iron preparations. Ferrous sulphate (200 mg three times daily, a total of 180 mg ferrous iron), ferrous gluconate (300 mg twice daily, only 70 mg ferrous iron), ferrous fumarate (325 mg two or three times daily), and others.
- **Parenteral iron therapy:**
  o Indications:
    - Intolerant to oral iron preparation
    - Severe malabsorption
    - Primary blood loss is uncontrollable

TABLE 11.4: Serum iron profile in iron-deficiency anaemia (IDA).

	Normal range	Value in IDA	Observation
Serum ferritin	15–300 µg/L	<15 µg/L	Low
Serum iron	50–150 µg/dL	10–15 µg/dL	Low
Serum transferrin saturation	30–40%	<15%	Reduced
Total plasma iron-binding capacity (TIBC)	310–340 µg/dL	350–450 µg/dL	Increased
Serum transferrin receptor (TFR)	0.57–2.8 µg/L	3.5–7.1 µg/L	Increased
Red-cell protoporphyrin	30–50 µg/dL	>200 µg/dL	Increased

TABLE 11.5: Differential diagnosis for microcytic hypochromic anaemia.

Iron deficiency	Anaemia of chronic disease
Thalassaemia	Sideroblastic anaemia
Lead poisoning	

- Chronic gastrointestinal (GI) tract disease (e.g., inflammatory bowel disease) which may worsen with oral iron.
  - Iron dose in mg = Body weight (kg) × 2.3 × (normal Hb-patient's haemoglobin, g/dL) + 500 or 1,000 mg (to provide body iron stores).
  - **Preparations:** Iron-sorbitol, iron-dextran (imferon), iron sucrose, or sodium ferric gluconate, ferric carboxymaltose, and iron isomaltoside
- Red cell transfusion:
  - **Indication:** It is reserved for patients who have symptoms of anaemia, cardiovascular instability, continued and excessive loss of blood loss from any site, and requires immediate intervention.
  - Transfusions correct the anaemia acutely as well as transfused red cells provide a source of iron for reutilisation.

■ MEGALOBLASTIC ANAEMIA

Megaloblastic anaemia has been explained in **Table 11.6.**

Pernicious Anaemia

Chronic autoimmune disorder characterised by atrophic gastritis with loss of parietal cells in the gastric mucosa which causes failure of production of intrinsic factor.

Presence of autoantibodies in most of the patients: **Two major types** of autoantibodies are found.
1. Anti-intrinsic factor (IF) antibody:
   ○ Type I (blocking) antibody: Blocks binding of vitamin B12 to IF, present in 50–75% of the cases, detected in both plasma and gastric juice.
   ○ Type II (binding) antibody attaches to IF–vitamin B12 complex and prevent its binding to receptors in the ileal mucosa, present in about 40% of patients.
2. **Parietal cell (type III) antibody:** Directed against α and β subunits of gastric proton pump (H^+, K^+-ATPase) in parietal cells but is neither specific for PA nor other autoimmune disorders, found in 90% of patients with PA as well as in older patients with chronic non-specific gastritis.

Diagnosis/laboratory findings of megaloblastic anaemia have been discussed in **Table 11.7**.

Test results on metabolites: serum methylmalonic acid and total homocysteine have been discussed in **Table 11.8.**

Clinical Features

Vitamin B12 Deficiency

- Classic triad: Weakness, sore throat, and paraesthesia.
- Painful red "beefy" tongue due to glossitis and atrophy of papillae. Loss of taste, appetite.
- Lemon-yellow color: Pallor and mild jaundice caused by excess breakdown of haemoglobin.
- Pigmentation of knuckles and palmar creases.

TABLE 11.6: Megaloblastic anaemia: Deficiency of vitamin B12 and folic acid.

Vitamin B12 deficiency	Folic acid deficiency
Decreased intake: Inadequate diet, "pure vegetarians"	**Decreased intake:** Inadequate diet: Alcoholism, malnutrition
Increased demand: Pregnancy, hyperthyroidism, disseminated cancer	**Increased loss:** Haemodialysis
Impaired absorption<ul><li>Gastric: Deficiency of gastric acid or pepsin or intrinsic factor<ul><li>Pernicious anaemia (PA)</li><li>Post-gastrectomy</li><li>Drugs: Prolonged use of H2-receptor blockers and proton-pump inhibitors</li></ul></li><li>Intestinal<ul><li>Loss of absorptive surface<ul><li>Malabsorption syndromes</li><li>Diffuse intestinal disease: Lymphoma, systemic sclerosis</li><li>Ileal resection, Crohn's disease</li></ul></li><li>Competition for vitamin B12: Bacterial overgrowth in blind loops and diverticula of bowel, *Diphyllobothrium latum*</li></ul></li></ul>	**Impaired absorption**<ul><li>Malabsorption states-non-tropical and tropical sprue, coeliac disease</li><li>Diffuse infiltrative diseases of the small intestine (e.g., lymphoma)</li><li>Drugs: Anticonvulsant phenytoin, oral contraceptives, metformin, cholestyramine</li></ul>**Increased demand:** Pregnancy, lactation, infancy, disseminated cancer, markedly increased haematopoiesis (haemolytic anaemias), chronic exfoliative skin disease, chronic inflammatory and infective diseases
Abnormal cobalamin transport: Transcobalamin II deficiency	**Impaired utilisation:** Folic acid antagonists (antifolate drugs), such as methotrexate, trimethoprim, pyrimethamine, pentamidine, 5-fluorouracil, hydroxyurea
Others—Antifolate drugs: For example, methotrexate; independent of either cobalamin or folate deficiency	

TABLE 11.7: Diagnosis/laboratory findings of megaloblastic anaemia.

Peripheral Blood	
Haemoglobin, haematocrit	Reduced
Red-cell indices	MCV raised above 100 fL
Peripheral smear	Pancytopaenia
• Red blood cells (RBCs)	• Macrocytic and oval (egg-shaped macro-ovalocytes) • Most macrocytes lack the central pallor • Marked variation in the size and shape of red cells (anisopoikilocytosis). • Dyserythropoiesis: Basophilic stippling, Cabot ring, Howell–Jolly bodies.
• White blood cells (WBCs)	• Decreased WBC count (leucopenia) • Hypersegmented neutrophils (more than five nuclear lobes): First and specific morphological sign of megaloblastic anaemia. These neutrophils are also larger than normal (macro polys).
• Platelets	Decreased
• Reticulocyte count	Normal—low. Reticulocytosis—response to small doses of parenteral vitamin B12

Continued

Continued

Bone marrow
- Markedly hypercellular
- Megaloblastic type of erythropoiesis
- Granulocytic precursors—nuclear-cytoplasmic asynchrony as giant metamyelocytes and band forms
- Megakaryopoiesis: Normal or increased in number

Bone marrow iron Moderately increased

Diagnostic/Specific tests for vitamin B12 deficiency
- **Serum vitamin B12 levels:** Reduced and levels are very low (< 200 pg/μL)
- **Serum methylmalonic acid (MMA) and homocysteine levels:** Raised
- **Urinary excretion of methylmalonic acid:** Raised
- **Schilling test** for vitamin B12 absorption, discontinued in 2003, once provided invaluable information on the locus and mechanism of cobalamin malabsorption

Diagnostic/Specific tests for folic acid deficiency
- **Serum folic acid levels:** Reduced
- **FIGLU in urine:** Excessively excreted

(FIGLU: formiminoglutamate; MCV: mean corpuscular volume)

TABLE 11.8: Test results on metabolites: Serum methylmalonic acid and total homocysteine.

Methylmalonic acid (Normal = 70–270 nM)	Total homocysteine (Normal = 5–14 μM)	Diagnosis
Increased	Increased	Cobalamin deficiency confirmed; folate deficiency still possible (i.e., combined cobalamin-folate deficiency)
Normal	Increased	Folate deficiency is likely; < 5% may have cobalamin deficiency
Normal	Normal	Cobalamin and folate deficiencies are excluded

- **Neurological features:**
  - **Peripheral nerves**—peripheral neuropathy: Glove and sock distribution of paraesthesia. Tingling begins in tips of toes and progresses proximally—bilateral and symmetric. Loss of ankle reflexes
  - **Spinal cord:** Subacute combined degeneration of the cord
    - Posterior columns—impaired/diminished vibration and position sensation
    - Corticospinal tracts—upper motor neuron signs -ataxia, uncoordinated gait
  - **Cerebrum:** Depression and loss of memory (dementia), optic atrophy
  - Positive Romberg sign, Lhermitte sign may be elicited.

Folate Deficiency

Similar to vitamin B12 deficiency without neurological features.

Management

Treat the underlying cause, whenever possible.
Vitamin B12/Cobalamin: Vitamin B12 therapy—cyanocobalamin, hydroxocobalamin, and methylcobalamin.
- **Dosage:**
  - **Initial dose:** Six intramuscular injection of hydroxycobalamin 1,000 μg at 3–7-day intervals.
  - **Maintenance dose:** 1,000 μg to be given intramuscularly every 3 months for rest of the patient's life. Methylcobalamin, metabolically active form of vitamin B12 can also be used.

Folate deficiency: Oral dose of 5 mg folate (folic acid) daily for 3 weeks will treat acute deficiency and 5 mg once weekly is adequate maintenance therapy.

Causes of non-megaloblastic macrocytic anaemia have been explained in **Table 11.9**.

TABLE 11.9: Causes of non-megaloblastic macrocytic anaemia.

Physiological causes	
Pregnancy	Newborn
Pathological causes	
Alcohol excess	Reticulocytosis
Chronic liver disease	Hypothyroidism
Post-splenectomy	Myeloproliferative disorders
Haematological disorders • Aplastic anaemia • Sideroblastic anaemia • Pure red cell aplasia	**Drugs** • Azathioprine • Hydroxycarbamide

■ HAEMOLYTIC ANAEMIA

Anaemias that result due to increase in the rate of red cell destruction.

Life span of red cells (normal life span is 90–120 days) is shortened.

Classification of Haemolytic Anaemias

The haemolytic anaemias are classified in a variety of ways.
- **Location of haemolysis:** Intravascular and extravascular haemolytic disorders
- **Source of defect:** Intracorpuscular defect or extracorpuscular mechanism
- **Mode of onset:** Hereditary and acquired disorders
- **Clinical point of view:** Acute or chronic

Classification of haemolytic anaemias has been described in **Table 11.10**.

Clinical Features of Haemolytic Anaemia

Depend on the severity, duration, and type of haemolytic anaemia.

Clinical features of haemolytic anaemia have been discussed in **Table 11.11**.

TABLE 11.10: Classification of haemolytic anaemias.

Hereditary	Acquired	
Defects in red-cell membrane	**Immunohaemolytic anaemias**	
• Hereditary spherocytosis • Hereditary elliptocytosis • Stomatocytosis • Abetalipoproteinemia (Acanthocytosis)	**Autoimmune haemolytic anaemias**	
	1. Due to warm antibodies • Idiopathic • Secondary	2. Due to cold antibodies • Cold agglutinin disease • Paroxysmal cold haemoglobinuria
	3. Haemolytic disease of the newborn	
Red-cell enzyme deficiencies	**Fragmentation syndromes**	
• Pyruvate kinase deficiency • Hexokinase deficiency • Glucose-6-phosphate dehydrogenase deficiency (G6PD)	• Haemolytic uraemic syndrome • Thrombotic thrombocytopenic purpura • Disseminated intravascular coagulation • Prosthetic cardiac valves	
Defects in globin synthesis: Haemoglobinopathies	**Miscellaneous**	
• Thalassaemia—quantitative • Sickle-cell syndromes—qualitative • Alpha thalassaemia • Unstable haemoglobin disease	• Drugs: Oxidant drugs (primaquine, dapsone) • Chemical (naphthalene, nitrites and nitrates, and oxidising chemicals) • Thermal injury: Burns	
	Paroxysmal nocturnal haemoglobinuria	

TABLE 11.11: Clinical features of haemolytic anaemia.

Symptoms/History	Physical findings/signs
• Mild jaundice • Symptoms due to anaemia • Urine color: Appears normal (acholuric), turns dark on standing due to oxidation of urobilinogen to urobilin. Black urine (haemoglobinuria) seen in intravascular haemolysis [malaria, mismatched blood transfusion, glucose-6-phosphate dehydrogenase (G6PD) deficiency] • Infections • Splenic pain: Enlargement or infarction of spleen • Acute crisis: Due to sudden fall in haemoglobin—fever, joint pains, and abdominal pain • Pigment gall stones: Chronic haemolysis • Leg ulcers manifest in adult males: Hereditary spherocytosis and sickle-cell anaemia • Family history: Congenital haemolytic anaemias	• Anaemia • Mild jaundice • Splenomegaly: Some cases of haemolytic anaemia—Thalassaemia, hereditary spherocytosis) • Chronic leg ulcers: Sickle-cell anaemia • Skeletal abnormalities: Expansion of bone marrow in some congenital haemolytic anaemias due to increased erythropoiesis, manifests as enlargement of maxillary bones and frontal bossing and malocclusion of the teeth due to overgrowth of upper jaw (thalassaemic facies) • Signs of systemic disease: Predisposing to haemolysis • Signs of cholelithiasis: Cholecystitis

TABLE 11.12: Extravascular and intravascular haemolysis.

Extravascular haemolysis	Intravascular haemolysis
Anaemia	
Unconjugated hyperbilirubinaemia (Jaundice)	
Increased urobilinogen in urine leading to high coloured urine	
Shortened red-cell lifespan (demonstrated by ^{51}Cr-labelled red-blood cells)	
Decreased plasma haptoglobin and haemopexin	
Splenomegaly	Increased plasma LDH, haemoglobinaemia, haemoglobinuria, haemosiderinuria (demonstrated by Prussian blue reaction) and methaemoglobinaemia (in some)

(LDH: lactate dehydrogenase)

Diagnosis of Haemolytic Anaemias

Extravascular and intravascular haemolysis has been described in **Table 11.12**.

Features of increased RBC production: Compensatory mechanism to haemolysis, there is increased production of red cells.
- **Bone marrow:** Compensatory erythroid hyperplasia

- **Peripheral smear:** Reticulocytosis. Other findings vary depending on the cause.
  ○ Nucleated red cells and polychromasia
  ○ Macrocytosis (due to increased reticulocyte count and folate deficiency)
  ○ Spherocytes [hereditary spherocytosis (HS) and autoimmune haemolytic anaemia]
  ○ Marked anisopoikilocytosis, hypochromic red cells, and target cells in thalassaemias
  ○ Fragmented red cells (microangiopathic anaemia and prosthetic cardiac valve)
- **Radiological changes:** Hair-on-end appearance in skull radiograph (thalassaemia and sickle-cell anaemia)

Tests for Cause of Haemolysis
- Common tests:
  ○ **Peripheral smear examination:** Red-cell morphology
    – Spherocyte (HS and autoimmune haemolytic anaemia)
    – Sickle cell (sickle-cell anaemia)
    – Target cell (thalassaemia)
    – Acanthocyte
    – Schistocyte (Intravascular haemolysis—fragmented red cells, helmet cells, and triangular cells)
    – Malarial parasite
  ○ Coomb's test

> **Box 11.1: Haemoglobinopathies: Qualitative and quantitative defect.**
>
> **Qualitative defect in (structurally abnormal) haemoglobins**
> - Haemoglobin S
> - Haemoglobin C
> - Haemoglobin D Punjab
>
> **Quantitative defect in haemoglobins**
> Thalassaemias (α, β-thalassaemia)
>
> **Combined qualitative and quantitative defects in haemoglobins**
> - Haemoglobin E
> - Sickle-cell β-thalassaemia
>
> **Acquired haemoglobinopathies**
> - Methaemoglobinaemia due to toxic exposures
> - Carboxyhaemoglobinaemia

TABLE 11.13: Description of sickle-cell anaemia.

Sickle-cell anaemia (SS)	Homozygous state in which both β-globin chains are abnormal.
Sickle-cell trait (AS)	Heterozygous state in which one gene is defective for HbS (abnormal) and other gene is for HbA (normal)
Compound heterozygous	Both β globin chains having different abnormalities, (HbSC, HbS-β-thalassaemia)

- o Osmotic fragility, sucrose lysis and Ham's test
- o Heinz body preparation
- o Haemoglobin electrophoresis
- o High performance liquid chromatography (HPLC)
- o Measurement of enzyme activity
- **Specific tests:** Identification of specific cause of haemolysis is dealt under individual diseases.

Treatment of Haemolytic Anaemias

- General supportive therapy:
  - o Blood transfusions
  - o Treatment of infections, leg ulcers, cholelithiasis, etc.
  - o Splenectomy: In some selected diseases
- **Specific therapy:** Dealt with under respective diseases.

■ HAEMOGLOBINOPATHIES

Box 11.1 explains about both qualitative and quantitative defect in haemoglobins.

■ SICKLE-CELL ANAEMIA

Sickle-cell anaemia has been shown in **Table 11.13**.

Aetiology and Pathogenesis

Caused by production of abnormal haemoglobin called sickle haemoglobin (HbS).

In HbS, there is an adenine (A) to thymidine (T) substitution (GAG→GTG) in codon 6 of the β-globin gene. This point mutation results in **replacement of the normal glutamic acid residue by a valine** and alters the solubility or stability of the haemoglobin.

Clinical Features (Figs. 11.2A to C)

Investigations

- **Evidences of haemolysis (see above)**
- **Blood count:** Haemoglobin is in the range 6–8 g/dL with a high reticulocyte count (10–20%).
- **Peripheral smear: Sickle cell**—long, curved cells with pointed ends.
- Hyposplenism: Howell–Jolly bodies (small nuclear remnants), **target cells** (due to red-cell dehydration) **and ovalocytes.**
- **Erythrocyte sedimentation rate (ESR) is low** because sickle cells do not form rouleaux.
- **Sickling test:** Sickling is induced by adding a reducing agent such as 2% sodium metabisulphite or sodium dithionite to blood sample.
- **Sickle solubility test:** A mixture of HbS in a reducing solution (e.g., sodium dithionite) gives a turbid appearance because of precipitation of HbS, whereas normal Hb gives a clear solution.

Haemoglobin electrophoresis: **No Hb-A, 80–95% Hb-SS and 2–20% HbF.** HbS—slow moving haemoglobin compared to HbA and HbF. In sickle-cell trait (heterozygous state) Hb-S is 20–40% and the rest is Hb-A.

Management

Anaemia

- **Blood transfusion:** Required to increase the oxygen carrying capacity, replace sickle-shaped RBCs with normal cells and to restore blood flow. Acute transfusions—life-saving,

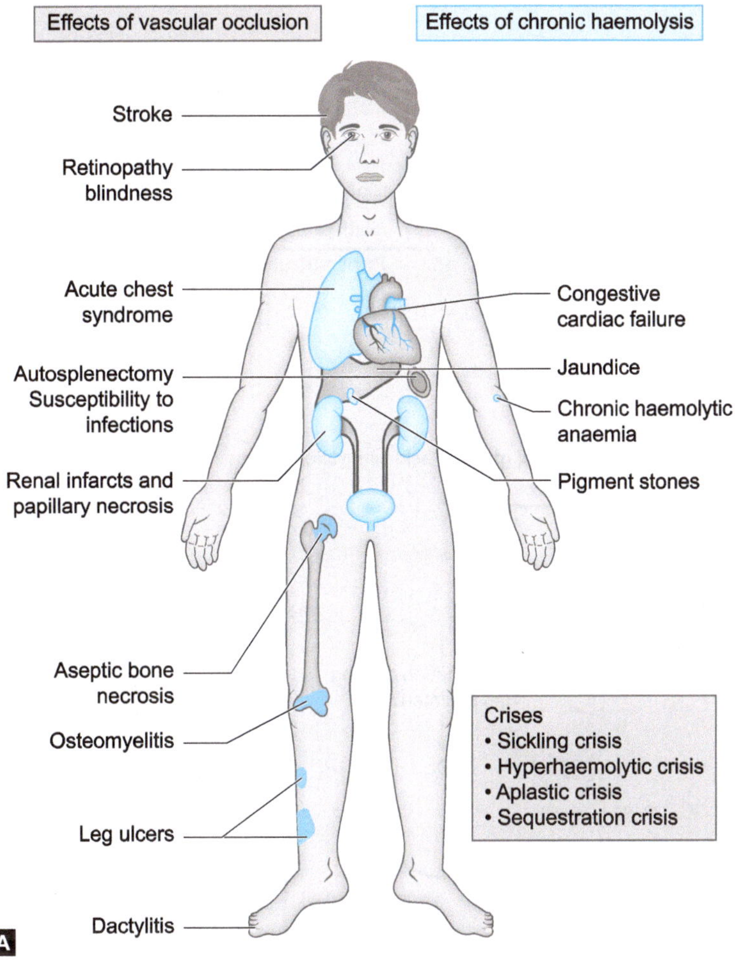

Effects of vascular occlusion
- Stroke
- Retinopathy blindness
- Acute chest syndrome
- Autosplenectomy Susceptibility to infections
- Renal infarcts and papillary necrosis
- Aseptic bone necrosis
- Osteomyelitis
- Leg ulcers
- Dactylitis

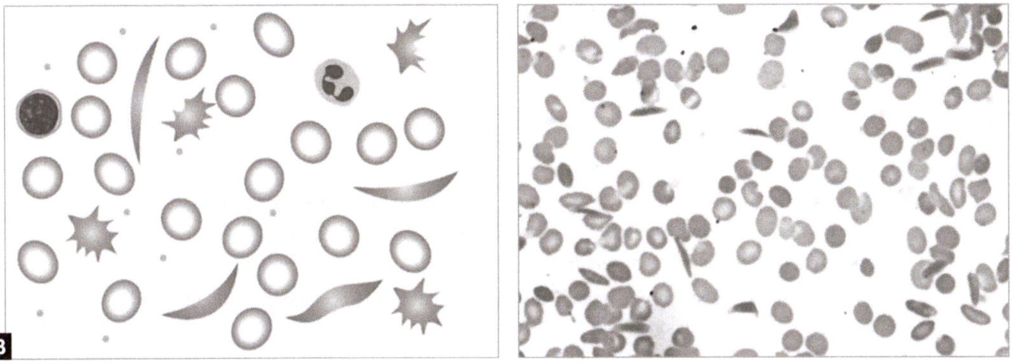

Effects of chronic haemolysis
- Congestive cardiac failure
- Jaundice
- Chronic haemolytic anaemia
- Pigment stones

Crises
- Sickling crisis
- Hyperhaemolytic crisis
- Aplastic crisis
- Sequestration crisis

Fig. 11.2A to C:

Continued

Continued

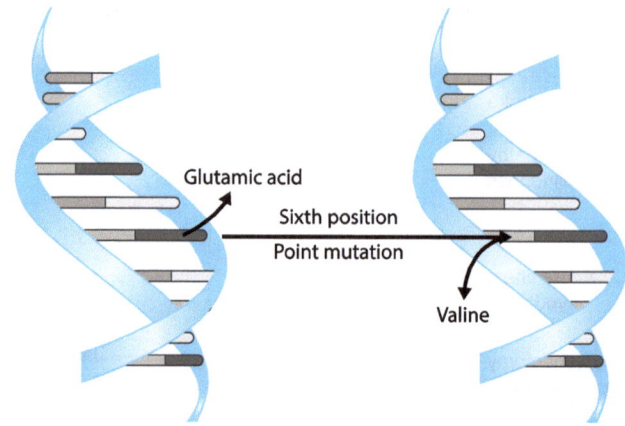

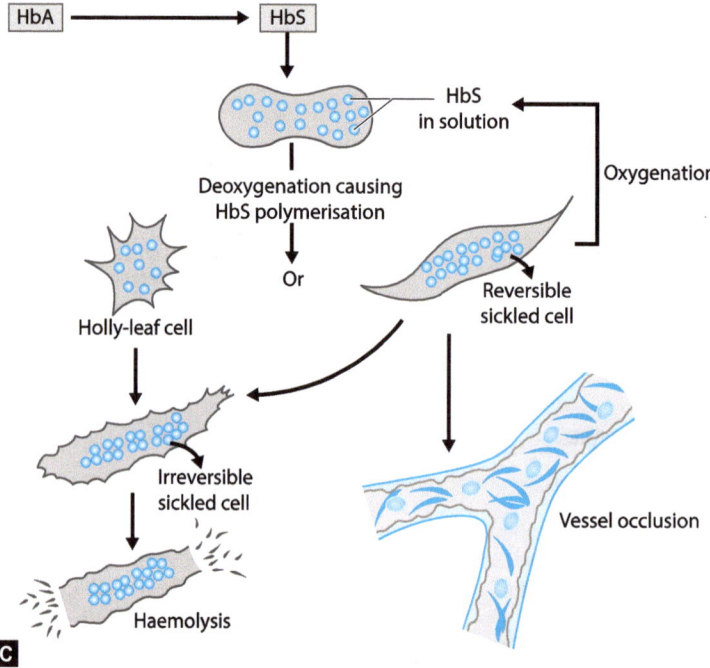

Fig. 11.2A to C: (A) Various effects of vascular occlusion and haemolysis in sickle-cell anaemia; (B) Peripheral smear with sickle cells; (C) Pathogenesis of sickle-cell anaemia. *(For color version, see plate 1)*

Courtesy: Exam Preparatory Manual for Undergradates—Medicine/Archith Boloor and Ramadas Nayak, 2nd edition.

chronic transfusions—reduce the incidence and severity of most complications.
- Heart failure, transient ischaemic attacks (TIAs), strokes, acute chest syndrome, and severe anaemia due to aplastic crises and acute splenic sequestration.
- **Repeated transfusions:** Reduce the proportion of circulating HbS to <20% to prevent sickling, before elective procedures and pregnancy. Chronic RBC transfusion reduces the chance of recurrent ischaemic stroke.

- **Exchange transfusions**: It may be necessary in patients with severe or recurrent crises, or before emergency surgery. Whether exchange transfusion is preferable to simple transfusion in the acute chest syndrome, stroke, or other acute complications have not been established by clinical trials.
- Infarction crises are managed with hydration, oxygen, analgesics and transfusion with RBC concentrate in selected cases.

Iron overload: Develops due to repeated transfusions, can result in heart and liver failure and other complications. Treated by using iron chelators (deferoxamine or deferasirox).

Hydroxycarbamide (hydroxyurea): Therapy for patients with severe symptoms. 10–30 mg/kg/day increases HbF and suppresses neutrophil and reticulocyte counts (sickle-cell crisis). This reduces episodes of pain, the acute chest syndrome, and need for blood transfusions.

Acute Painful Crisis

Supportive therapy with intravenous fluids, oxygen, antimicrobial agents and adequate analgesia.
- Acute severe pain—narcotic, analgesia (morphine); milder pain—codeine, paracetamol, and NSAIDs.
- **Inhaled nitric oxide** inhibits platelet function, reduces vascular adhesion of red cells and is also a vasodilator. Provides short-term pain relief and reduces opiate requirements in acute painful episodes. Avoid hypoxia and respiratory depression. Nasal oxygen should be employed as appropriate to protect arterial saturation.
- Acute chest syndrome is treated with antibiotics, maintenance of arterial oxygenation, pain relief, bronchodilators, and if required, exchange transfusion.

Curative:
- **Bone marrow/stem-cell transplantation:** In children and adolescents younger than 16 years of age with who have severe complications (strokes, recurrent chest syndrome, or refractory pain) can provide definitive cure.
- **Gene therapy:** It is intensively pursued, but no safe measures are currently available.

HEREDITARY SPHEROCYTOSIS

Red blood cells membrane defect due to cytoskeleton protein—ankyrin, band 3, spectrin, band protein 4.2 deficiency.

Clinical Features

- Present during anytime from the neonatal period to adulthood.
- **Family history:** About 75% HS inherited as autosomal dominant trait with strong family history of anaemia, jaundice, splenomegaly, and cholelithiasis.
- **Anaemia:** Anaemia is usually mild-to-moderate.
- **Jaundice:** Intermittent attacks of jaundice
- **Splenomegaly:** Moderate splenic enlargement is characteristic, constant (500–1,000 g) feature.

Complications

- Cholelithiasis (pigment gall stones)
- Chronic leg ulcers
- Aplastic crises due to parvovirus B19 infection
- Haemolytic crises (rare)

Investigations

- **Anaemia:** Usually mild, but occasionally can be severe.
- **Peripheral blood film** shows **spherocytes** and reticulocytes.
- **Demonstration of a haemolytic state:** Raised serum bilirubin and urinary urobilinogen.
- **Increased osmotic fragility:** It may be absent in mild cases and may be positive in autoimmune haemolytic anaemia.

Treatment

- *Splenectomy*: Treatment of choice, not to be done before 6 years. Corrects anaemia and its complications, increases infection risk. It should be preceded by pneumococcal and *Haemophilus influenzae* immunisation and followed by lifelong penicillin prophylaxis.
- *Folic acid supplementation*: In patients without splenectomy.
- Regular blood transfusions are required in few patients with severe disease.

THALASSAEMIAS

Alpha- and β-thalassaemia syndromes based on the genetic defect have been described in **Table 11.14**.

Clinical Features

- **Severe anaemia:** Infants are well at birth, develop moderate-to-severe anaemia 6–9 months after birth, when haemoglobin synthesis switches from HbF to HbA.
- **Retardation of growth and development:** Untreated/untransfused children **fail to thrive** and die early within 4–5 years of age from the effects of anaemia.
- They are susceptible to recurrent bacterial infections
- **Thalassaemic facies:** Enlargement and distortion of craniofacial bones (frontal bossing of the skull, prominent malar eminence, depression of bridge of nose, and hypertrophy of the maxillae, which tends to expose the upper teeth).
- **Hair-on-end (crew-cut) appearance:** In the skull X-ray due to new bone formation.
- **Splenomegaly:** Enlarges up to 1,500 g due to hyperplasia and extramedullary haematopoiesis.
- Liver (hepatomegaly) and lymph nodes also may show extramedullary haematopoiesis.
- **Haemosiderosis:** Blood transfusions improve the anaemia, but cause iron overload, haemosiderosis and secondary haemochromatosis. It may be due to increased gastrointestinal absorption of iron.
  - Cardiac haemosiderosis: Arrhythmias, heart blocks, and congestive heart failure.
  - Hepatic haemosiderosis: Cirrhosis
  - Pancreatic haemosiderosis: Diabetes
  - Pituitary: Hypogonadotropic hypogonadism.

Investigations

- **Peripheral smear:** Marked **microcytic hypochromic anaemia**, moderate-marked anisopoikilocytosis. Target cells nucleated red cells.
- **Haemoglobin F level is increased** (30–92%).
- **Markedly reduced or absent haemoglobin A** (HbA)
- Osmotic fragility test shows increased resistance to haemolysis.
- Skull radiograph: It shows a **"hair-on-end" appearance.**
- Evidence of thalassaemia minor in both parents.
- **Red-cell distribution width (RDW):** Within normal limits (in contrast to iron deficiency anaemia).

TABLE 11.14: Beta-thalassaemia syndromes—based on the genetic defect.

β-thalassaemia syndromes: Based on the genetic defect (β⁺ or β⁰)		
β-thalassaemia major	**β-thalassaemia intermedia**	**β-thalassaemia minor**
• Homozygous disorder. Most severe form • Either no production of β-chains (β⁰) or it is markedly reduced (β⁺) • Anaemia—severe, transfusion dependent. • High level of HbF in the blood	• Double heterozygous state • Anaemia—moderately severe, not transfusion dependent	• Also called β-thalassaemia trait • Heterozygous state • Asymptomatic with mild anaemia
α-thalassaemia syndromes		
• Each cell has four genes coding for α-globin, two on each chromosome. Each gene contributes to 25% of the total α-globin chains • Severity—depends on the number of genes deleted or affected. Deleted genes may vary from 1 to 4		

1 gene affected	2 genes affected	3 genes affected	4 genes affected
Silent carrier state	α–thalassaemia trait	HbH disease	Hb Bart's—hydrops fetalis • Incompatible with life—stillbirths or die shortly after birth • Pale, oedematous, hepatosplenomegaly

Management
- **Maintenance of Hb:** Long-term folate supplementation and blood transfusions to keep Hb > 10 g/dL.
- **Iron overload:** Chelating agent, desferrioxamine (parenterally)—indicated if serum ferritin > 1,500 µg/L. Ascorbic acid 200 mg daily along with desferrioxamine increases the urinary excretion of iron in response to desferrioxamine. Deferiprone and deferasirox are oral iron chelators.
- **Splenectomy:** It is indicated in children with massive symptomatic splenomegaly and those with progressively increasing requirement of blood transfusion.
- **Bone marrow transplantation**: In young patients

Management of associated complications: For example, congestive heart failure and endocrinopathies.

GLUCOSE-6-PHOSPHATE DEHYDROGENASE DEFICIENCY

X-linked disorder and is the most common enzyme deficiency. RBCs deficient in G6PD cannot keep glutathione in reduced state. RBCs are susceptible to injury by both exogenous and endogenous oxidants.

Pathogenesis of β-thalassaemia major and its consequences have been shown in **Figure 11.3**.

Clinical Features
- Most are clinically asymptomatic; however, all of them have an increased risk of developing acute haemolytic anaemia (AHA), neonatal jaundice (NNJ), and rarely, chronic non-spherocytic haemolytic anaemia (CNSHA).
- **Acute haemolytic anaemia:** Due to intravascular haemolysis is the most dramatic clinical presentation of G6PD deficiency. Develops after exposure to an oxidative stress and the triggers include:
    - **Drugs:** Antimalarials (primaquine, quinine, and chloroquine) sulphonamides (sulphamethoxazole), antibacterial/antibiotics (cotrimoxazole, nitrofurantoin), antipyretics/analgesics (acetanilide phenazopyridine) dapsone, quinidine, methylene blue, nitrofurantoin, etc.
    - **Fava beans** (favism)
    - **Infections:** Viral and bacterial
- **Neonatal jaundice:** It is a feature of Mediterranean type. Haemolytic anaemia is very rarely severe. Jaundice may be due to decreased hepatic elimination of bilirubin. Severe neonatal jaundice, if not adequately treated with phototherapy, may result in kernicterus or even death.
- **Chronic non-spherocytic haemolytic anaemia:** Develops in very small minority of patients. Seen in males and usually have a history of severe neonatal jaundice and chronic anaemia. The degree of chronic anaemia is variable and some patients may require intermittent transfusions. They have reticulocytosis, gallstones, and splenomegaly. Haemolysis is mainly extravascular.

Glucose-6-phosphate dehydrogenase deficiency (African variety) has a protective effect against *Plasmodium falciparum* (**Fig. 11.4**).

Laboratory Findings/Investigations
- **Intravascular haemolysis:** Raised unconjugated bilirubin, haemoglobinaemia, haemoglobinuria, high lactate dehydrogenase (LDH), and low or absent plasma haptoglobin.
- **Anaemia:** Moderate-extremely severe. Both intravascular and extravascular haemolysis.
- **Peripheral blood film:** Normocytic and normochromic with anisopoikilocytosis, reticulocytosis and spherocytes, bite (blister) cells, and Heinz bodies
- **Confirmation of diagnosis:** Estimating G6PD activity of the red cell. This should be estimated several days after the acute haemolytic episode. This is because if done during or immediately after acute haemolysis may give a falsely normal value as the young red cells and reticulocytes have near normal G6PD levels.

Treatment/Management of Glucose-6-phosphate Dehydrogenase Deficiency
- **Removal of triggering agent** and avoiding further exposure to triggering factors in previously screened patients. Once cause is recognised, in most cases no specific treatment is required.

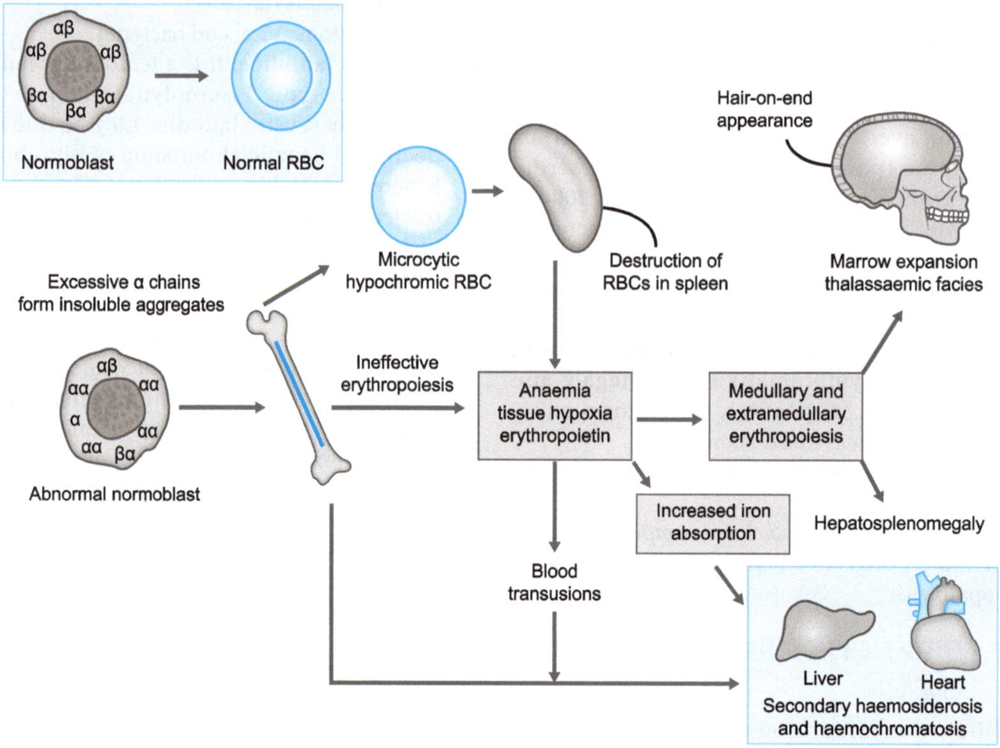

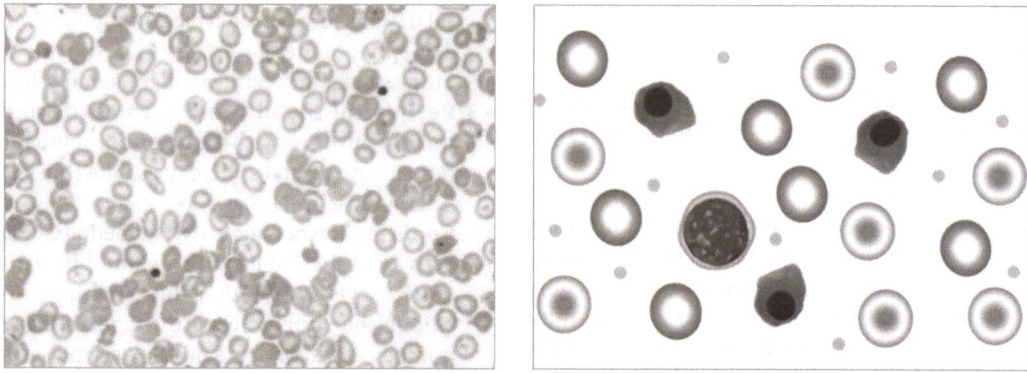

Peripheral blood smear in β-thalassaemia showing target cells and nucleated red cells.

(RBC: red blood cells)

Fig. 11.3: Pathogenesis of β-thalassaemia major and its consequences as well as peripheral blood smear in β-thalassaemia showing target cells and nucleated red cells. *(For color version, see plate 3)*
Courtesy: Exam Preparatory Manual for Undergradutes—Medicine/Archith Boloor and Ramadas Nayak, 2nd edition.

Haematology

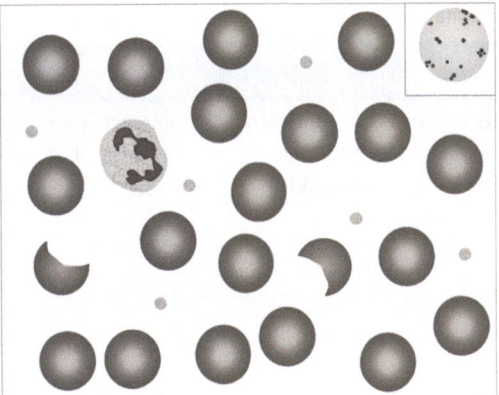

Fig. 11.4: Peripheral blood smear in glucose-6-phosphate dehydrogenase (G6PD) deficiency with "bite cells". Inset: Heinz bodies (supravital stain). *(For color version, see plate 4)*

Courtesy: Exam Preparatory Manual for Undergradates—Medicine/Archith Boloor and Ramadas Nayak, 2nd edition.

- Management of neonatal jaundice is similar to any other cause of neonatal hyperbilirubinaemia.
- Supportive therapy for anaemia: Blood transfusion and regular folic acid supplements in CNSHA
- Treatment of infection.

NORMOCYTIC AND NORMOCHROMIC ANAEMIA

Normocytic and normochromic anaemia have been discussed in **Table 11.15**.

DIFFERENTIATING HYPOCHROMIC MICROCYTIC ANAEMIAS

Differentiating hypochromic microcytic anaemias have been described in **Table 11.16**.

PANCYTOPAENIA

Table 11.17 describes about pancytopaenia.

SIDEROBLASTIC ANAEMIAS

Rare inherited or acquired disorders of refractory anaemia characterised by presence of ring sideroblasts, excess storage iron in the bone marrow and increased serum iron concentration.

Diagnostic feature is the presence of ring sideroblasts in the bone marrow.

Sideroblastic anaemias have been explained in **Table 11.18**.

Treatment

- Withdrawal of causative agent
- Occasional cases may respond to pyridoxine or folic acid
- Supportive treatment with transfusions
- Erythropoietin

PAROXYSMAL NOCTURNAL HAEMOGLOBINURIA

Stem cells and their progeny have **deficient synthesis of** glycosylphosphatidylinositol (GPI) **linked proteins** namely (1) decay–accelerating factor, or CD55, (2) membrane inhibitor of reac-

TABLE 11.15: Production of decreased red cell as well as destruction of increased red cell.

Decreased red cell production	Increased red cell loss or destruction

• Anaemia of chronic disease
• Chronic renal failure
• Chronic liver disease
• Endocrine disorders: Hypopituitarism, hypothyroidism, and hypoadrenalism
• Haematological disorders:
  ○ Marrow hypoplasia or aplasia
  ○ Myeloproliferative neoplasms
  ○ Myelofibrosis
  ○ Sideroblastic anaemia
	• Acute blood loss
	• Hypersplenism
	• Haematological disorders
	  ○ Haemoglobinopathies (sickle-cell disease)
	  ○ Hereditary spherocytosis
	  ○ Glucose-6-phosphate dehydrogenase deficiency
	  ○ Microangiopathic anaemias (disseminated intravascular coagulation, thrombotic thrombocytopenic purpura, and haemolytic uraemic syndromes)
	  ○ Autoimmune haemolytic anaemia
	  ○ Paroxysmal nocturnal haemoglobinuria

Expansion of plasma volume: Pregnancy	

TABLE 11.16: Differentiating hypochromic microcytic anaemias.

	Iron-deficiency anaemia	Thalassaemia trait	Anaemia of chronic disease	Sideroblastic anaemia
MCV	Reduced	Very low for degree of anaemia	Low normal or normal	Inherited: Low Acquired: High
Serum iron (normal 60–170 µg/dL)	Reduced	Normal to high	Reduced	Raised
Serum total iron binding capacity (normal 300–350 µg/dL)	Raised	Normal	Reduced	Normal
Serum ferritin (normal 15–300 µg/dL)	Reduced	Normal	Normal or raised	Raised
Serum soluble transferrin receptors	Increased	Normal or raised	Normal	Normal or raised
Iron in marrow	Absent	Present	Present	Present
Iron in erythroblasts	Absent	Present	Absent or reduced	Ring forms
Haemoglobin A$_2$ (normal <3%)	Reduced	Increased	Normal	Reduced

TABLE 11.17: Pancytopaenia: decreased bone marrow function as well as increased peripheral destruction.

Decreased bone marrow function	

Aplastic anaemia: Idiopathic, secondary, and inherited
Myelodysplastic syndromes (MDS)
• Bone marrow infiltration with:
  o Leukaemia (e.g., Hairy cell leukaemia)
  o Lymphoma, myeloma
  o Tumours (carcinoma)
  o Granulomatous diseases (e.g., TB, sarcoidosis)
	• Nutritional deficiencies: Megaloblastic anaemia
	• Paroxysmal nocturnal haemoglobinuria
	• Myelofibrosis (rare)
	• Haemophagocytic syndrome

Increased peripheral destruction: Hypersplenism	

TABLE 11.18: Characteristics of sideroblastic anaemias.

Inherited sideroblastic anaemia: X-linked disease—transmitted by females	

• Acquired sideroblastic anaemia
• Primary: Myelodysplasia
• Secondary:
  o Drugs, e.g., isoniazid, cycloserine, chloramphenicol, busulphan, D-penicillamine
  o Alcohol abuse
  o Lead toxicity
	• Myeloproliferative neoplasms
	• Myeloid leukaemia
	• Primary pyridoxine deficiency
	• Others (e.g., rheumatoid arthritis, carcinoma)

tive lysis, or CD59. This is a potent inhibitor of C3 and prevents activation of complement pathway on their membrane.

In paroxysmal nocturnal haemoglobinuria (PNH), the red cells are abnormally sensitive to complement-mediated intravascular haemolysis.

Intravascular haemolysis: Urine voided at night (nocturnal) and in the morning on waking it is dark in colour. Haemolysis is due to reduced pH of blood during sleep which enhances the activity of complement. Haemoglobin in acidic urine is converted into acid haematin which colours the urine dark brown. Urinary iron loss may be sufficient to cause iron deficiency.

Mild jaundice and mild hepatosplenomegaly often present.

Thrombosis: It is very common—Budd–Chiari syndrome. Portal or cerebral vein thrombosis is often the cause of death.

It may begin or progress to aplastic anaemia.

Diagnosis
- Ham's test and sucrose lysis test (cannot reliably detect small populations of affected red cells).
  - **Ham's acidified serum test:** Checks whether red blood cells become more fragile when they are placed in mild acid. Positive in congenital dyserythropoietic anaemia.
  - **Sucrose haemolysis test:** Red cell undergoes lysis when incubated low-tonic-strength solution of sugar sucrose. Positive in megaloblastic anaemia and autoimmune haemolytic anaemia.
- **Flow cytometry:** Detects red cells that are deficient in GPI-linked proteins (CD55 and CD59). Rapid and sensitive test diagnosis.

Treatment
- *Supportive measures*: Blood transfusions (severe anaemia) and control of infections.
- Iron therapy often necessary due to loss in urine.
- *Eculizumab*: Humanised monoclonal antibody that prevents cleavage of C5 and membrane attack complex), reducing intravascular haemolysis, haemoglobinuria, and transfusion requirements.
- Long-term anticoagulants may be necessary for patients with recurrent thrombotic episodes.
- Steroids may be useful in some cases.

■ METHAEMOGLOINAEMIA

Causes of methaemogloinaemia have been discussed in **Box 11.2**.

■ AUTOIMMUNOHAEMOLYTIC ANAEMIA

Autoimmunohaemolytic anaemia (AIHA) has been explained in **Box 11.3**.

Box 11.2: Causes of methaemogloinaemia.

Hereditary: deficiency of methaemoglobin reductase

Acquired: drugs and toxins (nitrites, nitrates, primaquine, dapsone, phenacetin, phenazopyridine, metoclopramide, and nitroglycerine)

Treatment:
- Methaemoglobin reductase deficiency: Oral methylene blue or ascorbic acid
- Severe methaemoglobinaemia: Intravenous methylene blue

Box 11.3: Autoimmunohaemolytic anaemia.

Based on antibody type

Warm antibody type (IgG antibodies active at 37°C)
- Primary (idiopathic)
- Secondary
  - Autoimmune disorders (systemic lupus erythematosus and others)
  - Drugs (e.g., methyldopa, penicillins, and quinidine)
  - Lymphomas: Hodgkin's lymphoma and chronic lymphocytic leukaemia

Cold agglutinin type (IgM antibodies active at 4–18°C)
- Acute
  - Mycoplasmal infection
  - Infectious mononucleosis
- Chronic
  - Idiopathic
  - Lymphomas

Cold haemolysin type (Donath–Landsteiner antibodies)

Rare; seen mainly in children; usually post-viral

Based on aetiology

Idiopathic (50%)

Secondary (50%)
- Drugs, e.g., methyldopa, penicillins, and quinidine
- Mycoplasmal infection
- Infectious mononucleosis
- Autoimmune disorders (systemic lupus erythematosus and others)
- Lymphomas

Investigations
- Evidence of haemolytic anaemia
- Spherocytosis (due to red-cell damage) and macrocytes in peripheral blood
- Direct antiglobulin (Coomb's) test is positive
- Autoantibodies may have specificity for the Rh blood group system (e.g., for the "e" antigen).
- **Autoimmune thrombocytopaenia** and/or neutropenia may also be present (Evans' syndrome).

Treatment
- **Corticosteroids** (e.g., prednisolone in doses of 1 mg/kg daily): Effective in about 80% of patients. Initially for first 2–4 weeks, prednisolone 60 mg daily, followed by gradual tapering of the dose.
  - **Avoid blood transfusion** (autoantibodies may cause difficulty in cross matching)
  - Danazol with prednisone as first-line therapy allowing for a shorter duration of prednisone therapy.
  - **Splenectomy** may be necessary.
    - If there is no response to corticosteroids, or
    - If the remission is not maintained when the dose of prednisolone is reduced, or
    - Require equivalent of > 10–15 mg/day prednisone to maintain haemoglobin levels.
- **Intravenous immunoglobulin:** Temporary treatment before splenectomy for those refractory to steroids.
- **Rituximab:** Monoclonal antibody directed against CD20 antigen expressed on B lymphocytes.

ANAEMIA OF CHRONIC DISEASE

Causes: It occurs in a wide variety of chronic diseases.
- **Chronic infections:** Infective endocarditis, tuberculosis, and osteomyelitis
- **Chronic immune disorders:** Crohn's disease, rheumatoid arthritis, and systemic lupus erythematosus
- **Associated with malignant tumours** (e.g., carcinoma of lung and breast)

Investigations
- **Peripheral smear:** Normocytic normochromic red cells
- **Increased storage iron** in the marrow (Prussian blue staining)
- **Raised serum ferritin** because of the inflammatory process
- **Reduced total iron-binding capacity** (TIBC). **Reduced serum iron.**
- Reduced transferrin levels. Normal serum soluble transferrin receptor level.

Management
- Treat the underlying disorder
- Recombinant EPO therapy may be tried if the anaemia is not corrected after treatment of the underlying disorder.

APLASTIC ANAEMIA

It is characterised by pancytopaenia (anaemia, neutropaenia, and thrombocytopaenia) with hypocellular bone marrow (< 30% cellularity), and no leukaemic, or other abnormal cells in the peripheral blood or bone marrow.

Causes of aplastic anaemia have been discussed in **Box 11.4**.

Treatment/Management
- **Removal of the causative factor**/agent wherever possible (refer causes of aplastic anaemia)
- **Providing supportive care** while awaiting bone marrow recovery
  - Prevention and treatment of infections
  - Treatment of haemorrhage
  - Treatment of anaemia by red cell transfusion
- **Severe aplastic anaemia**
  - **Stem-cell transplantation:** Treatment of choice for patients under 40 years who have an HLA-identical sibling donor. Patients over the age of 40 years—high risk of graft-versus-host disease (GVHD).
  - **Immunosuppressive therapy:** Patients without HLA-matched siblings and > 40 years of age.
    - Antilymphocyte globulin (ALG) and cyclosporine combination produces

haematological response rate of 60–80%. (Destroy activated suppressor cells)
- Androgens (e.g., oxymetholone) are sometimes useful in patients not responding to immunosuppression and those with moderately severe aplastic anaemia.

- *Steroids*: Little role in severe aplastic anaemia, useful for serum sickness induced by ALG. Steroids are used in children with congenital pure red cell aplasia (diamond-black fan syndrome) and in some adults with pure red cell aplasia associated with a thymoma.

■ PLATELET DISORDERS

Distinguishing patterns of bleeding in platelet and coagulation disorders have been explained in **Table 11.19**.

Laboratory Investigations

Evaluation of laboratory tests have been explained in **Table 11.20**.

■ THROMBOCYTOPAENIA

Causes of thrombocytopaenia have been explained in **Table 11.21**.

General Clinical Manifestations (Table 11.22)

- **Skin:** Purpura, petechiae, and ecchymoses.
- **Mucous membranes:** Epistaxis, haemorrhagic bullae in oral mucosa, genitourinary and GI bleeding.
- Severe thrombocytopaenia produces fundal haemorrhage and intracranial bleeding.

Laboratory Investigations

- **Platelet count:** Reduced and manifestations roughly correlate with the platelet count.

Box 11.4: Autoimmunohaemolytic anaemia.

Inherited:
- Fanconi anaemia
- Diamond-Blackfan anaemia
- Telomerase defects

Acquired

Idiopathic:
- Acquired defects in stem cell
- Immune mediated

Secondary
- **Chemical agents**
  - **Dose related:** Cytotoxic drugs (alkylating agents, antimetabolites), benzene, inorganic arsenicals, and chloramphenicol
  - **Idiosyncratic:** Chloramphenicol, phenylbutazone, penicillamine, carbamazepine, Gold salts, organic arsenicals, methylphenylethylhydantoin
- **Physical Agents:** Whole-body irradiation
- **Viral Infections**
  - Hepatitis (unknown type)
  - Epstein-Barr virus infections
  - Cytomegalovirus infections
  - Herpes zoster (Varicella zoster)
  - Human immunodeficiency virus (HIV)

TABLE 11.19: Distinguishing patterns of bleeding in platelet and coagulation disorders.

Characteristics	Platelet/vascular disorders	Coagulation disorders
Onset	Spontaneous and develops immediately after trauma/surgery	Delayed bleeding after trauma/surgery
Type of lesion	Petechiae, ecchymoses	Haematomas
Sites	Skin, mucous membrane	Deep tissues
Mucous membrane	Common from nose, mouth, gastrointestinal and genitourinary tracts	Uncommon except from gastrointestinal or genitourinary tract
Into the joint	Absent	Common in severe factor deficiencies
Into the muscle	Following trauma	Spontaneous
Local pressure	Effective	Ineffective

- **Hess test (capillary fragility test/tourniquet test) may be positive**
  - **Principle:** Measures the ability of capillaries to withstand the increased stress.

TABLE 11.20: Evaluation of laboratory tests.

Name of the test	Evaluation
Blood count and film	Number, morphology, blood disorder—leukaemia or lymphoma
Platelet count ($150–350 \times 10^3/mm^3$)	Platelets
Bleeding time (<9 min)	Platelet function, von Willebrand factor
Prothrombin time (12–14 s)	Extrinsic pathway, factors V, VII, X; factor II X, XII; factor II
Activated partial thromboplastin time (33–45 s)	Intrinsic pathway, factors I and II
Thrombin time (3–5 s > control)	Common pathway, factors I and II
Clot retraction	Platelets
Fibrinogen concentration	Fibrinogen
Fibrin degradation products (FDPs)	Lysis of fibrin

  - **Procedure**
    - Sphygmomanometer cuff is tied to the upper arm and the cuff is inflated to 80 mm for 5 minutes.
    - Release the pressure after 5 minutes and number of petechiae present in a circle of 5 cm diameter on the flexor aspect of forearm (below the bend of the elbow) is noted.
  - **Normal:** 0–5 petechiae.
  - **Interpretation:** Positive test—>10 petechiae and is observed in vascular purpura, defective platelet function, thrombocytopaenia, and scurvy
- **Bleeding time (BT):** Prolonged, and it bears a close relationship to platelet count.
- **Bone marrow:**
  - Normal or increased number of megakaryocytes indicates increased platelet

TABLE 11.22: Clinical features associated with decreased platelet count.

Platelet count/μL	Clinical features
30,000–50,000	Post-traumatic bleeding
<30,000	Spontaneous bleeding
<10,000	Intracranial bleeding

TABLE 11.21: Causes of thrombocytopaenia.

Increased platelet destruction	Decreased production of platelets

Immunemediated
• Primary: Idiopathic thrombocytopenic purpura—Acute and chronic
• Secondary:
  ○ Autoimmune: Systemic lupus erythematosus
  ○ Alloimmune: Post-transfusion or during pregnancy
  ○ Drugs: Quinidine, heparin, and sulpha compounds
  ○ Infections: Human immunodeficiency virus (HIV), infectious mononucleosis, cytomegalovirus (CMV)
Non-immune-mediated
• Disseminated intravascular coagulation
• Thrombotic thrombocytopenic purpura
• Haemolytic uraemic syndrome
• Mechanical destruction
• Microangiopathic haemolytic anaemias
	Generalised diseases of bone marrow
	• Aplastic anaemia: Congenital, acquired
	• Marrow infiltration: Leukaemia, disseminated cancer
	Selective impairment of platelet production
	• Drugs: Alcohol, thiazides, cytotoxic drugs, and alcohol
	• Infections: Measles, HIV
	Ineffective megakaryopoiesis
	• Megaloblastic anaemia
	• Myelodysplastic syndromes

Sequestration	**Dilutional**
Hypersplenism: Portal hypertension, lymphomas, myeloproliferative disorders	

destruction, hypersplenism or ineffective platelet production.
  o Decreased number of megakaryocytes indicates reduced production of platelets.

Management

Treatment of underlying cause. Severe, life-threatening bleeding (fundal haemorrhages and intracranial haemorrhage) can be temporarily treated by platelet transfusions.

■ QUALITATIVE PLATELETS DEFECTS

- Characterised by prolonged bleeding time and normal platelet count.
- It produces defects in the formation of haemostatic plug and thus results in bleeding. Classification of platelet function disorders has been discussed in **Table 11.23**.

■ IMMUNE (IDIOPATHIC) THROMBOCYTOPENIC PURPURA

Autoimmune disorder characterised by increased destruction of platelets by autoantibodies directed against platelet membrane GPIIb/III and GPIb/IX (**Fig. 11.5**).

Pathogenesis

- Antiplatelet antibodies demonstrated in approximately 80% of patients and are of the IgG type.
- Antibody-bound platelets are removed and prematurely destroyed by the spleen causing thrombocytopaenia.
- *Spleen*: Site of destruction of platelets and important site of autoantibody synthesis. Splenectomy shows improvement in about 75–80% of patients.
- Although destruction of sensitised platelets is the major mechanism responsible for thrombocytopaenia, the autoantibodies probably

TABLE 11.23: Classification of platelet function disorders.

Hereditary	Acquired
• **Disorders of adhesion:** Bernard–Soulier syndrome • **Disorders of secretion:** Storage pool deficiency • **Disorders of aggregation:** Glanzmann thrombasthaenia	• **Drugs:** Aspirin, non-steroidal anti-inflammatory drugs (NSAIDs), dipyridamole, sulphinpyrazone • **Renal failure** (Uraemia) • **Haematologic malignancies:** Myeloproliferative, myelodysplastic disorders

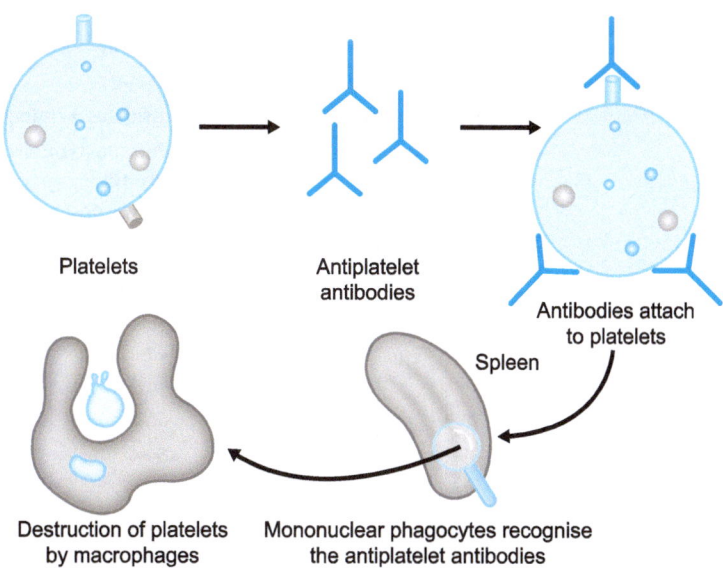

Fig. 11.5: Characterisation of immune (idiopathic) thrombocytopenic purpura.

also affect production of platelets by megakaryocytes and also impair platelet function.

Types of ITP 9 (Table 11.24)

Differences between acute and chronic idiopathic thrombocytopenic purpura have been shown in **Table 11.25**.

Clinical Features

- No physical signs other than those due to bleeding and anaemia (menorrhagia and epistaxis)
- May be associated with haemolysis (Evan's syndrome)

Investigations and diagnosis

- **Platelet count:** Thrombocytopaenia (below 80×10^9/L). Should be repeated using sodium citrate to exclude pseudothrombocytopaenia caused by platelet aggregation and clumping in ethylenediaminetetraacetic acid (EDTA) tubes.
- **Tourniquet test (Hess test):** Positive
- **Bleeding time (BT):** Prolonged
- **Bone marrow:** Moderate increase in number of immature and mature forms of megakaryocytes is usually not performed in acute ITP, unless treatment is necessary on clinical grounds. Important in chronic ITP to rule out thrombocytopaenias resulting from bone marrow failure. Decrease in number of megakaryocytes argues against the diagnosis of ITP.
- **Antiplatelet antibodies:** Not widely available but may be demonstrated in blood. Negative test does not exclude ITP.

TABLE 11.24: Types of immune (idiopathic) thrombocytopenic purpura.

Primary	Secondary
Most cases are primary. Subtypes: • **Acute:** more common in children • **Chronic:** Persistence of thrombocytopaenia for > 6 months, more common in adults	Observed in several diseases such as systemic lupus erythematosus, acquired immunodeficiency syndrome (AIDS), hepatitis C, following viral infections and as a complication of drug therapy

TABLE 11.25: Differences between acute and chronic idiopathic thrombocytopenic purpura.

	Children	Adults
Occurrence		
Peak age (years)	2–4	15–40
Sex (F:M)	Equal	1.2–1.7
Presentation		
Onset	Acute (< 1 week)	Insidious > 2 months
Symptoms	Purpura (< 10% with severe bleeding)	Purpura (typically bleeding not severe)
Platelet count	Most < 20,000/L	Most < 20,000/L
Antecedent infection	Usually follows an antecedent upper respiratory viral infection	Usually no preceding history of viral infection
Course		
Spontaneous remission	83%	2%
Chronic disease	24%	43%
Response to splenectomy	71%	66%
Eventual complete recovery	89%	64%
Morbidity and mortality		
Cerebral haemorrhage	< 1%	3%
Haemorrhagic death	< 1%	4%
Mortality of chronic refractory disease	2%	5%

Treatment (Box 11.5)

- **Children:** Mild acute ITP usually does not require treatment.
- **Adults:** Platelet counts $> 30 \times 10^9/L$ usually do not require treatment. Even lower platelet counts may require treatment, if they have spontaneous bruising or bleeding.
- **Indications for treatment:**
  - Overt haemorrhage (treated with platelet concentrates)
  - Platelet counts below 20,000/mm^3
  - Organ- or life-threatening bleeding irrespective of the circulating platelet count
- **First-line therapy:** Consists of treatment with **oral corticosteroids**.
  - 1–2 mg/kg of prednisolone/day, continued for at least 2 weeks (or if necessary 3–4 weeks), then reduced slowly and stopped.
  - 66% respond to prednisolone but relapse is common when the dose is reduced.
- **Second-line therapy: Splenectomy.**
- **Third-line therapy:** Patients who fail to respond to splenectomy, a wide range of other therapies are available. Major difficulties of these therapies are modest response rates and slow onset of action.

■ THROMBOCYTOSIS

Platelet count $> 4,50,000/mm^3$ is known as thrombocytosis (**Table 11.26**).

Box 11.5: Treatment of idiopathic thrombocytopenic purpura.

- High dose corticosteroids
- Intravenous immunoglobulin (i.e., IgG)
- Rho (D) immune globulin (anti-D)
- Immunosuppressive therapy
  - **Agents:** Vinca alkaloids (vincri0tine, vinblastine), azathioprine, cyclophosphamide, cyclosporine combination chemotherapy, mycophenolate mofetil
- **Plasmapheresis:** Emergency measure to remove antibodies from the plasma
- **TPO mimetic drugs:** eltrombopag or romiplostim
- **Specific immunomodulatory monoclonal antibodies:** Rituximab
- Other therapies
  - **Danazol:** androgen with low virilising activity has been tried in ITP
  - **Dapsone**
- **Platelet transfusions:** Reserved for intracranial or extreme haemorrhages, where emergency splenectomy may be justified
- **Emergency treatment:** Necessary in case of life-threatening bleeding. It consists of intravenous administration of methylprednisolone (30 mg/kg, maximum dose 1 g) over 20–30 min along with platelet transfusion. This is followed by intravenous immunoglobulin

(IgG: immunoglobulin G; ITP: idiopathic thrombocytopenic purpura; TPO: thrombopoietin)

TABLE 11.26: Causes of thrombocytosis.

Primary (autonomous production)	Secondary (reactive thrombocytosis)

• Myeloproliferative neoplasms:
  ○ Essential thrombocytosis
  ○ Polycythaemia vera
  ○ Chronic myeloid leukaemia
• Myelodysplastic syndrome
	• Iron deficiency
	• Malignancy (paraneoplastic feature)
	• Post-haemorrhage: Acute or chronic
	• Following splenectomy
	• Following major surgery
	• Inflammatory disorders: Rheumatoid arthritis and inflammatory bowel disease

CLOTTING ORDERS

■ HAEMOPHILIA A (FACTOR VIII DEFICIENCY)

It is the most common hereditary X-linked recessive disease with a reduction in the amount or activity of factor VIII (antihaemophilic factor). About 30% have no family history and may be due to acquired mutations.

- Antihaemophilic factor is secreted by the liver and has a half-life of 12 hours. In the blood, it is carried bound to the von Willebrand's factor (vWF).
- Factor VIII serves as a cofactor for factor IX in the activation of factor X in the coagulation cascade. Reduced amount or activity of factor VIII is associated with life-threatening bleeding.
- Bleeding is due to both inadequate coagulation and inappropriate clot removal (fibrinolysis).

Inheritance

- X-linked recessive disorder. Males are affected, females are carriers. Incidence: 1 in 10,000 males
- Females can be haemophilic if:
  o She is born to an affected father and a carrier mother (25% risk).
  o Inactivation of the X chromosome such as Turner's syndrome (45 X O)
  o Inactivation of normal X-chromosome due to unfavourable lyonisation (rare)
- A haemophiliac male's daughters will be carriers, while sons will be normal.
- A haemophilia female carrier can have: A haemophiliac boy, a carrier girl, and two normal children.
- Gene can be traced within families by using gene probes.
- Degree of deficiency of factor VIII and severity of bleeding tends to be similar in all the affected members of the same family.

Molecular genetics have detected a variety of defects in haemophilia. The mutations include deletions, inversions, point mutations, and insertions.

Normal level of factor VIII in the blood is 0.50–1.50 IU/mL.

Haemophilia A may be classified based on the factor VIII activity in blood (**Table 11.27**).

Clinical Features

- Clinical severity depends on the level of factor VIII activity and is presented in the **Table 11.27**.
- Excessive bleeding: Haemophilia A is characterised by excessive bleeding but is unusual until the child is about 6 months old.
- Post-traumatic bleeding: Bleeding following trauma is characteristically "delayed".
- Severity of bleeding: Range from mild to severe.
- Petechiae observed in platelet and vascular disorders are not seen in haemophilia.

Haemarthroses, bleeding into muscles, and other features have been discussed in **Table 11.28**.

Laboratory Investigations

- **Bleeding time:** Normal
- **Clotting time:** Prolonged
- **Platelet count:** Normal
- **Prothrombin time:** Normal
- **Activated partial thromboplastin time (APTT):** Increased (Normal 35–45 seconds) to 50 seconds—few minutes.

TABLE 11.27: Factor VIII level and clinical severity in haemophilia A.

Classification	Factor VIII Level	Clinical Features
Severe	≤1% of normal (≤0.01 U/mL)	• Spontaneous haemorrhage from early infancy • Frequent spontaneous haemarthroses and haemorrhages, requiring factor replacement
Moderate	1–5% of normal (0.01–0.05 U/mL)	• Haemorrhage secondary to trauma or surgery • Occasional spontaneous haemarthroses
Mild	6–30% of normal (0.06–0.3U/mL)	• Haemorrhage secondary to trauma or surgery • Rare spontaneous haemorrhage

TABLE 11.28: **Clinical features of haemophilia.**

Haemarthroses	Bleeding into muscles	Others

• Frequent, spontaneous haemorrhage into large joints—knee, elbow, ankle, wrist, and hip
• Spontaneous or follows minor trauma
• **Acute stage:** Affected joint is swollen, hot, and tender, movements severely restricted-gradually subside over a period of days
• **Consequences:** Recurrent bleeding into joints will lead to crippling deformities and disuse atrophy of muscles around the joint
	• **Commonly**—calf, psoas muscles
	• **Consequences:**
	  ○ **Psoas haematomas:** Femoral nerve compression resulting in sensory disturbances over thigh and weakness of quadriceps
	  ○ **Calf haematomas:** Contraction and shortening of the Achilles tendon
		• Easy bruising
		• Massive bleeding following trauma or procedures (dental extraction)
		• Cerebral haemorrhage
		• Haematuria, ureteric colic due to passage of blood clots

- **Factor VIII assay:** Confirmation of diagnosis, to assess factor VIII levels and severity of disease.

Management
- **Replacement therapy**
  ○ Factor VIII concentrate is available as plasma-derived and recombinant products.
  ○ **Indications of replacement therapy:**
    – Early treatment of spontaneous bleeding
    – Severe or prolonged wound and tissue bleeding
    – Control of bleeding during and after surgery and trauma
    – Prophylaxis: In all patients with severe haemophilia so as to prevent recurrent bleeding into joints and subsequent joint damage (arthropathy).
- **Non-tranfusion therapy in haemophilia**
  ○ D-amino D-arginine vasopressin (DDAVP) (1-amino-8-D-arginine vasopressin)
  ○ Antifibrinolytic drugs

Complications: About 15% of the patients receiving factor VIII therapy develop inhibitory antibodies that bind and inhibit factor VIII.
- **Treatment for patients with factor VIII inhibitors:** Immune tolerance induction (ITI) is the most effective strategy of eradication of inhibitor with steroids or other immunosuppressants.

- Antibodies to antihaemophilic globulin (AHG) may occur de novo in non-haemophiliacs as part of an immunological disorder such as systemic lupus erythematosus.

■ HAEMOPHILIA B (CHRISTMAS DISEASE)

Deficiency of factor IX.

Mode of inheritance: X-linked disorder.

Clinical Features
Similar to haemophilia A. Patients with severe disease present with muscle haematomas and haemarthroses which progress to crippling joint deformities.

Diagnosis
Factor IX assay shows deficiency of factor.

Management: Similar to haemophilia A.
- Replacement therapy:
  ○ Fresh frozen plasma (FFP) to treat mild-to-moderated bleeding
  ○ Recombinant factor IX: To treat moderate-to-severe bleeding.
- Gene therapy: This may be effective in managing severe disease.
- Desmopressin is ineffective.

■ VON WILLEBRAND'S DISEASE

Characterised by defective platelet function and factor VIII deficiency, due to a deficiency or dysfunction of von Willebrand factor (vWF).

Major categories: *vWF* gene—Chromosome 12 and numerous mutations of the gene produce von Willebrand's disease (vWD).
- **Quantitative deficiency in vWF:**
  - Type 1: Autosomal dominant, relatively mild disorder
  - Type 3: Autosomal recessive disorder and is a severe disorder.
- **Qualitative defects (dysfunction) in vWF:** Type 2 accounts for 25% of all cases and is usually an autosomal dominant disorder. There are several subtypes:
  - Type 2a is most commonly characterised by defective assembly of multimers.
  - Type 2b is caused by synthesis of an abnormal vWF with increased affinity for platelets which results in thrombocytopaenia.

von Willebrand factor: Protein synthesised by endothelial cells and megakaryocytes.
- **Main functions:**
  - Von Willebrand factor acts as a **carrier protein** which binds to **factor VIII** and forms plasma factor VIII-vWF complex. vWF protects factor VIII and is important for its stability. It has no role in the coagulation cascade, but deficiency of vWF causes a secondary reduction of factor VIII causing coagulation defect.
  - Von Willebrand factor is the most important co-factor for adhesion of platelets to the exposed subendothelial collagen matrix by GpIb/IX. Hence, the deficiency of vWF results in a defect of platelet function.

Clinical Features
- Variable and ranges from mild asymptomatic conditions to a severe haemorrhagic disorder.
- Spontaneous bleeding from mucous membranes (e.g. epistaxis), excessive bleeding from wounds or menorrhagia. In severe cases, manifestations may be similar to haemophilia A.

Laboratory Findings
- **Platelet count** is **normal**.
- **Bleeding time** is **prolonged** despite a normal platelet count because of defect in platelet function.
- **Tourniquet test** (Hess test): **Positive** due to defect in platelet adhesion.
- **Activated partial thromboplastin time: Prolonged** because vWF stabilises factor VIII by binding to it. A deficiency of vWF gives rise to a secondary decrease in factor VIII levels.
- **Von Willebrand factor assay:** Plasma level of active vWF is **decreased**.

Management
Mild bleeding: Desmopressin.

Severe bleeding: Intravenous cryoprecipitate or plasma-derived concentrates containing vWF and factor VIII. Recombinant activated factor VII (rFVIIa) has also been successfully used in vWD patients with severe haemorrhage refractory to VWF replacement therapy.

■ VITAMIN K DEFICIENCY
- Clinically, it manifests as ecchymoses, bleeding from injection sites, bruises, gum bleeding, haematemesis, melaena, or haematuria.
- Prothrombin time and activated partial thromboplastin time are prolonged.
- Administration of vitamin K in a dose of 5–10 mg stops bleeding within 1–2 days.
- If blood loss is severe or response to vitamin K is inadequate, transfusion of fresh blood or FFP is indicated.

Causes of excessive fibrinolysis (**Box 11.6**).

■ MICROANGIOPATHIC HAEMOLYTIC STATES
This syndrome consists of two closely related entities—**thrombotic thrombocytopaenic purpura (TTP) and haemolytic-uraemic syndrome (HUS)**. The underlying basic defects are:

Box 11.6: Causes of excessive fibrinolysis
- **Obstetric:** Abruptio placentae, amniotic fluid embolism
- **Surgical:** Gastrectomy, lung resection, nephrectomy, prostatectomy, cardiopulmonary bypass, splenectomy, and pancreatectomy
- **Medical:** Liver diseases (cirrhosis) Leukaemias (acute leukaemia, chronic granulocytic leukaemia type IV) anaphylactic shock, autoimmune diseases (SLE)

(SLE: systemic lupus erythematosus)

- Formation of microthrombi initiated and perpetuated by platelet adhesion and aggregation in the microcirculation of vital organs and consequently of thrombocytopaenia and organ dysfunction, and
- Microangiopathic haemolytic anaemia, resulting from damage to erythrocytes traversing the platelet thrombi and adhesion to endothelium of the affected vessels. Hallmark of microangiopathic haemolytic anaemia is presence of fragmented and damaged erythrocytes in circulation.
- Unlike in disseminated intravascular coagulation (DIC), there is no gross alteration in the process of coagulation and fibrinolysis.

THROMBOTIC THROMBOCYTOPAENIA PURPURA

It is a type of severe microangiopathic haemolytic anaemia (MAHA), characterised by systemic platelet aggregation, organ ischaemia, profound thrombocytopaenia (with increased marrow megakaryocytes), fragmentation of erythrocytes, fever, and renal failure.

Aetiology and Pathogenesis (Fig. 11.6)

- Normally endothelial cells and megakaryocytes secrete normal vWF multimers into the plasma. These multimers spontaneously develop into unusually large multimers which are effective in platelet adhesion.
- *Plasma protease enzyme*: ADAMTS-13 [a disintegrin and metalloproteinase with a thrombospondin type 1 motif, member-13 (vWF metalloprotease)] regulates activity of vWF by cleaving haemostatically active unusually large multimers into normal multimers. ADAMTS-13 regulates size of vWF multimers and prevents platelet adhesion.
- *Thrombotic thrombocytopaenia purpura*: Inherited or acquired deficiency of ADAMTS-13. Deficiency leads to accumulation of unusually large multimers of vWF in plasma.

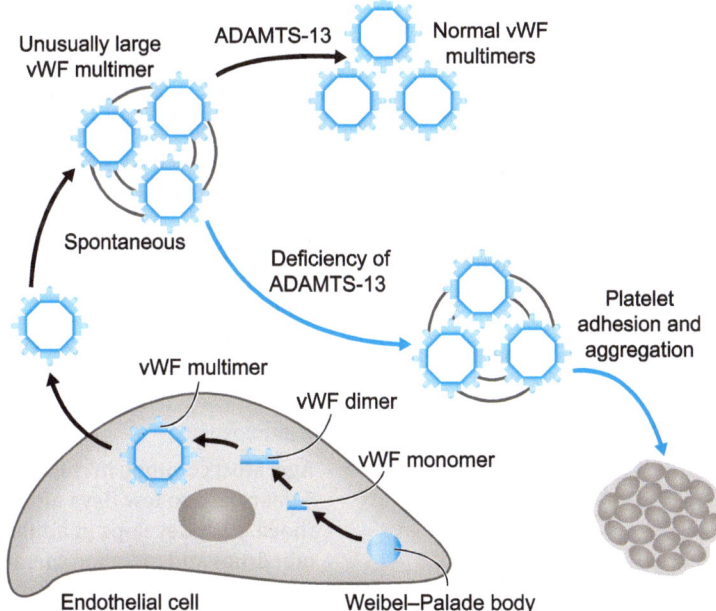

(ADAMTS-13: a disintegrin and metalloproteinase with a thrombospondin type 1 motif, member 13; vWF: von Willebrand factor)

Fig. 11.6: Aetiology and pathogenesis of thrombotic thrombocytopaenic purpura (TTP).

- These large multimers promote platelet adhesion or promote intravascular platelet aggregation and cause spontaneous activation of the coagulation cascade.
- This results in hyaline thrombi throughout the microcirculation, leading to tissue ischaemia and infarction that are characteristic of TTP.
- **Secondary causes:** These include pregnancy, oral contraceptives, SLE, infection and drugs (ticlopidine and clopidogrel). They may or may not have associated antibodies to ADAMTS-13.

Clinical Features

The classic five symptoms of TTP are: (1) Microangiopathic haemolytic anaemia (MAHA) with schistocytosis (at least 3 cells per 100), (2) severe thrombocytopaenia, (3) transient neurologic symptoms secondary to central nervous system (CNS) ischaemia, (4) fever, and (5) renal abnormalities including haematuria and/or proteinuria.

Laboratory Findings

- **Platelet count:** Markedly reduced often below 20,000/μL (thrombocytopaenia).
- Peripheral blood smear shows fragmented red cells (called **schistocytes**) and numerous reticulocytes.
- *Prothrombin time (PT), partial thromboplastin time (PTT), and fibrinogen concentration*: Normal, because the coagulation system is not activated.
- *Urine*: It shows moderate proteinuria and both gross and microscopic haematuria.
- **Serum LDH: Raised** due to release from ischaemic tissues.
- **ADAMTS-13 activity: Reduced** below 5–10% of normal.

Diagnosis: Schistocytes and elevated serum LDH (out of proportion to the degree of haemolysis) suggest the diagnosis of TTP.

Treatment

- **Plasma exchange**
- **Corticosteroids:** Pulsed intravenous methylprednisolone is given acutely and is generally added to plasma exchange to suppress formation of antibody.
- **Rituximab:** It is a monoclonal antibody against CD20 and suppresses antibody-producing cells. It is used in those patients who are refractory to plasma exchange and corticosteroids.
- **Splenectomy:** Performed in resistant cases which remove antibody-producing cells.
- **Platelet concentrates are contraindicated.**

Prognosis: Untreated cases have a mortality of up to 90% but with modern management it has been reduced to about 10%.

■ HAEMOLYTIC–URAEMIC SYNDROME

Haemolytic–uraemic syndrome is distinguished from TTP by the absence of fever and neurologic symptoms, the prominence of acute renal failure (uraemia), frequent affection of children, and different pathogenesis.

Aetiology and Pathogenesis

- Develops following damage to the endothelium by toxins, drugs, or radiation.
- A main cause of HUS in children and elderly is infectious gastroenteritis caused by *Escherichia coli (E. coli)* strain 0157:H7 (**Fig. 11.7**). *E. coli* produces a Shiga-like toxin which is absorbed from the inflamed gastrointestinal mucosa which enters circulation and damages endothelial cells of microvasculature, mainly in the renal glomerular capillaries and initiates platelet activation and thrombi formation.
- Red cells get trapped in the formed thrombi and undergo for fragmentation resulting in schistocytes.
- Splenic trapping of the fragmented red cells causes extravascular haemolysis.

Clinical Features

- **Age:** Most common in children between 1 and 5 years of age few days after a bloody diarrhoea. Also develops in adults following certain drugs and radiation therapy that damage endothelial cells.
- **Classical presentation:** Triad of microangiopathic haemolytic anaemia, thrombocytopaenia, and renal failure (oliguria). Haematuria and hypertension are also common. Despite

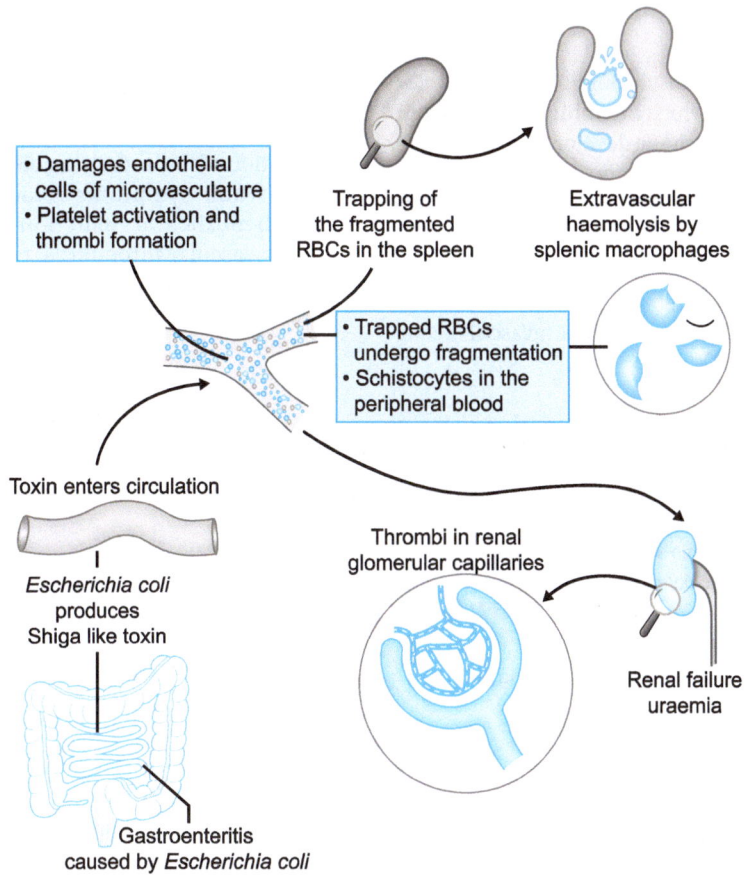

(RBC: red blood cell)

Fig. 11.7: Aetiology and pathogenesis of haemolytic-uraemic syndrome.

thrombocytopaenia, bleeding manifestations are rare.
- **Complications:** Fluid overload may result in pulmonary oedema and hypertensive encephalopathy.

Investigations

- *Haemoglobin levels*: Decreased (anaemia).
- *Platelet count*: Markedly reduced often below 20,000/μL (thrombocytopaenia).
- *Peripheral blood smear*: Fragmented red cells (schistocytes) and numerous reticulocytes.
- *Lactate dehydrogenase*: Elevated.
- *Blood urea and creatinine*: Elevated.
- *Urine*: May show proteinuria and red blood cells.
- *Prothrombin time and activated partial thromboplastin time*: Normal
- *Stool*: Culture for enterohaemorrhagic E. coli—positive; Shiga toxin—positive.

Treatment

- *Supportive care*: For the renal and haematological complications.
- *Antibiotics*: If shigellosis is suspected/detected.
- *Experimental*: Eculizumab, monoclonal antibody to C5.

Prognosis: With appropriate supportive care, they usually recover completely, but in more severe cases renal damage may result in death.

DISSEMINATED INTRAVASCULAR COAGULATION

Widespread acute or chronic thrombohaemorrhagic disorder in which a **combination of thrombosis and haemorrhage** develops as a secondary complication of wide variety of disorders.

Major disorders associated with DIC have been discussed in **Table 11.29**.

Pathogenesis

Pathogenesis of disseminated intravascular coagulation (**Fig. 11.8**).

Clinical Features (Table 11.30)

- Serious, often fatal, and important clinical condition which needs an immediate diagnosis and management. The symptoms of DIC depend on the nature, intensity, and duration of the underlying disorder.
- Signs and symptoms related to the tissue hypoxia and infarction caused by the microvascular thrombosis; or with bleeding diathesis due to the depletion of factors and the activation of fibrinolytic mechanisms; or both.

TABLE 11.29: Major disorders associated with disseminated intravascular coagulation.

Infections	Massive tissue injury
• Gram-negative bacterial sepsis	• Trauma, burns
• Meningococcaemia and other bacteria	• Fat embolism
• Fungi, viruses, rocky-mountain spotted fever, malaria	• Surgery

Neoplasms	Vascular disorders
• Carcinomas of pancreas, prostate, lung, and stomach	• Aortic aneurysm, giant haemangioma, vasculitis
• Acute promyelocytic leukaemia	

Obstetric complications	Miscellaneous
• Retained dead foetus	• Snake bite
• Septic abortion	• liver disease
• Abruptio placentae	• acute intravascular haemolysis
• Amniotic fluid embolism	• shock, heat stroke
• Toxaemia and pre-eclampsia	• hypersensitivity

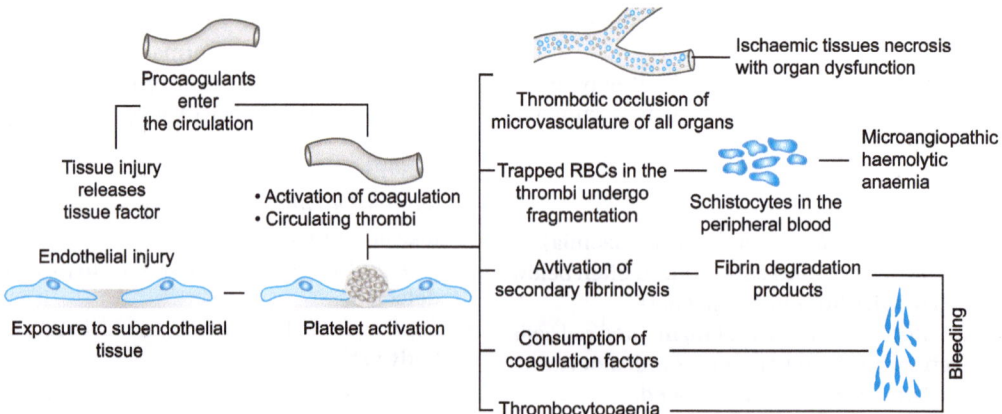

Fig. 11.8: Pathogenesis of disseminated intravascular coagulation.

TABLE 11.30: Effects and signs of disseminated intravascular coagulation (DIC).

Organ/site	Due to thrombi in microvasculature	Due to haemorrhagic diathesis
Central nervous system	Multifocal infarcts, delirium, and coma	Intracerebral bleeding
Renal system	Cortical necrosis—oliguria, and azotaemia	Haematuria
Skin	Focal ischaemic necrosis, and gangrene	Petechiae, ecchymoses, and bleeding at the sites of venipuncture
Gastrointestinal tract	Acute ulceration	Massive bleeding
Respiratory tract	Acute respiratory distress syndrome	
Mucous membranes		Epistaxis and gingival bleeding
Peripheral circulation	Fragmentation of trapped RBCs: Microangiopathic haemolytic anaemia	

- *Bleeding*: The most common clinical feature in acute **DIC**—ecchymoses, petechiae or bleeding from mucous membranes or at the sites of venipuncture.
- *Microvascular thrombi*: Ischaemic necrosis of the organ with resultant dysfunction of the involved organ and occur most often with chronic underlying diseases. Organ dysfunction may manifest as hepatic, renal, cardiac or respiratory failure, or neurological disturbances. It may also result in gangrene of extremities and haemorrhagic necrosis of the skin.
- **Waterhouse–Friderichsen syndrome:** Occult thrombosis of adrenal vein thrombosis resulting in adrenal haemorrhage.
- **Trousseau sign:** Migratory venous thrombosis in cancers.
- **Multiorgan dysfunction syndrome (MODS):** Frequent consequence of DIC and is usually due to bleeding into organs or thrombotic alterations in various organs (hepatic, cardiac, central nervous, renal, and pulmonary systems).

Laboratory Findings (Investigations) in Disseminated Intravascular Coagulation (Table 11.31)

- *Erythrocyte sedimentation rate*: Low
- *Peripheral smear*: Presence of schistocytes.
- **Screening assays**
  - **Platelet count:** Decreased because of utilisation of platelets in microthrombi.

TABLE 11.31: Routine Laboratory Value Abnormalities in disseminated intravascular coagulation (DIC).

Test	Abnormality
Platelet count	Decreased
Prothrombin time	Prolonged
aPTT	Prolonged
Fibrin degradation products	Elevated
Protease inhibitors (e.g. protein C, AT - antithrombin, protein S)	Decreased

(aPTT: activated partial thromboplastin time)

  - **Prothrombin time: Increased.**
  - **Activated partial thromboplastin time: Increased** because of consumption and inhibition of the function of clotting factors.
  - **Thrombin time (TT):** Increased because of decreased fibrinogen.
  - **Plasma fibrinogen:** Decreased.
  - Presence of schistocytes (fragmented RBCs) in the peripheral smear
- **Confirmatory tests**
  - **FDP** (fibrin degradation/split products): Secondary fibrinolysis results in generation of FDPs, which can be measured by latex agglutination.
  - **D-dimer** test: D-dimer is formed during fibrinolysis as a result of degradation of cross-linked fibrin by plasmin. D-dimer levels are elevated and are specific for diagnosing DIC.

Management

- *Control or elimination of the underlying cause*: For example, removal of a dead foetus, placenta, etc.
- Correction of precipitating factors: For example, acidosis, dehydration, and hypoxia.
- *Management of haemorrhagic symptoms*: It is necessary to maintain blood volume and tissue perfusion. Haemorrhagic symptoms are managed by transfusions of platelet concentrates, FFP, cryoprecipitate and red cell concentrates.
    - Platelet concentrates: 1–2 units/10 kg
    - Fresh frozen plasma: 15–20 mL/kg
    - *Cryoprecipitate*: 1 unit/10 kg
- Replacement of coagulation or fibrinolysis inhibitors
- Drugs to control coagulation such as heparin or antifibrinolytic drugs have been tried in DIC.
    - *Heparin*: Low doses of continuous infusion heparin (5–10 U/kg/h) are often used in patients with thrombotic manifestations. It should be given after the correction of bleeding. Major indications for heparin therapy are:
        - Purpura fulminans during the surgical resection of giant haemangiomas and during removal of a dead foetus.
        - Acute promyelocytic leukaemia
    - *Antifibrinolytic drugs*: For example, epsilon aminocaproic acid (EACA), or tranexamic acid prevent fibrin degradation by plasmin may reduce bleeding episodes. However, they increase the risk of thrombosis and concomitant use of heparin is indicated.

■ LEUKAEMIAS

Classification

Traditional classification (**Table 11.32**).
Revised French-American-British (FAB) classification of acute leukaemias (**Table 11.33**):
- According to French American-British (FAB), the marrow should show a blast count of 30% or more.
- It includes parameters which affect namely morphology, cytochemistry, immunophenotyping, cytogenetics, and molecular genetics.

TABLE 11.32: Traditional classification of leukaemias.

Acute	Chronic
• Acute myeloblastic/ myelocytic leukaemia (AML) • Acute lymphoblastic/ lymphocytic leukaemia (ALL)	• Chronic myeloid leukaemia (CML) • Chronic lymphocytic leukaemia (CLL)

TABLE 11.33: Revised FAB Classification of acute leukaemias (AML).

Type of AML	Type of ALL
M0 Minimally differentiated AML	L1
M1 AML without differentiation	L2
M2 AML with maturation	L3
M3 Acute promyelocytic leukaemia	
M4 Acute myelomonocytic leukaemia	
M5 Acute monocytic leukaemia	
M6 Acute erythroleukaemia (DiGugliemo's disease)	
M7 Acute megakaryocytic leukaemia	

(ALL: acute lymphoblastic/lymphocytic leukaemia; AML: acute myeloblastic/myelocytic leukaemia; FAB: French-American-British)

TABLE 11.34: Characteristics of chronic lymphocytic and myelocytic (myeloid).

Chronic lymphocytic	Chronic myelocytic (myeloid)
• B-cell CLL: Common • T cell CLL (rare), e.g. cell granular lymphocytic leukaemia • Hairy cell leukaemia • B-cell prolymphocytic leukaemia (PLL)	• Ph[X] positive • Ph[X] negative, BCR[XX] positive • Ph[X] negative, BCR[XX] negative • Eosinophilic leukaemia

(BCR[XX]: breakpoint cluster region; CLL: chronic lymphocytic leukaemia; Ph[X]: Philadelphia chromosome)

Characteristics of chronic lymphocytic and myelocytic (myeloid) have been shown in **Table 11.34**.
World Health Organization classification (2001) of acute myeloid and lymphoid leukaemia incorporates parameters namely

morphology, cytochemistry, cytogenetic, molecular genetics (which are related to prognosis), and clinical features (**Table 11.35**). The number of blasts necessary for the diagnosis is > 20% in bone marrow when compared to 30% in FAB classification.

Aetiology of Leukaemias

Risk Factors

In the majority of acute leukaemias the cause is not known. Numerous risk factors may cause mutations in the genes involved in regulating cell proliferation and differentiation. These genes include oncogenes and tumour suppressor genes. Sophisticated molecular techniques such as fluorescent in situ hybridisation (FISH) and gene array technology have led to the understanding of leukaemia at molecular level.

Environmental Factors

- **Ionising radiation:** Ionising radiation and X-rays are associated with increased risk of leukaemias. The evidences for this association are:
  o **Atomic bombing:** Survivors of atomic bomb explosions in Hiroshima and Nagasaki, who had high incidence of acute myeloblastic leukaemia (AML) and chronic myeloid leukaemia (CML).
  o **Therapeutic radiation:** Increased risk of AML (secondary leukaemia) in patients with malignancies/neoplasms treated by radiation.
  o **X-ray foetus during pregnancy**
- **Drugs:** Drugs can cause secondary haematopoietic neoplasms.
  o Leukaemia develops in patients who have been administered alkylating agents for neoplasms such as Hodgkin lymphoma (HL). The various drugs include nitrogen mustard, chlorambucil, etc.
  o Acute myeloid leukaemia in myeloma patients treated with melphalan.
  o Leukaemia follows chemotherapy of lung and ovarian cancer. Some anticancer drugs induce myelodysplastic changes with certain chromosomal abnormalities and subsequently develop AML.
- **Chemicals:**
  o Benzene is used in paint industry, plastic glues, etc. It causes chromosomal abnormalities resulting in higher incidence of acute leukaemia, myelodysplastic syndrome and aplastic anaemia.

TABLE 11.35: World Health Organization (WHO) Classification showing major subtypes of AML.

Acute myeloid leukaemia (AML)	
I. AML WITH GENETIC ABERRATIONS • AML with t(8;21) (q22; q22); *CBF-α/ETO* fusion gene • AML with inv(16) (p13; q22); *CBF-β/MYH11* fusion gene • AML with t(15;17) (q22;11-12); *RAR-α/PML* fusion gene • AML with t(11q23; v); diverse *MLL* fusion genes • AML with normal cytogenetics and mutated nucleophosmin (NPM)	**III. AML, THERAPY-RELATED** **IV. AML NOT OTHERWISE SPECIFIED** • AML minimally differentiated • AML without maturation • AML with myelocytic maturation • AML with myelomonocytic maturation • AML with monocytic maturation • AML with erythroid maturation • AML with megakaryocytic maturation
II. AML WITH MDS-LIKE FEATURES • With prior MDS • AML with multilineage dysplasia • AML with MDS-like cytogenetic aberrations: 5q-, 7q-, 20q-	
Acute lymphoid leukaemia	
Precursor T-cell acute lymphoblastic leukaemia Burkitt-cell leukaemia	Precursor B-cell acute lymphoblastic leukaemia • t(9;22) (q34; q11); *BCR/ABC* fusion gene • t(4;11) (q21; q23); *MLL-AF4* fusion gene • t(1;19) (q23; p13.3); *E2A/PBX1* fusion gene • t(12;21) (p13; q22); *TEL/AML1*

- **Viruses:** Leukaemias are often associated with human T cell lymphotropic virus type 1 (HTLV-1).
- **Immunological:** Immune deficiency states

Genetic Disorders

A few genetic disorders may be associated with acute leukaemias, e.g. Down's syndrome [acute lymphoblastic leukaemia (ALL) or AML], Fanconi's anaemia (AML), ataxia telangiectasia [ALL, non-Hodgkin lymphoma (NHL)], and Klinefelter syndrome.

Acquired Disorders

- Acquired stem-cell disorders such as PNH and aplastic anaemia may transform into acute leukaemia.
- *Myelodysplastic syndromes*: AML may develop de novo or secondary to MDS.

ACUTE LEUKAEMIA

Leukaemia is defined as a group of malignant stem cell neoplasms characterised by failure of cell maturation, proliferating of leucocyte precursors (blast/immature cells) which fill the bone marrow and abnormal numbers and forms of immature white blood cells ultimately spill over into the peripheral blood.

Clinical Features

Though ALL and AML are distinct (immunophenotypically and genotypically), they usually have similar clinical features. Patient usually presents with non-specific "flu-like" symptoms.

- **Bone marrow failure:** Replacement of normal marrow haematopoietic cells by leukaemic blast cells.
- **Anaemia:** Causes shortness of breath on effort, excessive tiredness/fatigue, and weakness.
- **Neutropaenia** results in life-threatening infections by bacteria or opportunistic fungi, *Pseudomonas* and commensals. Fever due to septicaemia. The infection may develop in the oral cavity, skin, lungs, kidneys, urinary bladder, and colon. The common presentations include respiratory infections (pneumonia), cellulitis, or sepsis.
- **Thrombocytopaenia** presents as bleeding manifestations in the form of petechiae, atraumatic ecchymosis, gum bleeding, epistaxis, urinary tract, and fundal haemorrhages. Intracranial bleeding is a serious and fatal complication and is usually associated with headache, fundal haemorrhages, and focal neurological deficits.
- Marrow expansion and infiltration of the subperiosteum causes bone pain (more common in ALL) and sternal tenderness.
- **Leucostasis:** Stasis of blood flow may develop when the blast count is above 50,000/mm^3.
- Cerebral leucostasis may cause headache, confusion, and visual disturbances.
- Pulmonary leucostasis can cause dyspnoea at rest, tachypnoea, chest pain, pulmonary infarction, and acute respiratory distress syndrome.
- **Coagulopathy:** Both disseminated intravascular coagulation (DIC) and primary fibrinolysis may lead to haemorrhagic diathesis. DIC is observed in AML-M3 (promyelocytic leukaemia).
- **Extramedullary leukaemic infiltration:**
  - Gingival hypertrophy and infiltration of skin (leukaemia cutis):
    - Hepatosplenomegaly
    - Generalised lymphadenopathy
  - Leukaemic meningitis is rare. It presents as headache and nausea. As the disease progresses papilloedema, cranial nerve palsies, seizures, and altered consciousness develop. Cerebrospinal fluid (CSF) characteristically shows leukaemic blast cells, elevated proteins, and reduced glucose levels.
  - *Chloromas*: Localised, solid, soft tissue tumour masses known as myeloblastomas, granulocytic sarcomas or chloromas.
- **Metabolic abnormalities:** Hyperuricaemia, elevated serum liver transaminases, and serum LDH are found in patients with acute leukaemia.

Investigations

- **Confirmation of diagnosis**
  - **Blood count**
    - *Haemoglobin*: Low
    - *Total leucocyte count*: Markedly raised, but usually < 100 × 10^9/L (range 1 × 10^9/L to 500 × 10^9/L). Leucopaenia is common in AML.
    - *Platelet count*: Markedly decreased.

- **Peripheral blood smear:**
  - Shows numerous blast cells and types of blasts can be identified morphologically and confirmed with immunophenotyping.
  - Auer rods are seen as rod-shaped red inclusion in the cytoplasm of myeloblast.
  - Severe normochromic anaemia
- **Bone marrow aspirate:** Hypercellular with reduced erythropoiesis and reduced megakaryocytes. Blast cells > 20% (often approaching 100%) and type of blast is confirmed by immuno-phenotyping (FISH), cytogenetic and molecular genetics.
- **Chest X-ray:** Mediastinal widening is often seen in T lymphoblastic leukaemia.
- *Cerebrospinal fluid examination*: To rule out occult CNS involvement
- **For planning therapy**
  - Biochemical parameters:
    - Serum urate
    - Liver function tests
    - Renal function tests
    - Coagulation studies
    - Plasma LDH
  - *Cardiac function*: ECG and direct tests of left ventricular function [echocardiogram or multiple-gated acquisition (MUGA) scan]

Management

At initial presentation, acute leukaemia may be:
- Probably curable (childhood ALL)
- Possibly curable (de novo low-risk AML)
- Probably incurable (AML with adverse cytogenetic features in the elderly, secondary AML, and recurrent acute leukaemia).
- **Palliative therapy:** Both chemotherapy and irradiation in addition to blood product support.
- **Curative therapy:** Implies that cure is possible and does not mean that cure is guaranteed or even expected. The failure rate may be high.
- **Active therapy:** The first and major decision to be taken is whether to give specific therapy or supportive therapy.
- **Supportive care/therapy:** Forms the basis of treatment for both curative and palliative therapy.
  - Treatment of anaemia with repeated transfusion of packed red cells to avoid symptoms of anaemia (haemoglobin > 10 g/dL).
  - Prevention or control of bleeding due to thrombocytopaenia with platelet transfusions.
  - Treatment of infection:
    - *Prophylactically*: Education about hand washing and isolation facilities. Use of selected antibiotics and antifungal agents.
    - *Therapeutically*: Management of fever by identifying the micro-organism and giving appropriate antimicrobial treatment in bacterial, fungal, protozoal, and viral infections.
  - Barrier nursing
  - Continuous monitoring of liver, kidney, and haemostatic functions
  - *Maintenance of fluid and electrolyte balance*: In patients receiving chemotherapy, rapid lysis of leukaemic cells may produce tumour lysis syndrome characterised by hyperuricaemia, hypokalaemia, and hyperphosphataemia. It can be prevented by close attention to hydration, urine alkalinisation, and prophylactic allopurinol before starting chemotherapy.
  - *Treatment of hyperleucocytosis*: Reduction in leucocyte counts can be achieved by using chemotherapy or hydroxyurea, and leukapheresis (removal of circulating cells and re-infusion of leucocyte—poor plasma).
  - Psychological support

Bone marrow transplantation has to be considered in following condition:
- Acute myeloblastic leukaemia in first remission in patients below 40 years of age
- Acute lymphoblastic leukaemia in first, second, or subsequent remission.

Specific Therapy

The specific therapy is intended to return the peripheral blood and bone marrow to normal [complete remission (CR)].

ACUTE LYMPHOCYTIC LEUKAEMIA

Specific therapy involves:
- **Remission induction** with combination chemotherapy (**Flowchart 11.1**)
  - *Goal of induction therapy*: To induce morphologic remission and to restore normal haematopoiesis in the bone marrow with <5% blasts.
  - Remission induction consists of combination chemotherapy including vincristine, prednisolone (dexamethasone), asparaginase (crisantaspase), and usually an anthracycline antibiotic, e.g. doxorubicin. It induces complete morphologic response within 4–6 weeks.
- **Consolidation phase (Flowchart 11.1)**—includes administration of high-dose systemic therapy and CNS-directed treatment.
  - *Aim*: To eliminate disease in the CNS and to reduce systemic minimal residual leukaemic burden.
  - Central nervous system-directed therapy consists of weekly or bi-weekly intrathecal therapy along with high-dose systemic therapy with methotrexate and 6-mercaptopurine. Cyclophosphamide and cytarabine (cytosine arabinoside) may also be used in consolidation phase.
- **Re-induction or re-intensification** (similar to induction phase) reduces chances of relapse.
- **Remission maintenance** to prevent relapse and effect cure. It involves administering drugs for 2 years or more and consists of daily 6-mercaptopurine and weekly methotrexate.

ACUTE MYELOID LEUKAEMIA

Initial therapeutic goal is to quickly induce CR and further therapy to prolong survival and achieve cure. Curative therapy is given to the majority of adults below the age of 60 years (without any significant co-morbidity).

Specific therapy of the newly diagnosed patient with AML is usually divided into two phases (1) induction and (2) maintenance (post-remission) therapy (**Flowchart 11.2**).
- **Induction chemotherapy:** Moderately intensive combination chemotherapy that includes an anthracycline (e.g. daunorubicin or idarubicin) and cytosine arabinoside (cytarabine) ± etoposide. "High-risk" patients (include patients <70 years with high-risk karyotype) may only be treated with curative intent if an HLA-identified sibling is available for stem-cell transplantation.

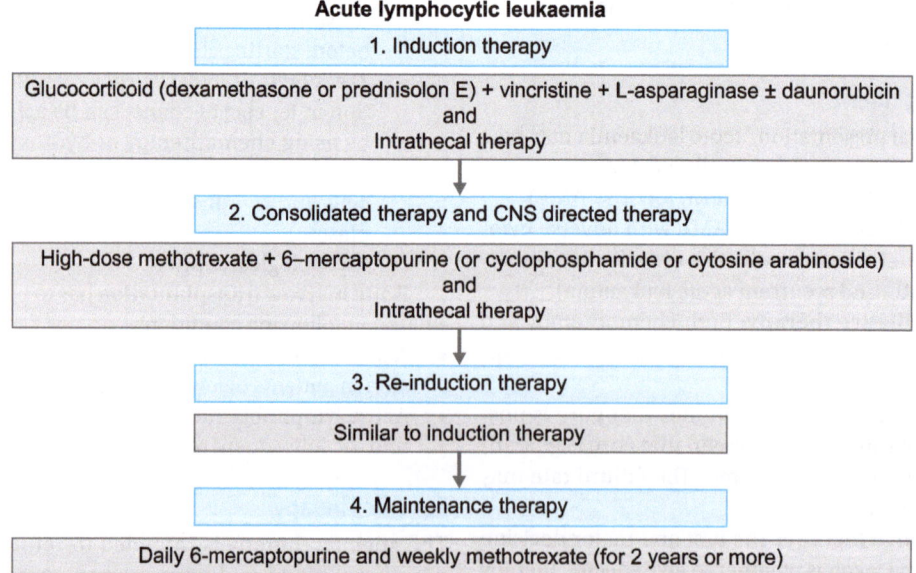

Flowchart 11.1: Steps of therapy of acute lymphocytic leukaemia.

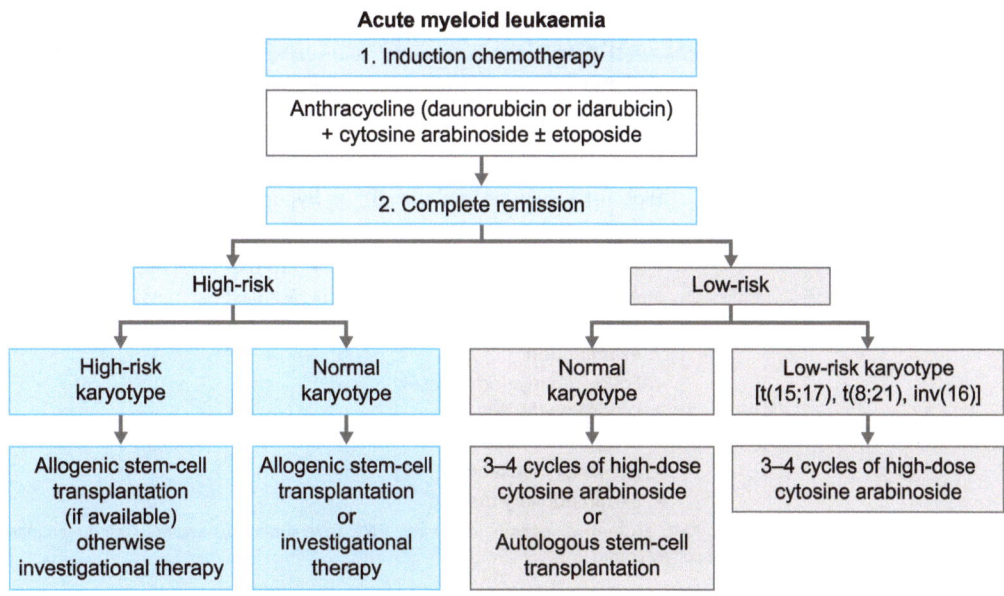

Flowchart 11.2: Steps of therapy of acute myeloid leukaemia.

- **Maintenance or post-remission therapy:** For patients achieving remission with induction therapy in young patients (<60 years) consists of 3–4 cycles of high-dose cytosine arabinoside.
  - Low risk patients in AML, patients with t(15;17) t(8;17) or inv(16) (i.e., low-risk karyotype) do not benefit from allogeneic stem-cell transplantation during their first complete remission.
  - Patients with high-risk karyotypes should have stem-cell transplantation because they respond poorly to conventional chemotherapy.

ACUTE PROMYELOCYTIC LEUKAEMIA (M3)

Uncommon variant of AML associated with severe coagulation complications. It has favourable prognosis. Responds well to combination of induction therapy plus all-trans-retinoic acid (ATRA). Alternatively, daunorubicin and cytarabine or idarubicin can be given.

Allogeneic transplantation: Necessary, if the leukaemia is not eliminated at the molecular level or following a second remission after recurrence.

In relapsed cases, arsenic trioxide (induces apoptosis via activation of the caspase cascade) has been also found to be effective.

Alternative chemotherapy: Used to curb excessive leucocyte proliferation and not for achieving remission.

Hydroxyurea up to 4 g daily and mercaptopurine up to 150 mg daily are used to reduce leucocyte count without inducing bone marrow failure.

Poor prognostic factors in AML and ALL have been shown in **Table 11.36** and differences between AML and ALL have been shown in **Table 11.37**.

HAIRY CELL LEUKAEMIA

Uncommon chronic malignant disorder of mature B cells with characteristic fine cytoplasmic projections. The term **hairy cell leukaemia** is derived from the appearance of fine hair-like cell membrane projections on the leukaemic cells, under the phase-contrast microscope.

Affects middle-aged to elderly men, with a male-to-female ratio of 5:1.

TABLE 11.36: Poor prognostic factors in AML and ALL.

Features	AML	ALL
Age	> 60 years	< 1 year or > 9 years
TLC	> 1,00,000/mm³	> 50,000/mm³
French-American-British (FAB) type	M0, M5, M6, M7	L3 type
Chromosomal abnormality	High-risk karyotype [t(6;9), inv(3)]	Hypodiploidy (<45 chromosomes)
Other features	• Secondary cause present • Presence of DIC • Auer rod absent • Fibrosis on bone marrow examination • Following myelodysplastic syndrome (MDS) • Relapsed disease • Secondary leukaemia • Extramedullary disease	• Male gender • Pro-B or T-cell ALL • Mediastinal mass • CNS involvement

(ALL: acute lymphoblastic leukaemia; AML: acute myelogenous leukaemia; CNS: central nervous system; DIC: disseminated intravascular coagulation; TLC: total leucocyte count)

TABLE 11.37: Clinical differences between acute myelogenous leukaemia (AML) and acute lymphoblastic leukaemia (ALL).

	Acute lymphoblastic leukaemia	Acute myelogenous leukaemia
Clinical features		
Age	Predominantly children	Predominantly adults
Coagulopathy (DIC)	Absent	Seen in M3
Gingival hypertrophy and dermal infiltrate	Absent	Seen in M4 and M5
Hepatosplenomegaly	In majority (50–75%)	Frequent
Lymphadenopathy	More common	Less common
Leukaemic meningitis	More common	Less common
Testicular involvement	In 10–20%	–
Eye involvement	More common	Less common
Investigations		
Leukaemic blasts	Lymphoblasts (10–15 μm) are smaller than myeloblasts, with a thin rim of agranular cytoplasm and round or convoluted nucleus	Myeloblasts (12–20 μm) are larger than lymphoblasts, with discrete nuclear chromatin and multiple nucleoli
Cytoplasmic Auer rods	Absent	Present in 10–20% (diagnostic)
Nuclear enzyme, terminal deoxynucleotidyl transferase (TdT) in leukaemic blasts	In > 90%	Rarely present
Cytochemical staining		
Myeloperoxidase	Negative	Positive
Sudan black B	Negative	Positive
Non-specific esterase	Negative	Positive in M4 and M5
Periodic acid Schiff (PAS)	Positive > 50% of cells (Block positivity)	Negative

Clinical Features

Mainly due to leukaemic infiltration of bone marrow, liver, and spleen.
- **Massive splenomegaly:** Common finding, hepatomegaly is less common, lymphadenopathy is rare.
- **Pancytopaenia:** Marrow failure and splenic sequestration and is found in >50% of cases.
- **Infections:** About one-third of patients present with infections especially with atypical mycobacteria, which may be due to monocytopaenia. Infections are the most common causes of death.
- **Risk of secondary malignancies:** Hodgkin's lymphoma, non-Hodgkin's lymphoma, and thyroid cancer.
    - **Chemotherapy:** The purine analogues 2-chloroadenosine acetate (2-CDA) (cladribine) and pentostatin are highly effective with just one cycle of treatment. Rituximab is used in patients who do not respond to the above drugs.
    - **Contraindicated drugs:** Corticosteroids and myelotoxic drugs.

Prognosis: Follows an indolent course and prognosis is excellent.

CHRONIC LEUKAEMIAS

■ CHRONIC MYELOID LEUKAEMIA

Myeloproliferative neoplasms (MPN) of **pluripotent haematopoietic stem-cell (HSC)** characterised by **overproduction** of cells of the **myeloid series** (results in marked splenomegaly and leucocytosis) and the presence of the Philadelphia chromosome.

Balanced reciprocal translocation between long arm of chromosome 9 and chromosome 22 resulting in shortened chromosome 22 known as "Philadelphia (Ph) chromosome" (**Fig. 11.9**).

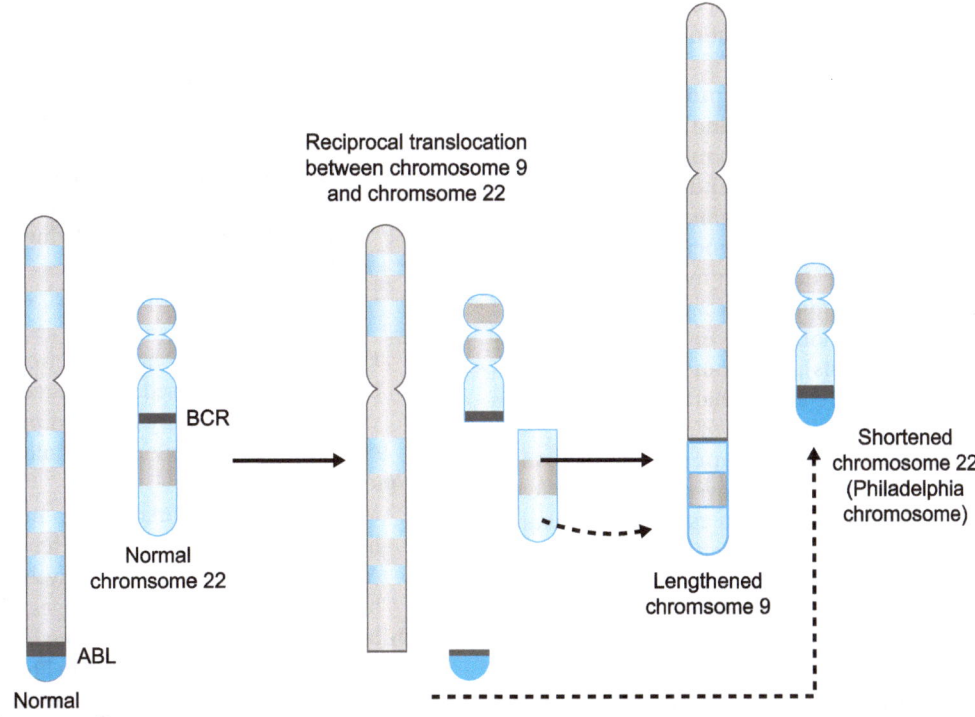

Fig. 11.9: Reciprocal translocation between chromosomes 9 and 22.

Molecular Pathogenesis

- **Philadelphia chromosome:** Acquired chromosomal abnormality of **HSCs. Balanced reciprocal translocation between the long arms of chromosomes 9 and 22 t(9;22)** increases the length of chromosome 9 and shortening of 22.

Natural course of CML: It has three phases.
1. **Chronic stable phase:** Most of the CML are diagnosed in this phase and lasts for about 3–5 years.
2. **Accelerated phase:** More aggressive and lasts for few months.
3. **Blast crisis phase:** It resembles acute (myeloid or lymphoid) leukaemia and has poor prognosis.

Symptoms

- *Age:* Usually occurs between 40 and 60 years of age.
- *Onset:* **Insidious**
- *Symptoms:* Many patients are asymptomatic during early stage of CML and may be diagnosed during routine peripheral blood examination.
  - **Non-specific symptoms:** Fatigue, weakness, weight loss, and anorexia.
  - **Symptoms due to massive splenomegaly: Fullness of abdomen** (abdominal distension, post-prandial fullness), reflux esophagitis, dyspnoea and dragging discomfort in the left hypochondrium due to splenomegaly (caused by leukaemic infiltration and extramedullary haematopoiesis). Splenomegaly is moderate-to-severe and is characteristic feature in majority (80–90%) of patients.
  - **Symptoms of hypermetabolic state:** Due to rapid turnover of cells may result in symptoms such as fatigue, weakness, fever, sweating, heat intolerance weight loss, and anorexia.
  - **Priapism:** Painful penile erection due to leucostasis (associated with marked leucocytosis or thrombocytosis).
  - Bleeding tendencies occur late in the disease.
- **Signs**
  - **Pallor** due to anaemia.
  - **Splenomegaly:** Moderate-to-massive, non-tender splenomegaly. It is due to leukaemia infiltration and extramedullary haematopoiesis. Presence of tender spleen and splenic friction rub indicate splenic infarction.
  - Mild **hepatomegaly** as a result of leukaemic infiltration may develop in 60–70% of cases.
  - **Sternal tenderness and bone pain:** It is due to hypercellularity of marrow and irritation of periosteum.

Investigations

- **Haemoglobin** is usually <11 g/dL.
- **Total leucocyte count** is markedly raising, almost always more than 20,000/μL, often exceeding 1,00,000/μL. In untreated patients, the leucocyte count progressively increases.
- **Peripheral smear (Figs. 11.10A and B):**
  - **Red blood cell** shows moderate degree of **normocytic normochromic anaemia**.
  - **White blood cells**
    - **Shift to left (shift to immaturity)** with granulocytes at all stages of development (neutrophils, metamyelocytes, myelocytes, promyelocytes, and occasional myeloblasts). **Predominant cells** are **neutrophils and myelocytes** in an untreated patient. **Blasts** are usually **<10%** of the circulating white blood cells.
    - Increase in basophils (<20%) and eosinophils
  - **Platelets:** Count may be normal, increased, or decreased. Automated analysers may give falsely elevated platelet counts due to disruption of granulocytes.
- **Bone marrow study:**
  - Markedly hypercellular due to marked hyperplasia of all granulocytic elements.
  - About 20–30% of the patients may develop bone marrow fibrosis in late stages.
- **Philadelphia chromosome** is positive in >95% of cases, in all three phases. In Ph negative cases, evidence of translocation can be demonstrated by cytogenetics, reverse transcription-polymerase chain reaction (RT-PCR) and FISH.

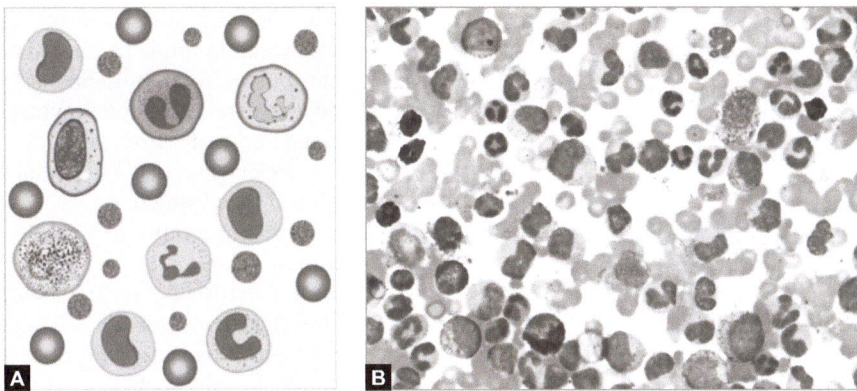

Figs. 11.10A and B: Peripheral blood picture in chronic stable phase of chronic myeloid leukaemia. *(For color version, see plate 4)*

TABLE 11.38: Drugs used and their dosage for induction and maintenance in chronic stable phase of CML.

Drug	Induction dose	Maintenance dose
Imatinib mesylate	300–400 mg/day	300–400 mg/day
Hydroxyurea (hydroxycarbamide)	0.5–2.0 g/day	0.5–2.0 g/day
Melphalan	4–12 mg/day	2–4 mg/day
Busulphan	4 mg/day	2–4 mg/day

(CML: chronic myelogenous leukaemia)

- **BCR-ABL fusion gene** can be demonstrated in peripheral blood or bone marrow.
- **Decreased neutrophil alkaline phosphatase (NAP)/leucocyte alkaline phosphatase (LAP) score:** It is usually below 20 (normal score range from 40 to 100) in majority of patients. This is helpful in differentiating CML from leukaemoid reaction.
- **Biochemical findings:**
  - Serum LDH and uric acid are increased.
  - Serum alkaline phosphatase is increased.
  - Serum vitamin B12 is markedly elevated due to production of binding protein (transcobalamin) by the granulocyte series.
  - Marked thrombocytosis may raise serum potassium spuriously as platelets release potassium during clotting.
  - Blood sugar may be falsely decreased due to glucose uptake and metabolism by leucocytes.

Treatment

- **Goal of therapy in CML:** Complete molecular remission and cure.
  - Achieve prolonged, durable, non-neoplastic, non-clonal haematopoiesis.
  - Eradication of any residual cells containing the *BCR-ABL1* transcript.
- **Chemotherapy**
  - First-line treatment for the chronic phase of CML.
  - If there is failure of response or progress on imatinib, options include: (1) second-generation tyrosine kinase inhibitors (such as dasatinib or nilotinib), (2) allogeneic bone marrow transplantation, or (3) classical cytotoxic drugs such as hydroxycarbamide (hydroxyurea) or interferon-α or melphalan, and busulphan (**Table 11.38**).
  - Hydroxyurea was widely used for initial control of disease and is still useful as palliative therapy. It does not decrease the frequency of the Ph chromosome or affect the onset of blast cell transformation but is used only to reduce leucocyte count. Chemotherapy is started with an induction dose, followed by a maintenance dose for a few months. The drug is reintroduced when the leucocyte counts rise.

Splenectomy
- Indicated to relieve the symptoms due to massive splenomegaly and in repeated splenic infarctions.

Stem cell transplantation (SCT) is the curative treatment

■ CHRONIC LYMPHOCYTIC LEUKAEMIA

Tumour of immature small round lymphocytes characterised by the accumulation of neoplastic mature looking lymphocytes in the peripheral blood, bone marrow, and lymphoid organs (spleen and lymph nodes).

Types
- **B-cell origin:** More than 95% of the cases of chronic lymphocytic leukaemia (CLL) express the pan-B-cell markers CD19 and CD20. And also, aberrant expression of T-cell antigen CD5 (found only in a small subset of normal B cells).
- **T-cell origin:** Constitutes <5%.

Clinical Features
- The most common form of chronic leukaemia.
- **Age:** Most of the patients at the time of diagnosis are over 50 years of age.
- **Sex:** More common in males than in females with a ratio of 2:1.
- **Asymptomatic:** In about 25% of patients and are detected either because of non-specific symptoms or routine blood examination for some other disease.
- **Non-specific symptoms:** This includes fatigue, loss of weight, and anorexia.
- **Painless generalised lymphadenopathy:** Initially the cervical lymph nodes are enlarged and in later stages there may be generalised lymphadenopathy. Involved nodes are rubbery, discrete, non-tender, small, and mobile.
- **Splenomegaly and hepatomegaly:** Mild degree is observed in very few cases.
- Transformation to diffuse large B-cell lymphoma (Richter syndrome).

Investigations
- **Haemoglobin:** Usually below 13 g/dL, as the disease progresses, it may decrease below 10 g/dL. This is due to marrow failure, but associated autoimmune haemolysis may also be contributory, when present.
- **Blood counts:** Total leucocyte count is increased and varies from 20×10^9/L to 50×10^9/L. Platelet count may be normal or low.
- **Peripheral blood smear**
    - Mild-to-moderate normocytic normochromic anaemia
    - Lymphocytosis is the characteristic feature which constitutes >50% of the white cells and absolute lymphocyte count should be $\geq 5.0 \times 10^9$/L.
    - Lymphocytes are of mature type in majority of the cases.
    - Smudge cells or basket cells are disintegrated lymphocytes and are due to the rupture of neoplastic lymphocytes while making the peripheral smear due to its fragile nature.
    - *Platelets*: Normal or reduced in number (autoimmune thrombocytopaenia).
- **Bone marrow:** Involved in all cases of CLL and its infiltration by mature lymphocytes results in hypercellular marrow.
- **Direct Coombs' test:** About 15–20% of patients manifest autoimmune haemolytic anaemia and have positive direct Coombs' test.
- **Lymph node** biopsy shows well-differentiated, small, non-cleaved lymphocytes.
- **Immunoglobulins:** Low or normal.
- Serum folic acid levels are low.

Diagnostic Criteria
Diagnostic criteria of CLL (**Table 11.39**).

TABLE 11.39: Diagnostic criteria of CLL.

Lymphocytosis	Immunophenotype
Absolute lymphocyte count should be >5,000 × 10^9//L	Positive for B-cell surface antigens (CD19, CD20, and CD23)
Lymphocytosis for >2 months	Aberrant expression of T-cell antigen CD5
Lymphoid cells ≤55% atypical immature	Weak expression of monoclonal surface immunoglobulin with κ or λ light chains

Clinical Staging

Clinical staging features of Binet and Rai staging (**Table 11.40**).

Treatment (Table 11.41)

Absolute indications for treatment—when any of the following features is present:
- Anaemia (due to haemolysis) and increasing anaemia or thrombocytopaenia due to bone marrow failure
- Recurrent infection and fever without evidence of infection, extreme fatigue, and night sweats weight loss
- Bulky or progressive lymphadenopathy; massive or progressive splenomegaly with discomfort
- Autoimmune cytopeni is not responsive to corticosteroids.
- Progressive disease manifests by doubling of the lymphocyte count in 6 months.

■ MYELOPROLIFERATIVE DISEASES

Clonal HSC disorders which are characterised by proliferation of one or more of the myeloid lineages (erythroid, granulocytic, megakaryocytic, and mast cells).

TABLE 11.41: Treatment options based on Binet staging.

Binet staging	Treatment
A	No specific therapy required
B	• No specific treatment if asymptomatic • Medically unfit elderly patients with symptoms: Chlorambucil (oral) • Young patients: Fludarabine (IV) • Local radiotherapy to troublesome lymph nodes
C	• Young patients: Fludarabine (IV) • Refractory cases: Combination chemotherapy with cyclophosphamide, hydroxydaunorubicin or doxorubicin, vincristine, and prednisolone (CHOP) • Rituximab in combination with fludarabine • Packed red-cell transfusion (for anaemia) with fludarabine • Prednisolone for patients with haemolytic anaemia and thrombocytopaenia • Splenectomy for symptomatic splenomegaly • Palliative total body irradiation

TABLE 11.40: Clinical staging features of Binet and Rai staging.

Binet staging		
Stage	Features	Survival
A	• No anaemia or thrombocytopaenia • < 3 lymphoid areas of enlarged	> 10 years
B	• No anaemia or thrombocytopaenia • Three or more lymphoid areas enlarged	7 years
C	• Anaemia (Hb < 10 g/dL) and or thrombocytopaenia (< 10,000/mm^3) present, regardless of the number of areas of lymphoid enlargement • Lymphoid enlargement includes cervical, axillary, and inguinal lymph nodes	2 years
Rai staging		
0	Lymphocytosis only in blood (> 5,000/mm^3) and bone marrow	> 10 years
I	Lymphocytosis with lymphadenopathy	9 years
II	Lymphocytosis with splenomegaly or lymphadenopathy or both	7 years
III	Lymphocytosis with anaemia (haemoglobin < 11 g/dL) and organomegaly	5 years
IV	Lymphocytosis with anaemia, thrombocytopaenia, and organomegaly	5 years

Seen in adults with a peak in the 5th to 7th decade. Splenomegaly and hepatomegaly occur commonly due to sequestration of excess haematopoietic cells or proliferation of abnormal haematopoietic cells (**Table 11.42**).

Classification of myeloid neoplasms: Includes five major entitles:
1. Acute myeloid leukaemia
2. Myelodysplastic syndromes
3. Myeloproliferative neoplasms
4. Myelodysplastic/myeloproliferative neoplasms overlap
5. Myeloid neoplasms associated with eosinophilia and specific molecular abnormalities

■ POLYCYTHAEMIA/ERYTHROCYTOSIS

Increase in the number of RBCs above normal in the circulating blood, usually with a corresponding increase in haemoglobin and PCV level. PCV is a more reliable indicator of polycythaemia than is haemoglobin. The increase in red cells can be absolute or relative.

Relative polycythaemia is characterised by decreased plasma volume with a normal red cell mass. They may result from dehydration following prolonged vomiting, diarrhoea or excessive use of diuretics.

Absolute polycythaemia is characterised by a true increase in total red cell mass and can be subclassified as primary and secondary (**Box 11.7**).
- **Primary polycythaemia** or polycythaemia vera (PV): Results from an intrinsic abnormality of the HSC. It is an autonomous, EPO independent proliferation of erythroid cells due to an acquired, clonal HSC disorder. PV is considered as one of the several neoplasms originating from myeloid stem-cells (chronic myeloproliferative neoplasm).
- **Secondary polycythaemia:** Results as a compensatory response of red-cell progenitors to an increase in EPO secretion. The EPO secretion may be physiological as a response to general chronic tissue hypoxia or it may be pathological like in paraneoplastic syndromes.

Clinical Features
- Usually appears insidiously, in late middle age (median age at onset: 60 years).
- Most symptoms are due to the increased red-cell mass and haematocrit.
- Plethora (excessive fullness of blood) and cyanosis due to stagnation and deoxygenation of

TABLE 11.42: World Health Organization (WHO) classification (2008) of myeloproliferative neoplasm (MPN).

• Chronic myelogenous leukaemia, BCR-ABL1 positive	• Chronic eosinophilic leukaemia not otherwise specified
• Chronic neutrophilic leukaemia	• Mastocytosis
• Polycythaemia vera (PV)	• Myeloproliferative neoplasm, unclassifiable
• Essential thrombocythaemia (ET)	
• Primary myelofibrosis (PMF)	

Box 11.7: Pathophysiologic classification of polycythaemia.

Relative
- Reduced plasma volume with normal red-cell mass (haemoconcentration) due to dehydration—low fluid intake, vomiting, diarrhoea, sweating, and acidosis
- Gaisböck syndrome (spurious polycythaemia)

Absolute (increased red cell mass)

Primary (low erythropoietin level)
- Polycythaemia vera (erythremia)

Secondary (high erythropoietin level)—erythrocytosis

Compensatory
- Lung disease [e.g. chronic obstructive pulmonary disease (COPD)]
- Living in high-altitude
- Cyanotic congenital heart disease (Tetralogy of Fallot, Eisenmenger's complex)
- Chronic carbon monoxide poisoning
- Sleep apnoea syndrome
- Smokers

As a consequence of local hypoxia: Renal artery stenosis, end-stage renal disease, hydronephrosis, renal cysts (polycystic kidney disease), post-renal transplant erythrocytosis

Paraneoplastic: Erythropoietin-secreting tumours—Renal cell carcinoma, hepatocellular carcinoma, cerebellar haemangioblastoma, uterine leiomyoma, and pheochromocytoma

blood in peripheral vessels are early findings. Headache, dizziness, and visual problems result from vascular disturbances in the brain and retina.
- Increased incidence of thrombotic episodes and bleeding.
- Secondary polycythaemia, in addition, shows manifestations of the underlying disease.

■ POLYCYTHAEMIA VERA

Acquired myeloproliferative neoplasm arising from malignant transformation of **HSC**.

Trilineage (erythroid, granulocytic, and megakaryocytic) **hyperplasia** in the bone marrow.

Leads to **uncontrolled production of red cells, granulocytes and platelets** (panmyelosis), **erythrocytosis** (polycythaemia), and/or granulocytosis and thrombocytosis. PV is generally dominated by an elevated haemoglobin concentration and polycythaemia is responsible for most of the clinical symptoms.

One of the chronic myeloproliferative neoplasm.

Aetiology

Not known. PV is partly due to a failure of apoptosis as a result of deregulation of the *Bcl-x* gene (anti-apoptotic gene), in addition a mutation in the **in-tyrosine** kinase **JAK-2 V617F** has been found; this stimulates low-grade erythropoiesis.

Clinical Features

- *Onset*: It is insidious.
- *Age and gender*: Late middle age (median age at onset is 60 years) and more common in males.
- Features due to increased viscosity and/or decreased cerebral perfusion
  ○ Plethora (excessive fullness of blood) and deep dusky cyanosis due to stagnation and deoxygenation of blood in peripheral vessels are early findings.
  ○ Headache, dizziness, vertigo, a sense of fullness in the head, rushing in the ears, visual problems, tinnitus, tiredness, syncope, and even chorea result from vascular disturbances in the brain and retina.
- Severe itching (pruritus) after a hot bath or when patient is warm is frequent and may be disabling.
- *Thrombotic episodes*: For example, deep venous thrombosis, myocardial infarction, and thrombosis of hepatic veins (producing Budd–Chiari syndrome).
- *Bleeding manifestations*: Include epistaxis, bleeding from peptic ulcer, bruising and intramuscular haemorrhages.
- Peptic ulcer is seen in few patients and is five times more frequent than general population.
- *Hyperuricaemia*: It may result in urate stones, gout, and uric acid nephropathy.
- Physical findings:
  ○ Injection of the conjunctivae, deep red palate, dusky red hands, and retinal venous engorgement.
  ○ Splenomegaly is very common (~70%) and is useful in distinguishing PV from secondary polycythaemia.
  ○ Hepatomegaly occurs in ~50%.

Diagnosis

- **Haemoglobin increased ranging from** 14 to 28 g/dL
- **Packed-cell volume (haematocrit)** increased to about 60%. However, in many patients, the plasma volume is also increased giving rise to near—normal haematocrit. Hence, it is important to determine the red cell mass.
- **Red cell count: Increased and usually about 6 million/mm³ (6×10^{12}/L)**
- **Increased red-cell volume and blood viscosity:** Red-cell volume is determined by isotope dilution using the patient's ^{51}Cr-tagged red cells (>36 mL/kg in males and 32 mL/kg in females).
- Total white cell count (~70%) and platelet count (~50%) usually increased.
- *Absolute basophil count*: Increased to >100/μL in majority of patients.
- **Arterial oxygen saturation** (PO_2) is normal and is useful for differentiating it from secondary polycythaemia.
- **Erythropoietin levels are decreased** in urine and serum, in contrast to secondary polycythaemia.

- **Bone marrow:** Shows either erythroid hyperplasia or hyperplasia of all elements (trilineage hyperplasia) and depletion of iron stores.
- **Leucocyte alkaline phosphatase (LAP):** Increased in majority of patients.
- **Serum vitamin B12 and vitamin B12-binding protein** transcobalamin-I (TC-I) levels: Increased (not routinely measured)
- **Serum uric acid:** Increased indicating increased cell turnover.
- Abnormal liver function tests
- **Janus kinase 2 (JAK2) mutations** (JAK2V617F mutation)
  - In ~95% patients with PV, and in ~50% of essential thrombocytosis (ET) and primary myelofibrosis.
  - Janus kinases belong to tyrosine kinase family located on chromosome 9
  - Janus kinase 2 is used by the EPO, thrombopoietin, and granulocyte colony-stimulating factor (G-CSF) receptors to transmit signals and is involved in haematopoiesis.
  - Janus kinase 2 inhibitors are used for managing these patients.

World Health Organization (WHO) diagnostic criteria for PV have been shown in **Table 11.43**.

The clinical course tends to proceed as a series of phases.

- **Proliferative phase:** Erythroid proliferation with increased red cell mass.
- **Spent phase:** Excessive proliferation of erythroid cells ceases, resulting in stable or decreased erythrocyte mass
- Progression to myelofibrosis
- Acute myelogenous leukaemia in 2–5% of cases.

Complications
- Thrombotic and bleeding episodes
- Peptic ulcer due to Helicobacter pylori
- Hyperuricaemia (gout)
- Sudden increase in splenic size
- Acute non-lymphocytic leukaemia
- Myelofibrosis and myeloid metaplasia
- Erythromelalgia (thrombocytosis, involving the lower extremities with erythema, warmth, and pain and occasionally digital infarction)

Treatment
Polycythemia vera generally has a very slow course (**Table 11.44**).
- **Aim:** To maintain a normal blood count, PCV below 0.45 L/L and the platelet count below 400×10^9/L and to prevent the complications (mainly thromboses and haemorrhage)
- **Venesection:** Repeated venesection (phlebotomy) is the treatment of choice and relieves many of the symptoms of PV.
- **Chemotherapy**
  - Indicated if patient is intolerant to venesection, or thrombocytosis occurs, or symptomatic or progressive splenomegaly develops.
  - Continuous or intermittent treatment with **hydroxycarbamide (hydroxyurea)** is

TABLE 11.43: World Health Organization (WHO) diagnostic criteria for polycythaemia vera (PV).

Major criteria	Minor criteria
Hb > 18.5 g/dL (men), > 16.5 g/dL (women) OR Hb or PCV > 99th percentile of reference range OR Hb > 17 g/dL (men) or > 15 g/dL (women) if associated with a documented and sustained increase of > 2 g/dL from baseline that cannot be explained otherwise. OR Elevated red cell mass > 25% above mean normal predicted value	• BM showing hypercellularity with trilineage (panmyelosis) myeloproliferation • Subnormal serum EPO level
Presence of JAF2V617F (a mutation in JAK2) or similar mutation	• Endogenous erythroid colony's (EEC's) growth

Diagnostic criteria for PV
Either both major criteria +1 minor criterion or first major criterion + 2 minor criteria

TABLE 11.44: Features of polycythaemia vera and secondary polycythaemia.

Feature	Polycythaemia vera	Secondary polycythaemia
Oxygen saturation	Normal	Low
Erythropoietin (EPO) levels	Decreased	Increased
Blood counts		
Total white cell count	Increased	Normal
Absolute basophil count	Increased	Normal
Platelet count	Increased	Normal
Leucocyte alkaline phosphatase (LAP)	Raised	Normal
Vitamin B12 levels	Increased	Normal
Bone marrow	Trilineage (panhyperplasia)	Erythroid hyperplasia
Splenomegaly	Present	Absent

the treatment of choice in patients above 40 years. It controls thrombocytosis and generally safer than alkylating agents (e.g. busulphan) and ^{32}P (phosphorus) which carry an increased risk of acute leukaemia.
- In younger patients, interferon-α is used.
- **Radioactive ^{32}P:** One dose may control for up to 1.5 years but carries an increased risk to acute leukaemia. In elderly patients, ^{32}P or low-dose of intermittent busulphan may be more convenient.
- **Other measures:**
  - *Low-dose aspirin*: It may be used to reduce thrombotic episodes.
  - *Anagrelide (inhibits platelet aggregation)*: It may be used if thrombotic features develop despite above treatment.
  - Itching should be treated with antihistamines. If antihistamines do not relieve, hydroxyurea, interferon-α, and psoralens with UV light in "A" range (PUVA) may be helpful.
  - Asymptomatic hyperuricaemia does not require treatment.

■ PRIMARY MYELOFIBROSIS

Clonal MPN characterised by increased fibrosis within the marrow, which replaces haematopoietic cells leading to cytopaenia's, splenomegaly, and extensive extramedullary haematopoiesis. The extramedullary haematopoiesis is seen in the spleen, liver, and at times in lymph nodes, kidneys, and adrenals.

It can arise from PV or ET.

Clinical Features
- Usually found in patients above 60 years of age.
- A significant number of cases develop acute myeloid leukaemia.

Symptoms
- *Due to progressive anaemia*: Fatigue, weakness, and anorexia.
- *Due to massive splenomegaly*: Abdominal distension, post-prandial fullness, reflux esophagitis, dyspnoea, and dragging discomfort in the left hypochondrium.
- *Hypermetabolic state*: Fever, fatigue, weight loss, night sweats, and heat intolerance.
- Bleeding tendencies due to thrombocytopaenia develop at late stages.
- Death usually occurs due to portal hypertension and infections. Median survival is about 5 years.

Signs
- Massive splenomegaly and hepatomegaly
- Anaemia, lymphadenopathy, bleeding manifestations, ascites, cardiac failure, and jaundice
- Hyperuricaemia and secondary gout due to a high rate of cell turnover
- *Extramedullary haematopoiesis*: It may produce paraspinal masses with spinal cord compression, ascites, and effusions (pleural and pericardial).

Investigations

- *Haemoglobin level*: Normal in the early stages, but markedly reduced in the late stages.
- *Total leucocyte count*: Normal/increased (early stages)/decreased (late stages)
- *Platelet count*: Increased in early stages and decreased in the late stages.
- **Peripheral smear:** Moderate-to-severe degree of normochromic normocytic anaemia accompanied by leucoerythroblastic blood picture (precursors of granulocytes and nucleated RBCs being present simultaneously). **Many tear drop-shaped red cells** (dacrocytes) probably due to damage in the fibrotic marrow. Basophilic stippling and giant platelets with vacuoles are also seen.
- **Bone marrow:** The peripheral smear findings are not specific and bone marrow biopsy is diagnostic.
    - *Cellularity*: Early stages (cellular phase), it is often hypercellular and in later stages (hypocellular phase), it becomes hypocellular and diffusely fibrotic.
    - Megakaryocytes are large, dysplastic and abnormally clustered.
- **LAP score:** Raised
- **Philadelphia chromosome:** Negative.
- JAK2 V617F mutation occurs in ~50% patients.
- **Serum vitamin B12:** Moderately increased.
- **Radiological examination: Shows** increased bone density of vertebrae and proximal ends of long bones.

Treatment

No specific therapy exists for primary idiopathic myelofibrosis (IMF).

- **Treatment of anaemia**
    - Correct other causes of anaemia such as gastrointestinal blood loss and folic acid deficiency (Folic acid 5 mg daily)
    - Packed red-cell transfusions
    - Neither recombinant EPO nor androgens (such as danazol) are consistently effective in controlling anaemia but can be tried in some patients.
    - Glucocorticoids (prednisolone) may control constitutional symptoms and autoimmune complications.
    - Combination with low-dose thalidomide (50–100 mg/day) with prednisolone can control anaemia and splenomegaly in a significant number of patients.
- **Treatment of splenomegaly**
    - **Patients with cellular bone marrow and marked leucocytosis:** Busulphan 2 mg daily.
    - Indications for splenectomy is selected cases:
        – With hypersplenism
        – If splenomegaly impairs alimentation, it should be performed before cachexia sets in.
    - *Splenic irradiation*: To reduce splenic size is reserved for patients who cannot undergo splenectomy. Patients often develop severe cytopaenias.
    - Hydroxyurea is useful to control splenomegaly but can produce myelosuppression that may exacerbate underlying anaemia.
- **Treatment of extramedullary haematopoiesis:** By low-dose irradiation.
- **Curative treatment: Allogeneic bone marrow transplantation** is the only curative treatment. It should be performed in younger patients as most patients in IMF are above 60 years of age.
- **Others:**
    - Allopurinol can control hyperuricaemia.
    - Etanercept (TNF-α antagonist) is used in patients with severe constitutional features.
    - JAK2 inhibitors are under trial.

Prognosis

Median survival varies from 27 to 135 months and depends on prognostic factors (**Box 11.8**).

■ MYELODYSPLASTIC SYNDROMES

World Health Organization classification (2008) of myelodysplastic syndromes has been shown in **Table 11.45**.

Box 11.8: Poor prognostic factors.

- Age > 65 years
- Haemoglobin level < 10 g/dL
- Total WBC count > 25,000/mm³
- Presence of blasts in peripheral blood
- Presence of constitutional symptoms

TABLE 11.45: World Health Organization (WHO) classification (2008) of myelodysplastic syndromes.

Disease	Peripheral smear	Bone marrow features
Refractory cytopaenia with unilineage dysplasia (RCUD): Refractory anaemia (RA), refractory neutropaenia (RN), refractory thrombocytopaenia (RT)	Unicytopaenia or bicytopaenia	• Unilineage dysplasia in > 10% of the cells in one myeloid lineage • < 5% blasts • < 15% ring sideroblasts
Refractory anaemia with ring sideroblasts (RARS)	• Anaemia • No blasts	• Dyserythropoiesis • > 15% ring sideroblasts • < 5% blasts
Refractory cytopaenia with multilineage dysplasia (RCMD)	• Bi/pancytopaenia • Rare blast • No Auer rods • < 1 × 10^9/L monocytes	• Dysplasia in > 10% of cells in two myeloid lineages (neutrophil and/or erythroid and/or megakaryocytes) • < 5% blasts • No Auer rods • ±15% ring sideroblasts
Refractory anaemia with excess blasts-1 (RAEB-1)	• < 5% blasts • Bi/pancytopaenia • No Auer rods • < 1 × 10^9/L monocytes	• 5–9% blasts • Unilineage or multilineage dysplasia • No Auer rods ±
Refractory anaemia with excess blsts-2 (RAEB-2)	• 5–19% blasts • Cytopaenia • Auer rods ± • < 1 × 10^9/L monocytes	• 10–19% blasts • Unilineage or multilineage dysplasia • Auer rods ±
MDS unclassified (MDS-U)	• < 1% blasts • Cytopaenia only	• < 5% blasts • Unequivocal dysplasia in < 10% of cells in one or more myeloid cell lines when accompanied by cytogenetic abnormalities considered as presumptive evidence for diagnosis of MDS
MDS with isolated del(5q)	• No or rare blasts • Anaemia • Platelets increased or normal	• < 5% blasts • No Auer rods • Increased to normal megakaryocytes with hypolobated nuclei • Isolated 5q deletion

(MDS: myelodysplastic syndrome)

Clinical Features

- Usually found in patients above 60 years of age and slightly more common in males.
- Detected incidentally on routine blood examination in about 50% of patients.
- Symptoms are due to cytopaenia's which may be single-lineage cytopaenia, bicytopaenia, or pancytopaenia. Symptoms include weakness (anaemia), infections (leucopenia), and haemorrhage (thrombocytopaenia).
- Extramedullary haematopoiesis may occur leading to hepatomegaly and splenomegaly but is uncommon.
- About 10–40% progresses to AML. MDS was referred to as preleukaemic syndrome.

Diagnosis

- *Minimal morphologic criterion for the diagnosis of an MDS*: Dysplasia in at least 10% of cells of any one of the myeloid lineages.

- *Complete blood count*: May give clues to this diagnosis.
- *Peripheral smear*:
  - Mild-to-moderate degree of macrocytic or dimorphic anaemia with evidence of dyspoiesis
  - **White blood cell count:** Normal or low. Neutropaenia with few blasts, number of blasts determines type of MDS. The cytoplasm of neutrophils is hypogranular or agranular. The nuclei may show hyposegmentation with only two nuclear lobes (pseudo–Pelger–Hüet cells), hypersegmenation or ringed neutrophils.
  - Variable thrombocytopaenia, presence of large hypogranular or giant platelets is seen.
  - **NAP score** is moderately or severely decreased.
- **Bone marrow:** Varying degree of dyspoietic (disordered) differentiation affecting all non-lymphoid lineages (erythroid, granulocytic, monocytic, and megakaryocytic) associated with cytopaenia's.
- **Cytogenic study of the marrow:** Most important for establishing the diagnosis.

Treatment

- *Therapy is supportive*: Packed red-cell transfusion for anaemia. Platelet transfusions for bleeding due to thrombocytopaenia. Antibiotic therapy for infections. Iron chelators to reduce iron overload from multiple transfusions.
- Erythropoietin and G-CSF may be useful in some patients to ameliorate symptoms.
- *Others*: Use of thalidomide, lenalidomide (a derivative of thalidomide), 5-azacytidine and decitabine. 5-azacytidine and decitabine (hypomethylating agents) may reduce requirements of blood transfusion and to retard the progression of MDS to AML. Lenalidomide is found useful in the 5q-syndrome.
- *Allogeneic HSC transplantation*: Curative. However, it may be performed in <5–10% of patients because MDS is the most common during seventh or eighth decade of life.

■ PLASMA CELL DYSCRASIAS

Classification of plasma cell proliferative disorders has been shown in **Table 11.46**.

■ MULTIPLE MYELOMA

Clinical Features (Table 11.47)

- Insidious in onset. Peak incidence is seen during sixth to seventh decade and males are more affected than females.
- Symptoms:
  - Bone pain: Most commonly backache due to involvement of vertebra (60%)

TABLE 11.46: Classification of plasma cell proliferative disorders.

Monoclonal gammopathies of undetermined significance (MGUS)	Malignant monoclonal gammopathies

• Benign (IgG, IgA, IgD, IgM, and rarely, free light chains)
• Associated neoplasms or other diseases not known to produce monoclonal proteins
• Biclonal gammopathies
• Idiopathic Bence–Jones proteinuria
	• Multiple myeloma (IgG, IgA, IgD, IgE, and free light chains)
	  ○ Overt multiple myeloma
	  ○ Smouldering multiple myeloma
	  ○ Plasma cell leukaemia
	  ○ Non-secretory myeloma
	  ○ Immunoglobulin D myeloma
	  ○ Osteosclerotic myeloma (POEMS syndrome)
	  ○ Solitary plasmacytoma of bone
	  ○ Extramedullary plasmacytoma
	• Waldenström's macroglobulinaemia
	• Other lymphoproliferative diseases

Heavy chain diseases (HCDs) • γ-HCD • α-HCD • C.μ-HCD	
Cryoglobulinaemia	**Primary amyloidosis (AL)**

(POEMS: polyneuropathy, organomegaly, endocrinopathy, monoclonal protein, and skin changes)

TABLE 11.47: Clinical features of multiple myeloma.

Involved system	Features
Bone	• Localised bony swellings over vertebrae, skull, sternum, ribs, and clavicle • Bone pain due to pathological fractures • Neurological symptoms: Sensory and/or motor loss due to lesion in the vertebra compressing the spinal cord nerve root
Bone marrow	Anaemia, leucopaenia, and thrombocytopaenia
Immune system	Humoural immune deficiency leading to increased susceptibility to infections, particularly of the respiratory system and urinary tract
Renal damage—multifactorial	• Bence–Jones proteinuria, hypercalcaemia, immune deficiency • Nephrocalcinosis, amyloidosis, renal insufficiency, infections or nephrotic syndrome
Bleeding tendency	Purpura, epistaxis, and gastrointestinal bleeding
Cryoglobulinaemia Hyperviscosity syndrome	• CNS: Confusion headache, vertigo, nystagmus, postural hypotension, and dizziness • Retina: Producing blurred vision, retinal venous congestion, and papilloedema • CVS: Congestive cardiac failure
Neurological manifestations	Amyloid peripheral neuropathy, carpal tunnel syndrome, and compressive myelopathy

(CNS: central nervous system; CVS: cardiovascular system)

- Symptoms of anaemia due to bone marrow infiltration
- Recurrent infections due to humoural immune deficiency
- Symptoms of renal failure (20–30%)
- Symptoms of hypercalcaemia following destruction of bone
- Symptoms of hyperviscosity and bleeding due to thrombocytopaenia (rare)
- Some patients may be asymptomatic and are accidentally detected during the preclinical phase.

■ OSTEOSCLEROTIC MYELOMA (POEMS SYNDROME)

This syndrome is characterised by polyneuropathy, organomegaly, endocrinopathy, M protein, and skin changes (POEMS).

The major clinical features are a chronic inflammatory-demyelinating polyneuropathy with predominantly motor disability and sclerotic skeletal lesions.

Diagnosis of Multiple Myeloma

Diagnosis of multiple myeloma (MM) requires at least two of the following:
- Monoclonal immunoglobulin (M protein) or light chains in the blood (>3 g/dL) and/or urine
- Infiltration of bone marrow with (clonal) plasma cells (≥10%), or plasmacytoma
- Evidence of myeloma-related organ or tissue impairment (≥1)—CRAB
  - **H**ypercal**c**aemia: Serum (ionised) > 5.5 mEq/L.
  - **R**enal insufficiency (creatinine > 2 mg/dL).
  - **A**naemia (haemoglobin < 10 g/dL)
  - Lytic **b**one lesions and/or osteoporosis

■ SMOULDERING (ASYMPTOMATIC) MULTIPLE MYELOMA

Presence of serum M protein level >3 g/dL and/or 10% or more plasma cells in bone marrow and patients are asymptomatic.

It lies in-between multiple myeloma (MM) and monoclonal gammopathy of uncertain significance. Patients with smouldering MM carry a much higher risk of progression to myeloma or related malignancy compared to monoclonal gammopathies of undetermined significance (MGUS).

Investigations

- **Peripheral blood:** Shows anaemia, leucopaenia, thrombocytopaenia, and raised ESR.
- *Peripheral smear*: May show rouleaux formation due to increased immunoglobulins.

- **Bone marrow examination: Hypercellular**, increased number of plasma cells and **myeloma cells** (neoplastic plasma cells), **> 30%** of the cellularity is diagnostic.
- **Urine:** Bence-Jones proteins may be present.
- **Serum findings:**
  - **Serum β_2-microglobulin:** Useful **prognostic marker** and **high values signify poor prognosis.**
  - **Hypercalcaemia:** Extensive osteolytic lesions and osteoporosis and there are also increased levels of serum phosphate.
  - *Serum alkaline phosphatase*: Usually normal in the absence of complications.
  - Blood urea and serum creatinine raised in 20% of cases and along with electrolytes are used to assess renal function.
  - *Serum proteins*: Total protein level increased, albumin decreases, globulins markedly increased.
  - *Serum uric acid*: Raised.
  - Serum immunoglobulin estimation reveals a reduction of normal immunoglobulins below normal levels.
- **Electrophoretic studies on serum and urine:** Raised levels of immunoglobulins in blood and/or light chains (Bence-Jones proteins) in the urine. The monoclonal immunoglobulin (M protein) is identified as abnormal protein "spikes" in serum or urine electrophoresis. The type of immunoglobulin can be determined by immunofixation. The most common M protein is IgG type, followed by IgA.
- **Radiological examination:**
  - Reveals generalised osteoporosis. Collapse of multiple vertebrates is a common finding.
  - **Radiographs** of flat bones: Skull, vertebral bodies, ribs, and pelvis show characteristic punched-out osteolytic lesions.
  - **MRI and positron emission tomography (PET):** May detect bone involvement when skeletal survey is normal.
  - **Bone scan:** Not required as it is often negative.

Staging systems have been shown in **Tables 11.48** and **11.49**.

TABLE 11.48: Modified from Durie–Salmon staging.

Stage	Criteria

I	- Low M-component:
	  - IgG < 5 g/dL
	  - IgA < 3 g/dL
	  - Urine BJ protein < 4 g/24 h
	- Normal haemoglobin, serum calcium, Ig levels (non-M protein)

II	Overall values between stages I and III

III	One or more of the following:
	- Haemoglobin < 8.5 g/dL, serum calcium > 12 mg/dL
	- High M-component:
	  - IgG > 7 g/dL
	  - IgA > 5 g/dL
	  - Urine light chain > 12 g/24 h
	- Advanced multiple lytic lesions on X-rays

Subclassification based on renal function
- Subclass A = Serum creatinine < 2 mg/dL
- Subclass B = Serum creatinine > 2 mg/dL

(BJ protein: Bence–Jones protein; Ig: immunoglobulin)

TABLE 11.49: International staging system.

Stage	Characteristic features	Median survival
I	Serum β_2 microglobulin <3.5 mg/dL and serum albumin >3.5 g/dL	62 months
II	Serum β_2 microglobulin <3.5 mg/dL and serum albumin < 3.5 g/dL and or serum β_2 microglobulin <3.5–5.5 mg/dL	44 months
III	Serum β_2 microglobulin <5.5 mg/dL	29 months

Treatment

- **Autologous stem-cell transplantation:** In young patients (<65 years) without renal failure: Standard treatment is first-line high-dose chemotherapy for myeloablation (melphalan 20 mg/m² intravenously) to maximum response and then an autologous stem-cell transplantation.

- **Chemotherapy: Older patients**
  - Thalidomide and alkylating agent (melphalan, cyclophosphamide, and chlorambucil) and prednisolone. Thalidomide is teratogenic. Recent studies have suggested that combination with thalidomide results in improved response rates and overall survival, albeit with increased toxicity.
  - Bortezomib-proteasome inhibitor, used in relapses, combined with doxorubicin, dexamethasone.
  - Lenalidomide in combination with steroids has been tried.
- **Younger patients (<65–70 years):**
  - Orally active cyclophosphamide, thalidomide, and dexamethasone (CTD)-based induction, followed by a high-dose melphalan autograft.
- **Radiotherapy:** Effective for local problems such as severe bone pain, pathological fractures, and tumourous lesions. As an emergency treatment of spinal cord compression complicating extradural plasmacytomas.

■ MONOCLONAL GAMMOPATHY OF UNCERTAIN SIGNIFICANCE

Presence of serum M protein concentration <3 g/dL, bone marrow clonal plasma cells <10% plasma cells, and no end-organ damage (CRAB: no hypercalcaemia, no renal impairment, no anaemia or no osteolytic lesions, or no evidence of other B-cell neoplasms).

It is one of the most common plasma cell dyscrasias, occurring in 3–5% of general population above the age of 50 years.

Progression: Considered as pre-neoplastic condition. It can progress to MM, Waldenström's macroglobulinaemia, primary amyloidosis, or a lymphoproliferative disorder at a rate of 1–1.5% per year. Risk of progression to MM and related disorders depends upon:
- Size of M component (risk of progression with an M protein value of 1.5 g/dL almost twice that of a patient with an M-Protein value of 0.5 g/dL)
- Type of M-component (IgM and IgA increased risk compared to IgG), and
- Abnormal free light chain ratio (kappa; lambda ratio-normal being 0.26–1.65)

Follow-up: Followed with serum protein electrophoresis at 6 months, if stable, follow every 1–2 years.

No treatment is indicated.

■ WALDENSTRÖM MACROGLOBULINAEMIA

Syndrome characterised by IgM monoclonal gammopathy sufficient to cause a hyperviscosity of the blood and bone marrow infiltration.

Most commonly occurs in association with lymphoplasmacytic lymphoma. The tumour cells undergo terminal differentiation to plasma cells and secrete monoclonal IgM.

It occurs in older adults (median age 60 years).

Clinical Feature

It may be asymptomatic.
- Usual presenting complaints are non-specific and include weakness, fatigue, and weight loss.
- Symptoms develop due to:
  - **Tumour infiltration:** Most patients present with weakness and fatigue due to anaemia caused by marrow infiltration. Other features include fever, night sweats, weight loss, lymphadenopathy, hepatomegaly, and splenomegaly.
  - **Monoclonal protein:** About 10% of patients have autoimmune haemolysis caused by cold agglutinins (monoclonal IgM binds to red cells at temperatures of <37°C). IgM may be associated with systemic amyloidosis. IgM-secreted by the tumour, because of its large size, at high concentrations increases the viscosity of the blood, giving rise to a hyperviscosity syndrome.
  - Features of **hyperviscosity syndrome** are:
    - Visual impairment associated with venous congestion (e.g. blurring or loss of vision)
    - Neurologic problems (e.g. dizziness, headache, vertigo, nystagmus, hearing loss, ataxia, paraesthesias, and diplopia)
    - Bleeding
    - Cryoglobulinaemia produces symptoms such as Raynaud phenomenon and cold urticarial

○ Tumour cells can infiltrate organs and result in hepatomegaly, splenomegaly, and lymphadenopathy in about 20% patients.

Diagnosis

- **Demonstration of monoclonal IgM:** Serum electrophoresis, sample may require warming to 37°C, to avoid interference of cold agglutinins. Immunofixation is required to characterise monoclonal protein.
- **Bone marrow aspirate and biopsy:** Shows >10% lymphoplasmacytic cells (CD20+).

Treatment

- It is a chemotherapy- and immunotherapy-sensitive disease curable with currently available therapies.
- No specific treatment is needed for patients who do not have systemic symptoms.
- Single agent therapy with rituximab is used in symptomatic patients with modest haematologic compromise, IgM-related neuropathy or haemolytic anaemia unresponsive to corticosteroids.
- *Combination of chemotherapy and rituximab*: With severe constitutional symptoms, profound haematologic compromise, bulky disease, and hyperviscosity syndrome should be treated with dexamethasone, rituximab, and cyclophosphamide.
- **Immunotherapy:** With anti-CD20 antibody.
- **Plasmapheresis:** Most of IgM secreted by tumour cells is intravascular. Patient with hyperviscosity syndrome and haemolysis to help in alleviating these symptoms.

Prognosis: Transformation to large-cell lymphoma occurs but is uncommon. Median survival is 4 years.

■ GENERALISED LYMPHADENOPATHY

Causes and diagnostic features of generalised lymphadenopathy have been shown in **Table 11.50**.

TABLE 11.50: Causes and diagnostic features of generalised lymphadenopathy.

Cause	Diagnostic feature
Malignant neoplasms	
Lymphomas: Hodgkin and non-Hodgkin	Histopathology of involved lymph node
Leukaemias: ALL, CLL, and CML in blast crisis	Peripheral smear and bone-marrow examination
Metastatic disease (head and neck cancers, lung and breast cancers, and GIT malignancies)	Fine-needle aspiration and biopsy
Infections	
Disseminated tuberculosis	Lymph node: Caseating granulomas
Human immunodeficiency virus infection	ELISA and Western blot
Infectious mononucleosis	Monospot test and Paul–Bunnell test
Brucellosis	Brucella agglutination test
Secondary syphilis	VDRL and TPHA
Local infections (cellulitis, pharyngitis)	Local examination
Plague	Inguinal nodes; FNAC—typical "safety pin" bacteria
Autoimmune diseases	
Systemic lupus erythematosus	ANA
Rheumatoid arthritis	Rheumatoid factor
Drugs induced	
Systemic disorders—Amyloidosis, sarcoidosis, serum sickness	
Rare—Castleman disease, Kikuchi–Fujimoto disease, Rosai–Dorfman disease	

(ALL: acute lymphoblastic leukaemia; ANA: antinuclear antibody; CLL: chronic lymphocytic leukaemia; CML: chronic myelogenous leukaemia; ELISA: enzyme-linked immunosorbent assay; FNAC: fine-needle aspiration cytology; GIT: gastrointestinal tract; TPHA: *Treponema pallidum* haemagglutination test; VDRL: venereal disease research laboratory)

BLOOD TRANSFUSION

RED CELL CONCENTRATES (PACKED RED CELLS)

General indications for RBC transfusion have been shown in **Box 11.9**.

PLATELET CONCENTRATE

Indications and contraindication of platelet concentrate have been shown in **Table 11.51**.

GRANULOCYTE CONCENTRATES

Prepared from single donors using cell separators.
Indications: Severe neutropaenia with definite evidence of bacterial infection.

FRESH FROZEN PLASMA

Indications: For replacement of coagulation factors in acquired coagulation factor deficiencies
- Patients on anticoagulant drug therapy (Coumarin)
- Antithrombin deficiency
- Coagulopathy of liver diseases
- Vitamin K deficiency
- *Microangiopathic haemolytic anaemia*: TTP, haemolytic uraemic syndrome, and HELLP (haemolysis, elevated liver enzymes, low platelet count) syndrome
- Disseminated intravascular coagulation

CRYOPRECIPITATE

Indications

Disseminated intravascular coagulation, other conditions where fibrinogen level is very low (hypofibrinogenaemia).

It was used for haemophilia, factor XIII deficiency, and von Willebrand disease. However, it is no longer used for these disorders because of the greater risk of virus transmission compared with virus-inactivated coagulation factor concentrates (**Table 11.52**).

FACTORS VIII AND IX CONCENTRATES

Freeze-dried preparations of coagulation factors prepared from large pools of plasma from many donors.

Box 11.9: General indications for RBC transfusion.

Replace acute blood loss due to haemorrhage or during surgery to relieve clinical features caused by insufficient oxygen delivery
Symptomatic anaemia
- β-thalassaemia major
- Sickle-cell anaemia
- Aplastic anaemia
- Severe anaemia of any cause

TABLE 11.52: Various coagulations factors and their amount in one unit of cryoprecipitate.

Coagulation factor	Quantity per unit
Fibrinogen	150–250 mg
Factor VIII	80–150 units
Von Willebrand factor	100–150 units
Factor XIII	50–75 units

TABLE 11.51: Indications and contraindication of platelet concentrate.

Indications	Contraindication

Bleeding due to:
Severe thrombocytopaenia (when platelet count is <20,000/mm^3)
• Immune-mediated: Autoimmune thrombocytopaenia—reserved for life-threatening bleeding.
• Secondary to bone marrow failure:
  ○ Chemotherapy-induced
  ○ Due to leukaemia
  ○ Dilutional
    – Abnormal platelet function
    – Disseminated intravascular coagulation (DIC)
Surgical or invasive procedures in thrombocytopenic patients
	• Thrombotic thrombocytopaenic purpura (TTP)
	• Heparin-induced thrombocytopaenia (HIT)
	
	Relative contraindication: Idiopathic thrombocytopenic purpura (ITP) or post-transfusion purpura (PTP) because the survival of transfused platelets is very brief

Indications

Haemophilia, von Willebrand's disease: When recombinant coagulation factors are unavailable. However, recombinant coagulation factor concentrates are the treatment of choice for patients with inherited coagulation factor deficiencies.

SALINE-WASHED RED BLOOD CELLS

Effective means of removing leucocytes and plasma (up to 99%). This product is largely restricted to patients with antibodies to IgA or IgE, and those requiring red cells with minimal plasma as in thalassaemia and PNH.

FROZEN RED BLOOD CELLS

Red blood cells can be frozen and stored up to 3 years by addition of glycerol as an endocellular cryoprotective agent. This procedure is used for storage of rare blood groups. Frozen red cells may be indicated for patients with history of severe allergic reactions to plasma or leucocyte factors, e.g. patients sensitised to IgA.

IRRADIATED BLOOD PRODUCTS

Cellular blood products (red cells, platelets, and granulocytes) can be irradiated to a dose of 1,500 rads before transfusion in order to minimise the risk of transfusion-acquired GVHD in immunocompromised individuals.

IMMUNOGLOBULINS—RH IMMUNE GLOBULIN

Indications

Known or suspected inoculation of Rh negative mother with unknown or Rh+ foetal red cells: Abortion, threatened abortion, ectopic pregnancy, amniocentesis, abdominal trauma in 2nd or 3rd trimester, and post-partum if newborn is Rh positive.

Following transfusion of Rh+ cellular blood products (e.g. platelets) to an Rh negative female of child-bearing age or younger

Acute ITP resistant to steroids.

COMPLICATIONS OF BLOOD TRANSFUSIONS

Complications of blood transfusion have been shown in **Table 11.53**.

Massive transfusion: Transfusion of >10 units of red cells or replacement of blood volume in 24 hours. The use of large quantities of stored blood may lead to complications such as dilutional coagulopathy, circulatory overload, hyperkalaemia, hypoglycaemia, hypothermia, and citrate-induced hypocalcaemia.

STEM-CELL THERAPY

Clinical Application

Clinical application of stem-cell therapy (**Table 11.54**).

BONE MARROW TRANSPLANTATION

Bone marrow transplantation is a type of HSC transplantation (**Table 11.55**).

COMPLICATIONS OF HAEMATOPOIETIC STEM-CELL TRANSPLANTATION

Autologous transplants: Fewer immunologic complications and higher relapse rates

Allogeneic HSC transplants: Lower relapse, more immunologic complications—GVHD, can be fatal.

Complications of HSC transplantation have been explained in detail in **Tables 11.56** and **11.57**.

TABLE 11.53: Complications of blood transfusion.

Immunological complications	Non-immunological complications
Immediate reactions	
• Acute haemolytic transfusion reactions • Febrile non-haemolytic reaction • Allergic reaction—urticaria • Anaphylactic reactions	• Transfusion-related acute lung injury (TRALI) • Circulatory overload • Air embolism
Delayed reactions	
• Alloimmunisation • Delayed haemolytic reactions (asymptomatic) • Transfusion associated graft-versus-host disease • Post-transfusion purpura	• Iron overload: Transfusion haemosiderosis • Thrombophlebitis • Infections: Hepatitis (HBV, HCV, HDV), HIV, malaria, cytomegalovirus, syphilis

(HIV: human immunodeficiency virus)

TABLE 11.54: Clinical application of stem-cell therapy.

Genetic diseases (allogeneic BMT)	Marrow failure syndromes
Red-cell disorders: Thalassaemia major and sickle-cell disease	**Allogeneic or syngeneic BMT**
Immunodeficiencies: Severe combined immunodeficiency and X-linked agammaglobulinaemia	Severe aplastic anaemia, Fanconi's syndrome, PNH
Enzyme deficiencies: Gaucher's disease, mucopolysaccharidoses, and leucodystrophies	**Malignant diseases**
Granulocyte disorders: Chediak–Higashi syndrome, chronic granulomatous disease, and Kostmann syndrome	**Autologous, syngeneic or allogeneic BMT**
Platelet disorders: Wiskott–Aldrich syndrome and Glanzmann's thrombasthaenia	Acute leukaemias, chronic leukaemias myelodysplastic syndromes Hodgkin's disease, non-Hodgkin lymphomas, breast cancer, and other solid tumours
Other: Osteopetrosis	

(BMT: bone marrow transplant; PNH: paroxysmal nocturnal haemoglobinuria)

TABLE 11.55: Indications for haematopoietic stem-cell transplantation.

Red blood cell disorders	White blood cell (WBC) disorders
• Severe aplastic anaemia • Thalassaemia major • Fanconi anaemia • Sickle-cell disease • Pure red-cell aplasia	• Leukaemias: Acute lymphoblastic leukaemia and chronic myeloid leukaemia • Myelodysplastic syndromes • Hodgkin and non-Hodgkin lymphoma • Multiple myeloma
Immunological disorders	**Solid tumours**
• Autoimmune diseases: Scleroderma, SLE • Immune-deficiency syndromes	Carcinoma breast, ovarian cancer, germ-cell tumours, and neuroblastoma

(SLE: systemic lupus erythematosus)

TABLE 11.56: Complications of haematopoietic stem-cell transplantation.

Infections
Susceptible to infections (bacterial, viral and fungal) due to lack of granulocytes and lack of a functioning immune system

First phase	Second phase	Third phase
Develops due to neutropaenia and damage to GI mucosal barrier induced by conditioning agents used during transplantation **Source:** Oral, skin, and GI flora	Develops during GVHD where T-cell function gets impaired **Causes:** Opportunistic viral and fungal infections	Develops in chronic GVHD where B- and T-cell functions are impaired **Causes:** Bacterial, opportunistic viral, and fungal infections

Organ toxicity: Damage to GI tract, liver and lungs

Interstitial pneumonitis	Veno-occlusive disease
Seen in 30–40% of patients, fatal in some. Toxicity of radiation and chemotherapy, GVHD and viral, and pneumocystis infections are responsible.	Injury to hepatocytes and endothelium in zone 3 of the liver acinus and obstruction of hepatic sinusoids and venules, often fatal in severe cases. **Features:** Jaundice, ascites, and painful hepatomegaly **Treatment:** Tissue plasminogen activator

Continued

Continued

Graft-versus-host disease

Major complication of allogeneic transplants caused by cytotoxic activity of donor T lymphocytes against the recipient's tissues/organs (foreign to donor T cells). Conditions for development of GVHD:
- An immunocompetent graft (i.e., one containing T cells)
- HLA mismatch (minor or major) between donor and recipient
- An immunosuppressed recipient who cannot mount an immune response to the graft.

Acute GVHD
- Occurs before 100 days. Due to production of cytokines by Th1 cells due to HLA mismatch.
- Affects skin, GI tract and liver simultaneously.
- Causes exfoliative dermatitis, diarrhoea, hepatitis, and cholestasis.

Treatment: Methotrexate, cyclosporine, steroids, antithymocyte globulin, T-cell monoclonal antibodies

Chronic GVHD
- Occurs after day 100. Develops due to cytokine production by Th2 cells.
- Affects the skin, GI tract, liver, eyes, lungs, joints.
- Difficult to treat, in severe cases it is usually fatal.

Treatment: Cyclosporine and corticosteroids

(GI: gastrointestinal; HLA: human leucocyte antigen)

TABLE 11.57: Complications of haematopoietic cell transplantation.

Vascular access complications	
Graft failure	Acute GVHD
Blood group incompatibilities, haemolytic complications	Chronic GVHD
Infectious complications	
Bacterial infections	Varicella-zoster virus infections
Fungal infections	Epstein-Barr virus infections
Cytomegalovirus infection	Adenovirus, respiratory viruses, HHV-6, -7, -8, and other viruses
Herpes simplex virus infections	
Gastrointestinal complications	
Mucosal ulceration/bleeding	Nutritional support
Hepatic complications	
Sinusoidal obstructive syndrome	Hepatitis: Infectious versus non-infectious
Lung injury	
Interstitial pneumonitis: Infectious, non-infectious	Engraftment syndrome
Diffuse alveolar haemorrhage	Bronchiolitis obliterans
Other complications	
Kidney and bladder complications	Drug–drug interactions
Endocrine complications	Growth and development
Late onset non-malignant complications	
Osteoporosis/osteopaenia, avascular necrosis	Secondary malignancies
Dental problems	Neurologic complications
Cataracts	Immunosuppression medication toxicities
Chronic fatigue	Psychosocial effects and rehabilitation

(GVHD: graft-versus-host disease; HHV: human herpesvirus)

LYMPHOMA

■ HODGKIN LYMPHOMA

Malignant lymphoma is characterised by a heterogeneous cellularity of specific **neoplastic cells** (Hodgkin cells and Reed–Sternberg cells) (1–3%) in a background of reactive non-neoplastic cells of various types.

Cell of origin: Neoplastic Reed–Sternberg cells derived from germinal centre or immediate post-germinal centre B cells indicating that most HLs are unusual tumours of B-cell origin.

Age: Bimodal incidence, one peak in young adults (15–35 years) and the other in older adults (45–75 years).

Reed–Sternberg Cell

Reed–Sternberg cells and its variants are **pathognomonic** and differentiate HL from NHL.

Histological diagnosis of HL should not be made in their absence. They are necessary but not sufficient for diagnosis of classical HL, should be found in cellular background for the specific subtype.

Appearance of diagnostic Reed–Sternberg cells: Giant cells with two large nuclei and nucleoli in each nucleus (owl-eye appearance).

Variants of Reed–Sternberg Cell

- *Mononuclear-variant*: Single, large, and round nucleus with a large eosinophilic inclusion-like nucleolus, also called as "Hodgkin cells".
- Lacunar cell variant
- Mummified cell (necrobiotic) variant
- Anaplastic/pleomorphic variant
- *Lymphohistiocytic variant (L&H cells/popcorn cell)*: Specific to lymphocyte predominance subtype.
- *Immunophenotype*: Classical forms of HL are CD15+ and CD30+. Lymphocyte predominant HL cells CD15 -ve and CD30 -ve.

Aetiology

- **Epstein-Barr virus (EBV):** Young adults who have had previous infectious mononucleosis have an increased risk of development and EBV genome is frequently identified in the Reed–Sternberg cells.
- **Genetic factors:** HLA-B18 is higher in patients with HL.
- **Immune status:** More in immunocompromised or with autoimmune diseases.

Classification of Hodgkin Lymphoma (Tables 11.58 and 11.59, Fig. 11.11)

Rye classification: The prognosis depends on the histological type. Nodular sclerosing type is most common.

Clinical Manifestations

- **The most common presentation:** Painless enlargement of one lymph node group (unifocal) usually cervical, which spreads in a predictable manner (contiguous spread).
- **Other presentation**
  - **Localised disease of mediastinum** (young women) cough due to mediastinal lymphadenopathy or axillary nodes, rarely in the abdominal, and pelvic, or inguinal nodes.
  - **Generalised disease:** Hepatosplenomegaly and constitutional "B" symptoms are uncommon in the beginning but

TABLE 11.58: Prognosis and histological type of Rye classification.

Histological type	Prognosis
Lymphocyte predominant	Very good
Nodular sclerosing	Good
Mixed cellularity	Fair
Lymphocyte depleted	Poor

TABLE 11.59: World Health Organization (WHO) classification of Hodgkin lymphoma (HL).

Classical HL (>95%)	Nodular lymphocyte predominance (LP) Hodgkin's lymphoma (<5%)
• Nodular sclerosis (NS): Classic HL • Mixed cellularity (MC): Classic HL (most common type in India) • Lymphocyte-rich (LR): Classic HL • Lymphocyte depletion (LD): Classic HL	

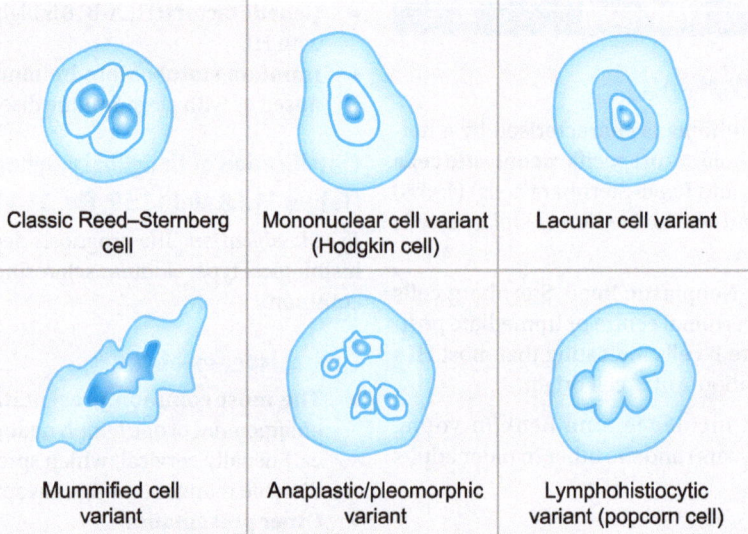

Fig. 11.11: Classification of Hodgkin lymphoma.

- may become prominent as the disease advances.
  - **Rare sites:** Waldeyer's ring, mesenteric epitrochlear, and popliteal nodes.
  - **Involvement of extralymphatic organs:** Not common, may occur in the later stages.
- **Classical Pel–Ebstein fever:** Cyclical pattern, characterised by several days or weeks of fever alternating with afebrile periods. Rarely seen.
- **Common symptoms:** Alcohol-induced pain at site of lymphadenopathy. Pruritus can be troubling.
- **Nephrotic syndrome:** Immune complex deposition, associated with depressed cell-mediated immunity and increases risk of infections such as herpes zoster, TB, cryptococcus, cytomegalovirus (CMV), and candida.
- **Compression** by lymph node masses or **infiltration** of various organs may develop with mediastinal involvement—dysphagia, dyspnoea, Horner's syndrome, hoarseness of voice, superior vena caval syndrome, and inferior vena caval obstruction.
- On examination, lymph nodes are discrete and non-tender and have a "rubbery" consistency.

Clinical Staging (Table 11.60)

Cotswold's modification of the Ann Arbor Classification.

Investigations

Investigations of peripheral blood, biopsy, and staging of Hodgkin lymphoma (**Table 11.61**)

Management

- **Aim:** Curative intent with expectation of success.
- Patients with localised disease receive a brief course of chemotherapy followed by radiotherapy to sites of node involvement and cured HD in >90% of cases.
- Presently, all stages of HL are treated initially with chemotherapy.
- With more extensive disease or those with B symptoms receive a complete course of chemotherapy.
- **Chemotherapy (Table 11.62):** Combination chemotherapy has been shown to be highly effective.

Treatment plan for adults with Hodgkin lymphoma has been shown in **Table 11.63**.

TABLE 11.60: Clinical staging: Cotswold's modification of the Ann Arbor Classification.

Stage	Definition
I	Involvement of a single lymph node region or lymphoid structure (e.g., spleen, Waldeyer's ring, and thymus) or involvement of a single extralymphatic site.
II	• Involvement of two or more lymph node groups on same side of diaphragm (mediastinum is a single site; hilar nodes, when involved on both sides, constitute stage II disease). • Localised contiguous involvement of only one extranodal organ or site and lymph-node region(s) on the same side of the diaphragm (IIE). • Number of anatomic sites should be indicated by suffix (e.g., II$_3$).
III	Involvement of lymph node regions or structures on both sides of the diaphragm, which may also be accompanied by involvement of the spleen (IIIS) or by localised involvement of only one extranodal organ site (IIIE) or both (IIISE).
III$_1$	With or without splenic, hilar, coeliac, or portal nodes
III$_2$	With para-aortic, iliac, or mesenteric nodes
IV	Diffuse or disseminated involvement of one or more extranodal organs or tissues, with or without associated lymph-node involvement

E: involvement of a single extra nodal site, or contiguous or proximal to known nodal site of disease.
A: No "B" symptoms
B: Place the patient in the "B" category when at least one of the following is observed:
- Unexplained weight loss > 10% of bodyweight during 6 months before staging
- Recurrent unexplained fever > 38°C during the previous month
- Recurrent heavy night sweats during the previous month

Lymphatic structures: Lymph nodes, spleen, thymus, Waldeyer's rings, appendix, and Peyer's patches. Liver and bone marrow are excluded.
Each stage is further divided into A or B based on the absence or presence of systemic symptoms (B symptoms), respectively.

TABLE 11.61: Investigations of peripheral blood, biopsy, and staging of Hodgkin lymphoma.

Peripheral blood	
Anaemia	• Normocytic normochromic anaemia • Advance stage: Microcytic anaemia due to defective utilisation of iron
Total leucocyte count	Normal, but sometimes neutrophil leucocytosis
Eosinophilia	Observed in ~20% of patients
Thrombocytosis	In some patients
Lymphopaenia	• Lymphocyte depletion and associated with bad prognosis • Terminal stages: Leucopaenia and thrombocytopaenia
Serum ALP	Raised usually indicate bone marrow or liver involvement
ESR	It may be raised
Biopsy	
Lymph node biopsy	Surgically or percutaneous needle biopsy under radiological guidance
Liver biopsy	Diagnosis in patients with hepatomegaly
PET scan	Staging management of Hodgkin lymphoma

Continued

Continued

Staging of Hodgkin lymphoma

- Predicts prognosis and guiding choice of therapy. Requires physical examination and investigations.
  - Chest radiographs
  - Liver function tests
  - Renal function tests
  - Abdominal ultrasound
  - Bone marrow trephine and aspirate (clinically advanced disease—stages III, IV, "B" symptoms, HIV-positive)
  - CT scans of neck, chest, abdomen, and pelvis
  - Staging laparotomy: Rarely required (stage IIA or less and in whom mantle radiation is planned).
- With current treatment protocols, tumour stage rather than histological type is the most important prognostic variable.
- The cure rate of patients with stages I and IIA is close to 90%.
- Even with advanced disease (IVA and IVB), 60–70% 5-year disease-free survival is obtained.

(ALP: alkaline phosphatase; ESR: erythrocyte sedimentation rate; HIV: human immunodeficiency virus; PET: positron emission tomography)

TABLE 11.62: Popular chemotherapy regimens used in the treatment of Hodgkin lymphoma.

Regimen	Drugs used
ABVD	Doxorubicin (adriamycin), bleomycin, vinblastine, and dacarbazine
MOPP	Mechlorethamine (mustine hydrochloride), vincristine, procarbazine, and prednisone
ABVD/MOPP	Alternating cycles of MOPP and ABVD
BEACOPP escalated	Bleomycin, etoposide, adriamycin, cyclophosphamide, vincristine, procarbazine, and prednisone in escalated dose

- *Early stage "low risk"*: "Moderate" chemotherapy, consisting of 2–4 cycles of ABVD followed by involved field irradiation (20–30 Gy). It has a 90% cure rate.
- **Advanced disease (including locally advanced unfavorable early stage):**
  - Cyclical chemotherapy with 6–8 cycles of adriamycin, bleomycin, vinblastine, and dacarbazine (ABVD) with involved field irradiation to sites which were initially bulky.
  - ***Stanford V* for ABVD:** Consists of weekly chemotherapy regimen of doxorubicin, vinblastine, mechlorethamine, etoposide, vincristine, bleomycin, and prednisone administered for 12 weeks and includes radiation therapy.
  - Escalated BEACOPP (bleomycin, etoposide, doxorubicin, cyclophosphamide, vincristine, prednisone, and procarbazine)
- Autologous bone marrow transplantation is successful in about 40% cases even after the failure of chemotherapy.

Late complications: Due to high cure rates achieved with modern treatment.
- *Second malignancies*: Acute leukaemia and solid organ cancers.
  - *Acute leukaemia*: Within 10 years of use of alkylating agents in combination with radiotherapy. The risk is higher with mechlorethamine (mustine hydrochloride), vincristine, procarbazine, and prednisone (MOPP) as compared to ABVD.
  - Solid organ cancers usually develop after 10 years of radiotherapy.
- Cardiac failure and accelerated coronary artery disease: Following radiotherapy.
- Pulmonary fibrosis
- Hypothyroidism

NON-HODGKIN LYMPHOMA

- Lymphomas represent solid tumours of the immune system.

TABLE 11.63: Treatment plan for adults with Hodgkin lymphoma.

Stage of Hodgkin lymphoma	Prognostic category	Choice of treatment
IA or IIA, no bulky disease*		ABVD × 4 if complete remission after 2 cycles or ABVD × 2 + involved-region radiation therapy (IRRT)
IB, IIB, or any stage III or IV or bulky disease, any stage	≤3 adverse factors**	ABVD until 2 cycles past complete remission (minimum 6, maximum 8)
	≥4 adverse factors**	BEACOPP escalated

*Bulky: largest diameter of any single mass ≥ 10 cm.
**Adverse factors: Male sex, older than 45 years of age, stage IV, haemoglobin < 10.5 g/dL, WBC count > 15,000/mL, lymphocyte count < 600/mL or <8% of the white blood cell count, or serum albumin < 4 g/dL.
(ABVD: adriamycin, bleomycin, vinblastine, and dacarbazine; BEACOPP: bleomycin, etoposide, adriamycin, cyclophosphamide, vincristine, procarbazine, and prednisone; WBC: white blood cell)

TABLE 11.64: Various factors associated with the development of non-Hodgkin lymphoma.

Genetic factors/inherited immune disorders	Acquired immune disorders
• Wiskott–Aldrich syndrome • Ataxia-telangiectasia	• Solid organ transplantation • Acquired immunodeficiency syndrome (AIDS) • Rheumatoid arthritis, SLE • Sjögren syndrome • Hashimoto thyroiditis
Infectious agents	**Occupational and environmental exposure**
• **Human T-lymphotropic virus type 1** with adult T-cell leukaemia/lymphoma. • **Human herpes virus 8** (Kaposi's sarcoma) associated with primary effusion lymphoma • **Hepatitis C virus:** :Lymphoplasmacytic lymphoma and splenic marginal zone lymphoma • *Helicobacter pylori*: Associated with gastric lymphoma of extranodal marginal zone/mucosa • **Epstein-Barr virus:** Associated with Burkitt lymphoma and Hodgkin lymphoma, mucosa associated lymphoid tissue (MALT).	• Ionising radiation • Herbicides • Organic solvents • Hair dyes • Ultraviolet light • High-fat diets and nitrates in drinking water • Heavy smoking associated with follicular lymphoma

- Can be divided into NHL and HL.
- About 80% of NHL are of B-cell origin and 20% of T-cell origin.

Aetiology (Table 11.64)

Not known in most of the cases. Genetic, environmental, and infectious agents implicated.

Immune disorders: Occurs in congenital or acquired immunodeficiency states.
- o **Genetic factors/congenital immunodeficiency:** Increased risk of lymphoma in—
  - *Family history*: Siblings, first-degree relatives with lymphoma or haematologic malignancies.
  - Certain inherited syndromes, e.g. ataxia-telangiectasia and Wiskott–Aldrich syndrome.
- o **Acquired immune disorders:** Immune suppression, immunosuppressant drugs, used for solid organ transplantation, and HIV infection are associated with an increased incidence of lymphoma.

Pathology and Classification

- **Grading of NHL (Table 11.65):**
  - Size of the lymphoid cells is a guide to prognosis. Small lymphoid cells (mature lymphocytes) are low-grade and those with large lymphoid cells (immature lymphoid cells) show high-grade disease.
  - **Follicular lymphomas:** Low grade with good prognosis. Most diffuse lymphomas are high grade with poor prognosis.
- **World Health Organization classification of lymphoid neoplasm**: It requires immunophenotyping, cytogenetics, FISH, and antigen receptor gene rearrangement studies (Table 11.66).

Clinical Features

- **Age:** Non-Hodgkin lymphoma can occur at any age, but the peak incidence is around 60 years.
- **The most common presentation:**
  - Painless firm, lymph node enlargement or symptoms due to lymph node mass.
  - *Extranodal involvement*: T-cell lymphoma, involves bone marrow, gut, thyroid, lung, skin, testis, brain and, more rarely, bone.
  - *Bone marrow involvement*: More common in low-grade (50–60%) than high-grade (10%) and can produce cytopaenias.
  - Primary extranodal lymphomas present with soft-tissue masses and symptoms relevant to the site. Waldeyer's ring and epitrochlear lymph nodes are frequently involved.
  - *Pressure effects*: Due to NHL includes gut obstruction, ascites, superior vena caval obstruction, and spinal cord compression.
  - Involvement of liver and spleen results in hepatosplenomegaly.

TABLE 11.65: Grading of non-Hodgkin lymphoma.

Indolent or low grade	Highly aggressive/high grade	Aggressive/intermediate grade
- Small lymphocytic - Follicular, predominantly small cleaved cells - Follicular, mixed, small-cleaved and large-cleaved cells	- Large cell, immunoblastic (B or T cell type) - Lymphoblastic - Small non-cleaved cell (Burkitt's and non-Burkitt's)	- Follicular, predominantly large cell, cleaved and/or non-cleaved - Diffuse, small-cleaved cell - Diffuse, large cell, cleaved or non-cleaved

TABLE 11.66: World Health Organization (WHO) classification of lymphoid neoplasm.

Precursor B-cell neoplasms (immature B cells)	**Precursor T-cell neoplasms** (immature T cells)
Precursor-B lymphoblastic leukaemia/lymphoma	Precursor-T lymphoblastic leukaemia/lymphoma
Peripheral B-cell neoplasms (mature B cells)	**Peripheral T-cell and natural killer (NK)-cell neoplasms** (mature T cells and NK cells)
Chronic lymphocytic leukaemia	T-cell prolymphocytic leukaemia
B-cell prolymphocytic leukaemia	Large granular lymphocytic leukaemia
Lymphoplasmacytic lymphoma	Mycosis fungoides/Sezary syndrome
Mantle cell lymphoma	Peripheral T-cell lymphoma, unspecified
Follicular lymphoma	Anaplastic large cell lymphoma
Marginal zone lymphoma	Angioimmunoblastic T-cell lymphoma
Hairy cell leukaemia	Adult T-cell leukaemia/lymphoma
Plasmacytoma/plasma cell myeloma	Extranodal NK/T-cell lymphoma
Diffuse large B-cell lymphoma	
Burkitt lymphoma	

- Patients with lymphoblastic lymphoma often present with an anterior mediastinal mass.
- Typically disseminates to the bone marrow and meninges and involves extranodal sites.
- It may be associated with "B" or systemic symptoms—weight loss, sweats, fever, and itching.
- Multicentric and spreads rapidly to non-contiguous areas, widespread at the time of diagnosis.
- Immunologic abnormalities—Autoimmune haemolytic anaemia and immune thrombocytopaenia
- *Paraneoplastic complications*: Neurological—demyelinating neuropathy, Guillain-Barré syndrome, autonomic dysfunction, peripheral neuropathy, skin—pemphigus, kidney—glomerulonephritis), and other systems—vasculitis, dermatomyositis, and cholestatic jaundice.

Clinical staging (Ann Arbor classification): Same staging system (**Table 11.67**) is used for both HL and NHL.

Investigations

Investigations required for staging disease are the same as that for HL. Laparotomy is rarely required, only when retroperitoneal nodes are involved.

- **Peripheral blood:**
    - *Anaemia*: Moderate anaemia may be observed when there is significant bone marrow involvement.
    - *Blood counts*: Usually normal, but few patients may show lymphocytosis.
    - Splenomegaly with hypersplenism or autoimmune haemolytic anaemia may lead to reduced haemoglobin level, reticulocytosis and positive Coomb's test.
- **Bone marrow aspiration and trephine biopsy:** Marrow involvement is common with NHL.

TABLE 11.67: Clinical staging (Ann Arbor classification) of low-grade and high-grade non-Hodgkin lymphoma.

Low-grade NHL	High-grade NHL
Radiotherapy	
Localised stage I disease	• In few stages I patients without bulky disease • Residual localised bulk disease after chemotherapy • Spinal cord and other compression syndromes
Chemotherapy	
Oral therapy—chlorambucil (not curative). Intensive IV chemotherapy in younger patients—better quality of life without any survival benefit	More than 90% of patients—IV combination chemotherapy—CHOP regimen (cyclophosphamide, doxorubicin, vincristine and prednisolone
Humanised monoclonal antibody therapy	
• Rituximab, 131I-Tositumomab, 90Y-Ibritumomab • Anti-CD20 antibody rituximab(R) alone or with chemotherapy, i.e., R-CVP-recommended as first-line therapy	• Combination with CHOP chemotherapy, rituximab (R) improves overall survival • R-CHOP: First-line therapy for those with stage II or greater diffuse large-cell lymphoma
Autologous bone marrow transplantation	
	In relapsed chemosensitive disease

CHOP-R	CVP-R	FCR
• Cyclophosphamide • Doxorubicin • Vincristine • Prednisone • Fixed dose rituximab	• Cyclophosphamide • Vincristine • Prednisone • Fixed dose rituximab	• Fludarabine • Cyclophosphamide • Rituximab

- **Other investigations**
  - **Immunophenotyping:** Distinguish T- and B-cell tumours, done on blood, marrow or lymph node material by flow cytometry and/or immunohistochemistry utilising a minimal antibody panel (CD45, CD20, and CD3) to identify B, T or NK subtypes.
  - **Immunoglobulin determination:** Associated with IgG or IgM paraproteins.
  - **Measurement of uric acid levels:** Few very aggressive high-grade NHLs are associated with very high urate levels that can precipitate renal failure when treatment is started.
  - Human immunodeficiency virus testing
  - Serum levels of LDH, β_2-macroglobulin, and serum protein electrophoresis are often needed.
  - **Diagnostic spinal tap:** Required when a prophylactic instillation of cytarabine, methotrexate is indicated in high-risk patients (involvement of CNS, orbit, bone marrow, testis, spine or skull base). Indicated in HIV-associated lymphoma and highly aggressive lymphoma.

Management

Characteristics of Hodgkin and non-Hodgkin lymphoma have been shown in **Table 11.68**.

BURKITT LYMPHOMA/LEUKAEMIA

- Highly aggressive, often extranodal B-cell lymphoma.
- The most common childhood malignancy worldwide and majority in children but can occur in all ages.
- Male:female ratio is 3:1.
- Often presents with extranodal involvement or as leukaemia.

Three categories of Burkitt lymphoma namely (**Table 11.69**):

About 80% of cases are associated with a chromosomal translocation involving MYC oncogene from chromosome 8 to the immunoglobulin (Ig) heavy chain region on chromosome 14. [t(8;14)].

TABLE 11.68: Characteristics of Hodgkin and non-Hodgkin lymphoma.

Characteristics	Hodgkin lymphoma	Non-Hodgkin lymphoma
Age	Bimodal peak incidence, 15–35 years and 45–70 years	Peak incidence around 60 years
"B" symptoms	More common	Less common
Alcohol-induced discomfort in lymph nodal region	Common	Does not observe
Disease at the time of diagnosis	Usually well-localised	Usually widespread
Site of involvement	Unifocal origin and arises in a single node or chain of nodes (cervical, mediastinal, para-aortic)	Mostly involves multiple peripheral nodes (multicentric origin)
Pattern of spread	Orderly spread by contiguity, predictable	Non-contiguous spread, unpredictable
Epitrochlear node involvement	Rare	Common
Mediastinal involvement	common	Uncommon
Mesenteric nodes, Waldeyer's ring	Rarely involved	Commonly involved
Bone marrow involvement	Late	Early
Extranodal involvement	Uncommon	Common
Neoplastic cells	Neoplastic cells—Hodgkin or Reed–Sternberg cells (1–5%)	Neoplastic cells form major tumour mass
Number of neoplastic cells	Few neoplastic cells (RS cells)	Majority of the cells are neoplastic

TABLE 11.69: Three categories of Burkitt lymphoma.

Endemic (African)	Sporadic (non-endemic)	Immunodeficiency-associated
• Affects children, adolescents • Associated with EBV infection, corresponds malaria distribution • Involves extranodal sites, particularly the jaw, gastrointestinal tract, gonads	• Burkitt lymphoma	• Human immunodeficiency virus (HIV) lymphomas

Clinical Features

- **Endemic form:** Presents as a rapidly growing jaw tumour in a young child (4–7 years). Mandibular and maxillary involvement leads to deformity, loosening of teeth, and extrusion of eye with loss of vision.
- **Sporadic form:** Presents as an abdominal mass.
- **Immunodeficiency-associated** (HIV) form usually occurs with CD4 counts above 200/mm^3. Presents with abdominal involvement.
- **Abdominal involvement:** Mass due to bilateral involvement of kidneys, adrenals, ovaries, bowel, and lymph nodes.
- **Other sites:** CNS (adults), long bones, salivary glands, thyroid, testes, heart, breast, and bone marrow.

Investigations

- **Histological examination:**
  - Distinctive, involved tissues are effaced by diffuse monotonous infiltrate of medium-sized lymphoid cells with round nuclei with clumped chromatin and multiple, centrally located nucleoli.
  - Mitoses—numerous, almost 100% of cells being in cell cycle.
  - Plenty of **apoptotic** tumour cells. Nuclear remnants of the apoptotic cells are phagocytosed by benign macrophages which are evenly and diffusely distributed among the tightly packed basophilic tumour cells, creating a **"starry sky" pattern** (Fig. 11.12).
- **Chromosome analysis (Fig. 11.13):** The most common translocation results in movement of MYC-containing segment of chromosome 8 to chromosome 14q32, placing it close to *IGH* gene. Genetic notation for translocation is t(8:14) (q24; q32). As a result, MYC protein is overexpressed resulting in cell proliferation and stimulates apoptosis.
- Antibodies to EB viral capsid antigen may be detected (most-endemic type, many with sporadic and HIV-associated tumours).

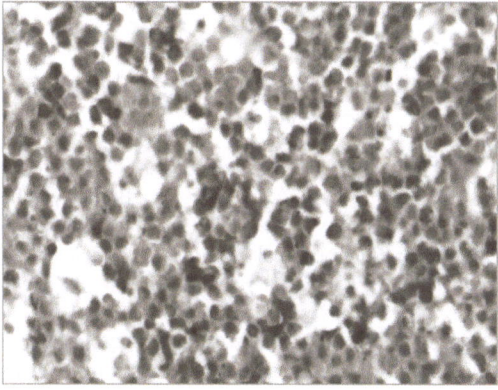

Fig. 11.12: Burkitt lymphoma composed of medium-sized lymphoid cells admixed with benign macrophages giving a "starry sky" appearance. *(For color version, see plate 4)*
Courtesy: Exam Preparatory Manual for Undergraduates—Medicine/Archith Boloor and Ramadas Nayak, 2nd edition.

Treatment

- Initiated urgently with curative intent whenever feasible
- Adequate hydration prior to the initiation of therapy to prevent the risk of tumour lysis syndrome.
- Standard treatment comprises of high-intensity, brief-duration cyclical combination chemotherapy
- Regimens include:
  - CHOP (cyclophosphamide, hydroxydaunorubicin or doxorubicin, vincristine, prednisolone)
  - Rituximab plus EPOCH (etoposide, prednisolone, vincristine, cyclophosphamide, doxorubicin)

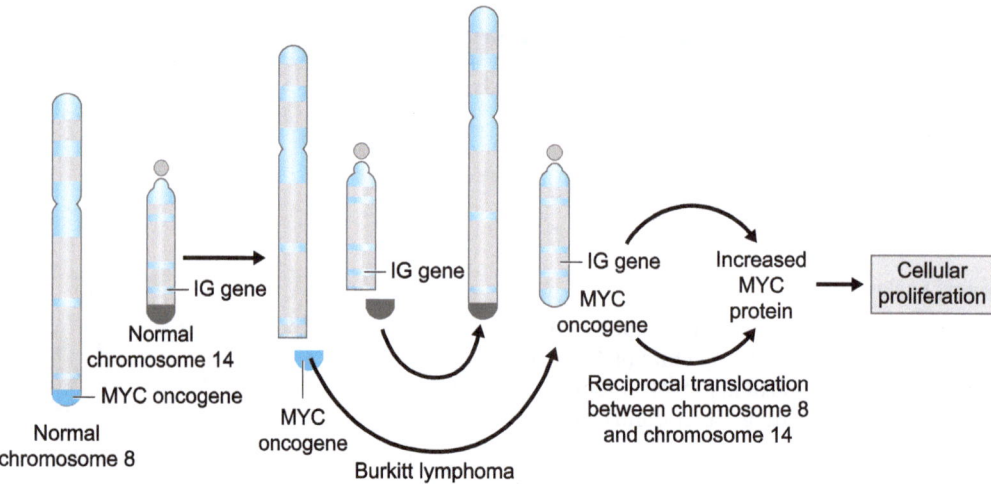

Fig. 11.13: Chromosomal translocation and activated mica oncogene in Burkitt lymphoma.

- ○ CODOX-M/IVAC regimen (cyclophosphamide, vincristine, doxorubicin, methotrexate/ifosfamide, etoposide or VP-16, and cytarabine)
- Prophylactic CNS therapy is essential, intrathecal methotrexate or cytosine arabinoside is given in addition to high-dose systemic administration.
- *Cure rates*: High as 70–80%.

BEST OF FIVES

1. A 79-year-old woman was admitted for elective hip replacement surgery. On examination, she was pale. There was a 2-cm splenomegaly and there were small discrete axillary lymph nodes.
Investigations reveal:
Haemoglobin 107 g/L (115–165)
White cell counts 15.5×10^9/L (4.0–11.0)
Platelet count 183×10^9/L (150–400)

What is the most likely diagnosis?
A. Acute myeloid leukaemia
B. Chronic lymphocytic leukaemia
C. Chronic myeloid leukaemia
D. Myelodysplasia
E. Myelofibrosis

2. Which of the following may be the best approach to a young patient with a fine needle aspiration (FNA) from an enlarged cervical lymph node showing possibility of Hodgkin's lymphoma?
A. Whole node-excision and immunohistochemistry (IHC) for confirmation of diagnosis. Upon confirmation, positron emission tomography/computed tomography (PET-CT) scan for staging
B. IHC is not mandatory for diagnosis of Hodgkin's lymphoma. The patient may be treated after staging
C. Proceed to PET-CT and treatment as delay in initiating therapy may be dangerous
D. Whole-body CT scan and bone marrow biopsy for staging followed by therapy
E. Start R-CHOP

3. A 33-year-old man presenting with favourable limited stage Hodgkin's lymphoma was assessed with interim positron emission tomography/computed tomography (PET-CT) scan after two cycles of ABVD. It shows residual activity in mediastinum. What would be the treatment plan?
A. Two more cycles of ABVD followed by an end of treatment PET-CT
B. Involved-field radiation therapy (IFRT) and observe

C. Two more cycles of ABVD plus IFRT
   D. Salvage therapy followed by PET-CT. If negative, proceed to HDT-auto SCT (high-dose therapy/autologous stem-cell transplant)
   E. No further therapy. PET-CT uptake in this patient is not clinically significant

4. Which of the following investigations may not be performed in a patient aged 65 years old presenting with pancytopaenia, platelet and red blood cell transfusion requirement, decreased reticulocyte count and absence of organomegaly?
   A. Paroxysmal nocturnal haemoglobinuria (PNH) by flow cytometry
   B. Chromosome breakage analysis
   C. Fluorescence in situ hybridisation (FISH) for myelodysplastic syndrome (MDS)
   D. Trephine biopsy
   E. Vitamin B12 assay

5. Following are known side effects of cyclosporine except:
   A. Hyperglycaemia
   B. Hepatic dysfunction
   C. Renal dysfunction
   D. Myelosuppression
   E. Hypertension

6. A patient of febrile neutropaenia responded to initial IV antibiotics and has become afebrile for >48 hours with persistent absolute neutrophil count (ANC) > 0.5×10^9/L. The next step-down approach will be:
   A. Low risk and no cause found: Consider changing to oral antibiotics
   B. High risk and no cause found: If on dual therapy, aminoglycoside may be discontinued
   C. High risk and no cause found: Consider changing to oral antibiotics
   D. When cause found: Continue on appropriate specific therapy
   E. Low risk and no cause found: Stop antibiotics

7. A 69-year-old man who has received repeated courses of chemoimmunotherapy for refractory mantle cell lymphoma presents with the gradual onset of cognitive impairment, dysphasia and dyspraxia. On lumbar puncture, there is only a slight increase in protein concentration, cell count is not increased and glucose is normal. Magnetic resonance imaging (MRI) of the brain shows multiple high-intensity signals on T2-weighted and FLAIR (fluid attenuation inversion recovery) sequences affecting mainly the white matter. The most likely organism implicated is:
   A. BK virus
   B. Herpes simplex
   C. John Cunningham (JC) virus
   D. *Treponema pallidum*
   E. Varicella zoster virus

8. A 77-year-old man presents with confusion and hypercalcaemia. A computed tomography (CT) scan shows generalised thoracic and abdominal lymphadenopathy. His complete blood count (CBC) shows white blood cell (WBC) 10.1×10^9/L, haemoglobin (Hb) 128 g/L and platelet count 127×10^9/L. The cells express CD10, CD19, CD20, BCL2 and focal, weak BCL6. Ki67 is 80%
   A. B-cell lymphoma, unclassifiable, with features intermediate between diffuse large B-cell lymphoma and Burkitt lymphoma
   B. Burkitt lymphoma
   C. Diffuse large B-cell lymphoma
   D. 'Double hit' lymphoma
   E. Mantle cell lymphoma

9. Haemoglobin E is a 'thalassaemic haemoglobinopathy'. That is, Hgb E is a structural or qualitative variant (β26 glu>lys) and its synthesis is also impaired. What primarily explains the quantitative reduction in the synthesis of this structurally abnormal globin?
   A. The β^E globin is unstable.
   B. The β^E mutation disrupts a promoter sequence.
   C. The β^E globin only forms tetramers with itself.
   D. The β^E mutation creates an abnormal cryptic splice site.
   E. The β^E globin is absent.

10. A 68-year-old man seeks evaluation for fatigue, weight loss and early satiety that have been present for ~4 months. On physical examination, his spleen is noted to be markedly enlarged. It is firm to touch and crosses the midline. The lower edge of the spleen reaches to the pelvis. His haemoglobin is 11.1 g/dL

and haematocrit is 33.7%. The leucocyte count is 6,200/μL and platelet count is 220,000/μL. The white cell count differential is 75% polymorphonuclear (PMN) leucocytes, 8% myelocytes, 4% metamyelocytes, 8% lymphocytes, 3% monocytes and 2% eosinophils.

The peripheral blood smear shows teardrop cells, nucleated red blood cells and immature granulocytes.

Rheumatoid factor is positive. A bone marrow biopsy is attempted, but no cells are able to be aspirated. No evidence of leukaemia or lymphoma is found on biopsy.

What is the most likely cause of the splenomegaly?
- A. Chronic idiopathic myelofibrosis [primary myelofibrosis (PMF)]
- B. Chronic myelogenous leukaemia
- C. Rheumatoid arthritis
- D. Tuberculosis
- E. Lymphoma

11. Which of the following monoclonal antibodies binds to both F VIII and F IX and holds promise as a future prophylaxis therapy for haemophilia?
- A. Concizumab
- B. Afutuzumab
- C. Emicizumab
- D. Caplacizumab
- E. Rituximab

12. A 48-year-old man whose parents were born in Jamaica presents with fever, night sweats and weight loss. On examination, he appears dehydrated but has no hepatosplenomegaly or lymphadenopathy. His full blood count (FBC) shows white blood cells (WBC) 90×10^9/L, haemoglobin (Hb) 155 g/L, mean corpuscular volume (MCV) 80 fl and platelet count 48×10^9/L. A blood film shows 80–90% abnormal lymphoid cells. On biochemical screening, there is a corrected calcium of 4.35 mmol/L (2.15–2.55) and a lactate dehydrogenase (LDH) of 1,395 IU/L (200–450). Immunophenotyping shows a lymphoid population expressing CD4, CD5, CD25 and CD45. There is no expression of surface membrane CD3, CD7, CD8 or CD10.

The most likely diagnosis is:
- A. Adult T-cell leukaemia/lymphoma
- B. Angioimmunoblastic T-cell lymphoma
- C. Gamma-delta T-cell lymphoma
- D. T-lineage prolymphocytic leukaemia
- E. Burkitt lymphoma

13. A 60-year-old man presents with multiple violaceous skin plaques. His full blood count (FBC) is normal.

A biopsy is performed and shows a dermal infiltrate without epidermotropism. Immunohistochemistry shows the infiltrating cells to express CD4, CD33, CD56 and CD123; negative for lysozyme.

The most likely diagnosis is:
- A. Blastic plasmacytoid dendritic cell neoplasm
- B. Granulocytic sarcoma
- C. Monocytic sarcoma
- D. Natural killer (NK) cell lymphoma
- E. Mycosis fungoides

14. In the anaemia of chronic disease, which of the following statements is true?
- A. The serum iron is high.
- B. The serum ferritin is low.
- C. The mean cell volume is raised.
- D. The hepcidin level is raised.
- E. The iron-binding capacity is raised.

15. All the following statements about iron deficiency are true except:
- A. It is usually microcytic hypochromic.
- B. The serum iron-binding capacity is raised.
- C. It is best treated with iron injections.
- D. It may be caused by aspirin.
- E. It is more common during pregnancy.

16. All the following are causes of neutrophil leucocytosis except:
- A. Myocardial infarction
- B. Erythropoietin therapy
- C. Still's disease
- D. Pneumococcal pneumonia
- E. Pregnancy

17. Which of the following is associated with massive splenomegaly?
- A. Polycythaemia vera
- B. Hereditary spherocytosis

C. Leishmaniasis
D. Portal hypertension
E. Typhoid

18. Which of the following statements about platelet transfusions is true?
    A. They are indicated in all patients with platelets <50 × 10⁹/L.
    B. They can transmit cytomegalovirus infection.
    C. They must be cross-matched.
    D. They are usually given as a pool of 10 individual donations.
    E. They will raise the platelet count in the recipient for 5–7 days.

19. A woman aged 25 years visits her GP complaining of night sweats and loss of weight. On examination, she is found to have an enlarged spleen but no other abnormality. The tests show a mild anaemia of 10.2 g/L and a raised white cell count of 95 × 10⁹/L with the differential showing predominant neutrophils and myelocytes. The platelet count is 539 × 10⁹/L. How will you treat this patient?
    A. Methylcobalamine
    B. Imatinib
    C. Rituximab
    D. Dapsone
    E. Amphotericin B

20. A 36-year-old man presented with a 2-day history of severe tiredness and jaundice. He has been passing dark urine over the past 12 hours. He had symptoms of a urinary tract infection and was treated with co-trimoxazole. He has had no serious illnesses in the past.
    On examination, he is pale and jaundiced. The liver and spleen are not palpable. Investigations show haemoglobin 67 g/L, white blood cells 11.1 × 10⁹/L and platelets 234 × 10⁹/L. Blood film shows abnormal red cells in which the haemoglobin has contracted away from the membrane ('bite cells'). There is polychromasia and anisocytosis. What is the diagnosis?
    A. Malaria
    B. Thalassaemia
    C. Glucose-6-phosphate dehydrogenase (G6PD) deficiency
    D. Sepsis
    E. Leptospirosis

Answers

1-B, 2-A, 3-C, 4-B, 5-D, 6-C, 7-C, 8-A, 9-D, 10-A, 11-C, 12-A, 13-A, 14-D, 15-C, 16-B, 17-C, 18-B, 19-B, 20-C

SUGGESTED READING

1. Price EA, Mehra R, Holmes TH, Schrier SL. Anemia in older persons: etiology and evaluation. Blood Cells Mol Dis. 2011;46(2):159-65.
2. Camaschella C. Iron-deficiency anemia. N Engl J Med. 2015;372(19):1832-43.
3. Lopez A, Cacoub P, Macdougall IC, Peyrin-Biroulet L. Iron deficiency anaemia. Lancet. 2016;387(10021):907-16.
4. Devalia V, Hamilton MS, Molloy AM, British Committee for Standards in Haematology. Guidelines for the diagnosis and treatment of cobalamin and folate disorders. Br J Haematol. 2014;166(4):496-513.
5. Carmel R. How I treat cobalamin (vitamin B12) deficiency. Blood. 2008;112(6):2214-21.
6. Peffault de Latour R, Peters C, Gibson B, Strahm B, Lankester A, de Heredia CD, et al. Recommendations on hematopoietic stem cell transplantation for inherited bone marrow failure syndromes. Bone Marrow Transplant. 2015;50(9):1168-72.
7. Killick SB, Bown N, Cavenagh J, Dokal I, Foukaneli T, Hill A, et al. Guidelines for the diagnosis and management of adult aplastic anaemia. Br J Haematol. 2016;172(2):187-207.
8. Malcovati L, Hellström-Lindberg E, Bowen D, Adès L, Cermak J, Cañizo CD, et al. Diagnosis and treatment of primary myelodysplastic syndromes in adults: recommendations from the European LeukemiaNet. Blood. 2013;122(17):2943-64.
9. Killick SB, Carter C, Culligan D, Dalley C, Das-Gupta E, Drummond M, et al. Guidelines for the diagnosis and management of adult myelodysplastic syndromes. Br J Haematol. 2014;164(4):503-25.
10. Swerdlow SH, Campo E, Harris NL, Jaffe ES, Pileri SA, Stein H, et al. (Eds). WHO Classification of Tumours of Haematopoietic and Lymphoid Tissues, revised 4th edition. International Agency for Research on Cancer (IARC). Lyon; 2017.
11. Rodeghiero F, Stasi R, Gernsheimer T, Michel M, Provan D, Arnold DM, et al. Standardization of terminology, definitions and outcome criteria in immune thrombocytopenic purpura of adults and children: report from an international working group. Blood. 2009;113(11):2386-93.

12. Cines DB, Bussel JB. How I treat idiopathic thrombocytopenic purpura (ITP). Blood. 2005;106(7):2244-51.
13. Laszik ZG, Kambham N, Silva FG. Thrombotic microangiopathies. In: Jennett JC, D'Agati VD, Olson JL, et al (Eds). Heptinstall's Pathology of the Kidney. Philadelphia: Lippincott Williams & Wilkins; 2014.
14. George JN, Nester CM. Syndromes of thrombotic microangiopathy. N Engl J Med. 2014;371(19):1847-8.
15. Engert A, Plütschow A, Eich HT, Lohri A, Dörken B, Borchmann P, et al. Reduced treatment intensity in patients with early-stage Hodgkin's lymphoma. N Engl J Med. 2010;363(7):640-52.
16. Radford J, Illidge T, Counsell N, Hancock B, Pettengell R, Johnson P, et al. Results of a trial of PET-directed therapy for early-stage Hodgkin's lymphoma. N Engl J Med. 2015;372(17):1598-607.
17. Dimopoulos MA, Sonneveld P, Leung N, Merlini G, Ludwig H, Kastritis E, et al. International Myeloma Working Group Recommendations for the Diagnosis and Management of Myeloma-Related Renal Impairment. J Clin Oncol. 2016;34(13):1544-57.
18. Vlaar AP, Oczkowski S, de Bruin S, Wijnberge M, Antonelli M, Aubron C, et al. Transfusion Strategies in Non-Bleeding Critically Ill Adults: A Clinical Practice Guideline From the European Society of Intensive Care Medicine. Intensive Care Med. 2020;46(4):673-96.
19. European Directorate for the Quality of Medicines and HealthCare (EDQM). Guide to the preparation, use and quality assurance of blood components, 19th edition. 2018.
20. Boer C, Meesters MI, Milojevic M, Benedetto U, Bolliger D, von Heymann C, et al. 2017 EACTS/EACTA guidelines on patient blood management for adult cardiac surgery. J Cardiothorac Vasc Anesth. 2018;32(1):88-120.
21. Kozek-Langenecker SA, Ahmed AB, Afshari A, Albaladejo P, Aldecoa C, Barauskas G, et al. Management of Severe Perioperative Bleeding: Guidelines From the European Society of Anaesthesiology: First Update 2016. Eur J Anaesthesiol. 2017;34(6):332-95.

CHAPTER 12

Pulmonology

NORMAL ARTERIAL BLOOD GAS LEVELS

Table 12.1 shows the normal arterial blood gas (ABG) levels.

CLUBBING

Clubbing is defined as a selective bulbous enlargement of the distal segment of a digit due to an increase in the soft tissue.

Grading of Clubbing

Grading of clubbing is given in **Box 12.1**.

Common Causes of Clubbing

Common causes of clubbing are given in **Box 12.2**.

PULMONARY FUNCTION TESTS

Pulmonary function tests are given in **Box 12.3**.

Ventilatory Capacity

- Forced expiratory volume in one second (FEV_1), forced vital capacity (FVC) and vital capacity (VC) are recorded using a spirometer. The patient inhales fully and then forcibly exhales as fast as possible into the mouth piece of the spirometer until no more air can be expelled.
  - FVC is the volume of air expired with a maximal effort after deep inspiration.
  - FEV_1 is the volume of air expired in the first second after deep inspiration.

TABLE 12.1: Normal arterial blood gas (ABG) levels.

Arterial oxygen tension	PaO_2	95 ± 5 mmHg
Arterial carbon dioxide (CO_2)	$PaCO_2$	40 ± 2 mmHg
Arterial oxygen saturation	SaO_2	$97 \pm 2\%$
Arterial blood pH	pH	7.40 ± 0.02
Arterial bicarbonate	HCO_3	24 ± 2 mmol/L
Base excess	BE	0 ± 2 mmol/L

Box 12.1: Grades of clubbing.
- Grade I: Increased fluctuation of the nail bed
- Grade II: Obliteration of the angle between nail and nail bed (lovibond angle; normal ≤ 160°)
- Grade III: Increased curvature of the nail resulting in a parrot beak or drumstick appearance
- Grade IV: Hypertrophic osteoarthropathy, characterised by painful, tender, swelling of wrists (most common), ankles, elbows and knees

Box 12.2: Common causes of clubbing.

Respiratory causes:
- Bronchogenic carcinoma
- Bronchiectasis
- Lung abscess
- Empyema
- Mesothelioma
- Interstitial lung diseases

Cardiac causes:
- Infective endocarditis
- Congenital cyanotic heart diseases

Alimentary causes:
- Ulcerative colitis
- Crohn's disease
- Cirrhosis of liver
- Hepatoma

Miscellaneous causes:
- Hereditary, idiopathic
- Thyrotoxicosis
- Acromegaly
- Unilateral clubbing in pancoast tumour, subclavian artery aneurysm and hemiplegia
- Undigital clubbing occurs in repeated trauma

- Two typical patterns of abnormalities can be found:
  - Obstructive ventilator defect, where there is narrowing of airways during expiration (e.g. bronchial asthma and chronic bronchitis). Here, FEV_1 is markedly decreased, VC is decreased or normal and FEV_1/VC is decreased.
  - Restrictive ventilator defect, where FEV_1 and VC are decreased, and FEV^1/VC is normal increased.

> **Box 12.3: Pulmonary function tests.**
> - Ventilatory capacity [forced expiratory volume in one second (FEV_1), forced vital capacity (FVC), peak expiratory flow rate (PEF)]
> - Reversibility of airflow limitation
>   - By administering inhaled bronchodilator
> - Flow-volume curves
> - Airway resistance
> - Gas transfer (diffusion)
> - Lung volumes [total lung capacity (TLC), residual volume (RV)]
> - Blood gases
> - Pulse oximetry
> - Exercise tests

- Peak expiratory flow rate (PEF) can be measured during forced expiration by a gauge or metre, which is simpler and cheaper than a spirometer. It measures the volume of forcibly expired air during the first 10 seconds after deep inspiration. Reduced values indicate airflow obstruction. It is of no use in restrictive ventilatory defect.
- Forced expiratory time (FET) is simple to measure, with just a watch and a stethoscope. Normal people can empty their chests from full inspiration in 4 seconds or less. Prolonged FET of > 6 seconds indicates air flow obstruction.

Reversibility of Airflow Limitation

When FEV_1 is disproportionately reduced resulting in FEV_1/FVC ratios of < 70%, spirometry should be repeated following inhaled short-acting β2-adrenoceptor agonists (e.g. salbutamol). A large improvement in FEV_1 (over 400 mL) is seen in bronchial asthma and, to some extent, in chronic bronchitis.

Table 12.2 lists the abbreviations that are used in pulmonary function tests.

Figure 12.1 shows the representation of various lung volume measurements in a diagram.

TABLE 12.2: Abbreviations used in pulmonary function tests.

Abbreviations	Explanation
FVC (forced vital capacity)	Volume of air expired with a maximal effort after deep inspiration
FEV_1 (forced expiratory volume in one second)	Volume of air expired in the first second after deep inspiration
VC (vital capacity)	• Maximum amount of air that can be expelled from the lungs after the deepest possible breath • TLC minus RV or maximum volume of air exhaled from maximal inspiratory level (60–70 mL/kg) (3100–4800 mL). VC decreases with age
PEF (peak expiratory flow)	Volume of forcibly expired air during the first 10 seconds after deep inspiration
TLC (total lung capacity)	Sum of all volume compartments or volume of air in lungs after maximum inspiration (4–6 L)
FRC (functional residual capacity)	• Sum of RV and ERV or the volume of air in the lungs at end-expiratory tidal position (30–35 mL/kg) (2300–3300 mL) • Measured with multiple-breath closed-circuit helium dilution, multiple-breath open-circuit nitrogen washout, or body plethysmography • It cannot be measured by spirometry

Continued

Continued

Abbreviations	Explanation
RV (residual volume)	• Volume of air remaining in lungs after maximum exhalation (20–25 mL/kg) (1700–2100 mL) • Indirectly measured (FRC-ERV) • It cannot be measured by spirometry. RV increases with age
IRV (inspiratory reserve volume)	Maximum volume of air inhaled from the end-inspiratory tidal position (1900–3300 mL)
ERV (expiratory reserve volume)	Maximum volume of air that can be exhaled from resting end-expiratory tidal position (700–1000 mL)
TV (tidal volume)	Volume of air inhaled or exhaled with each breath during quiet breathing (6–8 mL/kg)
IC (inspiratory capacity)	Sum of IRV and TV or the maximum volume of air that can be inhaled from the end-expiratory tidal position (2400–3800 mL)
EC (expiratory capacity)	TV + ERV
DLCO (diffusing capacity of lung for carbon monoxide)	Also known as transfer factor, DLCO measures the transfer of inhaled gases into the pulmonary capillaries

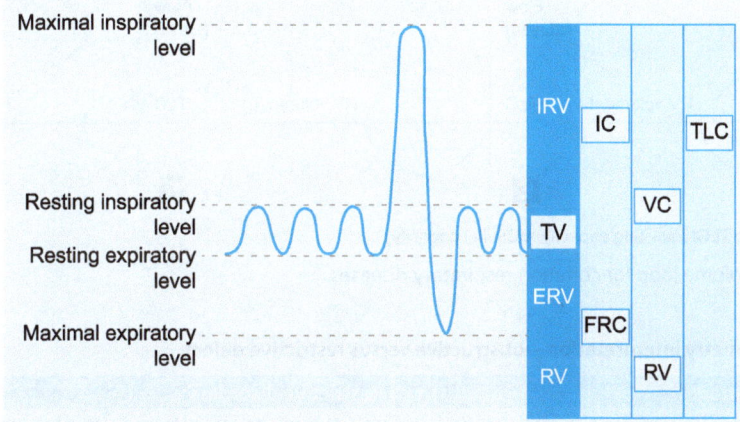

(ERV: expiratory reserve volume; FRC: functional residual capacity; IC: inspiratory capacity; IRV: inspiratory reserve volume; RV: residual volume; TLC: total lung capacity; TV: tidal volume; VC: vital capacity)

Fig. 12.1: Diagrammatic representation of various lung volume measurements.

Flow-volume Curves

Table 12.3 shows the flow-volume loops in various disorders and **Figure 12.2** shows the flow volume loop for common respiratory diseases.

Table 12.4 shows the interpretation of spirometry in terms of obstructive and restrictive defects.

Diffusing capacity of lung (DL): It is defined as the rate at which gas enters into blood divided by its driving pressure. It measures the ability of the lungs to transfer gas from inhaled air in the alveoli to the red blood cells in pulmonary capillaries.

Table 12.5 shows the diseases associated with reduced and increased diffusing capacity of lung for carbon monoxide (DLCO).

■ RESPIRATORY FAILURE

Definition

Respiratory failure is present when PaO_2 is 60 mmHg (8.0 kPa) and/or $PaCO_2$ is 50 mmHg (6.5 kPa).

TABLE 12.3: Flow-volume loops in various disorders.

Disease states	FVC	FEV$_1$	FEV$_1$/FVC
Obstructive	Normal	Reduced	Reduced
Stiff lungs	Reduced	Reduced	Normal
Respiratory muscle weakness	Reduced	Reduced	Normal

(FEV$_1$: forced expiratory volume in one second; FVC: forced vital capacity)

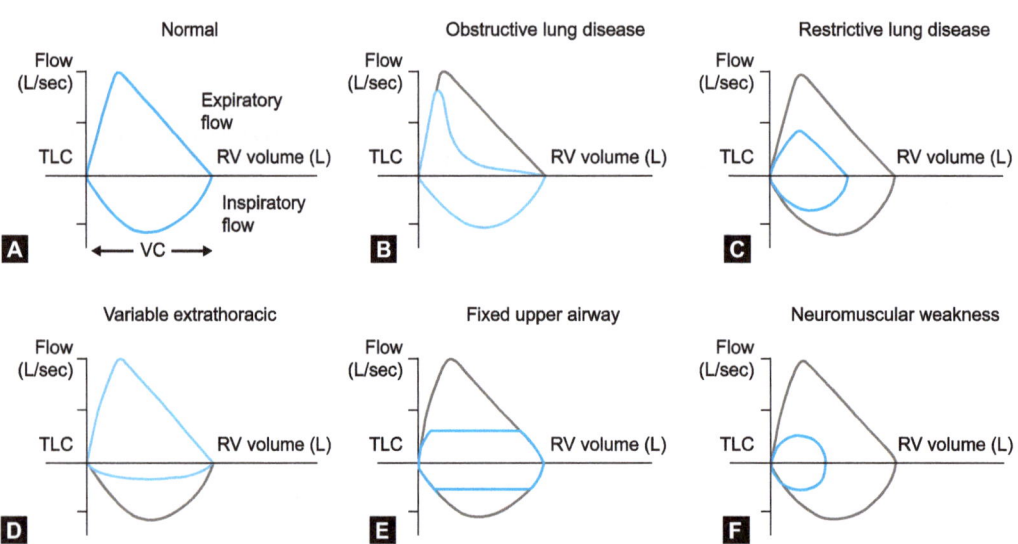

(RV: residual volume; TLC: total lung capacity; VC: vital capacity)

Fig. 12.2: Flow-volume loop for common respiratory diseases.

TABLE 12.4: Spirometry interpretation—obstructive versus restrictive defect.

Obstructive disorders	Restrictive disorders
Limitation of expiratory airflow as airways cannot empty as rapidly compared to normal (e.g. narrowed airways from bronchospasm, inflammation, etc.)	Characterised by reduced lung volumes/decreased lung compliance
• FVC normal or ↓ • FEV$_1$ ↓ (significantly decreased) • FEF 25–75% ↓ • FEV$_1$/FVC ↓ (> 0.7) • TLC normal or ↑	• FVC ↓ (significantly decreased) • FEV$_1$ ↓ • FEF 25–75% normal to ↓ • FEV$_1$/FVC normal to ↑ (> 0.7) • TLC ↓
Examples: Asthma, emphysema, cystic fibrosis	Examples: Interstitial fibrosis, scoliosis, obesity, lung resection, neuromuscular diseases, cystic fibrosis

(FEF: forced expiratory flow; FEV$_1$: forced expiratory volume in one second; FVC: forced vital capacity; TLC: total lung capacity)

Types of Respiratory Failure

- Acute hypoxaemia without hypercapnia (acute type I respiratory failure)
- Chronic hypoxaemia without hypercapnia (chronic type I respiratory failure)
- Acute hypoxaemia with hypercapnia (acute type II respiratory failure)
- Chronic hypoxaemia with hypercapnia (chronic type II respiratory failure)

TABLE 12.5: Diseases associated with reduced and increased diffusing capacity of lung for carbon monoxide (DLCO).

Reduced DLCO-ventilation is in excess of blood flow (a high VQ,-DEAD SPACE- 'wasted air')]	Increased DLCO [blood flow is in excess of ventilation (a low VQ, - SHUNT- 'wasted blood')]
• Emphysema, lung resection, pulmonary embolism, anaemia • Pulmonary fibrosis, sarcoidosis—increased thickness	Severe obesity, asthma, polycythaemia, supine position, exercise, and left to right shunt

TABLE 12.6: Causes of acute and chronic type I respiratory failure.

Acute type I respiratory failure	Chronic type I respiratory failure
• Pneumonia • Pulmonary oedema • Acute asthma • Pulmonary embolism • Acute respiratory distress syndrome (ARDS) • Pneumothorax	• Diseases with widespread pulmonary fibrosis • Chronic pulmonary oedema • Chronic disorders of chest wall or neuromuscular diseases • Chronic pulmonary thromboembolism

> **Box 12.4: Causes of acute and chronic type II respiratory failure.**
>
> **Acute type II respiratory failure**
> - Respiratory depressant drugs, e.g. diazepam, opiates, alcohol
> - Severe obstruction to the airflow, e.g. severe acute asthma, laryngeal and tracheal obstruction, acute exacerbation of chronic obstructive pulmonary disease (COPD)
> - Disorders of respiratory muscles, e.g. acute polymyositis
> - Injuries to chest, e.g. tension pneumothorax, massive haemothorax and flail chest
> - Brainstem damage, e.g. stroke, encephalitis, trauma
> - Disorders of spinal cord, nerves and neuromuscular transmission, e.g. spinal trauma, transverse myelitis, acute GB syndrome, poliomyelitis, myasthenia gravis and botulism
>
> **Chronic type II respiratory failure**
> - COPD (most common)
> - Chest wall abnormalities, e.g. marked kyphoscoliosis, marked obesity
> - Amyotrophic lateral sclerosis, muscular dystrophy
> - Central hypoventilation
>
> (GB: Guillain-Barré)

Table 12.6 and Box 12.4 show the causes of acute and chronic type I and type II respiratory failure, respectively.

OBSTRUCTIVE SLEEP APNOEA

Obstructive sleep apnoea (OSA) has been defined in **Box 12.5**.

Table 12.7 shows the risk factors for OSA.

Diagnosis

Table 12.8 shows the clinical features of OSA and **Table 12.9** shows the degree of OSA–hypoapnoea index.

Treatment

- Correction of treatable causes (obesity, acromegaly, hypothyroid, enlarged tonsils

> **Box 12.5: Types of obstructive sleep apnoea.**
>
> **Types of sleep apnoea:** (1) Obstructive sleep apnoea (OSA), (2) central sleep apnoea and (3) mixed sleep apnoea (combination of factors)
> - **Obstructive** sleep apnoea is characterised by continued thoracoabdominal effort in the setting of partial or complete airflow cessation.
> - **Central** sleep apnoea is characterised by the lack of thoracoabdominal effort in the setting of partial or complete airflow cessation.
> - **Mixed** sleep apnoea has both obstructive and central features. They generally begin without thoracoabdominal effort and end with several thoracoabdominal efforts in breathing.

TABLE 12.7: Risk factors for obstructive sleep apnoea.

Obesity (major)	Mandibular retrognathia and micrognathia
Male sex (major)	Family history
Enlarged tonsils (especially in children)	Endocrine diseases (e.g. acromegaly, hypothyroidism)
Menopause	Advancing age
Nasal obstruction (e.g. nasal deformities, rhinitis, polyps, adenoids)	Respiratory depressant drugs (e.g. alcohol, sedatives, strong analgesics)
Smoking	

TABLE 12.8: Clinical features of obstructive sleep apnoea.

Nocturnal features	Daytime features
• Snoring, usually loud, habitual • Witnessed apnoea, which often interrupt the snoring and end with a snort • Nocturnal gasping and choking sensations • Nocturia • Insomnia • Restless sleep	• Non-restorative sleep (i.e. waking up as tired as when they went to bed) • Morning headache, dry or sore throat • Excessive daytime sleepiness (EDS) • Daytime fatigue/tiredness • Cognitive deficits; memory and intellectual impairment (short-term memory, concentration) and impaired work performance • Decreased vigilance • Morning confusion • Personality and mood changes, including depression, anxiety and irritability

TABLE 12.9: Degree of obstructive sleep apnoea and apnoea-hypoapnoea index.

Degree of obstructive sleep apnoea	Apnoea-hypopnea index (AHI)
Mild	5–15
Moderate	16–30
Severe	> 30

- or adenoids) and removal of any respiratory depressants (alcohol and sedatives)
- Continuous positive airway pressure (CPAP) during sleep
- Non-invasive positive—pressure ventilation (bi-level nasal positive pressure or BiPAP)
- Oral appliances
- Surgery (uvulopalatopharyngoplasty)

Pulmonology

OXYGEN THERAPY

Table 12.10 shows the therapaeutic indications for oxygen therapy.

ACUTE RESPIRATORY DISTRESS SYNDROME

Table 12.11 shows the Berlin definition of acute respiratory distress syndrome (ARDS).

TABLE 12.10: Therapaeutic indications for oxygen therapy.

- Pulmonary oedema
- Acute attack of bronchial asthma
- Chronic obstructive pulmonary disease (COPD)
- Acute respiratory distress syndrome (ARDS)
- Respiratory paralysis
- Anaerobic infections
- High altitude
- Prevent development of severe pulmonary hypertension

TABLE 12.11: Berlin definition of acute respiratory distress syndrome (ARDS).

Timing	Within 1 week of a known clinical insult/new/worsening respiratory symptoms
Chest X-ray	Bilateral opacities–not fully explained by effusions, lobar/lung collapse or nodules
Origin of oedema	• Respiratory failure not fully explained by cardiac failure or fluid overload • Need objective assessment (e.g. echocardiography) to exclude hydrostatic oedema if no risk factor is present
Oxygenation	
Mild	200 mmHg < PaO_2/FiO_2 ≤ 300 mmHg with PEEP or CPAP ≥ 5 cm H_2O
Moderate	100 mmHg < PaO_2/FiO_2 ≤ 200 mmHg with PEEP ≥ 5 cm H_2O
Severe	PaO_2/FiO_2 ≤ 100 mmHg with PEEP ≥ 5 cm H_2O

(CPAP: continuous positive airway pressure; PEEP: positive end-expiratory pressure)

Aetiology of ARDS and Acute Lung Injury

Table 12.12 shows the disorders commonly associated with ARDS.

Clinical Features

- Development of acute dyspnoea and hypoxaemia within hours to days of an inciting event
- Tachypnoea, tachycardia, cyanosis and the need for a high fraction of inspired oxygen (FiO_2) to maintain oxygen saturation
- Bilateral rales/crepitations

Investigation

- Chest radiography: Diffuse, extensive bilateral interstitial and alveolar infiltrates appear

TABLE 12.12: Disorders commonly associated with acute respiratory distress syndrome (ARDS).

Direct lung injury	
Pulmonary infections	Pneumonia (viral, bacterial, fungal, *Pneumocystis jirovecii*, Mycoplasma)
Aspiration	Aspiration of gastric contents (vomitus)
Inhalation of toxic gas	Ammonia, chlorine, nitrogen dioxide, ozone, oxygen, smoke
Blunt chest trauma	Pulmonary contusion
Near drowning	
Indirect lung injury	
Systemic disorders	Shock, septicaemia, uraemia, eclampsia
Severe trauma	Multiple bone fractures (fat embolism), flail chest, head trauma, burns
Blood	Multiple transfusions
Drug overdose	
• Narcotic overdose	Heroin, methadone, morphine, dextropropoxyphene
• Non-narcotic drugs	Barbiturates, thiazides, nitrofurantoin
Others	Acute pancreatitis, cardiopulmonary bypass, trauma, Goodpasture's syndrome, SLE

(SLE: systemic lupus erythematosus)

('fluffy' or 'soft' shadowing). These are located more at the periphery of the lungs. Cardiac size is normal.
- ABG analysis:
  o In the early stages, the only abnormality is mild hypoxaemia (low PaO_2). As the disease progresses, hypoxaemia worsens and hypercapnia appears.
  o In the late stages, there occur severe hypoxaemia (low PaO_2) and severe hypercapnia (high $PaCO_2$).

Management

Treatment of the underlying cause.
- Correction of hypoxaemia:
  o Supplemental oxygen
  o Intubation and mechanical ventilation with low tidal volume (5–7 mL/kg) and positive end-expiratory pressure (PEEP) between 5 and 20 cm of H_2O
- Optimise systemic perfusion by judicious use of fluids, asopressors, inotropic agents and PEEP
- Treat pneumonia and other infections.
- Routine stress ulcer prophylactic therapy
- Role of steroids is controversial. Low-dose glucocorticoid treatment in early ARDS, not persistent ARDS, may be associated with reduction in duration of mechanical ventilation and intensive care unit (ICU) length stay but with no effect on mortality.

■ MECHANICAL VENTILATION

Box 12.6 shows the indications of mechanical ventilation.

Box 12.6: Indications of mechanical ventilation.
- Apnoea with respiratory arrest
- Acute lung injury
- Respiratory rate > 35 breaths per minute
- Vital capacity < 15 mL/kg
- PO_2 < 60 at FiO_2 0.6
- Respiratory muscle fatigue
- Obtundation or coma
- Bradypnoea
- PCO_2 of > 50 mmHg with pH < 7.25

Non-invasive Ventilation (NIV)

It is used to deliver bi-level positive airway pressure (BiPAP—different levels of positive pressure during inspiration and expiration) when there is a need for ventilator assistance, as indicated by such symptoms as worsened dyspnoea, acute respiratory acidosis and worsened oxygenation.

Indications for Non-invasive Ventilation

- Increased dyspnoea: Moderate to severe
- Tachypnoea (24 breaths per minute in obstructive, 30 breaths per minute in restrictive lung disease)
- Signs of increased work of breathing, accessory muscle use and abdominal paradox
- Acute/Chronic Ventilator Failure would be better.
- Hypoxaemia (PaO_2: FIO_2 ratio 200)

Contraindications for Non-invasive Ventilation

- Severe hypoxaemia PaO_2: FIO_2 ratio75
- Severe acidaemia
- Multiorgan failure
- Upper airway obstruction
- Anatomic abnormalities that interfere with gas delivery (e.g. facial burn and trauma)
- Respiratory arrest
- Cardiac arrest and haemodynamic or cardiac instability
- Uncooperative patient
- Encephalopathy with inability to protect airways and a high-risk of aspiration
- Increased risk of aspiration: Copious secretions, vomiting or severe gastrointestinal bleeding
- Recent airway or gastrointestinal surgery
- Inability to fit mask

Invasive Ventilation

- **Controlled mode ventilation**
  o Used for initiation of the ventilation
  o No patient contribution
  o All variables are independent (FiO_2, TV, RR, I/E)
- **Assist control mode ventilation**
  o Inspiratory cycle is initiated either by the patient or if no patient effort is present then by a timer signal within the ventilator
  o Also commonly used for initiation

- o Synchronisation of ventilator cycle with patient's inspiratory effort
- o Drawbacks: Respiratory alkalosis, myoclonus and seizures
- **Synchronised intermittent mandatory ventilation (SIMV)**
  - o Patient is allowed to breathe spontaneously without ventilator assist in between the ventilator breaths
  - o Ventilator breath is delivered in synchrony
  - o Mandatory are the number of present breaths
  - o Intermediate mode
  - o Helpful in weaning
- **Continuous positive airway pressure**
  - o Not a true mode of ventilation
  - o All ventilation occurs because of patients spontaneous efforts ventilator just gives fresh gas to the breathing circuit with operator dependent positive pressure
  - o Used to access the extubation potential in the patient who requires very little ventilator support or in patient with intact respiratory system function who requires an endotracheal (ET) tube for airway protection

Complications of Mechanical Ventilation

- Related to ET intubation (e.g. sinusitis, laryngeal injury, tracheomalacia, tracheal stenosis)
- Oxygen toxicity
- Barotrauma (pneumothorax, subcutaneous emphysema, pneumomediastinum)
- Reduced cardiac output (due to reduced venous return caused by positive pressure)
- Ventilator-associated pneumonia (VAP)

Criteria for Weaning

- Patient should have haemodynamic and cardiopulmonary stability
- PaO_2 60 mmHg
- $FiO_2 \leq 40\%$
- PEEP ≤ 5 cm H_2O
- Adequate and stable haemoglobin
- Stable renal function
- Conscious and alert status
- No need for vasoactive or sedative agents, or alert on a stable dose of vasoactive or sedative agents
- Intact respiratory drive
- Ability to protect airway and clear secretions

Positive End-expiratory Pressure

- PEEP maintains a positive pressure at the end of expiration thereby opening the closed alveoli. It improves oxygenations, enhances compliance and reduces work of breathing
- Deleterious effects of PEEP include barotraumas and reduced cardiac output due to reduced venous return. In addition, myocardial function may be compromised as a result of increased afterload to right ventricle that in turn causes shift of interventricular septum to the left side
- PEEP has been used in patients with pulmonary oedema (both cardiogenic and non-cardiogenic) and diffuse lung injury

INFLUENZA

- Influenza viruses type A and type B belong to the group of myxoviruses (RNA viruses)
- Haemagglutinin and neuraminidase are the major antigenic determinants of influenza A viruses. There are 16 haemagglutinin (H1 to H16) and 9 neuraminidase types (N1 to N9)
- Minor antigenic changes periodically occur in either the haemagglutinin or the neuraminidase component or both. This phenomenon is called antigenic drift. This 'drift' contributes to yearly seasonal epidemics, and is the basis for the yearly change in vaccine formulations
- Antigenic shift results in a virus of distinctly different antigenic character to which most or all of the population is susceptible. Generally, such shifts occur only every few decades and are the basis for influenza pandemics.
- Incubation period is 1–2 days.
- Clinical manifestations are sudden onset of fever, headache, generalised aches and pains, anorexia, nausea, vomiting and a harsh unproductive cough. The fauces are hyperaemic and chest is usually clear.
- In uncomplicated cases, the symptoms subside within 3–5 days.

Complications

- Tracheitis, bronchitis, bronchiolitis and bronchopneumonia (primary influenza pneumonia)
- Secondary bacterial pneumonia

- Exacerbation of underlying asthma and chronic obstructive pulmonary disease (COPD)
- Toxic cardiomyopathy, worsening of underlying congestive heart failure and coronary artery disease
- Encephalitis, post-influenzal demyelinating encephalopathy and peripheral neuropathy
- Post-influenzal asthenia and depression

Management
- Paracetamol 0.5–1 g every 4-6 hourly
- Aspirin should be avoided, particularly in adolescents and children, because of their association with the Reye's syndrome
- Oseltamivir and zanamivir (neuraminidase inhibitors) have been approved for the treatment of both influenzas A and B. Amantadine was earlier used.
- **Vaccination:**
  o Specific vaccination gives 70% protection
  o Two types of vaccines against seasonal influenza are available: Trivalent inactivated vaccine (injectable) and live attenuated influenza vaccine (nasal spray). Both vaccines contain three strains of influenza—an H3N2 virus, an H1N1 (seasonal) virus and an influenza B virus. Vaccine composition is adjusted yearly.
  o Annual winter vaccination is recommended for patients with chronic pulmonary, cardiac or renal disease.

■ SWINE FLU (H1N1 INFLUENZA)
- Like seasonal influenza, H1N1 is thought to be transmissible by three routes: Contact exposure (when a contaminated hand is exposed to facial membranes), droplet spray exposure (when infectious droplets are projected onto mucous membranes) and airborne exposure (via inhalation of infectious airborne particles)
- The incubation period for the H1N1 virus has been estimated to be between 1 and 7 days, similar to that of seasonal influenza.
- Usually, patients present with a mild disease characterised by fever (at least 100.4°F), cough and myalgias.
- Watery diarrhoea is common in H1N1 infection.

Groups at High risk of Influenza-related Complications
- Children < 5 years
- Adults ≥ 65 years
- Pregnant women
- Persons with certain chronic medical conditions (asthma, COPD, cardiac, haematologic, hepatic, neurologic and metabolic diseases)
- Immunosuppressed patients
- Adolescents < 19 years receiving long-term aspirin therapy

Diagnosis
Case Definitions
The Centers for Disease Control and Prevention (CDC) criteria for suspected H1N1 influenza have been given in **Box 12.7**.

Diagnostic Tests
- Rapid antigen tests: Not as sensitive as other available tests; does not differentiate between various types of influenza A viruses. Detect influenza viral nucleoprotein antigen and can provide results within 30 minutes
- Real-time reverse transcription-polymerase chain reaction (PCR)
- Virus isolation
- Four-fold rise in H1N1 influenza virus specific neutralising antibodies

Treatment
- **Oseltamivir** is recommended at a dosage of 75 mg twice daily for 5 days (for treatment) or 75 mg daily 7–10 days (for post-exposure

> **Box 12.7: The CDC criteria for suspected H1N1 influenza.**
> - Onset of acute febrile respiratory illness within 7 days of close contact with a person who has a confirmed case of H1N1 influenza A virus infection
> - Onset of acute febrile respiratory illness within 7 days of travel to a community (within the United States or internationally) where one or more H1N1 influenza A cases have been confirmed
> - Acute febrile respiratory illness in a person who resides in a community where at least one H1N1 influenza case has been confirmed
>
> (CDC: centers for disease control and prevention)

prophylaxis). It can cause nausea and vomiting and rarely confusion, hallucinations and self-injury.
- **Zanamivir** is recommended at two inhalations (10 mg) twice a day for similar periods. It is approved only for those without underlying pulmonary or cardiovascular disease.
- **Peramivir,** another neuraminidase inhibitor, is under clinical trials. It is given intravenously and may be useful for seriously ill patients.
- Supportive therapy

SEVERE ACUTE RESPIRATORY SYNDROME

- Severe acute respiratory syndrome (SARS) was described for the first time in 2002 from Southern China and rapidly spread to several countries within less than a year.
- A novel coronavirus (SARS CoV) is the pathogen responsible for SARS.
- It spreads by close person-to-person contact via droplet transmission or fomite.
- Incubation period is 2–10 days, but may be as long as 16 days.
- Persistent fever, chills/rigor, myalgia, malaise, dry cough, headache and dyspnoea. Less common symptoms include sputum production, sore throat, rhinorrhoea, nausea and vomiting and diarrhoea.
- About 20% of patients developed evidence of ARDS over a period of 3 weeks.
- Confirmation:
  - Detection of SARS CoV in urine, nasopharyngeal aspirate and stool specimen using reverse transcription polymerase chain reaction (RT-PCR) (positivity rates low in the first week).
  - Quantitative measurement of SARS CoV RNA in blood with RT-PCR technique.
  - Viral culture.
- Supportive treatment includes fluid and electrolyte balance, oxygenation and, if required, ventilation with proper protection of healthcare workers.
- High dose methylprednisolone (0.5 g daily) is given, if pneumonia or hypoxaemia develops.
- Interferon: It may be combined with steroids.
- Ribavirin or lopinavir/ritonavir, as the initial treatment option, reduces mortality and intubation rates.

PNEUMONIAS

Classification of pneumonia has been given in **Box 12.8**.

Box 12.9 shows the predisposing conditions for community-acquired pneumonia (CAP).

Table 12.13 lists the organisms causing primary pneumonia.

Box 12.8: Classification of pneumonia.

Classification depending on the anatomic distribution:
- Lobar pneumonia
- Bronchopneumonia
- Interstitial pneumonia

Aetiological classification:
- Primary
- Secondary
- Suppurative

Clinical setting in which the infection occurs (if no pathogen can be isolated):
- Community-acquired acute pneumonia
- Community-acquired atypical pneumonia
- Nosocomial pneumonia or hospital-acquired pneumonia
- Pneumonia in immunocompromised host
- Healthcare associated pneumonia

Box 12.9: Predisposing conditions for community-acquired pneumonia.

- Extremes of age
- Upper respiratory tract infections
- Comorbidities: For example, congestive heart failure, diabetes, chronic kidney disease, recent influenza infection and malnutrition
- Cigarette smoking
- Alcohol
- Corticosteroid therapy
- Congenital or acquired immune deficiencies, e.g. HIV
- Decreased or absent splenic function, e.g. sickle cell disease or post-splenectomy (risk for infection with encapsulated bacteria)
- Other respiratory conditions: Cystic fibrosis, bronchiectasis, COPD, obstructing lesion (endoluminal cancer, inhaled foreign body)
- Indoor air pollution

(COPD: chronic obstructive pulmonary disease; HIV: human immunodeficiency virus)

TABLE 12.13: List of organisms causing primary pneumonia.

Common	Less common
• *Streptococcus pneumoniae* (most common) • *Haemophilus influenzae* • *Moraxella catarrhalis* • *Staphylococcus aureus* • *Legionella pneumophila* • *Mycoplasma pneumonia*	• Enterobacteriaceae (*Klebsiella pneumoniae*) and *Pseudomonas* spp. • *Streptococcus pyogenes* • *Pseudomonas aeruginosa* • *Coxiella burnetii* (Q-fever) • *Chlamydia* spp. (*C. pneumoniae, C. psittaci, C. trachomatis*) • Viruses: Respiratory syncytial virus, H1N1 influenza virus, seasonal influenza virus, parainfluenza virus and human metapneumovirus (children); influenza A and B (adults); adenovirus (miliary recruits); corona virus producing severe acute respiratory syndrome (SARS) • *Actinomyces Israelii*

Clinical Features

- Sudden onset of rigors followed by fever, pleuritic chest pain, cough productive of purulent sputum and haemoptysis
- Patients with atypical pneumonia may have a dry cough. These patients often have extrapulmonary features that include myalgias, arthralgias, prominent headache, mental confusion, abdominal pain and diarrhoea.
- Respiratory rate is high and this may be the most sensitive sign in the elderly.
- Tachycardia is common.
- Chest examination reveals crepitation in the involved area. About one-third have bronchial breathing (**Table 12.14**).

General complications of pneumonia have been given in **Box 12.10**.

Investigations

Table 12.15 shows the investigations in CAP.

Indications for Hospitalisation

Box 12.11 shows the indications for hospitalisation.

Box 12.12 shows the CURB 65 rule.

Treatment

General Measures

- Check the airway, breathing and circulation.
- Treat shock with intravenous fluids initially.
- Correct hypoxia with oxygen inhalation. If hypoxia continues or patient develops increasing hypercapnia, ventilate the patient mechanically.
- Treatment of pleuritic pain with mild analgesics such as paracetamol or codeine.

TABLE 12.14: Extrapulmonary features of community-acquired pneumonia.

Extrapulmonary symptoms	Infectious agent
Myalgia, arthralgia and malaise	*Legionella* and *Mycoplasma*
Myocarditis and pericarditis	*Mycoplasma pneumoniae*
Headache, abdominal pain, diarrhoea and vomiting	*Legionella pneumoniae*
Labial herpes simplex reactivation	Pneumococcal pneumoniae
Skin rashes: Erythema multiforme and erythema nodosum	*Mycoplasma pneumoniae*

Box 12.10: General complications of pneumoniae.

- Respiratory failure ARDS
- Bacteraemic dissemination (bacteraemia): It can cause:
  ○ Endocarditis (heart valves)
  ○ Pericarditis (pericardium)
  ○ Meningitis (meninges)
  ○ Suppurative arthritis (joint)
  ○ Metastatic abscesses in kidneys or spleen
  ○ Sepsis—multisystem failure

TABLE 12.15: Investigations in community-acquired pneumonia (CAP).

Investigation	Significance
Complete blood count	
• Very high (> 20 × 10^9/L) or low (< 4 × 10^9/L) WBC count	Marker of severity. In viral and atypical pneumonias, total leucocyte count is often < 5000/mm^3
• Neutrophilic leucocytosis > 15 × 10^9/L	Suggests bacterial pneumonia
• Haemolytic anaemia	Occasionally complicates *Mycoplasma*
Urea and electrolytes	
• Urea > 7 mmol/L (~20 mg/dL)	Marker of severity
• Hyponatraemia	Marker of severity may occur in patients with Legionnaire's disease
Liver function tests	
• Abnormal transaminitis, raised bilirubin	When basal pneumonia inflames liver, or in atypical pneumonia
• Hypoalbuminaemia	Marker of severity
Erythrocyte sedimentation rate/C-reactive protein	Non-specifically elevated
Blood culture	Bacteraemia is a marker of severity. Causative organism may be grown (e.g. pneumococcal pneumonia). However, blood cultures are recommended only in hospitalised patients
Serological and antigen detection tests	• Pneumococcal antigens can be detected in the serum or urine in pneumococcal pneumonia • Acute and convalescent titres for *Mycoplasma*, *Chlamydia*, *Legionella* and viral infections
Cold agglutinins	Positive in 50% of patients with *Mycoplasma*
Arterial blood gases	Measure when SaO$_2$ < 93% or when severe clinical features to assess ventilatory failure or acidosis
HIV testing	Since pneumonia is common in previously undiagnosed HIV infection, a test should be offered to all patients with pneumonia
Sputum: It can be distinguished from saliva by microscopic examination. Sputum contain alveolar macrophages	Gram stain, culture, antimicrobial sensitivity testing and Ziehl–Neelsen staining
Oropharynx swab	PCR for *Mycoplasma pneumoniae* and other atypical pathogens
Urine	Pneumococcal and/or *Legionella* antigen. Haematuria may occur in patients with Legionnaire's disease
Chest X-ray	Essential for the confirmation of diagnoses, follow-up and detection of complications like parapneumonic effusion and empyema
• Lobar pneumonia	• Patchy opacification evolves into homogeneous consolidation of affected lobe • Air bronchogram (air-filled bronchi appear lucent against consolidated lung tissue) may be present
• Bronchopneumonia	Patchy and segmental shadowing
• Complications	Para-pneumonic effusion, intrapulmonary abscess or empyema
• *Staphylococcus aureus*	Multilobar shadowing, cavitation, pneumatoceles and abscesses
• *Mycoplasma*	Usually one lobe is involved but infection can be bilateral and extensive

Continued

Continued

Investigation	Significance
• Legionella	There is lobar and then multilobar shadowing, with the occasional small pleural effusion. Cavitation is rare
Aspiration	Percutaneous transtracheal aspiration of secretions Percutaneous transthoracic needle aspiration, preferable under CT guidance
Fibreoptic bronchoscopy with BAL and brushings	Gram stain, AFB stain, culture and cytology
Biopsy	A transbronchial biopsy of the lung tissue for culture and histopathology may be done in selected cases. Diagnostic open-lung biopsy, which carries a high-risk, is reserved for selected patients
Pleural fluid	Aspirate and culture when present in more than trivial amounts, preferably with ultrasound guidance

(AFB: acid-fast bacillus; BAL: bronchoalveolar lavage; CT: computed tomography; HIV: human immunodeficiency virus)

Box 12.11: Indications for hospitalisation.

Age over 65 years
Underlying diseases:
- Diabetes
- Renal failure
- Congestive heart failure
- Chronic lung disease
- Alcoholism
- Immunosuppression
- Post-splenectomy
- Malignancy

Signs:
- Respiratory rats > 30/min
- Systolic blood pressure < 90 mmHg
- Diastolic blood pressure < 60 mmHg
- Evidence of extrapulmonary involvement (meningitis, arthritis, etc.)
- Laboratory parameters
- White blood cell count < 4,000 or > 30,000/mm^3
- PaO$_2$ < 60 mmHg on room air
- Renal failure
- Haematocrit < 30%
- Multilobar involvement on chest X-ray

Box 12.12: CURB 65 rule.

- **Confusion:** New mental confusion
- **Urea** > 7 mmol/L (mg/dL)
- **Respiratory rate** > 30 breaths per minute
- **Blood pressure:** Diastolic BP < 60 mmHg or systolic blood pressure < 90 mmHg
- **Age ≥ 65** years of age (1 point for each)
  - Group 1: 0 or 1 of the above—mortality low—1.5%. Likely suitable for treatment at home
  - Group 2: 2 of the above—mortality—9.2%. Hospitalisation for treatment
  - Group 3: 3 or more of the above—mortality—22%. Likely requires admission to ICU

(BP: blood pressure; ICU: intensive care unit)

Antimicrobial Therapy

Empiric Regimens

- Administer antibiotics as soon as feasible once the diagnosis of CAP is established.
- Empiric therapy for CAP is based on providing coverage against the most likely pathogens, unless one can clinically differentiate these organisms.
- The antibiotic selected should therefore be active against common typical and atypical pathogens, unless one can clinically differentiate these organisms.
- Macrolides (erythromycin, clarithromycin and azithromycin) should not be used alone in moderately sick patients with CAP since nearly 25% of strains of *Streptococcus pneumoniae* are naturally resistant to macrolides.
- Newer fluoroquinolones such as levofloxacin, moxifloxacin and gemifloxacin have better gram-positive coverage than ciprofloxacin. These are effective against both typical and atypical pathogens and can be used as monotherapy, particularly if the patient is not severely ill.
- Ceftriaxone has no activity against atypical pathogens and should not be used alone in moderately sick patients.

- Doxycycline remains effective against atypical pathogens and should not be used alone in moderately sick patients.
- The approach for empiric antibiotics is shown below. The usual duration of therapy is 7–10 days. For *Mycoplasma* and *Chlamydia* pneumonia, the duration is 10–14 days. Patients initially treated with intravenous antibiotics can be switched to oral agents when afebrile.

Table 12.16 shows the empiric regimens for the treatment of pneumonia.

Unresolved Pneumonia

Table 12.17 shows the causes of unresolving or slow-resolving pneumonia.

Atypical Pneumonias

- Causes: *Mycoplasma pneumoniae*, *Legionella pneumophila*, *Chlamydia pneumoniae*, *Coxiella burnettii*, viruses [influenza, adeno respiratory syncytial virus (RSV), measles, varicella zoster virus (VZV), cytomegalovirus (CMV)]
- Evolve much more slowly than bacterial pneumonias
- Symptoms > Signs

Box 12.13 shows the parameters that favour the diagnosis of atypical pneumonias.

Hospital-acquired Pneumonia or Nosocomial Pneumonia

Hospital-acquired pneumonia (HAP) or nosocomial pneumonia is a new episode of pneumonia developing in hospital in a patient who is beyond

TABLE 12.16: Empiric regimens for the treatment of pneumonia.

Setting	Therapaeutic options
Ambulatory, not requiring hospitalisation, age under 60 years	Oral macrolide (erythromycin or azithromycin)
Ambulatory, not requiring hospitalisation, comorbidity or age over 60 years	Oral β-lactam/β-lactamase inhibitor + macrolide or oral antipneumococcal fluoroquinolone
Requiring hospitalisation	β-lactam (cefoperazone or ceftriaxone) + macrolide or antipneumococcal fluoroquinolone
Aspiration pneumonia requiring hospitalisation	β-lactam/β-lactamase inhibitor alone (ampicillin/sulbactam, piperacillin/tazobactam)

TABLE 12.17: Causes of unresolving/slow-resolving pneumonia.

Incorrect microbiological diagnosis (e.g. tuberculosis instead of classical organisms) or incomplete antimicrobial treatment	• Underlying antibiotic resistance • Inadequate dose/duration • Non-adherence • Malabsorption
Complication of CAP (community-acquired pneumonia)	• Parapneumonic pleural effusion (exudative), empyema, lung abscess
Underlying neoplastic lesion or other lung disease	• Bronchial obstruction causing partial or complete obstruction, bronchoalveolar cell carcinoma, bronchiectasis
Alternative diagnosis	• Pulmonary thromboembolic disease, cryptogenic organising pneumonia, eosinophilic pneumonia, pulmonary haemorrhage
Host factors	• Age especially > 50 years • Co-morbid illness: Diabetes, COPD (chronic obstructive pulmonary disease) • Others, e.g. alcoholism, immunosuppressive/cytotoxic therapy
Superinfection	• Fungi, *Mycobacterium tuberculosis*
Defects in defense	• For example, impaired cough (sedatives, neuromuscular illness, stroke), impaired mucociliary transport (chronic bronchitis), immune deficiency states—primary and secondary (B-cell and T-cell)

> **Box 12.13: Parameters that favour the diagnosis of atypical pneumonias.**
>
> - Age 60 years
> - Absence of any underlying co-morbid condition
> - Paroxysmal cough
> - No expectoration
> - Few clinical signs on examination of chest
>
> If total WBC count 10,000/mm³ is added to the above five parameters, then presence of four features indicates a strong likelihood of atypical pneumonia
>
> (WBC: white blood cells)

> **Box 12.14: Various aetiological agents causing hospital-acquired pneumonia.**
>
> - **Early onset (within 4 days of hospitalisation):** *Staphylococcus aureus*, EGNB, *S. pneumoniae* and *Haemophilus* influenzae
> - **Late onset:** *S. aureus, Pseudomonas, Enterobacter, Klebsiella, Acinetobacter*
>
> (EGNB: enteric Gram-negative bacilli)

2 days (> 48 h) of their initial admission to hospital, which was not incubating at the time of admission (**Box 12.14**).

■ PULMONARY INFILTRATES WITH EOSINOPHILIA

- Allergic bronchopulmonary aspergillosis (ABPA)
- Drug reactions (e.g. nitrofurantoin, sulphonamides, penicillins, thiazides, isoniazid, para-aminosalicylic acid, imipramine, chlorpropamide)
- Parasitic infestations (e.g. filarial, roundworm, hookworm)
- Loeffler's syndrome
- Acute eosinophilic pneumonia (AEP)
- Churg–Strauss syndrome
- Hypereosinophilic syndrome
- Tropical pulmonary eosinophilia

Tropical Pulmonary Eosinophilia

- Tropical eosinophilia is a hypersensitivity response to a helminthic parasite, particularly filarial parasite (*Wuchereria* and *Brugia*).
- The syndrome is characterised by pulmonary manifestations and peripheral blood eosinophilia of > 2,000/mm³.

Treatment

- Diethylcarbamazine 6 mg/kg/day in divided doses for 3 weeks
- Long-standing and resistant cases are treated with prednisolone and bronchodilators.

Aspiration Pneumonia

It occurs due to abnormal entry of fluid, particulate exogenous substances or endogenous secretions into the lower airways. It is of two types: Chemical aspiration pneumonia and bacterial aspiration pneumonia.

Predisposing Factors

- Reduced consciousness (including following anaesthesia)
- Dysphagia from neurologic deficits
- Disorders of the upper gastrointestinal tract including oesophageal disease, surgery involving the upper airways or oesophagus and gastric reflux
- Mechanical disruption of the glottis closure or cardiac sphincter due to tracheostomy, ET intubation, bronchoscopy, upper endoscopy and nasogastric feeding
- Miscellaneous conditions such as protracted vomiting, large volume tube feedings and feeding gastrostomy

Chemical Aspiration Pneumonia

- It occurs due to the aspiration of substances that are toxic to the lower airways, independent of bacterial infection. It includes chemical pneumonitis associated with the aspiration of gastric acid (Mendelson's syndrome).

■ TUBERCULOSIS

- Mycobacteria are divided into three groups.
  - *Mycobacterium tuberculosis* complex (*M. tuberculosis, M. bovis* and *M. africanum*)
  - *Mycobacterium leprae*
  - Atypical mycobacteria or non-tuberculous mycobacteria (NTM) or mycobacteria other than tuberculosis (MOTT). **Table 12.18** lists the atypical *Mycobacterium* and disease presentation.

Primary Pulmonary Tuberculosis

- From this primary site of infection, bacilli are carried to the hilar lymph nodes via lymphatic

TABLE 12.18: Atypical *Mycobacterium* and disease presentation

Agent	Disseminated disease	Localised disease			Treatment
		Lungs	Lymph nodes	Skin	
Mycobacterium avium intracellulare complex (N)	Yes; typical in AIDS with CD4 cells 50/L (fever, night sweat, diarrhoea, abdominal pain, weight loss with or without hepatosplenomegaly; blood and bone marrow cultures may be positive)	Cavities in cystic fibrosis and COAD	Yes (accounts for 80% cases of NTM-associated lymphadenitis)	Rare	Rifabutin, clarithromycin and ethambutol; add streptomycin in severe cases. For lymphadenitis, complete excision of involved lymph node, if feasible
M. marinum (P)	–	–	–	Yes	Cotrimoxazole
M. ulcerans (N)	–	–	–	Yes (Buruli's ulcer)	Debridement
M. xenopi (S)	Rare	Rare	–	–	Same as for *M. avium*
M. szulgai (S)	Rare	Rare	–	Yes	Rifampicin, INH, ethambutol
M. scrofulaceum (S)	Rare	Rare	–	–	Same as for *M. avium*
M. fortuitum (group IV)	Rare	Rare	Yes	Yes	Amikacin, ciprofloxacin, sulphonamides, clofazimine
M. chelonae (group IV)	Rare	Rare	–	Yes	Debridement, clarithromycin clofazimine, amikacin

(AIDS: acquired immunodeficiency syndrome; COAD: chronic obstructive airway disease; NTM: non-tuberculous mycobacteria)

channels, and the nodes enlarge. This parenchymal lesion (Ghon lesion) with its enlarged regional (hilar) lymph nodes and interconnecting lymphangitis is known as the primary complex of Ranke (Ghon's complex).
- The parenchymal lesion is subpleural and is usually located in lower part of the upper lobe, upper part of the lower lobe or the middle lobe.
- Vast majority are asymptomatic.
- A minority may experience a brief 'flu-like' febrile illness, which lasts no > 7–14 days. It occurs at the time of tuberculin conversion.
- Erythema nodosum may accompany primary pulmonary tuberculosis (TB).
- In great majority, the primary focus heals completely with or without calcification.
- In a few individuals, primary lesion in the lung may be actively progressive from the beginning (progressive pulmonary TB or progressive primary pulmonary TB).
- Tuberculin test is very valuable in children. A positive test in a previously non-immunised child strongly indicates the disease. A negative test makes the diagnosis very unlikely.

Post-primary (Secondary) Tuberculosis

Figure 12.3 shows the progress and complications of secondary TB of lung.

Complications of Pulmonary Tuberculosis

Table 12.19 shows the complications of pulmonary TB.

Investigations

Sputum Examination
- Microscopic examination of sputum smear
- Sputum culture for tubercle bacillus

Tuberculin test: A strongly positive test is a point in favour of TB, but a negative test does not exclude TB.

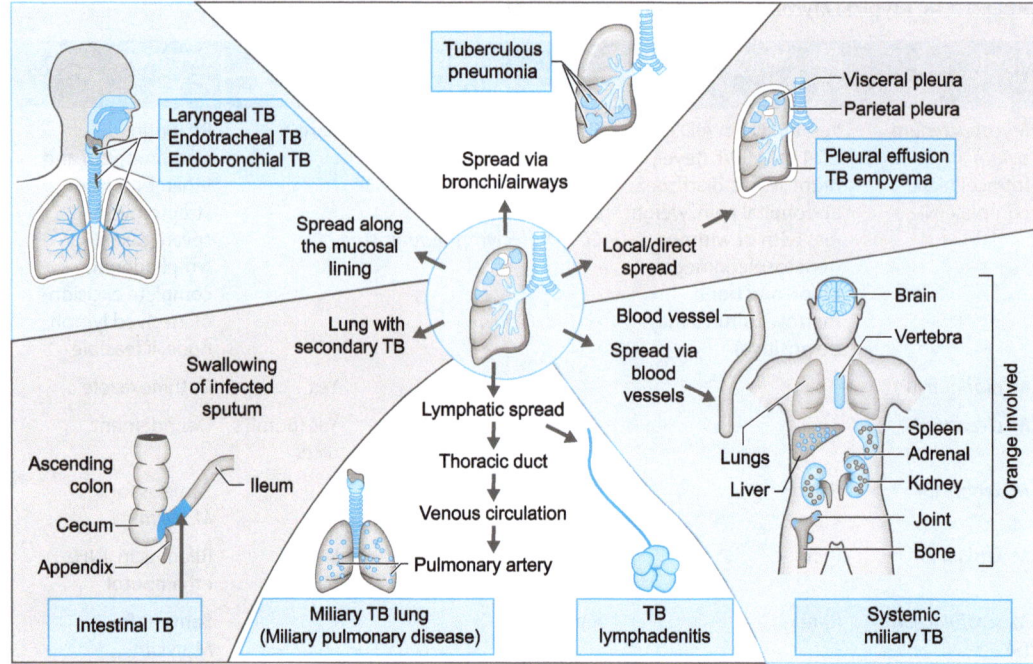

(TB: tuberculosis)

Fig. 12.3: Progress and complications of secondary tuberculosis of lung.

TABLE 12.19: Complications of pulmonary tuberculosis.

Pulmonary	Non-pulmonary
Exudative pleural effusion/empyema Spontaneous pneumothorax Massive haemoptysis pulmonary or bronchial arteritis and thrombosis, bronchial artery dilatation and Rasmussen aneurysm) Cor pulmonale Persistence of cavities even after treatment Pulmonary fibrosis/emphysema *Infection of cavities:* • Atypical mycobacterial infection • Aspergillus → aspergilloma Lung/pleural calcification Obstructive airways disease **Airway lesions:** These include bronchiectasis, tracheobronchial stenosis and broncholithiasis Bronchopleural fistula Bronchogenic carcinoma	Empyema necessitans Spread of tuberculosis to other organs (especially Addison's) Laryngitis *Following swallowing of infected sputum:* • Enteritis • Anorectal disease Amyloidosis Poncet's polyarthritis **Mediastinal lesions:** These include lymph node calcification and extranodal extension, esophagomediastinal or esophagobronchial fistula, constrictive pericarditis, and fibrosing mediastinitis Venous thromboembolism

T-cell Interferon- release assays (IGRAs)
Other methods of diagnosis
- In mycobacteria growth indicator tube (MGIT) method and growth
- BACTEC and radiometric growth detection
- Nucleic acid amplification tests (NAATs)

Latent Tuberculosis Infection
- Latent TB infection is a condition in which a person is infected with *M. tuberculosis*, but does not currently have active TB disease (**Box 12.15**)

Screening for Latent Tuberculosis
- Tuberculin test
- T-cell interferon-gamma release assays (IGRAs)

Antituberculous Drugs
Table 12.20 shows the side effects of the commonly used anti-tuberculous drugs.

Drug Resistance in Tuberculosis
- **Multiple drug resistance or multidrug-resistant TB**

> **Box 12.15: Groups at increased risk of progression to active tuberculosis.**
> - Children younger than 5 years of age
> - History of tuberculous infection
>   – Individuals infected with *Mycobacterium tuberculosis* within the past 2 years
>   – Past history of untreated or inadequately treated tuberculosis
> - Associated conditions
>   – Individuals with HIV infection
>   – Silicosis
>   – IV drug users
>   – Immunocompromised conditions
>   – Long-term use of corticosteroids or other immunosuppressants (including anti-TNF-α)
>   – Chronic renal failure
>   – Diabetes mellitus
>   – Malignancy
>
> (IV: intravenous; HIV: human immunodeficiency virus; TNF: tumour necrosis factor)

  o Multidrug resistant tuberculosis (MDR-TB) is a form of TB that is **resistance to at least both of isonicotinic acid hydrazide (INH) and rifampicin**, with or without other drug resistance. Hence, a patient should not be classified as multidrug-resistant disease if the patient has an infection with a bacterium susceptible to rifampicin but resistant to many other drugs.
  o MDR-TB can rarely be observed in new cases. It is more common in individuals in re-treatment cases [prior history of TB, particularly if treatment has been inadequate, and those with human immunodeficiency virus (HIV) infection]. It is a man-made phenomenon.
  o Chronic cases and MDR-TB cases are not synonymous. Chronic patients probably have MDR-TB because they have previously received at least two full courses of treatment with essential antituberculous drugs.
- **Extensive drug resistance TB (XDR-TB)**
  o Extensive drug resistance TB is a form of TB that is resistant to at least four of the core anti-TB drugs. These drugs include most important (core) anti-TB drugs, (1) isoniazid and (2) rifampicin and (3) injectable second-line aminoglycoside drugs (amikacin, capreomycin or kanamycin) + (4) fluoroquinolone (such as ofloxacin or moxifloxacin)
- **Totally drug resistant TB or (Extremely XXDR, TDR)**
  o Totally drug resistant tuberculosis (TDR-TB) is a form of TB strains that shows in-vitro resistance to all first and second line drugs tested (isoniazid, rifampicin, streptomycin, ethambutol, pyrazinamide, ethionamide, para-aminosalicylic acid, cycloserine, ofloxacin, amikacin, ciprofloxacin, capreomycin, kanamycin)

Extrapulmonary Tuberculosis
Table 12.21 shows the extrapulmonary sites of TB and their presentation.

TABLE 12.20: Side effects of the commonly used anti-tuberculous drugs.

Drug (daily dosages)	Adverse reactions	
	Major	Less common (rare)
Isoniazid (H) (5–10 mg/kg)	• Hepatitis • Peripheral neuropathy (preventable and treatable with pyridoxine) • Cutaneous hypersensitivity	Giddiness, seizures, optic neuritis, mental symptoms, haemolytic anaemia, aplastic anaemia, agranulocytosis, lupoid reactions, arthralgia, gynaecomastia
Rifampicin (R) (10 mg/kg)	Febrile reactions ('flu' syndrome; more common with intermittent therapy), hepatitis, cutaneous reactions, gastrointestinal disturbances	Shortness of breath, shock, haemolytic anaemia, interstitial nephritis, thrombocytopaenia
Pyrazinamide (Z) (20 mg/kg)	Anorexia, nausea, flushing, hepatitis, gastrointestinal disturbance, hyperuricaemia	Hepatitis (dose related), vomiting, arthralgia, cutaneous hypersensitivity, gout
Ethambutol (E) (15 mg/kg)	Retrobulbar neuritis (dose related), arthralgia	Peripheral neuropathy, rash
Streptomycin (S) and other aminoglycosides (15–20 mg/kg)	8th nerve damage, cutaneous hypersensitivity, giddiness, numbness, tinnitus	Vertigo, ataxia, deafness, hypokalaemia, renal damage, aplastic anaemia, agranulocytosis
Ethionamide (Etm) (10–20 mg/kg)	Anorexia, vomiting	Serious neurologic reactions, hepatitis
Cycloserine (Cys) (10–20 mg/kg)	Headache, somnolence	Psychosis, seizures, peripheral neuropathy
Quinolones (7.5–15 mg/kg)	GI intolerance, skin rashes	Phototoxicity (with sparfloxacin), dizziness, headache, insomnia
Thiacetazone (Tzn) (2.5 mg/kg)	Gastrointestinal reactions, cutaneous hypersensitivity, vertigo, conjunctivitis	Hepatitis, erythema multiforme, exfoliative dermatitis, haemolytic anaemia
Paraaminosalicylic acid (PAS) (8–12 g/day)	Gastrointestinal reactions, hepatitis, cutaneous hypersensitivity, hypokalaemia	Acute renal failure, haemolytic anaemia, thrombocytopaenia, hypothyroidism

(GI: gastrointestinal)

TABLE 12.21: Extrapulmonary sites of tuberculosis and their presentation.

Extrapulmonary site	Presentation
Pleural	Pleural effusion, pleuritis
Lymph nodes	Tuberculous lymphadenopathy (including mediastinal) non-healing sinuses
Skeletal system	Tuberculous osteomyelitis, cold abscess, vertebral tuberculosis, pyarthrosis
Nervous system	Tuberculous meningitis, tuberculous arteritis, cerebral tuberculoma
Gastrointestinal	Ulcerations of the tongue, intestinal tuberculosis, tuberculous peritonitis
Pericardium	Pericardial effusion and tamponade, constrictive pericarditis
Genitourinary	Renal tuberculosis, salpingitis, tubal abscess, tuberculous epididymitis
Miscellaneous	Addison's disease (tuberculous adrenalitis), skin tuberculosis (scrofuloderma, lupus vulgaris, tuberculids), phlyctenualr keratoconjunctivitis, choroiditis, iritis, erythema nodosum

Pulmonology

TUBERCULOSIS CHEMOPROPHYLAXIS: ISONIAZID PREVENTIVE THERAPY

Indications
- Close contacts of open case of TB who show recent Mantoux conversion
- Close contacts of children aged 5 years or below with strongly positive Mantoux and a TB patient in the family
- Breast-fed neonates/infants of sputum-positive mothers
- Newly infected patients as shown by recent change in tuberculin test from negative to positive
- Patient with old inactive disease who are assessed to have received inadequate treatment
- Certain diseases in which TB is more likely to develop. These include HIV infection, leukaemia, Hodgkin's disease, prolonged treatment with prednisolone, severe diabetes mellitus and patients on anti-malignancy drugs
- World Health Organization (WHO) recommends that partners of people living with HIV (PLHIV) who are unlikely to have active TB should receive at least 6 months of isoniazid preventive therapy (IPT) as part of a comprehensive package of HIV care.

BRONCHOPULMONARY ASPERGILLOSIS

Bronchopulmonary aspergillosis includes the bronchopulmonary diseases caused by *Aspergillus* species, the most common being *Aspergillus fumigatus*. Others in the group include *A. clavatus*, *A. niger* and *A. terreus*.

Classification
- Endobronchial saprophytic pulmonary aspergillosis
- Allergic bronchopulmonary (ABPA: Asthmatic pulmonary eosinophilia)
- Extrinsic allergic alveolitis (hypersensitivity pneumonitis)
- Intracavitary aspergilloma
- Chronic necrotising aspergillosis
- Invasive pulmonary aspergillosis

Allergic Bronchopulmonary Aspergillosis

Table 12.22 shows the main diagnostic criteria and other diagnostic features of allergic bronchopulmonary aspergillosis.

Management
- Oral prednisolone 40 mg daily for 7–10 days followed by gradual tapering to a maintenance dose of 5–10 mg/day for long-term.
- Oral itraconazole (200 mg twice a day) is helpful in reducing exacerbations and requirement of steroids.

BRONCHIAL ASTHMA

Definition: Asthma is a chronic inflammatory disorder of the airways (bronchial tree) in which breathing is periodically rendered difficult by widespread narrowing of the bronchi (reversible bronchoconstriction). It is clinically characterised by recurrent episodes (paroxysms) of wheezing, breathlessness (dyspnoea), tightness of the chest and cough.

Classification

Box 12.16 shows the classification of asthma.

TABLE 12.22: Main diagnostic criteria and other diagnostic features of allergic bronchopulmonary aspergillosis.

Main diagnostic criteria	Other diagnostic features
- Bronchial asthma - Pulmonary infiltrates - Peripheral eosinophilia > 1,000/mm^3 - Serum precipitins to *Aspergillus fumigatus* - Elevated serum IgE (> 1,000 ng/mL) - Central (proximal) bronchiectasis - Immediate wheal-and-flare response to *A. fumigatus*	- Brownish plugs in sputum - Culture of *A. fumigatus* from sputum - Elevated IgE (and IgG) class antibodies specific for *A. fumigatus*

> **Box 12.16: Classification of asthma.**
> **According to type of antigen**
> - Early-onset asthma (atopic/allergic/extrinsic)
> - Late-onset asthma (non-atopic/intrinsic/idiosyncratic) without evidence of allergen sensitisation
>
> **According to the agents or events that trigger bronchoconstriction**
> - Seasonal
> - Exercise-induced
> - Drug-induced (e.g. aspirin)
> - Occupational asthma
> - Asthmatic bronchitis in smokers
> - Cough variant asthma (CVA) in which cough is the only asthma symptom

Clinical Features

Episodic Asthma

- It occurs as episodes with asymptomatic intervening periods.
- It is characterised by paroxysms of wheeze and dyspnoea with relatively sudden onset.
- Episodes may be spontaneous in onset or triggered by allergens, exercise or viral infections.
- Attacks may be mild or severe and may last for hours, days or even weeks.

Severe Acute Asthma (Status Asthmaticus)

- It is a condition in which severe airway obstruction and asthmatic symptoms persist despite the initial administration of standard acute asthma therapy.
- Severe dyspnoea and unproductive cough.
- Patients adopt an upright position fixing the shoulder girdle to assist the accessory muscles of respiration.
- Physical signs include sweating, central cyanosis, tachycardia and pulsus paradoxus.

Chronic Asthma

- Symptoms are usually chronic unless controlled by appropriate therapy.
- Symptoms such as chest tightness, wheeze and breathlessness occur on exertion.
- Episodes of spontaneous cough and wheeze occur during the night.
- Repeated attacks of 'severe acute asthma' are common.

Investigations

- Pulmonary function tests useful in bronchial asthma are FEV_1, VC and PEF.
  - Asthma can also be diagnosed on the basis of demonstrating a > 15% improvement in FEV_1 (or PEF) following the inhalation of a bronchodilator: However, his degree of response may not be present in all cases.
- Sputum and blood eosinophilia
- Elevated serum IgE levels
- Others: Fractional exhaled nitric oxide to assess airway inflammation

Table 12.23 shows the classification of asthma severity and initiating treatment in persons ≥ 12 years of age.

TABLE 12.23: Classification of asthma severity and initiating treatment in persons ≥12 years of age.

Components of severity		Classification of asthma severity (≥12 years of age)			
		Intermittent	Persistent		
			Mild	Moderate	Severe
Impairment normal FEV_1/FVC:	Symptoms	≤ 2 days/week	> 2 days/week but not daily	Daily	Throughout the day
8–19 years: 85%	Night-time awakenings	≤ 2x/month	3–4x/month	> x/week but not nightly	Often 7x/week
20–39 years: 80%	Short-acting β2-agonist use for symptom control	≤ 2 days/week	> 2 days/week but not daily, and not more than 1x on any day	Daily	Several times per day

Continued

Continued

Components of severity		Classification of asthma severity (≥12 years of age)			
		Intermittent	Persistent		
			Mild	Moderate	Severe
40–59 years: 75% 60–80 years: 70%	Interference with normal activity	None	Minor limitation	Some limitation	Extremely limited
	Lung function	• Normal FEV_1 between exacerbations • FEV_1 > 80% predicted • FEV_1/FVC normal	• FEV_1 > 80% predicted • FEV_1/FVC normal	• FEV_1 > 60% but < 80% predicted • FEV_1/FVC reduced 5%	• FEV_1 < 60% predicted • FEV_1/FVC reduced > 5%
Risk	Exacerbations requiring oral systemic corticosteroids	0–1/year	←——————— ≥2/year ———————→ ← Consider severity and interval since last exacerbation → Frequency and severity may fluctuate over time for patients in any severity category Relative annual risk of exacerbations may be related to FEV_1		
Recommended step for initiating treatment		Step 1	Step 2	Step 3	Step 4 or 5 and consider short course of oral systemic corticosteroids
			In 2–6 weeks, evaluate level of asthma control that is achieved and adjust therapy accordingly		

(FEV_1: forced expiratory volume in one second; FVC: forced vital capacity)

TABLE 12.24: Drug useful in asthma.

Bronchodilators	Controllers	
β-adrenoreceptor agonists Methylxanthines Anticholinergics	Inhaled corticosteroids Systemic corticosteroids Steroid-sparing therapies, cromones antileucotrienes	Anti-IgE Immunotherapy Alternative therapies Miscellaneous agents, SLIT

(Ig: immunoglobulin; SLIT: sublingual immunotherapy)

Management of Bronchial Asthma

Management of bronchial asthma can be discussed under following broad headings:
- Avoidance of allergens
- Desensitisation or immunotherapy
- Drug therapy to control or suppress clinical manifestations
- Bronchial thermoplasty

Drug Therapy

Table 12.24 shows the drugs useful in asthma.

Figure 12.4 describes the stepwise management of asthma in adults.

Treatment of Severe Acute Asthma (Status Asthmaticus)

Flowchart 12.1 shows the management algorithm of acute asthma.

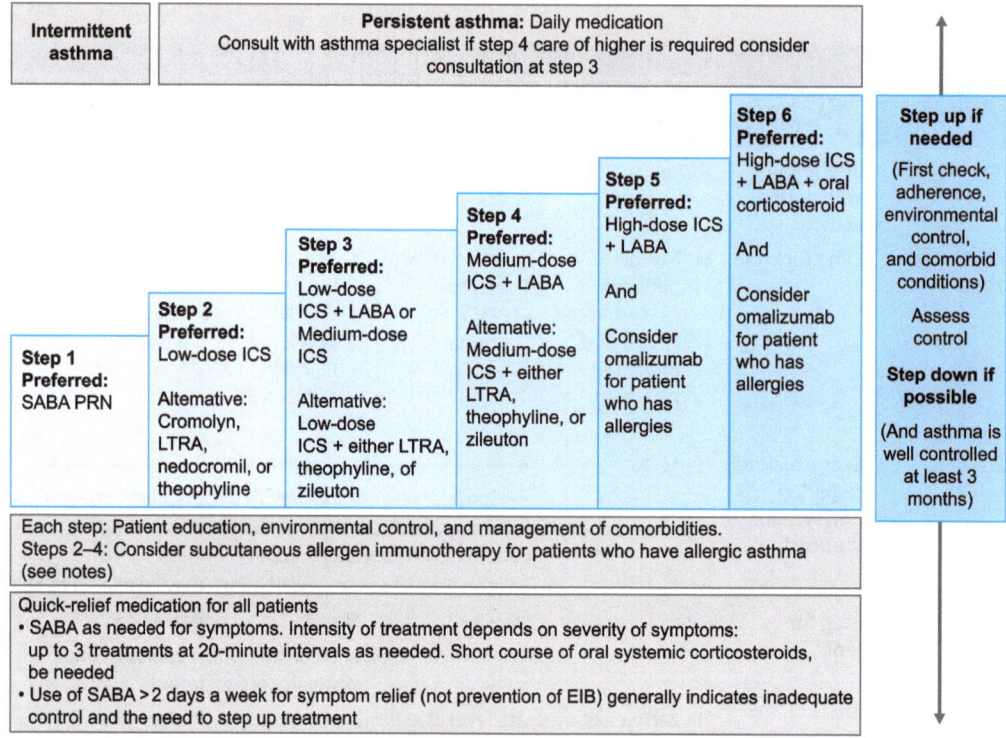

(ICS: inhaled corticosteroid; SABA: short-acting β2 agonists)

Fig. 12.4: Stepwise management of asthma in adults.

HYPERSENSITIVITY PNEUMONITIS (EXTRINSIC ALLERGIC ALVEOLITIS)

Hypersensitivity pneumonitis or extrinsic allergic alveolitis is an immune-mediated inflammation in the walls of alveoli and bronchioles secondary to inhalation of certain types of organic dusts including microbes (bacteria, fungi or protozoa, including amoebae contamination water in ventilation systems), animal or plant proteins, and several low-molecular weight chemicals.

Table 12.25 shows the examples of hypersensitivity pneumonitis.

BRONCHIAL OBSTRUCTION

Causes

Table 12.26 shows the causes of bronchial obstruction.

CHRONIC OBSTRUCTIVE PULMONARY DISEASE

Definition

- Chronic obstructive pulmonary disease, chronic obstructive lung disease (COLD) or chronic obstructive airway disease (COAD) is defined as a condition in which there is chronic obstruction to airflow due to chronic bronchitis and/or emphysema. The obstruction is not relieved (improvement < 15% of baseline) with bronchodilators.
- It is characterised by generalised airflow obstruction, the major site of obstruction being the small airways.
- Chronic bronchitis and emphysema are pathologically distinct, but usually co-exist in the same patient in varying proportions.

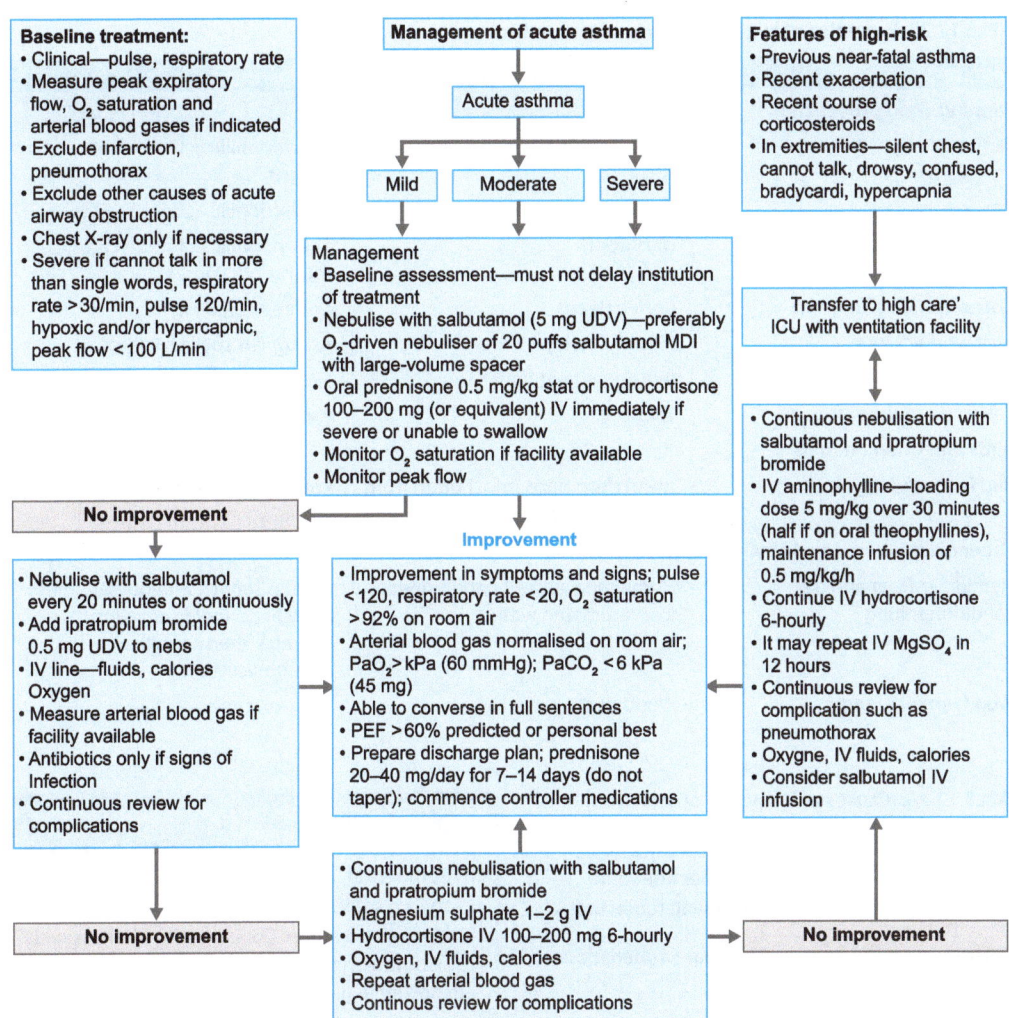

(ICU: intensive care unit; IV: intravenous; MDI: metered dose inhaler)

Flowchart 12.1: Management algorithm of acute asthma.

Chronic bronchitis is defined as a condition associated with excessive tracheobronchial mucus production to cause cough with expectoration for at least 3 months of the year, for > 2 consecutive years.

Emphysema (pulmonary) is a chronic lung disease characterised by abnormal irreversible (permanent) dilatation of the airspaces distal to the terminal bronchiole. This is associated with destruction of their walls but without obvious fibrosis.

Aetiology (Risk Factors)

Box 12.17 shows the risk factors for COPD.

Clinical Features

- The most striking features are an impressive history of cough with sputum production for many years and a relatively late onset of breathlessness.
- The sputum is usually scanty, mucoid and more in the mornings. Sputum is occasionally

TABLE 12.25: **Examples of hypersensitivity pneumonitis.**

Disease	Sources of antigen	Antigen
Farming/food processing		
Farmer's lung	Grain, moldy hay	Thermophilic actinomycetes, fungus
Bagassosis	Sugarcane	Thermophilic actinomycetes
Mushroom worker's lung	Mushroom	Thermophilic actinomycetes; mushroom spores
Coffee worker's lung	Coffee beans	Coffee bean dust
Malt worker's lung	Mouldy barley	*Aspergillus* species (clavatus)
Miller's lung	Infested wheat flour	*Sitophilus granarius* (wheat weevil)
Tobacco grower's lung	Tobacco	*Aspergillus* species
Birds and other animals		
Bird fancier's lung	Avian droppings (most often from pigeons and parakeets)	Protein in avian excreta, feathers
Other occupational and environmental exposures		
Humidifier fever and air-conditioner lung	Humidifiers and air conditioners (contaminated water)	*Bacillus subtilis, Aureobasidium pulluans; Candida albicans*, amoeba, thermophilic actinomycetes
Woodworker's lung	Wood dust	*Alternaria* species

TABLE 12.26: **Causes of bronchial obstruction.**

Tumours	Bronchial carcinoma, bronchial adenoma Malignant, tuberculous
Enlarged tracheobronchial lymph nodes	Malignant, tuberculous
Inhaled foreign bodies	–
Bronchial casts or plugs	Inspissated mucus, blood clots
Ineffective expectoration	Collection of mucus or mucopus in the bronchus
Rare cause	Congenital bronchial atresia, post-tuberculous bronchial stricture aortic aneurysm, giant left atrium, pericardial effusion

Box 12.17: **Risk factors for chronic obstructive pulmonary disease (COPD).**

Environmental
- Tobacco smoke
- Indoor air pollution. Cooking with biomass fuels
- Toxic industrial inhalants: Occupational dust exposure (e.g. coal dust, silica and cadmium)
- Respiratory infections: Recurrent infection; HIV infection (associated with emphysema), previous tuberculosis
- Low birth weight and bronchopulmonary dysplasia
- Lung growth: Childhood infections or maternal smoking may affect growth of lung during childhood
- Low socioeconomic status, antioxidant deficiency
- Cannabis smoking

Host factors
- Genetic factors: α1-antiproteinase deficiency TGF Beta 1 polymorphism, Serpine 2 gene expression
- Airway hyper-reactivity

(HIV: human immunodeficiency virus; TGF: transforming growth factor)

blood-stained (haemoptysis) and occasionally frankly purulent ('mucopurulent relapse').
- Breathlessness is relatively late in the onset in chronic bronchitis. It is due to airflow obstruction and is aggravated by infection, excessive smoking and adverse atmospheric conditions.
- Vesicular breath sounds with prolonged expiration
- Inspiratory and expiratory rhonchi
- Crepitations that either disappear or change in location and intensity after coughing

Box 12.18 shows the common comorbidities in COPD.

Investigations

- Radiological examination:
    - Chest radiograph does not show any characteristic abnormality in chronic bronchitis.
- Electrocardiography may show features of right atrial and ventricular hypertrophy (tall P waves P Pulmonale: right bundle branch block; Rs pattern in V_1)
- Pulmonary function tests:
    - FEV_1 is reduced.
    - FVC is decreased.
    - Ratio of FEV_1 to FVC is subnormal.
    - PEF is reduced.
    - RV is increased.
    - Functional residual capacity (FRC) is increased.
    - TLC is increased.

Box 12.18: Common comorbidities in chronic obstructive pulmonary disease (COPD).

Cardiovascular disorders
- Pulmonary hypertension
- Right heart failure, cor pulmonale
- Vascular disease: Coronary artery disease, cerebrovascular disease, peripheral vascular disease
- Systemic hypertension

Nutritional disorders: Cachexia

Musculoskeletal disorders
- Muscle dysfunction
- Osteoporosis

Cancer: Lung cancer

Other: Sleep disorders, sexual dysfunction, diabetes, depression, anxiety, anaemia, osteoporosis, peptic ulcer, glaucoma

---

- Gas transfer may be normal or mildly reduced.
- ABG studies in patients with $FEV_1 < 50\%$ of predicted, or those with respiratory failure or cor pulmonale.
    - PaO_2 is markedly reduced (hypoxaemia)
    - $PaCO_2$ is markedly raised (hypercarbia)

Complications

- **Mucopurulent relapses:** It may develop due to secondary bacterial infection by *S. pneumoniae*, *H. influenzae* or *M. catarrhalis*. It presents with fever and increased production of purulent sputum.
- **Carbon dioxide narcosis:** Persistent retention of CO_2 (hypercarbia: high $PaCO_2$) manifests as clouding of consciousness, altered behaviour, drowsiness, headache and papilloedema.
- **Respiratory failure:**
    - Type 1 respiratory failure (low PaO_2 normal $PaCO_2$): In mild-to-moderate COPD
    - Type II respiratory failure: Acute or chronic in severe COPD
- **Secondary polycythaemia:** Due to hypoxaemia which stimulates erythropoiesis
- **Pulmonary hypertension** and right ventricular failure (**cor pulmonale**)
- Pneumonia
- Tuberculosis
- Lung cancer
- Pneumothorax (emphysema)
- Deep vein thrombosis
- Pulmonary embolism

Management

- Regular exercises and nutritional management
- Weight loss in obese patients
- Reduction of bronchial irritation:
    - Stop smoking completely.
    - Dusty and smoke-laden atmospheres should be avoided.
- Treatment and prevention of respiratory infections:
    - Vaccination with pneumococcal and influenza vaccines.

Box 12.19 shows the drug therapy used in chronic bronchitis.

Figure 12.5 shows the pharmacotherapy which is based on the severity of COPD and **Figure 12.6**

> **Box 12.19: Drug therapy in chronic bronchitis.**
> - **β2-agonists**
>   - Short-acting beta-agonists (SABAs)
>   - Long-acting beta-agonists (LABAs)
> - **Anticholinergics/muscarinic antagonists**
>   - Short-acting anticholinergics (SAMAs)
>   - Long-acting anticholinergics (LAMAs)
> - Combination SABAs + anticholinergic in one inhaler
> - **Methylxanthines**
> - Inhaled corticosteroids (ICS)
> - Combination LABAs + corticosteroids in one inhaler
> - Systemic corticosteroids
> - Phosphodiesterase-4 inhibitors
> - Acebrophylline: An airway mucoregulator and anti-inflammatory agent

shows the Global initiative for chronic Obstructive Lung Disease (GOLD) staging for severity of COPD and management.

Table 12.27 shows the differences between emphysema and chronic bronchitis.

ASTHMA COPD OVERLAP SYNDROME

Major criteria for asthma COPD overlap syndrome (ACOS):
- It is characterised by persistent airflow limitation with several features usually associated with asthma and several features usually associated with COPD.

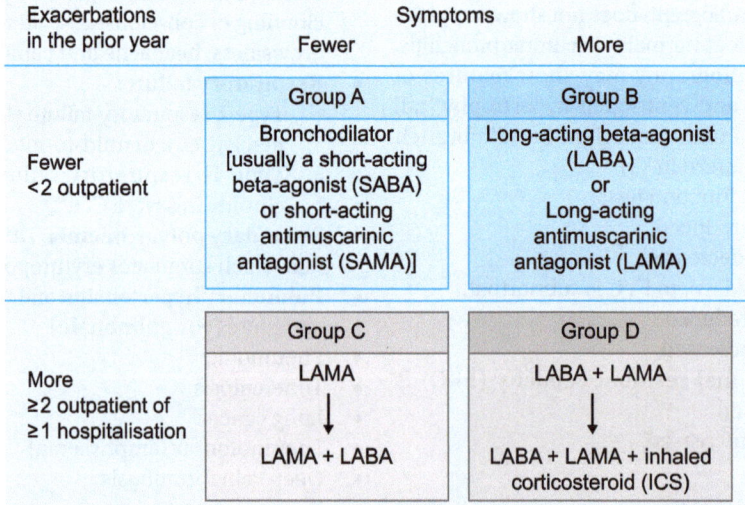

Fig. 12.5: Pharmacotherapy based on severity of chronic obstructive pulmonary disease (COPD).

Gold stage	I. Mild	II. Moderate	III. Severe	IV. Very severe
Spirometry findings	• $FEV_1/FVC < 0.70$ • $FEV_1 > 80\%$ of predicted	• $FEV_1/FVC < 0.70$ • FEV_1 50–79% of predicted	• $FEV_1/FVC < 0.70$ • FEV_1 30 to <49% of predicted	• $FEV_1/FVC < 0.70$ • FEV_1 30% of predicted or • FEV1 <50% of predicted, if respiratory failure present
Management	Short-acting beta-agonists (salbutamol, terbutaline, levosalbutamol) as needed	Long-acting beta-agonists [salmeterol, formoterol] ± anticholinergics (ipratropium, tiotropium)	Add inhaled glucocorticoids (beclomethasone, budesonide, fluticasone, ciclesonide) ± methylxanthines	Add oxygen therapy, ventilator assistance, management of right-sided heart failure, surgical options
	Avoid risk factors, influenza vaccination and use short-acting beta-agonists to all stages →			

(FEV_1: forced expiratory volume in one second; FVC: forced vital capacity)

Fig. 12.6: Global initiative for chronic Obstructive Lung Disease (GOLD) staging for severity of chronic obstructive pulmonary disease (COPD) and management.

TABLE 12.27: Differences between emphysema and chronic bronchitis.

Feature	Emphysema	Chronic bronchitis
Clinical features		
Dyspnoea	Severe	Mild-to-moderate
Cough	Develops after dyspnoea starts	Frequent, develops before dyspnoea starts
Sputum—amount and nature	Scanty, mucoid	Copious, purulent
Frequency of mucopurulent relapses	Less	More
Cyanosis	Absent	Present
Pulmonary hypertension	Late and mild	Early and severe
Right ventricular failure and respiratory failure	Late and often terminal	Repeated episodes
Mechanism of airway obstruction	Loss of elastic recoil	Decreased airway lumen due to mucus and inflammation
Investigations		
Haematocrit (PCV)	Normal	Increased
PaO_2	Normal to low 'pink puffer'	Low 'blue bloater'
$PaCO_2$	Normal mildly increased	High (> 40)
FEV_1	Decreased	Decreased
Diffusing capacity	Reduced	Normal
Chest X-ray	Features of hyperinflation, bullae and tubular heart	Increased bronchovascular markings and cardiomegaly
Elastic recoil	Decreased	Normal
Airway resistance	Normal to slightly increased	Increased
Cor pulmonale	Late, mild	Early, marked
Prognosis	Good	Poor

(PCV: packed cell volume)

- History or evidence of atopy (e.g. hay fever and elevated total IgE)
- Age 40 years or more
- Smoking > 10 pack-years, post-bronchodilator FEV_1 < 80% predicted and FEV_1/FVC < 70%.

A ≥ 15% increase in FEV_1 or ≥ 12% and ≥ 200 mL increase in FEV_1 post-bronchodilator treatment with albuterol would be a minor criterion.

■ BRONCHIECTASIS

Definition

- Bronchiectasis is defined as a permanent abnormal dilatation of one or more bronchi due to the destruction of elastic and muscular components of the bronchial wall.

Box 12.20 shows the causes of bronchiectasis.

Clinical Features

- The hallmarks of bronchiectasis are chronic cough with sputum production, haemoptysis and recurrent pneumonias.
- In some cases, the patient is asymptomatic or has non-productive cough 'bronchiectasis sicca'. It commonly occurs following upper lobe TB.
- General examination may reveal anaemia, clubbing of the digits (2–3% cases), fever, halitosis and sinusitis.
- The characteristics are 'bilateral, basal, coarse and leathery crepitations'.
- Chest radiograph is usually normal. Cystic or saccular bronchiectasis may be diagnosed by multiple 1–2 cm cystic-appearing lesions

> **Box 12.20: Causes of bronchiectasis.**
>
> **Congenital**
> - Cystic fibrosis (CF)
> - Ciliary dysfunction syndromes
>   - Primary ciliary dyskinesia (immotile cilia syndrome), Young's syndrome
>   - Kartagener's syndrome (sinusitis and transposition of the viscera)
> - Primary hypogammaglobulinaemia, alpha-1 antitrypsin deficiency
> - Others: Bronchial cysts, cul-de-sacs, bronchomalacia, atopic bronchial asthma, pulmonary sequestration, Mounier–Kuhn syndrome or tracheobronchomegaly, Williams–Campbell syndrome (bronchomalacia)
>
> **Acquired: Children**
> - Pneumonia (complicating whooping cough or measles)
> - Primary tuberculosis
> - Inhaled foreign body
>
> **Acquired: Adults**
> - Pulmonary tuberculosis, *Mycobacterium avium complex* (MAC)
> - Suppurative pneumonia
> - Allergic bronchopulmonary aspergillosis complicating asthma (ABPA)
> - Post-obstructive bronchiectasis: Partial or total obstruction of the bronchial lumen, e.g. endobronchial tumours or foreign bodies, enlarged hilar lymph nodes or tumour masses and bronchostenosis following endobronchial tuberculosis
> - Autoimmune diseases, e.g. rheumatoid arthritis, Sjögren's syndrome, systemic lupus erythematosus, inflammatory bowel disease
> - Others: Repeated aspiration of gastric juice, inhalation of toxic gas (ammonia), HIV infection, interstitial lung fibrosis (traction bronchiectasis), radiation fibrosis, sarcoidosis, chronic hypersensitivity pneumonitis, bronchiolitis obliterans after lung transplantation

(HIV: human immunodeficiency syndrome)

with or without fluid levels ('honey-comb' appearance or 'bird-nest' appearance). Less often, the chest film shows linear streaks (tram tracks), end-on thickened bronchi or signet-ring deformity, and groups of small curvilinear shadows called grape clusters.
- High-resolution computed tomography, in which the images are only 1 mm thick, has replaced bronchography for the diagnosis of bronchiectasis. Besides, some features on CT scan may suggest the aetiology of bronchiectasis (e.g. proximal bronchiectasis suggests ABPA).

> **Box 12.21: Complications of bronchiectasis.**
> - Haemoptysis
> - Pneumonia
> - Lung abscess
> - Empyema
> - Septicaemia
> - Osteomyelitis
> - Amyloidosis
> - Brain abscess
> - Aspergilloma
> - Cor pulmonale
> - Respiratory failure
> - Hypoproteinaemia

Complications
Box 12.21 shows the complications of bronchiectasis.

Management
- Postural drainage consists of adopting a position in which the lobe to be drained is uppermost. Postural drainage should be performed for a minimum of 5–10 minutes twice a day. Gentle percussion of the chest wall with cupped hands aids dislodgement of sputum.
- Antibiotic therapy
- Surgical treatment: Resection of areas of bronchiectatic lung

PRIMARY CILIARY DYSKINESIA

- Ciliary dysfunction syndromes or primary ciliary dyskinesia (PCD) are a group of genetically determined disorders characterised by dysfunction of cilia of the respiratory tract epithelium, sperms and other cells, causing impairment of mucociliary clearance, left-right body asymmetry and impaired sperm motility. Majority are autosomal recessive disorders.
- Kartagener's syndrome is one of the ciliary dysfunction syndromes. It is characterised by recurrent sinusitis, bronchiectasis, dextrocardia or situs inversus and infertility.
- Young's syndrome is characterised by recurrent sinopulmonary infections and obstructive azoospermia.

LUNG ABSCESS

Box 12.22 shows the causes of lung abscess.

LUNG CANCER

Table 12.28 shows the classification of tumours of the lung.

Box 12.22: Causes of lung abscess.

Infectious causes
- Bacteria
  - Usual: Mouth flora anaerobes, most frequently isolated anaerobes: *Peptostreptococcus, Fusobacterium nucleatum, Prevotella melaninogenica*
  - Less common: *Staphylococcus aureus, Streptococcus pyogenes, Pseudomonas aeruginosa, Klebsiella pneumoniae, Streptococcus pneumoniae*, gram-negative bacilli, such as *Escherichia coli, Haemophilus influenzae* type B, *Legionella, Nocardia asteroides*. Mixed infections occur when lung abscess develops due inhalation of foreign material
  - Mycobacteria: *M. tuberculosis, M. avium complex, M. kansasii*, other mycobacteria
- Fungi: *Aspergillus* spp., *Histoplasma capsulatum, Pneumocystis Jirovecii, Coccidioides immitis, Blastocystis hominis, Cryptococcus*
- Parasites: *Entamoeba histolytica, Paragonimus westermani, Strongyloides stercoralis* (post-obstructive)

Non-infectious causes
- Neoplasms: Primary lung cancer, metastatic carcinoma, lymphoma
- Pulmonary infarction: Due to bland embolus (may be secondarily infected in < 5%)
- Septic embolism: Tricuspid endocarditis due to *S. aureus* and others (typically with positive blood cultures), jugular venous septic phlebitis due to *Fusobacterium necrophorum* (Lemierre syndrome)
- Vasculitis: Wegener's granulomatosis, rheumatoid lung nodule
- Developmental: Pulmonary sequestration
- Airway disease: Bullae, blebs, or cystic bronchiectasis (usually thin-walled)
- Other: Sarcoidosis, transdiaphragmatic bowel herniation giving appearance of cavity with air fluid level

TABLE 12.28: Classification of tumours of the lung.

Benign tumours (5%)	Malignant tumours (95%)
Benign epithelial tumours	• **Non-small cell carcinoma** (75%)
• Papillomas	– Squamous or epidermoid carcinoma
• Adenomas	– Large-cell carcinoma
Mesenchymal tumours	– Adenocarcinoma
• Chondroma	♦ Bronchioloalveolar cell carcinoma (presently termed adenocarcinoma in situ)
• Lipoma	
Miscellaneous tumours	• Small-cell carcinoma (oat cell carcinoma) (25%)
• Pulmonary hamartoma	• Adenosquamous carcinoma/sarcomatoid carcinoma
• Sclerosing haemangioma	• Salivary gland tumour: Mucoepidermoid carcinoma, adenoid cystic carcinoma
	• Carcinoid tumour: Typical carcinoid, atypical carcinoid

Table 12.29 shows the clinical subgroups of lung cancer.

Table 12.30 shows the manifestation due to the location of the primary tumour.

Manifestations due to regional spread of tumour in the thorax (**Table 12.31**).

Manifestations of extrathoracic metastasis (**Table 12.32**).

Paraneoplastic Syndromes

- Paraneoplastic syndromes usually result from peptide hormone secretion by the tumour and may be in the first manifestations of lung cancers. They are often relieved by successful treatment of the primary tumour (**Table 12.33**).

Table 12.34 shows the tumour, node, metastasis (TNM) staging of non-small-cell carcinoma.

TABLE 12.29: Clinical subgroups of lung cancer.

Small cell lung carcinomas (SCLC) -highly metastatic, high response to chemotherapy	Non-small cell lung carcinomas (NSCLC) -less metastatic, less responsive
• Small-cell (oat cell) carcinoma	• Squamous (epidermoid) carcinoma • Adenocarcinoma (including bronchioloalveolar carcinoma) • Large cell carcinoma

TABLE 12.30: Manifestation due to the location of the primary tumour.

Due to a central or endobronchial growth	Due to a peripheral growth
• Cough • Haemoptysis • Wheeze and stridor • Breathlessness/dyspnoea • Post-obstructive pneumonitis presenting with fever and productive cough	• Chest pain from pleural or chest wall involvement • Dyspnoea on a restrictive basis • Symptoms of lung abscess due to cavitation of tumour

TABLE 12.31: Manifestations of lung cancer due to regional spread of tumour in the thorax.

Pathological basis	Local effects
• Obstruction of airway by tumour	Pneumonia, abscess, atelectasis, focal emphysema
• Tracheal obstruction	Stridor (a harsh inspiratory noise) and dyspnoea
• Local spread into pleura	Pleuritis and malignant effusion
• Local spread to pericardium	Pericarditis, effusion, tamponade
• Compression of superior vena cava (SVC) by tumour	Superior vena cava syndrome
Invasion of structure	**Its effects**
• Recurrent laryngeal nerve	Hoarseness of voice and 'bovine' cough
• Phrenic nerve	Diaphragm paralysis and dyspnoea
• Sympathetic ganglia	Horner syndrome
• Oesophagus	Dysphagia
• Chest wall (direct extension)	Destruction of rib producing rib pain, pathological fractures and intercostal neuralgia
• Superior sulcus tumour (destruction of the T1 and C8 roots in the lower part of the brachial plexus by an apical lung tumour)	Pancoast's syndrome (pain in the inner aspect of the arm, sometimes with small muscle wasting in the hand)
• Lymphatic obstruction	Pleural effusion
• Vascular obstruction	SVC syndrome
• Pericardial and cardiac extension	Pericardial effusion, cardiac tamponade, arrhythmias or cardiac failure

TABLE 12.32: Manifestations of extrathoracic metastasis.

Site of metastasis	Manifestations
Adrenal glands (~50%)	Usually asymptomatic, Addison's disease
Liver (30–50%)	Anorexia, nausea, biliary obstruction, weight loss, right upper quadrant pain and pain
Brain (20%)	Headache, vomiting, focal neurologic deficits, epileptic seizures confusion, and raised intracranial pressure
Bone (20%)	Bony pain, pathologic fractures or raised alkaline phosphatase
Bone marrow	Cytopenias or leucoerythroblastosis
Lymph node	Lymphadenopathy: Commonly to mediastinal, cervical, supraclavicular region (scalene node), and even axillary or intra-abdominal nodes
Epidural and bone metastases	Spinal cord compression (if spine is involved) syndromes

TABLE 12.33: Paraneoplastic syndromes in lung cancer.

System involved	Manifestations
Systemic	Anorexia, cachexia, weight loss, fever
Endocrine	• Syndrome of inappropriate secretion of antidiuretic hormone causing hyponatraemia (small-cell carcinoma) • Ectopic ACTH secretion resulting in hypokalaemia, rather than full-blown Cushing's syndrome (small cell carcinoma) • Hypercalcaemia due to ectopic production of parathyroid hormone or parathyroid hormone related peptide (squamous cell carcinoma) • Carcinoid syndrome, acromegaly, hypoglycaemia, hyperthyroidism • Gynaecomastia
Skeletal	• Clubbing of fingers (usually NSCLC) non-small cell carcinoma • Hypertrophic pulmonary osteoarthropathy (usually adenocarcinoma)-HPOA
Neuromyopathic	• Polyneuropathy • Myelopathy encephalomyelitis, opsoclonus-myoclonus, limbic encephalitis • Cerebellar degeneration • Myasthenia (Lambert–Eaton syndrome) and retinal blindness (small-cell carcinoma)
Haematological	• Migratory venous thrombophlebitis (Trousseau's syndrome) • Marantic endocarditis • Disseminated intravascular coagulation (DIC) • Anaemia, granulocytosis, leucoerythroblastosis
Cutaneous	• Dermatomyositis • Acanthosis nigricans
Renal	• Nephrotic syndrome • Glomerulonephritis

(ACTH: adrenocorticotropic hormone; HPOA: hypertrophic pulmonary osteoarthropathy; NSCLC: Non-small-cell lung carcinoma)

TABLE 12.34: TNM staging of non-small-cell carcinoma.

TNM	Description
Tx	Main tumour cannot be assesses, or cancer cells seen on sputum cytology or bronchial washing but no tumour can be found
T1	Tumour ≤ 3 cm in diameter; surrounded by lung or pleura; does not invade main bronchus
• T1a	Tumour 2 cm or less in greatest dimension
• T1b	Tumour > 2 cm but ≤ 3 cm
T2	Tumour > 3 cm in diameter; may invade pleura; may extend into main bronchus but remains 2 cm or more distal to carina
• T2a	Tumour > 3 cm but ≤ 5 cm
• T2b	Tumour > 5 cm but ≤ 7 cm
T3	Tumour > 7 cm, invasion of chest wall, diaphragm, pleura or pericardium; main bronchus < 2 cm distal to carina; atelectasis of entire lung
T4	Invasion of mediastinum, heart, great vessels, trachea, oesophagus, vertebral body or carina; separate tumour nodules; malignant pleural effusion
N0	No nodal metastasis
N1	Involvement of ipsilateral peribronchial or hilar nodes and intrapulmonary nodes
N2	Involvement of ipsilateral mediastinal or subcarinal nodes
N3	Involvement of contralateral nodes or any supraclavicular nodes
M0	No distant metastasis
M1	Distant metastasis

(TNM: tumour, node, metastasis)

Table 12.35 shows the staging of carcinoma of the lung.
- Treatment (**Box 12.23**)

Table 12.36 shows the general plan of treatment of small-cell carcinoma.

■ DIFFUSE PARENCHYMAL LUNG DISEASES/ INTERSTITIAL LUNG DISEASES

Aetiology

Table 12.37 shows the major causes of interstitial lung disease (ILD)/diffuse parenchymal lung diseases (DPLDs).

Clinical Features

- *Acute presentation:* Cough, dyspnoea and occasionally fever. Chest radiograph shows diffuse alveolar opacities and therefore can be confused with 'atypical' pneumonia.
- *Subacute presentation:* Gradually increasing symptoms of cough and dyspnoea over weeks to months
- *Chronic presentation:* Shortness of breath, especially with exertion

On physical examination—tachypnoea, clubbing, cyanosis, bilateral fine velcro crepitations (end-inspiratory).

TABLE 12.35: Staging of carcinoma of lung.

Stages of non-small-cell carcinoma based on TNM classification	
Occult carcinoma	TX, N0, M0
IA	T1a, bN0M0
IB	T2aN0M0
IIA	T2bN0M0; T1a, bN1M0; T2aN1M0
IIB	T2bN1M0; T3N0M0
IIIA	T1a, b, T2a, b, N2M0; T3N1, N2M0; T4N0, N1M0
IIIB	T4N2M0; any T N3M0
IV	Any T any N M1
Stage of small-cell carcinoma	**Description**
Limited stage	• 30–40% of small cell lung cancers • Confined to the haemithorax, mediastinum, and ipsilateral supraclavicular lymph node • Within the confines of radiation port
Extensive stage	• 60–70% of small cell lung cancers • Any distant spread

(TNM: tumour, node, metastasis)

Box 12.23: Treatment of non-small cell lung cancer.

Stage IA:
- Lobectomy is treatment of choice. T1N0, lobectomy has 70% 5 year recurrence free survival
- If inoperable:
  - 30% cure rate with XRT alone
  - Stereotactic radiosurgery (cyber knife)
  - Radiofrequency ablation

Stage 1B:
- Lobectomy
- Adjuvant chemotherapy adds a 4–12% survival benefit. Best in tumours > 4 cm

Stage II:
- Lobectomy is treatment of choice
- Adjuvant chemotherapy now standard
- Consider adjuvant XRT to mediastinum

Stage III:
- Combination chemotherapy with XRT is treatment of choice
- Surgery has yet to be established consistently as benefit in randomised trials
- Neoadjuvant therapy followed by surgical resection is option in IIIA

Stage IV:
- Chemotherapy

(XRT: X-ray telescope)

TABLE 12.36: General plan of treatment of small-cell carcinoma.

Stage	Status of patient	Treatment
Limited stage	• With good performance status of patient	• Chemotherapy + radiotherapy
	• With poor performance status of patient	• Modified chemotherapy and/or palliative radiotherapy
Extensive stage	• With good performance status of patient	• Chemotherapy ± local radiotherapy
	• With poor performance status of patient	• Modified chemotherapy and/or palliative radiotherapy

TABLE 12.37: Major causes of interstitial lung disease (ILD)/diffuse parenchymal lung diseases (DPLD).

ILD/DPLD due to known causes	ILD/DPLD due to unknown causes
Non-granulomatous interstitial inflammation (predominant inflammation and fibrosis)	
• Drugs: Antibiotics, gold, amiodarone, D-penicillamine, nitrofurantoin, chemotherapeutic (e.g. busulphan, bleomycin, methotrexate, CCNU) • Asbestos • Fumes and gases • Radiation • Aspiration pneumonitis • Residual of acute respiratory distress syndrome • Smoking related: Pulmonary Langerhans cell histiocytosis, respiratory bronchiolitis interstitial lung disease and desquamative interstitial pneumonia • Acute eosinophilic pneumonia	• Idiopathic interstitial pneumonias (IIPs) • Idiopathic pulmonary fibrosis • Pulmonary autoimmune rheumatic diseases (e.g. systemic lupus erythematosus, rheumatoid arthritis) • Pulmonary alveolar proteinosis • Eosinophilic pneumonias • Lymphangioleiomyomatosis (LAM) • Diffuse pulmonary haemorrhage • Goodpasture's syndrome • Idiopathic pulmonary haemosiderosis • Lymphocytic interstitial pneumonia (seen in HIV)
Granulomatous interstitial inflammation	
• Hypersensitivity pneumonitis (organic dusts) • Inorganic dusts: For example, silicosis, berylliosis	• Sarcoidosis • Pulmonary Langerhans' cell histiocytosis • Granulomatous lung disease with vasculitis (e.g. Wegener, Churg–Strauss)

(HIV: human immunodeficiency virus)

Investigations

Treatment

- Treatment of the underlying cause, if possible
- Removal of offending agent

Drugs

- Corticosteroids are the mainstay of treatment though they are not effective in majority of the patients, particularly those with significant fibrosis. Dose is 1 mg/kg for 6–12 weeks, which is then tapered to a maintenance level, if the patient improves.
- If the patient does not respond to steroids, another immunosuppressant (cyclophosphamide or azathioprine) is added.
- Other drugs include colchicine and cyclosporine.
- N-acetylcysteine is often combined with other medicines and has been found useful in some studies. It is a precursor to the naturally occurring antioxidant glutathione.
- Pirfenidone is an anti-fibrotic drug used for idiopathic pulmonary fibrosis (IPF).

■ OCCUPATIONAL LUNG DISEASES

Table 12.38 shows the occupational exposure and associated lung diseases.

■ SARCOIDOSIS

Definition

Sarcoidosis is a multisystem, chronic granulomatous inflammatory disorder of unknown aetiology.

Clinical Features

- Sarcoidosis can manifest in three forms:
  - Asymptomatic form (30–45%)
  - Acute or subacute form (10–15%)
  - Chronic form (40–60%)
    - Löfgren's syndrome is characterised by erythema nodosum, joint symptoms and radiographic evidence of bilateral hilar adenopathy. Uveitis may occur in some patients. It resolves over 6 months to 2 years with non-steroidal anti-inflammatory drugs (NSAIDs).
    - Heerfordt-Waldenström syndrome or uveoparotid fever characterised by anterior uveitis, parotid enlargement, fever and facial palsy

TABLE 12.38: Occupational exposure and associated lung diseases.

Occupational exposure	Disease associated with chronic exposure
Diseases due to inorganic (mineral) dusts: Common pneumoconiosis	
• Coal • Silica • Asbestos • Beryllium • Iron oxide • Tin dioxide	• Coal-worker's pneumoconiosis (CWP) • Silicosis • Asbestos-related diseases • Berylliosis • Siderosis • Stannosis
Diseases due to organic dusts	
• Cotton, flax or hemp dust • Mouldy hay, grain, straw • Mould malting • Contaminated bagasse (sugar cane)	• Byssinosis • Farmer's lung • Malt worker's lung • Bagassosis
Diseases due to gases and fumes	
• Irritant gases, isocyanates cadmium • Platinum salts	• Occupational asthma, bronchitis, ARDS • Occupational asthma
Diseases due to biological substances	
• Proteolytic enzymes, alllergens from animals and insects (excreta), contaminated grain dust	• Occupational asthma, bronchitis
Diseases due to chemicals and radioactive substances	
• Polycyclic hydrocarbons, radon	• Bronchial carcinoma

(ARDS: acute respiratory distress syndrome)

Pulmonary Manifestations

- Interstitial lung diseases
- Atelectasis
- Cavitation
- Unilateral pleural effusion
- Pulmonary nodules

Extrapulmonary Investigations

Table 12.39 shows the extrapulmonary investigations of sarcoidosis.

TABLE 12.39: Extrapulmonary investigations of sarcoidosis.

Lymph nodes	Hilar adenopathy (70–90%). Paratracheal and generalised lymphadenopathy
Skin	Erythema nodosum, plaques, maculopapular eruptions, subcutaneous nodules, lupus pernio, keloid, infiltration of previous scars by granuloma
Eyes	Uveitis, iridocyclitis, retinitis, phlyctenular conjunctivitis, lacrimal gland involvement (dry eyes)
Salivary glands	Parotid gland enlargement
Heart	Myocarditis, pericarditis, papillary muscle dysfunction, congestive heart failure (CHF) arrhythmias
Liver and spleen	Hepatosplenomegaly, hypersplenism, portal hypertension
Nervous system	Seventh nerve, cerebral, meningeal and peripheral nerve involvement, optic neuritis, diabetes insipidus due to hypothalamic involvement
Kidneys	Nephrocalcinosis, nephrolithiasis, tubule glomerular and renal artery disease
Musculoskeletal	Arthralgias, arthritis, phalangeal cysts, polymyositis, chronic myopathy
Endocrine	Diabetes insipidus, anterior pituitary dysfunction, Addison's syndrome

Investigations

- Blood examination shows lymphocytopaenia, anaemia, eosinophilia, raised erythrocyte sedimentation rate (ESR), hyperglobulinaemia, elevated serum alkaline phosphatase.
- Hypercalcaemia and hypercalciuria occur uncommonly (occur due to increased production of 1, 25-dihydroxyvitamin D by the granuloma).
- Plasma level of angiotensin-converting enzyme (ACE) is elevated in about 70% cases.
- Radiological features of sarcoidosis:
  - Hilar adenopathy, usually bilateral (70–90%)
  - Reticulonodular shadows in lung fields (usually upper lobes)
  - Paratracheal lymph nodal enlargement
  - Egg-shell calcification of hilar nodes (unusual)
  - Pleural effusion (very uncommon)
  - Large nodules
  - Cavitation
  - Atelectasis
  - Cardiomegaly
  - In addition to sarcoidosis, upper lobe involvement occurs with TB, pneumocystis pneumonia, hypersensitivity pneumonitis, silicosis and Langerhans cell histiocytosis.

Classic Radiographic Patterns of Pulmonary Sarcoidosis

Stage I: Bilateral hilar adenopathy with no parenchymal abnormalities (50% cases)
Stage II: Bilateral hilar adenopathy with diffuse parenchymal infiltrates (30% cases)
Stage III: Diffuse parenchymal infiltrates without hilar adenopathy (10% cases)
Stage IV: Evidence of diffuse pulmonary fibrosis

Treatment

- Prednisolone is given 20–40 mg daily for 4 weeks, followed by a maintenance dose of 7.5–10 mg daily for 6–18 months.
- Azathioprine and methotrexate as steroid-sparing agents are given if patient cannot be maintained on prednisolone dose of 10 mg/day or less.
- Hydroxychloroquine for skin, bone and joint involvement
- Other agents used include pentoxifylline, infliximab, etanercept (less effective than infliximab) and thalidomide.

■ PLEURAL EFFUSION

Table 12.40 shows the classification and causes of pleural effusion.

TABLE 12.40: Classification and causes of pleural effusion.

Types of effusion	Causes	
Transudative effusion	• Cardiac failure • Hypoproteinaemia (e.g. nephrotic syndrome, cirrhosis of liver, severe malnutrition) • Constrictive pericarditis	• Hypothyroidism • Meigs' syndrome (benign ovarian tumours with ascites and pleural effusion) • Peritoneal dialysis
Exudative effusion	• Tuberculosis • Bacterial pneumonia • Malignancy • Pulmonary infarction • Autoimmune diseases (e.g. rheumatoid arthritis, systemic lupus erythematosus) • Acute pancreatitis • Post-myocardial infarction syndrome (Dressler's syndrome)	• Drug-induced effusion • Benign asbestos-related effusion • Intra-abdominal abscess • Meigs' syndrome (can be transudative as well) • Ruptured amebic liver abscess, chylous pleural effusion • Acute rheumatic fever

Investigations

Radiological Examination
- Mediastinal shift to the opposite side
- Obliteration of costophrenic angle
- A dense uniform opacity in the lower and lateral part of haemithorax

Ultrasonography
- It can detect as little as 5 mL of effusion.
- It is useful in differentiating loculated pleural effusion from pleural tumour or pleural thickening.
- It detects septations within pleural fluid with greater sensitivity than CT scanning.
- It is useful in localisation of an effusion prior to aspiration and biopsy.
- Detection of solid pleural abnormalities may suggest pleural malignancy.

Pleural Aspiration and Fluid Analysis
Table 12.41 shows the differentiation of transudative from exudative effusion and **Table 12.42** shows the interpretation of pleural fluid parameters.

Light's criteria: Exudative pleural effusions must meet at least one of the following criteria, whereas transudative pleural effusions meet none.

Box 12.24 shows the Light's criteria for distinguishing pleural from exudate.

Other Investigations in Pleural Effusion
Management of Pleural Effusion
Flowchart 12.2 shows the approach to the diagnosis of pleural effusions.

■ EMPYEMA THORACIS

Empyema thoracic is in which pus and fluid from infection collects in the pleural cavity. It usually involves whole of the pleural space.

Aetiology
- Infection of pleural space from neighbouring structures, e.g. bacterial pneumonias, bronchiectasis, lung abscess, rupture of subphrenic abscess, oesophageal perforation, infection of haemothorax
- Infection of pleural space from a distant source, e.g. bacteraemia
- Infection of pleural space from external source, e.g. penetrating chest injury, chest tube placement and thoracic surgery
- The common organisms involved are *Pneumococcus, Streptococcus, Staphylococcus,*

TABLE 12.41: Differentiation of transudative from exudative effusion.

Characteristics	Transudative effusion	Exudative effusion
Cause and mechanism	Non-inflammatory process. Ultrafiltrate of plasma, due to increased hydrostatic pressure or decreased serum oncotic pressure with normal vascular permeability	Inflammation process and is rich in proteins due to increased vascular permeability
Appearance	Clear, serous	Cloudy/purulent/haemorrhagic/chylous
Colour	Straw yellow	Yellow to red
Specific gravity	< 1.018	> 1.018
Protein • Absolute value • Pleural fluid: Serum ratio	Low, < 2 g/dL, mainly albumin < 0.5	High, > 2 g/dL > 0.5
Clot	Absent	Clots spontaneously because of high fibrinogen
Leucocytes • Total leucocytes • Type of cells Differential leucocytes • Erythrocytes	< 1000/mm^3 > 50% lymphocytes or mononuclear cells and mesothelial cells < 500/mm^3	> 1000/mm^3 > 50% lymphocytes (tuberculosis, malignancy) > 50% polymorphs (acute inflammation) Variable
Bacteria	Absent	Usually present
Lactate dehydrogenase (LDH) • Absolute value • Pleural fluid LDH: Serum LDH ratio	< 200 IU/L < 0.6	200 IU/L > 0.6
Glucose	> 60 mg/dL (usually same as in blood)	< 60 mg/dL (variable)

TABLE 12.42: Interpretation of pleural fluid parameters.

Parameter	Interpretation
Appearance of pleural fluid	Putrid odour (anaerobic empyema), food particles (oesophageal rupture), bile stained (chylothorax/biliary fistula), milky (chylothorax/pseudo-chylothorax), anchovy sauce-like fluid (ruptured amebic abscess)
Pleural fluid glucose concentration • Low glucose concentration (< 60 mg/dL) • Very low glucose concentration (< 15 mg/dL)	• Suggests empyema, malignancy or tuberculosis. • Empyema, rheumatoid effusions

Continued

Continued

Parameter	Interpretation
Pleural fluid eosinophilia (> 10% of all cells)	May be observed in resolving infections, pneumothorax, hydropneumothorax, haemothorax and asbestos-related pleural effusion, dantrolene, bromocriptine, nitrofurantoin, paragonimiasis or Churg–Strauss syndrome
Pleural fluid erythrocyte counts > 100,000/mm^3	Most often in malignancy or pulmonary infarction/embolism, but may result from a traumatic tap
Low pH of pleural fluid < 7.2	Complicated parapneumonic effusion, oesophageal rupture, rheumatoid pleuritis, tuberculous pleuritis, malignant pleural disease, haemothorax, systemic acidosis, paragonimiasis, lupus pleuritis, urinothorax
Raised pleural fluid amylase	Pancreatic diseases and oesophageal rupture. However, routine amylase estimation is not recommended unless the clinical features suggest either of the two diseases
Pleural fluid antinuclear antibody titres or rheumatoid factor	No diagnostic significance and is not indicated in most cases
Mesothelial cells	• Absent: Tuberculosis • Markedly increased: Pulmonary embolism

Box 12.24: Light's criteria for distinguishing pleural transudate from exudate.

- Pleural fluid protein/serum protein > 0.5
- Pleural fluid LDH/serum LDH > 0.6
- Pleural fluid LDH more than two-thirds the normal upper limit for serum LDH levels

(LDH: lactate dehydrogenase)

Pseudomonas, M. tuberculosis, H. influenzae and anaerobes.

Clinical Features

- High-grade, remittent fever with chills and rigors, malaise and weight loss
- Respiratory symptoms such as pleuritic chest pain, breathlessness and dry cough are present. Copious, purulent sputum indicates the presence of a bronchopleural fistula.
- Physical examination reveals digital clubbing, oedema of the chest wall, intercostals tenderness and signs of fluid in the pleural space.
- Empyema necessitans: The pus may track through and point on the chest wall.

Management of Empyema Thoracis

- Acute antibiotics should be administered based on the sensitivity of the organism.
- The pus in the pleural cavity should be drained in all cases.
- Tuberculous empyema: Anti-tuberculous chemotherapy

■ PNEUMOTHORAX

Aetiology

Flowchart 12.3 shows the classification of pneumothorax.

Clinical Features

Sudden onset chest pain and dyspnoea are the most common symptoms.

Physical Signs

- General examination may reveal cyanosis, rapid thread pulse, pulsus paradoxus and signs of peripheral circulatory failure in severe cases.
- Inspection and palpation of the respiratory system reveal dyspnoea, shallow breathing, accessory muscles of respiration in actin, shift of trachea and mediastinum (apex beat) to the opposite side, fullness of the chest on the affected side, diminished chest movements and markedly diminished vocal fremitus on the affected side. Measurements show a reduction in total chest expansion, increase in the size of

Pulmonology

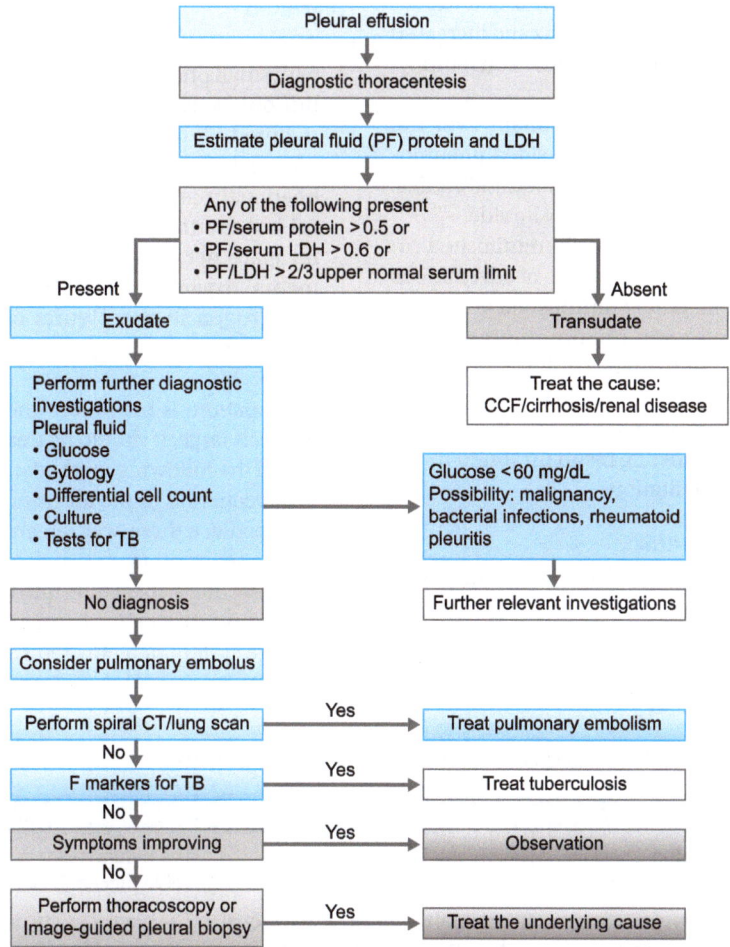

Flowchart 12.2: Approach to the diagnosis of pleural effusions.

(CCF: congestive cardiac failure; CT: computed tomography; LDH: lactate dehydrogenase; TB: tuberculosis)

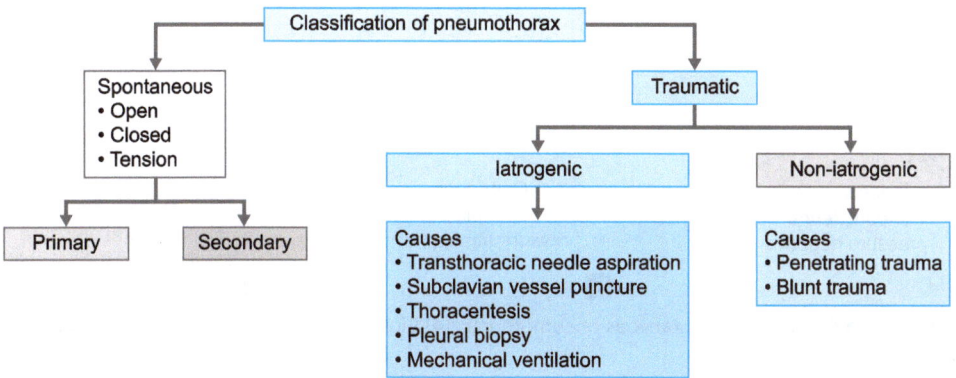

Flowchart 12.3: Classification of pneumothorax.

the affected haemithorax, diminished expansion of the affected haemithorax and increased spinoscapular distance. Subcutaneous emphysema may be present.
- Percussion is not hyper-resonant over the affected hemithorax. In right-sided pneumothorax, liver dullness is obliterated and cardiac dullness is shifted to the opposite side.
- Auscultation reveals markedly diminished-to-absent breath sounds, absence of adventitious sounds and markedly diminished vocal resonance. In an open pneumothorax with a bronchopleural fistula, amphoric bronchial breathing may be heard. Coin test may be positive. Two coins when tapped on the affected side produce a tinkling resonant sound that is audible on auscultation.

Types of Pneumothorax

Table 12.43 shows the differences between closed, open and tension pneumothorax and **Figures 12.7A to C** show the types of spontaneous pneumothorax.

Treatment

- Asymptomatic or slightly breathless patients with small pneumothorax need no treatment, but only serial radiographic monitoring is required till the lung re-expands. Spontaneous reabsorption of pneumothoraces has been estimated at 1.25–1.8% (about 50–70 mL) of the total volume of air in the pleural space per day. Administration of supplemental oxygen reduces the partial pressure of nitrogen in the pleural capillaries and increases air reabsorption from the pleural space
- If the patient is breathless and the pneumothorax is large, it should be treated actively by one of the following methods:
  o Evacuation of the air using a syringe and needle, a three-way tap and an underwater-seal system
  o Inserting a chest tube into the pleural cavity and connecting it to a water-seal drainage system or a non-return valve

TABLE 12.43: Differences between closed, open and tension pneumothorax.

Closed pneumothorax	Open pneumothorax	Tension pneumothorax
The pleural tear is **sealed**	The pleural tear is **open**	The pleural tear act as a **ball and valve** mechanism
The pleural cavity pressure is less than the atmospheric pressure	The pleural cavity pressure is equal to the atmospheric pressure	The pleural cavity pressure is more than the atmospheric pressure

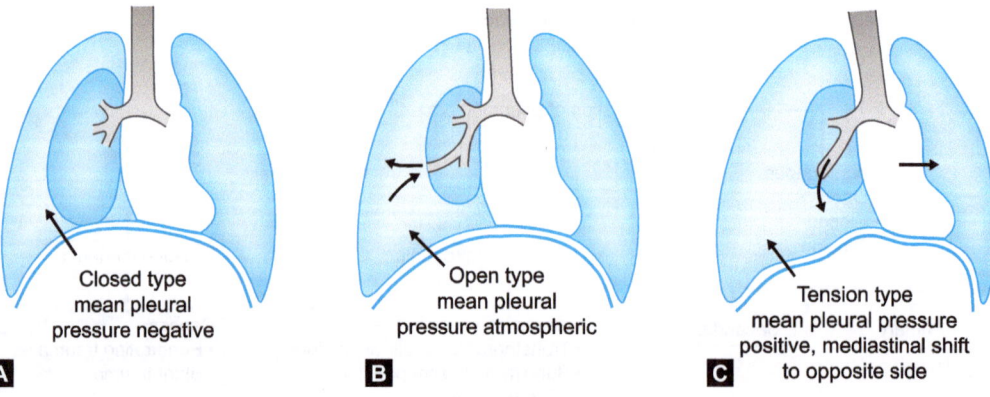

Figs. 12.7 A to C: Types of spontaneous pneumothorax. (A) Closed type; (B) Open type; (C) Tension (valvular) type.

Tension (Valvular) Pneumothorax

- The communication between pleura and lung persists. It acts as a one-way valve allowing air to enter the pleural space during inspiration, coughing, sneezing and straining, but not allowing it to escape. Large amounts of air get 'trapped' in the pleural space and the intrapleural pressure becomes much higher than the atmospheric pressure.
- Clinically, these patients present with rapidly progressive breathlessness, central cyanosis, raid thread pulse and signs of peripheral circulatory failure. Frank signs of pneumothorax are present. Death can occur within few minutes from asphyxia.
- Typical clinical situations where a tension pneumothorax may develop include the following:
    o Ventilated patients (invasive or non-invasive)
    o Traumatic chest injuries
    o During cardiopulmonary resuscitation patients
    o Lung disease, especially acute presentations of asthma and COPD
    o Blocked, clamped or displaced chest drains
    o Patients undergoing hyperbaric oxygen treatment

Treatment
Emergency treatment is the introduction of a wide-bore plastic cannula, the other end of which is attached to a long rubber tubing, the end of which is placed underwater in a bottle.

Recurrent Spontaneous Pneumothorax

- Recurrent episodes of pneumothorax are common in patients with emphysematous bullae, lymphangioleiomyomatosis (LAM) and Marfan's syndrome.
- The treatment includes obliteration of the pleural space by artificial pleurodesis using tetracycline hydrochloride of talc powder. Alternatively, pleural abrasion or parietal pleurectomy at thoracotomy may be attempted.

Catamenial Pneumothorax

- Repeated attacks of spontaneous pneumothorax occur, usually on the right side, in association with menstruation. Attacks usually occur within 48 hours before or after the onset of menstruation. Haemoptysis may also occur.
- Various treatment modalities attempted include ovulation-suppressing drugs, surgical exploration and pleurodesis.

■ HAEMOPTYSIS

- 'Potentially lethal' or 'massive' haemoptysis is defined as > 600–800 mL blood in 24 hours. A more clinical and practical definition of massive haemoptysis is any bleeding that results in a threat to life because of airway or haemodynamic compromise by bleeding.

Causes
Table 12.44 shows the causes of haemoptysis.

■ DIFFERENTIAL DIAGNOSIS OF DYSPNOEA
Table 12.45 shows the causes of acute and chronic dyspnoea.

■ BRONCHOSCOPY
Indications of bronchoscopy are given in Table 12.46.

■ MEDIASTINAL MASSES
Figure 12.8 shows the location of most common lesions of mediastinum.

TABLE 12.44: Causes of haemoptysis.

Structure involved	Common causes	Uncommon causes
Bronchial disease	Bronchial carcinoma, bronchiectasis, acute and chronic bronchitis	Bronchial adenoma, foreign body
Parenchymal disease of lung	Pulmonary tuberculosis (Rasmussen's aneurysm-dilation of a pulmonary artery in a tuberculous cavity), lung abscess, pneumonia (particularly *Klebsiella*), fungal infections (aspergilloma and invasive aspergillosis), pulmonary contusion/laceration (traumatic)	Parasites (e.g. hydatid disease, flukes), trauma, actinomycosis, mycetoma
Vascular diseases of lung	Pulmonary infarction	Goodpasture's syndrome, polyarteritis nodosa, idiopathic, pulmonary haemosiderosis, primary pulmonary hypertension
Cardiovascular disease	Acute left ventricular failure	Mitral stenosis, aortic aneurysm, pulmonary thromboembolism
Haematological disorders		Leukaemia, haemophilia, anticoagulants, haemorrhagic diathesis

TABLE 12.45: Causes of acute and chronic dyspnoea.

Acute dyspnoea	Chronic dyspnoea
Cardiovascular system	
Cardiogenic acute pulmonary oedema	Chronic heart failure, myocardial ischaemia
Respiratory system	
• Acute severe bronchial asthma • Acute exacerbation of COPD • Spontaneous pneumothorax • Pneumonia • Acute pulmonary embolism • ARDS • Inhaled foreign body (especially in children) • Lobar collapse • Laryngeal oedema (e.g. anaphylaxis) or obstruction • Metabolic acidosis (e.g. diabetic ketoacidosis, lactic acidosis, uraemia, overdose of salicylates, ethylene glycol poisoning) • Psychogenic hyperventilation (anxiety or panic-related)	• COPD • Chronic bronchial asthma • Bronchial carcinoma • Interstitial lung disease (e.g. sarcoidosis, fibrosing alveolitis, extrinsic allergic alveolitis, pneumoconiosis) • Chronic pulmonary thromboembolism • Lymphatic carcinomatosis • Large pleural effusion(s) • Severe anaemia • Obesity • Deconditioning

(ARDS: acute respiratory distress syndrome; COPD: chronic obstructive pulmonary disease)

Pulmonology

TABLE 12.46: Indications of bronchoscopy.

Diagnostic	Therapeutic
• Diagnosis of lung cancer • Chest radiographic abnormality (lung tumour or changes suggestive of bronchial obstruction, such as appearance of early volume loss or undoubted collapse, unresolved pneumonia or hemi-diaphragmatic paralysis) • Evaluation of haemoptysis • Evaluation of persistent or recurrent cough • Evaluation of paralysed vocal cord • To obtain positive sputum cytology • Staging of lung cancer • Diagnosis of diffuse lung disease • Identification of infecting agents	• Insertion of an endotracheal tube for general anaesthesia in patients in whom extension of neck may be dangerous (atlantoaxial subluxation) • Tamponade of endobronchial bleeding, either with end of bronchoscope itself or by using a fogarty • Removal of foreign bodies • Aspiration of secretions in acute inflammatory lobar atelectasis where physiotherapy has proved unsuccessful in achieving this end • Relief of tracheobronchial narrowing by laser treatment • Treatment of lung cancer by placement of stents or delivery of endobronchial radiotherapy (brachytherapy)

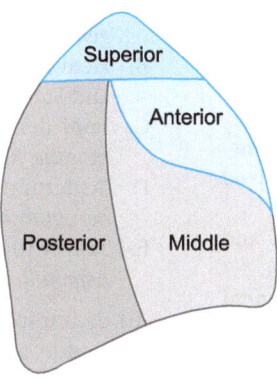

Superior:
- Thymoma and thymic cyst
- Malignant lymphoma
- Thyroid lesions
- Parathyroid adenoma

Posterior:
- Neurogenic tumours
- Most common mass of the posterior compartment schwannoma, neurofibroma malignant peripheral nerve sheath tumor (MPNST) neuroblastoma, ganglioneuroma, ganglioneuroblastoma

Meningoceles
Thoracic spine lesions:
- Pott's disease

Anterior
- **Thymus:** Thymoma, thymic cyst, thymic hyperplasia, thymic carcinoma
- **Lymphoma:** Hodgkin's lymphoma, lymphoblastic lymphoma mediastinal DLBCL
- **Germ cell tumors:** Teratoma, seminoma, non-seminematous tumours
- **Thyroid** (intrathoracic)
- **Others:** Parathyroid adenoma, hemangioma, lipoma, liposarcoma, hemangioma, fibroma, fibrosarcoma, paraganglioma, Foramen of morgagni hernia

Middle
- **Lymphadenopathy:** Most common mass of the middle compartment, lymphoma, metastatic lung cancer, metastatic breast cancer, sarcoidosis
- **Cysts:** Bronchogenic, pericardial, oesophageal duplication

Fig. 12.8: Location of most common lesions of mediastinum.

BEST OF FIVES

1. Which of the following statements regarding auscultation of the chest is TRUE?
   A. Absence of breath sounds in a haemithorax is almost always associated with a pleural effusion.
   B. An astute clinician should be able to differentiate 'fine' from 'coarse' crackles.
   C. 'Cardiac asthma' refers to wheezing associated with alveolar oedema in congestive heart failure.
   D. Rhonchi are a manifestation of obstruction of medium-sized airways.
   E. The presence of egophony can be used to distinguish pulmonary fibrosis from alveolar filling.

2. A 65-year-old male with a long history of tobacco use is seen in the clinic for 4 weeks of progressive dyspnoea on exertion and mild non-productive cough. On physical examination, he has normal vital signs and normal oxygen saturation on room air. Jugular venous pressure is normal.
The trachea is midline, and there is no associated lymphadenopathy. On pulmonary examination, the patient has dullness over the left lower lung field, decreased tactile fremitus and decreased breath sounds.
After obtaining chest X-ray, appropriate initial management at this point would include which of the following?
   A. Intravenous antibiotics
   B. Thoracentesis
   C. Bronchoscopy
   D. Deep suctioning
   E. Bronchodilator therapy

3. A 50-year-old man presents to his physician complaining of haemoptysis. He is ill for the past 4 days with a low-grade fever and cough.
The cough was initially productive of yellow-green sputum, but now it is sputum mixed with red blood.
He smokes one pack of cigarettes daily and has done so since 15 years of age.
Bilateral expiratory wheezing and rhonchi are heard on examination. Chest radiograph is normal. What is the most likely cause of haemoptysis in this individual?
   A. Acute bronchitis
   B. Infection with TB
   C. Lung abscess
   D. Lung cancer
   E. Medications

4. At what lung volume does the outward recoil of the chest wall equals the inward elastic recoil of the lung?
   A. Expiratory reserve volume
   B. Functional residual capacity
   C. Residual volume
   D. Tidal volume
   E. Total lung capacity

5. A 25-year-old woman is seen for follow-up of persistent asthma symptoms despite treatment with inhaled fluticasone 88 μg twice daily for the past 3 months. Which of the following changes in therapy can be considered?
   A. Addition of a leukotriene antagonist.
   B. Addition of a long-acting beta-agonist.
   C. Addition of low-dose theophylline.
   D. Increase the dosage of inhaled corticosteroid.
   E. Any of the above can be considered.

6. All of the following occupational lung diseases are correctly matched with their exposure EXCEPT:
   A. Berylliosis—high-technology electronics.
   B. Byssinosis—cotton milling.
   C. Farmer's lung—mouldy hay.
   D. Progressive massive fibrosis—shipyard workers.
   E. Metal fume fever—welding.

7. Which of the following associations correctly pairs clinical scenarios and CAP pathogens?
   A. Aspiration pneumonia: *Streptococcus pyogenes*
   B. Heavy alcohol use: Atypical pathogens and *Staphylococcus aureus*
   C. Poor dental hygiene: *Chlamydia pneumoniae, Klebsiella pneumoniae*
   D. Structural lung disease: *Pseudomonas aeruginosa, S. aureus*
   E. Travel to southwestern United States: *Aspergillus* spp.

8. All of the following individuals receiving tuberculin skin purified protein derivative (PPD) reactions should be treated for latent TB EXCEPT:
   A. A 16-year-old injection drug user who is HIV negative has a 12-mm PPD reaction.
   B. A 30-year-old fourth-grade teacher has a 7-mm PPD reaction and no known exposures to active TB. She has never been tested with a PPD previously.
   C. A 54-year-old individual in the Peace Corps working in sub-Saharan Africa has a 10-mm PPD reaction. Eighteen months ago, the PPD reaction was 3 mm.
   D. A 30-year-old man who is HIV positive has a negative PPD result. His partner was recently diagnosed with cavitary TB.
   E. A 46-year-old man who is receiving chemotherapy for non-Hodgkin's lymphoma has a 16-mm PPD reaction.

9. In March 2009, the H1N1 strain of the influenza A virus emerged in Mexico and quickly spread worldwide over the next several months. The genetic process by which this pandemic strain of influenza A emerged is an example of:
   A. Antigenic drift
   B. Antigenic shift
   C. Genetic reassortment
   D. Point mutation
   E. B and C

10. A 60-year-old woman presents with complaint of chronic cough that has worsened over a period of 6–10 months. The cough is present day and night and is productive of a thick green sputum.
    Over the course of the day, she estimates that she produces as much as 100 mL of sputum daily. Bilateral coarse leathery crackles are heard in the lower lung zones.
    What would you recommend as the next step in the evaluation of this patient?
    A. Bronchoscopy with bronchoalveolar lavage.
    B. Chest CT with intravenous contrast.
    C. High-resolution chest CT.
    D. Serum immunoglobulin levels.
    E. Treatment with a long-acting bronchodilator and inhaled corticosteroid.

11. Which of the following organisms is unlikely to be found in the sputum of a patient with cystic fibrosis?
    A. *Haemophilus influenzae*
    B. *Acinetobacter baumannii*
    C. *Burkholderia cepacia*
    D. *Aspergillus fumigatus*
    E. *Staphylococcus aureus*

12. What would be the expected finding on bronchoalveolar lavage in a patient with diffuse alveolar haemorrhage?
    A. Atypical hyperplastic type II pneumocytes
    B. Ferruginous bodies
    C. Hemosiderin-laden macrophages
    D. Lymphocytosis with an elevated CD4:CD8 ratio
    E. Milky appearance with foamy macrophages

13. All of the following would typically indicate a massive pulmonary embolism EXCEPT:
    A. Elevated serum troponin levels
    B. Initial presentation with haemoptysis
    C. Initial presentation with syncope
    D. Presence of right ventricular enlargement on CT scan of the chest
    E. Presence of right ventricular hypokinesis on echocardiogram

14. The most common cause of a pleural effusion is:
    A. Cirrhosis
    B. Left ventricular failure
    C. Malignancy
    D. Pneumoniae
    E. Pulmonary embolism

15. A 34-year-old male presents with dyspnoea and weight loss. CT of his chest reveals tree-in-bud appearance.

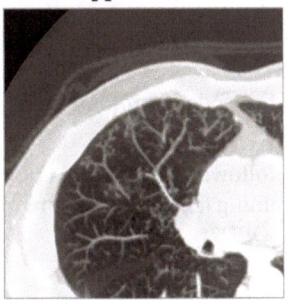

What is the likely diagnosis?
A. Sarcoidosis
B. Asbestosis
C. Tuberculosis
D. Emphysema
E. Bronchoalveolar carcinoma

16. The following flow–volume loop pattern is classical of:

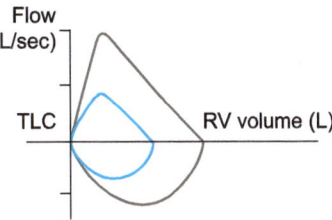

A. Obstructive pattern
B. Restrictive pattern
C. Neuromuscular weakness
D. Variable extrathoracic problem
E. Fixed upper respiratory problem

17. According to Light's criteria, a patient is considered to have an exudative effusion when
    A. Ratio of pleural fluid protein to serum protein is higher than 0.5.
    B. Ratio of pleural fluid lactate dehydrogenase (LDH) to serum LDH is higher than 0.6.
    C. Pleural fluid LDH is higher than two-thirds of the upper limit of normal range.
    D. Any of the above
    E. None of the above

18. Apnoea–hypopnoea index is calculated as
    A. Number of episodes/Number of hours of sleep.
    B. (Number of episodes × number of hours of sleep)/12.
    C. (Number of episodes × number of hours of sleep)/24.
    D. (Number of episodes/number of hours of sleep)/12.
    E. Number of episodes × number of hours of sleep × 24

19. Which of the following is the gold standard test for determining the need for supplemental oxygen in COPD?
    A. Spirometry
    B. Room-air resting ABG
    C. DLCO (diffusing capacity for carbon monoxide)
    D. Venous bicarbonate level
    E. Chest X-ray

20. A young male presents with high fever. Within a few hours, agonising left pleuritic pain and cough with rust-coloured sputum supervene. On examination, the man appears acutely ill with rapid shallow respiration. What clinical finding will you expect?
    A. Decreased movements in left haemithorax with increased vocal resonance.
    B. Increased movements in left haemithorax with decreased vocal resonance.
    C. Decreased movements in left haemithorax with decreased vocal resonance.
    D. Increased movements in left haemithorax with increased vocal resonance.
    E. Decreased movements in left haemithorax with normal vocal resonance.

21. Hyperuricaemia is an adverse effect of the following anti-TB drug:
    A. Ethambutol
    B. Isoniazid
    C. Rifampicin
    D. Pyrazinamide
    E. Streptomycin

22. All of the following cause transudative pleural effusions EXCEPT:
    A. Acute renal failure
    B. Congestive cardiac failure
    C. Cirrhosis
    D. Systemic sclerosis
    E. Beriberi

23. In diseases causing airflow obstruction, the ratio of forced expiratory volume in 1 second to the forced vital capacity, i.e. FEV1/FVC, is usually
    A. Less than 70%
    B. Less than 80%
    C. More than 70%
    D. More than 80%
    E. Between 70 and 80%

24. A 36-year-old lady presents to the OPD with complaint of cough since 15 years. The cough is more during the cooler months of the year and more on lying down on the right side. The cough is worst when the patient wakes up in the morning. It is productive and she brings out about three tablespoons of sputum. It is yellowish-green in colour and is aggravated by the same factors as cough. She also gives multiple episodes of blood in the sputum. There is a childhood history of chicken pox. What is the most likely diagnosis in this patient?
    A. Bronchiectasis
    B. Chronic bronchitis
    C. Lung abscess
    D. Tuberculosis
    E. Sarcoidosis

25. A patient with IPF typically has all the following features except
    A. Abnormal chest radiograph
    B. Exertional dyspnoea
    C. Fine bibasilar inspiratory crackles
    D. Productive cough
    E. Cyanosis and clubbing

26. Type 1 respiratory failure is characterised on ABG by:
    A. $PaO_2 < 60$ mmHg with $PaCO_2 > 50$ mmHg
    B. $PaO_2 < 50$ mmHg with $PaCO_2 > 60$ mmHg
    C. $PaO_2 < 60$ mmHg with $PaCO_2 < 50$ mmHg
    D. $PaO_2 > 60$ mmHg with $PaCO_2 > 50$ mmHg
    E. $PaO_2 > 80$ mmHg with $PaCO_2 > 50$ mmHg

27. All the following are components of CURB-65 criterion EXCEPT:
    A. Altered conscious levels
    B. Chest pain
    C. Hypotension
    D. Increased respiratory rate
    E. Age > 65 years

28. With respect to the definition of COPD, all the following terms are correct EXCEPT:
    A. Enhanced chronic inflammatory response
    B. Preventable and treatable
    C. Progressive
    D. Reversible airflow limitation
    E. Systemic disease

29. A patient who has a Modified Medical Research Council (mMRC) grade of 1 and COPD assessment test (CAT) score of 22 with one hospitalisation due to moderate exacerbation would be in Category ___ as per the refined ABCD assessment tool.
    A. A
    B. B
    C. C
    D. D
    E. E

30. Chronic obstructive pulmonary disease is associated with all EXCEPT:
    A. Skeletal muscle dysfunction
    B. Mean pulmonary arterial pressure of 25 mmHg
    C. Significant reversibility in airflow limitation with bronchodilator therapy
    D. FEV1/FVC ratio < 0.7
    E. Depression

Answers

1-E, 2-B, 3-A, 4-B, 5-E, 6-D, 7-D, 8-B, 9-E, 10-C, 11-B, 12-C, 13-B, 14-B, 15-B, 16-B, 17-D, 18-A, 19-B, 20-A, 21-D, 22-D, 23-A, 24-A, 25-D, 26-C, 27-B, 28-D, 29-D, 30-C

SUGGESTED READING

1. Global Initiative for Chronic Obstructive Lung Disease (GOLD). Global Strategy for the Diagnosis, Management and Prevention of Chronic Obstructive Pulmonary Disease: 2020 Report. [online] Available from: http://www.goldcopd.org. [Last accessed June, 2020].
2. Chalmers JD, Aliberti S, Blasi F. Management of bronchiectasis in adults. Eur Respir J. 2015;45:1446-62.
3. Polverino E, Goeminne PC, McDonnell MJ, Aliberti S, Marshall SE, Loebinger MR, et al. European Respiratory Society guidelines for the management of adult bronchiectasis. Eur Respir J. 2017;50(3):1700629.
4. National Heart, Lung, and Blood Institute. (2007). National Asthma Education and Prevention Program: Expert panel report III: Guidelines for the diagnosis and management of asthma. Bethesda, MD:(NIH publication no. 08-4051). [online] Available from: www.nhlbi.nih.gov/guidelines/asthma/asthgdln.htm. [Last accessed June, 2020].
5. Global Initiative for Asthma (GINA). Global Strategy for Asthma Management and Prevention. [online] Available from: www.ginasthma.org. [Last accessed June, 2020].
6. British Guideline on the Management of Asthma. [online] Available from: https://www.brit-thoracic.org.uk/guidelines-and-quality-standards/asthma-guideline. [Last accessed June, 2020].
7. Lupia T, Scabini S, Mornese Pinna S, Francesco GDP, De G, Corcione RS. 2019 novel coronavirus (2019-nCoV) outbreak: A new challenge. J Glob Antimicrob Resist. 2020; 21:22-7.
8. Schwartz M, King Jr TE. Interstitial Lung Disease, 5th edition. Shelton, CT: People's Medical Clearing House; 2011.
9. Raghu G, Collard HR, Egan JJ, Martinez FJ, Behr J, Brown KK, et al. An official ATS/ERS/JRS/ALAT statement: idiopathic pulmonary fibrosis: evidence-based guidelines for diagnosis and management. Am J Respir Crit Care Med. 2011;183(6):788-824.
10. American Thoracic Society, European Respiratory Society. American Thoracic Society/European Respiratory Society International Multidisciplinary Consensus Classification of the Idiopathic Interstitial Pneumonias. This joint statement of the American Thoracic Society (ATS), and the European Respiratory Society (ERS) was adopted by the ATS board of directors, June 2001 and by the ERS Executive Committee, June 2001. Am J Respir Crit Care Med. 2002;165(2):277-304.
11. King TE Jr, Pardo A, Selman M. Idiopathic pulmonary fibrosis. Lancet. 2011;378(9807):1949-61.
12. Mandell LA, Wunderink RG, Anzueto A, Bartlett JG, Campbell GD, Dean NC, et al. Infectious Diseases Society of America/American Thoracic Society consensus guidelines on the management of community-acquired pneumonia in adults. Clin Infect Dis. 2007;44 Suppl 2:S27-72.
13. File TM. Community-acquired pneumonia. Lancet. 2003; 362(9400):1991-2001.

14. Musher DM, Thorner AR. Community-acquired pneumonia. N Engl J Med. 2014;371(17):1619-28.
15. Sahn SA, Huggins JT, San Jose E, Álvarez-Dobaño JM, Valdes LFJ. The art of pleural fluid analysis. Clin Pulm Med. 2013;20(2):77-96.
16. Ferreiro L, Alvarez-Dobaño JM, Valdés L. Systemic diseases and the pleura. Arch Bronconeumol. 2011;47(7):361-70.
17. Sahn SA, Heffner JE. Spontaneous pneumothorax. N Engl J Med. 2000;342:868-74.
18. Light RW. Pleural Diseases, 6th edition. Philadelphia: Lippincott, Williams and Wilkins; 2013.
19. ARDS Definition Task Force, Ranieri VM, Rubenfeld GD, Thompson BT, Ferguson ND, Caldwell E, et al. Acute respiratory distress syndrome: the Berlin Definition. JAMA. 2012;307(23):2526-33.
20. Rubenfeld GD, Caldwell E, Peabody E, Weaver J, Martin DP, Neff M, et al. Incidence and outcomes of acute lung injury. N Engl J Med. 2005;353(16):1685-93.
21. Frutos-Vivar F, Nin N, Esteban A. Epidemiology of acute lung injury and acute respiratory distress syndrome. Curr Opin Crit Care. 2004;10(1):1-6.
22. Simonneau G, Montani D, Celermajer DS, Denton CP, Gatzoulis MA, Krowka M, et al. Haemodynamic definitions and updated clinical classification of pulmonary hypertension. Eur Respir J. 2019;53(1):1801913.

CHAPTER 13

Infectious Diseases

PYREXIA OF UNKNOWN ORIGIN

Fever of minimum 3 weeks duration with daily temperatures rising to above 101°F and the cause of which is not diagnosed even after investigating in a hospital for 1 week.

Types
- Classic pyrexia of unknown origin (PUO)
- Nosocomial PUO
- Neutropenic PUO
- Human immunodeficiency virus (HIV)-associated PUO

Common Causes of Prolonged Fever
Common causes of prolonged fever are given in **Table 13.1**.

Investigations for Pyrexia of Unknown Origin
Investigations for pyrexia of unknown origin are given in **Table 13.2**.

Treatment
- Treatment of underlying cause detected after investigations

TABLE 13.1: Common Causes of Pyrexia of Unknown Origin.

Infections:	Neoplasms:	Connective tissue disorders:
• Tuberculosis	• Lymphomas	• Systemic lupus erythematosus
• Malaria	• Leukaemias	• Rheumatoid arthritis
• Typhoid	• Gastrointestinal (GI) malignancies	• Temporal arteritis
• Infective endocarditis	• Metastatic tumours of liver	• Polyarteritis nodosa (PAN)
• Urinary tract infections	• Hypernephroma	
• Perinephric abscesses	• Atrial myxomas	
• Liver abscess		
• Abdominal abscesses		
• Pelvic inflammatory diseases		
• HIV infection		
Miscellaneous:	**Psychogenic fevers:**	**Periodic fevers:**
• Drug fevers (sulphonamides, aminoglycosides, and penicillins)	• Habitual hyperthermia	• Familial Mediterranean fever (polyserositis)
• Multiple pulmonary thromboembolism	• Factitious fever	
• Haemolytic anaemias	• Fabricated fever	
• Thyroiditis		
• Granulomatous hepatitis		
• Cyclic neutropaenia		

TABLE 13.2: Investigations for pyrexia of unknown origin.

Laboratory tests:	Serological tests:	Radiographic examination:
• Complete blood picture • Erythrocyte sedimentation rate (ESR) • Peripheral smear examination • Urine routine and microscopy • Blood and urine culture • Renal and liver function tests • Mantoux test	• Antistreptolysin O (ASO) titre • Rheumatoid factor • Antinuclear antibodies • Viral antibody titres • Brucella agglutination test	• Chest radiography • Barium gastrointestinal (GI) series • Echocardiography • Ultrasonography of abdomen and pelvis • Computed tomography (CT) scan of abdomen and thorax • Positron emission tomography (PET) scans
Biopsy:	**Diagnostic surgical procedures:**	
• Bone marrow biopsy • Liver biopsy • Lymph node biopsy	• Peritoneoscopy • Laparoscopy • Bronchoscopy • Exploratory laparotomy	

- Empirical broad-spectrum antibiotics
- Empirical antitubercular treatment

■ MEASLES (RUBEOLA)

- It is caused by a paramyxovirus (RNA virus) infection.
- Spread is by droplet transmission.
- Incubation period is of about 10 days.
- Period of infectivity is from 4 days before and 2 days after the onset of rash.

Clinical Features

- **Catarrhal stage:** Febrile onset with nasal catarrh, sneezing, conjunctival redness, watering of eyes and cough
- **Koplik's spots:** These are small, red, irregular lesions on the buccal mucosa with blue–white centres.
- **Exanthematous stage:** Red, maculopapular rashes are first seen over the back of the ears and forehead, later spreading downwards over the face, neck, trunk and feet.

Complications

- Bronchiolitis and bronchitis
- Interstitial giant cell pneumonia
- Conjunctivitis, keratitis and corneal ulcers
- Acute postinfectious measles encephalitis
- Subacute sclerosing panencephalitis (SSPE)— late complication (average of 7 years)
- Myocarditis
- Acute glomerulonephritis

Treatment

Supportive and symptomatic treatment only.

■ RUBELLA (GERMAN MEASLES)

- Rubella is caused by a togavirus infection
- Spread is by droplets
- Incubation period is about 2 weeks
- **The prodromal or catarrhal stage:** Malaise, headache, fever, mild conjunctivitis and lymphadenopathy (suboccipital).
- **The exanthematous stage:** Pink macular rashes first appearing behind the ears and on the forehead, later spreading downwards to the trunk and extremities, typically lasting 3 days.
- **Important complications:**
    o Postinfectious encephalitis
    o Thrombocytopaenia
    o Spontaneous abortion
    o Congenital rubella syndrome

Congenital Rubella or Rubella Syndrome

Congenital rubella results from the transplacental transmission of the virus to the foetus from an infected mother. The highest risk is during the first trimester of pregnancy.

Congenital Malformations Associated with Rubella Syndrome

- Congenital heart diseases
- Eye
- Deafness

- Mental retardation
- Microcephaly

■ MUMPS

- It is caused by a paramyxovirus.
- Incubation period is about 2–3 weeks.
- Spread is by droplet infection.

Clinical Features

Prodromal symptoms: Feverishness, generalised weakness and pain at the angle of the jaw. Progresses to parotitis which may be bilateral in two-third of the cases. Presents with dysphagia.

Complications

- Inflammation of testes (epididymo-orchitis) and inflammation of ovary (oophoritis).
- Pancreatitis
- Encephalomyelitis and mumps meningitis
- Myocarditis

■ INFECTIOUS MONONUCLEOSIS/GLANDULAR FEVER

Aetiology

- It is caused by Epstein–Barr Virus (EBV) that replicates in B lymphocytes and oropharyngeal epithelial cells. Transmission is largely by salivary contact, e.g., kissing.
- Incubation period is 7–10 days.

Clinical Features

- Constitutional symptoms, especially fever
- Severe pharyngitis and tonsillitis
- Lymphadenopathy (particularly posterior cervical lymph node enlargement but sometimes generalised).
- Hepatosplenomegaly
- Petechial rashes on palate
- Maculopapular rash on body

Investigations

- Peripheral blood lymphocytosis with atypical lymphocytes (> 20%)
- Deranged liver function test (LFT)
- Positive **Paul-Bunnell test**
- Positive **monospot test** (rapid screening test)—horse red cells agglutinate on exposure to heterophile antibodies

Complications

- Haemolytic anaemia and thrombocytopaenia
- Aplastic anaemia and thrombotic thrombocytopenic purpura
- Glomerulonephritis and interstitial nephritis
- Hepatitis
- Myocarditis and pericarditis
- Neurologic complications, e.g., meningoencephalitis, transverse myelitis and Guillain–Barré (GB) syndrome
- Airway obstruction due to severe pharyngeal oedema

Epstein–Barr virus-associated oncogenesis has been shown in **Box 13.1**.

Treatment

Symptomatic treatment includes rest, acetaminophen, etc.

■ CHICKEN POX (VARICELLA)

- Caused by Varicella zoster virus- Human alphaherpesvirus-3 (HHV-3)
- Spread by droplet infection or from secretions of skin lesions.
- The incubation period is about 2–3 weeks.
- The disease is contagious till pustules disappear.

Clinical Features

- The characteristic rash first appears on the trunk on the second day of illness and then the face, and finally on the limbs. The lesions

---

Box 13.1: EBV associated oncogenesis.

Benign EBV-associated proliferation
- Orally hairy leucoplakia, primarily in adults with AIDS
- Lymphoid interstitial pneumonitis in childrens with AIDS

Malignant EBV-associated proliferation
- Nasopharyngeal carcinoma
- Burkitt lymphoma
- Hodgkin disease
- Lymphoproliferative disorders
- Leiomyosarcoma immunodeficient including AIDS

(AIDS: acquired immunodeficiency syndrome; EBV: Epstein–Barr virus)

are maximum on the trunk and minimum on the periphery of the limbs.
- The characteristic lesions appear as macules and progress to papules, vesicles and pustules. The lesions finally dry up to form scabs.
- Low-grade fever is often present.
- In immunocompromised patients, the lesions are haemorrhagic and are numerous. Dissemination to other organs is quite frequent.

Complications
- Myocarditis
- Hepatitis
- Corneal lesions
- Perinatal varicella (affects foetus)
- Meningitis
- Acute glomerulonephritis
- Interstitial pneumonia
- Congenital varicella

Management
- No treatment is required in majority of cases.
- Symptomatic treatment includes antihistamines and local calamine lotion.
- **Acyclovir** can be used in adults or immunocompromised patients. It reduces complications of chicken pox, particularly if given within 24 hours.
- Other drugs that can be used include **valaciclovir** and **famciclovir**.
- Secondary bacterial infection on lesions is treated with local antiseptic or systemic antibiotics such as cloxacillin.

■ ARBOVIRAL DISEASES

Table 13.3 shows the examples of diseases caused by arthropod-borne and **Table 13.4** lists the diseases caused by arbovirus and their manifestations.

■ DENGUE FEVER
- It is caused by four distinct subgroups of dengue viruses, types 1, 2, 3 and 4 (DEN 1-4).
- Dengue infection of humans occurs from bites of *Aedes aegypti* mosquitoes.
- World Health Organisation (WHO) classifies dengue viral infections into non-severe dengue (with and without warning signs) and severe dengue (**Tables 13.5** and **13.6**). **Figure 13.1** describes manifestations of **Expanded Dengue syndrome**.

TABLE 13.3: Examples of diseases caused by arthropod-borne.

Family	Common diseases	Family	Common diseases
Arenaviridae	• Lymphocytic choriomeningitis • Lassa fever • Arenavirus	*Flaviviridae*	**Mosquito-borne** • Japanese encephalitis • West NILE encephalitis • St Louis encephalitis • Yellow fever • Dengue fever **Tick borne** • Kyasanur forest disease (KFD) **Direct contact:** Ebola disease
Bunyaviridae	• California encephalitis • Rift valley fever • Sandfly fever • Crimean-Congo haemorrhagic fever • Hanta virus: Haemorrhagic fever with renal/ cardiopulmonary syndrome	*Togaviridae*	• Chikungunya diseases • Sindbis diseases • Eastern equine encephalitis • Western equine encephalitis • Venezuelan encephalitis

TABLE 13.4: A few diseases caused by arbovirus and their manifestations.

	Flu-like syndrome	Encephalitis	Hepatitis	Haemorrhage	Shock
Dengue	+		+	+	+
Yellow fever	+		+	+	+
St Louis encephalitis	+	+			
West nile encephalitis	+	+			
Venezuelan encephalitis	+	+			
Western equine encephalitis	+	+			
Eastern equine encephalitis	+	+			
Japanese encephalitis	+	+			

(+: present; –: absent)

TABLE 13.5: WHO classification of dengue infections into non-severe dengue and severe dengue.

Non-severe dengue without warning signs	Non-severe dengue with warning signs	Severe dengue

Probable dengue:
• Travel to endemic area
• Fever with two of the following criteria:
  ◦ Nausea and vomiting
  ◦ Rashes
  ◦ Body pain
  ◦ Positive Tourniquet test
  ◦ Leucopaenia
  ◦ Absence of warning signs
  ◦ Laboratory-confirmed dengue
	Presence of warning signs:
	• Abdominal pain of tenderness
	• Persistent vomiting
	• Clinical fluid accumulation
	• Mucosal bleed
	• Lethargy and restlessness
	• Liver enlargement 2 cm
	• Laboratory: Increase in haematocrit concurrent with rapid decrease in platelet count
		• Severe plasma leakage leading to:
		  ◦ Dengue shock syndrome (DSS)
		  ◦ Fluid accumulation with respiratory distress
		  ◦ Severe bleeding
		As evaluated by clinician:
		• Severe organ involvement:
		  ◦ Liver: Aspartate aminotransferase (AST) or alanine aminotransferase (ALT) ≥ 1,000
		  ◦ Central nervous system (CNS): Impaired consciousness
		  ◦ Heart and other organs

Clinical Features

- After the incubation period of 5–8 days, the illness begins abruptly and is followed by the three phases:
  i. **Febrile phase:**
     - Presents with high-grade fever that usually lasts 2–7 days.
     - May have flushing of face, body ache, myalgia, arthralgia, severe backache ('break–bone' fever), retro-orbital pain and headache.
     - Sore throat and conjunctival redness in some patients.
     - Anorexia, nausea and vomiting.
     - Tenderness upon pressure on eyeball.
     - A positive tourniquet test may be present.
  ii. **Critical phase:**
     - Plasma leakage may happen which usually lasts 24–48 hours.
     - Fall in white blood cell (WBC) and platelet counts may precede plasma leakage.
     - May develop pleural effusion and ascites.
     - Shock and organ failure occurs when a critical volume of plasma is lost through leakage. It is often preceded by warning signs.

TABLE 13.6: WHO classification of dengue infections and grading of severity of DHF.

DF/DHF	Grade	Signs and symptoms	Laboratory
DF		Fever with two of the following: • Headache • Retro-orbital pain • Myalgia • Arthralgia/bone pain • Rash • Haemorrhagic manifestations • No evidence of plasma leakage	• Leucopaenia (WBC ≤ 5,000 cells/mm^2) • Thrombocytopaenia (platelet count < 150,000 cells/mm^2) • Rising haematocrit (Hct) (5–10%) • No evidence of plasma loss
DHF	I	Fever and haemorrhagic manifestation (positive tourniquet test) and evidence of plasma leakage	Thrombocytopaenia < 100,000 cells/mm^2; Hct rise ≥ 20%
DHF	II	As in Grade I plus spontaneous bleeding	Thrombocytopaenia < 100,000 cells/mm^2; Hct rise > 20%
DHF*	III	As in Grade I or II plus circulatory failure (week pulse, narrow pulse pressure (≤ 20 mmHg), hypotension, restlessness)	Thrombocytopaenia < 100,000 cells/mm^2; Hct rise ≥ 20%
DHF*	IV	As in Grade III plus profound shock with undetectable BP and pulse	Thrombocytopaenia < 100,000 cells/mm^2; Hct rise ≥ 20%

*DHF III and IV are DSS = dengue shock syndrome.
Source: https://www.who.int/csr/resources/publications/dengue/Denguepublication/en/
(ALT: alanine aminotransferase; AST: aspartate aminotransferase; BP: blood pressure; CNS: central nervous system; DF: dengue fever; DHF: dengue haemorrhagic fever)

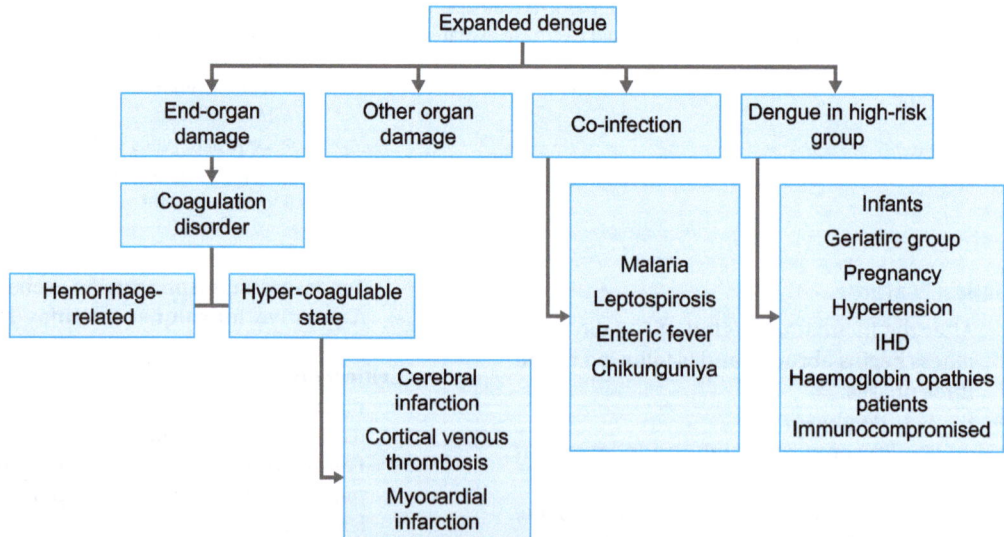

Fig. 13.1: WHO (2008) classification and levels of severity in dengue case.

iii. **Recovery phase:**
   - If the patient survives the 24–48 hours critical phase, a gradual reabsorption of extravascular fluid takes place in the following 48–72 hours.
   - Rash of 'isles of white in the sea of red.'
   - Some patients may experience pruritus, particularly on hands and feet.
   - Bradycardia

Severe Dengue

- Evidence of plasma leakage:
  ○ High or progressively rising haematocrit
  ○ Pleural effusions or ascites
- Circulatory compromise or shock significant bleeding.
- Altered level of consciousness (lethargy or restlessness, coma, convulsions).
- Severe gastrointestinal (GI) involvement (persistent vomiting, increasing or intense abdominal pain and jaundice).
- Severe organ impairment (acute liver failure, acute renal failure, encephalopathy or encephalitis and cardiomyopathy).

Diagnosis

- Leucopaenia, thrombocytopaenia and elevated liver enzymes
- Virus isolation from blood (within first 5 days)
- Serum onstructural protein 1 (NS1) antigen is highly specific and is positive early in the course of illness.
- Molecular methods such as reverse transcription polymerase chain reaction (RT-PCR) or nucleic acid sequence-based amplification (NASBA) to detect viral RNA.
- Rising viral antibody titres immunoglobulin G (IgG) and IgM (start after 5 days of onset)
- In patients with severe dengue, chest radiograph to look for pleural effusion, and ultrasound abdomen for ascites and gallbladder wall thickening.

Overview of Management

- Managing patients in early febrile phase of dengue—**antipyretics such as paracetamol.**
- Recognising early stage of plasma leakage or critical phase and initiating **fluid therapy— intravenous (IV) fluids** normal saline.

- Patients with warning signs need to be referred to a tertiary care hospital.
- Early **diagnosis and management** of complications such as shock, bleeding and organ impairment.
- During the early febrile phase, it is often not possible to predict clinically whether a patient with dengue will progress to severe disease. Therefore, **daily monitoring** of patients is crucial.

■ CHIKUNGUNYA

- It is caused by an alphavirus.
- Vector is *Aedes aegypti* **mosquitoe.**
- Incubation period varies from 1 to 12 days.

Clinical Features

- Fever: 2–5 days duration
- Maculopapular rash involving the limbs and trunk
- Arthralgia or arthritis affecting multiple joints
- Localised petechiae
- Headache
- Conjunctival injection

Diagnosis

- Thrombocytopaenia may occur but is uncommon.
- Molecular methods include RT-PCR to detect structural genes in the blood sample.

Treatment

- The treatment is symptomatic with antipyretics—paracetamol.
- Arthralgias and arthritis—ibuprofen, diclofenac or naproxen.

■ JAPANESE ENCEPHALITIS

- It is a zoonotic disease.
- It is caused by Arbovirus infection.
- It is transmitted by the bites of infected Culex mosquitoes.
- Incubation period is 6–8 days after the bite.
- Natural cycle of virus: Bird-mosquito-bird and pig-mosquito-pig. Humans are accidental hosts

Clinical features
- Fever
- Headache
- Nausea
- Diarrhoea
- Vomiting
- Myalgia
- Encephalitis—irritability, altered behavior, convulsion and coma.

Diagnosis
- Leucocytosis with neutrophilia.
- Cerebrospinal fluid (CSF) examination shows raised pressure, cell count and proteins. Lymphocyte predominant. CSF protein is moderately elevated in about 50% of case.
- Serological testing for antibodies to viral antigens.
- Virus isolation can be done from CSF.

Treatment
- Treatment is entirely symptomatic and includes control of fever, raised intracranial tension and convulsions.

■ DIPHTHERIA
- Diphtheria is caused by *Corynebacterium diphtheriae*.
- The disease is transmitted by droplet infection from active cases or carriers.
- The incubation period is about 1 week.

Clinical Features
- The usual presenting manifestations are fever and sore throat.
- The diagnostic feature is the typical **membrane on the tonsils**, with a surrounding area of inflammation (membranous tonsillitis). The membrane is firm and adherent.
- Oedema over the neck (**'bull-neck' appearance**)
- Tender enlarged cervical lymph nodes
- Nasal diphtheria is restricted to the nasal mucosa, and is characterised by nasal discharge, which is often blood-tinged.

Complications
- Extension of the membrane into larynx and trachea leads to laryngeal obstruction and bronchopulmonary diphtheria.
- Myocarditis can result in arrhythmias, cardiac failure and electrocardiographic (ECG) changes. It often occurs weeks after the initial episode of diphtheria.
- Peripheral neuropathy can occur in a 'glove and stocking' distribution.
- Cranial nerve palsies and diaphragmatic paralysis.

Diagnosis
- The diagnosis is based on the demonstration of the characteristic diphtheritic membrane.
- Demonstration of the organism by Albert Staining.
- Culture of the organism on Löeffler's medium

Management
- Isolation and strict bed rest
- Antidiphtheritic toxin should be given as early in the course of diphtheria as possible.
- Benzylpenicillin intravenously for 7 days to eradicate the organism
- Patients allergic to penicillin can be treated with erythromycin.
- Tracheostomy may become necessary for respiratory distress.
- Close contacts should be protected by erythromycin prophylaxis and immunisation.
- Vaccines include DPT (diphtheria, pertussis, tetanus), DTaP (Diphtheria-Tetanus-acellular Pertussis), Tdap and DT (diphtheria, tetanus).

■ PLAGUE
- Plague, known as 'black death,' is caused by *Yersinia pestis*, a gram-negative, non-motile bacillus.
- Three types of plague: Bubonic, septicaemic and pneumonic
- The most common route of infection in humans is after bite of a plague-infected rat flea.

Clinical Features
Bubonic Plague
- Presents in a week after exposure.
- Presents with fever with chills, weakness, nausea and vomiting.
- May have swollen painful lymph nodes of in the groin or axilla. These are called the buboes that are rarely fluctuant or suppurative.

- Complications include secondary septicaemia, pneumonia and meningitis
- The mortality rate for untreated bubonic plague is 60%.

Septicaemic Plague
- Septicaemic plague may occur as a complication of untreated bubonic plague or pneumonic plague (secondary septicaemic plague) and can develop in the absence of obvious signs of primary disease (primary septicaemic plague).
- Septicaemic plague presents with high fever, chills and malaise, but without any lymph node enlargement.
- Patients may develop septic shock and disseminated intravascular coagulation (DIC) with vasculitis.
- Gangrene of the tip of the nose or digits, due to small artery thrombosis may appear in advanced stages of the disease (black death).
- Left untreated, the mortality approaches 100%.

Pneumonic Plague
- Pneumonic plague may occur by primary respiratory infection, or as a complication of the bubonic and septicaemic forms of the disease (secondary pneumonia).
- Presents within 1–6 days of exposure
- It begins abruptly with intense headache, weakness, pyrexia, vomiting, abdominal pain and diarrhoea. Chest pain, cough, dyspnoea and haemoptysis develop thereafter.
- Complications are respiratory failure, septic shock, etc., and mortality is high.

Diagnosis
- Smears from blood, sputum, bubo aspirate and cerebrospinal fluid may be stained with Gram, Giemsa or Wayson stains to demonstrate bipolar staining coccobacilli (safety pin appearance).
- Cultures of various tissue fluids
- Serological tests for antibodies

Treatment
- With prompt use of antibiotics fatality rate decreases below 5% for bubonic plague and below 10% for septicaemic and pneumonic plague.
- Effective medications include **streptomycin, gentamicin and ciprofloxacin**. Total duration of treatment is 10 days.

BOTULISM
- It is caused by ***Clostridium botulinum***.

Classification
- **Food-borne botulism** occurs due to ingestion of preformed toxin in contaminated food. It is the most common form of botulism.
- **Wound botulism** develops from toxin produced by infection of a wound.
- **Infantile botulism** results from ingestion of spores, which on germination in the gut, produce toxin.

Clinical Features
- Incubation period varies from 2 hours to 8 days.
- Initial presentation includes gastro-intestinal (GI) symptoms followed rapidly by involvement of cranial nerves, causing diplopia, dysphagia and dysarthria.
- This is followed by progressive, descending motor paralysis, and then, diaphragmatic paralysis and death.
- Wound botulism is similar, except that GI upset does not occur.
- Infant botulism is characterised by the onset of constipation, followed by weakness in sucking, crying or swallowing. This is followed by progressive bulbar and extremity muscle weakness.

Diagnosis
- Diagnosis of botulism is based on clinical features.
- Conditions often confused with botulism include GB syndrome, myasthenia gravis, tick paralysis and diphtheria.

Treatment
- It includes supportive care with assisted ventilation prevention of secondary infection and administration of antitoxin (not available in India).

PERTUSSIS (WHOOPING COUGH)
- It is caused by *Bordetella pertussis*.
- Spread is by droplet infection.
- Incubation period: 1–2 weeks.

Clinical Features
- The first stage (catarrhal phase) is characterised by upper respiratory catarrh with conjunctivitis and dry cough.
- Followed by severe bouts of cough lasting for weeks.
- Characteristic whoop and may have cyanosis. Pertussis is the most contagious in the catarrhal and early paroxysmal stages.

Complications
- Bronchopneumonia
- Bronchiectasis
- Encephalitis
- Convulsions
- Conjunctival haemorrhage
- Prolapsed rectum.

Diagnosis
- Peripheral blood lymphocytosis may be seen in well-established cases.
- The diagnosis can be confirmed by the isolation of *B. pertussis*.
- Polymerase chain reaction (PCR) to detect *B. pertussis*
- Direct fluorescent antibody test.

Management
- Erythromycin for 7–14 days is the recommended treatment. Azithromycin and clarithromycin are equally effective and have lesser side effects than erythromycin.
- A cough suppressant such as methadone can reduce the severity of coughing paroxysms.

TYPHOID (ENTERIC FEVER)
- Enteric fevers include typhoid fever caused by *Salmonella typhi* (also known as *Salmonella enterica serovar typhi*) and paratyphoid fever caused by *S. paratyphi* A and B (*Salmonella enterica serovar paratyphi* A and B).
- These organisms are transmitted by faecal-oral route usually by carriers, often food handlers, through the contamination of food, mild or water.
- The incubation period of typhoid fever is about 2 weeks.

Clinical Features
- The disease usually presents with fever associated with headache, malaise and chills. A step-like daily increase in temperature to 40–41°C (**'step-ladder' pattern**) is seen in some cases. The hallmark of typhoid fever is prolonged, persistent fever, often lasting 4–8 weeks in untreated patients.
- Constipation, especially in adults, or mild diarrhoea in children, associated with abdominal tenderness.
- Mild hepatosplenomegaly may be present and the liver may be tender.
- There may be bradycardia relative to the height of the fever ('relative bradycardia').
- The characteristic 'rose-spots' or 'rose-red spots' may be seen on the chest and abdomen during the first week.
- Often, by the end of the first week, constipation is succeeded by diarrhoea and abdominal distension, with tenderness in the right iliac fossa. The stools are characteristically described as **'pea-soup'** because faeces are loose and greenish in colour.
- By the end of the second week, patient may become profoundly ill. By the third week, toxaemia increases and patient may pass into coma and die.
- Intestinal complications often occur in the third or fourth week of illness.

Complication of Typhoid
- General: Toxaemia, dehydration and peripheral circulatory failure.
- GI: Perforation of intestine and intestinal haemorrhage.
- Neurological: Delirium, meningitis and encephalopathy.

Diagnosis
- White cell count may show leucopaenia with relative lymphocytosis.
- Cultures: The maximum positivity of blood culture is during the first week of illness.

- Widal test: This test detects agglutinating antibodies to O, H and Vi antigens of *S. typhi*, and H antigens of *S. paratyphi* A and B. A fourfold rise antibody titre in paired samples is a good criterion, but of limited practical application.

Treatment
- General management includes bed rest, isolation and maintenance of nutrition and fluid intake.
- Antibiotic therapy: Several antibiotics are effective in enteric fever. Various regimens are given in **Table 13.7**.

■ FOOD POISONING
Causes of food poisoning are given in **Table 13.8**.

Clinical Features and Diagnosis
Table 13.9 shows various organisms causing food poisoning and their symptoms.

Management
- Non-specific therapy includes oral or IV fluid therapy and correcting electrolyte deficits
- Antibiotics should not be given routinely.

TABLE 13.7: Various antibiotic regimens in typhoid fever.

Drug	Dosage and duration of treatment
Ceftriaxone	75 mg/kg/day for 7–14 days
Chloramphenicol	3–4 g/day till the fever subsides, followed by 2 g/day, for a total duration of 14 days
Amoxicillin	4–6 g/day in four divided doses of 14 days
Cotrimoxazole	Trimethoprim 640 mg + sulphamethoxazole 3200 mg in two divided doses daily for 14 days
Ciprofloxacin	500–750 mg twice daily for 14 days
Ofloxacin	400–800 mg/day for 14 days
Cefotaxime	50–75 mg/kg/day for 7–14 days
Cefixime	20 mg/kg/day for 10–14 days
Azithromycin	1 g once a day for 7 days
Aztreonam	50–100 mg/kg/day for 14 days

■ CHOLERA
- Cholera is an acute illness that results from colonisation of the small intestine by *Vibrio cholerae*.
- The disease is characterised by its epidemic occurrence and explosive, severe diarrhoea with rapid depletion of extracellular fluid and electrolytes.
- The major pathogenic strain has a somatic antigen (O1). It is called serogroup O1.

Clinical Features
- The incubation period is about 12–48 hours.
- Explosive onset of watery diarrhoea without pain or colic follows vomiting (vomiting may be absent). The characteristic '**rice-water**' stool consists of clear fluid with flecks of mucus. Several litres of isotonic fluid may be lost within hours, leading rapidly to profound shock.
- In extreme cases, there may be signs of severe dehydration. The skin is cold, clammy and wrinkled ('washer women's skin') with loss of skin turgor. The blood pressure drops, and the pulse becomes rapid and thready.
- Occasionally, a very severe form of the disease occurs in which the loss of fluid into the

TABLE 13.8: Causes of food poisoning.

Infective	Non-infective

• Toxin-induced
  ○ Staphylococcus aureus
  ○ Bacillus cereus
  ○ Vibrio cholerae
  ○ Escherichia coli
  ○ Clostridium perfringens
  ○ Clostridium difficile
  ○ Changes in mucosa
	• Allergic
	  ○ Shellfish
	  ○ Strawberries

• Mucosal alteration with destruction
  ○ Shigella
  ○ E. coli
  ○ Campylobacter
  ○ Salmonella
  ○ Entamoeba histolytica
	• Non-allergic
	  ○ Scombrotoxin (fish)
	  ○ Ciguatoxin (tropical fish)
	  ○ Fungi (*Amanita phalloides*)
	  ○ Arsenic poisoning

TABLE 13.9: Various organisms causing food poisoning and their symptoms.

Organism	Incubation	Symptoms	Foods
Campylobacter jejuni	2–5 days	Diarrhoea, vomiting, headache, fever, muscle pain	Poultry, dairy products, water
Salmonella enteritidis	12–36 h	Abdominal cramps, headache, fever, nausea, diarrhoea	Poultry, meat, eggs and egg products, sliced melons
Escherichia coli	3–4 days	Diarrhoea, vomiting and mild fever	Undercooked ground beef, unpasteurised cider
Listeria monocytogenes	3–70 days	Flu-like, meningitis encephalitis, spontaneous abortion	Unpasteurised milk, ice cream, ready-to-eat lunch meats
Clostridium perfringens	10–12 h	Abdominal pain, nausea, diarrhoea, fever, headache, vomiting usually absent	Stews, gravies, beans
Clostridium botulinum (intoxication)	4 h to 8 days	Vomiting, constipation, diplopia, dysphagia, dysarthria, paralysis, death	Baked potatoes, fish, garlic/oil mixtures, low-acid canned foods
Staphylococcus aureus (intoxication)	1–7 h	Nausea, retching, abdominal cramps, diarrhoea	Ready-to-eat, reheated foods, dairy products, protein foods
Bacillus cereus (intoxication)	30 min to 6 h (emetic) or 6–15 h (diarrhoeal)	Nausea, vomiting, watery diarrhoea	Rice products, starchy foods, casseroles, pudding, soups
Hepatitis A	10–50 days	Sudden fever, vomiting, jaundice,	Water (ice), shellfish, ready-to-eat, fruit juice, vegetables
Norwalk virus	10–50 h	Nausea, diarrhoea, headache, mild fever	Water, shellfish, raw vegetables and fruits
Rotavirus	1–3 days	Vomiting, diarrhoea, mild fever	Ready-to-eat, water and ice
Giardia lamblia	3–25 days	Fatigue, nausea, weight loss, abdominal cramps,	Water, ice, raw vegetables
Cryptosporidium parvum	1–12 days	Severe diarrhoea, may have no symptoms	Water, raw foods, unpasteurised cider, ready-to-eat

dilated bowel kills the patient before typical GI symptoms appear. This is known as 'cholera sicca.'

Diagnosis

- 'Hanging drop' preparation of the stool demonstrates the characteristic motile organisms.
- Culture of the stool or a rectal swab can isolate and identify the organism.

Treatment

- Vigorous intravenous (IV) fluid and electrolyte therapy should be continued till the patient is haemodynamically stable and vomiting subsides.
- Oral rehydration also attempted along with IV fluids, if tolerated
- Tetracycline, cotrimoxazole and ciprofloxacin

LEPROSY (HANSEN'S DISEASE)

- Leprosy (Hansen's disease) is a chronic granulomatous disease, primarily affecting the peripheral nerves and secondarily involving the skin.
- The causative organism is *Mycobacterium leprae*, which is an acid- and alcohol-fast bacillus.
- The most important mode of spread of *M. leprae* is by droplets from the sneezes of lepromatous patients.
- Incubation period is generally 2–6 years.

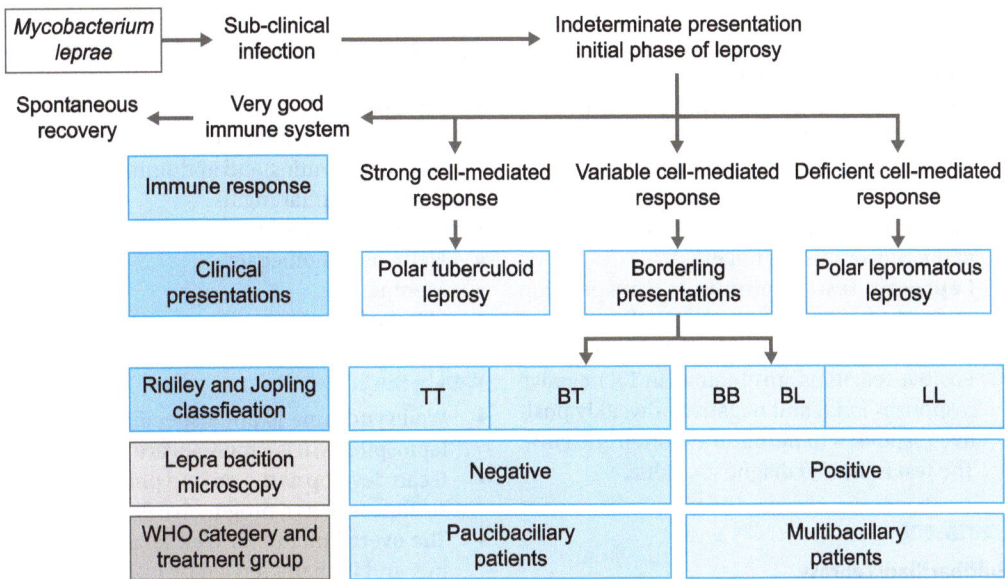

(BB: borderline-borderline; BL: borderline-lepromatous; BT: borderline tuberculoid; LL: lepromatous leprosy; TT: tuberculoid leprosy; WHO: World Health Organisation)

Fig. 13.2: Clinicopathological Classification of Leprosy.

Clinicopathological Classification

- In the early stage, the disease may be indeterminate, and may spontaneously remit or develop into overt leprosy.
- The determinate form of the disease may be classified as (**Fig. 13.2**):
  - **Tuberculoid leprosy (TT)**—when host resistance is good
  - **Borderline or dimorphic**
  - **Lepromatous leprosy (LL)**—when host resistance is poor

Clinical Features

Tuberculoid Leprosy (TT)

- **Skin involvement:** The early manifestation is a hypopigmented macule that is sharply demarcated and hypoaesthetic. Later, the lesions become larger, and the margins are elevated. The lesions show peripheral spread and central healing. Fully developed lesions are anaesthetic, with loss of sweat glands and hair follicles.

- **Nerve involvement:** Nerve involvement occurs early, and is usually asymmetric. Involved nerves are thickened and palpable. It leads to deformities in the hand and the foot.

Lepromatous Leprosy (LL)

- **Nasal symptoms:** Anosmia, nasal stuffiness, crust formation and blood-stained nasal discharge
- **Skin involvement:** The skin lesions are macules, nodules, plaques or papules. The macules are often hypopigmented. The borders of the lesions are ill-defined, and the centres indurated, raised and convex (**'inverted saucer' appearance**). Thickening and nodulation of ear and loss of lateral eyebrows are early manifestations. With advanced disease, the skin of the face and forehead becomes thickened and corrugated (**'leonine facies'**).
- **Nerve involvement:** Involvement of major nerve trunks is less prominent in LL, but a 'glove and stocking' anaesthesia is common in advanced disease. Mononeuritis multiplex can also occur.

Diagnosis of Leprosy
- Nasal secretions from patients with LL containing numerous bacilli.
- Demonstration of acid-fast bacilli in skin smears made by the scraped-incision method is useful in borderline lepromatous and LL. In TT, bacilli are not demonstrable. Smears are made from skin lesions, earlobes and dorsum of the ring or middle finger.
- **Lepromin test:** Lepromin is a suspension of dead *M. leprae*. The test is performed like the tuberculin test, but is read after 4 weeks. Positive reactions are obtained in TT, negative responses in LL and negative or weakly positive responses in borderline-borderline (BB). The test is limited diagnostic value.

Treatment

Multibacillary Leprosy
Two recommended regimens are given below. Treatment is 1 year for multibacillary and 6 months for paucibacillary.

Treatment of Multibacillary Leprosy (MB)
- Dapsone 100 mg daily (self-administered)
- Clofazimine 50 mg daily (self-administered) plus 300 mg once a month (supervised)
- Rifampicin 600 mg once a month (supervised)

Treatment of Paucibacillary Leprosy (PB)
- Dapsone 100 mg daily
- Rifampicin 600 mg once a month (supervised)
- The duration of treatment is 6 months, and the patient should be followed up for 5 years.

■ LEPTOSPIROSIS

Aetiology
- It is caused by *Leptospira interrogans*, which is pathogenic. The organism is a tightly coiled spirochete with one axial filament.
- Human infection can occur either by direct contact with urine or tissue of an infected animal or indirectly through contaminated water, soil or vegetation. Transmission may occur through cuts, mucous membranes (nasopharynx, conjunctiva and vagina) and possibly unabraded skin.

Clinical Features
- High-grade fever with chills and rigors
- Headache
- Myalgia
- Conjunctival suffusion
- Nausea, vomiting and abdominal pain
- Cough and pharyngitis
- Lymphadenopathy
- Hepatosplenomegaly
- Meningitis
- Skin rashes

Weil Syndrome
- Weil syndrome is not a specific subgroup of leptospirosis; it is simply **severe leptospirosis**.
- It can develop as the second phase of a biphasic illness or as a progressive illness.
- The overall picture in Weil syndrome is striking, and is characterised by intense jaundice, mental status changes, haemorrhage, purpura or petechiae and renal failure.
- Haemorrhagic manifestations are common.

Investigations
- Anaemia
- Neutrophilia
- Thrombocytopaenia
- Raised erythrocyte sedimentation rate (ESR)
- Deranged renal function: Urea and creatinine
- Deranged liver function
- Prolongation of prothrombin time
- Urine examination shows microscopic haematuria, pyuria and proteinuria.
- Levels of creatinine phosphokinase (CPK) are elevated in 50% of cases.
- Chest radiograph may show patchy bronchopneumonia and a small pleural effusion.
- CSF may be abnormal in up to 90% of cases.
- Serum IgM antibodies in the second phase of illness.

Treatment
- A variety of antimicrobial agents have been found to be effective in vitro, but the recommended drugs are given below.
- IV penicillin, ampicillin, ceftriaxone or doxycycline

- Renal failure and jaundice require meticulous attention of fluid and electrolyte therapy. Renal failure may require dialysis.
- Anaemia and thrombocytopaenia may require blood transfusion.

■ RICKETTSIAL DISEASES

- Rickettsiae are obligate intracellular gram-negative parasites.
- Most are zoonoses spread to humans by arthropods (except Q fever).

Table 13.10 shows the examples of rickettsial diseases and their features.

Treatment

- Tetracycline is the drug of choice or doxycycline 100 mg BID PO × 7–15 days.
- Chloramphenicol 500 mg QID PO × 7–15 days/IV chloramphenicol 150 mg/kg/day for 5 days.
- **Coxiella endocarditis:** Combination therapy—Tetracycline + Co-trimoxazole/Tetracycline + Rifampicin.

■ CANDIDIASIS (MONILIASIS)

- Infection of skin or mucous membranes (e.g., oral cavity and vagina) is called moniliasis.
- *Candida albicans* is the most common cause of candidiasis.
- It causes the following conditions of medical importance:
  - **Oral thrush:** Conditions that favor oral *Candida* infection include use of broad-spectrum antibiotics, xerostomia, immune dysfunction (e.g., diabetes,

TABLE 13.10: Examples of rickettsial diseases and their features.

Diseases	Rickettsial agent	Insect vector	Mammalian reservoir	Clinical features
Typhus group				
Epidemic typhus	R. prowazekii	Louse	Human	Fever/chills, myalgia, headache, rash (No eschar) all over body except palm, sole and face
Murine typhus (Endemic typhus)	R. typhi	Flea	Rodents	Fever, myalgia, headache, rash (No eschar), trunk, extremities, milder form of illness
Scrub typhus	R. tsutsugamushi	Mite	Rodents	Fever headache, **rash with eschar*** cigarette burn sign lymphadenopathy
Spotted fever group				
Indian tick typhus	R. conorii	Tick	Rodent, dog	Fever headache, **rash with eschar**, first appear on wrist and ankle
Rocky mountain spotted fever	R. rickettsii	Tick	Rodents, dogs	Fever, headache, rash (No eschar)—first appear on wrist and ankle, palms and soles involved, systemic complications—respiratory, cardiovascular, central nervous, renal, and hepatic system
Rickettsialpox	R. akari	Mite	Mice	Mild illness, fever, headache, vesicular rash with eschar, lymphadenopathy, resemblance to chicken pox
Others				
Q fever	C. burnetii	Nil	Cattle, sheep, goats	Fever, headache, fatigue, pneumonia, endocarditis, no rash
Trench fever	Rochalimaea/ bartonella quintana	Louse	Human	Fever, splenomegaly, bone pains, maculopapular rash

*In scrub typhus, the eschar begins as a small papule, then enlarges, undergoes central necrosis, and eventually acquires a blackened crust with an erythematous halo that resembles a cigarette burn.

immunosuppressive therapy, and HIV infection) or the presence of removable prostheses. Furthermore, about one in four patients with lichen planus will have superimposed candidiasis.
- **Vaginal candidiasis** occurs more commonly in diabetic patients.
- **Cutaneous candidiasis** presenting as intertriginous infection and paronychia.

Treatment

- Topical application of antifungal agents such as nystatin, clotrimazole or miconazole.
- Swallowing nystatin suspension or sucking on clotrimazole troches for oesophageal candidiasis.
- Systemic antifungal agent ketoconazole or itraconazole for 2 weeks.
- Severe systemic infections may require IV fluconazole or amphotericin B.
- Echinocandins are newer class of antifungals that include caspofungin, micafungin and anidulafungin. These agents have limited toxicity, are safe in presence of renal or hepatic impairment, have minimal drug interactions, and importantly, have broad-spectrum activity against most *Candida* species.

■ MALARIA

- Malaria is a protozoan disease transmitted by the bite of female *Anopheles* mosquitoes.
- Five species of the genus plasmodium infect humans. These are:
  - *P. falciparum*
  - *P. vivax*
  - *P. ovale*
  - *P. malariae*
  - **P. knowlesi** (new)
- *P. falciparum* causes the most severe forms of the disease. *P. vivax* infection is the most common in India.

Clinical Features

Vivax, Ovale and Malariae Malaria

- Incubation period:
  - *P. vivax:* 2 weeks
  - *P. ovale:* 2 weeks
  - *P. malariae:* 4–5 weeks

- Fever with chills and rigors: In vivax and ovale malaria infections, the characteristic tertian interval (48 h interval between spikes or fever on alternate days) may be seen. In *P. malariae* infections, the quartan interval (72 h interval between spikes or fever every third day) may be seen.
- Headache and body pain
- Jaundice
- Vivax and ovale malarias have a persistent hepatic cycle (hypnozoites) that may give rise to relapses.
- Occasionally, vivax malaria can produce complications similar to those of falciparum malaria.

Falciparum Malaria (Malignant Tertian or Subtertian Malaria)

- The incubation period: 1–2 weeks
- **Prodromal symptoms** such as malaise, headache, myalgia, anorexia and mild fever may last for several days before the onset of the classical 'malarial paroxysms.'
- In a **classical malarial paroxysm,** suddenly the patient feels inexplicably cold and apprehensive. Mild shivering follows, which quickly turns into violent shaking with teeth rattling. There is intense peripheral vasoconstriction and goose flesh. The rapid increase in temperature may trigger febrile convulsions. The rigor lasts up to 1 hour. This is followed by a hot flush with throbbing headache, palpitations, tachypnoea, prostration, postural syncope and vomiting. The temperature reaches its peak. Finally, a drenching sweat breaks off and the fever defervesce over the next few hours. The exhausted patient sleeps off. The whole paroxysm lasts about 8–12 hours.
- **Neurological complications of** falciparum malaria can manifest as acute headache, irritability, agitation, seizures, psychosis and impaired consciousness.

Severe Manifestations and Complications of Falciparum Malaria

Criteria for severe and complicated malaria are shown in **Table 13.11**.

TABLE 13.11: **Criteria for severe and complicated malaria.**

Complication	Definition
• Cerebral malaria	• Impaired consciousness, unrousable coma
• Repeated generalised convulsions	• Two convulsions within 24 h
• Severe anaemia	• Haemoglobin concentration < 5 g/dL
• Renal failure	• Serum creatinine > 3 mg/dL and oliguria
• Respiratory distress	• Acidotic breathing, pulmonary oedema, acute respiratory distress syndrome
• Hypoglycaemia	• Blood glucose < 40 mg/dL
• Circulatory collapse or shock	• Systolic blood pressure (BP) > 90 mmHg, rapid thready pulse
• Disseminated intravascular coagulation (DIC)	• Bleeding from different sites of the body
• Acidosis	• pH < 7.25
• Black water fever	• Macroscopic haemoglobinuria
• Jaundice	• Bilirubin > 3 mg/dL
• Hyperparasitaemia	• > 5% of erythrocytes infested by parasites

Investigations

Microscopy

- **Blood smears:** Diagnosis of malaria rests on the demonstration of asexual forms of the parasites in peripheral blood smears. Both thin and thick smears should be examined.
- **Quantitative buffy coat (QBC) analysis:** In this test, the centrifuged buffy coat is stained with a fluorochrome (e.g., acridine orange) that 'lights up' malarial parasites when viewed under ultraviolet (UV) light.

Other Laboratory Findings

- **Rapid diagnostic tests:** Detection of *P. falciparum*-specific histidine-rich protein-2 (HRP-2) and lactate dehydrogenase antigens in finger prick blood samples.
- Normochromic normocytic anaemia, thrombocytopaenia and raised ESR.
- Total leucocyte count is low to normal, but neutrophil leucocytosis may be seen in several infections.

Management

Management of Uncomplicated Malaria

P. Vivax Malaria

- Chloroquine is the drug of choice. It is given at a dose of 600 mg base (four tablets) stat, followed by 600 mg base (four tablets) on the second day, followed by 300 mg base (two tablets) on the third day.
- Primaquine is given at a dose of 15 mg daily for 14 days. It destroys the hypnozoite phase in the liver.

P. Falciparum Malaria

- Chloroquine resistance in falciparum malaria is common and therefore, WHO recommends combination therapy for *P. falciparum* malaria.
- Artemisinin derivatives produce faster relief. This is known as **artemisinin-based combination therapy or ACT.** These combinations can then be taken for shorter durations than artemisinin alone.
- These combinations include:
   o Artemether + Lumefantrine
   o Artesunate + Mefloquine
   o Dihydroartemisinin + Piperaquine
   o Artesunate + Sulfadoxine-pyrimethamine
- ACTs can be given in the second and third trimester of pregnancy. Recommended treatment in the first trimester of pregnancy is quinine.
- To prevent spread of disease, the patient should receive primaquine in a single dose of 45 mg.

KALA-AZAR OR VISCERAL LEISHMANIASIS

Aetiology

- Kala-azar (visceral leishmaniasis) is a generalised visceral infection by the organism *Leishmania donovani* (LD). It affects the

monocytes and macrophages of liver, spleen, bone marrow and lymph nodes.
- The flagellated forms (promastigotes) of the organism develop within the female sandflies (*Phlebotomus argentipes*), which convey the disease to humans.

Clinical Features
- Some patients present with a low-grade fever, whereas others present with a high-grade, intermittent fever showing a double rise of temperature in 24 hours ('camel hump fever').
- Generalised pigmentation, particularly over face is common (kala-azar means 'black fever').
- Anaemia and generalised lymphadenopathy.
- Massive splenomegaly and hepatomegaly.

Investigations
- Anaemia, granulocytopaenia and thrombocytopaenia.
- Low serum albumin and high serum globulin, especially IgG.
- Mild elevation in bilirubin, AST/ALT and alkaline phosphatase.
- Demonstration of amastigotes (LD bodies) in stained smears of aspirates of bone marrow, liver, spleen, lymph nodes or buffy coat of peripheral blood. Bone marrow is positive in 50–70% cases, while splenic aspirate is positive in 70–90% cases.
- Culture of the aspiration in the Novy-Mac-Neal-Nicolle (NNN) medium for the organism.

Treatment
- Pentavalent antimonials
- Pentamidine
- Amphotericin B
- Miltefosine

■ TOXOPLASMOSIS

Toxoplasmosis is caused by the protozoan *Toxoplasma gondii*.

Transmission
- Man is the intermediate host, while cat is the definitive host.
- Ingestion of oocysts from contaminated soil or bradyzoites from undercooked meat, contaminated vegetables or water.

Clinical Manifestations
Infection in Immunocompetent Host
- Most often, acute toxoplasmosis is asymptomatic.
- In symptomatic patients, the most common presentation is cervical lymphadenopathy. Some cases have generalised lymph node enlargement. Other features include fever, malaise and myalgias.
- It can cause congenital defects in newborn if pregnant women are affected.
- **Ocular infection**—chorioretinitis—occurs after congenital infection.

Infection in Immunocompromised Host
- Most common involvement is of the CNS.
- Encephalopathy, meningoencephalitis, seizures, headache and focal neurological deficits are common.
- Pneumonia and ocular involvement are also common.

Diagnosis
- Minimal lymphocytosis, elevated ESR and mild increase in liver enzymes.
- A rise in titre of IgM antibodies indicates acute infection.
- PCR for toxoplasma DNA in ocular secretions.

Management
- A combination of sulphadiazine and pyrimethamine for 4–6 weeks, along with leucovorin. In patients sensitive to sulphonamides, clindamycin or azithromycin can be used.
- Steroids are added for ocular toxoplasmosis.

■ CYSTICERCOSIS

- *Taenia solium*, the pork tapeworm, inhabits the intestinal lumen of **humans**, its only **definitive host**.
- **Pigs** are the usual **intermediate hosts**.
- Humans acquire the infection following eating of undercooked pork containing cysticerci.
- When human tissue is invaded by the larval form, the condition is referred to as

cysticercosis. The common locations are subcutaneous tissue, skeletal muscles, eyes and brain.

Clinical Features
- Presence of adult worm in the intestine is generally asymptomatic.
- The dead larvae may invoke marked tissue response with muscular pain, weakness, fever and eosinophilia.
- **Neurocysticercosis** results from brain cysts. It may manifest as meningoencephalitis, epilepsy, personality changes, staggering gait, space-occupying lesion, stroke (due to inflammatory changes in the wall of intracranial arteries located in the vicinity of cysticerci) or hydrocephalus.

Diagnosis
- Eggs and proglottids in stool.
- Soft tissue radiographs may show calcified cysts (cigar-shaped) in muscles.
- CT scan of the brain may show calcified spots, solid nodules, cystic lesions containing a scolex or hydrocephalus.
- Specific enzyme-linked immunoelectrodiffusion transfer blot (EITB)

Treatment
- For removal of the adult worm in the intestine, niclosamide (2 g as a single dose), praziquantel (5 mg /kg) or albendazole may be used.
- Neurocysticercosis should be treated on the following lines:
    - Albendazole for 2–4 weeks is the drug of choice.
    - Antiepileptic drugs should be given until the reaction in the brain has subsided.
    - Operative intervention may be required for internal hydrocephalus.

■ ECHINOCOCCOSIS
- Hydatid disease is a tissue infection of humans caused by the larval stage of *Echinococcus granulosus*.
- **Canines** (especially dogs) are the **definitive hosts**
    - **Sheep and cattle** are the common **intermediate hosts**.
    - **Man** is **accidental host**.

Clinical Features
- Mostly cyst in right lobe of the liver. These hepatic lesions often present as palpable masses or abdominal pain.
    - Obstruction of bile duct may result in obstructive jaundice.
    - Rupture of a hydatid cyst in the body may produce fever, pruritus, urticarial rash or an anaphylactic reaction that may be fatal.
- A pulmonary hydatid may rupture producing cough, chest pain or haemoptysis.
- Central nervous system (CNS) involvement may produce epilepsy or blindness.
- The disease can rarely involve heart, kidneys, spleen, ovary and thyroid.

Diagnosis
- Routine radiographs may pick up hydatid cysts. Pulmonary lesions are seen as round, irregular masses of uniform density.
- CT scan and ultrasonography can detect the hydatid lesions by showing scolices and daughter cysts.
- Complement fixation, immunofluorescent tests and enzyme-linked immunosorbent assay (ELISA) to detect antibodies.
- Specific echinococcal antigens by immunoblot assays for confirmation

Treatment
- Surgical excision of the cysts is the treatment of choice.
- In inoperable cases, 'high-dose' albendazole should be given for 1–3 months.
- In selected cases, percutaneous aspiration, infusion of scolicidal agents (e.g., 95% ethanol of hypertonic saline) and reaspiration (PAIR) can be done. It is followed by albendazole treatment for 1 month.

■ ASCARIASIS
Ascariasis is an infection of humans caused by *Ascaris lumbricoides*.

Clinical Features
- Ascaris bronchopneumonia characterised by fever, cough, dyspnoea, wheeze, eosinophilic leucocytosis and migratory pulmonary infiltrates may occur during the stage of larval migration through the lungs.

- The adult worm may be vomited or passed in the stool.
- Bolus of worms may result in volvulus, intussusception or intestinal obstruction.
- The adult worms may migrate into appendix, bile ducts or pancreatic ducts, causing appendicitis, cholangitis, liver abscess or pancreatitis.
- Diagnosis is by demonstrating typical eggs in the stools.

Treatment
- Ascaris bronchopneumonia is treated symptomatically.
- It is treated with oral albendazole or mebendazole.

■ ANCYLOSTOMIASIS
- Hookworm disease is a symptomatic infection caused by *Ancylostoma duodenale* or *Necator americanus*. It is one of the main causes of anaemia in the tropics.

Clinical Features
- Itching dermatitis ('ground itch dermatitis') occurs at the site of entry of the larvae. The lesions are maximum on the feet, particularly between the toes.
- The larval migration through the lungs causes cough with blood-stained sputum, fever and patchy pulmonary consolidation.
- The major clinical manifestations of hookworm disease are those of iron deficiency anaemia and hypoalbuminaemia.

Diagnosis
- The characteristic eggs can be demonstrated in the stool by microscopic examination.
- The stool test for occult blood is usually positive.
- A peripheral blood eosinophilia as high as 70–80% may be seen in some cases.
- The haemoglobin level is usually low, and the anaemia is characteristically hypochromic and microcytic.
- Hypoalbuminaemia is a common finding in severe disease.

Treatment
The drugs currently favoured for the treatment of hookworms are mebendazole, albendazole and pyrantel pamoate.

■ LYMPHATIC FILARIASIS
- Lymphatic filariasis is caused by *Wuchereria bancrofti* and Brugia malayi.
- These nematodes are conveyed to humans by the bites of infected Culex mosquitoes. The adult worms live in the lymphatics of humans.

Clinical Features
- During attacks of acute lymphangitis, there is fever with chills and sweats, headache, photophobia and muscle pain.
- Lymphangitis itself manifests as pain, tenderness and erythema along the course of inflamed lymphatics. The inguinal lymph nodes may become enlarged, painful and tender. Orchitis, epididymitis, funiculitis and hydrocele may also occur.
- The chronic stage of the disease is characterised by permanent lymphoedema ('elephantiasis') of legs, scrotal oedema, chylous ascites, chylous pleural effusion and chyluria.

Investigations
- In the early stages of lymphangitis, there may be peripheral blood eosinophilia.
- Microfilariae can be demonstrated in the peripheral blood at night.
- Serological tests demonstrating antibodies against filarial antigens are non-specific.

Treatment
- Diethylcarbamazine (DEC) for 12–21 days kills microfilariae and adult worms.
- Ivermectin is effective in killing microfilariae, but not the adult worms.

■ SEPSIS
- Body's response to a clinical insult (e.g., infection, inflammation and trauma).
- Must have **atleast two** of the following criteria:
  - Temperature > 38.5°C or < 36°C

- o Heart rate > 90 bpm
- o Respiratory rate > 20 breaths/min or $PaCO_2 < 32$ mmHg
- o WBC > 12,000 cells/mm³, < 4,000 cells/mm³, or > 10% immature forms
- Systemic inflammatory response syndrome (SIRS) + evidence of infections (via cultures, examination or imaging).
- **Definition:** Life-threatening organ dysfunction caused by dysregulated host response to infection.

Table 13.12 shows the risk factors for sepsis

TABLE 13.12: Risk factors for sepsis.

Genetic polymorphism	Intrinsic factors
• Cytokine response • Coagulation • Mannose-binding protein	• Age • Nutrition • Comorbidities • Vaccination
Procedures	**Community factors**
• Urinary catheters • IV cannula • Wound dressings	• Contacts • Disease outbreaks • Specific exposure
Surgeries	**Hospital Factors**
	• Duration of stay • Intensive care unit (ICU) stay • Local strain sensitivity patterns

Figure 13.3 shows the continuum of severity of sepsis.

Management of sepsis

- Initial resuscitation: IV fluid normal saline @30 mL/kg
- Send blood cultures
- Identify organ dysfunctions
- Control the source of sepsis
- Initiate broad-spectrum antibiotics
- Vasopressors and inotropes to combat hypotension.
- Steroids: If shock is not responding to initial fluid resuscitation
- Management of organ dysfunction (ventilator support and dialysis)

Early Goal-directed Therapy for Sepsis

Early goal-directed therapy (EGDT) has been shown in **Table 13.13**.

■ SCHISTOSOMIASIS

- Infection is mainly by *Schistosoma mansoni*, *S. japonicum* and *S. haematobium*.
- Mode of infection is by bathing in fresh water contaminated with cercariae.
- Acute infection can manifest with "**swimmer's itch**" or a systemic hypersensitivity reaction—**Katayama fever**.

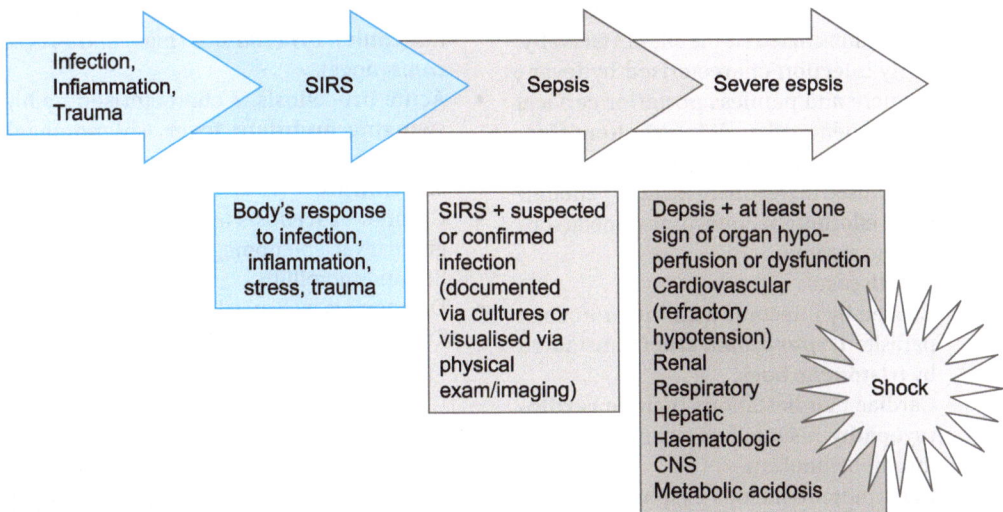

(CNS: central nervous system; SIRS: systemic inflammatory response syndrome)
Fig. 13.3: Continuum of severity of sepsis.

TABLE 13.13: Early goal-directed therapy (EGDT).

6-hour severe sepsis/septic shock bundle	24-hour severe sepsis and septic shock bundle

• **Early detection:** Obtain serum lactate level
• **Early blood culture/antibiotics:** Within 3 h of presentation
• Hypotension (SBP < 90 mmHg, MAP < 65 mmHg) or lactate > 4 mmol/initial fluid bolus 20–40 mL of **crystalloid** (or colloid equivalent) per kg of body weight
• **Vasopressors**
  ○ Hypotension not responding to fluid
  ○ Titrate to MAP > 65 mmHg
• **Septic shock or lactate > 4 mmol/L**
  ○ CVP and ScvO$_2$ measured
  ○ CVP maintained > 8 mmHg
  ○ MAP maintain > 65 mmHg
• **PRBCs (packed RBCs)** if haematocrit < 30%
• **Inotropes**
	• **Glucose control:** Maintained on average < 150 mg/dL
	• **Drotrecogin alfa (activated):** Administered in accordance with clinical situation
	• **Steroids:** For septic shock requiring continued use of vasopressors for ≥ 6 h
	• **Lung protective strategy:** Maintain plateau pressures < 30 cm H$_2$O for mechanically ventilated patients
	• DVT prophylaxis
	• Early enteral nutrition
	• Stress ulcer prophylaxis

(CVP: central venous pressure; DVT: deep vein thrombosis; MAP: mean arterial pressure; PRBC: packed red blood cell; RBC: red blood cell; SBP: systolic blood pressure)

- GI complications include **periportal fibrosis** and portal hypertension. Genitourinary complications include hematuria, bladder ulcers and polyps, obstructive uropathy and **bladder carcinoma**.
- **Praziquantel** is the drug of choice.

TRYPANOSOMIASIS

- **African trypanosomiasis (sleeping sickness)**
  ○ Caused by *Trypanosoma brucei gambiense* transmitted via the bite of a **tsetse fly**.
  ○ Early infection characterised by fever, chancre and painless posterior cervical lymphadenopathy—**Winterbottom sign**. Later meningoencephalitis develops.
  ○ Drugs used in treatment include pentamidine, eflornithine, nifurtimox, melarsoprol and suramin.
- **Chagas disease**
  ○ Caused by infection with the protozoan parasite *Trypanosoma cruzi* transmitted by **triatomine bugs**.
  ○ Cardiac manifestations include **cardiomyopathy**, heart failure, arrhythmias and thromboembolism.
  ○ GIT symptoms include dysphagia, odynophagia, regurgitation, constipation due to **megaoesophagus and megacolon**.
  ○ Treatment includes benznidazole and nifurtimox. More important is to treat the systemic complications.

BRUCELLOSIS

- Brucellosis (Malta fever, undulant fever, Mediterranean fever, Rock fever of Gibraltar) is a zoonotic disease caused by one of the four species of Brucella: *Brucella melitensis* (goats, sheep and camels), *Brucella abortus* (cattle), *Brucella suis* (pigs) and *Brucella canis* (dogs).
- Acute brucellosis is charecterised by high swinging **undulant fever**, splenomegaly, lymphadenopathy, hepatomegaly, sacroiliitis and arthritis.
- Chronic Brucellosis is charecterised by low grade fever, splenomegaly, arthritis, spondylitis and sacroiliitis.
- Diagnosis is by Brucella agglutination test.
- Treatment includes prolonged course of doxycycline with streptomycin/rifampicin.

CORONAVIRUS DISEASE 2019 (COVID-19)

- December 2019, a novel coronavirus caused pneumonia cases in Wuhan, a city in the Hubei Province of China which rapidly spread, resulting in a pandemic.

- It is a beta coronavirus that uses the receptor angiotensin-converting enzyme 2 (ACE2) for cell entry.
- Direct person-to-person transmission is the primary means of transmission.
- Duration of infectiousness is uncertain
- Incubation period ranges from 3–14 days
- Symptoms include fever, cough, dysponea, myalgias, diarrhoea, and loss of senses of smell or taste.
- Pneumonia, ARDS, thromboembolic events, acute cardiac injury, kidney injury cause mortality.
- Laboratory findings include lymphopenia, raised aminotransaminase levels, high LDH levels, and elevated inflammatory markers (ferritin, C-reactive protein, D-dimer).
- Management includes supportive therapy, oxygenation, thromboprophylaxis and management of complications.
- Drug therapy with hydroxychloroquine, remdesivir, dexamethasone, methyl prednisolone, tocilizumab, favipiravir, lopinavir-ritonavir have been tried.
- Convalescent plasma therapy has shown some benefit.
- Vaccines trials are underway.

BEST OF FIVES

1. A 44-year-old man returns from a trip to the jungles of northern Thailand with high-grade fever, body ache, severe myalgia and a rash which is on limbs and has now spread to involve the trunk. Malaria films are negative. What diagnosis fits best with this clinical picture?
   A. Dengue fever
   B. Malaria
   C. Hepatitis A
   D. Influenza
   E. Yellow fever

2. A 40-year-old patient presents with a slowly enlarging round erythema on her thigh. A few weeks later, she develops a lymphocytic meningitis and polyneuritis. What is the most likely diagnosis?
   A. Coxsackievirus infection
   B. Lyme disease
   C. Herpes simplex virus infection
   D. Generalised candida infection
   E. Relapse of a varicella zoster infection

3. A 35-year-old business traveller noticed some moderate diarrhoea. The diarrhoea lasted for 4 days. What is the most likely cause for his diarrhoea?
   A. *Legionella*
   B. *Staphylococcus*
   C. Enterotoxigenic *Escherichia coli*
   D. *Giardia lamblia*
   E. *Entamoeba histolytica*

4. A 78-year-old man presents with a 2-month history of cough with occasional haemoptysis, fever, night sweats and weight loss. Chest X-ray (CXR) shows bilateral apical cavitation. What is the most likely diagnosis?
   A. Lung cancer
   B. Chronic pulmonary disease (COPD)
   C. Asthma
   D. Tuberculosis
   E. Pneumonia

5. A 20-year-old man who has not received childhood vaccine presents with meningism, orchitis and unilateral parotitis. What is the most likely diagnosis?
   A. Epstein–Barr virus infection
   B. Human immunodeficiency virus (HIV)
   C. Measles
   D. Rubella
   E. Mumps

6. An 18-year-old woman presents with fever, diarrhoea and myalgia. She currently has her menstruation. On examination, her temperature is 40°C, blood pressure 90/50 mmHg and pulse 140/minute. What is the most likely organism responsible for the toxins?
   A. Staphylococci
   B. Streptococci
   C. *Escherichia coli*
   D. Herpes simplex virus
   E. HIV

7. A young female presents with lymphangitis and fever. Blood films for malaria parasites are negative, but an eosinophilia is noted. Blood films at night demonstrate microfilariae. What is the likely aetiological agent?
   A. *Brugia malayi*
   B. *Loa loa*
   C. *Onchocerca volvulus*

D. *Schistosoma haematobium*
E. *Wuchereria bancrofti*

8. A sewage worker presents with a high temperature and myalgia, especially in his legs. After a short improvement, he develops jaundice 6 days later. On examination, his temperature is 39°C, he is jaundiced and has hepatosplenomegaly. Investigations revealed-leucocytes 17 × 109/L, bilirubin 325 mmol/L, aspartate aminotransferase (AST) 70 U/L, alanine aminotransferase (ALT) 45 U/L, creatinine 248 mmol/L and HbsAg-negative. What is the most likely diagnosis?
   A. Hepatitis A
   B. Infectious mononucleosis
   C. Cytomegalovirus infection
   D. Leptospirosis
   E. Budd–Chiari syndrome

9. A 19-year-old woman who has just returned from a holiday is severely dehydrated and gives a history of passing voluminous watery stools that look like rice water, mixed with mucus and blood. Blood testing reveals a raised haemoglobin, markedly raised urea and raised creatinine. What diagnosis fits best with this clinic picture?
   A. Cholera
   B. Typhoid fever
   C. Shigella
   D. Salmonella
   E. Amoebic dysentery

10. A patient with stable sickle-cell anaemia presents with an erythematous rash all over her body, which is associated with painful swollen joints. On examination, she has clinical signs of anaemia. The full blood count shows absent reticulocytes in the peripheral blood. Infection with which pathogen is most likely to have caused her symptoms?
    A. Hepatitis C virus
    B. Hepatitis B virus
    C. HIV
    D. Rubella virus
    E. Parvovirus B19

11. A patient has been diagnosed with chlamydia pneumonia. What is the most appropriate antibiotic therapy?
    A. Ampicillin
    B. Erythromycin
    C. Imipenem
    D. Cefuroxime
    E. Amikacin

12. A 14-year-old student presents with a 1-day history of rash, which has followed a 3-day history of cold-like symptoms and conjunctivitis. The rash began as a maculopapular eruption in the postauricular region but has rapidly spread to his face and upper body. On examination, white papules are visible inside his mouth. What diagnosis fits best with this clinical picture?
    A. Scarlet fever
    B. German measles
    C. Measles
    D. Enterovirus infection
    E. Adenovirus infection

13. A 34-year-old farm labourer presents with an aching, stiff lower back and an inability to open his mouth fully. He subsequently suffers from what is described as a generalised rigid spasm. He was treated with intravenous diazepam. What is the next most important step?
    A. Broad-spectrum antibiotic treatment
    B. Immunoglobulin treatment
    C. Lumbar puncture
    D. Brain computed tomography (CT) scan
    E. Call the police

14. Post total right knee replacement surgery undertaken 3 weeks ago, a patient develops chills and a fever of 39.2°C. On examination, the right knee is red, hot and very tender. Synovial fluid aspirate reports the growth of gram-positive cocci. Which of the following is the most likely organism?
    A. *Staphylococcus epidermidis*
    B. *Pseudomonas aeruginosa*
    C. *Streptococcus pneumoniae*
    D. *Staphylococcus aureus*
    E. *Haemophilus influenzae*

15. A 50-year-old patient noticed an abscess from which sulphur granules were found microscopically. What is the most likely diagnosis?
    A. Leprosy
    B. Tuberculosis
    C. Acquired immunodeficiency syndrome (AIDS)
    D. Syphilis
    E. Actinomycosis

16. Which of the following statements is true with regard to Legionnaires' disease?
    A. Legionella pneumophila is a gram-positive rod
    B. The urinary antigen test for *Legionella* species has low sensitivity and is not particularly specific
    C. The infection is generally confined to immunocompromised patients
    D. The beta-lactam group of drugs is now regarded as the drug of choice against *Legionella* species
    E. Hyponatraemia occurs significantly more often in Legionnaires' disease than in other pneumonias

17. A 30-year-old patient presents with a sudden collapse. On recovering, she recalls having had a tick bite followed by a prolonged local rash. What is the likely cause of the collapse?
    A. Meningoencephalitis
    B. Acute Bell's palsy
    C. Atrioventricular (AV) heart block
    D. Bannwarth syndrome
    E. Acute large joint arthritis

18. A patient is hospitalised with cavitary pulmonary tuberculosis. Combination chemotherapy is started and he is placed in isolation. How long should the patient remain in isolation?
    A. 2 weeks
    B. For the duration of treatment
    C. Until the patient shows clinical improvement and has three negative sputum samples
    D. If there is improvement on the chest X-ray
    E. 3 months

19. A Thai woman was diagnosed with multibacillary leprosy. What is the appropriate treatment?
    A. Intravenous benzylpenicillin and flucloxacillin
    B. Isoniazid, rifampicin, pyrazinamide and ethambutol
    C. Prednisolone
    D. Clindamycin and ciprofloxacin
    E. Dapsone, clofazimine and rifampicin

20. Which degenerative disease of the central nervous system is caused by an infectious protein called a prion?
    A. Alzheimer's disease
    B. Parkinson's disease
    C. Creutzfeldt–Jakob disease
    D. Guillain–Barré syndrome
    E. Amyotrophic lateral sclerosis

21. A 44-year-old patient presents with nausea, diarrhoea and headache because of a 3-day history of general malaise. On examination, the patient looks well but red/bluish petechiae can be seen on the extensor surfaces of both legs. Given the likely clinical diagnosis, what is the most important prehospital treatment?
    A. Cefuroxime
    B. Erythromycin
    C. Ampicillin
    D. Gentamicin
    E. Benzylpenicillin

22. A previously well 65-year-old man who had travelled to a congregation organised in the summer months presents with a community-acquired pneumonia and mild, watery diarrhoea. He is slightly confused and disorientated but has no clinical evidence of meningitis. The peripheral white cell count is on the upper limit of normal and Na is 125 mmol/L. Two fellow members are also ill with a similar illness. What is the most likely causative organism?
    A. Mycoplasma pneumoniae
    B. Legionella pneumophila
    C. Influenza A virus
    D. Chlamydia pneumoniae
    E. Penicillin-resistant *Streptococcus pneumoniae*

23. A 16-year-old student with fever and sore throat has grey plaques on his tonsils, cervical lymphadenopathy and splenomegaly. What is the most likely diagnosis?
    A. *Streptococcus* infection
    B. Borrelia vincentii infection
    C. Diphtheriae
    D. Infectious mononucleosis
    E. Toxoplasmosis

24. A 17-year-old intravenous drug user comes with high spiking fevers. On examination, he is hypotensive, his jugular venous pressure (JVP) is raised with giant cv waves and there is a pansystolic murmur. Blood cultures are taken and empirical antibiotics are started. What is the most likely organism?
    A. *Candida* species
    B. *Enterococcus* species
    C. *Haemophilus, Aggregatibacter, Cardiobacterium hominis, Eikenella corrodens,* and *Kingella* (HACEK) group
    D. *Staphylococcus aureus*
    E. Viridans group streptococci

25. A young man with epilepsy presents with a 3-day history of cough with foul-smelling sputum. Chest X-ray shows a right upper lobe infiltration. What is the most likely cause?
    A. *Mycoplasma pneumonia*
    B. Chemical pneumonitis
    C. Pneumonia due to gram-negative aerobes
    D. Pneumonia due to gram-positive aerobes
    E. Pneumonia due to anaerobes

26. A 70-year-old diabetic developed a foot infection with osteomyelitis, which has been treated with several different antibiotics for the last 4 weeks. Suddenly, she developed watery diarrhoea and stomach cramps. Now, 2 days later, she has fever associated with diarrhoea. What is the most likely diagnosis?
    A. Salmonella gastroenteritis
    B. *Clostridium difficile* enterocolitis
    C. Enteritis due to enterohaemorrhagic *Escherichia coli* (EHEC)
    D. Shigella infection
    E. Acute mesenteric ischaemia

27. A young lady has been scratched by a cat and develops axillary lymphadenopathy. Which organism is most likely responsible for this?
    A. *Bartonella henselae*
    B. *Staphylococcus aureus*
    C. *Streptococcus pyogenes*
    D. *Toxoplasma gondii*
    E. *Pasteurella multocida*

28. A 17-year-old male presents with cervical lymphadenopathy. An acid-fast bacilli (AFB) stain from a fine-needle aspiration proved positive and he was commenced on quadruple antituberculous therapy. Now, 2 weeks later, his liver function tests (LFTs) have become deranged with an alanine aminotransferase (ALT) of 400 U/L and bilirubin of 50 µmol/L. What is the most important management step?
    A. Liver ultrasound
    B. Blood cultures
    C. Stop the tuberculosis medication
    D. HIV test
    E. Give prednisolone

29. On returning to UK last week from a walking trip in the United States, a young male developed fever with rash. He had a history of tick bite there. What diagnosis fits best with this clinical picture?
    A. Infectious mononucleosis
    B. Rocky Mountain spotted fever
    C. Reiter's syndrome
    D. Influenza
    E. Typhoid fever

30. On return from South America, a young executive developed abdominal pain, diarrhoea and fevers 1 week prior to his return. On examination, he has a fever of 38.5°C relative bradycardia and diffuse abdominal pain. Stool microscopy shows pus cells and red blood cells; culture is awaited. What is the most likely organism?
    A. *Plasmodium falciparum*
    B. *Norwalk* virus
    C. *Rotavirus*
    D. *Salmonella* species
    E. *Vibrio cholerae*

31. A traveller returned from the tropics 5 days ago. He felt unwell on the plane, complaining of headache, loss of appetite and sweats. His temperature was 39.5°C 2 days ago; however, it is now normal. What is the most important investigation to conduct?
    A. Repeated thick and thin blood smears
    B. Blood cultures
    C. Lumbar puncture
    D. Coombs' test
    E. Erythrocyte sedimentation rate

32. A 45-year-old woman presents with a widespread nodular rash, loss of eyebrows and burns on her hands. Her ulnar nerves are

thickened and exquisitely tender. Skin biopsy shows the presence of numerous AFBs. What is the most likely diagnosis?
A. Tuberculosis
B. Leprosy
C. Scleroderma
D. Motor neurone disease
E. HIV

33. A 30-year-old teacher presents with features suggestive of meningitis. The cerebrospinal fluid (CSF) is clear, with 24 white blood cells/μL (50% lymphocytes), protein 0.4 g/L, glucose 3.5 mmol/L (serum glucose 5.0 mmol/L) and no organisms on the Gram stain. What is the most likely causative organism?
A. *Enterovirus* species
B. *Listeria monocytogenes*
C. *Mycobacterium tuberculosis*
D. *Neisseria meningitidis*
E. *Streptococcus pneumoniae*

34. A 30-year-old male following a recent trip to Egypt presents with dysuria, urinary frequency and haematuria which he notices particularly at the end of stream. What is the diagnosis?
A. Gonorrhoea
B. Tuberculosis
C. Schistosomiasis
D. Herpes
E. Chancroid

35. In a patient who is aged over 60 years or below 3 months, what is an appropriate addition to ceftriaxone for the empirical management of meningitis?
A. Rifampicin
B. Amoxicillin 1 g 8 hourly
C. Vancomycin
D. Amoxicillin 2 g 6 hourly
E. Gentamicin

36. A week after return to the UK from India, a 45-year-old man develops fevers and a blood test confirms the presence of falciparum malaria. What is the most appropriate treatment?
A. Erythromycin
B. Quinidine
C. Chloroquine
D. Artesunate
E. Praziquantel

Answers

1-A, 2-B, 3-C, 4-D, 5-E, 6-A, 7-E, 8-D, 9-A, 10-E, 11-B, 12-C, 13-B, 14-A, 15-E, 16-E, 17-C, 18-C, 19-E, 20-C, 21-E, 22-B, 23C, 24-D, 25-E, 26-B, 27-A, 28-C, 29-B, 30-D, 31-A, 32-B, 33-A, 34-C, 35-D, 36-D

■ SUGGESTED READING

1. Yang X, Yu Y, Xu J, Shu H, Xia J, Liu H, et al. Clinical course and outcomes of critically ill patients with SARS-CoV-2 pneumonia in Wuhan, China: a single-centered, retrospective, observational study. Lancet. 2020;8:475-81.
2. Arentz M, Yim E, Klaff L, Lokhandwala S, Riedo FX, Chong M, et al. Characteristics and outcomes of 21 critically ill patients with COVID-19 in Washington State. JAMA. 2020;323(16):1612-4.
3. Nahid P, Dorman SE, Alipanah N, Barry PM, Brozek JL, Cattamanchi A, et al. Official American Thoracic Society/Centers for Disease Control and Prevention/Infectious Diseases Society of America Clinical Practice Guidelines: Treatment of Drug-Susceptible Tuberculosis. Clin Infect Dis. 2016;63:e147-95.
4. Dheda K, Barry CE 3rd, Maartens G. Tuberculosis. Lancet. 2016;387(10024):1211-26.
5. Kariuki S, Gordon MA, Feasey N, Parry CM. Antimicrobial resistance and management of invasive Salmonella disease. Vaccine. 2015;33 Suppl 3:C21-9.
6. Yan M, Li X, Liao Q, Li F, Zhang J, Kan B. The emergence and outbreak of multidrug-resistant typhoid fever in China. Emerg Microbes Infect. 2016;5(6):e62.
7. Wang A, Gaca JG, Chu VH. Management considerations in infective endocarditis: A review. JAMA. 2018;320(1):72-83.
8. Baddour LM, Wilson WR, Bayer AS, Fowler Jr VG, Tleyjeh IM, Rybak MJ, et al. Infective endocarditis in adults: Diagnosis, antimicrobial therapy, and management of complications: A scientific statement for healthcare professionals from the American Heart Association. Circulation. 2015;132(15):143-86.
9. Centers for Disease Control and Prevention. Malaria Information and Prophylaxis, by Country [A]. [online] Available from: http://www.cdc.gov/malaria/travelers/country_table/a.html. [Last accessed June, 2020].
10. Bonell A, Lubell Y, Newton PN, Crump JA, Paris DH. Estimating the burden of scrub typhus: A systematic review. PLoS Negl Trop Dis. 2017;11:e0005838.
11. Balcells ME, Rabagliati R, García P, Poggi H, Oddó D, Concha M, et al. Endemic scrub typhus-like illness, Chile. Emerg Infect Dis. 2011;17(9):1659-63.
12. Stevens DL, Bisno AL, Chambers HF, Dellinger EP, Goldstein EJC, Gorbach SL, et al. Practice guidelines for the diagnosis and management of skin and soft tissue infections: 2014 update by the infectious diseases society of America. Clin Infect Dis. 2014;59(2):e10-52.
13. Lyu C, Jewell MP, Piron J, Ehnert K, Beeler E, Swanson A, et al. Burden of Bites by Dogs and Other Animals in Los Angeles County, California, 2009-2011. Public Health Rep. 2016;131(6):800-8.

14

CHAPTER

HIV Infection and AIDS

◾ AETIOLOGY

Acquired immunodeficiency syndrome (AIDS) is caused by human immunodeficiency virus (HIV), which is a **non-transforming human retrovirus** belonging to the *Lentivirus* family.

Retroviruses are RNA viruses having an enzyme called reverse transcriptase, which prepares a DNA copy of the RNA genome of the virus in host cell.

Genetic forms: HIV occurs in two genetically different but related main forms, **HIV-1 and HIV-2**.

1. **HIV-1** is the most common in the United States, Europe and Central Africa. Four major groups of HIV-1 are:
   i. Group M ('major', 98% of infections worldwide): Group M subtypes exhibit a high degree of diversity and consists of nine subtypes: A–D, F–H, J and K (subtypes E and I were subsequently shown to be recombinants of other subtypes).
      a. Subtype C (Africa and India) accounts for half of strains and more readily transmitted.
      b. Subtype B predominates in Western Europe, North America and Australia.
      c. In Europe, the prevalence of non-B subtypes is increasing because of the migrants (predominantly from Africa).
      d. Subtypes A and D are associated with slower and faster disease progression, respectively.
   ii. Group O ('outlier') subtypes are highly divergent from group M and are largely confined to small numbers centred on Cameroon.
   iii. Group N (new—'non-major and non-outlier') is mostly restricted to West Central Africa (e.g. Gabon).
   iv. Group P related to gorilla strains of SIV has been identified from a patient from Cameroon.
2. **HIV-2 is common** in West Africa and India.

Structure of HIV

- **Viral core:** It contains:
  ○ **Major capsid protein p24:** This viral antigen and the antibodies against this are **used for the diagnosis of HIV infection** in enzyme-linked immunosorbent assay (**ELISA**).
  ○ **Nucleocapsid protein p7/p9**
  ○ **Two identical copies of single-stranded RNA genome**: The inner cone-shaped protein core (p24) houses two copies of the single-stranded RNA genome and viral enzymes (mentioned below).
  ○ **Three viral enzymes: (1) protease, (2) reverse transcriptase** (RNA-dependent DNA polymerase) and **(3) integrase**. **When the virus infects a cell**, the retroviral **RNA is not translated; instead it is transcribed by reverse transcriptase into DNA**. The **DNA form of the retroviral genome** is called a **provirus** which can be **integrated into the chromosome of host cell**.
- **Nucleocapsid:**
  ○ The **viral core is surrounded by a matrix protein p24 and p17**, which lies underneath the lipid envelope of the virion.

- **Lipid envelope:**
  - The virus contains a lipoprotein envelope/membrane, which **consists of lipid derived from the host cell and two viral glycoproteins**. These glycoproteins are: **(1) gp120** which projects as numerous external (on the surface) knob-like spikes, and **(2) gp41** anchoring transmembrane pedicle. These glycoproteins are essential for HIV infection of cells.

HIV Genome

The HIV genome contains two main groups of genes and their products act as antigens.
1. **Standard genes:** HIV-1 RNA genome **contains three** characteristic standard retroviral genes, which are typical of retroviruses. These include: **Gag** (encodes the structural proteins of the core including p24), pol [(codes for the enzymes crucial for viral replication, i.e. reverse transcriptase (that converts viral RNA into DNA), integrase (that incorporates the viral DNA into host chromosomal DNA) and protease (that cleaves large gag and pol protein precursors into their components)] and env (codes for envelope glycoproteins gp120 and gp41). Initially, the protein products of the **gag** and **pol** genes are translated into **large precursor proteins** and are later cleaved by the viral enzyme protease to form → **mature proteins**.

2. **Six regulatory/accessory genes:** HIV contains accessory genes, e.g. tat, rev, vif, nef, and vpr and vpu. They regulate the synthesis and assembly of infectious viral particles and the pathogenicity of the virus.

The structure of HIV has been shown in **Figure 14.1**.

■ MODES/ROUTES OF TRANSMISSION

Modes/routes of transmission are given in **Table 14.1**.

Routes by which HIV is not transmitted
- Close personal contact (including kissing and hugging)

TABLE 14.1: Modes/routes of transmission.

Exposure route	HIV transmission
Blood transfusion	90–95%
Perinatal	20–40%
Sexual intercourse	0.1–1%
Vaginal	0.05–0.1%
Anal	0.065–0.5%
Oral	0.005–0.01%
Injecting drugs use	0.67%
Needle-stick exposure	0.3%
Mucous membrane splash to eye, oro-nasal	0.09%

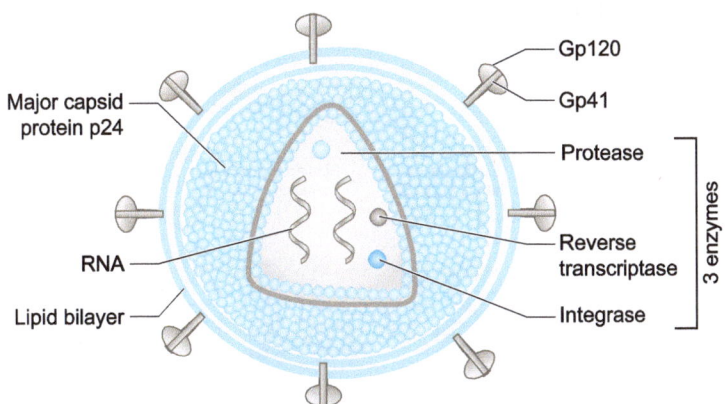

Fig. 14.1: Diagrammatic representation of structure of the human immune deficiency virus (HIV)–1 virion. The viral particle is covered by a lipid bilayer derived from the host cell and studded with viral glycoproteins (gp), gp41 and gp120.

- Sharing of utensils and insect bites
- Household contact
- Contact at school, swimming pool, etc.

PATHOGENESIS OF HIV INFECTION AND AIDS

- The interrelationship between HIV and the host immune system is the basis of the pathogenesis of HIV disease.
- **Major targets:** HIV can infect many tissues, but can only infect cells bearing the **CD4 receptor**. These are T-helper lymphocytes, monocyte–macrophages, dendritic cells and microglial cells in the central nervous system (CNS).

Lifecycle of HIV

Various molecular steps involved in the life cycle of HIV are as follows (**Fig. 14.2**):
- **Infection of cells by HIV:**
    - **Cell tropism:** HIV has **selective affinity** for host cells with **CD4 molecule receptor**. The cells with such receptors include **CD4+ T cells** which are present in **the mucosal lymphoid tissue** (largest reservoir of T cells and where majority of memory cells are lodged) and other CD4+ cells such as **monocytes/macrophages** and **dendritic cells**. The HIV envelope contains two glycoproteins, surface gp120 non-covalently attached to a transmembrane protein, gp41.
    - **Gp120 of HIV binding to CD4 molecule receptor** on the host cell is the first step in HIV infection. Binding alone is not enough for infection and **requires participation of a co-receptor molecule**.
    - **Conformational change:** Binding to CD4 leads to a conformational change in the HIV that results in the formation of a new recognition site on gp120 for the co-receptors, **CCR5 or CXCR4**. Inhibition of this binding will inhibit viral replication. T-cell tropic HIV strains mainly use CXCR4 as a co-receptor and are called X4 strains whereas macrophage-tropic strains, responsible for host-to-host transmission, use CCR5 as a co-receptor and are referred to as R5 strains. Individuals homozygous for mutations within *CCR5* gene are resistant to infection by HIV-1.
    - **Gp120 binding to chemokine receptor:** New recognition site on gp120 of HIV bind to **chemokine receptors,** i.e. CCR5 and CXCR4.
    - **Penetration of host cell membrane by gp41:** Binding of gp120 to the chemokine co-receptors leads to **conformational changes in gp41**.
    - **Membrane fusion:** The conformational change in gp41 allows **HIV to penetrate the cell membrane of the target cells** (e.g. CD4+ T cells or macrophages) **leading to fusion of the virus with the host cell**.
    - **Entry of viral genome into cytoplasm of host cell:** Once internalised, the virus core containing the HIV genome enters the cytoplasm of the host cell.

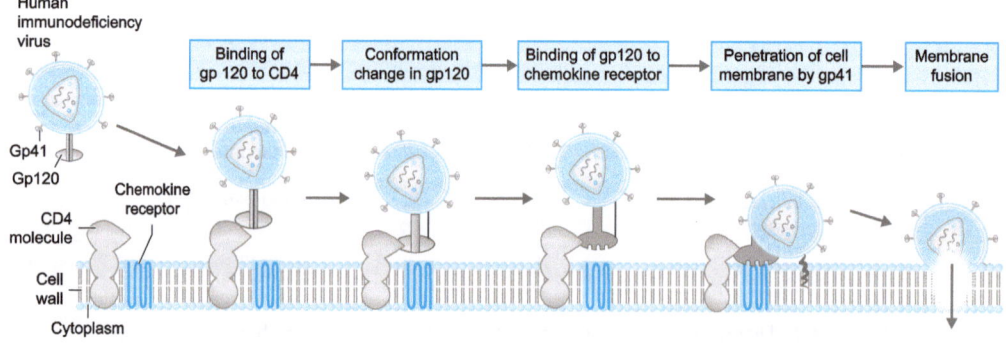

Fig. 14.2: Various molecular steps involved in the life cycle of human immunodeficiency virus (HIV).

- **Integration of the proviral DNA into the genome of the host cell:**
  - After the internalisation of the virus core, reverse transcriptase enzyme initiates copying of the viral RNA into double-stranded DNA→leading to the **synthesis of double-stranded complementary DNA (cDNA/proviral DNA)**.
  - **Episomal form:** In quiescent T cells, HIV cDNA may remain as a linear episomal form in the cytoplasm of infected cell.
  - **Integration of cDNA:** In dividing T cells, HIV cDNA enters the nucleus and becomes integrated into the genome of the host cell with the help of the enzyme viral integrase. The provirus can then remain latent or be active, generating products for the generation of new virions.
- **Viral replication:** After the integration of proviral DNA, it can either be latent or productive infection.
  - **Latent infection:** During this, the **provirus remains silent** for months or years.
  - **Productive infection:** In this, the **proviral DNA is transcribed** → leading to **viral replication** → formation of **complete viral particles**.
- **Production and release of infectious virus:** The complete **virus particle** formed **buds from the cell membrane** and **releases new infectious virus**. This productive infection when extensive leads to death of infected host cells. **HIV causes death of CD4+ cells** resulting in **significant depletion of T cells**.

The virus infection remains latent for long periods in lymphoid tissues. Active viral replication is associated with more infection of cells and progression to AIDS.

Dissemination: Virus disseminates to other target cells. This occurs either by fusion of an infected cell with an uninfected one or by the budding of virions from the membrane of the infected cell.

HIV CLINICAL STAGING AND CLASSIFICATION

Viral transmission→acute retroviral syndrome: 2–3 weeks→seroconversion: 2–4 weeks →asymptomatic chronic HIV infection: 8 years (average)→symptomatic HIV infection/AIDS: 1.3 years (average)

Two clinical staging systems, namely the World Health Organization (WHO) and Centers for Disease Control and Prevention (CDC) are being used. In both systems, patients are staged according to the most severe manifestation.

HIV clinical staging and classification are given in **Box 14.1** and **Table 14.2**.

NATURAL HISTORY OF HIV INFECTION

Virus usually enters the body through mucosal epithelia and clinical course can be divided into three main phases:

1. **Early acute phase:** Primary HIV infection (PHI) refers to the first 6-month period following acquisition of HIV. HIV infection starts as an acute infection, usually **self-limited non-specific illness**. During this period, uncontrolled viral replication resulting in high levels of HIV circulating in the plasma (**viraemia**) and genital tract and consequently of high infectiousness. The 2–4 weeks immediately following the infection may be silent, both clinically and serologically. It may be followed by **acute HIV syndrome** (non-specific signs and symptoms similar to many viral diseases). **These symptoms include sore throat,** mucosal ulcers, arthralgia, **myalgias, fever, weight loss,** lethargy, lymphadenopathy **and fatigue**. Other features such as transient faint pink maculopapular rash, diarrhoea and vomiting may also occur. Neurological symptoms are common including myelopathy, neuropathy, headache and photophobia. The illness lasts up to 3 weeks and followed by complete recovery.
   - Laboratory findings:
     - Early diagnosis: By **detecting HIV-RNA on polymerase chain reaction (PCR) or p24 antigenaemia**.
     - **Specific anti-HIV antibodies in serum:** They may be absent during this early stage of infection. Their appearance in serum (seroconversion) occurs 2–12 weeks after the development of symptoms. The window period during which antibody tests may be false negative is prolonged

Box 14.1: The World Health Organization (WHO) clinical staging classification of HIV infection.

Primary HIV infection
- Asymptomatic
- Acute retroviral syndrome

Clinical stage 1
- Asymptomatic
- Presistent generalised lymphadenopathy

Clinical stage 2
- Unexplained moderate weight loss (<10% of body weight)
- Recurrent upper respiratory tract infections (sinusitis, tonsillitis, otitis media, pharyngitis)
- Herpes zoster
- Angular cheilitis
- Recurrent oral ulceration
- Papular pruritic eruptions
- Seborrhoeic dermatitis
- Fungal nail infections

Clinical stage 3
- Unexplained severe weight loss (>10% of body weight)
- Unexplained chronic diarrhoea for longer than 1 month
- Unexplained persistent fever (above 37.5°C for >1 month)
- Persistent oral candidiasis
- Oral hairy leukoplakia
- Pulmonary tuberculosis
- Severe bacterial infections
- Acute necrotising ulcerative stomatitis, gingivitis or periodontitis
- Unexplained anaemia (<8 g/dL), neutropaenia (<500/μL) or HIV-associated immune thrombocytopaenia (<50,000/μL)

Clinical stage 4
- Candidiasis of oesophagus, trachea, bronchi or lungs
- Cryptococcosis—extrapulmonary
- Cytomegalovirus disease (outside liver, spleen and nodes)
- HIV encephalopathy
- Isosporiasis, chronic (>1 month)
- Lymphoma (cerebral or B-cell non-Hodgkin's)
- Mycosis-disseminated endemic (coccidiodomycosis or histoplasmosis)
- Pneumocystis pneumonia
- Progressive multifocal leucoencephalopathy
- Tuberculosis—extrapulmonary (CDC includes pulmonary)
- Symptomatic HIV-associated nephropathy
- Symptomatic HIV-associated cardiomyopathy
- Cervical carcinoma–invasive
- Cryptosporidiosis, chronic (>1 month)
- Herpes simplex chronic (>1 month) ulcers or visceral
- HIV wasting syndrome
- Kaposi's sarcoma
- Mycobacterial infection, non-tuberculous, extrapulmonary or disseminated
- Pneumonia, recurrent bacterial
- Toxoplasmosis—cerebral
- Septicaemia, recurrent (including non-typhoidal *Salmonella*) (CDC only includes *Salmonella*)
- Leishmaniasis, atypical disseminated

TABLE 14.2: Centers for Disease Control (CDC)—case definition for HIV infection among adolescents and adults.

Stage	CD4 count	CD4 %	Clinical evidence
Stage 0	Early HIV infection		
Stage 1	≥500 cell/mm³	26	No AIDS-defining condition
Stage 2	200–499 cell/mm³	14–25	No AIDS-defining condition
Stage 3	<200 cell/mm³	<14	or documentation of AIDS-defining condition
Stage unknown	No data	No data	No information on presence of AIDS-defining condition

(AIDS: acquired immunodeficiency syndrome; HIV: human immunodeficiency virus)

when post-exposure prophylaxis (PEP) is used.
- **Other laboratory abnormalities**: Lymphopaenia with atypical reactive lymphocytes in peripheral blood film, thrombocytopaenia and raised liver transferases. There may be marked depletion of CD4 lymphocytes and reversal of CD4:CD8 ratio.

2. **Middle chronic phase (clinical latency period):** Following acute phase, a prolonged period of clinical latency during which the infected individuals are asymptomatic for a substantial but variable length of time. This period is called the clinical latency period (middle chronic phase) **(Fig. 14.3)**.
   - **Minimal/no symptoms:** This phase is **characterised by dissemination of virus, viraemia, continuous viral replication in the lymph nodes and spleen** and **development of immune response by host.** The host immune response can handle most infections with opportunistic microbes with no or minimal clinical symptoms. It may have **few or no clinical manifestations.** The **symptoms may be due to minor opportunistic infections (OIs)** such as oral candidiasis (thrush), vaginal candidiasis, herpes zoster and perhaps mycobacterial tuberculosis (TB).
   - **Persistent generalised lymphadenopathy (PGL):** A subgroup of patients may develop PGL. PGL is defined as lymphadenopathy (>1 cm) at two or more extra-inguinal sites for >3 months in the absence of causes other than HIV infection. Biopsy reveals non-specific lymphoid hyperplasia. The lymph nodes are usually symmetrical, firm, mobile and non-tender. Nodes may disappear as the disease progresses.
   - **Progressive decrease of CD4+ T cells:** There is **continuous destruction of CD4+ T cells in the lymphoid tissue** accompanied by steady **decrease in their number in the peripheral blood**. During the early course of disease, the loss of CD4+ T cells can be replaced by new T cells. However, over a period of years, the continuous cycle of viral infection and death of T cells → leads to steady decrease in the number of CD4+ T cells both in the lymphoid tissue and in circulation. **Direct killing of T cells by the virus** is the major **mechanism of T-cell depletion.**
   - **Inversion of CD4+/CD8+ ratio:** Normal CD4+/CD8+ ratio is 1:2. Loss of CD4+ cells in AIDS patient leads to inversion of ratio of 0.5 or less **(Fig. 14.4)**.
   - **HIV infection of non-T cells:** HIV can infect non-T cells such as macrophages

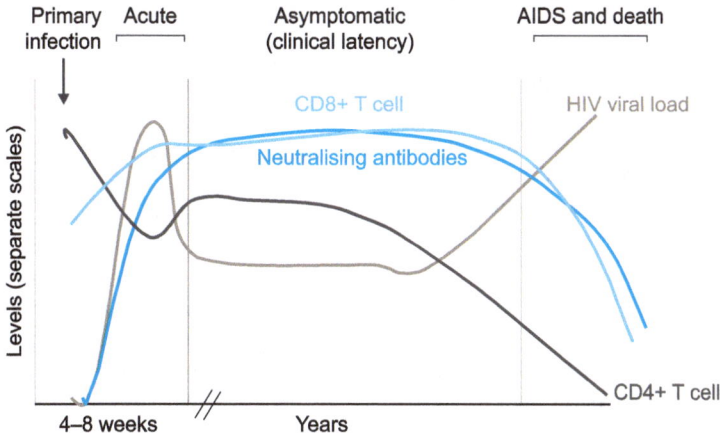

(AIDS: acquired immunodeficiency syndrome)

Fig. 14.3: Human immunodeficiency virus (HIV) disease progression.

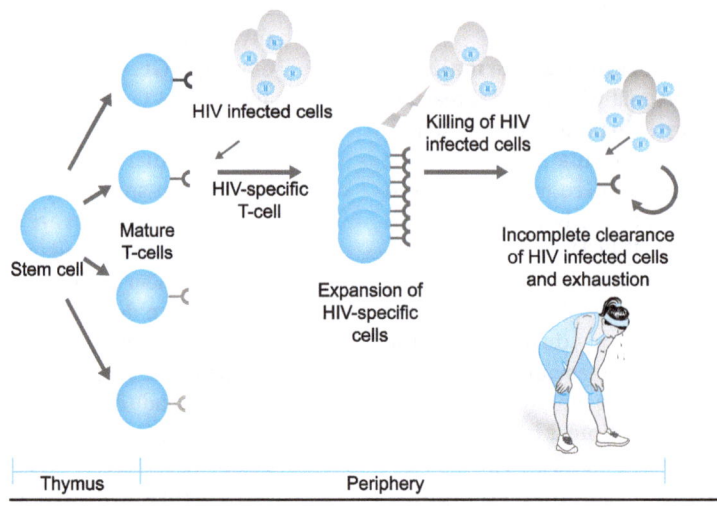

Fig. 14.4: Human immunodeficiency virus (HIV)-specific T-cell responses.

and dendritic cells (**mucosal and follicular**).
- ○ ***Abnormalities of B-cell function:***
  - Polyclonal activation of B cells → hypergammaglobulinaemia → circulating immune complexes.
  - Impaired humoral immunity → disseminated infections caused by capsulated bacteria such as *Streptococcus pneumoniae* and *Haemophilus influenzae*.
3. **Final crisis phase:** It is **final phase of HIV with progression to AIDS**. Within an average of 7–8 years, the patients present with fever, weight loss, diarrhoea, generalised lymphadenopathy, multiple OIs, neurologic disease and secondary neoplasms. Most of the untreated (but not all) patients with HIV infection **progress to AIDS after a chronic phase lasting from 7–10 years**.

■ PRIMARY HIV INFECTION

Definition:
- High-risk exposure within previous 6 weeks
- Detectable virus in plasma (p24 Ag and/or HIV-RNA) and/or
- Evolving anti-HIV antibody reactivity (negative or indeterminate to positive)
- With or without clinical symptoms

Classification:
- Acute infection: HIV detection (p24 Ag and/or HIV-RNA) in the absence of HIV antibody
- Recent infection: HIV antibody detection; up to 6 months after infection

Treatment of PHI is recommended for all people living with HIV (PLWH). Several circumstances indicate immediate treatment initiation:
- Acute symptomatic infection
- Severe or prolonged symptoms
- Neurological disease
- Age ≥50 years
- CD4 count <350 cells/μL
- Pregnancy

■ PATTERNS OF HIV PROGRESSION

- **Typical progressors** have a drop of 35–50 CD4 cells/year.
- **Rapid progressors** ('CD4 crash') have a drop of 50 CD4 cells per month after seroconversion. In these patients, the middle, **chronic phase is shortened to 2–3 years** after primary infection, and they **rapidly progress to AIDS**.
- **Slow progressors** have a CD4 decline, i.e. these are very slow compared to the typical progressors.
- **Long-term non-progressors** have CD4 counts that are stable at a baseline for many years. It is defined **as untreated patient who**

is asymptomatic for 10 years or more, with stable CD4+ T-cell counts and low levels of plasma viraemia.

AIDS-DEFINING OPPORTUNISTIC INFECTIONS IN PATIENTS WITH HIV INFECTION

AIDS-defining opportunistic infections in patients with HIV infection are given in **Table 14.3**.

Relation between CD4+ cell count and common illness in HIV patients has been shown in **Figure 14.5** and **Table 14.4**.

PRESENTING PROBLEMS IN HIV INFECTION

Respiratory System

- Acute bronchitis and sinusitis (encapsulated organisms such as *H. influenzae* and *S. pneumoniae*; Low CD4+ T cell counts—mucormycosis)
- The most common manifestation of pulmonary disease is pneumonia. (*S. pneumoniae* and *H. influenzae*, *Staphylococcus aureus* and *Pseudomonas aeruginosa*)
- **Pulmonary TB:** TB progresses more rapidly and may present sub-acutely or even acutely. It involves lower lobes of the lungs and cavities are rarely seen. Pleural effusions and hilar or mediastinal lymphadenopathy are common.
- ***Pneumocystis jirovecii* infection:**
  - It is the single most common cause of pneumonia in patients with HIV and is likely the aetiologic agent in 25% of cases of pneumonia in patients with HIV infection.
  - Key presenting feature is progressive dyspnoea. Fever and dry (non-productive) cough or productive cough with only scant amounts of white sputum are common. Extra-pulmonary sites may be involved (e.g. skin, meninges, brain, eyes, heart, liver, spleen and kidneys).
  - Diagnosis:
    - Chest X-ray: Bilateral interstitial infiltrate spreading out from the hilar regions. Pneumatocoeles may occur and may rupture resulting in a pneumothorax.

TABLE 14.3: AIDS-defining opportunistic infections (OIs) in patients with HIV infection.

OIs	Organ or site involved or type of damage
Protozoal and helminthic infections	
Cryptosporidiosis or isosporidiosis	Enteritis
Toxoplasmosis	Pneumonia or central nervous system (CNS) infection
Fungal infections	
Pneumocystosis	Pneumonia or disseminated infection
Candidiasis	Oesophageal, tracheal or pulmonary
Cryptococcosis	Infection of CNS
Coccidioidomycosis	Disseminated
Histoplasmosis	Disseminated
Bacterial infections	
Mycobacteriosis	
Atypical, e.g. *M. avium-intracellulare*	Disseminated or extra-pulmonary
M. tuberculosis	Pulmonary or extra-pulmonary
Nocardiosis	Pneumonia, meningitis, disseminated
Salmonella infections	Disseminated
Viral infections	
Cytomegalovirus	Pulmonary, intestinal, retinitis or CNS infections
Herpes simplex virus	Localised or disseminated
Varicella zoster virus	Localised or disseminated
Progressive multifocal leucoencephalopathy	CNS
Neoplasms	**Cause**
Kaposi's sarcoma (KS)	KS herpes virus
Non-Hodgkin B-cell lymphoma—primary lymphoma of the brain	Epstein–Barr Virus
Cervical cancer in women	Human papillomavirus

(AIDS: acquired immunodeficiency syndrome; HIV: human immunodeficiency virus)

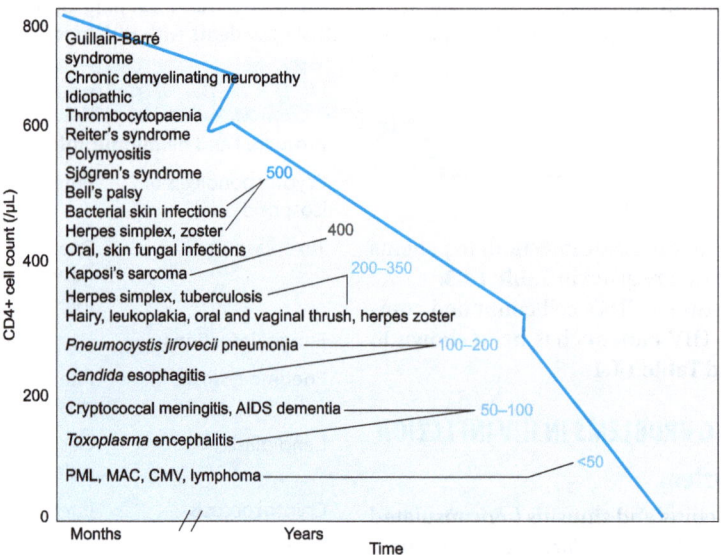

(PML: progressive multifocal leucoencephalopathy; MAC: *Mycobacterium avium* complex; CMV: cytomegalovirus)

Fig. 14.5: Relation between CD4+ cell count and common illness in human immunodeficiency virus (HIV) patients.

TABLE 14.4: Relation between CD4+ cell count and common illness in human immunodeficiency virus (HIV) patients.

CD4+ count	Illnesses
200–350/µL	• Herpes simplex • Tuberculosis • Oral and vaginal thrush • Herpes zoster
100–200/µL	• *P. jirovecii* pneumonia • *Candida* oesophagitis
50–100/µL	• Cryptococcal meningitis • AIDS dementia • *Toxoplasma* encephalitis
<50/µL	• Progressive multifocal leucoencephalopathy • *Mycobacterium avium* complex • Cytomegalovirus infection

- High-resolution computed tomography (CT) scan: It is more sensitive than chest X-ray and usually shows typical 'ground-glass' interstitial infiltrates.
- Arterial blood gas:
  - Mild cases: Room air arterial oxygen (pO_2) >70 mmHg or alveolar–arterial O_2 difference <35 mmHg.
  - Moderate-to-severe cases: pO_2 <70 mmHg or alveolar-arterial O_2 difference >35 mmHg.
- Serum LDH: Elevated
- Diagnosis: It is made by examination of induced (hypertonic saline nebulisation) sputum stained with silver stains, PCR or immunofluorescence of bronchoalveolar lavage or transbronchial biopsy.
• Management of *Pneumocystis jirovecii* infection has been shown in **Table 14.5**.
  - Primary prophylaxis is indicated in patients with CD4 cell count <200/mm³ or if there is a history of oropharyngeal candidiasis.
  - Secondary prophylaxis is indicated in all patients who have recovered from PCP.
    - Trimethoprim 160 mg + sulphamethoxazole 800 mg/day OR

TABLE 14.5: Management of *Pneumocystis jirovecii* infection.

Mild cases	Moderate-to-severe cases (PaO$_2$ < 70 mmHg)
Trimethoprim 5 mg/kg 6 hourly + sulphamethoxazole 25 mg/kg 6 hourly orally OR	Trimethoprim 5 mg/kg 6 hourly + sulphamethoxazole 25 mg/kg 6 hourly intravenous (IV) OR
Trimethoprim 5 mg/kg 6 hourly + dapsone 2 mg/day OR	Pentamidine 4 mg/kg/day IV OR
Pentamidine 4 mg/kg/day IV OR	Clindamycin (600 mg qid) + primaquine (30 mg od)
Atovaquone 750 mg tid	In all cases, add prednisolone 40 mg bid for 5 days, then 40 mg/day for 5 days and then 20 mg/day for 11 days

- Aerosolised pentamidine 300 mg once a month OR
- Dapsone 50 mg bid
- Others include atovaquone, dapsone plus pyrimethamine plus leucovorin

- **Atypical mycobacterial infections:**
  - *Mycobacterium avium* complex (MAC) infection is a late complication of HIV infection, occurring predominantly in patients with CD4+ T cell counts of <50/μL.
  - Common presentation is disseminated disease with fever, weight loss, night sweats, abdominal pain, diarrhoea and lymphadenopathy.
  - Alveolar or nodular infiltrates and hilar and/or mediastinal adenopathy
  - Anaemia and elevated liver alkaline phosphatase are common.
  - Treatment includes use of clarithromycin + ethambutol + rifabutin.
- **Other respiratory infections:**
  - ***Rhodococcus equi*** is a gram positive, pleomorphic, acid-fast non-spore forming bacillus that can cause pulmonary and disseminated infection in HIV-infected patients.
  - ***Coccidioides immitis*** is a mould that is endemic in the southwest United States.
    - It can cause a reactivation pulmonary syndrome in patients with HIV infection.
    - Most patients with this condition will have CD4+ T cell counts <250/4.
    - Patients present with fever, weight loss, cough, and extensive, diffuse reticulonodular infiltrates on chest X-ray.
    - Nodules, cavities, pleural effusions and hilar adenopathy are also seen.
  - **Invasive aspergillosis** is not an AIDS-defining illness and is generally not seen in patients with AIDS in the absence of neutropaenia or administration of glucocorticoids.
    - Primary pulmonary infection of the lung may be seen with **histoplasmosis.**
  - **Idiopathic interstitial pneumonia** is benign infiltrate of the lung, is due to the polyclonal activation of lymphocytes is and common.

Gastrointestinal Disease

Oesophageal diseases:
- Oesophagitis develops in as many as 90% of the patients with AIDS. It is usually due to *Candida*, cytomegalovirus (CMV) and herpes simplex virus.
- Oesophageal candidiasis is the most common cause of pain on swallowing (odynophagia), dysphagia and regurgitation in HIV patients. Systemic azole therapy (e.g. fluconazole 200 mg daily for 14 days) is usually curative.

Diarrhoea

Causes of diarrhoea in HIV patients are given in **Table 14.6.**

Protozoal, CMV and mycobacterial infections usually produce protracted diarrhoea, and fluid and electrolyte imbalance. Nitazoxanide is the treatment of choice for *Cryptosporidium* infection. Co-trimoxazole (TMP-SMX) is drug of choice for treatment of isosporiasis.

Mucocutaneous Diseases

- Mucocutaneous manifestations are extremely common in HIV. These include warts, *Mollus-*

TABLE 14.6: Causes of diarrhoea in human immunodeficiency virus (HIV) patients.

Infections	HIV related
• Bacterial: *Salmonella, Shigella, Campylobacter, Escherichia coli* • Fungal: Histoplasmosis, coccidioidomycosis and penicilliosis • Protozoa: Cryptosporidia, microsporidia, and *Isospora belli, Giardia, Entamoeba histolytica* • Viral: Cytomegalovirus • *Mycobacterium avium* complex	HIV invading gut epithelium
	Gastrointestinal malignancies
	• Lymphoma • Kaposi's sarcoma

cum contagiosum, herpes simplex, varicella zoster and KS.
- KS presents as red or purple, flat or raised skin lesion.

Neurological Disease

Acute meningitis: During acute infection, CNS invasion occurs in >90% cases. The clinical spectrum ranges from silent cerebrospinal fluid (CSF) pleocytosis, aseptic meningitis, infectious mononucleosis-like syndrome, multiple cranial nerve palsies to acute encephalopathy.

Aseptic meningitis may occur any time in the course of HIV infection; however, it is rare following the development of AIDS. This appears to be an immune-mediated disease.

HIV-Associated Dementia
- HIV-associated dementia (HAD) is also called as **AIDS dementia complex (ADC)** or HIV encephalopathy.
- Most HIV patients have some neurologic disorder during the course of their disease.
- It precedes the lesions in white matter of lateral and posterior columns.

Vacuolar Myelopathy
It involves the white matter of lateral and posterior columns of the spinal cord resulting in spastic paraparesis and sensory ataxia. It is subacute in onset.

Progressive Multifocal Leucoencephalopathy
Progressive multifocal leucoencephalopathy (PML) is a progressive disease caused by JC virus (JCV). It presents with stroke-like episodes and cognitive impairment is characterised by focal neurological abnormalities including impairment of vision (blindness due to involvement of the occipital cortex), aphasia, hemiparesis and ataxia that progresses to altered sensorium and death within 6 months.

Herpes Simplex Encephalitis
It may be insidious in onset as compared to an immunocompetent host. Despite treatment with acyclovir, prognosis is poor.

Herpes zoster may also produce myelitis or radiculitis.

Cytomegalovirus Encephalitis
This presents as slowly progressive disease with behavioural disturbance, cognitive impairment and a reduced level of consciousness. Identification of CMV DNA in the CSF supports the diagnosis. Response to anti-CMV therapy is poor. CMV may also cause myelitis and retinitis (retinal haemorrhage resulting in blindness).

Cryptococcal Meningitis
- *Cryptococcus neoformans* is the most common cause of meningitis in AIDS patients.
- Patients usually present with headache, vomiting and mild confusion.
- CSF pleocytosis may be mild or even absent, and protein and glucose concentrations are variable. However, CSF cryptococcal antigen tests and culture are usually positive and this test has a sensitivity and specificity of almost 100%. India ink staining on CSF may show the *Cryptococcus neoformans*.
- Treatment is with amphotericin B (0.7 mg/kg/day) (plus flucytosine 25 mg/kg qid, if available) for 2 weeks, followed by fluconazole (400 mg/day) for 8–10 weeks. Relapse rates are high and hence, continuous therapy with fluconazole (200 mg/day) is recommended.

Tuberculosis Meningitis
It is common in AIDS patients. It may present in a manner similar to cryptococcal meningitis. CSF findings of tuberculous meningitis are similar to those in HIV-uninfected patients. It usually shows elevated cell counts (lymphocytes) and protein along with low glucose. CT scan may show multiple ring lesions suggestive of tuberculomas.

Syphilis
It may present as neurosyphilis, manifestations of which include optic neuritis, uveitis, meningitis, encephalitis and cerebral infarction.

Cerebral Toxoplasmosis
- It is the most common opportunistic infection of CNS caused by *Toxoplasma gondii*. It presents with headache, confusion, seizures, ataxia and focal deficits. The characteristic findings on contrast CT scan are multiple contrast-enhancing lesions and space-occupying lesions with ring enhancement on contrast and surrounding oedema.
- *Toxoplasma* serology shows evidence of previous exposure [positive immunoglobulin (Ig) G antibodies].
- Treatment is sulphadiazine with pyrimethamine together with folinic acid, to reduce the risk of bone marrow suppression. However, co-trimoxazole is also effective and less toxic.
- Definitive diagnosis is by brain biopsy but this is usually not necessary.

Primary CNS lymphoma (PCNSL) is high-grade B-cell lymphoma associated with EBV infection. It occurs in about 5% of cases and may present with encephalopathy, focal deficits and seizures of lymphomatous meningitis. Characteristically, CT scan demonstrates a single, homogeneously enhancing, peri-ventricular lesion with surrounding oedema. PCR for EBV DNA in the CSF has a high sensitivity and specificity for PCNSL.

Ocular Diseases
Retinopathy:
- Ocular toxoplasmosis usually presents with vitritis and retinitis without retinal haemorrhages.
- HIV retinopathy is a microangiopathy that causes cotton wool spots, which are of benign in nature.
- Herpes zoster may lead to ocular pain, conjunctival infection and corneal opacification.
- Varicella zoster virus can also cause rapidly progressive outer retinal necrosis.
- CMV retinitis is the most serious infection of the eyes. It occurs when the CD4 count is <100 cells/mm^3.
  - Fundoscopy: Haemorrhages and exudates are seen in the retina which follow the vasculature of the retina (so-called 'pizza pie' appearances/'frosted branch angiitis').
  - Treatment: It should be started immediately, with either oral valganciclovir (900 mg twice daily), IV ganciclovir (5 mg/kg twice daily) or foscarnet (90 mg/kg twice daily) given intravenously for at least 3 weeks or until retinitis is quiescent.

Cardiovascular Diseases
- The most common heart disease is coronary heart disease.
- Dilated cardiomyopathy associated with congestive heart failure (CHF) in a HIV-infected patient is referred to as HIV-associated cardiomyopathy.
- Pericardial effusions may be seen in the setting of advanced HIV infection. Predisposing factors include TB, CHF, mycobacterial infection, cryptococcal infection, pulmonary infection, lymphoma and KS.

Psychiatric Disease
- Anxiety and mood disturbance may be caused by pre-test issues such as worries about being infected and disclosure, receiving a positive result.
- Mild cognitive dysfunction is a common occurrence in later-stage disease and usually improves with highly active antiretroviral therapy (HAART).
- Disorders of mental state may also result from drugs directly (e.g. depression with EFV) or indirectly.

Diseases of Kidney and Genitourinary System
- Due to direct consequence of HIV infection, due to opportunistic infection, neoplasms or due to drug toxicity
- HIV-associated nephropathy presents with proteinuria.

- Ultrasound examination shows enlarged and hyperechoic kidneys.
- Focal segmental glomerulosclerosis is seen in 80%, and mesangial proliferation in 10–15% of the cases.

Haematological Conditions

- Anaemia is caused by bone marrow infiltration with opportunistic infections, neoplasms, bone marrow suppression with drugs, as a direct effect of HIV, blood loss from KS or malabsorption as a result of a GI infection.
- Leucopoenia results from bone marrow infiltration or due to drug toxicity. Lymphopaenia is a good marker of HIV.
- Thrombocytopaenia occurs very early and may be the first indicator of HIV in some cases.

Cancers in HIV

Types of cancers in HIV are given in **Box 14.2**.

Diagnosis of HIV Infection or AIDS

- **Detection of virus-specific antibodies (anti-HIV):** Antibodies against the virus are detectable within 3–12 weeks after infection.
  - Detection of IgG antibody to envelope
  - IgG antibody to p24 (antip24): This antibody can be found during the earliest weeks of infection and during the asymptomatic phase.
  - Viral p24 antigen (p24ag): This is detectable shortly after infection but has usually disappeared by 8–10 weeks after exposure.

Box 14.2: Cancers in HIV.	
AIDS defining	**Virus**
• KS	HHV-8
• Non-Hodgkin's lymphoma (systemic and CNS)	EBV, HHV-8
• Invasive cervical carcinoma	HPV
Non-AIDS defining	
• Anal cancer	HPV
• Hodgkin's disease	EBV
• Leiomyosarcoma (paediatric)	EBV
• Squamous carcinoma (oral)	HPV
• Merkel cell carcinoma	MCV
• Hepatoma	HBV, HCV

- **Western blot assays: Most specific** or the **confirmatory test** for HIV.
- Direct detection of viral material/**infection:**
  - **p24 antigen capture assay**
  - **Reverse transcriptase-polymerase chain reaction (RT-PCR)**
  - **DNA-PCR:** For measuring the amount of viral particles (HIV-RNA) in the blood (viral load)
- **Haematological abnormalities:** Normochromic, normocytic anaemia, lymphopaenia, leucopoenia, thrombocytopaenia and decrease in T-helper cells (CD4+ counts)

■ MANAGEMENT OF A PATIENT WITH HIV INFECTION

Treatment of common opportunistic infections in AIDS is given in **Table 14.7**.

■ ANTIRETROVIRAL DRUGS

Combination antiretroviral therapy (cART), also called as HAART, is the cornerstone of management of patients with HIV infection (**Fig. 14.6, Box 14.3** and **Table 14.8**).

Indications for Antiretroviral Therapy

- ART should be initiated in all adults living with HIV, regardless of the WHO clinical stage and at any CD4 cell count.
- As a priority, ART should be initiated in all adults with severe or advanced HIV clinical disease (WHO clinical stage 3 or 4) and adults with CD4 count ≤350 cells/mm^3.
- ART at any CD4 count in PLHIV:
  - Active TB disease
  - Hepatitis B virus (HBV) co-infection with severe chronic liver disease
  - HIV-positive partners in serodiscordant couples
  - Pregnant and breastfeeding women
  - Children younger than 5 years of age
  - Infants diagnosed in the first year of life

Antiretroviral Regimens

Antiretroviral regimens are given in **Tables 14.9** and **14.10**.

TABLE 14.7: Treatment of common opportunistic infections (OI) in AIDS.

OI	First-line treatment	Alternate treatment
P. jirovecii	See text	See text
Toxoplasma	Pyrimethamine 50–100 mg/day + sulphadiazine 2 g qid	Pyrimethamine 5–100 mg/day + clindamycin 500 mg qid
Cryptococcus	Amphotericin 0.3 mg/kg/day + flucytosine 25–37 mg/kg qid	Amphotericin 0.7 mg/kg/day
Isospora belli	Co-trimoxazole 7 mg/kg	
Candida (mucosal)	Co-trimoxazole 200–600 mg OR fluconazole 50–100 mg/day	Ketoconazole 200 mg/day
Candida (systemic)	Amphotericin 0.3 mg/kg/day	
Cytomegalovirus	Ganciclovir 5 mg/kg bid IV	Foscarnet 60 mg/kg tid
Herpes simplex (oral)	Acyclovir 200–400 mg 5 times/day	
Herpes simplex (encephalitis)	Acyclovir 10 mg/kg tid IV	Vidarabine 15 mg/kg/day
Herpes zoster (local)	Acyclovir 30 mg/kg/day in five doses	
Herpes zoster (disseminated)	Acyclovir 10 mg/kg tid	Vidarabine 10 mg/kg/day

(AIDS: acquired immunodeficiency syndrome)

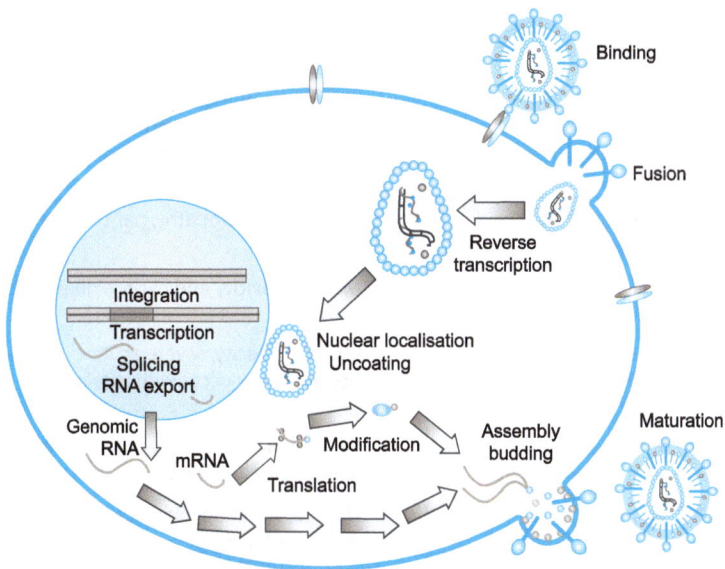

Fig. 14.6: Possible sites for chemotherapeutic intervention in the human immunodeficiency virus (HIV) life cycle.

> **Box 14.3: Antiretroviral drug.**
> - Drugs that inhibit the viral reverse transcriptase enzyme:
>   - **Nucleoside reverse transcriptase inhibitors (NRTIs):**
>   - Zidovudine (AZT, ZDV)
>   - Zalcitabine (ddC)
>   - Didanosine (ddI)
>   - Abacavir (ABC)
>   - Stavudine (d4T)
>   - Lamivudine (3TC)
>   - Emtricitabine (FTC)
>   - **Nucleotide reverse transcriptase inhibitor (nRTI):**
>   - Tenofovir disoproxil fumarate (TDF)
>   - **Non-nucleoside reverse transcriptase inhibitors (NNRTIs):**
>   - Nevirapine (NVP)
>   - Delavirdine (DLV)
>   - Efavirenz (EFV)
> - **Protease inhibitors (PIs):**
>   - Indinavir (IDV)
>   - Ritonavir (RTV)
>   - Saquinavir (SQV)
>   - Nelfinavir (NFV)
>   - Amprenavir (APV)
>   - Lopinavir (LPV)/ritonavir (RTV)
>   - Atazanavir (ATV)
>   - Fosamprenavir (FOSAPV)
>   - Tipranavir (TPV)
>   - Darunavir (TMC114)
> - **Integrase inhibitors:**
>   - Raltegravir and dolutegravir
> - Drugs that interfere with viral entry:
>   - **Fusion inhibitors:** Enfuvirtide (eT20)
>   - **CCR5 antagonists (CCR5 inhibitors):** Maraviroc
> - Pharmacokinetic enhancers (CyP3A inhibitors)
>   - Cobicistat: PIs and integrase inhibitor elvitegravir are administered in combination with another agent (e.g. low-dose ritonavir or cobicistat) to increase trough plasma drug concentrations, increase drug half-lives and increase maximum plasma concentrations.)

TABLE 14.8: Common antiretroviral drugs, dosages and adverse events.

Name	Adult dose	Adverse events
Abacavir	600 mg PO qid OR 300 mg PO bid	Hypersensitivity reaction (may include fever, rash, nausea, vomiting, diarrhoea, malaise, shortness of breath, cough, pharyngitis); patients positive for HLA-B5701 are at highest risk for hypersensitivity (perform HLA screening before initiating)
Didanosine	• > 60 kg: 400 mg PO qid • < 60 kg: 250 mg PO qid	Peripheral neuropathy, pancreatitis, nausea and lactic acidosis
Emtricitabine	200 mg PO qid OR 240 mg (24 mL) oral solution PO qid	Minimal toxicity and hyperpigmentation
Lamivudine	300 mg PO qid OR 150 mg PO bid	Minimal toxicity, severe acute exacerbation of hepatitis may occur with HBV co-infection upon discontinuation
Stavudine	• > 60 kg: 40 mg PO bid • < 60 kg: 30 mg PO bid	Peripheral neuropathy, pancreatitis, lactic acidosis, lipoatrophy and hyperlipidaemia
Tenofovir	300 mg PO qid	Nausea, vomiting, diarrhoea, headache, asthenia and renal insufficiency
Delavirdine	400 mg PO tid	Rash and headache
Efavirenz	• 600 mg PO qid • Take on empty stomach	Rash, CNS (e.g. somnolence, vivid dreams, confusion, visual hallucinations) and hyperlipidaemia

Continued

Continued

Name	Adult dose	Adverse events
Etravirine	200 mg PO bid	Rash and nausea
Nevirapine	• 200 mg PO bid • XR: 400 mg PO qid	Rash and hepatitis
Rilpivirine	25 mg PO qid with meal	Depressive disorders, insomnia, headache and rash
Atazanavir	400 mg PO qid OR 300 mg + ritonavir 100 mg PO qd	Indirect hyperbilirubinaemia, prolonged PR interval, hyperglycaemia, skin rash (20%) and hyperlipidaemia
Darunavir	800 mg qd + ritonavir 100 mg PO qd OR 600 mg bid + ritonavir 100 mg PO bid	Rash, nausea, diarrhoea, hyperlipidaemia and hyperglycaemia
Fosamprenavir	700 mg bid + ritonavir 100 mg PO bid OR 1400 mg PO bid or 1400 mg + ritonavir 100–200 mg PO qd	Rash, nausea, vomiting, diarrhoea, hyperlipidaemia and hyperglycaemia
Indinavir	• 800 mg PO qid • 800 mg PO bid + ritonavir 100–200 mg PO bid	Nephrolithiasis, nausea, indirect hyperbilirubinaemia, hyperlipidaemia and hyperglycaemia
Lopinavir/ ritonavir	• 400 mg/100 mg PO bid OR 800 mg/200 mg PO qd • Oral solution: Take with meals	Nausea, vomiting, diarrhoea, asthenia, hyperlipidaemia and hyperglycaemia
Nelfinavir	1250 mg PO bid OR 750 mg PO tid (cannot be boosted); take with food	Diarrhoea, hyperlipidaemia and hyperglycaemia
Ritonavir	• Boosting dose for other PIs: 100–400 mg/day • Non-boosting dose: 600 mg bid	Nausea, vomiting, diarrhoea, asthenia, hyperlipidaemia, oral paresthesias and hyperglycaemia
Saquinavir	• 1000 mg + ritonavir 100 mg PO bid • Unboosted not recommended • Take with food	Nausea, diarrhoea, headache, hyperlipidaemia, hyperglycaemia, PR and QT interval prolongation
Tipranavir	• 500 mg + ritonavir 200 mg PO bid • Unboosted not recommended	Hepatotoxicity, rash, hyperlipidaemia, hyperglycaemia and intracranial haemorrhage

TABLE 14.9: Antiretroviral regimens.

Regimen	Main requirements	Additional guidance (footnotes)
Recommended regimens		
2 NRTIs + INSTI (preferred)		
ABC/3TC + DTG ABC/3TC/DTG	HLA-B*57:01 negative HBsAg negative	I (ABC: HLA-B*57:01, cardiovascular risk)
TAF/FTC or TDF/FTC or TDF/3TC + DTG		II (TDF: Prodrug types. Renal and bone toxicity. TAF dosing)
TAF/FTC/BIC		III Weight increase

Continued

Continued

Regimen	Main requirements	Additional guidance (footnotes)
TAF/FTC or TDF/FTC or TDF/3TC + RAL qd or bid		II (TDF: Prodrug types. Renal and bone toxicity. TAF dosing) IV (RAL: Dosing)
1 NRTI + INSTI		
DGT + 3TC	HBsAg negative HIV-VL <500,000 copies/mL CD4 count >200 cells/µL	
2 NRTIs + NNRTI		
TAF/FTC or TDF/FTC or TDF/3TC + DOR TDF/3TC/DOR		II (TDF: Prodrug type. Renal and bone toxicity. TAF: Dosing) V (DOR: HIV-2)
TAF/FTC or TDF/FTC or TDF/3TC + RPV TAF/FTC/RPV TDF/FTC/RPV	CD4 count >200 cells/µL HIV-VL <100,000 copies/mL Not on proton pump inhibitor with food	II (TDF: Prodrug types. Renal and bone toxicity. TAF dosing) VI (RVP: HIV-2)
2 NRTIs + PI/r or PI/c		
TAF/FTC or TDF/FTC or TDF/3TC + DRV/c or DRV/r TAF/FTC/DRV/c	With food	II (TDF: Prodrug types. Renal and bone toxicity. TAF dosing) VII (DRV/r: Cardiovascular risk)
Alternative regimens		
2 NRTIs + INSTI		
ABC/3TC + RAL qd or bid	HBsAg negative HLA-B*57:01 negative	I (ABC: HLA-B*57:01, cardiovascular risk) IV (RAL: Dosing)
TDF/FTC/EVG/c TAF/FTC/EVG/c	With food	II (TDF: Prodrug types. Renal and bone toxicity) VIII (EVG/c: Use in renal impairment)
2 NRTIs + NNRTI		
ABC/3TC + EFV	HLA-B*57:01 negative HBsAg negative HIV-VL <100,000 copies/mL At bed time or 2 h before dinner	I (ABC: HLA-B*57:01, cardiovascular risk) IX (EFV: Sucidality. HIV-2 or HIV-1 group 0)
TAF/FTC or TDF/FTC or TDF/3TC + EFV TDF/FTC/EFV	At bed time or 2 h before dinner	II (TDF: Prodrug types. Renal and bone toxicity. TAF dosing) IX (EFV: Sucidality. HIV-2 or HIV-1 group 0)
2 NRTIs + PI/r or PI/c		
ABC/3TC + ATV/c or ATV/r	HLA-B*57:01 negative HBsAg negative HIV-VL <100,000 copies/mL Not on proton pump inhibitor with food	I (ABC: HLA-B*57:01, cardiovascular risk) X (ATV/b and renal toxicity)

Continued

Continued

Regimen	Main requirements	Additional guidance (footnotes)
ABC/3TC + DRV/c or DRV/r	HLA-B*57:01 negative HBsAg negative With food	I (ABC: HLA-B*57:01, cardiovascular risk) VII (DRV/r and cardiovascular risk)
TAF/FTC or TDF/FTC or TDF/3TC + ATV/c or ATV/r	Not on proton pump inhibitor with food	II (TDF: Prodrug types. Renal and bone toxicity. TAF dosing) X (ATV/b: Renal toxicity)
Other combination		
RAL 400 mg bid + DRV/c or DRV/r	HBsAg negative HIV-VL <100,000 copies/mL CD4 count >200 cells/μL With food	VII (DRV/r: Cardiovascular risk)

TABLE 14.10: When to start ART in PLWH with opportunistic infections.

	CD4 count	Initiation of ART	Comments
General recommendation	Any	As soon as possible and within 2 weeks after starting treatment for the opportunistic infection	–
Tuberculosis (TB)	• <50 cells/μL • >50 cells/μL	• As soon as possible and within 2 weeks after starting TB treatment • Can be delayed up to 8 weeks after starting tuberculosis (TB) treatment, especially if difficulties with adherence, drug-drug interactions or toxicity	• A threshold of 100 cells/μL may be more appropriate due to variability in CD4 count assessments • CD4 thresholds also apply for TB meningitis – with close monitoring due to increased risk of adverse effects • For details, see ART in TB/HIV Co-infection section
Cryptococcal meningitis	Any	Defer initiation of ART for at least 4 weeks (some specialists recommend a delay of 8–10 weeks in severe cryptoccocal meningitis)	
Cytomegalovirus and organ disease	Any	A delay of maximum of 2 weeks might be considered	Especially for persons with chorioretinitis and encephalitis due to risk of IRIS

(ART: antiretroviral therapy; PLWH: people living with HIV)

■ SWITCH STRATEGIES FOR VIROLOGICALLY SUPPRESSED PERSONS

Indications:
- Documented toxicity caused by one or more of the antiretrovirals included in the regimen. Examples of these reactive switches: Lipoatrophy (d4T, AZT), CNS adverse events (EFV, DTG), diarrhoea (PI/r) and jaundice (ATV), proximal renal tubulopathy and low bone mineral density (TDF).
- Prevention of long-term toxicity. Example of this proactive switch: Prevention of lipoatrophy in persons receiving d4T or AZT and prevention of proximal renal tubulopathy with TDF.

- Avoidance of drug–drug interactions: This includes ART switch when starting hepatitis C virus (HCV) treatment to avoid DDIs.
- Planned pregnancy or women wishing to conceive.
- Ageing and/or comorbidity with a possible negative impact of drug(s) in current regimen, e.g. on cardiovascular (CVD) risk and metabolic parameters.
- Simplification: To reduce pill burden, adjust food restrictions, improve adherence and reduce monitoring needs.
- Protection from HBV infection or reactivation by including TDF in the regimen.
- Regimen fortification: Increasing the genetic barrier of a regimen in order to prevent resistance (e.g. in persons with reduced adherence).
- Cost reduction: Switching to the generic form of their current regimen, if available.

Treatment Failure

Table 14.11 shows the types of treatment failure.

IMMUNE RECONSTITUTION INFLAMMATORY SYNDROME

- Immune reconstitution inflammatory syndrome (IRIS) is a pathologic inflammatory immune recognition of antigens associated with a known or unknown replicating infection or persistent non-replicating antigens from a previous infection.
- Categories:
  - Related to underlying opportunistic infection:
    - Inflammatory 'unmasking' of a previously untreated infection
    - Paradoxical clinical deterioration of an infective process for which patient is on appropriate treatment
  - Autoimmune, e.g. Graves' disease
  - Malignancies, e.g. worsening of KS
- Management:
  - In general, OI–IRIS resolves within a few weeks with continuation of specific treatment for the OI, without discontinuing ART and without anti-inflammatory treatment.
  - TB–IRIS: Start of systemic corticosteroids is recommended (e.g. oral prednisone 1.5 mg/kg/day for 2 weeks, then 0.75 mg/kg/day for 2 weeks).
  - Cryptococcal meningitis: Start therapy with amphotericin B plus flucytosine and defer start of cART for at least 4 weeks.
  - PML: Intravenous (IV) methylprednisolone (1 g/day for 3–5 days or IV dexamethasone 0.3 mg/kg/day for 3–5 days), then oral tapering.

TABLE 14.11: Treatment failure.

Failure	Definition
Clinical failure	**Adults and adolescents** New or recurrent clinical event indicating severe immunodeficiency (WHO clinical stage 4 condition) after 6 months of effective treatment **Children** New or recurrent clinical event indicating advanced or severe immunodeficiency (WHO clinical stage 3 and 4 clinical condition with exception of tuberculosis) after 6 months of effective treatment
Immunological failure	**Adults and adolescents** CD4 count falls to baseline (or below) or persistent CD4 <100 **Children:** • Less than 5 years: Persistent CD4 <200 or <10% • More than 5 years: Persistent CD4 <100
Virological failure	Plasma viral load >1,000 based on two consecutive viral load measurements after 3 months, with adherence support

(WHO: World Health Organization)

HIV Infection and AIDS

POST-EXPOSURE CARE OF A HEALTHCARE WORKER

Risk of transmission:
- HIV: 0.3%, HBV: 2–40%, HCV: 2.7–10%
- PEP 80% effective
  - Decontamination:
    - Wash the area with soap and water.
    - Avoid squeezing or milking the wound.
    - Do not use caustic agents such as bleach.
- **Type of exposure:**
  - Less severe: Solid needle or superficial injury
  - More severe: Large-bore hollow needle, deep puncture, visible blood on device, needle used in patient's artery or vein
- **Infection status of source:**
  - Class 1: Asymptomatic HIV infection or known low viral load (<1,500 copies/mL)
  - Class 2: Symptomatic HIV, AIDS, acute seroconversion or known high viral load
- **Initiating PEP:**
  - Start within 72 hours.
  - 2–3-drug regimen based on risk
  - PEP should be given for 28 days, if tolerated.

Post-exposure prophylaxis (PEP) regimens are shown in **Table 14.12**.

- **Basic regimen for PEP:**
  - One nRTI and one NRTI (tenofovir + emtricitabine), or
  - Two NRTIs (zidovudine + lamivudine, zidovudine + emtricitabine, lamivudine + stavudine, lamivudine + tenofovir, stavudine + didanosine).

- Expanded regimen includes an additional third drug (ritonavir/lopinavir, indinavir, nelfinavir or efavirenz). Most commonly used third drug is ritonavir/lopinavir.
- The Medical Care Criteria Committee now recommends:

Preferred HIV PEP regimen:
Raltegravir 400 mg PO twice daily

PLUS

Tenofovir DF 300 mg + emtricitabine 200 mg fixed-dose combination 1 PO once daily.

PRE-EXPOSURE PROPHYLAXIS

Guidelines for pre-exposure prophylaxis (PrEP):
- Were released in May, 2014
  - Addresses the role of PrEP in the following adult populations
    - Men who have sex with men
    - Heterosexual men and woman
    - Injection drug users
    - Serodiscordant couples

ONLY medication to be used in this setting is tenofovir/emtricitabine.

TUBERCULOSIS IN PEOPLE LIVING WITH HIV

Table 14.13 shows the dosage of drugs for the treatment of tuberculosis.

Latent Tuberculosis

- Tuberculin skin test (TST) > 5 mm or positive interferon-gamma release assay (IGRA) or close contacts to persons with sputum smear-positive TB

TABLE 14.12: Post-exposure prophylaxis (PEP) regimens.

Exposure type	Infection status of	Source
	HIV+, class 1	**HIV+, class 2**
Less severe	Recommend basic two-drug PEP	Recommend expanded ≥3-drug PEP
More severe	Recommend expanded three-drug PEP	Recommend expanded ≥3-drug PEP
	Unknown HIV status	**Unknown source**
Less severe	Generally, no PEP warranted; consider basic two-drug PEP if source has HIV risk factors	Generally, no PEP warranted; consider basic two-drug PEP if exposure to HIV-infected persons is likely
More severe	As above	As above

TABLE 14.13: Dosage of drugs for the treatment of diseases.

Disease	Drug	Dose	Comments
Initial phase	Rifampicin + isoniazid + pyrazinamide + ethambutol	Weight based	Initial phase for 2 months, then continuation phase (rifampicin + isoniazid) according to tuberculosis (TB) type (see below) Possibility to omit ethambutol, if *M. tuberculosis* is known to be fully drug sensitive
Alternative	Rifabutin + isoniazid + pyrazinamide + ethambutol	Weight based	Initial phase for 2 month, then continuation phase according to TB type (see below) Possibility to omit ethambutol, if *M. tuberculosis* is known to be fully drug sensitive
Continuation phase	Rifampicin/rifabutin + isoniazid according to TB type		Total duration of therapy: • Pulmonary, drug susceptible TB: 6 months • Pulmonary TB and positive culture at 8 weeks of TB treatment: 9 months • Extrapulmonary TB with CNS involvement or disseminated TB: 9–12 months • Extrapulmonary TB with bone joint involvement and in other sites: 6–9 months

- Isoniazid 5 mg/kg/day (maximum 300 mg) po + pyridoxine (vitamin B6) 25 mg/day po for 6–9 months
  OR
- Rifampicin 600 mg/day po or rifabutin po for 4 months

BEST OF FIVES

1. An internee has a needlestick injury after taking blood from a patient known to be HIV positive. What is the most appropriate immediate management after hand washing for 10 minutes?
   A. Continue hand washing for a further 20 minutes
   B. Antiretroviral therapy
   C. Test for hepatitis B and C
   D. Blood cultures
   E. Broad-spectrum antibiotics

2. A 40-year-old HIV-positive patient presents with a history of altered sensorium. A computed tomography (CT) scan of the brain shows two 3-cm ring-enhancing lesions in the left cerebral hemisphere with surrounding oedema and midline shift.
   Which is the most likely cause?
   A. Toxoplasmosis
   B. Tuberculosis
   C. Herpes simplex virus infection
   D. Brain metastasis
   E. Brain tumour

3. HIV patients with a CD4 count <200/mm^3 should receive appropriate prophylaxis against *Pneumocystis jiroveci* (formerly called *Pneumocystis carinii*) pneumonia. What is the most appropriate medication?
   A. Ampicillin
   B. Erythromycin
   C. Co-trimoxazole
   D. Corticosteroids
   E. Cefaclor

4. An HIV-positive patient presents with diarrhoea for 1 month and fever. On examination, he looks dehydrated. What is the most likely diagnosis?
   A. Toxoplasmosis
   B. Cryptosporidiosis
   C. Salmonellosis
   D. Pneumocystis infection
   E. Ulcerative colitis

5. An HIV-positive woman on antiretrovirals with an undetectable viral load becomes pregnant. Which of the following courses of action is recommended to reduce the risk of vertical transmission?
   A. Admit to hospital for close monitoring.
   B. Arrange an elective caesarean section.
   C. Change the antiretroviral regimen to zidovudine, lamivudine and efavirenz.
   D. Stop antiretroviral therapy immediately and recommence at the time of birth.
   E. Take vitamin supplements.

6. An HIV-positive patient was admitted after having had a generalised tonic-clonic seizure (GTCS). Which finding favours infection with *Toxoplasma* sp. over *Cryptococcus* sp.?
   A. Mass on brain computerised tomography scan
   B. Cotton-wool spots
   C. Serum *toxoplasma* antibodies
   D. CD4 count <80/mm^3
   E. Raised C-reactive protein

7. A 24-year-old homosexual, known to be HIV-seropositive, presents with left hemiplegia and dysarthria. The CD4 T-lymphocyte count is 50 cells/μL. A magnetic resonance imaging (MRI) scan of the brain demonstrates a large ring-enhancing lesion in bilateral hemispheres. What is the most likely diagnosis?
   A. HIV encephalopathy
   B. Lymphoma
   C. Progressive multifocal leucoencephalopathy (PML)
   D. Toxoplasmosis
   E. Tuberculosis

8. A HIV positive patient has been commenced on antiretroviral therapy 1 year ago. Initial follow-up blood tests at 3 and 6 months demonstrated an undetectable viral load; however, the latest results show a viral load of 2,000 copies/mL. What is the most likely cause for the virological failure?
   A. Co-morbidity
   B. Drug interaction
   C. Poor compliance
   D. Re-infection with a new strain of virus
   E. Viral resistance

9. A 22-year-old commercial sex worker is diagnosed as being HIV-positive. Her CD4 count is above 200. In addition to highly active antiretroviral therapy (HAART), against which of the following organisms would prophylaxis be most useful?
   A. *Toxoplasma gondii*
   B. Cytomegalovirus
   C. *Pneumocystis jiroveci*
   D. Salmonellae
   E. Cryptococci

10. A 54-year-old smoker presents with cough and weight loss. Blood testing reveals that he is HIV-positive. Chest X-ray reveals multiple calcified lymph nodes, fibrosis and thick-walled cavity. What is the most likely diagnosis in this case?
    A. Bronchial carcinoma
    B. Sarcoidosis
    C. Silicosis
    D. Pulmonary tuberculosis
    E. Histoplasmosis

11. An HIV-positive patient but in the stable phase of the disease is best monitored with which biomarker?
    A. C-reactive protein
    B. CD4 lymphocyte count
    C. Erythrocyte sedimentation rate
    D. Polymerase chain reaction
    E. Blood cultures

12. A patient with HIV complains of visual impairment. On examination, he has haemorrhages. What is the most likely diagnosis?
    A. Cytomegalovirus retinitis
    B. Toxoplasmosis
    C. Aspergillosis
    D. Tuberculosis
    E. Herpes keratitis

13. A patient with acquired immune deficiency syndrome (AIDS) has been complaining of a 2-month history of increasingly sized, purplish, nodular skin lesions. What is the most likely diagnosis?
    A. Malignant melanoma
    B. Tuberculosis
    C. Papillomavirus infection
    D. Keratosis
    E. Kaposi's sarcoma

14. An acquired immune deficiency syndrome (AIDS) patient on combination antiretroviral therapy (cART) was brought into casualty because he had a fit lasting approximately 15 minutes at home. The day before, he had complained of headaches and fever. On examination, he is confused but has no localising neurological signs. Cerebrospinal fluid (CSF) shows lymphocytic pleocytosis with India ink stain-positive organism. What is the most likely diagnosis?
    A. Tuberculosis
    B. *Toxoplasma gondii* cysts
    C. Cerebrovascular accident
    D. *Pneumocystis jiroveci* infection
    E. *Cryptococcus* infection

15. A 34-year-old male HIV-positive patient is suffering weight loss, night sweats, a chronic cough and shortness of breath on exercise. Laboratory testing reveals a relative lymphopaenia, with the CD4 lymphocyte subfraction reduced at only 85/mm^3 (normal 200–800). There is desaturation on blood gas monitoring associated with exercise. Other blood tests reveal a raised lactate dehydrogenase level. Chest X-ray reveals diffuse pulmonary infiltrates. What diagnosis fits best with this clinical picture?
    A. Tuberculosis
    B. *Pneumocystis jiroveci* pneumonia
    C. Histoplasmosis
    D. Cryptococcosis
    E. Mycoplasma pneumonia

16. A patient with HIV presents after noticing several lesions on his legs and his mouth. The lesions are nodular and brown in colour. Given the most likely diagnosis, what is the causative agent?
    A. Human herpes virus 1
    B. Human papilloma virus 6
    C. Human T-lymphotropic virus (HTLV) 4
    D. Human papilloma virus 16
    E. Human herpes virus 8

17. A patient with HIV presents with a sudden onset of confusion. Cytomegalovirus (CMV) encephalitis is suspected. What treatment should be commenced?
    A. Ganciclovir
    B. Aciclovir
    C. Ceftriaxone
    D. Dexamethasone
    E. Nil required

18. A 40-year-old homosexual with AIDS (acquired immunodeficiency syndrome) presents with generalised tonic-clonic seizure (GTCS). A computed tomography (CT) scan of his brain shows ring-enhancing masses with surrounding oedema. Given the likely diagnosis, what is the most appropriate treatment?
    A. Erythromycin
    B. Ampicillin
    C. Aspirin and clopidogrel
    D. Sulfadiazine and pyrimethamine
    E. Fluconazole

19. Given the most common organism to lead to watery diarrhoea, nausea and abdominal cramps in a patient with HIV, what treatment is most useful?
    A. Metronidazole
    B. Azithromycin
    C. Clarithromycin
    D. Nitazoxanide
    E. Ciprofloxacin

20. A male with AIDS (acquired immunodeficiency syndrome) with CD4 <50/cumm presents with a 2-week history of confusion and lethargy. His Mini-Mental State Examination (MMSE) is 20/30. A computed tomography (CT) scan shows atrophy and magnetic resonance imaging (MRI) reveals diffuse white matter hyperintensity. Which of the following is the most likely diagnosis?
    A. Cytomegalovirus (CMV) encephalitis
    B. AIDS dementia complex
    C. Toxoplasmosis
    D. Progressive multifocal leucoencephalopathy
    E. Cryptococcosis

21. Which of the following is not an AIDS (acquired immunodeficiency syndrome) defining illness?
    A. Aspergillosis
    B. Cytomegalovirus retinitis
    C. Candidiasis
    D. Kaposi's sarcoma
    E. *Mycobacterium tuberculosis*

22. An HIV patient presents with a 1-week's history of profuse watery, non-bloody diarrhoea, approximately 10–20 episodes per day. Modified acid-fast staining of stools reveals red-stained oocysts. Which of the following is the most likely causative agent?
    A. *Cryptosporidium parvum*
    B. *Entamoeba histolytica*
    C. *Giardia intestinalis*
    D. *Shigella dysenteriae*
    E. Cytomegalovirus

23. A patient with HIV presents with fever, malaise, dyspnoea, diarrhoea, generalised lymphadenopathy and significant weight loss. His CD4 count is 20. There is evidence of tender hepatosplenomegaly. What is the most likely causative agent?
    A. Histoplasmosis
    B. *Mycobacterium avium* complex
    C. *Cryptococcus*
    D. Toxoplasmosis
    E. Cryptosporidiosis

24. A 39-year-old HIV-positive patient has declined antiretroviral therapy. On examination, there was a soft pericardial rub at the left sternal border. His chest was clear. Abdominal examination was normal.
    What is the most likely cause of the pericardial effusion?
    A. Autoimmune disease
    B. Lymphoma
    C. Pyogenic infection
    D. Tuberculosis
    E. Viral infection

Answers

1-B, 2-A, 3-C, 4-B, 5-B, 6-A, 7-D, 8-C, 9-C, 10-D, 11-B, 12-A, 13-E, 14-E, 15-B, 16-E, 17-A, 18-D, 19-D, 20-D, 21-A, 22-A, 23-B, 24-D

■ SUGGESTED READING

1. Panel on Antiretroviral Guidelines for Adults and Adolescents. Guidelines for the use of antiretroviral agents in HIV-1-infected adults and adolescents. Department of Health and Human Services. [online] Available from: http://aidsinfo.nih.gov/contentfiles/lvguidelines/AdultandAdolescentGL.pdf. [Last accessed June, 2020].
2. Braun DL, Kouyos RD, Balmer B, Grube C, Weber R, Günthard HF, et al. Frequency and Spectrum of Unexpected Clinical Manifestations of Primary HIV-1 Infection. Clin Infect Dis. 2015;61(6):1013-21.
3. Crowell TA, Colby DJ, Pinyakorn S, Fletcher JLK, Kroon E, Schuetz A, et al. Acute retroviral syndrome is associated with high viral burden, CD4 depletion, and immune activation in systemic and tissue compartments. Clin Infect Dis. 2018;66(10):1540-9.
4. Samji H, Cescon A, Hogg RS, Modur SP, Althoff KN, Buchacz K, et al. Closing the gap: increases in life expectancy among treated HIV-positive individuals in the United States and Canada. PLoS One. 2013;8(12):e81355.
5. World Health Organization. WHO case definitions of HIV for surveillance and revised clinical staging and immunologic classification of HIV-related disease in adults and children. Geneva, Switzerland: World Health Organization; 2007. pp. 1-48.
6. Centers for Disease Control and Prevention (CDC). Revised surveillance case definition for HIV infection--United States, 2014. MMWR Recomm Rep. 2014;63(RR-03):1-10.
7. Brooks JT, Kaplan JE, Holmes KK, Benson C, Pau A, Masur H. HIV-associated opportunistic infections--going, going, but not gone: the continued need for prevention and treatment guidelines. Clin Infect Dis. 2009;48(5):609-11.
8. Aberg JA, Gallant JE, Ghanem KG, Emmanuel P, Zingman BS, Horberg MA, et al. Primary care guidelines for the management of persons infected with HIV: 2013 update by the HIV medicine association of the Infectious Diseases Society of America. Clin Infect Dis. 2014;58(1):e1-34.
9. Djawe K, Buchacz K, Hsu L, Chen MJ, Selik RM, Rose C, et al. Mortality Risk After AIDS-Defining Opportunistic Illness Among HIV-Infected Persons--San Francisco, 1981-2012. J Infect Dis. 2015;212(9):1366-75.
10. Saag MS, Benson CA, Gandhi RT, Hoy JF, Landovitz RJ, Mugavero MJ, et al. Antiretroviral Drugs for Treatment and Prevention of HIV Infection in Adults: 2018 Recommendations of the International Antiviral Society-USA Panel. JAMA. 2018;320(4):379-96.
11. Cahn P, Andrade-Villanueva J, Arribas JR, Gatell JM, Lama JR, Norton M, et al. Dual therapy with lopinavir and ritonavir plus lamivudine versus triple therapy with lopinavir and ritonavir plus two nucleoside reverse transcriptase inhibitors in antiretroviral-therapy-naive adults with HIV-1 infection: 48 week results of the randomised, open label, non-inferiority GARDEL trial. Lancet Infect Dis. 2014;14(7):572-80.
12. Emu B, Fessel J, Schrader S, Kumar P, Richmond G, Win S, et al. Phase 3 Study of Ibalizumab for Multidrug-Resistant HIV-1. N Engl J Med. 2018;379:645-54.
13. Huesgen E, DeSear KE, Egelund EF, Smith R, Max B, Janelle J. A HAART-breaking review of alternative antiretroviral administration: Practical considerations with crushing and enteral tube scenarios. Pharmacotherapy. 2016;36(11):1145-65.

CHAPTER 15

Sexually Transmitted Diseases

Sexually transmitted diseases (STDs) are a group of communicable diseases that are transmitted predominantly by sexual contact and caused by a wide range of bacterial, viral, protozoal and fungal agents and ectoparasites (**Box 15.1**).

■ GONORRHOEA

Gonorrhoea is a sexually transmitted infection (STI) due to the gram-negative diplococcus *Neisseria gonorrhoeae*.

Mode of transmission: Genito-genital, ano-genital, oro-genital and oro-anal contact or from mother-to-child transmission during delivery

Incubation period: Usually 2–10 days following exposure

Box 15.1: Sexually transmitted infections.

Bacterial agents
- *Neisseria gonorrhoeae*
- *Chlamydia trachomatis*
- *Haemophilus ducreyi*
- *Mycoplasma hominis*
- *Ureaplasma urealyticum*
- *Calymmatobacterium granulomatis*
- *Shigella* species
- Group B *Streptococcus*
- Bacterial vaginosis-associated organisms

Viral agents
- Human (alpha) herpesvirus
- Human (beta) herpesvirus
- Hepatitis B virus
- Human papillomavirus
- Molluscum contagiosum virus
- Human immunodeficiency virus

Protozoal agents
- *Entamoeba histolytica*
- *Giardia lamblia*
- *Trichomonas vaginalis*

Fungal agents
- *Candida albicans*

Ectoparasites
- *Phthirus pubis*
- *Sarcoptes scabiei*

Clinical Features

- Gonococcal infections in men: Acute urethritis
- Gonococcal infections in women: Gonococcal cervicitis and vaginitis. It may be asymptomatic in up to 80% of women.
- Anorectal and pharyngeal gonorrhoea are usually asymptomatic.
- Ocular gonorrhoea
- Disseminated gonococcal infection (DGI): Arthritis of one or more joints (asymmetric and migratory), pustular skin lesions, fever and tenosynovitis. Gonococcal endocarditis or meningitis may rarely occur.
- Acute perihepatitis (Fitz-Hugh–Curtis syndrome) is a rare complication of pelvic inflammatory disease (PID) and is thought to occur through direct extension of *Neisseria gonorrhoeae* from fallopian tube to liver capsule and peritoneum along the paracolic gutters. Patients present with sharp pleuritic right upper quadrant pain.

Diagnosis

- **Gram's staining and culture** of urethral exudates, genital, rectal, pharyngeal or ocular secretions show gram-negative intracellular monococci and diplococci.
- **Sterile pyuria:** Urine may show polymorphonuclear leucocytes with a negative urine culture report.

Complications

If untreated, infections can develop following complications

Treatment

Treatment of gonorrhoea is given in **Box 15.2**.

■ NON-GONOCOCCAL URETHRITIS

Causes of non-gonococcal urethritis (NGU) are given in **Box 15.3**.

Treatment
- Doxycycline 100 mg twice daily for 7 days OR
- Azithromycin 1 g orally

Alternatives
- Erythromycin base 500 mg four times for 7 days OR
- Ofloxacin 300 mg twice daily for 7 days OR
- Levofloxacin 500 mg once daily for 7 days
- All sex partners in last 60 days should be evaluated and treated.

Box 15.2: Treatment of gonorrhoea.

- One of the following regimens is recommended at present:
  - Cefixime, 400 mg orally (single dose)
  - Ceftriaxone, 250 mg intramuscularly (single dose)
  - Spectinomycin, 2 g intramuscularly (single dose)
- If quinolone and azithromycin resistance is not a problem:
  - Ciprofloxacin, 500 mg orally (single dose)
  - Ofloxacin, 400 mg orally (single dose)
  - Levofloxacin, 250 mg orally (single dose)
  - Azithromycin, 2 mg orally (single dose)
- For epididymo-orchitis doxycycline 100 mg twice daily for 14 days along with one dose of ceftriaxone

---

Box 15.3: Causes of non-gonococcal urethritis.

Chlamydia trachomatis (15–40%)
- Others (20–50%)
  - *Trichomonas vaginalis*
  - *Ureaplasma urealyticum*
  - Herpes simplex virus (in absence of skin lesions)
  - Adenovirus
  - Haemophilus

Mycoplasma genitalium (15–25%)
- Miscellaneous
  - In association with urinary tract infection, bacterial prostatitis, urethral stricture, phimosis, secondary to instrumentation of the urethra, congenital abnormalities, chemical irritation, tumours

---

- Sexual abstinence till completion of treatment.
- Patients with NGU reviewed 2–3 weeks after treatment to confirm resolution of symptoms and treatment of sexual contacts.
- Should be checked for other STIs including syphilis and HIV (human immunodeficiency virus); results of tests checked during review.

■ CHANCROID

Chancroid or soft chancre is an acute STI caused by *Haemophilus ducreyi*. It is characterised by painful genital ulcerations and inguinal adenitis.

- **Lesion in the external genitalia:**
  - **Sites of lesions:** Prepuce and frenulum in men and vaginal entrance and the perineum in women. At the site of inoculation (the external genitalia), an initial erythematous papule appears which then breaks down within 2–3 days into a classic chancroidal ulcer which is superficial, circumscribed and painful. Ulcers have ragged and undermined edges, and necrotic base, bleeds easily and generally not indurated.
- **Lymphadenopathy:** About 50% of patients develop enlarged, painful, tender inguinal lymph nodes (usually unilateral). The involved nodes become matted and progress to form large unilocular buboes which suppurate.

Diagnosis
- It is based on the microscopic identification and culture isolation of *H. ducreyi* in scrapings from ulcer or pus from bubo.
- Polymerase chain reaction (PCR) technique is not commercially available.
- Detection of antibody to *H. ducreyi* using enzyme immunoassay (EIA) may be useful.

Treatment options for chancroid are given in **Box 15.4**.

Box 15.4: Treatment options for chancroid.

- Azithromycin, 1 g orally as a single dose, OR
- Ceftriaxone, 250 mg by intramuscular injection as a single dose, OR
- Ciprofloxacin, 500 mg orally, twice daily for 3 days, OR
- Erythromycin base, 500 mg orally 4 times daily for 7 days

LYMPHOGRANULOMA VENEREUM

It is a sexually transmitted disease caused by *Chlamydia trachomatis* (types LGV 1, 2 and 3).

Clinical Features

Incubation period: 3–30 days.

Stages: Three characteristic stages—
1. **Primary genital lesion:** Lymphogranuloma venereum (LGV) starts as a small asymptomatic painless papule. at the site of inoculation (external genitalia) which tends to ulcerate.
2. **Regional lymphadenopathy**
3. **Buboes:** Later in the course, the lymph nodes may become matted, fluctuant (buboes) and rupture. The overlying skin becomes thinned, inflamed and fixed. Extensive enlargement of inguinal lymph nodes above and below the inguinal ligament ('groove sign') can develop.

Diagnosis

- **Detection of nucleic acid (DNA):** Direct immunofluorescence antibody and nucleic acid amplification tests are positive which should be confirmed by real time PCR for LGV-specific DNA.
- **Isolation of the LGV (L1–3 serotypes) strain of *Chlamydia*:** Tissue culture from swab obtained from the ulcer, aspirated pus from the bubo or swabs from infected tissue such as the rectum, urethra or the endocervix or from other infected tissue is the most specific test; however, sensitivity is only 75–85%.
- **Serological tests:** For example, microimmunofluorescence (micro-IF) test, complement fixation test (CF) to detect antibodies
- Frei skin test is not useful.

Treatment

Treatment options for LGV are given in **Box 15.5**.

Box 15.5: Treatment options for lymphogranuloma venereum.

- Doxycycline, 100 mg orally, twice daily for 14 days, OR
- Erythromycin, 500 mg orally, 4 times daily for 14 days, OR
- Tetracycline, 500 mg orally, 4 times daily for 14 days

GRANULOMA INGUINALE (DONOVANOSIS)

Granuloma inguinale is a genital ulcerative disease caused due to intracellular gram-negative bacterium *Klebsiella granulomatis* (Donovan bodies).

Clinical Features

Incubation period: 3–40 days

Genital lesions:
- Painless, progressive ulcerative lesions without regional lymphadenopathy
- Genital lesions are highly vascular, produce 'beefy-red appearance' and bleed easily on touch. However, they can also produce hypertrophic granulomatous, necrotic or sclerotic lesions.

Diagnosis

Microscopy examination of material from the lesion (tissue crush preparation or biopsy) shows dark, bipolar-staining intracellular Donovan bodies. The causative organism is difficult to culture.

Treatment

Treatment options for granuloma inguinale are given in **Box 15.6**.

SYPHILIS

Syphilis (lues), a **chronic,** systemic infection **caused by spirochaete *Treponema pallidum,*** is usually **sexually transmitted**. Spirochaetes are slender, cork-screw shaped gram-negative bacteria.
- **Mode of transmission:**
  - *Sexual contact:* It is the usual mode of spread.

Box 15.6: Treatment options for granuloma inguinale.

- Azithromycin, 1 g orally on the first day, then 500 mg orally, once a day, OR
- Doxycycline, 100 mg orally, twice daily, OR
- Erythromycin, 500 mg orally, 4 times daily, OR
- Tetracycline, 500 mg orally, 4 times daily, OR
- Trimethoprim 80 mg/sulphamethoxazole 400 mg, 2 tablets orally, twice daily

- *Transplacental transmission:* From mother with active disease to the foetus (during pregnancy) → congenital syphilis
- *Blood transfusion*
- *Direct contact:* Open lesion is a rare mode of transmission.

Classification

Classification of syphilis is given in **Box 15.7**.

Fig. 15.1 describes the Course of syphilis (if untreated).

Acquired Syphilis
- **Primary syphilis**
  - *Primary chancre:* It is the classical lesion of primary syphilis.
    - Location: The primary chancre develops at the site of inoculation.
      - In males: **Penis or scrotum** in males (in heterosexual) and in homosexual males, it may occur in the anal canal, rectum or within the mouth.
      - In females: **Cervix, vulva** and **vaginal** wall.
    - Primary chancre is single, firm, **nontender (painless)**, slightly raised, **red papule** (chancre) up to several centimetres in diameter. It rapidly becomes eroded to create a clean-based shallow ulcer. Because of the induration surrounding the ulcer, it is designated as **hard chancre**.
  - *Regional lymphadenitis*
- **Secondary syphilis**
  - *Mucocutaneous lesions:* These are painless, superficial lesions and contain spirochaetes and are infectious.
  - *Skin rashes (75%):* They begin as **discrete red-brown macules**.
  - *Condylomata lata (10%):* In moist, warm, intertriginous areas of the skin, such as the **anogenital region (perineum, vulva and scrotum)**, inner thighs and axillae
  - *Mucosal lesions (30%):* Usually occurs in the mucous membranes of **oral cavity (lip, oral** mucosa, tongue, palate and pharynx) **or** vulva, vagina or glans penis **as silvery-grey superficial** mucosal **erosions**. They are surrounded by a red serpiginous periphery and are usually painless. Rarely, they may coalesce to produce characteristic 'snail track' ulcers in the mouth.

> **Box 15.7: Classification of syphilis.**
>
> **Acquired syphilis**
> - Primary syphilis
> - Secondary syphilis
> - Latent syphilis
> - Late syphilis (tertiary)
>   - Late latent
>   - Benign tertiary
>   - Quaternary syphilis (cardiovascular and neurosyphilis)
>
> **Congenital syphilis**
> - Intrauterine death and perinatal death
> - Early (infantile)
> - Late (tardive)

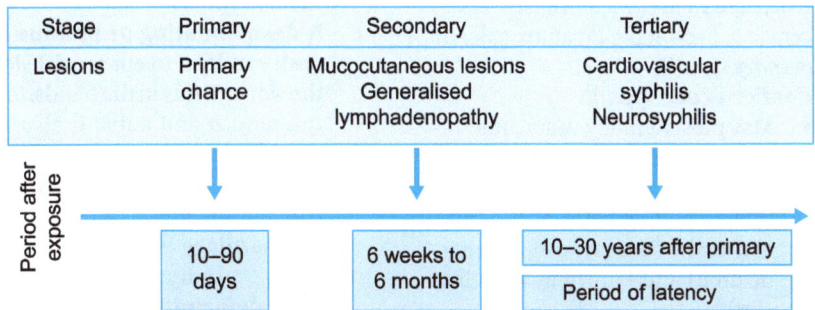

Fig. 15.1: Course of syphilis (if untreated).

Generalised painless lymphadenopathy: Generalised, firm non-tender lymphadenopathy occurs in about 50% of patients. They involve especially **epitrochlear nodes.**

Less common manifestations include meningitis, cranial nerve palsies, anterior or posterior uveitis, hepatitis, gastritis, glomerulonephritis (proteinuria, nephrotic syndrome or haemorrhagic glomerulonephritis) or arthritis and periostitis.

- **Latent syphilis**
  - *Early latency (within 1 year of infection):* During this period, syphilis may be transmitted sexually.
  - *Late latency (begins at 1 year of infection):* During this, the patient is no longer sexually infectious. Pregnant women with latent syphilis may infect the foetus in utero.
- **Late (tertiary) syphilis**
  - *Late latent syphilis*
    - This phase may persist for many years or for life.
    - No symptoms or signs of syphilis
    - More than 60% of patients suffer little or no ill health even without treatment.
  - *Benign tertiary (gummatous) syphilis*
    - It is called benign because of its response to therapy rather than its clinical manifestations.
    - It may develop after 3–10 years after initial infection.
    - Structures involved: Skin (frequently at sites of trauma as nodules or ulcers), mucous membranes (mouth, pharynx, larynx or nasal septum appear as punched-out ulcers), bone (e.g. skull, tibia, fibula and clavicle), muscle or viscera (e.g. liver-hepar lobatum, spleen)
  - *Quaternary syphilis*
    - *Cardiovascular syphilis*
      - May present many years after initial infection
      - Most frequently involves the aorta (the ascending aorta, aortic valve and/or the coronary ostia, the aortic arch) and known as syphilitic aortitis
      - Clinical features include angina, features of aortic incompetence and aortic aneurysm.
    - *Neurosyphilis:* It may take years to develop. It may be asymptomatic or symptomatic.
      - *Asymptomatic neurosyphilis:* It is detected by cerebrospinal fluid (CSF) examination, which shows pleocytosis (increased numbers of inflammatory cells), elevated protein levels or decreased glucose. Antibodies can also be detected in the CSF, which is the most specific test for neurosyphilis.
      - *Symptomatic disease:* Takes one of several forms:
        ◊ *Chronic meningo-vascular disease:* Chronic meningitis → involves base of the brain, cerebral convexities and spinal leptomeninges.
        ◊ *Tabes dorsalis:* It is characterised by **demyelination of posterior column, dorsal root and dorsal root ganglia**.
        ◊ *General paresis of insane:* Shows generalised brain parenchymal disease with **dementia**; hence called general paresis of insane.

Congenital Syphilis

- **Intrauterine death and perinatal death**
- **Early (infantile) congenital syphilis:** It manifests within the **first 2 years of life** and is often manifested by **nasal discharge** (rhinitis) and congestion (**snuffles**). It resembles features of secondary syphilis.
  - A **desquamating or bullous eruption/rash** can lead to epidermal sloughing of the skin, mainly in the hands, feet, around the mouth and anus. It also may show condylomata lata.
  - **Skeletal abnormalities:** Syphilitic osteochondritis (inflammation of bone and cartilage is more distinctive in the nose → produces characteristic **saddle nose deformity**), **syphilitic periostitis**

(involves the tibia and leads to anterior bowing, or **saber shin**).
- Others organs involved include **liver** (diffuse fibrosis) and **lungs** (airless-pneumonia)
- **Late (tardive) congenital syphilis**
  - Manifests **2 years after birth**, and about 50% of untreated children with neonatal syphilis will develop late manifestations and take the form of 'stigmata' relating to early damage to developing structures, particularly teeth and long bones (**Box 15.8**).

- Distinctive manifestation is **Hutchinson's triad**: (1) **interstitial keratitis**, (2) **Hutchinson's teeth** (small widely spaced screwdriver or peg-shaped upper central incisors, with notches in the enamel) and (3) **eighth-nerve deafness**. Stigmata of congenital syphilis are listed in **Box 15.6**.

Laboratory Diagnosis
- Demonstration of *Treponema pallidum*
  - **Dark-field microscopy**
  - Direct fluorescent antibody *T. pallidum* (DFA-TP) test
- **Serological tests (Table 15.1)**

Management
Management of syphilis is given in **Table 15.2**.

■ APPROACH TO A CASE OF GENITAL ULCER [GENITAL ULCER DISEASE (GUD)]

Definition
Ulcerative, erosive, pustular or vesicular lesions on the genitalia with or without lymphadenopathy

Aetiology
Aetiology given in **Box 15.9**.
Table 15.3 describes the epidemiology and natural course of common GUDs.

Box 15.8: Stigmata of congenital syphilis.
- Hutchinson's incisors (anterior–posterior thickening with notch on narrowed cutting edge)
- Mulberry molars (imperfectly formed cusps/deficient dental enamel)
- High-arched palate
- Maxillary hypoplasia
- Saddle nose
- Rhagades (radiating scars around mouth, nose and anus following rash)
- Salt and pepper scars on retina (from choroiditis)
- Corneal scars (from interstitial keratitis)
- Sabre tibia (from periostitis)
- Bossing of frontal and parietal bones (healed periosteal nodes)

TABLE 15.1: Sensitivity of serological tests in untreated syphilis.

Test	Stage of disease [percent positive (range)]			
	Primary	Secondary	Latent	Tertiary
VDRL	78 (74–87)	100	95 (88–100)	71 (37–94)
RPR	86 (77–99)	100	98 (95–100)	73
FTA-ABS*	84 (70–100)	100	100	96
Treponemal Agglutination*	76 (69–90)	100	97 (97–100)	94
EIA	93	100	100	

*FTA-ABS and TP-PA are generally considered equally sensitive in the primary stage of disease.
(EIA: enzyme immunoassay; FTA-ABS: fluorescent treponemal antibody absorption; RPR: rapid plasma reagin; TP-PA: Treponema pallidum particle agglutination; VDRL: venereal disease research laboratory)

TABLE 15.2: Management of syphilis.

Stage	Drug	Regimen
Primary	Procaine penicillin	6,00,000 units IM once daily for 12 days
	Oxytetracycline	500 mg orally four times daily for 15 days
	Doxycycline	100 mg orally two times daily for 15 days
	Benzathine penicillin	2.4 mega (million) units IM single dose (1.2 million units in each buttock)
Secondary	Procaine penicillin	6,00,000 units IM once daily for 15 days
	Benzathine penicillin	2.4 million units IM single dose
Early latent	Benzathine penicillin	2.4 million units IM single dose
Late latent/tertiary	Benzathine penicillin	2.4 million units IM weekly for 3 weeks
Cardiovascular	Benzathine penicillin	0.4 million units IM weekly for 3 weeks
Neurosyphilis	Crystalline penicillin	18–24 million units/day for 10–14 days
	Procaine penicillin PLUS Probenecid	2.4 million units/day IM for 10–14 days PLUS 500 mg QID for 10–14 days

(IM: intramuscular)

> **Box 15.9: Aetiology of GUD.**
>
> **STD-related aetiologies and organisms:**
> - Genital herpes: Herpes simplex virus Type 1 and Type 2
> - Primary syphilis: *Treponema pallidum* var. pallidum
> - Chancroid: *Haemophilus ducreyi*
> - Lymphogranuloma venereum (LGV): *Chlamydia trachomatis* serovars L1-L3
> - Granuloma inguinale (Donovanosis): *Calymmatobacterium granulomatis*
>
> **Non-STD-related aetiologies:**
> - Non-STD infections: *Candida*, CMV, EBV, mycobacteria, *Staphylococcus*
> - Noninfectious: Behcet's, Reiter's, cancer, trauma, aphthous and fixed-drug eruptions
>
> **No aetiology is found in 20% to 30–50% of GUD cases**
>
> (CMV: cytomegalovirus; EBV: Epstein–Barr virus; GUD: genital ulcer disease; STD: sexually transmitted disease)

TABLE 15.3: Epidemiology and natural course of common GUDs.

Disease	Incubation period	% of STI-related GUD	Spontaneous healing time	On treatment
Primary syphilis	9–90 days (average 3 weeks)	>1	• 3–8 weeks • Never exceeds 3 months	1–2 weeks
Chancroid	1–14 days	<1	Self-limiting but may persist for years	1–2 weeks
Herpes genitalis	5–21 days	80–95	14–21 days	6–12 days
LGV	3–30 days	<1	2–5 days	–
Donovanosis	1–180 days	<1	No tendency for healing	3 weeks

(GUD: genital ulcer disease; LGV: lymphogranuloma venereum; STI: sexually transmitted infection)

TABLE 15.4: Clinical manifestations of common GUDs.

Characteristic	Syphilis	Herpes	Chancroid	LGV	Donovanosis
Primary lesion	Papule	Vesicle	Pustule	Papule, vesicle pustule	Papule
Number of lesions	Usually one	Multiple	Multiple	Single	Variable
Diameter	5–15 mm	1–2 mm	Variable	2–10 mm	Variable
Edges	Sharply demarcated elevated	Erythematous Polycyclic	Undermined Ragged	Elevated Round or oval	Elevated Irregular
Depth	Superficial or deep	Superficial	Excavated	Superficial or deep	Elevated
Base	Smooth Non-purulent Covered with serous exudate	Erythematous	Purulent Dirty grey Base	Variable	Red Velvety Bleeds easily
Induration	Button hole	None	Not indurated	Not indurated	Not indurated
Pain	Absent	Present	Present	Absent	Absent
Lymph nodes	Bilateral Non-tender Firm, lead-shot, non-suppurative	Bilateral Tender Firm Non-suppurative	Unilateral Tender Suppurative Unilocular	Unilateral Tender Suppurative Multilocular	None Pseudo-bubo seen

(LGV: lymphogranuloma venereum)

Table 15.4 describes the clinical manifestations of common GUDs.

BEST OF FIVES

1. A 23-year-old man who lives with his male partner consults you for an opinion. He has been suffering from anal discharge and pruritis for the past 3 days. There are also some symptoms of dysuria. A urethral smear reveals intracellular diplococci. What is the most likely infective agent to fit with this clinical picture?
   A. *Neisseria gonorrhoeae*
   B. *Chlamydia trachomatis*
   C. *Treponema pallidum*
   D. Herpes simplex-type 1
   E. Herpes simplex-type 2

2. A 24-year-old homosexual man has been diagnosed with anal carcinoma. Which pathogen is responsible for this?
   A. Human herpesvirus 8 (HHV8)
   B. Human T-cell lymphotropic virus type I (HTLV-I)
   C. Hepatitis C virus (HCV)
   D. Cytomegalovirus (CMV)
   E. Human papillomavirus (HPV)

3. An 18-year-old woman has been diagnosed with human papillomavirus infection. What is the most significant long-term risk following this infection?
   A. Coronary artery disease
   B. Endometriosis
   C. Infertility
   D. Cervical cancer
   E. Carcinoma of the endometrium

4. A 23-year-old student taking the oral contraceptive pill develops pain and soreness around the genitals. On examination there are multiple, shallow and tender ulcers at the skin and mucous membrane of the vagina. The most probable diagnosis is:
   A. Genital herpes

B. Chancroid
C. Granuloma inguinale
D. Primary syphilis
E. Lymphogranuloma venereum

5. A 36-year-old woman presents complaining of a yellowish-green vaginal discharge that started 1 week ago. On examination, her vagina is swollen and erythematous. What is the most likely diagnosis?
   A. Candidiasis
   B. Trichomoniasis
   C. Acquired immunodeficiency syndrome (AIDS)
   D. Papillomavirus infection
   E. Lactobacilli infection

6. A 22-year-old male has recently had unprotected sex and has noticed the development of a firm lesion on his penis. He states that it began as a small bump which then ulcerated and became a firm lesion. It is not painful. He has associated inguinal lymphadenopathy which is not painful. You suspect syphilis; however, his enzyme-linked immunosorbent assay (EIA), fluorescent treponemal antibody absorption (FTA-ABS), Treponema pallidum haemagglutination (TPHA) and Venereal Disease Research Laboratory (VDRL) tests are negative. Which other test if positive will confirm early primary syphilis?
   A. Cerebrospinal fluid (CSF) sample
   B. Positive dark ground microscopy
   C. Repeat VDRL in a few weeks
   D. Negative dark ground microscopy
   E. Blood cultures

7. A 22-year-old male has just returned from Africa and presents with painful inguinal lymphadenopathy. He states that he had noticed a painless ulcer on his penis about 1 week ago and then he noticed very tender lumps in his groins. The lymph nodes on examination are tender and fixed and the skin overlying is a dusky erythematous colour. Some of them are fluctuant. What is the most likely diagnosis?
   A. Chancroid
   B. Genital warts
   C. Lymphogranuloma venereum
   D. Herpes simplex virus
   E. Syphilis

8. A 21-year-old man was admitted to a hospital with a 5-day history of fever and vomiting. He also complained of knee and ankle pains. He was homosexual and had last had receptive anal intercourse 6 weeks ago. On examination, he had a widespread erythematous macular rash. His temperature was 37.5°C, pulse was 85 beats per minute and blood pressure was 115/60 mmHg. There was no joint swelling. What is the most likely diagnosis?
   A. Acute hepatitis B
   B. Acute hepatitis C
   C. Acute HIV (human immunodeficiency virus) infection
   D. Gonococcal bacteraemia
   E. Secondary syphilis

9. A 19-year-old female presents with vaginal discharge. She has also noticed dysuria and post-coital bleeding. On examination, the cervix has a cobblestone appearance and there is contact bleeding. Given the most likely diagnosis, what treatment is most useful?
   A. Single dose 1 g azithromycin
   B. Single dose IM 250 mg ceftriaxone
   C. 200 mg Doxycycline 1-week course
   D. 200 mg Doxycycline single dose
   E. 400 mg Ofloxacin 1-week course

10. The Centers for Disease Control and Prevention has recommended gonorrhoea treatment with an injectable third-generation cephalosporin and azithromycin. Which of the following answers is the correct rationale for this recommendation?
    A. Azithromycin should be used in conjunction with an injectable third-generation cephalosporin to provide therapy with two different mechanisms of action, thereby delaying emergence of resistance
    B. There is a high rate of concomitant chlamydial infection as well as an increasing recognition of *Mycoplasma genitalium* coinfection that should be treated
    C. Cefixime and azithromycin may be used in some settings without further follow-up
    D. Moxifloxacin may be used to treat *M. genitalium* as well as *Neisseria gonorrhoeae*
    E. Synergistic action causing early clearance

11. Male circumcision is currently recommended by the World Health Organization/Joint United Nations Programme on HIV and AIDS (WHO/UNAIDS). Which of the following statements is incorrect regarding male circumcision?
    A. The long-term effectiveness of male circumcision is well described and has been demonstrated in several studies.
    B. Sexually transmitted infection (STI) prevention trials that incorporate interventions such as circumcision may lead to a bias/blunting of effect compared with community standards of care.
    C. Male circumcision demonstrated greater than 75% reduction in human immunodeficiency virus (HIV) acquisition during a 5-year period in at least two African trials.
    D. Circumcision was not accepted by men after completion of the trial.
    E. Circumcised men were more likely to engage in risky sexual behaviours compared with uncircumcised men.

12. A 27-year-old male with recent unprotected anal and oral sex with anonymous male partners presents for evaluation of a diffuse rash and low-grade fever. Identify the appropriate clinical response(s).
    A. Thorough history and physical examination, fourth-generation HIV (human immunodeficiency virus) test, HIV viral load, rapid plasma reagin (RPR), admission for lumbar puncture (LP) and ophthalmological examination
    B. Sexually transmitted disease (STD) testing and empiric benzathine penicillin; it is too soon for another HIV test
    C. Post-exposure prophylaxis for HIV
    D. HIV and STD testing to include RPR and instructions to follow up in the clinic next week
    E. Reassurance and review after 3 weeks

13. Which of the following statements regarding granuloma inguinale is correct?
    A. It is transmitted efficiently and only by sexual contact.
    B. The initial lesion is typically painful and associated with fever.
    C. Lesions are associated with buboes.
    D. Diagnosis requires demonstration of intracellular Donovan bodies.
    E. Diagnosis requires serologic confirmation.

14. A 17-year-old woman comes to your office requesting contraception. She recently started a new relationship with a man and sometimes uses condoms. Her test result comes back positive for both gonorrhoea and chlamydial infection. You call the patient to give her the results and arrange her follow-up. Which of the following would be part of your initial management of this patient?
    A. Have the patient return to your office for treatment with ceftriaxone 250 mg IM plus azithromycin 1 g PO as a single dose.
    B. Arrange for the patient to return to your office for follow-up testing in 3 months.
    C. Ask the patient to bring her partner to your office with her so that he can be treated.
    D. Talk to the patient and her partner about condoms and risk reduction when she returns to see you and advise them to abstain from sex for 1 week after the completion of both of their treatment.
    E. All of the above

15. A 29-year-old man comes to your clinic with pain and swelling affecting his right knee. He did have unprotected vaginal sex with two sex workers during his trip. About 1 week ago, he developed pain in his wrists, fingers and ankles. You perform an arthrocentesis, which reveals 30,000 white blood cells (90% polymorphonuclear neutrophils) with no crystals and no organism seen on Gram stain. Synovial fluid culture is pending. Which of the following is not indicated?
    A. Call orthopaedics to perform open drainage of the knee.
    B. Obtain culture specimens and nucleic acid amplification test (NAAT) specimens for gonorrhoea from all anatomic sites of potential sexual exposure to gonorrhoea and a synovial fluid sample for NAAT.

C. Obtain blood culture samples.
D. Initiate therapy with ceftriaxone and vancomycin while awaiting additional laboratory information.
E. Test the patient for HIV (human immunodeficiency virus) infection and syphilis.

Answers

1-A, 2-E, 3-D, 4-A, 5-B, 6-B, 7-C, 8-D, 9-A, 10-A, 11-C, 12-A, 13-D, 14-E, 15-A

SUGGESTED READING

1. Workowski KA, Bolan GA, Centers for Disease Control and Prevention. Sexually transmitted diseases treatment guidelines, 2015. MMWR Recomm Rep. 2015;64(RR-03):1-137.
2. LeFevre ML, U.S. Preventive Services Task Force. Screening for Chlamydia and gonorrhea: U.S. Preventive Services Task Force recommendation statement. Ann Intern Med. 2014;161(12):902-10.
3. U.S. Preventive Services Task Force. Bibbins-Domingo K, Grossman DC, Curry SJ, Davidson KW, Epling Jr JW. Final recommendation statement: Syphilis infection in nonpregnant adults and adolescents: Screening. June 2016. [online] Available from: http://www.uspreventiveservicestaskforce.org/Page/Document/RecommendationStatementFinal/syphilis-infection-in-nonpregnant-adults-and-adolescents. [Last accessed June, 2020].
4. US Preventive Services Task Force, Bibbins-Domingo K, Grossman DC, Curry SJ, Davidson KW, Epling Jr JW, et al. Serologic Screening for Genital Herpes Infection: US Preventive Services Task Force Recommendation Statement. JAMA. 2016;316(23):2525-30.
5. Aberg JA, Gallant JE, Ghanem KG, Emmanuel P, Zingman BS, Horberg MA, et al. Primary care guidelines for the management of persons infected with HIV: 2013 update by the HIV medicine association of the Infectious Diseases Society of America. Clin Infect Dis. 2014;58(1):e1-34.
6. Committee on Adolescence, Society for Adolescent Health and Medicine. Screening for nonviral sexually transmitted infections in adolescents and young adults. Pediatrics. 2014;134(1):e302-11.
7. Ghanem KG, Workowski KA. Management of adult syphilis. Clin Infect Dis. 2011;53 Suppl 3:S110-28.
8. Gottlieb SL, Berman SM, Low N. Screening and treatment to prevent sequelae in women with Chlamydia trachomatis genital infection: how much do we know? J Infect Dis. 2010;201 Suppl 2:S156-67.
9. Manhart LE, Broad JM, Golden MR. Mycoplasma genitalium: should we treat and how? Clin Infect Dis. 2011;53 Suppl 3:S129-42.
10. Ross JD, Lewis DA. Cephalosporin resistant Neisseria gonorrhoeae: time to consider gentamicin? Sex Transm Infect. 2012;88(1):6-8.
11. Unemo M, Bradshaw CS, Hocking JS, de Vries HJC, Francis SC, Mabey D, et al. Sexually transmitted infections: challenges ahead. Lancet Infect Dis. 2017;17(8):e235-79.

CHAPTER 16

Diseases of the Nervous System

■ UPPER MOTOR VERSUS LOWER MOTOR NEURON LESION

Differences between upper motor neuron (UMN) and lower motor neuron (LMN) lesion are given in **Table 16.1**.

Apraxia
- Disorder of learnt motor act in the absence of weakness, in co-ordination, sensory loss of failure to comprehend commands
- Ideomotor apraxia seen with left parietal lobe lesions
- In dressing apraxia seen with right parietal lobe lesions

Agnosia
Lack of recognition of objects, individuals, sounds, forms or smells despite the sensory system being intact. It is caused by contralateral parietal lobe lesions.

■ APHASIA
Aphasia is loss or defective language content of speech resulting from damage to the speech centres within the dominant (usually left in 97%) hemisphere (**Table 16.2**).

■ SUMMARY OF FUNCTIONS OF LOBES
The functions of lobes are summarised in **Table 16.3**.

TABLE 16.1: Differences between upper motor neuron (UMN) and lower motor neuron (LMN) lesion.

Signs	UMN	LMN
Weakness	Voluntary movements are disturbed.	Paralysis of muscles supplied by the segment or nerve
Tone	Hypertonia (clasp-knife spasticity)	Hypotonia
Deep tendon reflexes	Increased, ± clonus	Decreased or absent
Superficial reflexes	Absent or decreased	Absent or decreased
Plantar response	Extensor	Flexor or absent
Muscle nutrition	Disuse atrophy	Marked atrophy
Fasciculations	Absent	Present

TABLE 16.2: Types of aphasias.

Type of aphasia	Site of lesion	Compre-hension	Fluency	Repetition	Reading	Writing	Naming
Wernicke's/ sensory/receptive/ posterior	Infarction of inferior division of middle cerebral artery	Absent	Preserved	Absent	–	–	–
Broca's/ motor/ expressive/ anterior	Infarction of superior frontal branch of middle cerebral artery	Preserved	Absent	Absent	–	–	–
Global	Dominant frontal, parietal and superior temporal lobe	Absent	Absent	Absent	–	–	–
Conduction/ arcuate	Arcuate fascile	Preserved	Preserved	Absent	–	–	–
Transcortical sensory	Posterior watershed zone	Absent	Preserved	Preserved	–	–	–
Transcortical motor	Anterior watershed zone	Preserved	Absent	Preserved	–	–	–
Alexia without agraphia	Occipitotempo-ral region	Preserved	Preserved	Preserved	Lost	Preserved	–
Alexia with agraphia	Left angular gyrus	Preserved	Preserved	Preserved	Lost	Lost	–
Nominal/anomic/ amnesic	Temporoparietal	Preserved	Preserved	Preserved	Preserved	Preserved	Absent

TABLE 16.3: Functions and effects of damage to various lobes of cerebral hemispheres.

Lobe	Function	Cognitive/Behavioural effects of damage
Frontal Please **SMILE** (MNEMONIC)	**P**ersonality	Disinhibition
	Social behaviour	Lack of initiation
	Micturition	Anti-social behaviour
	Intelligence	Impaired memory
	Language	Expressive dysphasia
	Emotional response	Incontinence
Parietal: Dominant side	Language	Dysphasia, dyslexia
	Calculation	Acalculia
	Others	Apraxia, agnosia
Parietal: Non-dominant side	Spatial orientation	Spatial disorientation, neglect of contralateral side
	Constructional skills	Constructional apraxia, dressing apraxia

Continued

Continued

Lobe	Function	Cognitive/Behavioural effects of damage
Temporal: Dominant side	Auditory perception	Receptive aphasia
	Language	Dyslexia
	Verbal memory	Impaired verbal memory
	Smell	
	Balance	
Temporal: Non-dominant side	Auditory perception	Impaired non-verbal memory
	Melody/pitch perception	Impaired musical skills (tonal perception)
	Non-verbal memory	
	Smell	
	Balance	
Occipital	Visual processing	Visual inattention, visual loss, visual agnosia (Anton–Babinski syndrome)

Box 16.1: Causes of dementia.

Dementia without additional neurological deficits:
- Alzheimer's disease
- Pick's disease

Dementia with additional neurologic deficits:
- Multiple infarct dementia or vascular dementia
- Parkinson's disease
- Wilson disease
- Chronic infections (tuberculosis, fungal, HIV, progressive multifocal leucoencephalopathy, syphilis)
- Hydrocephalus (obstructive and non-obstructive)
- Normal pressure hydrocephalus
- Chronic subdural haematoma
- Lewy body dementia
- Brain neoplasms

Metabolic disorders:
- Dialysis dementia
- Hypothyroidism
- Hyperparathyroidism
- Uraemia
- Hepatic encephalopathy
- Porphyria
- Vitamin B12 deficiency
- Adrenal insufficiency
- Cushing's syndrome
- Chronic hypoglycaemia

Toxic causes:
- Heavy metal poisoning
- Chronic drug abuse

■ DEMENTIA

Dementia is a global deterioration of the higher mental functions.

Causes

Causes of dementia are given in **Box 16.1**.

Clinical Features

Mild Cognitive Impairment

Impairment of memory in relation to age and education of the patient, but preservation of overall cognitive function and intact daily operations. On MMSE, the patients generally score in the range of 26-28. It precedes to several types of dementia.

- Symptoms include memory lapses, reasoning and judgement.
- There are prevalent mood disorders such as sadness, rage and frustration.
- There are dysphasia, apraxia, agnosia, urinary incontinence and neurological focal deficits.
- Mood disorders such as sadness, anger and frustration are common.
- Dysphasia, apraxia, agnosia, urinary incontinence and focal neurological deficits occur.

ALZHEIMER'S DISEASE

It is the most common cause of cognitive impairment in elderly persons.

Potential acquired risk factors are given in **Box 16.2**.

Clinical Features

- A gradual decrease in activities of daily life leads to a deep disability and reliance on others.
- Patients have memory, language and visual disturbances: Impaired capacity to perform motor functions despite intact motor function (dyspraxia)
- Lack of object recognition or identification despite of intact sensory function (agnosia)

Other characteristics include behavioural issues, psychotic symptoms and depression; psychotic symptoms are not presenting characteristics but grow later during illness. Occurrence of psychosis during the original phases of dementia indicates other diagnoses such as Lewy bodies dementia. About 50% of patients experience persecutory delusions.

Laboratory Investigations

- These are carried out to exclude a treatable cause of dementia.
- Common laboratory tests are blood chemistry, a complete blood count, tests for syphilis, serum levels of vitamin B12 and thyroid functions.
- A computed tomography (CT) head is usually done to exclude an intracranial pathology.
- A magnetic resonance imaging (MRI) may show atrophy in the hippocampus, mesial and lateral temporal, isthmus cingulate and orbitofrontal areas. It is also required to detect presence of white matter ischaemic lesions indicating vascular dementia.

Management

Cognitive deficits: Inhibitors of cholinesterase are madepezil, rivastigmine, galantamine and tacrine. Although their precise function is not evident, other agents include vitamin E, statins and non-steroidal anti-inflammatory drugs (NSAIDs).

Co-morbid conditions:
- Optimal management of all co-morbid circumstances, including visual or hearing deficiencies, dental issues and other prevalent medical conditions should be given.
- Atypical antipsychotic medicines (risperidone and olanzapine) are preferred for psychosis management. Serotonin-reuptake inhibitors (e.g. citalopram, escitalopram and sertraline) are used for depression.

LUMBAR PUNCTURE

Indications

Indications of lumbar puncture are given in **Box 16.3**.

Contraindications

- Raised intracranial pressure (ICP)
- Spinal deformity
- Local infections
- Coagulation disorders

Box 16.2: Potential acquired risk factors of Alzheimer's disease.

- Ageing
- Family history of Alzheimer's disease
- Reduced reserve capacity of brain
- Low educational and occupational levels
- Low mental ability to early life
- Reduced mental and physical activity during old age
- Diet:
  - Reduced consumption of fish
  - Increased consumption of dietary fat
- Head injury
- Risk factors associated with vascular disease:
  - Hypercholesterolaemia
  - Hypertension
  - Smoking
  - Obesity
  - Diabetes

Box 16.3: Indications of lumbar puncture.

- Meningitis
- Encephalitis
- Guillain–Barré syndrome
- Acute demyelinating diseases
- Therapeutic indications
  - Methotrexate in leukaemia
  - Spinal anaesthesia
  - Benign intracranial hypertension

Common Cerebrospinal Fluid Abnormalites

- High cerebrospinal fluid (CSF) pressure: Raised ICP
- Blood stained: Traumatic puncture, subarachnoid haemorrhage (SAH)
- Xanthochromia: SAH, Froin's syndrome (spinal block), high serum bilirubin level
- Cobweb formation: Tuberculous meningitis (TBM)
- Low sugar: Pyogenic, tuberculous, fungal and carcinomatous meningitis, rheumatoid arthritis
- Raised protein: Inflammatory, infective, neoplastic and ischaemic disorders, Guillain-Barré syndrome (GBS)
- Polymorphonuclear reaction: Acute inflammation, mainly pyogenic meningitis
- Lymphocytic reaction: Chronic infective disorders such as TBM and fungal meningitis
- Oligoclonal Ig bands in multiple sclerosis

■ TRIGEMINAL NEURALGIA (TIC DOULOUREUX)

Clinical Features

Paroxysmal, sharp, shooting, electric shock-like pain and limited to the nerve distribution

- Commonly impacted are the maxillary and mandibular divisions. Rarely affects ophthalmic division.
- Touching trigger areas such as cold wind blowing on the face, washing the face, chewing or speaking, precipitates pain.
- Touch and vibration are more likely to cause more attacks than pinprick.
- Small regions around the face, nose and lips are the trigger zones.

Treatment

- Carbamazepine, phenytoin, clonazepam and gabapentin
- Injection of phenol or alcohol
- Radiofrequency thermal rhizotomy—heat lesion of trigeminal ganglion or nerve

■ BELL'S PALSY

Aetiology

Herpes simplex virus and herpes zoster are suspected.

Clinical Features

It is acute in onset. There is sometimes history of cold exposure. For a few days, mild pain in stylomastoid foramen may precede the paralysis. Examination displays isolated lower motor neuron type of facial palsy with or without hyperacusis and loss of taste sensation of anterior two-thirds of the tongue.

Investigations

- No specific confirmatory diagnostic procedure
- Electrophysiological tests [electromyography (EMG)] may help in prognostication.
- To rule out alternate diagnosis, appropriate diagnostic procedures may be necessary.

Treatment

- If patient is seen early (within 1 week), a short course of prednisolone may be given. Usually, prednisolone is given at 1 mg/kg/day for the 1st week, with the dosage tapering off over the 2nd week.
- Acyclovir
- Adhesive tape to maintain your eye shut to avoid ulceration of the cornea

■ RAMSAY HUNT SYNDROME (GENICULATE HERPES)

Aetiology

Herpes zoster of geniculate ganglion

Clinical Features

- Starts with severe pain in external ear, followed by appearance of vesicles in the external auditory canal, and occasionally tongue and pharynx, along with LMN facial paralysis. Eighth nerve palsy may be associated.
- Complete recovery is less likely than in Bell's palsy.

Treatment

- Analgesics
- Oral acyclovir 800 mg five times a day is useful if started early (within 72 h)
- Other agents are famciclovir (500 mg thrice daily) and valacyclovir (1 g thrice daily).
- Idoxuridine (5% solution) may be applied over the vesicles in early stages.

RAISED INTRACRANIAL PRESSURE

Causes
The causes of raised intracranial pressure are given in **Box 16.4**.

Clinical Features
- There is diffuse anterior headache and vomiting characteristics due to increased ICP.
- If ICP has increased sharply, the pulse rate may be slower and BP (**Cushing's reflex**) may be increased. Respiratory depression (Cushing's triad) is another element.
- More than a few days of raised ICP will lead to papilloedema.
- Other characteristics are drowsiness and coma.

Investigations
- Relevant to possible underlying pathology
- CT head may show midline shift and compressed basal cisterns.
- ICP monitoring in selected cases (e.g. those with Glasgow Coma Scale ≤ 8 with CT scan showing haematoma, contusion, oedema, herniation or compressed basal cisterns)

Treatment
- Medical:
    - Assisted ventilation to correct hypoxia and hypercarbia.
    - Administering normal saline to achieve a central venous pressure of 5–10 mmHg.
    - Osmotic diuretics:
        - Mannitol 0.25–1 g/kg dose
        - Glycerol 30 mL orally three to four times a day.
        - Frusemide 20 mg thrice daily
    - Steroids—dexamethasone 4 mg 6th hourly
    - Elevation of head by 15–30°C
- Surgical management:
    - Management of underlying cause
    - Removal of the space-occupying lesion
    - Ventriculo-atrial or ventriculo-peritoneal shunting to be done in hydrocephalus
    - Decompressive craniectomy
    - Surgical decompression to be done as a life-saving procedure by limited frontal or temporal lobectomies

HEADACHE

Classification of headache is given in **Table 16.4**.

Migraine
Migraine is characterised by periodic headaches, typically unilateral, often associated with visual disturbance and vomiting.

Classification
- **Classical migraine:** Visual or sensory symptoms can precede or accompany the headache
- **Common migraine:** There are no visual or sensory features
- **Basilar migraine:** Brain-stem symptoms
- **Hemiplegic migraine:** Hemiparesis that recovers slowly over days
- **Retinal migraine:** Monocular visual disturbance scintillations and scotomata

Precipitating Factors
- Commonly, these are stress, exposure to bright light, loud noises, smoke or strong scents, menstruation, lack or excess of sleep, cheese, caffeine, alcohol, chocolate, citrus fruit, food additives such as monosodium glutamate, vasodilators, exercise and contraceptive pills.
- Familial tendency is usual.

Clinical Features
- Attacks are episodic and start at puberty and continue till late middle life.

Box 16.4: Causes of raised intracranial pressure.

Primary or intracranial causes:
- Brain tumour
- Trauma (epidural and subdural haematoma, cerebral contusion)
- Non-traumatic intra-cerebral haemorrhage
- Ischaemic stroke
- Hydrocephalus
- Idiopathic or benign intracranial hypertension
- Post-neurosurgery

Secondary or extracranial causes:
- Hypoxia or hypercarbia (hypoventilation)
- Hyperpyrexia
- Seizure
- Drug and toxins (e.g. tetracycline, valproate sodium, lead intoxication)
- Hepatic failure
- Reye syndrome
- High-attitude cerebral oedema

TABLE 16.4: Classification of headache.

Primary headache		Secondary headache	
Type	%	Type	%
• Tension-type	69	• Systemic infection, meningitis, encephalitis	63
• Migraine	16	• Head injury–post-traumatic	4
• Idiopathic stabbing	2	• Vascular disorders, e.g. giant cell arteritis	1
• Exertional	1	• Subarachnoid haemorrhage	<1
• Cluster	0.1	• Brain tumour	0.1

• Other primary headache
   ○ Paroxysmal hemicrania
   ○ Short-lasting unilateral neuralgiform headache attacks with conjunctival injection and tearing (SUNCT)
		Other secondary causes
		Headaches associated with metabolic disorders
		• Hypoxia
		• Hypercapnia
		• Dialysis
		• Substance abuse
		• Venous thrombosis	

- Headache is typically hemicranial, throbbing in character, and associated with nausea and vomiting.
- In classical migraine, headache is preceded by an aura that is a focal neurologic, disturbance manifesting as visual aura (flashing lights or scintillating spots that may cross visual field over minutes, scotoma), sensory aura or language aura.
- Allodynia (production of pain from normally non-painful stimuli) is an extremely common phenomenon in migraine, occurring in about two-thirds of patients.
- Severe attacks are associated with photophobia and prostration.

Treatment
The drugs used in the treatment of migraine are given in **Box 16.5**.

Red flags of headache are listed in **Box 16.6**.

Cluster Headache
Usually occurs in young adult males.

Clinical Features
- Characterised by repeated, short-lived attacks (15–180 min) of excruciating peri-orbital unilateral pain.
- Often followed by autonomous ipsilateral signs (lacrimation, nasal congestion, ptosis, miosis, lid oedema and eye redness)

Box 16.5: Drugs used in the treatment of migraine.

Drugs useful in acute migraine:
- Paracetamol/Aspirin/Ibuprofen
- Ketorolac
- Ergotamine
- Dihydroergotamine
- Prochlorperazine
- Metoclopramide
- Sumatriptan
- Rizatriptan

Drugs used for prophylaxis:
- Propranolol
- Pizotifen
- Amitriptyline
- Flunarizine
- Gabapentin
- Valproate
- Topiramate

- Circadian periodicity with clustered attacks in bouts that may happen during particular months of the year.

Treatment
- Treatment is not curative.
- Acute treatment by using sumatriptan and high-flow oxygen
- Prophylaxis by verapamil, lithium, methysergide, prednisone, topiramate or greater occipital nerve block
- Deep-brain stimulation in refractory cases

> **Box 16.6: RED flags of headache.**
> - 'Worst' headache ever
> - First severe headache
> - Subacute worsening over days or weeks
> - Altered level of sensorium/consciousness
> - Abnormal neurologic examination
> - Fever or unexplained systemic signs
> - Significant weight loss
> - Vomiting that precedes headache
> - Pain induced by bending, lifting, cough, worsens with Valsalva manouevres
> - Pain which disturbs sleep or presents immediately upon awakening
> - Known systemic illness, history of trauma, cancer or HIV
> - New-onset headache in a patient > 50 years of age
> - Focal neurologic deficits, jaw claudication
> - Morning headache associated with nausea and vomiting
> - Pain associated with local tenderness (e.g. region of temporal artery)
>
> (HIV: human immunodeficiency virus)

EPILEPSY

Classification

Classification of epilepsy is given in **Table 16.5**.

Aetiology

- **Primary**
  - In majority of cases, epilepsy is idiopathic. This forms the group of idiopathic epilepsy. There may be a positive family history, childhood onset and has a genetic background.
- **Secondary (symptomatic)**
  - Any intracranial disease such as cerebral tumours, head injury, cerebrovascular accidents, central nervous system (CNS) infections.
  - Hypoglycaemia and hyperglycaemia
  - Uraemia and heart block
  - Ingestion or withdrawal of alcohol or drugs

Clinical Features

- **Tonic-clonic seizures:**
  - There is an altered consciousness at the onset that may be associated with an epileptic cry.
  - Fit starts simultaneously with generalised tonic state that lasts for few seconds to minutes.
  - Patient is unconscious and cyanose, does not breathe (as glottis is closed and respiratory muscles are in tonic contraction) and pupils are dilated.
  - Tongue may be bitten and urinary or bowel incontinence may occur.
  - This is followed by post-ictal phase where patient passes off into sleepy state.
- **Absent seizures (petit mal):**
  - The most common variety—transient loss of consciousness. An interruption occurs in current activity and patient may stare blankly ahead.
  - Brief loss of consciousness associated with myoclonic jerking of arms.
  - 'Akinetic seizure': Patient falls to ground, loses consciousness, recovers and rises up immediately.
- **Complex absent seizures:**
  - Usually absent attacks last for a few seconds. When an attack lasts longer, occasional jerks, automatic behaviour, and chewing and smacking movements resembling complex partial seizure may be seen.

TABLE 16.5: Classification of epilepsy.

Partial (focal) seizures	Primary generalised seizures	Status epilepticus

- Simple partial seizures
  - Simple partial motor seizures
  - Simple partial sensory seizures
- Complex partial seizures
- Secondary generalised partial seizures
	- Tonic-clonic (grand Mal)
	- Tonic
	- Absence
	- Atypical absence
	- Myoclonic
	- Atonic
	- Clonic
		- Tonic-clonic status
		- Absence status (simple)
		- Focal status (complex)
		- Epilepsia partialis continua

- **Juvenile myoclonic epilepsy (JME):**
  - Myoclonic jerks happen as the only form of seizure in about 17% of JME patients; the remainder have generalised tonic-clonic seizures (GTCSs) (80%) or absence seizures or both.
- **Partial seizures (focal seizures):**
  - Partial or focal seizure is a term used to describe abnormal electric activity only in a localised part of the brain.
- **Simple partial seizures:**
  - Symptoms at onset may be motor (jerking of muscles at one area, head turning), sensory (paraesthesia), visual (flashes of light), auditory (ringing sound), gustatory, olfactory or autonomic. Further symptoms depend on the spread of seizure activity.
- **Jacksonian seizures**
  - March of symptoms occur where it is motor, clonic jerking starts at a point, say face, and spreads to upper limb, then to lower limb and then on to opposite side to become a generalised fit
- **Complex partial seizures**
  - Complex symptoms at onset and is associated with altered awareness of the surroundings. Psychomotor (automatic, repetitive and non-purposeful behaviour such as lip smacking, chewing, walking—automatism).
  - Typically last for < 3 minutes
- **Secondary generalised seizures**
  - Attack starts with an aura (which actually denotes the site of onset of seizure discharge) that may be simple or complex, and is soon followed by loss of consciousness and generalised tonic-clonic seizures. Time taken from the onset of aura to generalised seizure may be variable but is usually very brief.
  - Post-ictal motor paralysis is called **Todd's palsy.**
- **Reflex epilepsy:** Occasionally, a sensory stimulus may precipitate an epileptic attack and can be readily reproduced. The following are common instances:
  - TV epilepsy (happens during close quarters watching TV)
  - Musicogenic (the attack is caused by certain musical tones)
  - Hot water (only over the vertex poured warm water)

Causes of Seizures

Causes of seizures are given in **Box 16.7**.

Diagnosis of Epilepsy

- **Electroencephalography (EEG):**
  - Helps in differentiating primary generalised attacks from focal epilepsies
  - Confirms the clinical diagnosis
  - Video EEG: Prolonged EEG-video monitoring provides information about electrographic seizures and seizure activity (actual events recorded on video).

Box 16.7: Causes of seizures.

Infancy:
- Anoxia (or post-anoxic)
- Hypocalcaemia
- Hypoglycaemia
- Hyponatraemia
- Fever (febrile seizures)
- Meningitis, birth trauma

Early childhood:
- Genetically determined metabolic disorders of brain
- CNS infections
- Idiopathic

Late childhood and adolescence:
- Idiopathic (genetically determined)
- Sequelae of previous injury
- Infections
- Drugs and toxins including lead poisoning

Adult life:
- Tumours
- Current or previous brain injury (traumatic or post-operative)
- CNS infections, including HIV
- Metabolic
- Drugs and toxins (cocaine, amphetamines, theophylline, alcohol, organophosphates); alcohol or benzodiazepine withdrawal
- Idiopathic

Late life:
- Metabolic
- Tumours
- Current or previous brain injury (traumatic or post-surgical)
- Ischaemia to the brain
- Drugs and toxins

(HIV: human immunodeficiency virus; CNS: central nervous system)

- CSF examination (if an infection is suspected):
  - Metabolic parameters such as blood sugar, sodium, calcium urea, creatinine, acid–base balance and magnesium.
- **Neuroimaging:**
  - MRI is better than CT scan for the detection of cerebral lesions associated with epilepsy.

Treatment of Various Types of Epilepsies

Treatment of various types of epilepsies is shown in **Figure 16.1**.

Newer Anti-epileptic Agents

Felbamate, gabapentin, lamotrigine, levetiracetam, oxcarbazepine, pregabalin, tiagabine, topiramate and vigabatrin

Status Epilepticus

Status epilepticus denotes sustained epileptic activity, and is clinically diagnosed with one of the following two:
1. Two fits occur without recovery of consciousness in between.
2. A single fit lasts longer than 30 minutes with or without loss of consciousness.
3. Status epilepticus can be classified into partial and generalised.

Treatment

Treatment of status epilepticus is given in **Box 16.8**.

■ CEREBROVASCULAR ACCIDENT

Cerebrovascular accident or stroke is defined as abrupt onset neurological disorder of vascular aetiology. Types of strokes are discussed in **Flowchart 16.1**.

Types of Haemorrhagic Strokes

- Primary intracerebral haemorrhage
- Subarachnoid haemorrhage
- Primary intraventricular haemorrhage

Types of Ischaemic Strokes

- Transient ischaemic attacks (TIA)
- Completed stroke
- Lacunar infarcts
- Watershed infarcts

Risk Factors

The risk factors of cerebrovascular accident are given in **Table 16.6**.

■ TRANSIENT ISCHAEMIC ATTACKS

A brief episode of neurological dysfunction caused by focal brain or retinal ischaemia with clinical symptoms typically lasting <1 hour and without neuroimaging evidence of acute infarction

Symptoms and Signs

Transient ischaemic attacks imply an active plaque in the major feeding artery and is a warning sign of a major stroke. The risk of recurrence

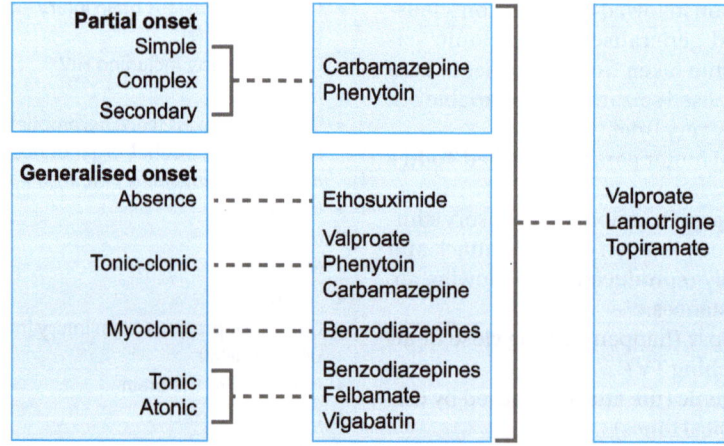

Fig. 16.1: Treatment of various types of epilepsies.

Box 16.8: Treatment of status epilepticus.

First 5 minutes
- Check emergency ABC's
- Give O_2
- Obtain IV access
- Begin ECG monitoring
- Check finger stick glucose
- Draw blood for serum electrolytes. RFT, magnesium, calcium, phosphate, CBC, LFTs, AED levels, ABG, troponin
- Toxicology screen (urine and blood)

6–10 minutes
- Thiamine 100 mg IV; 50 mL of D50 IV unless adequate glucose known
- Lorazepam 4 mg IV over 2 minutes; if still seizing, repeat × 1 in 5 minutes
- If no rapid IV access give diazepam 20 mg PR or midazolam 10 mg intranasally, buccally or IM

10–20 minutes
- If seizures persist, begin fosphenytoin 20 mg/kg IV at 150 mg/min, with blood pressure and ECG monitoring.

OR
- Phenytoin 15–20 mg/kg at 30–50 mg/min

Reasonable to bypass this step, or perform subsequent step simultaneous with fosphenytoin loading

10–60 minutes: One (or more) of the following 4 options (intubation usually necessary except for valproate):

1. Continuous IV midazolam: Load: 0.2 mg/kg; repeat 0.2–0.4 mg/kg boluses every 5 min until seizures stop, up to a maximum total loading dose of 2 mg/kg. Initial rate: 0.1 mg/kg/h. Continuous IV dose range: 0.05 – 2.9 mg/kg/h.

OR

2. Continuous IV propofol: Load: 1 mg/kg; repeat 1–2 mg/kg boluses every 3–5 minutes until seizures stop, up to maximum total loading dose of 10 mg/kg. Initial continuous IV rate: 2 mg/kg/h. Continuous IV dose range: 1–15 mg/kg/h. Avoid >48 hours of >5 mg/kg/h (increased risk of propofol infusion syndrome).

OR

3. IV valproate: 40 mg/kg over ~10 minutes. If still seizing, additional 20 mg/kg over ~5 minutes.

OR

4. IV phenobarbital: 20 mg/kg IV at 50–100 mg/min.

60 minutes
- Continuous IV pentobarbital. Load: 5 mg/kg at up to 50 mg/min; repeat 5 mg/kg boluses until seizures stop. Initial continuous IV rate: 1 mg/kg/h. Continuous IV-dose range: 0.5–10 mg/kg/h; traditionally titrated to suppression-burst on EEG.

Perform neuroimaging when convulsive activity is controlled.
- Begin continuous EEG, if patient does not awaken rapidly or if continuous IV Rx is used.
- Treat metabolic abnormalities and hypothermia.
- Lumbar puncture and antibiotics can be considered if infection is suspected.

and stroke is about 10% within first 7 days of a TIA, with most of them occurring within 48 hours. More than 30% of patients with recurrent TIAs will suffer from completed stroke if untreated.

Carotid Territory

Ipsilateral mono-ocular blindness (amaurosis fugax), contralateral hemiparesis, hemianaesthesia, dysarthria and rare hemianopia, monoparesis, isolated facial weakness or sensory symptoms may occur in the face or limbs alone.

Vertebrobasilar Territory

Ataxia, dysarthria, hemianopia, diplopia, sudden fall (drop attacks), weakness on both sides, paraesthesia on both sides, swallowing trouble, vertigo and tinnitus.

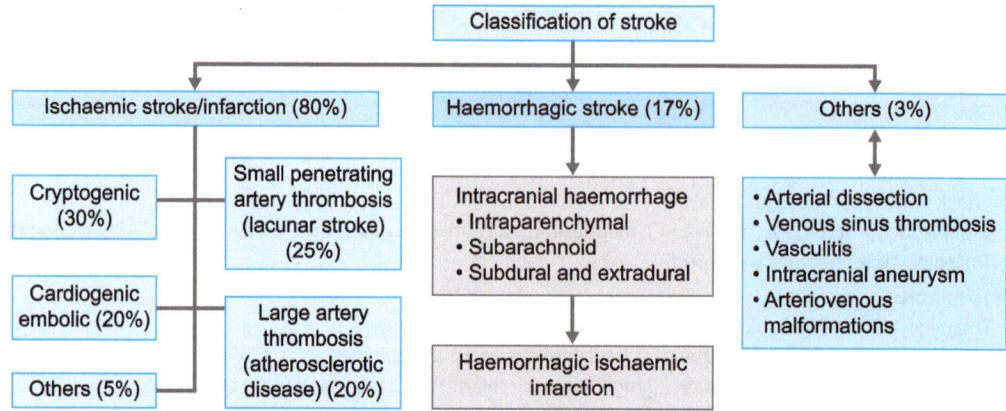

Flowchart 16.1: Classification of stroke.

TABLE 16.6: Risk factors of cerebrovascular accident.

High risk	Low risk	Risk factors that are more common in young patients
• Hypertension • Diabetes mellitus • Atrial fibrillation • Smoking • Use of cocaine or amphetamines • Vasculitis (polyarteritis nodosa, Wegener's, Takayasu's arteritis, primary CNS vasculitis, vasculitis related to meningitis) • Dilated cardiomyopathy • Endocarditis	• Migraine • Use of oral contraceptives or alcohol • Patent foramen ovale • Recent myocardial infarction • Prosthetic valve	• Protein C and S deficiencies • Antithrombin III deficiency • Anti-phospholipid syndrome • Factor V Leiden • Sickle cell anaemia • Hyperhomocysteinaemia • Thrombotic thrombocytopaenic purpura • Arterial dissection • Infections (e.g. syphilis, HIV)

(CNS: central nervous system; HIV: human immunodeficiency virus)

Investigations

Routine tests for TIA:
- Full blood count, erythrocyte sedimentation rate (ESR)
- Serological tests for syphilis
- Blood glucose, urea, proteins
- Chest X-ray, electrocardiography (ECG)

In younger patients:
- Antinuclear factors
- Cholesterol
- Coagulation studies (anti-cardiolipin antibodies, protein C and S, antithrombin III)

Additional tests in vertebrobasilar TIAs:
- Lying and standing BP
- 24-hour ECG monitoring
- X-ray of cervical spine
- MRI angiography

In carotid TIAs:
- CT scan or diffusion-weighted MRI of head
- Carotid Doppler study
- Arteriography, CT or MR angiography.

Diagnosis

Work-up in a case of TIA should include evaluation for risk factors for stroke. They are the following:
- Hypertension
- Diabetes
- Hyperlipidaemia
- Arterial disease affecting the heart and limbs
- Cardiac disease (valvular and ischaemic)
- Smoking

Risk assessment for occurrence of stroke:
Calculate **ABCD2 score:** high risk of early stroke if ABCD2 score > 4 points.
- Age > 60 years, 1 point
- BP > 140/90 mmHg, 1 point
- Clinical features
    o Speech disturbance, 1 point
    o Unilateral weakness, 2 points
- Duration
    o ≥ 10 minutes, 1 point
    o ≥ 1 hour, 2 points
- Diabetes, 1 point

Treatment

- Patients who score 4 and above on ABCD2 are at elevated risk of recurrent stroke and should receive instant aspirin and be referred to a greater centre for evaluation and inquiry within 24 hours of the start of symptoms.
- If the ABCD2 score is < 4, start aspirin and have specialist assessment within 7 days.
- Correction of risk factors: This includes treatment of hypertension, diabetes and hyperlipidaemia, correction of valvular heart diseases and cessation of smoking.

Haemorrhagic, Thrombotic and Embolic Strokes

Classification of stroke is given in **Table 16.7**.

Clinical Features

Clinical features of cerebral ischaemia on neuroanatomic basis are given in **Table 16.8** and clinical features of stroke depending on localisation are shown in **Figure 16.2** and **Table 16.9**.

Structures involved in leiomyosarcoma and their associated symptoms are given in **Table 16.10**.

Management

Initial evaluation:
- Metabolic status:
    o Blood sugar
    o Presence or absence of hypoxia
    o Renal functions
    o Electrolyte status
    o Haemoglobin
    o Coagulation parameters
- CT scan: To confirm infarct and to rule out haemorrhage, tumour and subdural haematoma.

Treatment

General measures:
- Maintain adequate airway with periodic clearance of secretion and chest physiotherapy in unconscious patients.
- Treat hypoglycaemia with 50% dextrose; treat hyperglycaemia with insulin if serum glucose > 200 mg/dL.

TABLE 16.7: Classification of stroke.

Feature	Haemorrhagic	Thrombotic	Embolic
Time of onset	During activity	In sleep	Any time
Progression	Over minutes and hours	On waking up or over hours	Within seconds
TIAs	Absent	Present	Present
Vomiting	Recurrent	Absent or occasional	Absent or occasional
Headache	Prominent	Mild or absent	Mild or absent
Early resolution	Unusual	Variable	Possible
Meningeal irritation	May be present	Absent	Absent
Carotid bruit	Not seen	Highly supportive	Possible
Valvular heart disease and atrial fibrillation	Not seen	Unusual	Highly supportive
CT scan	Haemorrhage	Pale infarct (normal in early stage)	Pale infarct (normal in early stage)

(CT: computed tomography; TIA: transient ischaemic attack)

TABLE 16.8: Features of cerebral ischaemia depending on the neuroanatomic basis.

Vascular territory	Signs and symptoms
Internal carotid artery	• Combined ACA + MCA • Ipsilateral monocular visual loss (amaurosis) secondary to CRAO
Left anterior cerebral artery (ACA)	• Right leg numbness and weakness • Transcortical motor aphasia • Ideomotor apraxia
Right ACA	• Left leg numbness and weakness • Motor neglect • Possibly ideomotor apraxia
Left middle cerebral artery (MCA)	• Right face/arm > leg numbness and weakness • Aphasia • Left gaze preference
Right MCA	• Left face/arm > leg numbness and weakness • Left hemispatial neglect • Right gaze preference • Agraphesthesia/astereognosia

(CRAO: central retinal artery occlusion)

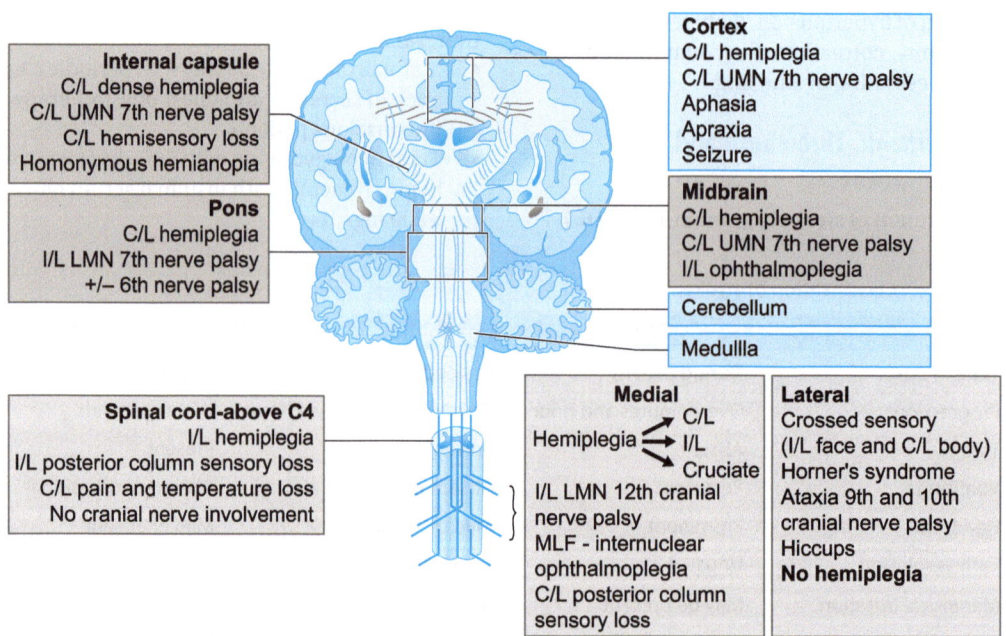

(I/L: ipsilateral; C/L: contralateral; LMN: lower motor neuron; UMN: upper motor neuron)

Fig. 16.2: Localisation of lesion in hemiplegia.

TABLE 16.9: Clinical features of stroke depending on localisation.

Syndrome	Clinical features	Localisation
Middle cerebral artery [MCA (M1)] syndrome	Produces pure motor or sensory motor stroke contralateral (C/L) to the side of lesion. If ischaemia of putamen, pallidus-predominantly parkinsonian features	Internal capsule, caudate nucleus, putamen and outer pallidus
MCA-M2 syndrome	• Brachial syndrome: Weakness of hand and arm • Frontal opercular syndrome: Broca's aphasia with facial weakness with or without arm weakness	Superior division of MCA-M2 involved
	• If dominant hemisphere: Wernicke's aphasia without weakness with C/L homonymous superior quadrantanopia • If non-dominant hemisphere: Hemispatial neglect, spatial agnosia without weakness	Inferior division of MCA-M2 involved
Complete MCA syndrome	• Contralateral hemiplegia, C/L hemianaesthesia, C/L homonymous hemianopia, gaze preference to the ipsilateral side • If dominant hemisphere involved-global aphasia • If non-dominant hemisphere involved-hemispatial neglect, anosognosia and constructional apraxia	
Unpaired anterior cerebral artery syndrome	Profound abulia and bilateral pyramidal signs with paraparesis or quadriparesis and urinary incontinence	Frontal lobe, entire medial part of cerebral hemispheres
Anterior choroidal artery occlusion syndrome	Contralateral hemiplegia, C/L hemianaesthesia, C/L homonymous hemianopia	Posterior limb of internal capsule, retrolentiform and sublentiform parts
Claude's syndrome	3rd nerve palsy + C/L ataxia	Red nucleus/cerebral peduncle
Weber's syndrome	3rd nerve palsy + C/L hemiplegia	Medial midbrain/cerebral peduncle
Benedict's syndrome	Weber's + tremors + ataxia	Red nucleus/medial midbrain
Dejerine–Roussy syndrome	Contralateral hemisensory loss and agonising pain	Thalamus
Parinaud's syndrome	Loss of up gaze, convergence-retraction nystagmus on attempted up gaze, downward ocular deviation ('setting sun' sign), lid retraction nystagmus (Collier's sign), mydriasis	Dorsal midbrain
Marie–Foix syndrome	• Ipsilateral ataxia—arm and leg • Contralateral hemiparesis and hemisensory loss	Lateral pontine (middle cerebellar peduncle, corticospinal tract and spinothalamic tract)
Raymond–Cestan syndrome	Ipsilateral lateral gaze palsy (VI nerve), C/L hemiparesis	Ventral pons
Millard–Gubler syndrome	Ipsilateral lateral gaze palsy (VI nerve) and LMN facial palsy, C/L hemiparesis	Ventral pons

Continued

Continued

Syndrome	Clinical features	Localisation
Medial medullary syndrome (Dejerine syndrome)	• Ipsilateral XII nerve palsy, C/L hemiparesis • Internuclear ophthalmoplegia (involvement of medial longitudinal fascicle), loss of posterior column sensation	Medial medulla
Hemimedullary syndrome (Babinski–Negolette)	Lateral medullary syndrome + C/L hemiparesis	Involve both lateral and medial medulla
Top of basilar syndrome	Parinaud's syndrome features+ oculomotor palsy, behavioural features, abulia	• Basilar artery occlusion • Involves thalamus, midbrain, occipital lobes, cerebellum (superior cerebellar artery)

(LMN: lower motor neuron)

TABLE 16.10: Localisation/structures involved and associated symptoms of Lateral Medullary syndrome (LMS).

Localisation/structures involved	Symptoms
• Vestibular nuclei and connections • Inferior cerebellar peduncle (restiform body)	• Dizziness and imbalance • Hypotonia ipsilateral side • Diplopia/oscillopsia • Nystagmus, limb ataxia
• Spinal nucleus of fifth cranial nerve (CNV) • Spinothalamic tract	• Loss of pain and temperature sensation in ipsilateral face • Loss of pain and temperature contralateral trunk (crossed sensory loss)
• Nucleus ambigus (CN IX and X)	• Ipsilateral paralysis palate, pharynx, and larynx • Absent gag reflex
• Descending sympathetic fibres • Dorsomotor nucleus of Vagus	• Ipsilateral Horner's syndrome • Autonomic signs—labile BP/tachycardia/sweating/arrhythmias
• Ventrolateral medullary tegmentum and the medullary reticular zone (respiratory centres)	• Failure of automatic respirations • Hiccoughs
• Corticospinal tracts, medial lemniscus NOT involved	• No pyramidal tract signs. Posterior column sensations preserved

- Skin care by changing position once in 2 hours to prevent bed sore.
- Bladder catheterisation, if incontinence or retention has occurred.
- Passive movements of limbs to prevent contractures, oedema of the limb, venous stasis and pulmonary embolism.

Specific measures:
- Control of BP: Drugs most often used include IV labetalol, enalapril or sodium nitroprusside.

- Anti-oedema measures:
  ○ Mannitol 20% IV over 20 minutes (0.25 g/kg) three to four times a day
  ○ Glycerol 30 mL orally three to four times a day
  ○ Frusemide 20 mg IV three times a day

Anticoagulants

Recommended only when cerebral ischaemic event occurs in presence of:

- Recent myocardial infarction where anticoagulants are recommended for a period of 3 months
- Previous myocardial infarction with ventricular akinetic segment or ventricular aneurysm
- Presence of other cardiac conditions as noted above
- Presence of prosthetic valves

Thrombolytic Therapy
- Recombinant tissue plasminogen activator (rTPA)
- **Contraindications:**
  - Blood on CT scan
  - Possible SAH
  - A large hypodense lesion in a distribution consistent with the neurologic examination
  - Active internal bleeding
  - Bleeding diathesis
  - Systolic blood pressure > 185 mmHg, diastolic blood pressure > 110 mmHg.
  - Major neurosurgery or head injury within 3 months
  - History of intracranial haemorrhage or AV malformation
- Dose: About 0.9 mg/kg (maximum 90 mg) with 10% of total dose as bolus and rest over 1 hour
- Intra-arterial (through carotid artery) rTPA can be given in selected patients up to 6 hours after onset

Secondary Prophylaxis
Anti-platelet agents should be started within 48 hours. In patients receiving thrombolysis, aspirin should be started within 24 hours.

■ LACUNAR INFARCTION
- Small deep infarcts, usually <15 mm in size secondary to diseases of small perforating branches of brain. May or may not present with symptoms or signs.
- Occlusion may be caused by microatheroma and lipohyalinosis linked with hypertension, smoking and diabetes, or heart or carotid artery microembolism.

The signs and symptoms of lacunar stroke on the basis of the location of lesion are given in **Table 16.11**.

■ CEREBRAL VENOUS THROMBOSIS
- Cerebral venous thrombosis is the cause of approximately 1–2% of strokes which occur in young adults.
- Superior sagittal sinus is most commonly involved.

The causes of cerebral venous thrombosis are given in **Box 16.9**.

Clinical Features
- Develops slowly or subacutely
- Nausea and vomiting are common.
- Papilloedema due to elevated ICP
- Some patients experience seizures or sensory focal or motor deficits
- Cranial nerve palsies can happen, especially when petrosal sinuses are involved.
- CT or MR venography
- CT or MRI to detect secondary parenchymal lesions
- CSF examination in appropriate clinical context to rule out meningitis or SAH
- Coagulation studies in appropriate patients

Treatment
- Supportive measures such as hydration, adequate antimicrobials, anticonvulsant seizure control and ICP control.
- IV heparin to halt progression of thrombosis; can be given even if haemorrhage is present.
- Intra-dural thrombolysis in patients whose clinical status worsens while on anticoagulation
- Mechanical thrombectomy

■ STROKE IN YOUNG
The term 'young stroke' is used to denote stroke in individuals <45 years of age (**Box 16.10**).

■ MOVEMENT DISORDERS
An algorithmic approach to movement disorders is shown in **Flowchart 16.2**.

Parkinsonism
Classification
Primary parkinsonism:
Paralysis agitans or Parkinson's disease or idiopathic parkinsonism

TABLE 16.11: Signs and symptoms of lacunar stroke depending on location of lesion.

Syndrome	Signs/Symptoms	Localisation	Vascular supply
Pure motor	• Contralateral hemiparesis or hemiplegia • Affects face, arm and leg equally	• Posterior limb of internal capsule • Corona radiata–Basis pontis	Lenticulostriate branches of the middle cerebral artery (MCA) or perforating arteries from basilar artery
Pure sensory	• Contralateral hemisensory loss • Persistent or transient numbness and/or tingling on one side of the body	• Ventral posterolateral (VPL) nucleus of thalamus	Lenticulostriate branches of MCA. Small thalamoperforators of posterior cerebral artery (PCA)
Mixed sensorimotor	• Contralateral weakness and numbness • Hemiparesis or hemiplegia with ipsilateral sensory impairment	Thalamus and adjacent posterior limb of internal capsule	Lenticulostriate branches of MCA
Dysarthria-clumsy hand	Slurred speech and weakness of contralateral hand (fine motor)	Basis pontis	Basilar artery perforators
Ataxia-hemiparesis	Combination of cerebellar and motor symptoms. Contralateral hemiparesis and ataxia out of proportion to weakness	• Internal capsule-posterior limb • Basis pontis • Corona radiata	• Lenticulostriate branches of MCA • Perforating arteries of basilar artery
Hemiballismus/hemichorea	Contralesional limb flailing/dyskinesis	Subthalamic nucleus	Perforating arteries of anterior choroidal or posterior communicating artery (PCOM)

Box 16.9: Causes of cerebral venous thrombosis.

Local causes:
- Trauma to the dural sinuses
- Infection near the dural sinuses
- Otitis media
- Mastoiditis
- Sinusitis
- Tonsillitis
- Invasion by neoplastic processes

Systemic causes:
- Hyper-coagulable states
- Oral contraceptive use
- Pregnancy
- Malignancy
- Protein C or protein S deficiency
- Presence of lupus anticoagulant
- Dehydration

Secondary parkinsonism (symptomatic):
- Post-encephalitic (post-encephalitis lethargica)
- Toxins, e.g. methylphenyltetrahydropyridine (MPTP), manganese, carbon monoxide
- Drugs, e.g. reserpine, phenothiazines, butyrophenones, α-methyldopa, metoclopramide
- Ischaemic (vascular parkinsonism)
- Tumours in basal ganglion
- Punch-drunk syndrome in boxers
- Infections, e.g. HIV, influenza

Parkinsonism plus (degenerative disorders with prominent additional neurological features):
- Progressive supra-nuclear palsy
- Diffuse Lewy body disease, Wilson's disease, Huntington's disease (HD) in children
- MSA includes variable combination of parkinsonism (poor response of L-dopa), cerebellar, pyramidal and autonomic degeneration. MSA can have a predominance of parkinsonian features (MSA—P subtype) or cerebellar ataxia (MSA—C subtype). Autonomic dysfunction results in urinary symptoms (urge incontinence and incomplete bladder emptying), erectile dysfunctions in males, orthostatic hypotension and chronic constipation.

Box 16.10: Causes for young stroke.

- **Cardiac**
  - Congenital heart disease, patent foramen ovale
  - Atrial myxoma
  - Atrial fibrillation and other arrhythmia
  - Cardiomyopathy, myocarditis, myocardial infarction
  - Cardiac surgery, cardiac catheterisation
  - Endocarditis, rheumatic heart disease
  - Prosthetic valve
- **Haematologic**
  - Sickle cell disease, iron deficiency anaemias, polycythaemia vera
- **Hypercoagulable states**
  - Inherited prothrombotic states, protein C and S deficiency, antithrombin III deficiency, factor V Leiden gene mutation, prothrombin gene mutation
  - Anti-phospholipid syndrome
  - Hyperhomocysteinaemia
  - Myeloproliferative disorders (e.g. leukaemia, lymphoma)
  - Pregnancy exposure to hormonal treatments such as anabolic steroids and erythropoietin, nephrotic syndrome
- **Vascular**
  - **Non-inflammatory**
    - Arterial dissection
    - Secondary to connective tissue disease (Ehlers-Danlos, Marfan)
    - Moyamoya disease
    - Hypertension
    - Radiation vasculopathy
    - Vasculitis and post-infectious vasculopathy
    - Migraine
    - Cerebral autosomal dominant arteriopathy with subcortical infarcts and leukoencephalopathy (CADASIL), Fibromuscular dysplasia, Susac's syndrome, Sneddon's syndrome, Fabry's disease
  - **Inflammatory**
    - Takayasu arteritis
    - Giant cell arteritis
    - Kawasaki disease
    - Polyarteritis nodosa
    - Human immunodeficiency virus (HIV)
    - Bacterial meningitis

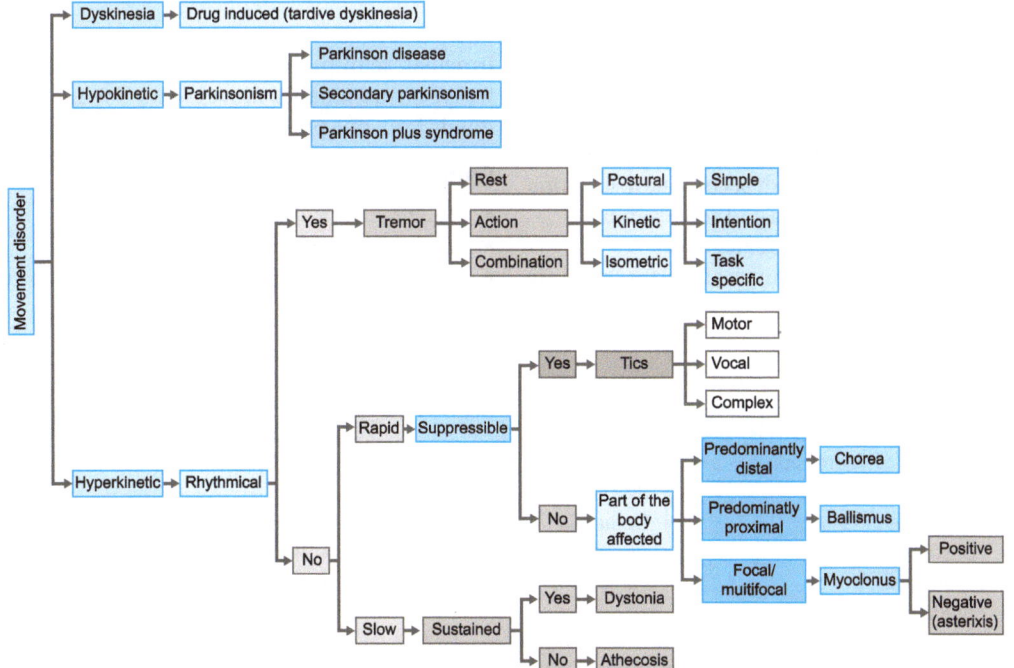

Flowchart 16.2: Algorithmic approach to movement disorders.

Clinical Features
- **Tremors:** It is classically a tremor at rest and is compound (called **pill-rolling tremor**), occurring at wrist and fingers on one side first that decreases with action. At times, action or postural tremor may also be present. Tremor may also occur at head, jaw or lower limbs.
- **Rigidity:** Hypertonia is due to rigidity. When tremor is present, it adds cog wheeling character to the basic lead pipe hypertonia (cogwheel rigidity). It is unilateral in the beginning of disease.
- **Hypokinesia/Akinesia/Bradykinesia**
    - It is the paucity or slowness of movements. There is reduced movement in acts such as getting up, adjusting posture walking; two common features are reduced arm swing on one and repetitive supination/pronation of hands.
    - Face looks blank and expressionless ("mask-like face"). Amplitude of writing declines near the end of a sentence.
- **Disturbed postural reflexes:** Speech is of low volume and dis-monotonous. Micrographia is present with a tendency of tail off at the end of a line. Stance is stooped, gait becomes shuffling (festinant), associated arm swinging is absent, and turning about becomes slow and laborious.
  With advancing disease, patient assumes fixed-flexed postures, remains curled in bed unable to move. Death occurs due to infection (bronchopneumonia and septicaemia).
- **Others (non-motor features)**
  Other non-motor features of parkinsonism are given in **Table 16.12**.

Diagnosis
- CT scan or MRI is required if these additional signs are present.
- In typical cases, PET and SPECT

Management
Drug therapy:
- Anti-cholinergics: Trihexyphenidyl, benzhexol and orphenadrine
- Amantadine
- L-dopa:
    - L-dopa + carbidopa (4:1 or 10:1 ratio)
    - L-dopa + benserazide (4:1 ratio).
- Dopamine receptor agonists: Bromocriptine, pergolide, cabergoline, apomorphine, pramipexole, ropinirole and rotigotine.
- Selegiline and rasagiline
    - Catechol-O-methyltransferase (COMT) inhibitors: Tolcapone and entacapone
    - Rivastigmine

Surgery:
- Stereotacic thalamotomy (ventrolateral nucleus of thalamus)
- Deep brain stimulation (sub-thalamic nucleus and globus pallidus interna)

Chorea
Irregular, semi-purposeful, abrupt, quick, short, jerky, unsustainable movements flowing randomly from one portion of the body to the next

Causes
- Rheumatic (Sydenham's chorea)
- Huntington's chorea
- Encephalitis, e.g. Japanese encephalitis, measles, mumps

TABLE 16.12: Non-motor features of parkinsonism.

Autonomic dysfunction	Neuropsychiatric symptoms	Sensory problems
- Orthostatic hypotension	- Depression	- Reduces smell
- Urinary incontinence	- Psychosis	- Pain
- Impotence	- Dementia	- Sleep disorders
- Constipation	- Anxiety	- Restless legs
- Sialorrhoea	- Panic attacks	- Insomnia
- Anhidrosis		- Daytime somnolence

- Vascular, e.g. HIV-related (toxoplasmosis, progressive multifocal leuco-encephalopathy, HIV and encephalitis)
- Pregnancy

Treatment
- Sodium valproate
- Haloperidol

Athetosis
Athetosis is slow writhing distal movements affecting fingers, hands, toes and feet (snake charmer's movement).

Causes
- Kernicterus
- Encephalitis
- Previous cerebral infarcts
- Degenerative brain disorders

Treatment
Haloperidol, tetrabenazine

Dystonia
Dystonia is sustained abnormal posture of limbs, neck or trunk. May be focal or generalised

Causes
- Kernicterus
- Previous brain injury
- Familial
- Degenerative disorders

Treatment
- Tetrabenazine, a dopamine-depleting drug
- High-dose anti-cholinergics
- Sodium valproate
- Botulinum toxin A and dB for cervical dystonias
- Stereotactic thalamotomy or deep brain stimulation may be required if the disease is severe and distressing.

Hemiballismus
It is violent flinging movements of the limbs. It is usually unilateral, and hence called hemiballismus.

Cause
Stroke affecting sub-thalamic nucleus (on contralateral side)

Treatment
- Haloperidol 0.5–2.5 mg tid
- Tetrabenazine 25–50 mg tid

Myoclonus
Myoclonus is a rapid, brief, irregular movement of a part of body caused by muscle contraction. It may occur at two or more sites.

Causes
- Metabolic disturbances
- Post-hypoxic brain injury
- Chronic renal failure
- Chronic liver disease
- Respiratory failure
- Electrolyte imbalance
- Encephalitis
- Tricyclic antidepressants
- Lipid storage diseases
- Creutzfeldt–Jakob disease
- Myoclonic epilepsy

Treatment
- Correction of underlying disease
- Sodium valproate
- Clonazepam

TICS
- Abrupt, generally short and often repetitive and stereotypical movements, varying in intensity and repeating at uneven intervals.
- Tourette syndrome is present in childhood. Drug treatment includes neuroleptic drugs (e.g. fluphenazine, risperidone), tetrabenazine (a monoamine-depleting drug), topiramate and clonazepam.

Tremors
- Tremor is rhythmic alternate movement at a joint due to synchronous or alternate contraction of antagonistic muscles.
- Tremor may be simple (when it occurs in a single plane) or compound (when it is multiplanar, e.g. pill-rolling tremor of Parkinson's disease).
- It may be physiological or pathological.

Rest or static tremor:
- Rest tremor (static tremor) is maximal at rest and becomes less prominent or disappears with activity.

- It is typically seen in parkinsonism where it may be of pill-rolling type. It is often associated with bradykinesia and rigidity.

Postural tremor:
- Tremor is maximal when limb posture is actively maintained against gravity.
- It is reduced by rest and is not markedly enhanced during voluntary movements toward a target.

Intention tremor:
- Intention tremor is a cerebellar sign.
- Classic intention tremor is produced by lesions in the cerebellum.

CEREBELLAR DISEASES/ATAXIA

Signs
Signs of cerebellar diseases are given in **Box 16.11**.

Classification of Ataxia
Classification of ataxia is given in **Table 16.13**.

Acute Bacterial Meningitis/Pyogenic Meningitis

Aetiology
- **Common organisms:**
  - *Streptococcus pneumoniae* (30–50%)
  - *Neisseria meningitidis* (10–35%)
  - *Haemophilus influenzae* type B (1–3%)
- **Uncommon organisms:**
  - *Staphylococcus aureus*
  - *S. epidermidis*
  - *Listeria*

Clinical Features
- Fever, headache and vomiting are the cardinal features.
- Seizures, impairment of consciousness, photophobia, stiff neck and stiff back
- In elderly, immunocompromised and debilitated patients, the classic signs of meningitis may be minimal, where low-grade fever and changes in mental status may occur without headache or neck rigidity.
- Meningococcal meningitis:
  - The evolution is extremely rapid and the onset is attended by petechial or purpuric skin eruptions, large ecchymoses and lividity of the skin of the lower parts of the body.
  - Circulatory collapse may occur.

Box 16.11: Signs of cerebellar diseases.
- Dysynergia
- Dysmetria
- Rebound phenomenon
- Pendular knee jerk
- Dysdiadochokinesia
- Intention tremor
- Hypotonia
- Nystagmus
- Titubation
- Gait ataxia
- Scanning or staccato speech

TABLE 16.13: Classification of ataxia.

Acquired or sporadic ataxias	Hereditary ataxias

• Stroke
• Toxin-induced ataxias
• Ethanol
• Drugs (antiepileptic agents, lithium, antineoplastic, cyclosporine, metronidazole)
• Heavy metals
• Multiple sclerosis
• Miller-Fisher syndrome
• Paraneoplastic syndrome
• Cerebellar abscess
• Neoplastic disorder
• Hypothyroidism
	• Autosomal dominant cerebellar ataxias:
	  ○ Spinocerebellar ataxias
	  ○ Episodic ataxias
	• Autosomal recessive cerebellar ataxias:
	  ○ Friedreich ataxia
	  ○ Abetalipoproteinaemia
	  ○ Ataxia telangiectasia

- Pneumococcal meningitis is usually preceded by an infection in the lung, ear or sinuses. Heart valves may be affected.
- *H. influenzae* meningitis follows upper respiratory tract infections and ear infections in young.

Signs of Meningeal Irritation

- **Neck stiffness (neck rigidity):** The examiner is unable to put the patient's chin on the chest by passive flexion of the neck (due to neck muscle spasm).
- **Kernig's sign:** If the patient's thigh is flexed to 90° from the abdomen, it is then impossible to straighten the knee to >135° passively owing to spasm of hamstrings.
- **Brudzinski's neck sign:** With the patient supine, the physician places one hand behind the patient's head and places the other hand on the patient's chest.

Investigations

- Total leucocytes increased, polymorphonuclear leucocytosis and raised ESR
- Cerebrospinal fluid studies

Cerebrospinal Fluid Findings in Pyogenic (Bacterial) Meningitis

- Appearance is turbid
- Pressure is elevated above 180 mm H_2O.
- Cell count is raised, ranging from 5,000 to 20,000/mL, neutrophil leucocytes predominate
- Protein level is elevated (> 45 mg/dL)
- Sugar level is decreased (< 40 mg/dL or < 40% of blood sugar)
- Gram's stain of the sediment of CSF may show meningococci as gram-negative, kidney-shaped, intracellular diplococci (inside neutrophils)
- Culture of CSF grows the pathogen in 70–80% of cases.
- Measurement of bacterial antigen in the CSF (latex agglutination test)

Treatment

Initial management includes:
- Airway protection and oxygenation
- Volume resuscitation
- Prevention of hypoglycaemia
- Control of seizures
- Reduction of hyperthermia and measures to reduce ICP and maintain CBF

Antibiotics

Empiric antibiotic therapy for bacterial meningitis is given in **Table 16.14**.
- **Pneumococcal and meningococcal meningitis**
  - Penicillin G, 20–24 million units/day in 4–6 divided doses IV for 10 days
  - Chloramphenicol 4–6 g/day in divided doses IV
- ***H. influenzae* meningitis**
  - Ampicillin 8–12 g/day in divided doses plus chloramphenicol 3–4 g/day divided doses, both IV.

Steroids

- Despite antibiotics, serious complications can occur in patients with meningitis.
- Corticosteroids have been found to decrease the incidence of hearing impairment in children with *H. influenzae* meningitis.
- Dexamethasone is given in a dose of 0.15 mg/kg every 6th hourly for a period of 4 days.

Complications

- CNS complications include cerebrovascular involvement, cranial nerve palsies, focal neurological deficits, cerebral oedema and hydrocephalus.
- Pneumonia and otitis media are frequently seen in patients with meningitis.

Aseptic Meningitis

- Aseptic meningitis is inflammation of the meninges with CSF lymphocytic pleocytosis,

TABLE 16.14: Empiric antibiotic therapy for bacterial meningitis.

Age group	Likely organisms	Empirical treatment (dose/day)
Adults	*N. meningitidis, S. pneumoniae*	Ceftriaxone (or cefotaxime) plus vancomycin (40 mg/kg)
Elderly or immunocompromised	*S. pneumoniae, Listeria,* gram-negative organisms	Ampicillin plus ceftriaxone or cefotaxime or ceftazidime plus vancomycin

with no apparent cause after routine CSF stains and cultures.
- Viruses (e.g. herpes simplex virus, varicella zoster virus, HIV, enteroviruses) are the most common cause.
- Other causes may be infectious (rickettsiae, spirochetes, parasites, etc.)
- Non-infectious [vaccine reactions—rabies, pertussis: Drugs—azathioprine, carbamazepine, etc.; sarcoidosis, Behcet's disease, systemic lupus erythematosus (SLE), reaction to intrathecal drugs, etc.]
- Some may be asymptomatic but with CSF abnormalities.
- Symptoms include fever, headache, vomiting and meningeal signs.
- Treatment is symptomatic.

Tuberculous Meningitis

Clinical Features

- It has a subacute or chronic course.
- Classical symptoms of meningitis are fever, headache and vomiting that appear over a couple of days.
- Signs include neck rigidity and positive Kernig's and Brudzinski's signs.
- Furthermore, hemiparesis or paraplegia follow cranial nerve palsies (frequently blindness, ophthalmoplegia diplopia, facial paralysis and deafness).
- Because of vasculitis, these deficits may happen abruptly.
- Increased ICP characteristics due to hydrocephalus will lead to intellectual modifications, altered consciousness, urinary incontinence, and gait ataxia.
- Seizures are common.

Investigations
- CT scan and MRI

Cerebrospinal Fluid Findings in Tuberculosis Meningitis

- Pressure is increased.
- A fine cot or cobweb may form on allowing CSF to stand for some time.
- Protein levels are elevated (100–800 mg/dL). Very high levels indicate block to CSF flow.
- Sugar is lowered (to <40% of blood sugar).
- Cell counts are elevated and predominantly lymphocytic.
- Ziehl–Neelsen staining or fluorescent staining of the coagulum may show mycobacteria.
- Adenosine deaminase levels (ADA) are elevated; however, no cut-off has been defined to differentiate TBM from pyogenic meningitis.
- Nucleic acid amplification tests (NAATs) on CSF-polymerase chain reaction (PCR) tests to detect mycobacterial nucleic acids

Management
- Anti-tubercular chemotherapy should be started at the earliest.
- Early phase (first 2 months) involves intensive therapy combining rifampicin, isoniazid [isonicotinic acid hydrazide (INH)], pyrazinamide and streptomycin.
- After a period of 2 months, rifampicin with INH is continued for another 7–10 months.
- Ethambutol does not penetrate blood-brain barrier effectively.
- All patients should receive prednisolone 40 mg a day to reduce meningeal adhesions and severity of arteritis.

■ DEMYELINATING DISODERS

Common Causes of Demyelination

Common causes of demyelination are given in **Box 16.12**.

■ SPINAL CORD DISEASES

Spinal Causes of Paraplegia

Spinal causes of paraplegia are given in **Box 16.13**.

Transverse Myelitis

A heterogeneous group of inflammatory illnesses is characterised by acute or subacute motor, sensory and autonomic dysfunction of the spinal cord (bladder, intestine and sexual).

Causes
- Para infectious: Herpes simplex, herpes zoster, cytomegalovirus, Epstein–Barr virus, enteroviruses, *Mycoplasma*, Lyme borreliosis
- Post-vaccinal (rabies)
- Systemic autoimmune disease: SLE
- Multiple sclerosis

- Para-neoplastic syndrome
- Vascular:
  - Thrombosis of spinal arteries

Clinical Features

- Over several hours to several weeks, the symptoms of transverse myelitis (TM) evolve quickly.
- Due to several more days of deficit, full transverse sensorimotor myelopathy may advance.
- Common TM symptoms include weakness of the limb, sensory disturbance, dysfunction of the bowel and bladder.
- Recovery may be absent, partial or complete and usually commences within 1–3 months.
- Diagnosis requires MRI and CSF analysis.
- MRI typically shows cord swelling and gadolinium-enhancing lesions (single or multiple).
- CSF usually contains monocytes; protein content is slightly increased and IgG index is elevated.

Treatment

- Directed at the cause or associated disorder but is otherwise supportive
- In idiopathic cases, high-dose corticosteroids and plasma exchange may be tried.

Compressive Myelopathy

Features of compressive myelopathy are given in **Table 16.15**.

Box 16.13: Spinal causes of paraplegia.

Acute:
- Trauma, transverse myelitis, multiple sclerosis
- Infarction of spinal cord vasculitis
- Anterior spinal artery thrombosis
- Spinal epidural abscess

Subacute or chronic:
- Spinal cord compression (extra-dural)
- Intra-spinal tumours (intra-dural extra-medullary)
- Intra-medullary tumours (intra-dural intra-medullary)

Features Cauda equina and Conus medullaris lesions are given in **Table 16.16**.

Syringomyelia

Syringomyelia is a disorder where cavitations (syrinxes) occur within spinal cord.

Clinical Features

- Numbness in upper limbs with frequent burns and injuries that are painless
- Later, spastic weakness in lower limbs with urinary bladder involvement occurs.

Signs

- LMN signs in upper limbs, usually at C8-T1 myotomes with wasting of muscles in the neck, shoulders, arms and hands with absent reflexes in the upper limb.

Box 16.12: Common causes of demyelination.

Demyelinating diseases of central nervous system
- Multiple sclerosis
- Neuromyelitis optica
- Infectious: Acute disseminated encephalomyelitis (ADEM)
- Human immunodeficiency virus encephalitis
- Progressive multifocal leucoencephalitis, subacute sclerosing pan-encephalitis, Creutzfeldt–Jakob encephalitis
- Nutritional: Wernicke encephalopathy, subacute combined degeneration
- Toxic: Radiation, chemotherapeutic agents, toluene, mercury, methanol
- Hypoxic/ischaemic: Vasculitis, posterior reversible encephalopathy syndrome

Demyelinating diseases of peripheral nervous system
- Dry beriberi
- Guillain-Barré syndrome
- Chronic inflammatory demyelinating polyneuropathy
- Charcot-Marie-Tooth disease
- Vitamin B12 deficiency
- Organophosphate poisoning
- Copper deficiency

- Dissociated suspended anaesthesia
  - There is loss of pain and temperature sense bilaterally with intact touch and proprioception (dissociated) over dermatomes of upper limbs and intact sensations above and below (suspended)
  - This is due to lesion at anterior commissure of spinal cord. This disrupts crossing pain and temperature fibres at midline.
- Pyramidal signs in lower limbs

Investigations
MRI is the most sensitive method. It shows fluid-filled cavitation and dilated central canal. MRI of brain and entire spinal cord should be done.

Treatment
Surgical removal of obstruction of CSF flow, if any, along with syringe—subarachnoid shunt

BROWN–SÉQUARD SYNDROME
- Brown-Séquard syndrome refers to findings which are seen in hemi-section of the spinal cord.
- In diseased states, it is never seen in its pure form, except may be in stab injuries.

Clinical Manifestations
Clinical manifestations of Brown-Séquard syndrome are given in **Table 16.17**.

Subacute Combined Degeneration
- It is nutritional disorder of CNS due to vitamin B12 deficiency, including pernicious anaemia
- Condition is characterised by demyelination of corticospinal tracts and posterior column. It is usually associated with peripheral neuropathy, optic neuritis and mental changes.

TABLE 16.15: Features of compressive myelopathy.

Extra-dural myelopathy	Intra-dural extra-medullary myelopathy	Intra-dural intra-medullary myelopathy
• Localised pain common and early • Local deformity • Root pains common • LMN involvement localised to the site of involvement • Pyramidal signs late • Bladder involvement late • Early sacral sensory loss	• Root pains less common compared to extra-dural • LMN involvement localised • Bladder involvement rare • Early onset of pyramidal signs producing spasticity • Early sacral sensory loss	• Root pains uncommon • LMN involvement spreads over many segments • Bladder involvement common • Pyramidal signs late in onset • Dissociated sensory loss may be present, e.g. syringomyelia • May have 'sacral sparing' (sacral sensory loss delayed)

(LMN: lower motor neuron)

TABLE 16.16: Features of Cauda equina and Conus medullaris lesions.

Features	Cauda equina	Conus medullaris
Onset	Asymmetrical and gradual	Symmetrical and acute
Dissociated sensory loss	Absent	Present
Root pain	Common	Rare
Low backache	Common	Rare
Fasciculations	Common	Rare
Bladder and bowel involvement	Early or late (depends on root involvement)	Early
Muscle tone	Decreased	Increased
Knee and ankle reflexes	Both absent	Knee present but ankle absent
Anal reflex	Absent or diminished	
Peri-anal (saddle) numbness	Yes (saddle anaesthesia)	Normal (peri-anal sparing)

- Paraesthesia in lower limbs, associated with sensory ataxia
- Examination shows impaired tactile sensation in glove and stocking distribution.
- Impaired joint position and vibration senses.
- Absent ankle jerks (due to associated peripheral neuropathy) with extensor plantar response and brisk knee jerks.
- Megaloblastic anaemia is usually present.
- Associated optic neuritis and dementia may be seen.
- MRI of spinal cord shows abnormally increased T2-signal hyperintensity in posterior columns and occasionally in lateral columns.

Treatment and Prognosis

Injection hydroxocobalamin or cyanocobalamin 1 mg daily for 5 days followed by 1 mg once in 1–3 months.

■ MOTOR NEURON DISEASE

Classification

- **Hereditary**
  - Werdnig–Hoffmann disease (infantile spinal muscular atrophy [infantile spinal muscular atrophy (SMA)]
  - Kugelberg–Welander disease [adolescent spinal muscular atrophy (adolescent SMA)]
  - Others
- **Sporadic**
  - Amyotrophic lateral sclerosis (most common)
  - Progressive muscular atrophy (PMA) or SMA
  - Progressive bulbar palsy
  - Primary lateral sclerosis (PLS)
  - Multifocal motor neuropathy with conduction block

- **Progressive bulbar palsy**
  - Dysarthria, dysphagia and dysphonia
  - Impaired articulation occurs early with low volume of speech.
  - Difficulty in swallowing and hoarseness occur later.
  - Wasting and fasciculations of tongue along with spasticity.
  - Jaw jerk is exaggerated.
  - Emotional lability with uncontrolled laughter and crying.

Amyotrophic lateral sclerosis (ALS)

The most common mode of onset

- 'Amyotrophic' implies muscle atrophy and 'lateral sclerosis' relates to pathological modifications in the spinal cord (and brain stem) involving lateral column degeneration where the corticospinal tract is situated.
- Starts in the limbs of approximately two thirds of patients (spinal form); bulbar onset in one-third of patients.
- **In the extremities:**
  - Generally, LMN signs in upper limbs and UMN signs in lower limbs.
  - Cervical onset of lateral amyotrophic sclerosis with symptoms of the upper limb, either bilateral or unilateral.
  - Proximal weakness may present as trouble with shoulder-related abduction duties
  - Distal weakness causes the loss of tiny muscles of the hands that manifests with impairment of activity requiring pincer grip.
  - Later, wasting and fasciculation spread to proximal arm muscles. In upper limbs, both UMN and LMN signs can occur.
  - Thus, deep tendon reflexes (DTR) in upper limbs become exaggerated (UMN involvement) in spite of atrophic muscles.

TABLE 16.17: Clinical manifestations of Brown–Séquard syndrome.

Features	Ipsilateral	Contralateral
At level of lesion	• LMN signs (atrophy with depressed jerks) • All modalities of sensations are lost with or without hyperaesthesia • UMN signs (hypertonia, exaggerated DTR and extensor plantar response)	Impaired pain and temperature sense
Below level of lesion	Impaired joint position and vibration sense	

(LMN: lower motor neuron; UMN: upper motor neuron; DTR: deep tendon reflexes)

Lower limbs would have UMN sings (spasticity of legs, extensor plantar response and exaggerated DTR in lower limbs).

Treatment

- No curative medical treatment—walking aids, wheelchair and physiotherapy.
- Symptomatic treatments include use of botulinum toxin to control drooling
- Gastrostomy to reduce aspiration
- Baclofen or tizanidine for spasticity
- Death occurs from pneumonia or respiratory failure.
- The only drug that has a modest effect on survival is riluzole, a sodium-channel blocker that inhibits glutamate release

Multiple Sclerosis

Most frequently affects young and middle-aged people

Classification

- Relapsing remitting multiple sclerosis (RRMS)
- Primary progressive multiple sclerosis (PPMS)
- Secondary progressive multiple sclerosis (SPMS)
- Progressive relapsing multiple sclerosis (PRMS)

Clinical Features

- **Motor features:**
    - Predominantly UMN weakness of muscles (brisk deep tendon reflexes, Babinski's sign, loss of abdominal reflexes)
    - Wasting of muscles of hands and spasticity in advanced cases
- **Sensory features:**
    - Tingling, numbness common
    - Objective sensory loss including posterior column features. Loss of pain and temperature sensation less common
- **Other features:**
    - Cerebellar signs common
    - Optic neuritis usually occurs at the onset of disease.
    - Bladder and bowel involvement
    - Uhthoff's phenomenon is worsening of symptoms on exposure to heat (hot water bath) or exercise, and occurs due to conduction block.
    - Disequilibrium, truncal or limb ataxia, scanning speech and intention tremor are common cerebellar findings.
    - Emotional changes, delusions
    - Lhermitte sign (shooting electric pain in the neck with radiation to the shoulders on flexing the neck and occurs due to posterior column involvement)

Investigations

- Cerebrospinal fluid: Increased cells (< 75/μL), raised protein (< 1,000 mg/dL) and increased IgG. Electrophoresis of CSF shows oligoclonal bands.
- CSF analysis is very useful for ruling out infectious or neoplastic conditions that mimic MS.
- Visual, auditory and somatosensory evoked potentials show prolongation, and help in diagnosing involvement of clinically silent lesions.

Treatment

- **Acute exacerbation**
    - Methylprednisolone 1 g IV daily for 3 days is the standard therapy. It is followed by oral prednisolone 60 mg for 5 days and then tapered off.
- **Disease-modifying drugs**
    - These include interferon β-1b, interferon β-1a, mitoxantrone, glatiramer acetate and natalizumab. These are used to reduce disease progression and relapses.
    - May be used in RRMS and SPMS varieties.

■ Neuromyelitis Optica (Devic's Disease)

- More common in females
- Optic neuritis can be unilateral or bilateral.
- It is almost always acute, usually severe and may or may not be associated with retro-orbital pain.
- Fatal autonomic disorders may happen owing to autonomic outflow involvement in thoracic myelitis.
- Lower brain-stem involvement can occur from contiguous cervical myelitis, and produces nausea, intractable hiccups and respiratory failure.
- MRI of spinal cord helps in diagnosis. The spinal cord lesions are central, contiguous and longitudinally extensive (involving more than three spinal vertebral segments

- CSF oligoclonal bands are uncommon, whereas a neutrophilic pleocytosis ($\geq$ 50 cells/mm^3 and $\geq$ 5 neutrophils/mm^3) occurs commonly during acute attacks.

Treatment
- Neuromyelitis optica attacks are more serious, less frequently sensitive to steroids, and often result in important morbidity and mortality from respiratory failure due to cervical myelopathy.
- IV steroids for acute attack
- Immunosuppressives for prophylaxis (oral steroids + azathioprine or mycophenolate mofetil; rituximab)

Differences between multiple sclerosis and neuromyelitis optica are given in **Table 16.18**.

Peripheral Neuropathy
- Polyneuropathy is a definite clinical syndrome consisting of involvement of all peripheral neurons symmetrically to result in a characteristic clinical picture.
- Mononeuropathy is involvement of one nerve.
- Mononeuritis multiplex is involvement of multiple peripheral nerves, separated both in anatomic location as well as temporally. Diabetes mellitus is the most common cause.

Types of Peripheral Neuropathy and Their Causes
Types of peripheral neuropathy and their causes are given in **Box 16.14**.

Classification and Causes of Polyneuropathy
Classification and causes of polyneuropathy are given in **Box 16.15**.

Small Fibre Polyneuropathy
- Diabetes mellitus (burning feet syndrome)
- Alchoholism
- Vitamin B12 deficiency
- Amyloidosis

Causes of Thickened Nerves
- Leprosy
- Acromegaly
- Amyloidosis
- Neurofibromatosis
- Infiltration of nerves by lymphoma

TABLE 16.18: Differences between multiple sclerosis (MS) and neuromyelitis optica (NMO).

Features	Devic's disease (NMO)	Multiple sclerosis
Age	Adults	Young adults
F:M	>3:1	<3:1
Distribution of signs and symptoms	Restricted to optic nerves and spinal cord	Any white matter
Attack severity	Usually severe	Usually mild
Brain MRI	Usually normal (rarely lesion around area postrema +)	Multiple periventricular white matter lesions
Cord MRI	Longitudinally extensive transverse myelitis (LETM) central necrotic lesions, 3 or more spinal cord segments involved	Multiple small peripheral lesions
CSF cells	Pleocytosis during attack	Rarely >25 cells
Oligoclonal bands	Usually absent	Usually present
Antibodies	Anti NMO antibody (46%), antiQP4 (aquaporin) (85%) present	No antibodies
Co-existing autoimmunity	Frequent (30–40%) (Sjögren's syndrome)	Less common
Recurrence rate	Higher (90%)	Lower
Recurrence interval	Shorter	Longer

(CSF: cerebrospinal fluid; MRI: magnetic resonance imaging)

> **Box 16.14: Types of peripheral neuropathy and their causes.**
>
> **Focal neuropathy (mononeuropathy):**
> - Leprosy
> - Entrapment
> - Myxoedema
> - Rheumatoid arthritis
> - Amyloidosis
> - Acromegaly
> - Trauma
> - Ischaemic lesions
> - Diabetes mellitus
> - Vasculitis
> - Sarcoidosis
>
> **Mononeuritis multiplex:**
> - Leprosy
> - Diabetes mellitus
> - Vasculitis
> - Polyarteritis nodosa
> - Systemic lupus erythematosus
> - Sjögren's syndrome
> - Temporal arteritis
> - Sarcoidosis
> - HIV infection
> - Paraneoplastic syndrome
> - Lead poisoning
> - Polycythaemia
> - Cryoglobulinaemia

> **Box 16.15: Classification and causes of polyneuropathy.**
>
> **Acute:**
> - Guillain-Barré syndrome
> - Polyarteritis nodosa
> - Diphtheria
> - Dapsone
> - Acute intermittent porphyria
>
> **Subacute:**
> - Nutritional deficiency
> - Toxins:
>   - Arsenic, lead
>
> **Drugs:**
> - Chloroquine, phenytoin
> - Vincristine
>
> **Industrial toxins:**
> - Carbon tetrachloride
>
> **Chronic:**
> - Diabetes
> - Carcinoma
> - Chronic inflammatory demyelinating polyradiculoneuropathy (CIDP)
> - Hypothyroidism
> - Hereditary

- Chronic inflammatory demyelinating polyradiculoneuropathy
- Charcot-Marie-Tooth diseases
- Refsum disease

Guillain–Barré Syndrome/Acute Inflammatory Demyelinating Polyradiculoneuropathy

- GBS is the most common acute demyelinating polyneuropathy that is presumed to be autoimmune in nature.
- It affects people at any age.
- It usually follows viral infection, rarely after surgery or immunisation.

Clinical Features

- It is an acute disorder.
- It usually progresses for a new day and rarely up to 1 month.
- It is a predominant motor neuropathy.
- Sensory findings are minimum.
- Motor paralysis is more striking and is symmetrical, involving proximal muscles more than distal. It begins in the legs, progressing over several days to involve arms, face and eyes (ascending paralysis).
- Reflexes are absent.
- About 50% show bifacial weakness.
- Respiratory paralysis occurs in a few.
- Autonomic disturbances occur in a few, resulting in sudden fluctuations in BP and heart rate.
- Bladder involvement is rare, and even when seen in mild it hardly lasts longer than 1 week.

Miller Fisher Syndrome

- It is a variant of GBS and is characterised by areflexia, ataxia and ophthalmoplegia without significant limb weakness.
- Often preceded by *Campylobacter jejuni* infection (usually producing diarrhoea)

Other Variants

- Acute motor axonal neuropathy
- Acute motor and sensory axonal neuropathy

Course
Muscle weakness gradually progresses over 1–3 weeks and then plateaus over next several days to weeks before gradual recovery.

Investigations
- CSF becomes abnormal after 1 week of illness and shows raised proteins (> 45 mg/dL) with normal cell count (albumin—cytological dissociation).
- Nerve conduction velocity studies show slowing of velocities (demyelination pattern).

Treatment
- Immediate management of a patient with GBS consists of maintenance of airway, breathing and circulation
- Ventilate if patient develops respiratory failure.
- Monitor pulse, BP and cardiac activity using a cardiac monitor as these patients have autonomic instability.
- Plasmapheresis and IV immunoglobulin (0.4 g/kg/day for 5 days or 2 g/day for 2 days) have been shown to accelerate recovery.

Myasthenia Gravis
Myasthenia gravis (MG) is an autoimmune disorder in which antibodies are produced against acetylcholine receptors located at motor end plates in myoneural junctions.

Clinical Features
- Age of onset is 15–50 years.
- Females are more affected than males.
- Characteristic feature is easy fatigability associated with paresis of muscles.
- Repeated contractions worsen the weakness.
- Rest improves the muscular strength.
- Reflexes and sensations are normal.
- Diurnal variation is present.
- Ocular muscles are mostly affected resulting in ptosis and diplopia.
- Pupils are spared.
- The involvement of bulbar muscles leads to dysphagia, nasal regurgitation and speech (nasal voice) difficulty.
- Limb muscle participation is a proximal group resulting in difficulty in raising the arm above the knee and difficulty in getting out of squatting or sitting positions.
- Respiratory muscle involvement leads to myasthenic crisis and can lead to death.

Myasthenia gravis is referred to as ocular MG when eyelid and extra-ocular muscle weakness is exclusive, and generalised MG when weakness extends beyond these ocular muscles.

Investigations
- Tensilon test (edrophonium test)
- Chest radiography and CT scan for thymic enlargement.
- Thyroid function tests (10% may have associated hyperthyroidism).
- Acetylcholine receptor antibody levels (present in > 90% patients with generalised myasthenia).
- Anti-muscle-specific protein (tyrosine) kinase (anti-MuSK)
- Electro-diagnostic studies (nerve-conduction testing, repetitive nerve stimulation, exercise testing and in certain instances singled fibre EMG).
- Ice pack test: A small ice cube is put over the eyelid for about 2 minutes in a patient with ptosis. Improving the ptosis following this operation indicates a neuromuscular transmission disorder.

Management
- Anti-cholinesterases are effective in providing symptomatic relief.
  - Neostigmine (15 mg) one to two tablets, three to six times a day or pyridostigmine 60–120 mg three to six times a day may be used.
  - Cholinergic pyridostigmine is generally better tolerated than neostigmine due to fewer gastrointestinal side effects.
- Corticosteroids are useful in induction and maintenance of remission.
- Thymectomy can induce remission when the disease is generalised and has not been chronic.

- Immunosuppression with azathioprine cyclophosphamide, cyclosporine or mycophenolate mofetil is recommended when the dosage of steroid requirement is too high to maintain remission.
- Plasma exchange and IV immunoglobulin are useful for inducing a short-term remission like prior to surgery or during myasthenic crisis.

MUSCULAR DYSTROPHIES OR HEREDITARY MYOPATHIES

Classification
- X-linked muscular dystrophies:
  - Duchenne muscular dystrophy (DMD)
  - Becker muscular dystrophy
  - Emery-Dreifuss muscular dystrophy
- Autosomal muscular dystrophies (can be dominant or recessive):
  - Limb-girdle muscular dystrophy
  - Others
- Autosomal dominant muscular dystrophies:
  - Facioscapulohumeral muscular dystrophy
  - Ocular muscular dystrophy
  - Oculopharyngeal muscular dystrophy
  - Myotonic dystrophy
- Sporadic:
  - Congenital muscular dystrophy

Duchenne Muscular Dystrophy
- X-linked recessive disorder caused by absence of dystrophin due to mutation of DMD dystrophin gene.
- Onset between 3 and 5 years
- Proximal muscles of lower limbs are affected first followed by proximal muscles of upper limbs. Boys fall frequently.
- On getting up from the floor, patient uses his hands to climb up himself (Gower's sign).
- Later, neck muscles, extra-ocular muscles, diaphragm and facial muscles involved
- Patient is bed-ridden by the age of 10 years.
- Pseudo-hypertrophy of calf muscles and occasionally deltoid muscles.
- Other features include contractures, macroglossia, absence of incisor teeth, mental retardation, skeletal atrophy and cardiac involvement (tachycardia, tall R-waves in right pre-cordial leads, deep Q-waves in limb leads and left pre-cordial leads).
- EMG shows myopathic pattern (small, short-duration, polyphasic muscle action potentials).
- Muscle biopsy shows muscle fibres of varying sizes as well as small groups of necrosis and regenerating fibres. It also shows deficiency of dystrophin.
- Treatment with prednisolone may slow progression for up to 3 years. Others include physiotherapy, management of respiratory and cardiac complications and maintenance of nutrition.

Becker Muscular Dystrophy
- X-linked recessive disorder resulting from partial dystrophin deficiency
- Onset between 5 and 25 years
- Pelvic and pectoral muscles predominantly involved
- Patient unable to walk after about 25 years of onset
- Significant facial weakness is not common.
- Associated features include cardiac involvement, contractures and hypertrophy of muscles.
- Serum creatine kinase (CK) is raised.
- EMG shows myopathic pattern.

Myotonic Dystrophy
- Type 1 more common than type 2
- Autosomal dominant
- Onset during second decade of life
- Typical 'hatchet-faced', appearance due to atrophy and weakness of temporalis, masseter and facial muscles
- Neck flexors, sternocleidomastoid and distal limb muscles affected early
- Dysarthria, nasal voice and swallowing difficulties due to palatal, pharyngeal and tongue involvement
- Proximal muscles remain strong.
- Myotonia:
  - Percussion of thenal muscles or tongue produces contraction without immediate relaxation
  - Slow relaxation of hand grip after a forced voluntary closure
- Frontal baldness

- Cardiac conduction defects; may produce sudden death
- Mitral valve prolapsed
- Others include cataract, gonadal atrophy, insulin resistance and intellectual impairment.
- Serum CK normal or mildly elevated
- EMG shows evidence of myotonia
- Myotonia usually requires no treatment. If it is severe, phenytoin or mexiletine may be used.
- Cardiac pacemaker, if cardiac conduction defects produce symptoms.

COMA

It is defined as a state of altered consciousness from which a person cannot be aroused easily. Stupor is defined a disturbed consciousness from which the patient can be aroused by vigorous external stimuli.

Causes of Coma

Causes of coma are given in **Box 16.16**.

Box 16.16: Causes of coma.

Primary neurological disorders:
- Cerebral hemispherical lesions
- Brain tumours
- Abscess
- Cerebral infarcts (large)
- Cerebral haemorrhage
- Subarachnoid haemorrhage
- Subdural haematoma
- Hydrocephalus
- Posterior fossa mass lesions
- Wernicke encephalopathy

Metabolic encephalopathies:
- Hypoglycaemia
- Hyponatraemia
- Hyperglycaemia with or without ketosis
- Anoxia
- Hypercapnia
- Hyperpyrexia
- Hepatic and uraemic encephalopathy

Miscellaneous
- Toxic encephalopathies secondary to systemic infections
- Hypertensive encephalopathy
- Poisoning

Evaluation of Severity of Coma

Glasgow coma score:

Eye opening (E) score:
- Spontaneous — 4
- To speech — 3
- To pain — 2
- None — 1

Best motor response (M)
- Obeys — 6
- Localises — 5
- Withdraws — 4
- Abnormal flexion — 3
- Abnormal extension — 2
- None — 1

Verbal response (V):
- Oriented — 5
- Confused conversation — 4
- Inappropriate words — 3
- Incomprehensible sounds — 2
- None — 1

Coma Score:
- Fully conscious — 15
- Deeply comatose — 3

FACIAL PALSY: DIFFERENTIAL DIAGNOSIS

Causes of facial nerve palsy are given in **Table 16.19**.

TABLE 16.19: Causes of facial nerve palsy.

Unilateral	Bilateral
UMN	**UMN**
• Vascular (stroke)	• Vascular (multi-infarct dementia)
• Tumour	• Motor neuron disease
• Multiple sclerosis	
LMN	**LMN**
• Bell's palsy	• Guillain-Barré syndrome
• Ramsay Hunt syndrome	• Sarcoidosis (uveoparotid tumour)
• Parotid tumour	• Leprosy
• Head injury	• Lyme's disease
• Skull base tumour	• Leukaemia
• Basal meningitis	• Lymphoma
• Diabetes mellitus	• Moebius
• Hypertension	• Melkersson Rosenthal
• Chronic suppurative otitis media	• Toxin: Thalidomide
	• Bilateral Bell's palsy

(UMN: upper motor neuron; LMN: lower motor neuron)

BEST OF FIVES

1. You are doing a neurologic examination on a patient with a history of transient weakness. You ask the patient to stand with both arms fully extended and parallel to the ground with his eyes closed for 10 seconds. What is the name of this test?
   A. Babinski sign
   B. Dysdiadochokinesis
   C. Lhermitte symptom
   D. Pronator drift
   E. Romberg sign

2. A patient has been recently diagnosed with small-cell lung cancer. She is now complaining of headaches. Metastatic disease to the brain is suspected. A mass lesion on magnetic resonance imaging (MRI) is demonstrated in the right parietal lobe. Which MRI technique would best identify the extent of the oedema surrounding the lesion?
   A. Magnetic resonance angiography
   B. Fluid-attenuated inversion recovery (FLAIR)
   C. 1-weighted
   D. 2-weighted
   E. Both B and D

3. A 70-year-old man has been diagnosed with mild cognitive impairment. He asks you to prescribe something that will decrease his likelihood to progress to Alzheimer disease. What treatment do you recommend?
   A. Brain training exercises
   B. Donepezil
   C. Gingko biloba
   D. Memantine
   E. No treatment at this time has been demonstrated to delay the progression of mild cognitive impairment to Alzheimer disease

4. Which of the following statements regarding Parkinson disease is true?
   A. Cigarette smoking reduces the risk of developing the disease.
   B. Older age at presentation is more likely to be associated with genetic predisposition.
   C. Parkinson disease has been identified as a monogenetic disorder related to mutations in the α-synuclein protein.
   D. The typical age of onset of symptoms is about 70 years.
   E. The hallmark pathologic feature of Parkinson disease is the presence of neurofibrillary tangle and tau protein in the substantia nigra pars compacta.

5. A 46-year-old woman presents with complaints of very sharp pain lasting for about 1 minute over her right cheek and lips. These pain episodes occur in clusters with intense pain during the episode. When an episode occurs, it is present both day and night and can recur over a period of about a week. Paroxysms of pain can be elicited by washing her ace. On physical examination, there is no sensory or motor loss in the right face. What is the apprpiate next step?
   A. Initiate treatment with carbamazepine 100 mg with a goal dose of 200 mg qid.
   B. Perform a magnetic resonance imaging (MRI)/magnetic resonance angiography (MRA) of the brain.
   C. Refer patient for a temporal artery biopsy.
   D. Refer patient for electromyography and nerve conduction study.
   E. Refer patient for microvascular decompression surgery.

6. A young man presents for evaluation of foot drop. Both his father and paternal aunt have had some weakness in their lower extremities. He does not remember his grandparents having any symptoms. The patient's examination is notable or distal leg weakness with reduced sensation to light touch in both lower extremities. Knee and ankle jerk reflexes are unobtainable. Upper extremity examination is normal. Which of the following is the most likely diagnosis?
   A. Charcot-Marie-Tooth syndrome
   B. Fabry disease
   C. Guillain–Barré syndrome
   D. Hereditary neuralgic amyotrophy
   E. Hereditary sensory and autonomic neuropathy

7. A 34-year-old woman is seen for complaints of weakness for the past month. She notes this to be particularly worse in the late afternoon and evening. Initially, she attributed the weakness

to stress from her job. On physical examination, you note the appearance of mild ptosis and a nasal, breathy tone to her voice. Which of the following tests would be most sensitive and specific for making a diagnosis in this patient?
   A. Acetylcholine receptor (AChR) antibodies
   B. Edrophonium test
   C. Muscle-specific kinase (MuSK) antibodies
   D. Repetitive nerve stimulation test
   E. Voltage-gated calcium channel antibodies

8. The following endocrine conditions are associated with myopathy:
   A. Hypothyroidism
   B. Hyperparathyroidism
   C. Hyperthyroidism
   D. Acromegaly
   E. All of the above

9. All of the following antidepressant medications are correctly paired with their class of medication except:
   A. Duloxetine—selective serotonin reuptake inhibitor
   B. Fluoxetine—selective serotonin reuptake inhibitor
   C. Nortriptyline— tricyclic antidepressant
   D. Phenelzine—monoamine oxidase inhibitor
   E. Venlafaxine—mixed norepinephrine/serotonin reuptake inhibitor and receptor blocker

10. Which of the following statements best reflects the effect of alcohol on neurotransmitters in the brain?
    A. Decreases dopamine activity
    B. Decreases serotonin activity
    C. Increases γ-aminobutyric acid activity
    D. Stimulates muscarinic acetylcholine receptors
    E. Stimulates N-methyl-D-aspartate excitatory glutamate receptors

11. A 48-year-old woman is recovering from alcohol dependence and requests medication to help prevent relapse. She has a medical history of stroke occurring during a hypertensive crisis. Which of the following medications could be considered?
    A. Acamprosate
    B. Disulfiram
    C. Naltrexone
    D. Both A and C
    E. A, B and C

12. Allodynia refers to:
    A. Pain on imagination
    B. Fear of pain
    C. Painful response to non-painful stimulus
    D. Non-painful response to painful stimulus
    E. Absence of pain sensation

13. In Dejerine–Roussy syndrome, the lesion is in:
    A. Spinal cord
    B. Brainstem
    C. Thalamus
    D. Cortex
    E. Cerebellum

14. A chronically spinally injured patient becomes hypertensive and sweaty during general anaesthesia for urinary sphincterotomy. His level of spinal cord injury is T4 and it is complete. You consider the diagnosis of autonomic hyperreflexia. Autonomic hyperreflexia:
    A. Could have been prevented by performing subarachnoid anaesthesia
    B. Is unlikely with a T4 lesion
    C. Should be treated by administration of a beta-blocker
    D. Should be treated by administration of an opioid analgesia
    E. Will resolve once the surgical stimulus ceases

15. Cerebellar hemisphere lesions are characterised by:
    A. Cogwheel rigidity
    B. Intention tremor
    C. Absent deep tendon reflexes
    D. Dysphagia
    E. Loss of sensations

16. Finger agnosia occurs as a part of:
    A. Gertmann's syndrome
    B. Central cord syndrome
    C. Brown– Séquard syndrome
    D. Wallenberg syndrome
    E. Weber syndrome

17. The basal ganglia, cerebellum and supplementary motor area are critical for:
    A. Episodic memory
    B. Semantic memory

C. Procedural memory
D. Working memory
E. Functional memory

18. Damage to optic radiation in the temporal lobe (Meyer's loop) produces:
    A. Bitemporal hemianopia
    B. Superior quadrantic homonymous hemianopia
    C. Inferior quadrantic homonymous hemianopia
    D. Total homonymous hemianopia
    E. Uniocular blindness

19. Migraine is associated with release of:
    A. Neurotensin
    B. Substance P
    C. Calcitonin gene-related peptide (CGRP)
    D. Cholecystokinin
    E. Serotonin

20. Waxy flexibility is a feature of which of the following?
    A. Abulia
    B. Akinetic mutism
    C. Catatonia
    D. Locked-in state
    E. Schizophrenia

21. Which of the following is a feature of acute Wernicke's disease?
    A. Global confusion
    B. Impairment of eye movements
    C. Gait ataxia
    D. All the above
    E. A and B

22. Which of the following occurs as a bilateral motor sign in typical absence seizures?
    A. Small amplitude, clonic movements of hands
    B. Large amplitude, clonic movements of hands
    C. Small amplitude, tonic movements of hands
    D. Large amplitude, tonic movements of the hands
    E. Medium amplitude, tonic-clonic movements

23. Insular ribbon sign is the earliest indicator of:
    A. Meningitis
    B. Subarachnoid haemorrhage
    C. Cerebral infarction
    D. Encephalitis
    E. All the above

24. Sentinel bleed is the term used for small aneurysmal rupture into:
    A. Subarachnoid space
    B. White matter
    C. Grey matter
    D. Thalamus
    E. Pons

25. Eye of the tiger in magnetic resonance imaging (MRI) best relates to:
    A. Restless leg syndrome
    B. Wilson's disease
    C. Hallervorden–Spatz disease
    D. Machado–Joseph disease
    E. Charcot–Marie disease

26. The percentage of diabetic patients with autonomic neuropathy is reported to be:
    A. <5%
    B. 10–20%
    C. 20–40%
    D. 60–80%
    E. >80%

27. A patient with a head injury who has eye opening to speech, no verbal responses and withdrawal motor responses would have a Glasgow Coma Scale score of:
    A. 4
    B. 5
    C. 6
    D. 7
    E. 8

Answers
1-D, 2-E, 3-E, 4-A, 5-A, 6-A, 7-A, 8-E, 9-A, 10-A, 11-D, 12-C, 13-C, 14-A, 15-B, 16-A, 17-C, 18-B, 19-C, 20-C, 21-D, 22-A, 23-C, 24-A, 25-C, 26-C, 27-E

■ SUGGESTED READING

1. Powers WJ, Rabinstein AA, Ackerson T, Adeoye OM, Bambakidis NC, Becker K, et al. Guidelines for the Early Management of Patients With Acute Ischemic Stroke: 2019 Update to the 2018 Guidelines for the Early Management of Acute Ischemic Stroke: A Guideline for Healthcare Professionals From the American Heart Association/American Stroke Association. Stroke. 2019;50(12):e344-418.
2. Demaerschalk BM, Kleindorfer DO, Adeoye OM, Demchuk AM, Fugate JE, Grotta JC, et al. Scientific Rationale for the Inclusion and Exclusion Criteria for Intravenous Alteplase in Acute Ischemic Stroke: A Statement for Healthcare

Professionals From the American Heart Association/American Stroke Association. Stroke. 2016;47(2):581-641.
3. Hemphill JC 3rd, Greenberg SM, Anderson CS, Becker K, Bendok BR, Cushman M, et al. Guidelines for the Management of Spontaneous Intracerebral Hemorrhage: A Guideline for Healthcare Professionals From the American Heart Association/American Stroke Association. Stroke. 2015;46(7):2032-60.
4. Bijlsma MW, Brouwer MC, Kasanmoentalib ES, Kloek AT, Lucas MJ, Tanck MW, et al. Community-acquired bacterial meningitis in adults in the Netherlands, 2006-14: a prospective cohort study. Lancet Infect Dis. 2016;16(3):339-47.
5. Carteaux G, Maquart M, Bedet A, Contou D, Brugières P, Fourati S, et al. Zika virus associated with meningo-encephalitis. N Engl J Med. 2016;374(16):1595-6.
6. Kupila L, Vuorinen T, Vainionpää R, Hukkanen V, Marttila RJ, Kotilainen P. Etiology of aseptic meningitis and encephalitis in an adult population. Neurology. 2006;66(1):75-80.
7. Fokke C, van den Berg B, Drenthen J, Walgaard C, van Doorn PA, Jacobs BC, et al. Diagnosis of Guillain-Barré syndrome and validation of Brighton criteria. Brain. 2014;137(Pt 1):33-43.
8. Liu J, Wang LN, McNicol ED. Pharmacological treatment for pain in Guillain-Barré syndrome. Cochrane Database Syst Rev. 2015;CD009950.
9. Headache Classification Committee of the International Headache Society (IHS) The International Classification of Headache Disorders, 3rd edition. Cephalalgia. 2018;38(1): 1-211.
10. Chou DE. Secondary Headache Syndromes. Continuum (Minneap Minn) 2018;24(4, Headache):1179-91.
11. Galea I, Ward-Abel N, Heesen C. Relapse in multiple sclerosis. BMJ. 2015;350:h1765.
12. Díaz-Manera J, Rojas García R, Illa I. Treatment strategies for myasthenia gravis: an update. Expert Opin Pharmacother. 2012;13(13):1873-83.
13. Sanders DB, Wolfe GI, Benatar M, Evoli A, Gilhus NE, Illa I, et al. International consensus guidance for management of myasthenia gravis: Executive summary. Neurology. 2016;87(4):419-25.
14. Morrison B, Chaudhry V. Medication, toxic, and vitamin-related neuropathies. Continuum (MinneapMinn). 2012; 18(1):139-60.
15. Hanewinckel R, Drenthen J, van Oijen M, Hofman A, van Doorn PA, Ikram MA. Prevalence of polyneuropathy in the general middle-aged and elderly population. Neurology. 2016;87(18):1892-98.
16. Krishnan C, Kaplin AI, Pardo CA, Kerr DA, Keswani SC. Demyelinating disorders: update on transverse myelitis. Curr Neurol Neurosci Rep. 2006;6(3):236-43.
17. Ostrom QT, Gittleman H, Truitt G, Boscia A, Kruchko C, Barnholtz-Sloan JS, et al. CBTRUS Statistical Report: Primary Brain and Other Central Nervous System Tumors Diagnosed in the United States in 2011-2015. Neuro Oncol. 2018;20 (Suppl 4):iv1-86.

CHAPTER 17

Nutrition and Metabolism

VITAMIN A

Clinical Features of Deficiency

- Eye signs
  - Night blindness
  - Xerophthalmia
  - Conjunctival xerosis
  - Bitot's spots
  - Corneal xerosis
  - Corneal ulcer covering less than one-third of the cornea
  - Keratomalacia
  - Corneal scarring

Diarrhoea, decreased growth rate, infertility. Increased susceptibility to infections (respiratory, urinary).

Treatment: About 60 mg of vitamin A, 3 doses—day 0, 1 and 14.

SCURVY

Ascorbic acid deficiency (vitamin C).

Types

Types of scurvy are given in **Table 17.1**.

Management

Investigations

- Low vitamin C levels
- Bones—white line of Frankel, Wimberger ring sign

Treatment

- Consumption of citrus fruits and vegetables
- Ascorbic acid 500 mg daily initially

THIAMINE

Deficiency

- **Wet beriberi**
  High output cardiac failure:
  - Peripheral vasodilatation
  - Tachycardia

TABLE 17.1: Types of scurvy.

Adult scurvy	Infantile scurvy (Barlow's disease)
• Scorbutic gingiva—gingivitis, loosening of teeth, bleeding gums • Perifollicular haemorrhages • Deformed 'corkscrew' hair projects out of a follicle • Petechial haemorrhages, ecchymoses, epistaxis and gastrointestinal bleeding • Nail beds—splinter haemorrhages • Haemorrhages into muscles of arms and legs with secondary phlebothrombosis • Haemorrhages into joints • Poor wound healing	• Subperiosteal haemorrhage into shafts of long bones • Scorbutic rosary denotes enlargement of costochondral junctions • Purpura or ecchymotic skin lesions • Gingival bleeding • Retrobulbar, subarachnoid and intracerebral haemorrhages • Lassitude • Anorexia • Painful limbs giving rise to 'pseudoparalysis'

- o Raised jugular venous pressure (JVP) and tender hepatomegaly
- o Hyperdynamic circulation with a rapid circulation time
- o Dyspnoea and cardiovascular collapse
  - Marked cardiomegaly

Treatment: About 100 mg thiamine IM for 7 days, then 10 mg/day orally for many months.

- **Dry beriberi**
  Polyneuropathy → symmetric impairment of sensory, motor and reflex functions that affect the distal segments of limbs more than the proximal ones.
- **Wernicke's encephalopathy**
  - o Global confusional state, profound listlessness, inattentiveness and disorientation
  - o Ophthalmoplegia: Sixth nerve palsy, diplopia, nystagmus
  - o Ataxia of gait: This affects stance and gait predominantly

Treatment: About 500 mg of thiamine IV, three times daily for two consecutive days and 250 mg IV or IM once daily for the next 5 days.

- **Korsakoff's psychosis**
  - o Apathy, drowsiness, global confusion
  - o Confabulation
  - o Amnesic state characterised by large gaps in memory (both antegrade and retrograde memory loss)
  - o Treatment—thiamine (100 mg IM daily for 7 days)
- **Leigh syndrome** is a progressive subacute necrotising encephalomyopathy.

■ PELLAGRA

- Metabolic encephalopathy caused by niacin (nicotinamide) deficiency
  - o Dermatitis—symmetric erythema over body parts exposed to sunlight, especially neck (**Casal's necklace** or collar rash)
  - o Diarrhoea
  - o Dementia
  - o Insomnia, anxiety, disorientation, tremor, delusions, depression, encephalopathy

Management

- Oral 100 mg nicotinamide every 6 hours

■ CALCIUM, VITAMIN D, PARATHYROID HORMONE AND CALCITONIN

Physiology of vitamin D is shown in **Figure 17.1**.

Rickets

Types of rickets are given in **Table 17.2**. Disorders affecting bone metabolism are compared in **Table 17.3**. Role of vitamin D in health and disease is listed in **Table 17.4**.

Clinical Features

- Infants younger than 6 months → hypocalcaemia tetany or seizures
- Older children → failure to thrive or skeletal deformities
- Prone to infections (respiratory and gastrointestinal)
- Retardation of skeletal growth
  - o Craniotabes
  - o 'Rickets rosary' on costal cartilage
  - o Pectus carinatum
  - o Harrison's groove
  - o Frontal bossing of skull
  - o Poor dentition
  - o Epiphyses enlargement of long bones
  - o Delayed closure of fontanelle
  - o Kyphosis, genu valgum or varum
  - o Triradiate pelvis

Investigations

- Lower ends of the shaft of radius and ulna become splayed ('saucer' deformity)
- Low serum calcium
- Low serum phosphate
- Increased alkaline phosphatase
- Low 25-hydroxyvitamin D3 levels

Treatment

- Correction of underlying cause
- Supplementation of calcium and vitamin D
- Ergocalciferol, 150,000–600,000 IU orally or intramuscularly as a single dose

Osteomalacia

Defective mineralisation of the organic matrix of the skeleton in adults.

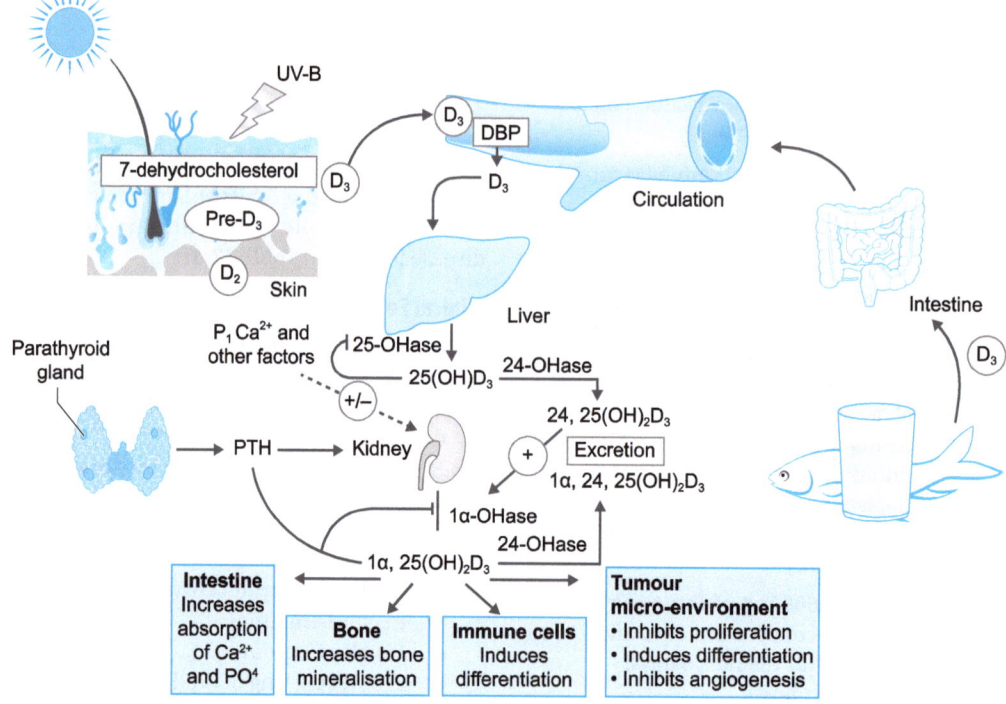

Fig. 17.1: Physiology of vitamin D.

TABLE 17.2: Types of rickets.

Types of rickets	Features
Secondary rickets	Malabsorption states, e.g. coeliac disease, intestinal resection; inadequate intake of calcium, vitamin D, inadequate sunlight exposure
Renal rickets	Seen in cases of chronic renal failure
Drug-induced rickets	Anticonvulsants such as phenytoin sodium
Tumour-induced rickets	Due to underlying malignancy
Resistant rickets	Familial hypophosphataemic rickets and vitamin D dependent rickets

Aetiology
- Dietary deficiency of vitamin D
- Malabsorption
- Chronic kidney disease (CKD), phenytoin, steroids
- Parenteral nutrition, distal renal tubular acidosis, nephrotic syndrome

Clinical Features
- Bone pains
- Proximal muscle weakness → waddling gait
- Fractures of bones
- Deformities due to softening of skeleton and include kyphosis and coxa vera

Investigations
- Low or normal serum calcium and serum phosphorus
- Elevated serum alkaline phosphatase
- Low serum 25-hydroxyvitamin D3 levels
- Elevated parathyroid hormone (PTH) levels
- Radiological features:
  o Osteopaenia
  o Looser's zones
  o Bone mineral density (BMD) using dual-energy X-ray absorptiometry is reduced at spine, hip and forearm

TABLE 17.3: Comparison of conditions involving bone metabolism.

Condition	Calcium	Phosphorous	Vitamin D	Alkaline phosphatase	Parathormone	Bone
Rickets/osteomalacia	Decreased	Decreased	Low	Elevated	Elevated	Softening, Looser's zones
Osteopaenia	Normal	Normal	Normal	Normal/decreased	Normal	Decrease bone mass
Osteoporosis	Normal	Normal	Normal/decreased	Normal/mild elevation	Normal	Degeneration of bone matrix
Hyperparathyroidism	Increased	Decreased	Normal	Elevated	Elevated	Brown tumour Lytic lesions
Paget's disease	Normal	Normal	Normal	Variable	Variable	Osteolytic/sclerotic lesion

TABLE 17.4: Role of vitamin D in health and disease.

Parathyroid hormone	• Hypovitaminosis D causes secondary hyperparathyroidism which increases the risk of MI, HTN and stroke
Malignancy	• Transcription of oncogenes involved with cell differentiation and proliferation is controlled: For example, c-myc, c-fos, c-sis • There is an inverse relationship between sun exposure and cancer mortality. 10 ng/mL rise in vitamin D level or associated with 17% reduction in cancer incidence, 29% reduction in all cancer mortality and 45% reduction in GI cancer mortality
Nervous system function	• Vitamin D modulates neurotransmitter and neurological function • Has anticonvulsant and antidepressant effect. 50% of multiple sclerosis patients are vitamin D deficient • Seizures are common with vitamin D deficiency
Anti-inflammatory function	• Suppresses and may prevent autoimmune diseases • Seems to reduce severity and frequency of childhood pneumonia
Calcium homeostasis	• Calcium absorption increases as 25 (OH) D blood levels increase
Cardiovascular function	• Risk of myocardial infarction doubles in patients with vitamin D deficiency • Heart failure patients have much lower vitamin D levels. HTN patients given UV light treatments 3 times per week for 6 weeks have shown mild decreases in BP
T1DM	• Infants and children who were supplemented with Vitamin D had decreased incidence of T1DM by 80%
T2DM	• Low vitamin D levels associated with insulin resistance and β-cell dysfunction • Postprandial glucose and insulin sensitivity: Better in healthy adults with highest vitamin D levels • Highest vitamin D levels associated with 60% improvement in insulin sensitivity
Respiratory system	• Vitamin D supplementation provides significant protective effect against influenza • It is also associated with decrease in FEV1 and an increased incidence of rhinobronchial atopy
Osteoarthritis (OA)	• Vitamin D deficiency hastens the progression of OA hip and knee
Mood disorders	• Vitamin D supplementations improve general mood and hasten recovery in seasonal affective mood disorders

Continued

Continued

Polycystic ovary syndrome	• Deficiency exists in 60% of cases with normalisation of menses and/or fertility within 3 months of supplementation
Pain	• Persistent, non-specific musculoskeletal pain in 93% of patients had vitamin D deficiency • Low back pain patients (53%) have vitamin D deficiency
Autoimmune disease	Vitamin D insufficiency in: • Half of the patients with fibromyalgia + SLE, Graves' disease, ankylosing spondylitis and rheumatoid arthritis
Falls in the elderly	• Vitamin D deficiency reported to affect predominantly the weight-bearing antigravity muscles of the lower limb, which are necessary for postural balance and walking • Improvement in lower extremity muscle strength and balance with vitamin D supplementation thought to explain the reduced number of fall-related fractures

(T1DM: type 1 diabetes mellitus; T2DM: type 2 diabetes millitus; FEV1: forced expiratory volume in the first second; GI: gastrointestinal; HTN: hypertension; MI: myocardial infarction; OA: osteoarthritis; SLE: systemic lupus erythematosus)

Treatment

- About 1,000–4,000 IU of vitamin D2 or vitamin D3 for 3 months
- Malabsorption → 50,000–100,000 IU of vitamin D along with calcium supplementation

Disorders associated with vitamin D deficiency are given in **Box 17.1**.

■ PROTEIN-ENERGY MALNUTRITION

- Underweight: Being underweight for one's age
- Stunted: Being too short for one's age
- Wasted: Being dangerously thin
- Micronutrient malnutrition: Being deficient in vitamins and minerals

Wellcome classification

Parameter: → Weight for age ± oedema
- Almost 80–60% without oedema → underweight
- Almost 80–60% with oedema → Kwashiorkor
- Less than 60% with oedema → Marasmic-kwashiorkor
- Less than 60% without oedema → Marasmus

Complications of Protein-energy Malnutrition

- Water, electrolyte and mineral imbalance
- Hypothermia
- Hypoglycaemia

Box 17.1: Disorders associated with vitamin D deficiency.

- Type 1 diabetes mellitus (T1DM) and type 2 diabetes mellitus (T2 DM)
- Systemic lupus erythematosus (SLE)
- Ischaemic heart disease
- Increased cancer mortality
- Rhinobronchial atopy
- Hypothyroidism
- Rheumatoid arthritis
- Atherosclerosis
- Increased susceptibility to infections
- Depression
- Graves' disease
- Polycystic ovary disease (PCOD)
- Multiple sclerosis
- Osteoarthritis
- Infertility

- Superadded infections
- Vitamin deficiency
- Cardiac failure
- Renal impairment
- Long-term—growth and mental retardation

■ OBESITY

Causes

The causes of obesity are mentioned in **Box 17.2**.

Box 17.2: Causes of obesity.

- Physical inactivity
- Eating habits
- Psychological factors
- Genetic factors
- Hypothyroidism
- Cushing's syndrome
- Hypothalamic disorders
- Diabetes mellitus
- Pickwickian syndrome
- Laurence–Moon–Biedl syndrome
- Drugs: Insulin, Pioglitazone
- Atypical antipsychotics
- Steroid hormones: Progestational steroids, corticosteroids, hormonal contraceptives

Leptin
- A defect in leptin gene or its receptor may produce obesity.

TABLE 17.5: BMI categories and classes of obesity.

	BMI (kg/m^2)	Obesity Class
Underweight	< 18.5	–
Normal	18.5–24.9	–
Overweight	25.0–29.9	–
Obesity	30.0–34.9	I
	35.0–39.9	II
Extreme obesity	40.0+	III

(BMI: body mass index)

BMI categories and classes of obesity are listed in **Table 17.5**.

Risks associated with obesity
Risks associated with obesity are given in **Table 17.6**.

Treatment

Dietary therapy
- Low-fat diet
- Very low carbohydrate diet or Atkins diet
- High-protein diet

Physical exercise
- Moderate exercise should be done for 30–45 min/day, 3–5 days a week

Pharmacotherapy
- Drugs may be used if body mass index (BMI) ≥ 30 kg/m^2
  - Sibutramine
  - Orlistat
  - Rimonabant
  - Other drugs
  - Phentermine, diethylpropion, metformin, pramlintide, liraglutide, lorcaserin, bupropion

Surgery
Bariatric Surgery:
- Adjustable gastric banding, vertical banded or sleeve gastroplasty, duodenal switch, Roux-en-Y gastric bypass, intragastric balloon, biliopancreatic diversion
- Useful if BMI ≥ 35–40 kg/m^2 when other methods have failed

METABOLIC DEFECTS IN AMINO ACID METABOLISM

Nine amino acids (histidine, isoleucine, leucine, lysine, methionine, phenylalanine, threonine, tryptophan and valine) are considered 'essential' in the diet because humans are not able to synthesise them endogenously.

Most of the non-essential amino acids, such as alanine, arginine, asparagine, aspartate, glutamate, glutamine, glycine, proline and serine, are synthesised from glucose while tyrosine is synthesised from the metabolism of phenylalanine and cysteine from the metabolism of methionine.

Phenylketonuria
- Phenylketonuria (PKU) is a disease caused by a deficiency of phenylalanine hydroxylase.
- It is one of the commonest inborn errors of amino acid metabolism encountered in clinical practice (prevalence is 1 in 15,000).
- Biochemically, it is characterised by an accumulation of the amino acid phenylalanine and often a deficiency of tyrosine.
- A newborn with PKU rarely presents with immediate symptoms, though he or she might sleep or eat poorly. If left untreated, it may

TABLE 17.6: Conditions and complications associated with obesity.

Risk factors/system involved	Outcomes
Metabolic syndrome	
• Type 2 diabetes mellitus	Coronary heart disease, Ischaemic heart disease
• Hypertension	Stroke
• Hyperlipidaemia	Diabetes complications
Cardiovascular	Heart failure
Gastrointestinal	Gastroesophageal reflux, disease, hiatus hernia
Hepatobiliary	Liver fat accumulation, nonalcoholic steatophepatitis, cirrhosis, gallstones
Pulmonary disease Restricted ventilation	Exertional dyspnoea, breathlessness
	Obstructive sleep apnoea
	Obesity hypoventilation syndrome (Pickwickian syndrome)
Mechanical effects of weight	Urinary incontinence, osteoarthritis of knees and hips, varicose veins, back strain
Endocrine manifestations (Increased peripheral steroid interconversion in adipose tissue)	Menstrual abnormalities Hormone-dependent cancers (breast, uterus) Polycystic ovarian syndrome (infertility, hirsutism)
Increased morbidity and mortality	
Psychological problems	Lack self-confidence, depression, more physical and sexual abuse, lack of attention, low education and low self-esteem
Others	Accident proneness, socioeconomic disadvantage (lower income, less likely to be promoted), post-operative problems, increased cancer risk (e.g. colorectal cancer), skin infections (groin and submammary candidiasis; hidradenitis)

cause mental retardation over the first few years of life in infants, which eventually will progress further.
- Infants may also often give off a 'mousy' odour from their bodies as well as from their urine which is due to the by-product of phenylalanine (Phenyllactate, Phenylacetate and Phenylpyruvate) in their urine and sweat.
- Failure to walk or speak, seizures, tremor, microcephaly, nausea and vomiting, an eczema-like rash, aggressive or self-injurious behaviour, hyperactivity and sometimes psychiatric symptoms are also symptoms of PKU in infants.

Maple Syrup Urine Disease

It is an autosomal recessive disorder characterised by partial or complete deficiency in Branched-chain α-keto acid dehydrogenase.

- The enzyme complex that decarboxylates Leucine, isoleucine and valine
  Various clinical features of the disease are feeding problems, vomiting, dehydration, severe metabolic acidosis and characteristic maple syrup odour to the urine
- In case the disease is left untreated, it can cause mental retardation, physical disabilities and sometimes death in severe cases
- These by-products also cause body fluids, such as urine and sweat, to smell like maple syrup.

Albinism

This condition is a resultant of a biochemical pathway which converts phenylalanine to melanin.
- The main clinical feature includes problems in the eye; however, people affected by albinism are expected to have a normal lifespan.

- Albinism is a heterogeneous condition inherited through either autosomal recessive or sex-linked recessive genes that affect approximately 1 in 17,000 people.
- It is characterised by a lack of the pigment melanin due to an error in the biochemical pathway that converts phenylalanine to melanin.

People with albinism may lack melanin in their hair, skin and eyes, while others may only have problems with their eyes—Oculocutaneous albinism and Ocular albinism.

Alkaptonuria

- Alkaptonuria is a rare autosomal recessive metabolic disorder resulting from loss of homogentisate 1,2-dioxygenase activity.
- Affected individuals accumulate large quantities of homogentisic acid, an intermediary product of the catabolism of tyrosine and phenylalanine, which darkens the urine and deposits in connective tissues (Ochronosis) causing a debilitating arthritis.

Homocystinuria

Autosomal recessive illness with a defect in the enzyme cystathionine β-synthase which converts homocysteine to cystathionine.

Characterised by ectopia lentis, skeletal abnormalities, marfanoid habitus, thromboembolism, mental retardation, behavioural abnormalities.

Hartnup Disease

Defect transport in intestine and kidney of large neutral amino acid (Tryptophan).

Pellagra like symptoms, diarrhoea, dermatitis, dementia

Cystinuria

Defect transport in intestine and kidney of basic amino acids causing urinary tract infections (UTIs) and renal stones.

Glycine Encephalopathy

Disorder of the glycine cleavage system. Glycine accumulates in cerebrospinal fluid and other body tissues presenting in the newborn period with intractable seizures.

BEST OF FIVES

1. A 75-year-old male with liver disease and poor nutrition develops alopecia, dermatitis and paronychia. Which vitamin deficiency can lead to these symptoms?
   A. Calcium
   B. Selenium
   C. Zinc
   D. Magnesium
   E. Thiamine

2. What food is a good source of vitamin D?
   A. Red meat
   B. Green leafy vegetables
   C. Herring
   D. Salmon
   E. Eggplant

3. A 3-year-old child was born at term, with no congenital anomalies. She is now only 70% of normal body weight. On examination, she shows dependent oedema of the lower extremities as well as an enlarged abdomen with palpable fluid wave. Her desquamating skin shows irregular areas of depigmentation, and hyperpigmentation. Which of the following nutritional problems is most likely present in this child?
   A. Marasmus
   B. Scurvy
   C. Vitamin A toxicity
   D. Niacin deficiency
   E. Kwashiorkor

4. A 24-year-old man has a history of multiple and recurrent pulmonary infections since childhood. He has also noted foul-smelling stools for the past 10 years. Laboratory studies show an elevated sweat chloride test. He has a quantitative stool fat of 10 g/day. A deficiency state involving which of the following nutrients is most likely to develop in this patient?
   A. Vitamin B1
   B. Vitamin D
   C. Iron
   D. Calcium
   E. Folic acid

5. A 60-year-old woman has developed red, roughened skin in sun-exposed areas over the past 2 years. She also has a chronic, watery

diarrhoea. On physical examination, she exhibits memory loss with confusion. These findings are most consistent with which of the following vitamin deficiencies?
A. Vitamin A
B. Thiamine
C. Niacin
D. Pyridoxine
E. Vitamin E

6. A 6-year-old child has complained of pain in his legs for the past year. On physical examination, there is bowing deformity of his lower extremities. Plain film radiographs of his lower legs show widened epiphyses and bowing of tibiae. BMD appears normal, consistent with failure of osteoid matrix formation. Which of the following vitamin deficiencies is this child most likely to have?
A. D
B. E
C. C
D. B3
E. B6

7. It is observed that pregnant women who do not get a diet that includes green, leafy vegetables develop a specific nutritional deficiency that affects their developing foetuses. Which of the following abnormalities is most likely to be found with increased frequency in these foetuses?
A. Anencephaly
B. Diaphragmatic hernia
C. Low birth weight
D. Congenital cytomegalovirus
E. Neuroblastoma

8. A clinical study is performed involving dietary iron metabolism in adults. It is observed that intestinal absorption of iron can be enhanced in patients with iron deficiency anaemia by supplementing their diet with another nutrient. Which of the following vitamins is most likely to have this effect?
A. A
B. B1
C. C
D. D
E. E

9. A 50-year-old chronic alcoholic man has had increasing dyspnoea for the past year. On physical examination, his temperature is 37°C, pulse 106/min, respiratory rate 20/min and blood pressure 90/60 mmHg. He has diffuse crackles at lung bases. A chest X-ray shows pulmonary oedema and cardiomegaly. Echocardiography shows an ejection fraction of 40%. Laboratory studies show glycosylated haemoglobin (HbA1c) 14 g/dL, haematocrit 42% and white blood cell (WBC) count 8,320/µL. A deficiency in which of the following vitamins is most likely to produce these findings?
A. A
B. B1
C. B2
D. K
E. D

10. A 50-year-old man has a 15-year history of chronic alcohol abuse. He has had worsening problems with ambulation for the past year. On physical examination, his gait is ataxic. Magnetic resonance (MR) imaging of the brain shows diminished size of the mamillary bodies and of the cerebellar vermis. He is most likely to have a deficiency of which of the following vitamins?
A. A
B. B1
C. C
D. D
E. E

11. A 30-year-old primigravida is in her 8th month of gestation. She is feeling increasingly tired and weak. Laboratory studies include a complete blood count (CBC) which shows HbA1c 9.7 g/dL, haematocrit (Hct) 28.8%, mean corpuscular volume (MCV) 71 fL, platelet count 289,000/µL and WBC count 5,600/µL. On the peripheral blood smear, the red blood cells (RBCs) show increased variation in size and shape, with many that are hypochromic and microcytic. Which of the following dietary deficiencies is she most likely to have?
A. Folic acid
B. Vitamin B12
C. Iron
D. Calcium
E. Nicotinic acid

12. A 30-year-old man with a 10-year history of chronic alcohol abuse has noted during the

past year that he has bruising with minimal trauma. On physical examination, he has abdominal enlargement with a fluid wave. He has pitting oedema to the knees. He has palmar erythema. Laboratory studies show that he has a prothrombin time of 30 seconds (control 12). His HbA1c is 13.8 g/dL, haematocrit 44.4%, MCV 94 fL, platelet count 229,000/μL and WBC count 6,630/μL. Which of the following nutrients is most likely to be of benefit in treating this man?
A. Thiamine
B. Vitamin C
C. Niacin
D. Vitamin K
E. Folic acid

13. It is observed that some commonly available foods have more vitamin A than others. Which of the following is most likely to provide the best source for vitamin A in the diet?
A. Milk
B. Bread
C. Meat
D. Beer
E. Carrots

14. A 14-year-old girl has been under a physician's care for the past year after diagnosis of anorexia nervosa. Her BMI (BMI) is now 17.8 kg/m². On physical examination, she has cheilosis. Laboratory studies show HbA1c 13.7 g/dL, haematocrit 41.0%, MCV 88 fL, platelet count 191,055/μL and WBC count 4,930/μL. Her serum glucose is 66 mg/dL. Which of the following nutrient deficiencies is most likely to cause her findings?
A. Riboflavin
B. Ascorbic acid
C. Folic acid
D. Iron
E. Niacin

15. A 40-year-old woman goes to the health food store to buy dietary supplements that she is convinced will help her to be more healthy and live longer. Instead, a year later she has increasing headaches, joint pain, nausea, vomiting and weight loss. On physical examination she is noted to have dryness of the oral mucosa, and a mild degree of papilloedema is noted on funduscopic examination. An excessive intake of which of the following nutrients is most likely responsible for her findings?
A. Calcium
B. Fluoride
C. Vitamin A
D. Alpha-tocopherol
E. Niacin

16. A 44-year-old woman has been on and off diets for the past 10 years trying to lose weight. She has had no major illnesses during this time. Her BMI has ranged from 25 to 31 kg/m² over that time. Which of the following problems is her pattern of dieting most likely to cause?
A. Vitamin deficiencies
B. Increased risk for osteoporosis
C. Decreased risk for atherosclerosis
D. Greater weight gain
E. Anorexia nervosa

17. A 7-year-old child develops gradual loss of vision over the past 2 years resulting in blindness. On physical examination, there is bilateral keratomalacia and corneal scarring. This child's blindness could most likely have been prevented by an adequate dietary intake of which of the following vitamins?
A. A
B. B1
C. B6
D. B12
E. K

18. An 11-month-old infant is only 60% of ideal body weight. The baby is proportionately small in size. Upon physical examination, the baby is listless and does not respond with vocalisation when touched. A small purplish contusion is noted over the right lower extremity. Which of the following is the most likely diagnosis?
A. Physical abuse
B. Marasmus
C. Hypocalcaemia
D. Premature birth
E. Vitamin C deficiency

19. A 45-year-old woman has felt increasingly fatigued. On physical examination, she has decreased sensation to touch in her lower

extremities bilaterally. Laboratory studies show HbA1c 10.1 g/dL, haematocrit 31.2% and MCV 126 fL. Microscopic examination of her peripheral blood smear shows RBC that have macrocytosis and neutrophils with hypersegmentation of nuclei. Laboratory testing for which of the following nutrients is most likely to show a deficiency state?
A. Folate
B. Ascorbic acid
C. Iron
D. Cobalamin
E. Pyridoxine

20. A 32-year-old woman has been having particularly heavy menstrual periods for the past year. She is becoming progressively fatigued. She then becomes pregnant. She receives no prenatal care. She delivers a term baby. During the delivery, bleeding is excessive. Which of the following nutrient deficiencies is most likely to be present in both mother and baby post-partum?
A. Niacin
B. Magnesium
C. Calcium
D. Vitamin K
E. Iron

Answers

1-C, 2-C, 3-E, 4-A, 5-C, 6-C, 7-A, 8-C, 9-B, 10-B, 11-C, 12-D, 13-E, 14-A, 15-C, 16-D, 17-A, 18-B, 19-D, 20-E

■ SUGGESTED READING

1. Food and Nutrition Information Center, Dietary Reference Intake Reports. [online] Available at: https://fnic.nal.usda.gov/dietary-guidance/dietary-reference-intakes/dri-nutrient-reports. [Last accessed June, 2020].
2. Institute of Medicine. Dietary Reference Intakes for Thiamin, Riboflavin, Niacin, Vitamin B6, Folate, Vitamin B12, Pantothenic Acid, Biotin, and Choline, 1998. [online] Available at: https://www.ncbi.nlm.nih.gov/books/NBK114310/. [Last accessed June, 2020].
3. Bemeur C, Butterworth RF. Thiamin. In: Modern Nutrition in Health and Disease, 11th edition, Ross AC, Caballero B, Cousins RJ, TUcker KL, Ziegler TR, (Eds). Philadelphia: Lippincott Williams and Wilkins; 2014. p.317.
4. Vieth R. What is the optimal vitamin D status for health? Prog Biophys Mol Biol. 2006;92(1):26-32.
5. Dawson-Hughes B, Mithal A, Bonjour JP, Boonen S, Burckhardt P, Fuleihan GEH, et al. IOF position statement: vitamin D recommendations for older adults. Osteoporos Int. 2010;21(7):1151-4.
6. American Geriatrics Society Workgroup on Vitamin D Supplementation for Older Adults. Recommendations abstracted from the American Geriatrics Society Consensus Statement on vitamin D for Prevention of Falls and Their Consequences. J Am Geriatr Soc. 2014;62(1):147-52.
7. Black RE, Victora CG, Walker SP, Bhutta ZA, Christian P, de Onis M, et al. Maternal and child undernutrition and overweight in low-income and middle-income countries. Lancet. 2013;382(9890):427-51.
8. GBD 2015 Child Mortality Collaborators. Global, regional, national, and selected subnational levels of stillbirths, neonatal, infant, and under-5 mortality, 1980-2015: a systematic analysis for the Global Burden of Disease Study 2015. Lancet. 2016;388(10053):1725-74.
9. World Health Organization. (2017). Joint child malnutrition estimates - Levels and trends (2017 edition). [online] Available from: https://www.who.int/nutgrowthdb/estimates2016/en/. [Last accessed June, 2020].
10. Jensen MD, Ryan DH, Apovian CM, Ard JD, Comuzzie AG, Donato KA, et al. 2013 AHA/ACC/TOS guideline for the management of overweight and obesity in adults: a report of the American College of Cardiology/American Heart Association Task Force on Practice Guidelines and The Obesity Society. Circulation. 2014;129:S102-38.
11. Centers for Disease Control and Prevention. Overweight & obesity. [online] Available from: https://www.cdc.gov/obesity/index.html. [Last accessed June, 2020].
12. Look AHEAD Research Group, Gregg EW, Jakicic JM, Blackburn G, Bloomquist P, Bray G, et al. Association of the magnitude of weight loss and changes in physical fitness with long-term cardiovascular disease outcomes in overweight or obese people with type 2 diabetes: a post-hoc analysis of the Look AHEAD randomised clinical trial. Lancet Diabetes Endocrinol. 2016;4(11):913-21.
13. Mingrone G, Panunzi S, De Gaetano A, Guidone C, Iaconelli A, Nanni G, et al. Bariatric-metabolic surgery versus conventional medical treatment in obese patients with type 2 diabetes: 5 year follow-up of an open-label, single-centre, randomised controlled trial. Lancet. 2015;386(9997):964-73.

CHAPTER 18

Psychiatry

HALLUCINATIONS

- Hallucinations mean things that are not really there.
- Auditory hallucinations: Hearing voices of people talking to the patient even when there is no one nearby
- Thought insertion: Feeling that thoughts are being put into patient's mind
- Thought withdrawal: Feeling that thoughts are being taken out of patient's mind
- Thought broadcasting: Feeling that other people are aware of patient's thoughts

DELUSIONS

- Delusions are beliefs that are maintained despite obvious evidence to contrary.
- Delusion of control or passivity: Feeling of under the control or influence of an outside force
- Delusions of reference: Feeling that programmes on television or radio hold special meaning for the patient
- Delusions of persecution: Feeling that patient is being singled out for special treatment or there is a conspiracy against the patient
- Delusions of grandeur: Feeling special, with unusual abilities or power

Table 18.1 presents differences between psychosis and neurosis.

SCHIZOPHRENIA

Schizophrenia is a group of disorders characterised by perturbations in language, perception, cognition, and behaviour.

TABLE 18.1: Differences between psychosis and neurosis.

Feature	Psychosis	Neurosis
Contact with reality	Lost	Preserved
Interpersonal behaviour	Marked disturbance in reality and behaviour	Preserved
Empathy	Absent	Present
Insight	Absence of understanding current symptoms	Present symptoms are recognised as undesirable
Organic causative factor	Present	Absent
Symptoms	Delusions, illusions and hallucinations	Usually physical or psychic symptoms
Dealing with reality	Capacity is grossly reduced	Preserved
Examples	Schizophrenia	Anxiety, phobia and depression

Types:
- There are four major types of schizophrenic disorders: Catatonic, disorganised, paranoid, and undifferentiated.
- Schizophrenic patients may also be classified as type I and type II (**Box 18.1**).

Clinical Features

Bleuler's criteria for the diagnosis of schizophrenia are given in **Box 18.2**.

Box 18.1: Two types of schizophrenia.

Type I (reactive or acute schizophrenia) patients:
- They have 'positive' symptoms, normal ventricular size and a good response to antipsychotic drugs.
- It is usually sudden and seems to be a reaction to some life crisis.
- It is a more treatable form of the illness than process or chronic.

Type II (process schizophrenia) patients:
- They have 'negative' symptoms, increased ventricular size and a poor response to antipsychotic drugs.
- It is also referred to as poor premorbid schizophrenia.
- It is characterised by lengthy periods of its development with a gradual deterioration and exclusively negative symptoms.
- It does not seem to be related to any major life change or negative event.
- Usually this type of schizophrenia is associated with 'loners' who are rejected by society, tend not to develop social skills and do not excel out of high school.

Box 18.2: Bleuler's criteria (4 As) for the diagnosis of schizophrenia.

- **Autism:** Totally engorged in thinking, not at all affected by external stimuli
- **Association loosening**
- **Ambivalence:** Simultaneous opposite action/thought, do/do not (**Ambitendency:** Inability to choose between two opposite action)
- **Affective blunting**/(Snap prop) inappropriate facial expressions of mood

Table 18.2 presents negative and positive symptoms of schizophrenia.

Schneider's 11 first rank symptoms are given in **Box 18.3**.

Major types of schizophrenic disorders are described in **Box 18.4**.

Management
- Neuroleptic drugs (antipsychotic drugs)
- It is conventional to start with chlorpromazine 100 mg thrice daily, gradually building up the dose to a maximum of 1,500 mg daily or until symptoms subside. Higher doses may be required if the patient is aggressive or agitated.

TABLE 18.2: Negative and positive symptoms of schizophrenia.

Negative symptoms	Positive symptoms
Alogia: 'Lack of words' including poverty of speech and of speech content in response to a questions	Hallucinations
Affective flattering Decreased expression of emotion, such as lack of expressive gestures	Delusions
Avolition-apathy • Loss of function • Impaired concentration • Diminished social engagement	• Bizzare behaviour • Conceptual disorganisations • Aggressive/agitated, odd clothing or appearance, odd social behaviour, repetitive stereotyped behaviour
Anhedonia-asociality Few friends, activities, interests; impaired intimacy, little sexual interest	**Formal thought disorder:** Loosening of association
Attention impairment	

Box 18.3: Schneider's 11 first rank symptoms of schizophrenia.

3 Thought phenomenon
- Thought insertion
- Thought withdrawal
- Thought broadcasting

3 Made phenomenon
- Made volition
- Made affect
- Made impulse

3 Disorders of thought perception
Auditory hallucinations:
- 1st person (Thought Echo)
- 2nd person (Command Hallucination)
- 3rd person (Running commentary)

2 Special phenomenon
- Somatic passivity phenomenon
- Primary delusions: Of persecution, of reference, of infidelity, of control, somatic hypochondriac delusions

> **Box 18.4: Major types of schizophrenic disorders.**
>
> **Paranoid schizophrenia**
> - Most common type of schizophrenia with best prognosis
> - Additional features include
>   - Delusions of persecution, reference, grandeur, control, infidelity
>   - Hallucinations have a persecutory or grandiose content, and
>   - Disturbance of affect, volition, speech and motor behaviours
>
> **Disorganised (hebephrenic) schizophrenia**
> - Additional features include
>   - Marked thought disorder, incoherence, loosening of associations
>   - Emotional disturbances-blunted effect, and senseless giggling
>
> **Catatonic schizophrenia**
> - In addition has marked disturbance of motor behaviours
> - Clinical forms:
>   - Excited catatonia: Increase in psychomotor activity (restlessness, agitation, excitement, aggressiveness) and increase in speech production
>   - Stuporous (retarded) catatonia: Extreme retardation of psychomotor function
>   - Catatonia alternating between excitement and stupor: Features of both the above forms
>
> **Schizophrenia undifferentiated type**
> - Meets criteria for schizophrenia. Do not meet the criteria for other schizophrenia types. Mainly has negative symptoms

- Newer antipsychotics include clozapine, risperidone and olanzapine. Though efficacy is similar to older drugs, these are better tolerated.
- Indications for hospital admission: Include suicide/violent, severe psychosis, severe depression, catatonic schizophrenia, non-compliance and failure of outpatient treatment.
- Electroconvulsive therapy (ECT) is for catatonic schizophrenia.
- Psychotherapy:
  - Psychoeducation can prevent relapse by enhancing insight.
  - Cognitive behavioural therapy (CBT) to challenge delusions
  - Social skill training: Improve relationship
  - Behavioural: Positive reinforcement of desirable behaviour
  - Family therapy: To reduce expressed emotion (EE) (High EE include hostility, overinvolvement, critical comments from family; hence reduce relapse rate).

■ MOOD DISORDERS

Spectrum of mood disorders is presented in **Figure 18.1** and classification of mood disorders is given in **Table 18.3**.

Depression

Depressive disorders are characterised by persistent low mood, loss of interest and enjoyment, and reduced energy. They often impair day-to-day functioning.

Box 18.5 gives diagnostic criteria for major depressive episode.

Management

- Mood stabilisers with proven antidepressant effects in bipolar depression include lithium, lamotrigine, quetiapine and olanzapine.
- Tricyclic antidepressant (e.g. amitriptyline) drug was the first choice followed by monoamine oxidase inhibitor (MAOI) or mianserin.
- Now, selective serotonin reuptake inhibitors (SSRIs) are better tolerated and are relatively safer if taken in overdose. SSRIs include fluoxetine, sertraline, fluvoxamine and citalopram.
- Another agent is Desvenlafaxine that inhibits reuptake of nor-epinephrine and serotonin.
- Other effective agents include venlafaxine lithium, valproate, olanzapine and lamotrigine.
- Cognitive therapy in combination with anti-depressants may be beneficial in some cases.

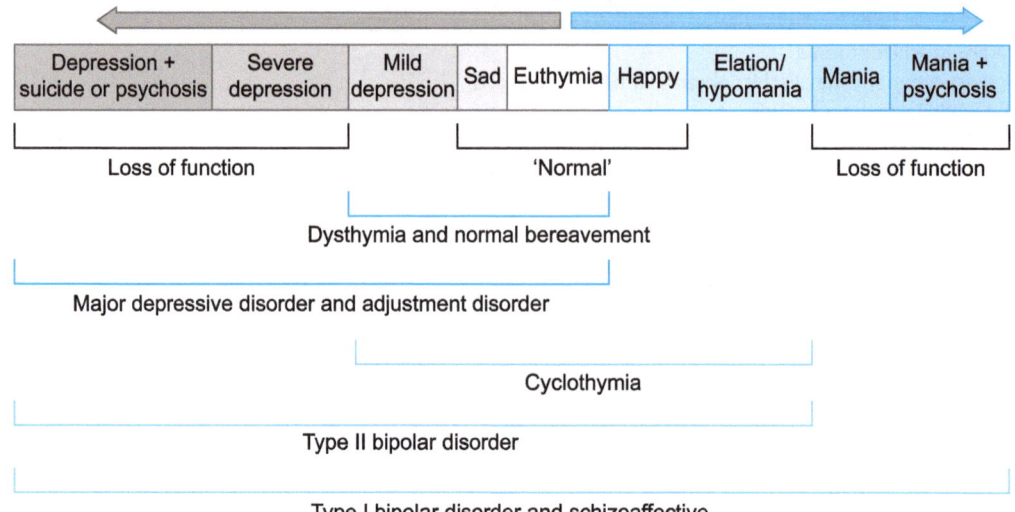

Fig. 18.1: Spectrum of mood disorder.

TABLE 18.3: Classification of mood disorder.

Unipolar	Bipolar	Mood disorders with known aetiology
Major depressive disorder	Bipolar I disorder	Substance-induced mood disorder
Dysthymic disorder	Bipolar II disorder	Mood disorder due to general medical condition
	Cyclothymic disorder	Depression, mania, bipolar disorders, depression-affect, mood, syndrome

- Imipramine and sertraline are useful in patients with psychotic depression.
- ECT is indicated in selected situations, e.g. in those with a high risk of suicide, depressive stupor, psychotic symptoms, and when antidepressants have been ineffective.

Mania

Clinical features of acute mania are presented in **Box 18.6** and diagnostic criteria for manic episode are given in **Box 18.7**.

Elevated mood: It has four stages depending on severity of manic episodes (**Table 18.4**).

Box 18.5: Diagnostic criteria for major depressive episode.

Mood: Depressed mood most of the day, nearly everyday (dysphoria)
Sleep: Insomnia or hypersomnia
Interest: Marked decrease in interest and pleasure in most activities (anhedonia)
Guilt: Feelings of worthlessness or inappropriate guilt
Energy: Fatigue or low energy nearly everyday
Concentration: Decreased concentration or increased indecisiveness
Appetite: Increased or decreased appetite or weight gain or loss
Psychomotor: Psychomotor agitation or retardation
Suicidality: Recurrent thoughts of death, suicidal ideation, suicidal plan, suicide attempt

General criteria for a major depressive episode require five or more of the above symptoms to be present for at least 2 weeks; one symptom must be *depressed mood or loss of interest or pleasure*. The symptoms must also cause *distress or impairment*.

Management

- Manic attacks can be suppressed with lithium, valproate, carbamazepine or atypical antipsychotic (e.g. olanzapine, aripiprazole, quetiapine or risperidone).

Box 18.6: Clinical features of acute mania.

- **Changes in mood:** Irritability, excitability, exhilaration, hostility, anxious, hyper, wound-up
- **Changes in perceptions:** Inflated self-esteem, feeling superior, hallucinations, paranoia, increased appetite
- **Changes in speech:** Rapid, pressured speech, incoherent speech, clang associations
- **Increased social behaviour:** Unnecessary phone calls, increased sexual activity, talkative and sociable
- **Increased energy:** Little fatigue, despite decreased sleep, insomnia, increased productivity, doing several things at once, making lots of plans, taking on too many responsibilities, others seem slow, restlessness, difficulty staying still
- **Impaired judgement:** Lack of insight, inappropriate humour and behaviours, impulsive or thrill-seeking behaviours: Increased alcohol consumption, financial extravagance, dangerous driving, sexual promiscuity
- **Changes in thought patterns:** Distractibility, inability to concentrate, creative thinking, flight of ideas, racing thoughts, disorientation, disjointed thinking, grandiose thinking

Box 18.7: Diagnostic criteria for manic episode.

Three to four of the following criteria are required during the elevated mood period
- **Self-esteem:** Highly inflated, grandiosity
- **Sleep:** Decreased need for sleep, rested after only a few hours
- **Speech:** Pressured
- **Thoughts:** Racing thoughts and flight of ideas
- **Attention:** Easy distractibility
- **Activity:** Increased goal-directed activity
- **Hedonism:** High excess involvement in pleasurable activities (sex, spending, travel)

TABLE 18.4: Stages of elevated mood.

Stage	Features
Euphoria (stage-I) hypomania	Increased sense of psychological well-being and happiness not in keeping with ongoing events
Elation (stage-II)	Moderate elevation of mood with increased psychomotor activity
Exaltation (stage-III)	Intense elation of mood with delusions of grandeur
Ecstasy (stage-IV)	Severe elevation of mood, intense sense of rapture, or blissfulness seen in delirious or stuporous mania

- Also add neuroleptic drugs (haloperidol, chlorpromazine) or benzodiazepines to calm or sedate the mood until the mood stabiliser agent takes effect (about 1 week).
- ECT in resistant cases
- Lithium carbonate and carbamazepine are useful prophylactically.

■ ANXIETY DISORDERS

Anxiety States

- Panic disorder
- Generalised anxiety disorder
- Post-traumatic stress disorder (PTSD)

Phobic Disorders

- Agoraphobia
- Social phobia
- Simple phobia

Panic Disorder

There are recurrent attacks of severe anxiety that are sudden and unpredictable. During attacks, physical symptoms are prominent and include palpitations, chest pain, breathlessness, sweating, chills, nausea, trembling, fear of dying or losing control, numbness, and feeling of detachment. These last for 10–15 minutes.

It may be accompanied by agoraphobia, an avoidance of situations where a person may feel trapped and unable to escape.

In between attacks, the patient is free of anxiety.

Generalised Anxiety Disorder

- Patients have persistent, excessive and/or unrealistic worry associated with other features including muscle tension, impaired concentration, autonomic arousal, restlessness and insomnia. Complaints of tachycardia, dyspnoea, and palpitations are rare.
- Symptoms of anxiety are prominent in psychiatric disorders such as depressive illness and schizophrenia. Many physical illnesses such as hyperthyroidism, phaechromocytoma, hypoglycaemia, alcohol withdrawal and temporal lobe epilepsy can mimic anxiety disorders. Hence, these conditions should be excluded before making a diagnosis of generalised anxiety disorder.

Post-traumatic Stress Disorder

- PTSD is characterised by recurrent bouts of severe anxiety accompanied by vivid reminiscences (or 'flashbacks') of the initial traumatic event.
- PTSD stems from exposure to a traumatic event (e.g. a military experience, a physical or sexual assault, a motor vehicle accident and a natural disaster) that involved actual or threatened death or serious injury to oneself or others.
- Typically, patients re-experience the traumatic event (e.g. nightmares, flashbacks), engage in avoidance of stimuli associated with the sentinel trauma (e.g. impaired recall of events related to the trauma) and experience increased autonomic reactivity (e.g. hypervigilance, irritability, insomnia, heightened startle response).

Phobic Disorders

- Phobic disorders comprise a group of disorders having in common persistently recurring, irrational severe anxiety of specific objects, activities or situations with secondary avoidance behaviour of the phobic stimulus.
- Agoraphobia: The individual has marked fear of and thus avoids being alone or being in public places, e.g. crowds, tunnels and bridges.
- Social phobias: These are persistent irrational fears and the need to avoid any situation where one might be exposed to scrutiny by others and potentially be embarrassed or humiliated.

Treatment

- Use of a selective serotonin–norepinephrine reuptake inhibitor (e.g. venlafaxine).
- Anxiolytic agents such as benzodiazepines (e.g. lorazepam, alprazolam, clonazepam) can be used as a temporary adjunct to aid in minimising anxiety, in particular when starting a medication therapy. Their long-term use should be avoided since it may lead to tolerance and increase risk of abuse of dependence.
- Cognitive behavioural therapy that involves addressing cognitive distortions, psychoeducation, breathing exercises, progressive muscle relaxation and progressive exposure.

■ OBSESSIVE-COMPULSIVE DISORDER

- Obsessions are persistent intrusive thoughts. Compulsions are intrusive behaviours. Attempt made to ignore or suppress the obsessive thought is usually not successful. The compulsives act is performed with a sense of subjective compulsion coupled with a desire to resist the compulsion. The individual generally recognises the senselessness of the behaviour and does not derive pleasure from carrying out the activity, although it provides a release of tension.
- Examples are repeated checking to be assured that the door was looked, repeated hand washing and extreme neatness.

Treatment

- Psychotherapy
- Pharmacotherapy
   - SSRIs including fluoxetine, fluvoxamine and citalopram.
   - Tricyclic antidepressants, particularly clomipramine.

■ ORGANIC PSYCHIATRY

Delirium

It is an acute organic mental disorder characterised by confusion, restlessness, incoherence, inattention, anxiety or hallucinations which may

Box 18.8: Causes of delirium.

- Metabolic causes
  - Hypoxia, CO_2 narcosis
  - Hypoglycaemia
  - Hepatic encephalopathy
  - H_2O and electrolyte imbalance
- Drugs and poisons
  - Digitalis
  - Alcohol
  - Tricycle antidepressants
  - Salicylates, penicillin, etc.
- Nutritional deficiencies
  - Thiamin, niacin
  - Proteins
- Endocrine causes
  - Hypo- and hyperpituitarism
  - Hypo- and hyperthyroidism
  - Hypo- and hyperparathyroidism
  - Hypo- and hyperadrenalism
- Intracranial cause
  - Epilepsy
  - Head injury
  - Meningitis
  - Migraine
- Miscellaneous
  - Post-operative states
  - Sleep deprivation
  - Acute and chronic systemic infections
  - Febrile delirium in children

TABLE 18.5: Differences between delirium, dementia and psychosis.

Condition	Onset	Pattern	Orientation	Attention	Memory	Duration
Delirium	Acute	Fluctuating	Usually impaired	Impaired/fluctuating	Impaired	Hours or days
Dementia	Insidious	Progressive	Normal or impaired	~Normal	Impaired	Months or years
Psychosis	Variable	Variable	~Normal	Normal or impaired	Normal or impaired	Variable

be reversible with treatment. Causes of delirium are given **Box 18.8**.

Differences between delirium, dementia and psychosis are presented in **Table 18.5**.

Differences between delirium and dementia are presented in **Table 18.6**.

■ ALCOHOL DEPENDENCE

Consequences of chronic alcohol misuse are described in **Box 18.9**.

Treatment

Two phases: Detoxification and rehabilitation

Detoxification
- Deals with acute withdrawal symptoms and, therefore, requires use of medications
- Approved medications include naltrexone, disulfiram and acamprosate.

Rehabilitation
- Helps to prevent relapse and development of lifestyle compatible with long-term abstinence
- Requires psychotherapeutic interventions

■ NICOTINE DEPENDENCE

Health Effects of Chronic Smoking

Complications of tobacco use are given in **Box 18.10**.

Nicotine Withdrawal

- Withdrawal symptoms in chronic users begin to appear approximately 30 minutes after every dose.
- Features include confusion, restlessness, anxiety, insomnia, dizziness, depression, feelings of frustration and anger, nightmares, poor concentration, headache and increased appetite.

TABLE 18.6: Difference between delirium and dementia.

Features	Delirium	Dementia
Onset	Rapid (hours to days)	Gradual (years)
Course	Wide fluctuations; may continue for weeks if cause is not found	Slow but continuous decline
LOC (loss of consciousness)	Hyper-alert to difficult to arouse	Normal
Orientation	Disoriented, confused	Disoriented, confused
Attention	Always impaired	May be intact; may focus on one thing for long periods
Sleep	Always disturbed	Usually normal
Behaviour	Agitated, restless	May be agitated or apathetic, may wonder
Memory	Especially recent memory impairment	Especially recent memory impairment
Cognition	• Disordered reasoning • Thought content: Incoherent, confused, delusional	Disordered reasoning and calculation
Perception	Illusions, hallucinations	No change
Judgement	Poor	Poor, socially inappropriate

Box 18.9: Consequences of chronic alcohol misuse.

Acute alcohol intoxication
- Disturbances in emotional and behavioural state
- Medical symptoms: Due to hypoglycaemia, aspiration of vomit, respiratory depression
- Complication of other medical problems
- Accidents, injuries developed in fights

Consequences of harmful alcohol use

Medical
- Neurological: Peripheral neuropathy, dementia, cerebral haemorrhage, cerebellar degeneration, Marchiafava–Bignami syndrome, subacute combined degeneration of the cord myopathy, ventricular enlargement and cognitive impairment
- Hepatic: Fatty change and cirrhosis, hepatocellular carcinoma
- Gastrointestinal: Oesophagitis, oesophageal varices, Mallory-Weiss syndrome, oesophageal carcinoma, gastritis, malabsorption, pancreatitis, parotid enlargement
- Skin: Palmar erythema, spider naevi, Dupuytren's contracture, telangiectasia
- Cardiac: Cardiomyopathy, hypertension
- Respiratory: Pneumonia, tuberculosis
- Musculoskeletal: Myopathy, fractures

Features of alcohol withdrawal syndrome
- Psychological: Restlessness, anxiety, panic attacks
- Autonomic: Tachycardia, sweating, pupil dilatation, nausea, vomiting
- Delirium tremens: Agitation, hallucinations, illusions, delusions
- Seizure

- Endocrine and metabolic: Pseudo-Cushing's syndrome, hypoglycaemia, gout
- Reproductive: Hypogonadism, infertility, foetal alcohol syndrome

Psychiatric and cerebral
- Depression
- Alcoholic hallucinosis
- Alcoholic 'blackouts'
- Wernicke's encephalopathy
  - Nystagmus
  - Opthalmoplegia
  - Ataxia
  - Confusion
- Korsakoff's syndrome
  - Short-term memory deficit
  - Confabulation

Smoking Cessation
- Nicotine replacement therapy
- Use of nicotine patches, nicotine gums, lozenges and nasal sprays
- Bupropion: Dose is 75–150 mg twice a day.
- Varenicline: A nicotine receptor partial agonist is possibly more effective than nicotine and bupropion.
- Other drugs: Clonidine, nortriptyline

ANTIPSYCHOTIC DRUGS
Classification of antipsychotic drugs is given in **Box 18.11**.

ANTIDEPRESSANT DRUGS
Types of antidepressant drugs and their side effects are mentioned in **Table 18.7**.

ELECTROCONVULSIVE THERAPY
ECT involves the administration of high voltage, brief, direct current impulses to the head to induce seizures in brain while the patient is anaesthetised and paralysed. Electrodes can be placed bilaterally or unilaterally over the non-dominant hemisphere.

Box 18.10: Complications of tobacco use.

Cardiovascular disease
- Premature coronary artery disease
- Peripheral vascular disease and erectile dysfunction
- Cerebrovascular disease
- Aortic aneurysm

Gastrointestinal
- GERD
- Peptic ulceration
- Gallstones and cholecystitis in women
- Pancreatitis
- Crohn's disease

Renal
- Increase risk of CKD

Infections: Increased risk of several types of infections including tuberculosis, pneumococcal pneumonia, Legionnaire's disease, meningococcal disease, influenza and the common cold

Neurological
- Dementia and cognitive decline
- Increased risk of amyotrophic lateral sclerosis

Drug interactions
- Induces hepatic microsomal enzyme systems, e.g. increased metabolism of propranolol and theophylline

Other cancers
- Larynx
- Oral cavity and lip
- Nasopharynx, oropharynx and hypopharynx
- Nasal cavity and paranasal sinuses
- Oesophagus
- Stomach
- Pancreas

Respiratory disease
- Chronic obstructive pulmonary disease
- Cancer of lung, bronchus and trachea
- Increased incidence of post-operative respiratory complications
- Increased incidence of respiratory infections including tuberculosis
- ILD
- Pneumothorax

Pregnancy
- Spontaneous abortion
- Abruptio placentae
- Premature rupture of membranes
- Foetal death
- Neonatal death
- Sudden infant death syndrome
- Post-partum venous thromboembolism

Endocrine
- Increased risk of diabetes mellitus

Osteoporosis and hip fracture: Smoking accelerates bone loss and is a risk factor for hip fracture in women

Ophthalmological
- Age-related macular degeneration
- Increased risk of cataract

- Colorectal
- Kidney
- Bladder
- Uterine
- Cervix
- Acute myeloid leukaemia

(CKD: chronic kidney disease; GERD: gastroesophageal reflux disease; ILD: interstitial lung disease)

> **Box 18.11: Classification of antipsychotic drugs.**
>
> **Typical antipsychotic/first generation**
> - Phenothiazines (chlorpromazine, perphenazine, fluphenazine, thioridazine)
> - Thioxanthenes (flupenthixol, clopenthixol)
> - Butyrophenones (haloperidol, droperidol)
>
> **Atypical antipsychotics/second generation**
> - Aripiprazole, asenapine, brexpiprazole, cariprazine, clozapine, iloperidone, lurasidone, olanzapine, paliperidone, pimavanserin, quetiapine, risperidone, ziprasidione
>
> **Mechanism of action** of most first and second generation antipsychotic: It appears to be post-synaptic blockade of brain dopamine D2 receptors.
> Exceptions
> - Aripiprazole and brexpiprazole are D2 receptor partial agonists
> - Cariprazine is a D3 preferring D3/D2 receptor partial agonist
> - Pimavanserin is a serotonin 5-HT2A inverse agonist and antagonist with no dopamine D2 affinity

Indications for ECT in Depressive Illness

- Severe depression with paranoid or nihilistic delusion
- High suicidal risk where quick response is needed
- Failure to respond to a tricyclic and an alternative antidepressant
- Depressive stupor
- Inability to tolerate the side effects of antidepressants

Contraindications

- Absolute: Increased intracranial pressure (ICP), aortic aneurysm
- Relative:
  - Cardiovascular diseases: Coronary artery disease, hypertension, aneurysms, arrhythmias
  - Cerebrovascular disease: Recent strokes, space-occupying lesions, aneurysms
  - Severe pulmonary diseases: Tuberculosis, pneumonia, asthma
  - Deep vein thrombosis (DVT)

TABLE 18.7: Various types of antidepressant drugs and their side effects.

Group and drug	Side effects
Tricyclic antidepressants (TCAs) NA + 5-HT reuptake inhibitor • Imipramine, amitriptyline, trimipramine, doxepin, dothiepin, clomipramine, dosulepin Predominantly NA reuptake inhibitor • Desipramine, nortriptyline, amoxapine, reboxetine	• Anticholinergic: Dry mouth, bad taste, constipation, epigastric fullness, urinary retention (more common in elderly male), blurred vision, palpitation • Sedation, mental confusion, weakness • Increased appetite and weight, sweating, fine tremors, precipitation of seizures, postural hypotension, cardiac arrhythmias, rashes and jaundice
Selective serotonin reuptake inhibitors (SSRIs) • Fluoxetine, fluvoxamine, paroxetine, sertraline, citalopram, escitalopram	Gastric upset, nausea, interfere with ejaculation, nervousness, restlessness, insomnia, anorexia, headache, diarrhoea, epistaxis, ecchymosis, serotonin syndrome
Reversible inhibitor of MAO-A (RIMAs) • Moclobemide, clorgyline (isocarboxazid, phenelzine, tranylcypromine)	• ↑appetite (phenelzine) • ↓appetite (tranylcypromine) • Hepatotoxicity, SLE, drug and food interactions (cheese reaction)
Atypical antidepressants Trazodone, mianserine, mirtazapine, venlafaxine, duloxetine, tianeptine, aminoptine, bupropion	Priapism (trazodone), bone marrow suppression, hepatotoxicity

(5-HT: 5-hydroxytryptamine; MAO: monoamine oxidase; NA: noradrenaline; SLE: systemic lupus erythematosus)

Risks and side effects: ECT is safe with few side effects.
- Impairment of cognition: Period of confusion immediately after ECT and generally lasts for few minutes to several hours
- Memory loss: May forget weeks/months before treatment, during treatment or after treatment has stopped. Usually improves within couple of months. Permanent loss of memory is rare.
- Myalgia, dislocation and fractures
- Medical complications: Nausea, vomiting, headache, aspiration and jaw pain

■ SLEEP DISORDERS

Insomnia

- Inability to sleep or maintain sleep despite the patient having adequate opportunity and circumstances to sleep, when associated with impairment of daytime functioning or mood symptoms
- Patients may complain of difficulty falling asleep (sleep-onset insomnia) or difficulty remaining asleep (sleep-maintenance insomnia) with frequent nocturnal awakenings or early morning awakenings associated with non-restorative sleep.
- Insomnia can heighten the perception of pain and may be associated with development of endocrine disturbances. It also has an association with increased risk for hypertension or cardiovascular disease. Insufficient sleep can lead to increased risk for motor vehicle accidents and occupational errors.

Common causes of insomnia are given in **Box 18.12**.

Treatment
- Cognitive behavioural therapy
- Pharmacologic therapy:
  - Triazolam, zolpidem and ramelteon for sleep-onset insomnia
  - Estazolam and eszopiclone for sleep-maintenance insomnia
  - Zaleplon and sustained-release zolpidem for both sleep-onset and sleep-maintenance insomnia

> **Box 18.12: Common cause of insomnia.**
> **Primary sleep disorders:**
> - Idiopathic insomnia
> - Periodic leg movements
> - Restless legs syndrome
>
> **Secondary sleep disorders:**
> - **Psychiatric or psychological problems:** Mood disorders (e.g. mania, depressive and anxiety disorders); delirium and dementia
>
> **Use or misuse of drug/substance abuse:** Consumption or discontinuation of drugs/substances. Withdrawal of addictive drug (e.g. alcohol, benzodiazepines), stimulant drugs (e.g. caffeine, nicotine, amphetamines), prescribed drugs (corticosteroids, dopamine agonists)
> - **Physical/medical disorders:** Chronic pain (e.g. carpal tunnel syndrome); nocturia (e.g. prostatism); malnutrition, chronic obstructive pulmonary disease, asthma, menopause and neurologic disorders

Narcolepsy

It is excessive daytime sleep that a patient cannot resist.

Diagnosis
- Severe excessive daytime sleepiness occurring almost daily for at least 3 months that interferes with functioning
- Rapid eye movement (REM) intrusion phenomena that includes:
  - Cataplexy: Sudden self-limited episodes of loss of muscle tone when patient is awake, which is usually triggered by laughter or other strong emotions
  - Hypnagogic hallucinations: Vivid and often frightening perceptual hallucinatory experiences, which occur during the transition between waking and sleep
  - Sleep paralysis: Occurs as the patient transitions from sleep to waking, and consists of episodes up to several minutes in duration of inability to move and occasionally feeling unable to breathe despite being awake

Treatment
- Modafinil, a wakefulness-promoting drug, is useful. It has low addiction potential.

- Sodium oxybate, a sodium salt of y-hydroxybutyrate, is administered at night to help consolidate REM sleep and increase slow-wave sleep. It significantly reduces daytime sleepiness and also improves cataplexy.
- Others: Selegiline (MAO-B inhibitor), clomipramine, fluoxetine and venlafaxine

Circadian Rhythm Sleep Disorders
Common Types
- Delayed sleep phase type: Sleep and wake times are later than desired, often resulting in daytime sleepiness when conventional waking times are enforced.
- Jet lag: Transient symptoms of difficulty falling asleep at the appropriate time and daytime sleepiness following rapid change in time zones altering the timing of exogenous light stimuli

Parasomnias
Types of parasomnias and their features are given in **Table 18.8**.

Treatment
- Avoid serotonin reuptake inhibitors, MAO inhibitors, caffeine or alcohol.
- Remove dangerous objects from the sleep environment.
- Drugs include clonazepam, tricyclic antidepressants dopamine agonists or levodopa, carbamazepine and melatonin.

Restless Leg Syndrome
- Willis–Ekbom disease
- An overwhelming urge to move legs, usually accompanied by an uncomfortable sensation.
- May disrupt sleep initiation.
- Rest or inactivity exacerbates the urge to move the legs.
- Physical activity temporarily relieves the urge to move the legs.
- Symptoms are more prominent in the evening or night-time that may disrupt sleep initiation.
- It may be secondary to pregnancy, end-stage renal disease, iron or folate deficiency, peripheral neuropathy, radiculopathy, rheumatoid arthritis or fibromyalgia.

TABLE 18.8: Types and features of parasomnias.

Type of parasomnias	Features
Non-REM sleep parasomnias	
Confusional arousals	Sudden arousals, associated with confusion and disorientation
Sleep terrors	Sudden arousal with fearful agitated behaviour, often with screaming or crying; patients may be disoriented, unresponsive to the enviroment and typically do not remember the event afterward
Sleepwalking	Arousal with complex motor behaviour, walking, running, talking, and eating
REM sleep-associated parasomnias	
Nightmare disorder	Recurrent, distributing dreams not associated with autonomic activity or amnesia
REM sleep behaviour disorder (RBD)	Abnormal persistance of muscle tone during REM sleep, permitting vigorous movements while dreaming. Also include screaming, punching and kicking for up to several minutes, sometimes resulting in an injury to the patient or bed partner

(REM: rapid eye movement)

- First-line drugs are dopaminergic medications (ropinirole, pramipexole). Others include gabapentin, benzodiazepines, clonidine or opiates.

■ EATING DISODERS
Anorexia Nervosa (AN)
Diagnostic Criteria
- Marked weight loss: Refusal to maintain body weight at or above a minimally normal weight for age and height.
- Avoidance of high-calorie foods: Weight loss arising from food avoidance because of intense fear of gaining weight or becoming fat, even though underweight.
- Distortion of body image so that patients regard themselves as fat even when they appear grossly underweight.

- In post-menarcheal females, amenorrhoea, i.e., the absence of at least three consecutive menstrual cycles (or 3 months)

Major Subtypes
- Restricting type: Fasting, introverted, decreased risk of substance abuse, family conflict is covert
- Bulimic type: Binge eating or purging, more volatile, family frequently disengaged, prone to substance abuse

Bulimia Nervosa

Diagnostic Criteria
- Recurrent episodes of binge eating
- Absence of self-control over eating during binges
- Self-induced vomiting, purgation or dieting after binges
- Weight maintained within normal range

Major Subtypes
- Purging type: Self-induced vomiting or use of laxatives, diuretics or enemas
- Non-purging type: Use of other compensatory mechanisms, such as fasting or excessive exercise

Clinical features of anorexia nervosa and bulimia nervosa are listed in **Table 18.9**.

TABLE 18.9: Clinical features of anorexia nervosa (AN) and bulimia nervosa (BN).

AN	BN or AN (purging type)
• Dry skin, lanugo, hair, scalp hair loss	• Perioral acne
• Cold intolerance, hypothermia	• Parotid gland enlargement
• Cyanotic hands and feet	• Dental caries and erosion (lingual surface of teeth)
• Weakness, fatigue (despite high physical activity)	• Orthostatic hypotension and dehydration
• Sinus bradycardia, orthostatic hypotension	• Presyncopal and syncopal symptoms
• Presyncopal and syncopal episodes	• Heartburn, gastroesophageal reflux
• Early satiety	• Muscle cramps and paraesthesias (from electrolyte abnormalities)
• Bloating	
• Constipation	• Diarrhoea and constipation (laxative abusers)
• Primary or secondary amenorrhoea	• Cardiac arrhythmias
• Peripheral neuropathy	• Oligomenorrhoea or amenorrhoea
• Decreased bone density, fractures	
• Muscle wasting and cachexia	
• Nose bleeds, bruising (thrombocytopaenia)	

BEST OF FIVES

1. A 65-year-old man comes to the outpatient clinic with his wife. Over the last 2 months, he complains of auditory hallucinations. His sleep quality is poor. His appetite has decreased and he has lost about 10 kg in the last 3 months. He admits drinking one a half bottles of whisky a day. There is no clouding of consciousness or suggestion of delusions and paranoid symptoms. What is the likely diagnosis in this man?
   A. Alcoholic hallucinosis
   B. Korsakoff's psychosis
   C. Major depression psychosis
   D. Psychotic depression
   E. Schizophrenia

2. A 24-year-old student presents with sleepiness, weakness and vivid dreams since the last 2 months. She is a type 1 diabetic using basal bolus insulin. What is the likely explanation of her symptoms?
   A. Hypoglycaemic episodes
   B. Narcolepsy syndrome
   C. Schizophrenia
   D. Sleep apnoea
   E. Temporal lobe epilepsy

3. A 65-year-old man who had undergone aortic valve replacement with a mechanical valve

complains of difficulty in sleeping, which he says started when his wife died suddenly 1 year ago. He is very tearful and says that he often cries without any apparent reason. What would be the best choice of antidepressant in this gentleman?
A. Amitriptyline
B. Citalopram
C. Fluoxetine
D. St John's wort
E. Venlafaxine

4. A 45-year-old chronic alcohol abuse man presented in the accident and emergency department with confusion, agitation and ataxia. On examination, he was disoriented in time and place and had bilateral 6th nerve palsies, gaze-evoked nystagmus and gait ataxia. What treatment should this patient receive?
A. Diazepam
B. Immunoglobulins
C. Penicillin
D. Steroids
E. Thiamine

5. A 17-year-old man collapsed after taking some unidentified tablets at a nightclub. On examination, his temperature was 40.2°C, pulse was 136 beats per minute and regular and blood pressure was 176/112 mmHg. He was tremulous and agitated. His abdomen was soft, but he had increased bowel sounds. Neurological examination showed dilated pupils, hyper-reflexia and myoclonus of his limbs. His Glasgow coma score was 14. Investigations reveal serum creatine kinase 31,000 U/L (24–195). What is the most likely diagnosis?
A. Amphetamine poisoning
B. Anticholinergic poisoning
C. Malignant hyperthermia
D. Neuroleptic malignant syndrome
E. Serotonin syndrome

6. Which of the following is more suggestive of vascular dementia than other dementias?
A. Early loss of insight
B. Sleep-wake cycle disturbance
C. Seizures
D. Increased creativity
E. Slow onset

7. Which of the following is a contraindication to electroconvulsive therapy (ECT)?
A. Immunocompromised
B. Pregnancy
C. Cardiac pacemaker
D. Epilepsy
E. Raised intracranial pressure

8. You are asked to see a 45-year-old man with memory problems. He has problems recalling past events from his life and he is unable to recall a list of everyday items. He cannot tell you where he is or the month of the year and gives bizarre answers to many of your questions. What is the diagnosis?
A. Post-ictal state
B. Early signs of Alzheimer's disease
C. Stroke
D. Vascular dementia
E. Korsakoff's syndrome

9. A 35-year-old female presents to her GP with low mood, poor concentration, problems in sleeping and no interest in any of her hobbies. She does not appear as well dressed as she normally would be. Blood tests including thyroid function are normal. Which of the following is most likely?
A. Depression
B. Anxiety disorder
C. Alcohol excess
D. Early onset dementia
E. Pick's disease

10. A 37 year old male was brought to the accident and emergency department. He was found wandering the streets of a city and was unsure of where he was or who he was. Which of the following is the most likely diagnosis?
A. Transient global amnesia
B. Multiple personality
C. Fugue state
D. Transient ischaemic attack
E. Malingering

11. A patient with a 6-month history of low mood and some suicidal thoughts is discussing her treatment options. Which of the following is the best pharmacological treatment?
A. Lorazepam
B. Amitriptyline

C. Fluoxetine
D. Selegiline
E. Haloperidol

12. A patient describes a sensation in which some of her thoughts are repeated by a voice in her head. How is this normally described?
    A. Thought broadcasting
    B. Echophonia
    C. Thought echo
    D. Thought revolving
    E. Thought multiplication

13. A 24-year-old female attends her GP with her mother due to anxiety. Her mother states that her daughter is worried that her mother will leave. She is unemployed and does not have any hobbies. She hates confrontation. She moves from one relationship to the other very rapidly as she does not like to be on her own for any length of time. Which of the following is the most likely diagnosis?
    A. Obsessive-compulsive disorder
    B. Anxiety disorder
    C. Dependent personality disorder
    D. Avoidant personality disorder
    E. Borderline personality disorder

14. Which of the following is false regarding obsessive-compulsive disorder (OCD)?
    A. Clomipramine may be trialled if selective serotonin reuptake inhibitors (SSRIs) do not prove effective.
    B. Surgery on the cingulate cortex is the last resort but effective treatment in 30% of patients.
    C. Cognitive behavioural therapy (CBT) is an effective treatment.
    D. The dose of SSRIs needed to treat OCD is lower than depression.
    E. The chance of developing OCD is increased if you have a first-degree relative.

15. A 34-year-old male presents to his GP to talk about the messages that he receives through a chip in his fillings. He believes that he is being used by an unknown power for an unknown mission. What is the diagnosis?
    A. Normal
    B. Personality disorder
    C. Bipolar syndrome
    D. Schizophrenia
    E. Depression

16. A 50-year-old male complains of low mood and problems in sleeping which get a lot worse during the winter months. The rest of the history and examination reveal nothing of note. What is the likely diagnosis?
    A. Dysthymia
    B. Seasonal affective disorder
    C. Normal
    D. Depression
    E. Bipolar

17. Which of the following is not commonly found in a manic episode of bipolar disorder?
    A. Hypersexuality
    B. Visual hallucinations
    C. Pressured speech
    D. Elevated mood
    E. Low attention span

18. A 24-year-old woman complains of headaches, upset stomach, jaw pain, sore muscles and difficulty in sleeping. Full examination reveals no medical issues. She does not accept that nothing was found during the investigations and seeks a second opinion. What is the diagnosis?
    A. Personality disorder
    B. Conversion disorder
    C. Hypochondriac
    D. Somatisation disorder
    E. Psychosis

19. A young female presents to her GP with feelings of anxiousness. On further questioning, she states that she is constantly ruminating about things. On numerous occasions, she constantly obsesses about whether or not she has locked the doors or switched off the gas and she has to go back three or four times to check if this is the case. What is the most likely diagnosis?
    A. Anxiety
    B. Schizophrenia
    C. Obsessional personality
    D. Depressive disorder
    E. Obsessive-compulsive disorder

20. An elderly man is on the ward due to a left-sided pneumonia. He becomes acutely distressed and punches a nurse. His notes state that he drinks 4 pints of beer a day. On examination, his temperature is 38.1°C, blood pressure is 100/60 mmHg and pulse is 100/min and regular. There is consolidation at his left

lung base His white cell count is raised significantly and renal function is impaired. What has caused his symptoms?
A. Undiagnosed dementia
B. Delirium secondary to infection
C. Wernicke's encephalopathy
D. Korsakoff's psychosis
E. Delirium tremens

21. A 20-year-old male has slept rough since leaving home when he was 15 years old and freely admits to heroin use. He describes three unknown voices that talk about plans they are making to hurt him and is convinced that cigarette packets contain messages that only he can see. What is the most likely diagnosis?
A. Personality disorder
B. Schizoaffective disorder
C. Drug-induced psychosis
D. Bipolar disorder
E. Schizophrenia

22. A 40-year-old former soldier presents with insomnia, low mood and nightmares that wake him. He has been formally discharged at his own request from the army for 6 months and has been unable to hold down a job since. He describes witnessing a series of bomb explosions in which many of his colleagues lost their lives or were brutally injured and cannot stop repeating them in his head. What is the most likely diagnosis?
A. Depression
B. Acute stress disorder
C. Post-traumatic stress disorder
D. Schizophrenia
E. Personality disorder

23. Which of the following gives the strongest indication that a suicide attempt was serious and not a cry for help?
A. Phoned the Samaritans during the act
B. Did not make any final plans such as making a will or leaving a note
C. Timed so that intervention is highly unlikely and takes measures to prevent discovery or intervention
D. Taking excessive amounts of paracetamol as the method
E. Drug addiction

24. Which of the following would describe delirium rather than dementia?
A. No tearfulness
B. Low Montreal Cognitive Assessment (MoCA) score
C. Confused more about the present than the past
D. Shouting
E. Fluctuating level of consciousness

25. Which of the following is not commonly found in a manic episode of bipolar disorder?
A. Pressured speech
B. Elevated mood
C. Hypersexuality
D. Low attention span
E. Visual hallucinations

26. Which of the following is common secondarily to alcohol abuse?
A. Morbid jealousy
B. Depression
C. Increased creativity
D. Lower levels of bipolar syndrome
E. Agoraphobia

27. Which of the following supports a diagnosis of alcohol dependence syndrome?
A. Continued drinking despite physical harm
B. Drinking a variety of alcohol types
C. History of falls
D. Morbid jealousy
E. Drinking despite criminal convictions related to drink

28. Which of the following suggests a good prognosis for anorexia?
A. Short duration
B. They do not exercise excessively
C. Adult onset
D. Weight loss has not been severe
E. No history of psychological problems

Answers

1-A, 2-A, 3-C, 4-E, 5-E, 6-C, 7-E, 8-E, 9-A, 10-C, 11-C, 12-C, 13-C, 14-D, 15-D, 16-B, 17-B, 18-D, 19-E, 20-B, 21-E, 22-C, 23-C, 24-E, 25-E, 26-A, 27-A, 28-A

SUGGESTED READING

1. American Psychiatric Association. Diagnostic and Statistical Manual of Mental Disorders (DSM-5), 5th edition. Arlington, VA: American Psychiatric Association; 2013.
2. American Psychiatric Association. Diagnostic and Statistical Manual of Mental Disorders, 4th edition, Text Revision. Washington, DC: American Psychiatric Association; 2000.
3. Cermolacce M, Sass L, Parnas J. What is bizarre in bizarre delusions? A critical review. Schizophr Bull. 2010;36(4):667-79.
4. Olfson M, Blanco C, Wang S, Laje G, Correll CU. National trends in the mental health care of children, adolescents, and adults by office-based physicians. JAMA Psychiatry. 2014;71(1):81-90.
5. Soria-Saucedo R, Walter HJ, Cabral H, England MJ, Kazis LE. Receipt of Evidence-Based Pharmacotherapy and Psychotherapy Among Children and Adolescents With New Diagnoses of Depression. Psychiatr Serv. 2016;67(3):316-23.
6. Stein MB, Sareen J. CLINICAL PRACTICE. Generalized anxiety disorder. N Engl J Med. 2015;373(21):2059-68.
7. Ruscio AM, Stein DJ, Chiu WT, Kessler RC. The epidemiology of obsessive-compulsive disorder in the National Comorbidity Survey Replication. Mol Psychiatry. 2010;15(1):53-63.
8. American Academy of Sleep Medicine. International Classification of Sleep Disorders, 3rd edition. Darien, IL: American Academy of Sleep Medicine; 2014.
9. Sateia MJ. International classification of sleep disorders-third edition: highlights and modifications. Chest. 2014;146(5):1387-94.
10. Wildes JE, Marcus MD. Incorporating dimensions into the classification of eating disorders: three models and their implications for research and clinical practice. Int J Eat Disord. 2013;46(5):396-403.
11. Lavender JM, Crosby RD, Wonderlich SA. Dimensions in the eating disorders: past, present, and future. Commentary on Wildes and Marcus: Incorporating dimensions into the classification of eating disorders. Int J Eat Disord. 2013;46(5):404-7.
12. World Health Organization (WHO). WHO global status report on alcohol 2004. Geneva: WHO; 2004.
13. Fiellin DA, Reid MC, O'Connor PG. New therapies for alcohol problems: application to primary care. Am J Med. 2000;108(3):227-37.
14. Case BG, Bertollo DN, Laska EM, Price LH, Siegel CE, Olfson M, et al. Declining use of electroconvulsive therapy in United States general hospitals. Biol Psychiatry. 2013;73(2):119-26.
15. Wilkinson ST, Agbese E, Leslie DL, Rosenheck RA. Identifying Recipients of Electroconvulsive Therapy: Data From Privately Insured Americans. Psychiatr Serv. 2018;69(5):542-8.

CHAPTER 19

Fluid, Electrolytes and Acid-base Disorders

Table 19.1 shows the normal ranges of different serums and plasmas.

■ ANION GAP (FIG. 19.1)

- It denotes the concentration of the unmeasured anions in the plasma, namely phosphates, sulphates, organic acids and protein anions.

  Anion gap = $Na^+ - (Cl^- + HCO_3^-)$

- The normal anion gap is 10–12 mmol/L.
- An increased anion gap is usually seen in some forms of metabolic acidosis.
  - Diabetic ketoacidosis
  - Lactic acidosis
  - Uraemic acidosis
  - Salicylate poisoning
  - Methanol poisoning
  - Ethylene glycol poisoning

TABLE 19.1: Normal ranges of different serums and plasmas.

Investigation	Normal range	Investigation	Normal range
• Sodium (serum)	• 136–145 mmol/L	• Magnesium (serum)	• 1.7–2.2 mg/dL (0.85–1.10 mmol/L)
• Potassium (serum)	• 3.5–5.0 mmol/L	• pH of blood	• 7.38–7.44
• Chloride (serum)	• 98–106 mmol/L	• Bicarbonate (blood)	• 21–28 mmol/L
• Calcium (plasma)	• 8.5–10.5 mg/dL (4.3–5.3 mEq/L or 2.2–2.7 mmol/L)	• Osmolality (serum)	• 285–295 mOsm/kg water
• Phosphorus (serum)	• 3.4–4.5 mg/dL (1.12–1.45 mmol/L)		

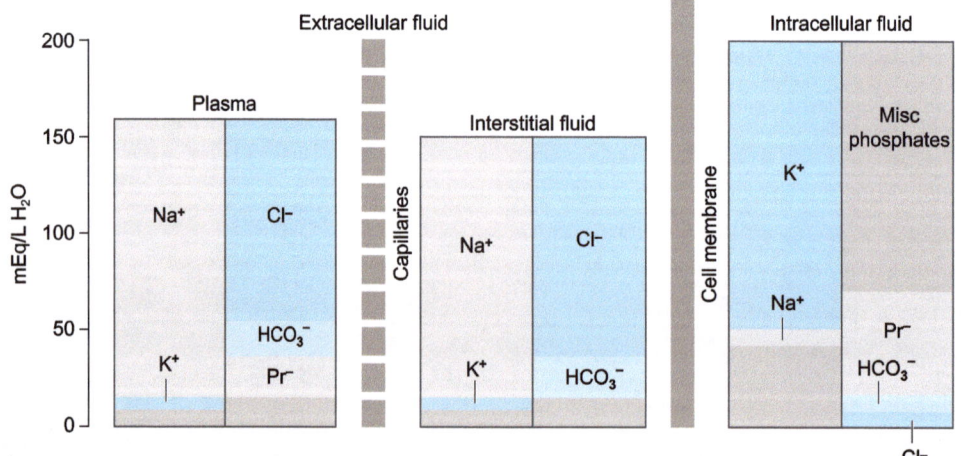

Fig. 19.1: Anion gap: extracellular and intracellular fluid.

HYPOVOLAEMIA

Extrarenal and renal losses in hypovolaemia are shown in **Table 19.2**.

Clinical Features
- Signs of volume depletion are dry skin and mucous membranes, reduced or absent tears, reduced skin turgor, tachycardia, shock, and altered mental status.
- In patients with extrarenal losses, the urine output is reduced.

Treatment
- Mild-to-moderate volume depletion is often due to gastroenteritis. This should be corrected by increasing oral intake of sodium and water, usually in the form of an oral rehydration solution.
- In severe cases, administer intravenous fluids, usually as normal saline or Ringer's lactate.

HYPONATRAEMIA

It is defined as serum sodium < 135 mEq/L.

Causes
Table 19.3 shows the causes of hyponatraemia and **Flowchart 19.1** shows the types and causes of hyponatraemia.

Clinical Features
- Hyponatraemia per se does not produce any significant clinical features.
- These include muscle cramps, weakness and fatigue, mental confusion, disorientation, coma and convulsions.
- Speed of development and severity of hyponatraemia determine its clinical significance (**Table 19.4**).

Treatment
- Dangers of rapid correction of hyponatraemia are vascular overload, shrinkage of brain → central pontine myelinolysis
- Correction of hyponatraemia requires either addition of sodium or removal of water, if indicated.
    - Loop diuretic
    - Hypertonic saline: 3% saline
    - Vasopressin V_2-receptor antagonists: Tolvaptan (**Flowchart 19.2**)

TABLE 19.2: Extrarenal and renal losses.

Extrarenal losses	Renal losses

• Gastrointestinal losses
• Vomiting
• Diarrhoea
• Gastric aspiration
• Sequestration in the abdomen
  ○ Peritonitis
• Loss from skin
  ○ Excessive sweating
  ○ Burns
	• Excessive use of diuretics:
	  ○ Osmotic diuresis
	  ○ Glycosuria as seen in uncontrolled diabetes
	  ○ Excessive use of mannitol
	• Renal diseases:
	  ○ Salt-wasting tubular diseases
	  ○ Chronic renal failure
	• Deficiency of mineralocorticoids:
	  ○ Addison's disease

TABLE 19.3: Causes of hyponatraemia.

Hyponatraemia with low osmolality		
Increased extracellular fluid (ECF) volume (oedema states) • Congestive heart failure • Nephrotic syndrome • Cirrhosis of liver	Reduced ECF volume (no oedema) • Renal loss of sodium (diuretics, ketonuria and Addison's disease) • Extrarenal sodium loss (sweating, vomiting, diarrhoea, peritonitis and pancreatitis)	Normal or increased effective blood volume: • Syndrome of inappropriate secretion of antidiuretic hormone (SIADH) • Primary polydipsia • Chronic renal failure
Hyponatraemia with raised osmolality • Hyperglycaemia • Mannitol administration		

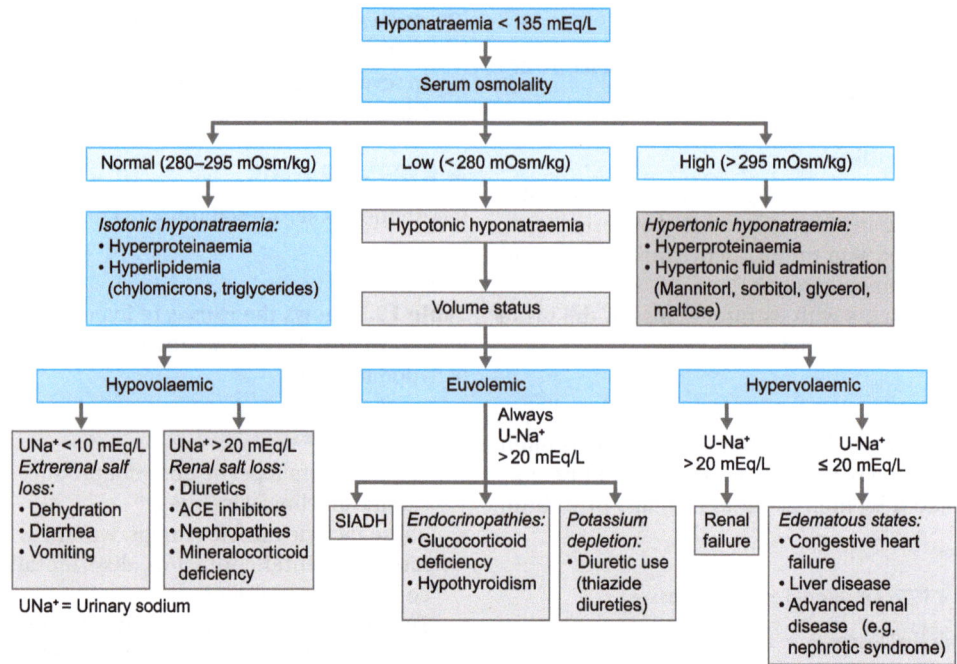

(ACE: angiotensin-converting enzyme; SIADH: syndrome of inappropriate antidiuretic hormone; UNa+: urinary sodium)

Flowchart 19.1: Algorithm for types and causes of hyponatraemia.

TABLE 19.4: Clinical findings of hyponatraemia.

Clinical findings	Type I, hypervolaemic	Type II, hypovolaemic	Type IIIA, euvolaemic	Type IIIB, euvolaemic (SIADH)
History				
Congestive heart failure (CHF), cirrhosis or nephrosis	Yes	No	No	No
Salt and water loss	No	Yes	No	No
Adrenocorticotropic hormone (ACTH)—cortisol deficiency and/or nausea and vomiting	No	No	Yes	No
Physical examination				
Generalised oedema and ascites	Yes	No	No	No
Postural hypotension	Maybe	Maybe	Maybe	No
Laboratory				
Blood urea nitrogen (BUN) and creatinine	High-normal	High-normal	Low-normal	Low-normal
Uric acid	High-normal	High-normal	Low-normal	Low-normal
Serum potassium	Low-normal	Low-normal	Normal	Normal
Serum albumin	Low-normal	High-normal	Normal	Normal
Serum cortisol	Normal-high	Normal-high	Low	Normal
Plasma renin activity	High	High	Low	Low
Urinary sodium (mEq unit of time)	Low	Low	High	High

(SIADH: syndrome of inappropriate antidiuresis hormone)

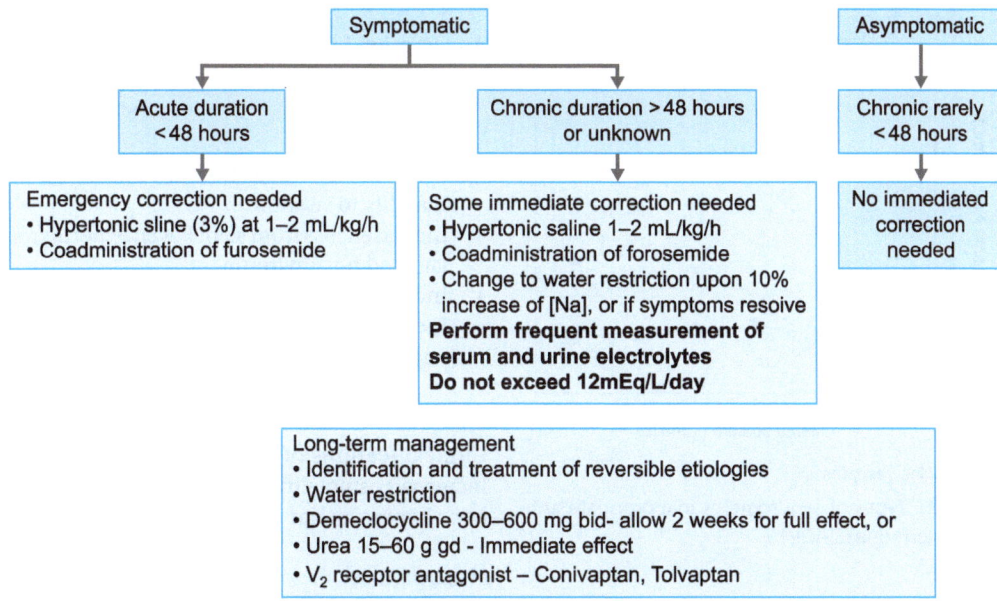

Flowchart 19.2: Treatment of severe hyponatraemia.

SYNDROME OF INAPPROPRIATE ANTIDIURETIC HORMONE SECRETION

- Hyponatraemia due to excessive water retention
- Urine osmolality exceeds plasma osmolality.
- Plasma urea and creatinine are normal or low.
- Continued urinary sodium excretion

Causes

- Neoplasm: Carcinomas—lungs, duodenum, ovary and bladder.
- Infection: Abscess, cavitation, pneumonias, tuberculosis (TB), acquired immunodeficiency syndrome (AIDS) and meningitis.
- Vascular: Cerebrovascular accident (CVA) and cavernous sinus thrombosis.
- Neurological: Guillain-Barré syndrome (GBS), multiple sclerosis (MS), amyotrophic lateral sclerosis (ALS) and hydrocephalus.
- Respiratory: Positive-pressure ventilation (PPV), pneumothorax and asthma.
- Drugs: Chlorpropamide, selective serotonin reuptake inhibitor (SSRI), monoamine oxidase inhibitor (MAOI), oxytocin, desmopressin and carbamazepine.

Clinical Features

Clinical features include nausea, irritability, confusion, seizures and coma. There is no oedema.

Four types syndrome of inappropriate antidiuretic hormone (SIADH) (**Fig. 19.2**):
1. Type A: Characterised by unregulated secretion of vasopressin.
2. Type B: Elevated basal secretion of vasopressin despite normal regulation by osmolality.
3. Type C: A 'reset osmostat'.
4. Type D: Undetectable arginine vasopressin (AVP) levels (these patients may have a gain of function mutation of the V_2-receptor).

Treatment

- The underlying cause should be corrected.
- Fluid intake should be restricted to 500–1,000 mL/day.
- Hypertonic saline: 3% saline.
- Vasopressin V_2-receptor antagonists: Tolvaptan.
- Demeclocycline [antidiuretic hormone (ADH) antagonist].

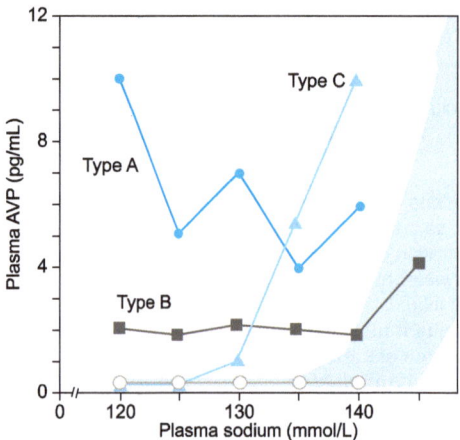

(AVP: arginine vasopressin)

Fig. 19.2: Types of syndrome of inappropriate antidiuretic hormone (SIADH)

CEREBRAL SALT WASTING

Causes

Central nervous system (CNS) damage
- Closed head injury
- CNS surgery
- CNS tumours
- CNS infections and meningitis.

Signs/Symptoms

- Polyuria
- Weight loss
- Dehydration/hypovolaemia
- Hypotension
- Low central venous pressure (CVP)

Laboratory Values

- Hyponatraemia due to excessive renal Na loss
- High urine Na > 20 mmol/L
- Increased plasma atrial natriuretic peptide (ANP), ANP, because of low volume status
- Inappropriately normal or low aldosterone and ADH levels despite high ANP

Treatment

- Volume for volume replacement of urinary Na losses
- Salt supplementation to the diet

HYPERNATRAEMIA

An elevation in the serum sodium concentration > 145 mEq/L.

Causes

- Decreased intake: Coma, depression and inability to swallow.
- Increased loss from skin: Fever, hyperthyroidism and hot environment.
- Increased respiratory loss: Hyperventilation.
- Increased loss in urine: Diabetes insipidus and medullary cystic disease.

Clinical Features and Investigations

Clinical features of hypernatraemia are due to increased osmolality and are same as that of diabetic hyperosmolar state (**Table 19.5**).

Management

In patient with gradual onset of water depletion over > 2 days, correction should be done slowly.

When hypernatraemia is associated with hypotension due to volume depletion, the initial solution should be isotonic saline so as to increase the ECF volume.

If neurological features are also present, therapy should be started with 1/2 normal saline or 5% dextrose.

Management of hyponatraemia has been shown in **Table 19.6**.

TABLE 19.5: Clinical features and investigations of hypernatraemia.

Clinical features	Investigations
• Marked thirst	• Haematocrit usually 50%
• Muscle weakness and rigidity	• Raised blood urea levels
• Dry mouth	
• Mental confusion and coma	• Raised plasma sodium
• Intracranial haemorrhage (in acute hypernatraemia)	• Urine specific gravity 1.010
• Tachycardia and low systolic blood pressure	

TABLE 19.6: Management of hyponatraemia.

Severity	Fluid and route of administration	Quantity and time for replacement
Mild depletion (1–2 L deficit)	Water by mouth or 5% glucose intravenous (IV)	2 L, over 6–12 h
Moderate (2–4 L deficit)	5% Glucose IV	2–4 L, over 24 h
Severe (4–10 L deficit)	0.9% NaCl IV	1 L, over 1 h
	5% dextrose IV	3 L, over 2 h
	5% dextrose IV	4 L, over 24–48 h

■ OSMOTIC DEMYELINATION SYNDROME OR CENTRAL PONTINE MYELINOLYSIS

- Risk factors: Alcoholism, chronically ill patients, elderly/malnourished, cirrhosis predisposes to demyelination (due to depletion of intracellular organic solutes).
- Hypokalaemia is a strong predictor.
- Demyelination can be diffuse and not involving the pons. Extrapontine areas include cerebellar and neocortical white/grey junctional areas, thalamus, sub-thalamus, amygdale, globus pallidus, putamen, caudate and lateral geniculate bodies.
- Rate of correction over 24 hours more important than rate of correction in any one particular hour.
- More common, if sodium increases by > 20 mEq/L in 24 hours.
- Very uncommon, if sodium increases by 12 mEq/L or less in 24 hours.
- Symptoms generally occur 2–6 days after elevation of sodium and usually either irreversible or only partially reversible.

Clinical Features

- Dysarthria, dysphagia, Parkinsonism, catatonia, locked-in syndrome, lethargy and coma, seizures, nystagmus, ataxia, emotional lability, akinetic mutism, gait disturbance, myoclonus, behavioural disturbances, paraparesis or quadriparesis.
- MRI (magnetic resonance imaging) with diffusion-weighted imaging will be helpful in early detection.

■ HYPOKALAEMIA

Causes

- Loss from gastrointestinal (GI) tract: Vomiting, diarrhoea, villous adenoma, ureterosigmoidostomy and intestinal obstruction
- Loss of urine: Primary and secondary hyperaldosteronism, Cushing's syndrome, diuretics.
- Intracellular shift of K^+: Alkalosis, high-dose insulin and periodic paralysis.
- Reduced intake: Diet containing inadequate potassium, potassium free IV fluids.

Clinical Features

- Generalised muscle weakness and depression of tendon reflexes
- Paralytic ileus
- Electrocardiogram (ECG) changes: Flattering and inversion of T waves, sagging of the ST segment and appearance of **U wave**.
- Atrial and ventricular arrhythmias may occur, especially in patients receiving digitalis.
- Death may occur due to respiratory paralysis or cardiac arrest.

Treatment

- Treatment must be directed at correcting the hypokalaemia and eliminating the cause of potassium loss.
- Potassium supplementation can be given orally or intravenously in the form of potassium chloride (KCl).
- Mild hypokalaemia—3.0–3.5 mEq/L—treat with diet rich in potassium.

- Moderate hypokalaemia—2.5–3 mEq/L—treat with oral potassium supplementation.
- Potassium < 2.5 mEq/L—treat with intravenous potassium supplementation.

■ HYPERKALAEMIA

Causes

- Impaired excretion: Acute kidney injury (AKI), severe chronic renal failure (CRF), Addison's disease, hypoaldosteronism, type 4 renal tubular acidosis, potassium-sparing diuretics, angiotensin-converting enzyme (ACE) inhibitors, NSAIDs.
- Excessive intake: Intravenous fluids containing K^+ and high K^+ foods.
- Tissue breakdown: Haemolysis, rhabdomyolysis, crush injury, burns and tumour lysis syndrome.
- Shift of K^+ out of cells: Acidosis, insulin deficiency, and hyperkalaemic periodic paralysis.
- Pseudohyperkalaemia: Haemolysed blood sample and marked thrombocytosis.

Clinical Features

- Cardiac arrhythmias, muscular weakness progressing to flaccid paralysis and respiratory embarrassment.
- ECG changes of hyperkalaemia are (**Fig. 19.3**):
  o Tall, peaked T waves
  o Prolongation of PR interval
  o Reduced height of P wave
  o Widening of QRS complex
  o 'Sine wave' pattern
- Terminally ventricular fibrillation and standstill may occur.

Management

- Identification and elimination of the underlying cause.
- '10 mL of 10% calcium gluconate' solution is given intravenously slowly over 2–5 minutes. It stabilises the myocardial cells.
- Intravenous glucose along with insulin encourages shift of potassium from extracellular compartment to intracellular compartment.
- Intravenous administration of sodium bicarbonate.

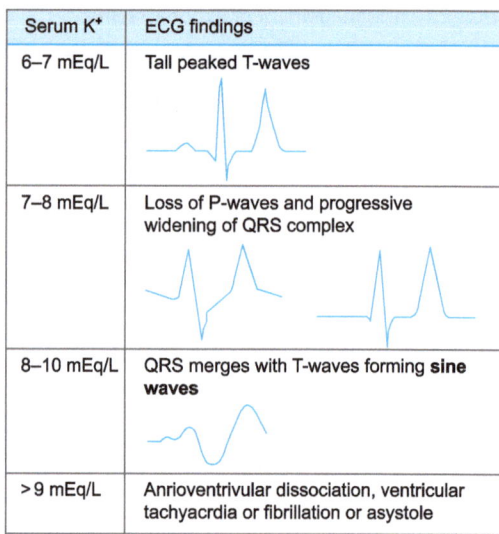

Serum K^+	ECG findings
6–7 mEq/L	Tall peaked T-waves
7–8 mEq/L	Loss of P-waves and progressive widening of QRS complex
8–10 mEq/L	QRS merges with T-waves forming **sine waves**
> 9 mEq/L	Anrioventrivular dissociation, ventricular tachyacrdia or fibrillation or asystole

(ECG: electrocardiogram)

Fig. 19.3: ECG changes in hyperkalaemia in relation to serum potassium.

- Nebulisation of β-agonists (salbutamol and terbutaline) also can reduce potassium levels by producing shift of potassium to intracellular compartment.
- Cation exchange resins such as sodium polystyrene sulphonate are helpful in the removal of K^+. The resins can be given orally or as enema.
- If these measures fail, haemodialysis is indicated.

Table 19.7 shows the drugs that are used in the treatment of hyperkalaemia.

■ METABOLIC ACIDOSIS

Causes of metabolic acidosis are shown in **Table 19.8**.

Clinical Features

- Kussmaul's breathing or 'air hunger'.
- Peripheral vasodilatation and fall in cardiac output may result in a fall in blood pressure.
- Severe acidosis may be associated with drowsiness, confusion, and coma.
- Serum bicarbonate is low, blood pH is low, and partial pressure of carbondioxide is low.

TABLE 19.7: Drugs used in the treatment of hyperkalaemia.

Therapeutic goal	Intervention	Dose and method of administration
Myocardial membrane stabilisation, if ECG changes are +ve	Calcium chloride or	• 1 g IV over 10 minutes non-emergent setting
	Calcium gluconate	• 1 g IV push in cardiac arrest or significant dysrhythmia
Intracellular potassium shifting	Dextrose/insulin	• Dextrose 50 g IVP (intravenous push) • Insulin (regular) 10 units IVP
	Sodium bicarbonate	• 1 mEq/kg ideal body weight • IVP over 10–20 minutes non-emergent setting • IVP in cardiac arrest or significant dysrhythmia
	Magnesium sulphate	• 1–2 g IV over 10 minutes non-emergent setting • IVP in cardiac arrest or significant dysrhythmia
	Sympathomimetic agents	• Albuterol-standard metered 'respiratory dose' via nebuliser non-emergent/emergent (significant dysrhythmia) setting • Epinephrine-**cardiac arrest only:** 1 mg IVP (1:10,000 concentration)
Potassium removal from body (excretion from the body)	Sodium polystyrene	• 30–60 g PO or PR
	Normal saline	• Volume determined by clinical setting
	Furosemide	• 20 g IV for furosemide-naïve patients
	Haemodialysis	• Best way of removal

(ECG: electrocardiogram; IV: intravenous; IVP: intravenous push)

TABLE 19.8: Causes of metabolic acidosis.

Increased anion gap	Normal anion gap

• Severe renal failure
• Increased production of organic acids
  o Diabetic ketoacidosis
  o Alcoholic ketosis
  o Starvation ketosis
  o Poisoning: Methanol, salicylates and ethylene glycol
• Increased lactic acid production:
  o Cardiorespiratory arrest
  o Shock
  o Septicaemia
	• Diarrhoea
	• Renal tubular acidosis

Treatment

- Main aim of treatment is to correct the underlying disorder.
- Sodium bicarbonate may be given in severe acidosis.
- In renal failure with metabolic acidosis, dialysis may be necessary.

METABOLIC ALKALOSIS

Metabolic alkalosis is characterised by increased plasma bicarbonate, a fall in hydrogen ion concentration and a small compensatory rise in partial pressure of carbon dioxide.

Causes

- Loss of hydrogen and chloride ion, e.g., vomiting or aspiration of gastric contents.
- Administration of diuretics such as thiazides and furosemide.
- Hyperaldosteronism
- Excessive alkali intake

Clinical Features

- Specific clinical disturbances are rare. Acute alkalosis may induce tetany due to increased neuromuscular activity.
- The underlying cause should be corrected.
- Potassium chloride supplementation is necessary in cases of alkalosis associated with hypokalaemia

RESPIRATORY ACIDOSIS

Causes of respiratory acidosis have been shown in Table 19.9.

Clinical Features
Confusion and obtundation

Treatment
The underlying causes should be corrected.

RESPIRATORY ALKALOSIS

- This occurs when there is excessive loss of carbon dioxide by hyperventilation of the lungs.
- Partial pressure of carbon dioxide and hydrogen ion concentration fall. Plasma bicarbonate is decreased.

  Causes of respiratory alkalosis are shown in Table 19.10.
- In severe respiratory alkalosis, hyperventilation may be present. Sometimes, there may be manifestations of tetany.

TABLE 19.9: Causes of respiratory acidosis.

Disorders of gas exchange	Disorders of musculoskeletal system
• Acute severe asthma • Acute exacerbation of obstructive lung disease • Foreign body inhalation • Chronic obstructive lung disease	• Flail chest • Tension pneumothorax • Myasthenia gravis • Poliomyelitis
Others	
• Overdose with opiates and sedatives • Brain stem and cervical cord lesions	

TABLE 19.10: Causes of respiratory alkalosis.

Central	Pulmonary
• Anxiety • Fever • CNS infections • Cerebrovascular accident • Metabolic encephalopathy • Septicaemia • Salicylate poisoning • Hepatic failure	• Interstitial lung disease • Asthma • Pneumonia • Congestive heart failure • Pulmonary embolism

- In acute respiratory alkalosis, patients may complain of paresthesia, numbness, tingling and light-headedness.
- Treatment is elimination of the underlying disorder.
- In acute hyperventilation syndrome, sedation and rebreathing into a bag may terminate the attack.

BEST OF FIVES

1. A patient with a history of Sjögren's syndrome has the following laboratory findings: Plasma sodium 139 mEq/L, chloride 112 mEq/L, bicarbonate 15 mEq/L, and potassium 3.0 mEq/L; urine studies show a pH of 6.0, sodium of 15 mEq/L, potassium of 10 mEq/L, and chloride of 12 mEq/L. The most likely diagnosis is:
   A. Type I renal tubular acidosis (RTA)
   B. Type II RTA
   C. Type III RTA
   D. Type IV RTA
   E. Chronic diarrhoea

2. Type II RTA is associated with all the following except:
   A. Normal anion gap (AG) acidosis
   B. Hypercalciuria
   C. Decreased urinary citrate
   D. Minimum urinary pH < 5.5
   E. Bone demineralisation

3. All are used in the management of hyperkalaemia except:
   A. Calcium gluconate
   B. Insulin with dextrose
   C. Beta-2 antagonist
   D. Dialysis
   E. Furosemide

4. A patient on amphotericin B has weakness and cramps. Serum potassium = 2.3 mEq/dL. Calculate the total parenteral potassium supplementation to be given to the patient over the next 24 hours.
   A. 40 mEq
   B. 80 mEq
   C. 100 mEq
   D. 140 mEq
   E. 200 mEq

5. Tolvaptan is useful for:
   A. Hyponatraemia
   B. Hypernatraemia
   C. Nephrogenic diabetes insipidus
   D. Decreased water clearance
   E. Hyperkalaemia

6. Tetany may be a feature of the following except:
   A. Hyperventilation
   B. Hypokalaemic alkalosis
   C. Thyroid surgery
   D. Hyponatraemia
   E. Hypomagnesaemia

7. A 40-year-old man comes with complaints of vomiting for the last 3 days. Arterial blood gas (ABG) shows a pH of 7.22 with pCO_2 of 21 mmHg and HCO_3 of 9 mEq/dL. What is the diagnosis?
   A. Mixed metabolic acidosis and respiratory alkalosis
   B. Metabolic acidosis
   C. Respiratory alkalosis
   D. Mixed respiratory acidosis and metabolic alkalosis
   E. Respiratory alkalosis

8. All of the statements regarding calcium homeostasis are true except:
   A. Calcium balance is controlled by parathyroid hormone (PTH) and calcitonin
   B. PTH activates osteoblasts to break down bone matrix
   C. PTH enhances intestinal absorption of calcium
   D. Calcitonin is a PTH antagonist, but its contribution to calcium and phosphate homeostasis is minor to negligible
   E. In the kidney, calcium reabsorption and phosphate excretion go hand in hand

9. Arterial blood gas (ABG) showing pH of 7.46 with pCO_2 of 57 mmHg and HCO_3 of 42 mEq suggests:
   A. Metabolic alkalosis with compensatory respiratory acidosis
   B. Metabolic acidosis with compensatory respiratory alkalosis
   C. Respiratory acidosis with compensatory metabolic alkalosis
   D. Respiratory alkalosis with compensatory metabolic acidosis
   E. Mixed respiratory and metabolic acidosis

10. All of the following are causes of metabolic acidosis with a normal anion gap except:
    A. Proximal RTA
    B. Salicylate poisoning
    C. Diarrhoea
    D. Pancreatitis
    E. Distal renal tubular acidosis (RTA)

11. All the following are true about sodium except:
    A. It contributes 280 mOsm of the total 300 mOsm extracellular fluid (ECF) solute concentration
    B. It is the only cation exerting significant osmotic pressure
    C. Sodium ions leak into cells and are pumped out against their electrochemical gradient
    D. It accounts for 90–95% of all solutes in the ECF
    E. It is the chief cation in the intracellular fluid (ICF)

12. Urine osmolality is calculated with which of the following formula?
    A. 2 × (urine sodium) + (urine potassium) + (urinary urea nitrogen/2.8) + (urine glucose/18)
    B. 2.8 × (urine sodium) + (urine potassium) + (urinary urea nitrogen/2.8) + (urine glucose/18)
    C. 3 × (urine sodium) + (urine potassium) + (urinary urea nitrogen/2.8) + (urine glucose/18)
    D. 3.8 × (urine sodium) + (urine potassium) + (urinary urea nitrogen/2.8) + (urine glucose/18)
    E. 1.8 × (urine sodium) + (urine potassium) + (urinary urea nitrogen/2.8) + (urine glucose/18)

13. An 85-year-old man admitted to the intensive care unit (ICU) for sepsis was recently given a diagnosis of SIADH (syndrome of inappropriate antidiuretic hormone secretion). His serum sodium acutely fell from 130 to 115 mEq/L during the past 3 days, and he recently developed seizures due to this problem. Which would be the most appropriate treatment option?
    A. Intravenous 0.9% sodium chloride
    B. Intravenous DDAVP (desmopressin acetate)
    C. Intravenous 3% sodium chloride

D. Intravenous conivaptan
E. Intravenous furosemide

14. A 40-year-old man (weight 60 kg) is admitted to the trauma ICU after a motor vehicle accident. He is noted to have a serum magnesium concentration of 1.2 mg/dL, and his family states that he has a history of alcohol abuse. He is given magnesium sulphate 6 g intravenously over 4 hours by the primary service. His repeat serum magnesium concentration on the following day is 1.8 mg/dL. Which would be the most appropriate treatment for this patient?
    A. No treatment is necessary because his serum magnesium concentration is normal
    B. If a repeat serum magnesium concentration is 2 mg/dL or greater, no additional magnesium therapy is indicated
    C. Supplemental calcium therapy should be given concurrently with the magnesium therapy
    D. Additional magnesium therapy should be given daily over the next 4–5 days
    E. Supplement phosphorous concurrently with magnesium

15. Saline responsive (urinary chloride <10 mEq/L) is seen in all except:
    A. Excessive gastric fluid losses
    B. Diuretic therapy (especially loop diuretics)
    C. Dehydration (contraction alkalosis)
    D. Hypokalaemia
    E. Excessive mineralocorticoid activity (e.g. hydrocortisone)

16. Delta ratio = $\Delta AG/\Delta HCO_3$ = (measured AG – normal AG)/(normal HCO_3 – measured HCO_3) <0.4 is seen in:
    A. Metabolic alkalosis
    B. Hyperchloraemic normal AG acidosis
    C. High AG acidosis and normal AG acidosis
    D. High AG acidosis and concurrent metabolic alkalosis
    E. Compensated respiratory alkalosis

17. Which is the most appropriate replacement fluid for a patient with significant nasogastric (NG) fluid drainage?

    A. 0.9% sodium chloride and potassium chloride 20 mEq/L
    B. 0.45% sodium chloride and potassium chloride 20 mEq/L
    C. 5% dextrose in 0.225% sodium chloride and potassium chloride 20 mEq/L
    D. Lactated Ringer solution
    E. 1.8% sodium chloride with potassium chloride 40 mEq/L

18. Renal glutaminase activity is increased in:
    A. Metabolic acidosis
    B. Respiratory acidosis
    C. Both A and B
    D. Metabolic alkalosis
    E. Respiratory alkalosis

19. The greatest buffering capacity at physiological pH would be provided by a protein rich in which of the following amino acids?
    A. Lysine
    B. Histidine
    C. Aspartic acid
    D. Leucine
    E. Glutamine

20. A young woman is found comatose, having taken an unknown number of sleeping pills an unknown time before. An arterial blood sample yields the following values: pH – 6.90, HCO_3 13 mEq/L and $PaCO_2$ 68 mmHg. This patient's acid–base status is most accurately described as:
    A. Uncompensated metabolic acidosis
    B. Uncompensated respiratory acidosis
    C. Mixed respiratory and metabolic acidosis
    D. Respiratory acidosis with partial renal compensation
    E. Compensated respiratory alkalosis

Answers

1-A, 2-C, 3-C, 4-D, 5-A, 6-D, 7-B, 8-B, 9-A, 10-B, 11-E, 12-A, 13-C, 14-D, 15-E, 16-B, 17-B, 18-C, 19-B, 20-C

■ SUGGESTED READING

1. Sterns RH. Treatment of severe hyponatremia. Clin J Am Soc Nephrol. 2018;13(4):641-9.
2. Halawa I, Andersson T, Tomson T. Hyponatremia and risk of seizures: a retrospective cross-sectional study. Epilepsia. 2011;52(2):410-3.

3. Rose BD, Post TW. Clinical physiology of acid-base and electrolyte disorders, 5th edition. New York: McGraw-Hill; 2001. p. 775.
4. Adrogué HJ, Madias NE. Hypernatremia. N Engl J Med. 2000;342(20):1493-9.
5. Mount DB. Disorders of Potassium Balance. In: Brenner and Rector's The Kidney, 10th edition. London: Elsevier; 2016.
6. Rose BD, Post TW. Hypokalemia. In: Clinical Physiology of Acid-Base and Electrolyte Disorders, 5th edition. Rose BD, Post TW (Eds). New York: McGraw-Hill; 2001. p. 836.
7. Kamel KS, Wei C. Controversial issues in the treatment of hyperkalaemia. Nephrol Dial Transplant. 2003;18(11):2215-8.
8. Littmann L, Gibbs MA. Electrocardiographic manifestations of severe hyperkalemia. J Electrocardiol. 2018; 51(5):814-7.
9. Garibotto G, Sofia A, Robaudo C, Saffioti S, Sala MR, Verzola D, et al. Kidney protein dynamics and ammoniagenesis in humans with chronic metabolic acidosis. J Am Soc Nephrol. 2004;15(6):1606-15.
10. Corey HE. Stewart and beyond: new models of acid-base balance. Kidney Int. 2003;64(3):777-87.
11. Emmett M. Anion-gap interpretation: the old and the new. Nat Clin Pract Nephrol. 2006;2(1):4-5.
12. Galla JH. Metabolic alkalosis. J Am Soc Nephrol. 2000;11(2):369-75.
13. Maier JD, Levine SN. Hypercalcemia in the intensive care unit: A review of pathophysiology, diagnosis, and modern therapy. J Intensive Care Med. 2015;30(5):235-52.

CHAPTER 20

Dermatology

PRIMARY AND SECONDARY SKIN LESIONS

Description of primary and secondary skin lesions are given in **Figures 20.1** and **20.2**, respectively.

Macule	Description: A circumscribed flat, coloured lesion, <2 cm in diameter, with sharp borders, not raised above the surface of the surrounding skin. Examples: Freckle, rashes of rickettsial infections, rubella	**Vesicle**	Description: A small, fluid-filled lesion, <0.5 cm in diameter, raised above the plane of surrounding skin. Examples: Herpes infections, acute allergic contact dermatitis, dermatitis herpetiformis	
Patch	Description: A large (>2 cm) flat lesion with a colour different from that of surrounding skin. Example: Vitiligo	**Bulla**	Description: A fluid-filled, raised, often translucent lesion >0.5 cm in diameter. Examples: Burns, pemphigus vulgaris and bullous pemphigoid	
Papule	Description: A small, solid, <0.5 cm in diameter, without fluid, raised lesion above the surface of the surrounding skin with sharp borders. Examples: Naevi, warts, lichen planus, seborrheic and actinic keratosis	**Wheal**	Description: An evanescent elevated lesion with erythaema and oedema frequently with central pallor. Example: Urticaria	
Nodule, tumour	Description Nodule: Palpable, large (0.5–5.0 cm), firm/solid lesion with distinct border raised above the surface of the surrounding skin. Tumour: A solid, raised growth >5 cm in diameter. Examples: Cysts, lipomas and fibromas.	**Pustule**	Description: A vesicle filled with pus (leucocytes). Examples: Folliculitis	
Plaque	Description: A large (>1 cm), flat-topped, raised area of skin. Examples: Psoriasis and granuloma annulare	**Telangiectasia**	Description: A visible dilatation of small cutaneous blood vessels Examples: Hereditary haemorrhagic telangiectasia	

Fig. 20.1: Schematic representation of common primary skin lesions.

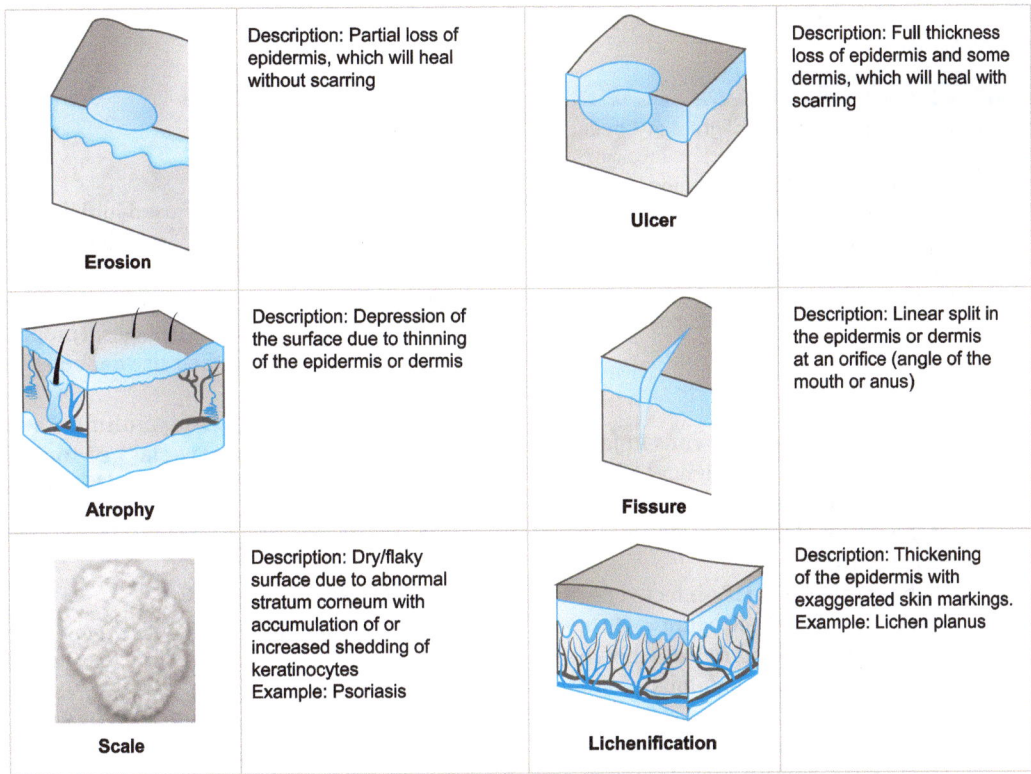

Fig. 20.2: Schematic representation of common secondary skin lesions.

ECZEMA/DERMATITIS

Characteristic inflammatory response of the skin to both exogenous and endogenous agents

Types

Exogenous
- Irritant contact eczema is due to detergents, alkalis, acids, solvents and abrasive dust. Strong irritants often cause acute eczema, whereas weak irritants often cause chronic eczema.
- Allergic contact eczema is due to delayed hypersensitivity reaction following contact with antigens or haptens. Face, neck and hands are the most common body parts involved. Forehead and ears are commonly affected by hair dyes and shampoos; ears are susceptible to metals from earrings; eyelids are particularly affected by airborne allergens and nail polish; the cheeks and lips are prone to reaction to facial cosmetics.

Endogenous
- **Atopic eczema** is due to a genetic predisposition to form excessive IgE antibodies to inhaled, injected or ingested antigens.
  - Patients with atopic eczema have a tendency to develop other allergic diseases such as asthma, allergic rhinitis, hay fever, urticaria and food and other allergies.
  - The cardinal features of atopic eczema are itch, xerosis, scratching and lichenification.
  - Usually chronic or relapsing
  - Primarily flexural (antecubital and popliteal fossae) in its distribution in children and adults, but facial and truncal involvement predominates in infants.
  - By adulthood, 40–80% of patients will experience either a decrease or complete resolution of their disease.

Table 20.1 gives cutaneous and vascular stigmata of atopic dermatitis.

TABLE 20.1: Cutaneous and vascular stigmata of atopic dermatitis.

Cutaneous stigmata	Vascular stigmata
• Dennie–Morgan infraorbital fold • Pityriasis alba • Keratosis pilaris • Hertoghe's sign—thinning of the lateral eyebrows	• Headlight sign—perinasal and periorbital pallor • White dermographism—balancing of the skin at the site of stroking with a blunt instrument—cause oedema and obscure colour of underlying vessels

- **Seborrhoeic eczema** often runs in families, and is associated with a tendency to dandruff.
  - Possible due to excessive growth of fungi of the genus *Malassezia* (formerly called *Pityrosporum*).
  - High prevalence in HIV-infected persons particularly if CD4 cell count < 400/mm^3.
  - Patient has characteristic 'seborrhoeic look'—oily skin with patulous, prominent follicular orifices.
  - Involves areas rich in sebaceous glands—scalp, retro-auricular folds, eyebrows, nasolabial folds, beard area, inter-scapular and pre-sternal regions, axillae, public region, groin, umbilicus and folds under pendulous breasts
  - Scalp area—diffusely involved with greasy scales on a dull red background
  - Eyebrows—fine scaling of eyelid margins
  - An infantile form, which usually involves the scalp (cradle cap), the face and the diaper area, affects as many as 70% of newborns during the first 3 months of life but usually disappears by 1 year of age.
- **Discoid eczema (nummular eczema)** is seen most often on the limbs of elderly males and is of uncertain aetiology.
- **Asteatotic eczema** is commonly seen on the lower legs, in hospitalised elderly patients.
- **Gravitational (stasis) eczema** occurs on the lower legs and is often associated with signs of venous insufficiency.
- **Pompholyx (dyshidrotic eczema)** describes a form of eczema in which bouts of recurrent vesicles or bullae affect the palms, fingers and soles.

General Management

General:
- Emollients for moisturising.

Atopic Eczema
- Oral antihistamines
- Topical steroids should be used judiciously. The various preparations available are 1% hydrocortisone (mildly potent), clobetasone butyrate (moderately potent), betamethasone valerate (potent) and 0.05% clobetasol propionate (very potent) and their use depends on severity of lesions.
- Calcineurin inhibitors (tacrolimus and pimecrolimus) are a new class of topical immunomodulators and are useful if steroids are not effective. However, these agents cannot be used for erosions and ulcers.

Seborrhoeic Eczema
- Ordinary shampooing in mild cases with scalp involvement
- In severe cases, medicated shampoos containing selenium sulphide (2.5%), zinc pyrithione (1%) or ketoconazole (2%)
- In severe cases, medicated shampoos containing selenium sulphide (2.5%), zinc pyrithione (1%) or ketoconazole (2%)
- Topical lithium succinate and lithium gluconate are effective alternative agents for the treatment of seborrhoeic eczema in areas other than the scalp.
- In acute state, topical steroids of low potency to control erythema and itching

XEROSTOMIA

Aetiology
- Anticholinergic drugs (reduce volume of saliva)—anticholinergics, antidepressants, antiemetics, antihistamines, antihypertensives, antiparkinsonian drugs, antipsychotics, antispasmodics, diuretics
- Sympathomimetic drugs (produce viscous saliva)—amphetamines, appetite suppressants, bronchodilators, decongestants.
- Systemic causes—Addison's disease, Alzheimer's diseases, alcoholic cirrhosis, diabetes mellitus, HIV/AIDS (human immunodeficiency virus/acquired immunodeficiency

syndrome), radiation to head and neck area (e.g. for cancer therapy), salivary gland infection, severe dehydration, Sjögren's syndrome.
- Others—elderly persons, sleep-related xerostomia (due to mouth-breathing during sleep).

■ PRURITUS

Systemic causes and dermatological causes of pruritus are mentioned in **Boxes 20.1** and **20.2**, respectively.

Treatment

General measures:
- Controlling xerosis with moisturisers and humidification of indoor environment
- Use of antihistamines such as diphenhydramine

Specific measures:
- Treatment of underlying cause
- Ursodeoxycholic acid (UDCA) in cholestasis
- Cholestyramine, rifampicin and opioid antagonists (e.g. naltrexone) in primary biliary cirrhosis
- Ultraviolet (UV) B phototherapy and ondansetron in uraemic patients
- Corticosteroids in patients with Hodgkin's disease
- Paroxetine, a selective serotonin reuptake inhibitor, is useful in itching produced as paraneoplastic manifestation of malignancies.

■ PSORIASIS

- The main abnormality in psoriasis is the increased epidermal proliferation due to excessive division of cells in the stratum basale and a shorter cell cycle.
- Commonly presents before the age of 35 years. It is equally common in both males and females.
- May be a presenting sign of HIV infection.
- The characteristic lesions are pink-red, sharply demarcated papules and rounded plaques covered by silvery scales.
- The most common areas of involvement are the extensor body areas (elbows, knees), gluteal cleft and the scalp. Trunk is also

> **Box 20.2: Dermatological causes of pruritus.**
> - Atopic dermatitis
> - Scabies
> - Xerosis
> - Lichen simplex chronicus
> - Contact dermatitis
> - Insect bites
> - Sunburn
> - Ichthyoses
> - Dermatitis herpetiformis
> - Psoriasis
> - Lichen planus
> - Fungal infections
> - Pediculosis
> - Plaster of Paris casts

> **Box 20.1: Systemic causes of pruritus.**
>
> **Autoimmune**
> - Dermatitis herpetiformis
> - Dermatomyositis
>
> **Haematological**
> - Haemochromatosis
> - Mastocytosis
> - Polycythaemia vera
>
> **Infectious diseases**
> - AIDS
> - Infectious hepatitis
> - Parasitic diseases (e.g. giardiasis, ascariasis)
>
> **Neurologic**
> - Cerebral abscess
> - Cerebral tumour
>
> **Hepatobiliary**
> - Biliary cirrhosis
> - Drug-induced cholestasis
>
> **Metabolic and endocrine**
> - Carcinoid syndrome
> - Chronic renal disease
> - Diabetes mellitus
>
> **Malignancy**
> - Leukaemia, lymphoma
> - Multiple myeloma
> - Solid tumours with paraneoplastic syndrome
>
> **Others**
> - Drug
> - Pregnancy
>
> (AIDS: acquired immunodeficiency syndrome)

commonly involved. Traumatised areas are often involved (**Koebner or isomorphic phenomenon**) and this explains common involvement of elbows and knees. About half of the patients have finger nail involvement. The characteristic nail changes are punctuate pitting, onycholysis (separation of nail from the nail bed) and subungual hyperkeratosis.
- On scrapping a psoriatic lesion with a microscopic slide, silvery scales come out first. After that, pin-point bleeding appears at the base of the lesion. The latter is known as **Auspitz sign**.
- Psoriatic arthritis is seen in 5–10% of psoriatic patients and usually occurs several years after appearance of skin lesions. It is a form of seronegative spondyloarthropathy.

Types of psoriasis are mentioned in **Box 20.3**.

Treatment

Most patients with psoriasis have skin lesions limited to localised areas. For these patients, topical therapy remains a part of their therapeutic regimen.
- **Local treatment:** Application of emollients, coal tar preparations, dithranol and topical steroids, and UV radiation [(narrow band UV-B and PUVA (psoralens with UV-A)]. Topical steroids range in strength from weak steroids such as 1% hydrocortisone to superpotent corticosteroids, such as clobetasol propionate and betamethasone dipropionate. Other local agents include vitamin D analogues—calcipotriol, calcitriol and tacalcitol. Local retinoid, tazarotene, is also useful.
- **Systemic treatment:** PUVA, retinoids (etretinate and acitretin), methotrexate and cyclosporine

Box 20.3: Types of psoriasis.
- Plaque psoriasis (psoriasis vulgaris), chronic plaque psoriasis
- Guttate psoriasis (small rain drop-like psoriatic lesions)
- Inverse psoriasis (flexural psoriasis)
- Localised pustular psoriasis
- Generalised pustular psoriasis
- Erythrodermic psoriasis
- Von Zumbusch psoriasis-pustular + erythroderma

- **Biological therapy:** Includes alefacept (causes apoptosis of T cells), efalizumab (inhibits T-cell activation) and etanercept, infliximab and adalimumab [tumour necrosis factors (TNF)-inhibitors]

■ LICHEN PLANUS

Lichen planus (LP) is a pruritic inflammatory dermatosis, i.e. commonly associated with mucosal involvement. Rarely, it may be associated with involvement of nail (nail dystrophy) and hair (scarring alopecia).

The typical rash of LP is well-described by the 5 P's: **Well-defined pruritic, planar, purple, polygonal papules or plaques**.

Sites involved: Flexor surfaces especially wrists, flanks, medial thighs, shins of tibia, glans penis, nails, scalp and oral mucosa.
- There may be a characteristic fine lacy-white pattern (network) on the surface of lesions (Wickham's striae).
- Koebner phenomenon is seen.

Treatment

Topical steroids, PUVA, immunosuppressive agents (azathioprine)

■ ERYTHEMA NODOSUM

- Erythema nodosum is inflammation of subcutaneous fat (panniculitis) of skin.
- Most often idiopathic; common identifiable causes include streptococcal infection and tuberculosis (usually primary tuberculosis).
- It develops as a result of a non-specific cutaneous reaction to a variety of antigens, with many immune-mediated mechanisms implicated including immune-complex mediated reaction and type IV delayed hypersensitivity response to antigens.

Triggering factors associated with erythema nodosum are mentioned in **Box 20.4**.

Clinical Features

- More common in females (male-to-female ratio—1:6).
- Presents with painful, symmetrical, erythematosus nodules and plaques ranging in size

Dermatology

> **Box 20.4: Triggering factors associated with erythema nodosum.**
>
> **Infections**
> - Bacteria, e.g. β-**haemolytic streptococci**, mycobacteria (usually primary **tuberculosis**, leprosy), Brucella, Mycoplasma, Rickettsia, Chlamydia, Salmonella, Yersinia
> - Viruses, e.g. hepatitis B and infectious mononucleosis
> - Fungi, e.g. coccidioidomycosis, histoplasmosis, blastomycosis
> - Parasitic, e.g. amebiasis, giardiasis
>
> Drug administration, e.g. **sulphonamides**, sulphonylureas, oral contraceptives
>
> Systemic disease, e.g. **sarcoidosis**, inflammatory bowel disease, Behçet's disease
>
> Malignancies: Lymphoma, leukaemia, renal cell carcinoma
>
> Idiopathic: > 50% cases

from 1 to 10 cm. Nodules are poorly demarcated due to their subcutaneous location and are most commonly located on the anterior aspect of legs, particularly shins, ankles and knees. Within a few days, the nodules become livid red or purplish colour.

Treatment

- Treat any underlying disorders.
- Rest and analgesics with NSAIDs. However, NSAIDs should be avoided in treating erythema nodosum secondary to Crohn's disease because they may trigger a flare-up of the underlying Crohn's disease.

ACNE VULGARIS

This is a disorder characterised by chronic inflammation of blocked pilosebaceous follicles. It predominantly affects teenagers.

Aetiopathogenesis

- There is an increase in sebum excretion, which is probably androgen mediated.
- Increased and abnormal keratinisation at the exit of the pilosebaceous follicle causes obstruction to the flow of sebum.
- Colonisation by pathogenic *Propionibacterium acnes* causing inflammation at a later stage of the disease.

Clinical Features

- Lesions are limited to the face, shoulders, upper chest and back.
- Open comedones (blackheads) are due to plugging of the pilosebaceous orifice by keratin and sebum.
- Closed comedones (whiteheads) are due to accretions of sebum and keratin deeper in the pilosebaceous ducts.
- Later in the course, inflammatory lesions occur that tend to lead to more scarring. The lesions may include papules, pustules, nodules and cysts, and any combination of these. Severe forms of inflammatory acne include nodular cystic disease with all its potentially destructive sequelae.

Clinical variants listed in **Box 20.5**.

> **Box 20.5: Clinical variants of Acne.**
>
> - **Acne conglobata** is rare and commonly affects adult males. It is a severe form of acne characterised by numerous comedones, large abscesses with sinuses, grouped inflammatory nodules associated with suppuration. It may be associated with hidradenitis suppurativa (a chronic, inflammatory disorder of apocrine glands, mainly affecting axillae and groins), folliculitis and pilonidal sinus.
> - **Acne fulminans** is a rare, severe variant of acne, usually affecting the trunk in adolescent males. It presents with fever, arthralgias and systemic inflammation, with leucocytosis and raised plasma viscosity.
> - **Acne excoriée** (also known as 'picker's acne') is self-inflicted excoriations produced by compulsive picking of pre-existing or imagined acne lesions. It is usually observed in teenage girls with psychological problems.
> - **SAPHO syndrome:** Synovitis, acne, pustulosis, hyperostosis and osteitis syndrome.
> - **Acne venenata:** Contact with acnegenic chemicals can produce comedones. For example, chlorinated hydrocarbons, cutting oils, petroleum oil, coal tar.
> - **Acne aestivalis** (Mallorca acne): Rare, seen in females 25–40 years. Starts in spring, resolves by fall characterised by small papules on cheeks, neck, upper body. Comedones and pustules are sparse and absent.

Management

- **General measures:**
  - Regular washing with soap and water.
  - Antibacterial skin cleansers containing chlorhexidine.
- **Local measures:**
  - Keratolytics include α-and β-hydroxy acids, azelaic acid and retinoids. Tretinoin is the most potent keratolytic agent. Other retinoids include isotretinoin (less effective), adapalene (less irritating) and tazarotene. Topical retinoids may produce skin irritation, sun sensitivity and initial flaring of acne.
  - Reducing infection by *P. acnes* by using benzoyl peroxide and local antibiotics. Benzoyl peroxide commonly causes dry skin and occasionally allergy. It has mild but significant keratolytic effect. It inactivates topical retinoic acid when used concurrently and may cause skin bleaching. Topical antibiotics include clindamycin and erythromycin.
  - Usually, topical benzoyl peroxide or antibiotic is applied in the morning and a keratolytic preparation at night.
- **Systemic measures:**
  - Long-term antibiotic therapy with doxycycline, minocycline or erythromycin for duration of 3 months to 2 years. Erythromycin is less effective due to development of resistance in *P. acnes* but is used if tetracyclines cannot be used.
  - Isotretinoin (13-cis-retinoic acid) given orally in a 4-month course can reduce sebum excretion and may be required in severe acne.
- **Physical measures:**
  - Incision and drainage of cysts
  - Intralesional injections of triamcinolone acetonide
  - Light (blue light with wavelength of 407–420 nm) and laser treatment
  - Photodynamic therapy using aminolevulinic acid or indocyanine green dye application

■ ERYTHEMA MULTIFORME

- Erythema multiforme (EM) is an acute, self-limiting and sometimes recurring skin condition considered to be a hypersensitivity reaction associated with certain infections and medications.
- Previously, EM was thought to be part of a clinical spectrum of disease that included erythema minor, erythema major [often equated with Stevens–Johnson syndrome (SJS)] and toxic epidermal necrolysis (TEN).

Causes

Precipitating factors in erythema multiforme are given in **Box 20.6**.

- Individual lesions begin acutely as numerous sharply demarcated red or pink macules than then become papular. The papules may enlarge gradually into plaques several centimetres in diameter. The central portion of the papules or plaques gradually becomes darker red, brown, dusky or purpuric. Crusting or blistering sometimes occurs in the centre of the lesions.

Box 20.6: Precipitating factors in erythema multiforme.

Infections
- Viral, e.g. herpes simplex, Orf, infectious mononucleosis, hepatitis B, HIV
- *Mycoplasma* and other bacterial infections (e.g. typhoid)
- Fungal, e.g. histoplasmosis, coccidioidomycosis
- Rickettsia

Exposure to drugs
For example, sulphonamides, penicillins, barbiturates salicylates, hydantoins, antimalarials and carbamazepine

Systemic disease
- Sarcoidosis
- Malignancy (carcinomas and lymphomas)
- Collagen vascular diseases [systemic lupus erythematosus (Rowell's syndrome), Wegener's granulomatosis, dermatomyositis, and polyarteritis nodosa)]

Others
Radiotherapy, pregnancy

- The characteristic **'target' or 'iris' lesion** has a regular round shape and three concentric zones: A central dusky or darker red area, a paler pink or oedematous zone and a peripheral red ring.
- Common sites of involvement are hands, extensor forearms, palms, soles and mucous membranes of mouth, nose, eyes and genitalia.
- Mucosal lesions may occur but usually are limited to the oral cavity.

Stevens–Johnson Syndrome

- Characterised by confluent purpuric macules, sometimes blisters, on the face and trunk and severe mucosal erosions. Target lesions are not seen and the epidermal detachment does not involve > 10% surface area. Usually, it is accompanied by severe constitutional symptoms in the form of fever, tachycardia and hypotension. Electrolyte imbalance is frequent.
- Involvement of oral and/or mucous membranes may be severe enough that patients may not be able to eat or drink.
- Patients with genitourinary involvement may complain of dysuria or an inability to void.
- Severe ophthalmic involvement may lead to permanent scarring and blindness.
- Epithelial loss results in vulnerability to bacterial infections and predisposes to septicaemia.
- Mortality approximately 5%

Toxic Epidermal Necrolysis

- Begins with severe mucosal erosions and progresses to diffuse, generalised detachment of the epidermis. Nikolsky sign is often positive.
- Target lesions are not seen.
- More than 30% skin is involved.
- Mortality as high as 30%.

Management

- Management of the primary causes (discontinuation of medications and treatment of infection)
- Mild cases do not require any specific treatment. Antihistamines and local corticosteroids may provide symptomatic relief.
- Severe cases may require systemic corticosteroids.
- Oral acyclovir early in herpes-associated outbreaks of EM is useful to lessen the number and duration of lesions.
- In SJS and TEN, fluid and electrolyte balance must be maintained. Manage oral lesions with mouthwashes. Topical anaesthetics are useful in reducing pain and allowing the patient to take in fluids. Areas of denuded skin must be covered with compresses of saline. Role of systemic steroids and intravenous immunoglobulins is controversial.

VITILIGO

- Occurs due to selective destruction of the skin melanocytes that results in development of unsightly de-pigmented patches.
- Onset before the age of 18 years in >50% cases.
- Vitiligo can be separated into segmental and non-segmental types. Segmental vitiligo has important differences in aetiology, prevalence of associated illnesses and therapy compared to other forms of vitiligo.

Clinical Features

- Presents as small, de-pigmented lesions that may enlarge and coalesce into larger patches.
- Vitiligo is most striking around the body orifices; eyes, nostrils, mouth, nipples, umbilicus and genitalia.
- Vitiligo can affect melanocytes in the hair roots resulting in patches of white hair. De-pigmentation can affect mucosal areas such as in the mouth or genitalia.
- In non-segmental vitiligo, lesions are usually symmetrical and new patches may appear throughout the patient's life. It may be either generalised or localised. The overlying hair may remain pigmented or turn white. This type of vitiligo is often associated with a number of immune system aberrations. Childhood, non-segmental vitiligo is frequently associated with autoimmune thyroiditis. To the contrary, vitiligo in adults is quite strongly associated with a number of autoimmune disorders, including alopecia areata, diabetes mellitus, pernicious anaemia, Addison's disease and Hashimoto's thyroiditis.
- Segmental vitiligo usually has unilateral involvement and a dermatomal distribution.

Without treatment, lesions are typically persistent throughout developing within 2 years of onset. It has no association with autoimmune thyroiditis and is in fact rarely associated with any autoimmune disease.
- Koebner phenomenon: Non-segmental vitiligo can spread by Koebner phenomenon. Other skin conditions that can also spread by Koebner phenomenon include psoriasis, molluscum contagiosum, warts and LP. The Koebner phenomenon is the initiation of new lesions that occur as a result of trauma, particularly mechanical trauma such as scratching.

Treatment
- Topical PUVA therapy
- Narrow-band UV-B phototherapy
- Local application of corticosteroids along with UV-A exposure is effective in many patients.
- Autologous skin grafting is a method of choice for treating stable, focal vitiligo.
- Bleaching creams used for this purpose include monobenzylether of hydroquinone and 4-methoxy-phenol. Another option is to give oral psoralen given after a meal followed 2-3 hours later by exposure to long UV rays.

PITYRIASIS ALBA
- Pityriasis alba is a common dermatologic disorder in children that is usually evident before puberty.
- Its cause is unclear; however, these patients often have a history of atopy.
- Presents with hypopigmented patches or macules with slight scale, primarily on the face and less frequently on the neck, trunk and extremities.
- It does not create any permanent damage to the skin.
- Often improves after puberty.
- Treatment includes use of lubricants and mild topical steroids.

SCABIES
- An intensely itchy dermatosis caused by the mite Sarcoptes scabiei var hominis.
- Occurs at all ages but particularly in children.

Mode of Transmission
- Highly contagious, and person-to-person spread occurs via direct contact with the skin
- Transfer from clothes and bedding if contaminated by infested people immediately beforehand.

Clinical Features
- Incubation period is 3 weeks. In cases of re-infestation, symptoms develop in 1-3 days.
- Patients with scabies complain of itching, which is most severe at night.
- Other skin manifestations include papules, blisters, nodules and eczematous changes.
- These lesions commonly involve web spaces, flexor surface of wrists, axillae, waist, feet, ankles, lower portions of buttocks and genital areas.
- The pathognomonic sign is **burrow**, the linear tunnel in which the mites live. These occur as short, wavy, scaly, grey lines on the skin surface and are most easily found on hands and feet, particularly in the finger web spaces, thenar and hypothenar eminences, and on the wrists. They are often missed if the skin has been scratched, has become secondarily infected or if eczema is present.
- Secondary infection can occur with *Staphylococcus*, *Streptococcus* or both.

Crusted or Norwegian Scabies
Crusted scabies, also known as Norwegian scabies (because of its initial description in Norwegian patients with leprosy), occurs in patients with neurological disorders or immunosuppression including HIV.

Diagnosis
- Scabies is usually diagnosed on history and examination.
- Definitive diagnosis relies on microscopic identification of mites or eggs from skin scrapings of a burrow.

Treatment
- It is important to treat all members of the affected household at the same time.
- All clothes and bed linen should be washed at temperatures above 50°C.

Topical treatment:
- Sulphur
- Benzyl benzoate is used as a 25% emulsion
- Crotamiton is used as 10% cream or lotion.
- Malathion
- Lindane: A single 6-hour application of 1% cream is effective in treatment of scabies.
- Permethrin 5% dermal creams

Oral therapy:
Ivermectin

PEDICULOSIS

- **Head louse (*Pediculus humanus capitis*):**
  - Transmission occurs person-to-person and indirectly through hats, clothes or pillow covers.
  - Presents with rash and pruritus
  - Persistent infection is often associated with secondary infection of the scalp and is an important cause of impetigo.
  - Because of pruritus and subsequent sleep disturbances and difficulties in concentration, infested children may perform poorly in school.
- **Body louse (*Pediculus humanus humanus*):**
  - Transmission occurs person-to person through infested clothes.
  - A vector for epidemic typhus, relapsing fever and trench fever.
- **Public louse (*Pthirus pubis*):**
  - Infests pubic hair and occasionally other hairy areas, such as eye lashes.
  - Usually transmitted during sexual intercourse
  - Treatment must therefore include the patient's partner.

Treatment
- Physical removal by wet combing is suboptimal.
- Topical application of lindane, malathion and permethrin.
- Treatment of secondary bacterial infection.

WARTS

- Warts are the cutaneous manifestations of human papillomavirus (HPV).
- Warts may exist in different forms:
  - **Common warts** (verruca vulgaris), appear as firm, irregular verrucous surfaced papules that vary in size, shape and number. These are distributed anywhere on the body and are asymptomatic.
  - **Plantar warts** (verruca plantaris) occur on the plantar aspects and are painful keratotic plaques with a central depressed area.
  - **Flat or planar warts** (verruca plana) are smooth, skin-coloured, flat-topped papules that are more frequently seen in children on the face or hands.
  - Warts located in ano-genital region are due to sexual transmission of virus and are known as venereal warts. Condyloma acuminata is a type of venereal wart that shows vegetative or cauliflower-like growth.

Treatment
- No single therapy has been proven effective at achieving complete remission in every patient.
- These can be destroyed by local salicylic acid (10–20%) application, imiquimod (5% cream), cryotherapy with liquid nitrogen, chemical cauterisation (50–100% trichloroacetic acid or phenol), electric cauterisation or surgical removal.
- Podophyllin resin 25% in alcohol is effective in condyloma acuminata.
- Bleomycin injection into the wart may be used as a second-line agent if others fail.
- Systemic retinoids have the ability to alter keratinisation and accelerate the clearing of warts by inducing an irritant—dermatitis.

PEMPHIGUS VULGARIS

- Pemphigus vulgaris (PV) is a chronic vesicular and erosive disease that may lead to systemic involvement due to fluid exudation or infection.
- PV affects both sexes equally.
- The disease is most prevalent between the fourth and sixth decades of life.

Aetiology

- While the precise aetiology of PV is not clear, it is known to involve an autoimmune mechanism with IgG antibodies that alter the epithelial intercellular junctions. These antibodies target desmoglein 1 and 3, which belong to subfamily of cellular adhesion molecules found within desmosomes.
- Pemphigus can also be drug-induced. Some known PV-inducing agents are sulphonamides, penicillins and antiepileptic drugs.

Clinical Features

In most cases (75%), oral lesions are the first manifestation of the disease.

Oral Cavity

- The lesions at first comprise small asymptomatic blisters that are very thin-walled and easily rupture giving rise to painful and haemorrhagic erosions.
- The lesions may persist within the mouth for a number of months before progressing to the skin and other mucosal membranes (nose, pharynx, larynx, oesophagus, vulva, penis or anus).

Skin Lesions

- The primary lesion of PV is a flaccid blister filled with clear fluid that arises on normal skin or on an erythematous base.
- The blisters are fragile; therefore, intact blisters may be sparse.
- **Nikolsky's sign** is positive—apply pressure to the affected skin (e.g. where a blister is located), or rub sideways the peri-lesional skin or normal skin with a cotton swab or finger; a positive response is indicated by extension of the blister and/or removal of epidermis in the area immediately surrounding the blister. It is also positive in patients with TEN, staphylococcal scalded skin syndrome, bullous impetigo and epidermolysis bullosa. This sign is usually negative in bullous pemphigoid.

Treatment

- Anaesthetic mouth lozenges may reduce the pain of mild-to-moderate mouth ulcers.
- Antibiotics may be required to control infections.
- To inhibit production of the aggressor antibodies, moderate doses of corticosteroids via oral or intravenous route are required.
- Immunosuppressors such as azathioprine, methotrexate, cyclosporine, cyclophosphamide or mycophenolate mofetil can be used if steroids do not help.

■ BULLOUS PEMPHIGOID

Bullous pemphigoid (BP) or pemphigoid is a chronic, autoimmune, sub-epidermal, blistering skin disease that rarely involves mucous membranes.

Aetiology

- BP is characterised by the presence of IgG autoantibodies specific for the hemidesmosomal antigens present in the basement membrane.
- BP may be precipitated by UV irradiation, X-ray therapy and exposure to some drugs (furosemide, ibuprofen and other non-steroidal anti-inflammatory agents, captopril, penicillamine and antibiotics).

Clinical Features

- The patient often presents with generalised bullous lesions on erythematous or urticarial background.
- Tense bullae arise on any part of the skin surface with a prediction on the flexural areas of the skin. The bullous lesions may contain haemorrhagic fluid.
- Oral and ocular mucosa involvement rarely occurs, and when seen, it is of minor clinical significance.
- The bullae usually heal without scarring.
- Relapses occur less frequently than PV.

Diagnosis

- Direct immunofluorescence studies demonstrate deposits of antibodies and complements in a linear band at the dermal–epidermal junction.
- Indirect immunofluorescence shows the presence of circulating IgG autoantibodies in the serum.

Treatment

The most commonly used medications are anti-inflammatory agents (e.g. corticosteroids, tetracyclines, dapsone) and if required, immunosuppressants (e.g. azathioprine, methotrexate, mycophenolate mofetil, cyclophosphamide).

■ DERMATOPHYTOSES

Dermatophytosis, also known as ringworm or tinea, is a chronic infection of the skin, hair or nails by dermatophytes (a group of fungi that invades the superficial layer of the epidermis and survives on the keratin of skin, hair and nails). Species of *Trichophyton, Microsporum* and *Epidermophyton* are called dermatophytes.

Types

- Dermatophytosis of the glabrous skin is called **tinea corporis**. The lesions are circulate (hence the term 'ringworm'), erythematous pruritic papules that enlarge to form a ring. The borders are irregular, raised and active. The centre is relatively normal.
- In **tinea cruris**, the lesions start at the apex of the groin and extend to the inner aspect of the thighs, genitalia, perineum or gluteal regions.
- Dermatophytosis of the fool is called **tinea pedis** (athlete's foot). This may present as fissuring of the toe webs, scaling of the plantar surfaces or vesicles around the toe webs and soles.
- Scalp dermatophytosis is known as **tinea capitis**. This commonly presents as circular areas of alopecia and scaling. The 'kerion' type is characterised by intense inflammatory reaction. In the so-called 'endothrix infection', the hair shaft breaks off at the skin surface, leaving the hairs visible as black dots on the scalp.
- Dermatophytosis of the bearded area is known as **tinea barbae**.
- **Tinea unguium** (onychomycosis) presents as white-discoloured nails or thickened, chalky crumbling nails. Subungual hyperkeratosis may be present. Risk factors for developing onychomycosis (fungi causing nail involvement) include atopy, diabetes mellitus, immunosuppression, peripheral vascular insufficiency, occlusive footwear and nail trauma.

Treatment

- For tinea capitis and barbae, ketoconazole cream or shampoo can be used as an adjunct. Systemic therapy is often required.
- For tinea corporis, cruris and pedis, topical therapy using clotrimazole, ketoconazole or miconazole applied twice a day for 4 weeks.
- For distal tinea unguium, amorolfine 5%, tioconazole 28% or ciclopirox olamine 8% may be tried.
- More severe and unresponsive lesions are treated with griseofulvin 500–1,000 mg daily, ketoconazole 200–400 mg daily, fluconazole 400 mg daily, itraconazole 200 mg daily or terbinafine 250 mg daily. The period of treatment is 4–8 weeks.

■ TINEA VERSICOLOR OR PITYRIASIS VERSICOLOR

- Tinea versicolor is caused by non-dermatophyte fungus, *Malassezia furfur* (also known as *Pityrosporum ovale*), which is a normal inhabitant of the skin. Infection is promoted by heat and humidity.
- The typical lesions consist of oval scaly macules, papules and patches concentrated on the chest, shoulders and back and rarely on the face. On dark skin, they appear as hypopigmented areas, while on light skin they are slightly hyper-pigmented.
- Other diseases have been associated with tinea versicolor. These include Cushing's syndrome, hyperhidrosis and altered immune status such as HIV.
- A KOH preparation from scaling lesions will demonstrate spores and characteristic short, cigar-butt hyphae.
- Treatment includes topical application of solutions containing sulphur, salicylic acid or selenium sulphide or imidazoles (miconazole, clotrimazole, ketoconazole) and traizoles (fluconazole, itraconazole).
- Oral therapy is also effective for tinea versicolor and is often preferred by patients because it is more convenient and less time consuming. Ketoconazole (200 mg daily for 10 days or 400 mg/day for 2 days, though less effective), fluconazole (150–300 mg weekly for 2–4 weeks) and itraconazole (200 mg daily for 7 days) are the preferred oral agents.

ACANTHOSIS NIGRICANS

- Presents with symmetric, darkened areas of skin that are thickened and described as 'velvety' in texture and located in areas and creases such as the axillae, neck and groin.
- Other locations include the face, elbows, knees and hands.
- Acanthosis nigricans can be divided into three types:
  o Type I is associated with malignant diseases, particularly gastric and lung carcinomas; may develop acutely.
  o Type II is familial, inherited as autosomal dominant and is usually apparent at birth or may develop later in childhood.
  o Type III is the most common form and is associated with obesity, insulin-resistant disorders and other endocrine disorders, including diabetes mellitus, Cushing's disease, Addison's disease, pinealoma, and hyperandrogenic and hypogonadal states. Some medications have been linked to the development of acanthosis nigricans including oral contraceptives, insulin, glucocorticoids, nicotinic acid and methyltestosterone.

Treatment
- Treat the underlying disease.
- Loss of weight in obesity-related acanthosis nigricans
- Some patients may benefit from medications such as metformin, oral isotretinoin, topical retinoic acid, topical salicylic acid and oral fish oil.

SKIN MALIGNANCIES

Box 20.7 lists malignant skin tumours.

Basal Cell Carcinoma
- At least three times more common than squamous cell carcinoma
- Usually occurs on sun-exposed areas of skin. Sun exposure between 10 AM and 4 PM is thought to be most harmful.
- Nose is the most frequent site.
- High-risk areas for tumour recurrence include periorbital region, eyelids, nasolabial fold,

> **Box 20.7: List of malignant skin tumours.**
> **Common malignant tumours:**
> - Basal cell carcinoma
> - Squamous cell carcinoma and its precursor Bowen's diseases
>
> **Uncommon malignant tumours:**
> - Primary
>   o Malignant melanoma
>   o Cutaneous T-cell lymphomas (e.g. mycosis fungoides)
>   o Kaposi sarcoma
>   o Apocrine carcinoma of the skin
> - Metastasis

post-auricular region, pinna, ear canal, forehead and scalp.
- Most characteristic presentation is the asymptomatic nodular or nodular-ulcerative lesion that has a pearly quality and contains telangiectatic vessels. Crusting and bleeding in the centre of the tumour frequently develop.
- Has a tendency to be locally destructive

Treatment
- Basal cell carcinoma rarely metastasises, and thus, a metastatic work-up is usually not necessary.
- Options for treatment include Mohs micrographic surgery (using microscopic control to evaluate the extent of tumour invasion before surgical excision), cryosurgery, radiation therapy, electro-desiccation and curettage, and simple excision. These methods have cure rates ranging from 85 to 95%.
- Other options include topical application of 5-fluorouracil, intra-lesional interferon-α and photodynamic therapy using photosensitisers.

Squamous Cell Carcinoma
- Also tends to occur on sun-exposed portions of the skin such as ears, lower lip and dorsal aspect of hand
- Chronic sun damage, sites of prior burns, chronic arsenic exposure, chronic cutaneous ulcers and sites of previous X-ray therapy predispose to the development of squamous cell carcinoma.

- Squamous cell carcinoma in-situ, also known as Bowen's disease, also has invasive malignant potential. These lesions present clinically as pink, well-defined, erythematosus papules and plaques anywhere on the body including the trunk, eyelids, hands, feet, face and genital area. The lesions may have scale and may bleed.
- Tumours arising in non-sun-exposed areas or those originating de novo on areas of sun-exposed skin are prognostically worse due to greater tendency to metastasise.
- Presents commonly as a red, scaling, thickened patch on sun-exposed skin. Ulceration and bleeding may occur. If not treated, it may develop into a large mass.

Management

- In squamous cell carcinoma, regional lymph nodes should be routinely examined particularly for high-risk tumours appearing on lips, ears, peri-genital regions, or if the tumour arises at sites of chronic ulceration, burn scars or sites of previous radiation therapy treatment.
- The options for treatment are similar to those for basal cell carcinoma.

Malignant Melanoma

- Risk factors include sun sensitivity, white skin, fair hair, light eyes, tendency to freckle, family history of melanoma (8–12 times increased risk), dysplastic naevi and immunosuppression.
- In a patient with pigmented lesions, important clinical features suggesting a diagnosis of malignant melanoma are:
  - Asymmetrical lesion
  - Border irregular
  - Colour irregular
  - Diameter > 6 mm
  - Elevation irregular
- Since nearly 30% of melanomas develop in pre-existing moles, a change in any naevus should be considered suspicious of malignant transformation.

Treatment

- Patients with non-ulcerated melanoma < 1-mm deep are unlikely to have nodal metastasis and do not require further surgical evaluation of the lymph nodes.
- For local disease, surgical excision is curative.
- Sentinel lymph nodal biopsy is important in patients diagnosed with a melanoma with intermediate thickness (1–4 mm) and clinically negative nodes. In this technique, draining lymph node is identified by injecting radioisotope adjacent to the primary tumour. The node is then identified using radioscintigraphy and then removed to look for any histological evidence of metastasis.
- No additional therapy is required for patients with a tumour-free sentinel lymph node.
- Patients with metastatic tumour in the sentinel lymph node and those who have clinically evident nodal metastasis should undergo lymph node resection with post-surgical adjuvant therapy (interferon-α-2b) as an optional therapy.

Mycosis Fungoides

- Mycosis fungoides (MF) is a cutaneous lymphoma of mature CD4+ T-cells. The most common cutaneous T-cell lymphoma.
- MF patches are usually distributed in sun-shielded areas such as those covered by a bathing suit or intertriginous regions
- The cardinal features of MF are infiltration of epidermis and then dermis by atypical cerebriform lymphoid cells—**Pautrier microabscess**. It is a chronic, slowly progressive disease that evolves from patch stage to plaque stage and subsequently to nodule/tumour stage.
- A diagnosis of **Sézary syndrome** is made when there is a high number of these cells circulating in the peripheral blood in the presence of a lymphadenopathy and cutaneous erythroderma occupying >80% of the body surface area.
- Chemotherapy, retinoids, electron beam therapy, photo-chemotherapy are used in the treatment.

■ NEUROCUTANEOUS SYNDROMES

Box 20.8 lists common neurocutaneous syndromes.

Box 20.8: Common neurocutaneous syndromes.

- Neurofibromatosis I and II
- Tuberous sclerosis
- Von Hippel–Lindau disease
- Sturge–Weber syndrome
- Klippel–Trenaunay–Weber syndrome
- Osler–Weber–Rendu syndrome
- Wyburn–Mason syndrome
- Linear naevus sebaceous syndrome
- Neurocutaneous melanosis
- Waardenburg syndrome types I and II
- Fabry's disease
- Lentiginosis, deafness, cardiopathy syndrome
- Hypomelanosis of Ito
- Ataxia–telangiectasia (Louis–Bar syndrome)
- Xeroderma pigmentosum
- Cockayne's syndrome
- Rothmund–Thomson syndrome
- Sjögren–Larsson syndrome
- Neuroichthyosis
- Werner syndrome and Progeria
- Incontinentia pigmenti
- Neurocutaneous melanosis
- Retinal-neurocutaneous cavernous haemangioma syndrome [Weskamp–Cotlier syndrome]

Box 20.9: Diagnostic criteria for neurofibromatosis type 1.

Two or more of the following clinical features must be present:

- Six or more café-au-lait macules of > 5 mm in greatest diameter in prepubertal individuals, and > 15 mm in greatest diameter in post-pubertal individuals.
- Two or more neurofibromas of any type or one plexiform neurofibroma
- Freckling in the axillary or inguinal regions
- Optic glioma
- Two or more iris hamartomas (Lisch nodules)
- Distinctive bony lesions, such as sphenoid dysplasia, or thinning of the long bone cortex with or without pseudo-arthrosis
- A first-degree relative (parent, sibling, or offspring) with NF1 based on the above criteria

Box 20.10: Diagnostic criteria for neurofibromatosis type 2.

- Bilateral vestibular schwannomas
- A first-degree relative with NF2 and
  - Unilateral vestibular schwannoma or
  - Any two of: Meningioma, schwannoma, glioma, neurofibroma, posterior subcapsular lenticular opacities*
- Unilateral vestibular schwannoma and
  - Any two of: Meningioma, schwannoma, glioma, neurofibroma, posterior subcapsular lenticular opacities*
- Multiple meningiomas and
  - Unilateral vestibular schwannoma or
  - Any two of: Schwannoma, glioma, neurofibroma, cataract

* 'Any two of' - Two individuals tumours or cataract
(NF2: neurofibromatosis type 2)

Neurofibromatosis Type 1

- Synonyms: von Recklinghausen disease, Watson disease
- An autosomal dominant neurogenetic disorder. Neurofibromatosis type I (NF1) is caused by mutation in the *neurofibromin* gene located on chromosome 17, at the band q11.2.

Diagnostic criteria of NF1 are given in **Box 20.9**.

Neurofibromatosis Type 2

Neurofibromatosis type 2 (NF2) is associated with abnormalities of the *NF2* gene, which is located on chromosome 2.

Diagnostic criteria of NF1 are given in **Box 20.10**.

Tuberous Sclerosis

- Called as Bourneville disease
- Clinical triad of Vogt—**EPI-LOI-A**: Epilepsy, low intelligence and adenoma sebaceum.

Diagnostic criteria of tuberous sclerosis complex are given in **Table 20.2**.

ALOPECIA

Table 20.3 gives classification and causes of alopecia.

TABLE 20.2: Diagnostic criteria of tuberous sclerosis complex (TSC).

Major features	Minor features
• Facial angiofibromas or forehead plaque • Non-traumatic ungual or periungual fibroma • Hypomelanotic macules (more than three) • Shagreen patch (connective tissue nerves) • Multiple retinal nodular hamartomas • Cortical tuber • Subependymal nodule • Subependymal giant cell astrocytoma • Cardiac rhabdomyoma, single or multiple • Lymphangiomyomatosis • Renal angiomyolipoma	• Multiple randomly distributed pits in dental enamel • Hamartomatous rectal polyps • Bone cysts • Cerebral white matter migration lines • Gingival fibromas • Non-renal hamartoma • Retinal achromic patch • 'Confetti' skin lesions • Multiple renal cysts

Definite TSC: Either 2 major features or 1 major feature with 2 minor features
Probable TSC: One major feature and 1 minor feature
Possible TSC: Either 1 major feature or 2 or more minor features

TABLE 20.3: Classification and causes of alopecia.

Localised	Diffuse
\multicolumn{2}{c}{Non-scarring}	

• **Abnormality of cycling**
  ○ Alopecia areata
  ○ Syphilitic alopecia
• **Production decline**
  ○ Androgenetic alopecia
  ○ Triangular alopecia
• **Hair breakage**
  ○ Trichotillomania
  ○ Tinea capitis
  ○ Traction alopecia
  ○ Primary or acquired hair shaft abnormality
	• Abnormality of cycling
	  ○ Alopecia areata
	  ○ Telogen effluvium
	  ○ Anagen effluvium
	  ○ Loose anagen syndrome
	• Hair shaft abnormality
	  ○ Hair breakage
	  ○ Unruly hair
	• Failure of follicle production
	  ○ Congenital universal atrichia
	  ○ Atrichia with papular lesions
	  ○ Hereditary vitamin-D-resistant rickets
	Androgenetic, hypothyroidism, hyperthyroidism, hypopituitarism, diabetes mellitus, HIV, nutritional (especially iron) deficiency, liver disease, post-partum, alopecia areata, syphilis, drug-induced (e.g. chemotherapy, retinoids)

\multicolumn{2}{c}{Scarring}	

• Lymphocytic
  ○ Chronic cutaneous lupus erythematosus, discoid lups, erythematosus (DLE)
  ○ Lichen planopilaris
  ○ Classic pseudopelade of Brocq
  ○ Alopecia mucinosa
• Neutrophilic
  ○ Folliculitis decalvans
  ○ Dissecting folliculitis/cellulitis
• Mixed
  ○ Folliculitis (acne) keloidalis
  ○ Folliculitis (acne) necrotica
  ○ Erosive pustular dermatitis
	• Discoid lupus erythematosus
	• Radiotherapy
	• Folliculitis decalvans
	• Lichen planus

(HIV: human immunodeficiency syndrome)

BEST OF FIVES

1. A 19-year-old woman presented with a widespread skin eruption 2 weeks after a sore throat. On examination, there were multiple 5-mm diameter, scaly, erythematous papules over her trunk and limbs. What is the most likely diagnosis?
   A. Atopic eczema
   B. Dermatitis artefacta
   C. Guttate psoriasis
   D. Lichen planus
   E. Pityriasis rosacea

2. All of the following are seen in tuberous sclerosis except:
   A. Civatte bodies
   B. Koenen tumours
   C. Ash leaf macules
   D. Shagreen patch
   E. Adenoma sebaceum

3. Which of the following is not a cutaneous marker of internal malignancy?
   A. Bullous pemphigoid
   B. Acanthosis nigricans
   C. Dermatomyositis
   D. Erythema chronicum migrans
   E. Seborrheic keratosis

4. The most common type of vitiligo is:
   A. Segmental vitiligo
   B. Focal vitiligo
   C. Generalised vitiligo
   D. Mucosal vitiligo
   E. Lip-tip vitiligo

5. An 18-year-old young girl presented a pruritic rash. This rash had started as a single lesion on her abdomen 2 weeks ago and later developed to multiple smaller lesions. The likely diagnosis is:

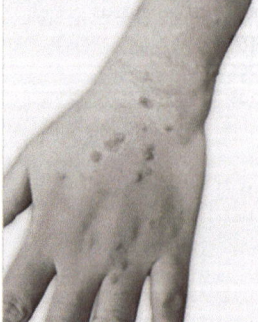

(For color version, see plate 5)

A. Eczema
B. Erythema multiforme
C. Erythema migrans
D. Guttate psoriasis
E. Lichen planus

6. A 36-year-old factory worker developed itchy, annular scaly plaques in both groins. Application of a corticosteroid ointment led to temporary relief, but the plaques continued to extend at the periphery.

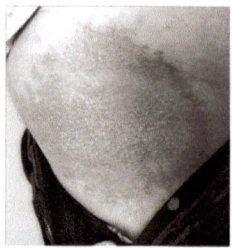 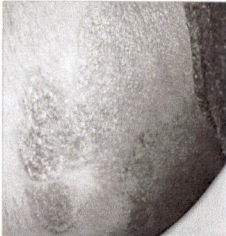

(For color version, see plate 5)

The most likely diagnosis is:
A. Erythema annulare centrifugum
B. Granuloma annulare
C. Annular lichen planus
D. Tinea cruris
E. Psoriasis

7. A 24-year-old unmarried woman has multiple nodular, cystic, pustular and comedonal lesions on face, upper back and shoulders for 2 years.

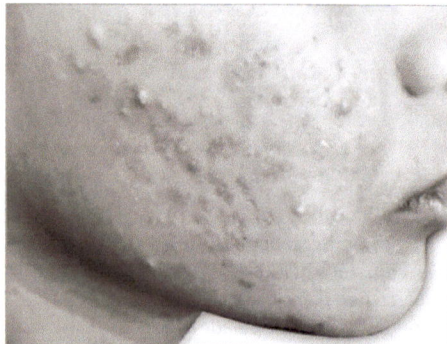

(For color version, see plate 5)

The drug of choice for her treatment would be:
A. Acitretin
B. Isotretinoin
C. Doxycycline
D. Azithromycin
E. Penicillin

8. Pterygium of nail is characteristically seen in:

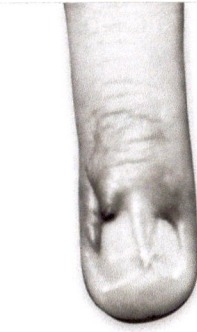

(For color version, see plate 6)
A. Lichen planus
B. Psoriasis
C. Tinea unguium
D. Alopecia areata
E. Eczema

9. A 40-year-old male presents with arthralgia and syncopal episodes. An electrocardiogram (ECG) reveals complete heart block. He returned from a hill-walking holiday 3 months ago and has noticed an annular, indurated erythematous area on his legs. What is the most likely diagnosis?
A. Psoriasis
B. Lyme disease
C. Systemic lupus erythematosus (SLE)
D. Granuloma annulare
E. Tuberculosis

10. A 25-year-old woman who has just been diagnosed with acute myeloid leukaemia (AML) presents to her GP feeling unwell and feverish and has tender plum-coloured plaques, nodes and pseudovesicles on her head, neck and arms. Her bloods reveal a neutrophilia. Which of the following is the most likely diagnosis?
A. Erythema multiforme
B. Adverse drug reactions
C. Nodular vasculitis
D. Sweet's syndrome
E. Erythema nodosum

11. A 35-year-old female with ulcerative colitis presents with lesions on her legs. On examination, there are lesions of palpable purpura which are approximately 3 mm in diameter on her shins. Bloods reveal an elevated erythrocyte sedimentation rate (ESR) and low complement. Which of the following is the most likely diagnosis?

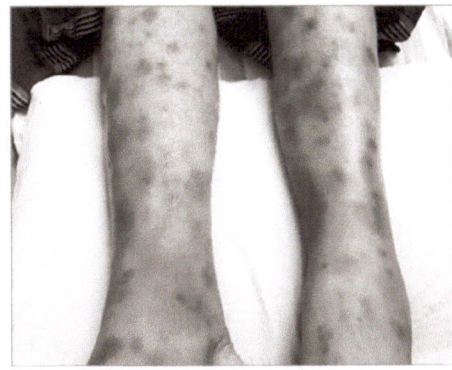

(For color version, see plate 6)
A. Leucocytoclastic vasculitis
B. Systemic lupus erythematosus (SLE)
C. Idiopathic thrombocytopaenic purpura
D. Pyoderma gangrenosum
E. Erythema nodosum

12. What disorder would you most commonly associate with this skin lesion?

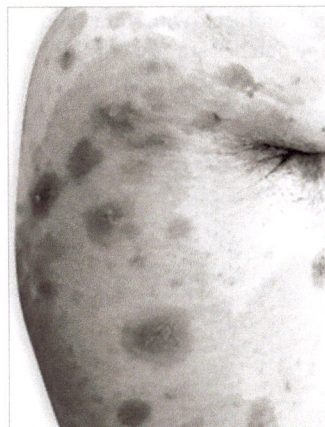

(For color version, see plate 6)
A. Infective endocarditis
B. Sarcoidosis
C. Penicillin use
D. Herpes simplex infection
E. Streptococcal infection

13. A 28-year-old soldier presents with an itchy rash. He is itchy in his finger webs, wrists and groin and there is evidence of excoriation in these areas. What is the most likely diagnosis?

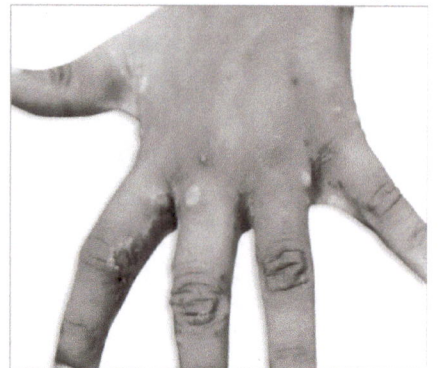

(For color version, see plate 6)

A. Lichen planus
B. Tinea corporis
C. *Sarcoptes scabiei* infection
D. Psoriasis
E. Contact dermatitis

14. A 35-year-old presents with red scaly patches on her face, scalp and hands. On examination, there is evidence of red plaques on her face, hands and scalp with some bald patches. Some of the patches are scarring and discoloured.

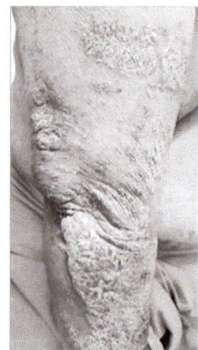

(For color version, see plate 6)

What is the diagnosis that fits best with this clinical picture?
A. Psoriasis
B. Systemic lupus erythematosus (SLE)
C. Drug-induced lupus
D. Chronic discoid lupus erythematosus
E. Seborrhoeic dermatitis

Answers

1-E, 2-A, 3-D, 4-C, 5-E, 6-D, 7-B, 8-A, 9-B, 10-D, 11-E, 12-C, 13-C, 14-A

■ SUGGESTED READING

1. Michalek IM, Loring B, John SM. A systematic review of worldwide epidemiology of psoriasis. J Eur Acad Dermatol Venereol. 2017; 31(2):205-12.
2. Parisi R, Symmons DP, Griffiths CE, Darren M Ashcroft, Identification and Management of Psoriasis and Associated ComorbidiTy (IMPACT) project team. Global epidemiology of psoriasis: a systematic review of incidence and prevalence. J Invest Dermatol. 2013;133(2):377-85.
3. Rachakonda TD, Schupp CW, Armstrong AW. Psoriasis prevalence among adults in the United States. J Am Acad Dermatol. 2014;70(3):512-6.
4. Schwager Z, Stern M, Cohen J, Femia A. Clinical epidemiology and treatment of lichen planus: A retrospective review of 2 tertiary care centers. J Am Acad Dermatol. 2019;81(6):1397-9.
5. Stern RS, Divito SJ. Stevens-Johnson syndrome and toxic epidermal necrolysis: Associations, outcomes, and pathobiology-thirty years of progress but still much to be done. J Invest Dermatol. 2017;137(5):1004-8.
6. Ezzedine K, Eleftheriadou V, Whitton M, van Geel N. Vitiligo. Lancet. 2015;386(9988):74-84.
7. Mohammed GF, Gomaa AH, Al-Dhubaibi MS. Highlights in pathogenesis of vitiligo. World J Clin Cases. 2015;3(3):221-30.
8. Salmi TT, Hervonen K, Kautiainen H, Collin P, Reunala T. Prevalence and incidence of dermatitis herpetiformis: a 40-year prospective study from Finland. Br J Dermatol. 2011;165(2):354-9.
9. Reyes MA, Eisen DB. Inherited syndromes. Dermatol Ther. 2010;23(6):606-42.
10. Brougham ND, Dennett ER, Cameron R, Tan ST. The incidence of metastasis from cutaneous squamous cell carcinoma and the impact of its risk factors. J Surg Oncol. 2012;106(7):811-5.
11. Eichenfield LF, Tom WL, Chamlin SL, Feldman SR, Hanifin JM, Simpson EL, et al. Guidelines of care for the management of atopic dermatitis: section 1. Diagnosis and assessment of atopic dermatitis. J Am Acad Dermatol. 2014;70(2):338-51.
12. Zuberbier T, Aberer W, Asero R, Abdul Latiff AH, Baker D, Ballmer-Weber B, et al. The EAACI/GA²LEN/EDF/WAO guideline for the definition, classification, diagnosis and management of urticaria. Allergy. 2018;73(7):1393-1414.
13. Patterson JW, Requena L. Panniculitis. In: Bolognia JL, Schaffer JV, Cerroni L, (Eds). Dermatology, 4th edition. London: Elsevier; 2018. p. 1733.

CHAPTER 21

Immunological Factors in Disease

IMMUNITY

Immunity is the ability of an organism to recognise and defend itself against *specific* pathogens or antigens.

Defence mechanisms in the body are listed in **Table 21.1**.

Immune Response

Immune response involves production of antibodies and generation of specialised lymphocytes against specific antigens.

Innate or Genetic Immunity

Immunity with which an organism is born with is called the innate or genetic immunity
- It is determined genetically.
- Possibly because of lack of other molecules or receptors which are required for infection. For instance:
  o Human beings have innate immunity to canine distemper.
  o Mice have innate immunity to poliovirus.

Acquired Immunity

This is a kind of immunity which is acquired or developed due to external factors during an organism's lifetime.

- It is not determined genetically.
- It is possibly acquired naturally or artificially. For instance:
  o Development of immunity to measles in response to infection or vaccination.

Types of Acquired Immunity

- Naturally acquired immunity: Developed during the course of life
  o Naturally acquired active immunity:
    – The entrance of antigens or pathogens in the body occurs naturally.
    – Body generates an immune response to antigens.
    – Immunity may be lifelong (chickenpox or mumps) or temporary (influenza or intestinal infections).
  o Naturally acquired passive immunity:
    – Antibodies are transferred from mother to foetus via placenta or breastfeeding (colostrum).
    – There is no immune response towards antigens.
    – Immunity is usually short-lived (weeks to months).
    – It offers protection until child's immune system is strong or is fully developed.

TABLE 21.1: Types of defence mechanism.

Non-specific defence mechanisms		Specific defence mechanisms (immune system)
First line of defence • Skin • Mucous membranes • Secretions of skin and mucous membranes	Second line of defence • Phagocytic white blood cells • Antimicrobial proteins • The inflammatory response	Third line of defence • Lymphocytes • Antibodies

- Artificially acquired immunity: Obtained by receiving a vaccine or immune serum
  - Artificially acquired active immunity:
    - Antigens are introduced in vaccines (immunisation).
    - Body generates an immune response to antigens.
    - Immunity can be lifelong (oral polio vaccine) or temporary (tetanus toxoid).
  - Artificially acquired passive immunity:
    - Preformed antibodies (antiserum) are introduced into body by injection.
    - Snake antivenom injection from horses or rabbits
    - Immunity is short-lived (half-life 3 weeks).
    - Host immune system does not respond to antigens.

Duality of Immune System

- **Humoral (antibody-mediated) immunity**
  - Involves production of antibodies against foreign antigens
  - Antibodies are produced by a subset of lymphocytes called B cells.
  - B cells that are stimulated will actively secrete antibodies and are called *plasma cells*.
  - Antibodies are found in extracellular fluids (blood plasma, lymph, mucus, etc.) and the surface of B cells.
  - Defence against bacteria, bacterial toxins and viruses that circulate freely in body fluids, *before* they enter cells
  - Also cause certain reactions against transplanted tissue
- **Cell-mediated Immunity**
  - Involves specialised set of lymphocytes called T cells that recognise foreign antigens on the surface of cells, organisms or tissues:
    - Helper T cells
    - Cytotoxic T cells
  - T cells regulate proliferation and activity of other cells of the immune system: B cells, macrophages, neutrophils, etc.
  - Defence against:
    - Bacteria and viruses that are inside host cells and are inaccessible to antibodies
    - Fungi, protozoa and helminths
    - Cancer cells
    - Transplanted tissue

■ ANTIGENS

- Most are proteins or large polysaccharides from a foreign organism.
  - Microbes: Capsules, cell walls, toxins, viral capsids, flagella, etc.
  - Non-microbes: Pollen, egg white, red blood cell surface molecules, serum proteins and surface molecules from transplanted tissue.

■ HAPTEN

It is a small foreign molecule which is not antigenic. It must be coupled to a carrier molecule to be antigenic. Once antibodies are formed, they will recognise hapten.

Epitope

- Small part of an antigen that interacts with an antibody
- Any given antigen may have several epitopes.
- Each epitope is recognised by a different antibody.

■ ANTIBODIES

- Proteins that recognise and bind to a particular antigen with very high *specificity*
- Made in response to exposure to the antigen
- One virus or microbe may have several *antigenic determinant sites*, to which different antibodies may bind.
- Each antibody has at least two identical sites that bind antigen: *Antigen binding sites*.
- Valence of an antibody: Number of antigen binding sites. Most are bivalent.
- Belong to a group of serum proteins called immunoglobulins (Igs)

Antibody Structure

- Monomer: A flexible Y-shaped molecule with four protein chains:
  - Two identical *light* chains
  - Two identical *heavy* chains
  - Variable regions: Two sections at the end of Y's arms. They contain the antigen-binding sites (Fab) and are identical on

the same antibody, but vary from one antibody to another
- Constant regions: Stem of monomer and lower parts of Y arms.
- Fc region: Stem of monomer only. Important because they can bind to complement or cells
- Fab region: For antigen binding (**Figs. 21.1A** and **B**)

Functions of Immunoglobulins/Antibodies
- Acts as opsonins: Immunoglobulins coat bacterial surface and act as opsonins. This facilitates phagocytosis by cells possessing Fc receptor (e.g. neutrophils).
- Antibody-dependent cell-mediated cytotoxicity (ADCC): In this, antibodies bind to microbes via their Fab region. Cytotoxic natural killer (NK) cells attach via Fc receptors and kill these organisms by releasing toxic substances called perforins.
- Activation of complement system: Binding of antibodies to antigen can trigger activation of the classical complement pathway. Complement components can function as opsonins (C3b component and aid in phagocytosis), chemotaxis (recruitment of leucocytes by C3a and C5a) and cause death of microbes (by MAC—membrane attack complex—C5–9).
- Neutralisation: Some antibodies may directly neutralise the biological activity of their antigen target or toxins released by bacteria. This is an important feature of IgA antibodies at mucosal surfaces.
- Processing of antigen: Antibodies present on B lymphocytes help in internalisation of antigen and further processing it for presentation to other cells.
- Agglutination: Antibodies (e.g. IgM) help in agglutination of particulate matter including bacteria and viruses.
- Immobilisation of microbes: Antibodies against bacterial cilia or flagellae may immobilise their movement and ability to escape the phagocytosis.
- Protection of mucosal surface: This is observed with IgA type of antibodies.
- Immune-complex formation: Antibodies combine with antigen to form immune complexes. The size of immune complexes varies depending upon the ratio between antigen and antibody. Larger immune complexes can be removed by the phagocytic cells in the reticuloendothelial (RE) system.
- Transplacental passage: Maternal antibodies can pass through placenta from mother to foetus conferring immunity to the foetus.

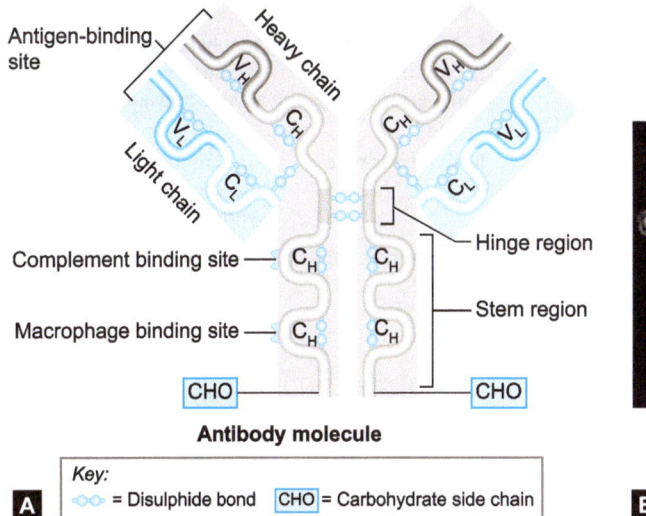
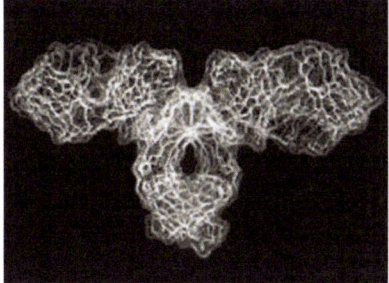

Figs. 21.1A and B: Structure of immunoglobulin molecule.

TABLE 21.2: Features of immunoglobulin (Ig) classes.

Features	IgG	IgM	IgA	IgD	IgE
Structure	Monomer	Pentamer, hexamer	Dimer	Monomer	Monomer
Subtypes	G1, G2, G3, G4	Other chains: J chain	A1, A2		
Percentage serum antibodies	75–85% (IgG1 = 45–53%, IgG2 = 11–15%)	5–10%	7–15%, (IgA1 = 11–14%, IgA2 = 1–4%)	0.04%	0.003%
Location	Blood, lymph, intestine	Blood, lymph, B-cell surface (monomer)	Secretions (tears, saliva, intestine, milk), blood and lymph	B-cell surface, blood and lymph	Bound to mast cells and basophils throughout body
Half-life in serum	23 days	5 days	6 days	3 days	2.5 days
Complement fixation	Yes (classsical, alternate)	Yes (classical)	No	Alternate pathway	No
Placental transfer	Yes	No	No	No	No
Known functions	Enhances phagocytosis, neutralises toxins and viruses, protects foetus and newborn	First antibodies produced during an infection. Effective against microbes and agglutinating antigens	Localised protection of mucosal surfaces. Provides immunity to infant digestive tract	In serum function is unknown. On B-cell surface, initiate immune response. Marker of mature B-cell	Allergic reactions and antiparasitic action

Characteristic features of individual antibody classes are listed in **Table 21.2**.

TYPES OF IMMUNE REACTIONS

Types of immune reactions are given in **Table 21.3**.

Allergy

Common reactions include asthma, rhinitis, urticaria, angioedema, eczema, food hypersensitivity and anaphylaxis.

Urticaria or Hives

- Formation of wheal-and-flare cutaneous lesions involving only the superficial portions of the dermis. This results in circumscribed wheals with erythematous, raise, serpiginous borders with blanched centres.
- Almost always pruritic and usually last for a few to 24 hours

TABLE 21.3: Types of immune reactions.

I - Anaphylactic type or immediate hypersensitivity type	Anaphylaxis, urticaria, angioedema, bronchial asthma and allergic rhinitis
II - Cytotoxic type	Autoimmune haemolytic anaemia and Goodpasture syndrome
III - Immune-complex type	Serum sickness, Arthus reaction, systemic lupus erythematosus (SLE), Henoch–Schönlein purpura, immune-complex type of glomerulonephritis and transfusion reactions
IV - Cell-mediated (delayed) type	Tuberculosis and transplant rejection
V - Stimulatory antibody-mediated	Graves' disease

- Those lasting up to 6 weeks are classified as acute urticaria while those persisting beyond 6 weeks are classified as chronic urticaria.
- Pathogenesis involves degranulation of mast cells and subsequent release of histamine and various cytokines leading to oedema

Angioedema
- An IgE-mediated reaction
- Well-demarcated oedema involving the deeper layers of skin as well as subcutaneous and submucosal tissues.
- Due to insect sting, drug reaction and food allergy
- Angiotensin-converting enzyme (ACE) inhibitors can cause angioedema.
- **Hereditary angioedema:** Deficiency of production of CI-esterase inhibitor

Clinical Features
- Well-defined, non-pitting swelling, usually non-pruritic
- Characteristically, the periorbital, perilabial and genital areas are involved
- Involvement of tongue and pharynx → dysphagia
- Stridor, hoarseness and dysphagia → impending airway compromise

Treatment
- Remove the offending agent, if possible
- Control an acute attack with epinephrine
- Diphenhydramine in a dose of 50 mg four times a day
- Glucocorticosteroids and other immunomodulating agents (e.g. methotrexate, cyclosporine, intravenous and immunoglobulins) may be considered.
- Hereditary angioedema; fresh frozen plasma provides C1-esterase inhibitor
- Newer therapy for hereditary angioedema: Purified C1 inhibitor concentrate, recombinant C1 INH—**conestat alfa**, bradykinin receptor antagonist—**icatibant** and kallikrein inhibitor—**ecallantide**

ANAPHYLACTIC REACTIONS
- Type 1 hypersensitivity immunologic reaction, i.e. IgE-mediated
- Common allergens (**Box 21.1**)

Box 21.1: Common allergens.

Drugs
- Antibiotics (penicillins, cephalosporins tetracyclines and trimethoprim-sulphamethoxazole)
- Chemotherapeutic agents
- Insulin
- Vitamin B1 and folic acid
- Diuretics and β-blockers
- Intravenous anaesthetic agents

Biological agents
- Blood
- Tetanus, rabies and diphtheria antitoxins
- Antithymocyte globulin

Proteins
- Foods (peanuts, fish, egg, milk and soy products)
- Food additives (aspartame and monosodium glutamate)

Insect bites and stings
- Honey bee
- Wasps

Box 21.2: Anaphylactoid reactions.

Cutaneous
- Pruritus
- Flushing
- Urticaria
- Angioedema
- Conjunctival injection

Respiratory
- Bronchospasm → dyspnoea and wheeze
- Laryngeal oedema → stridor
- Pulmonary oedema

Gastrointestinal
- Nausea and vomiting
- Abdominal cramps
- Diarrhoea

Cardiovascular
- Tachycardia
- Hypotension
- Arrhythmias
- Shock and collapse

- Anaphylactoid reactions → involve IgG and IgM antibodies and not IgE antibodies (**Box 21.2**)

Treatment
- Oxygen 4–6 L/min
- Endotracheal intubation or tracheostomy and intermittent positive ventilation

- 0.2–0.5 mL of a 1:1,000 solution epinephrine is given intramuscularly
- Hypotension is managed with intravenous fluids and vasopressors
- Bronchodilators—nebulised salbutamol
- Hydrocortisone 200 mg IV stat
- Diphenhydramine (H_1 blocker), 50–80 mg IM/IV
- Ranitidine (H_2 blocker), 50 mg IV

Serum Sickness

- This is a type III hypersensitivity immune reaction where IgG is produced in response to the injection of foreign antigen in large quantities.
- Fever, glomerulonephritis, arthritis and cardiac involvement
- Treatment is antihistamines and corticosteroids

CHARACTERISTIC FEATURES OF HYPERSENSITIVITY REACTIONS

Characteristic features of hypersensitivity reactions are given in **Table 21.4**.

COMPLEMENT IN HEALTH AND DISEASE

See **Figure 21.2** and **Table 21.5**.

Major Histocompatibility Complex

- These antigens are encoded by a segment of chromosome 6 (6p21.3) known as the major histocompatibility complex (MHc).
- Human leucocyte antigen (HLA) and disease association (**Table 21.6**)

TABLE 21.4: Characteristic features of hypersensitivity reactions.

Type	I (immediate)	II (cytotoxic)	III (immune complex)	IV (delayed)
Antigens	Pollens, moulds, mites, food drugs and parasites	Cell surface or tissue bound	Exogenous (viruses, bacteria fungi, parasites) Autoantigens	Cell/tissue bound
Mediators	IgE and mast cells	IgG, IgM and complement	IgG, IgM, IgA and complement	Cyotoxic T-cells, activated macrophage
Time taken for reaction to develop	5–10 min	6–36 h	4–12 h	48–72 h
Pathological feature	Oedema, vasodilatation, mast cell degranulation, eosinophils	Antibody-mediated damage to target cells	Acute inflammatory reaction (neutrophils), vasculitis	• Perivascular inflammation, mononuclear cells, fibrin • Granulomas: Caseation and necrosis in TB
Prototype disorder/dieases produced	• Asthma (extrinsic) • Anaphylaxis (systemic and localised) • Ulticaria, eczema • Angioedema • Allergic rhinitis • Food allergies	• Autoimmune haaemolytic anaemia, transfusion reaction, hemolytic diease of newborn • Goodpasture's syndrome • Pernicious anaemia • Myasthenia gravis	Autoimmune disease (e.g. SLE, glomerulonephritis rheumatoid arthritis) serum sickness, arthus reaction	• Tuberculosis • Contact dermatitis • Leprosy • Transplant rejection

Continued

Immunological Factors in Disease

Continued

Type	I (immediate)	II (cytotoxic)	III (immune complex)	IV (delayed)
Diagnostic tests	• Skin-prick tests • Specific IgE in serum	• Coombs' test • Indirect immunofluorescence	Immune complexes, complement levels	Skin test-erythema induration (e.g. tuberculin test)
Treatment	• Antigen avoidance • Antihistamines, corticosteroids (usually topical) • Leucotriene receptor antagonists • Sodium cromoglicate • Epinephrine (adrenaline) for life-threatening anaphylaxis	• Exchange transfusion • Plasmapheresis • Immuno-suppressives/cytotoxic drugs	• Corticosteroids • Immuno-suppressive/cytotoxic drugs • Plasmapheresis • Anti-TNF antibody, anti-B-cell antibody, anti-CTLA-4 antibody	• Immuno-suppressives • Corticosteroids, removal of antigen

(CTLA: cytotoxic T-lymphocyte-associated protein; Ig: immunoglobulin; SLE: systemic lupus erythematosus; TB: tuberculosis; TNF: tumour necrosis factor)

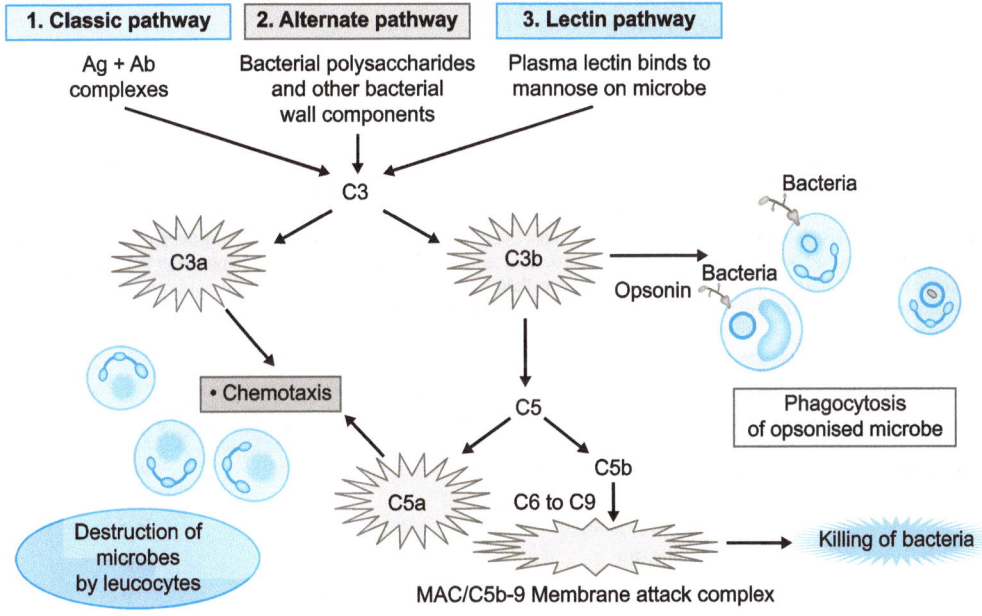

Fig. 21.2: Different pathways of activation and functions of the complement system. All pathways of activation lead to cleavage of C3.

■ PRIMARY IMMUNODEFICIENCY DISORDERS

Classification of primary immunodeficiency disorders is given in **Box 21.3**.

■ ADULT IMMUNISATION SCHEDULE

Adult immunisation schedule is given in **Table 21.7**.

TABLE 21.5: Genetic deficiencies of plasma complement components and associated clinical findings.

Deficiency	Infection	Autoimmune disease
Classical Pathway		
C1q	Pneumococcal B/M, Other pyogenic	SLE, GN, DV/DLE
C1rs	Other pyogenic, pneumococcal B/M, DGI	SLE, GN
C4	Other pyogenic	SLE, GN, other AD
C2	Other pyogenic, pneumococcal B/M, meningococcal M	SLE, GN, DV/DLE, other AD
C3	Other pyogenic, pneumococcal B/M, meningococcal M	GN, DV/DLE, SLE, other AD
C5, C6, C7, C8, C9	Meningococcal M, DGI, Other pyogenic	SLE, GN, other AD
Lectin Pathway		
MBL	Other pyogenic, fungal, HIV	SLE
MASP-2	Pneumococcal pneumonia	SLE
Alternative Pathway		
Factor D	DGI, meningococcal M, Other pyogenic	
Control Proteins		
C1 INH	Hereditary angioedema	SLE
Factor I	Other pyogenic, mningococcal M pneumococcal B/M	
Factor H	Meningococcal B/M, other pyogenic	GN, HUS, SLE
Properdin	Meningococcal M, pneumococcal B/M, other pyogenic	DV/DLE
C4-binding protein		Other AD

[B/M: bacteraemia or meningitis; DGI: disseminated gonococcal infection; DV/DLE: dermal vasculitis or typical discoid lupus erythematosus; GN: glomerulonephritis invarious forms, often membranoproliferative; HIV: human immunodeficiency virus; HUS: haemolytic-uraemic syndrome; M: meningitis; MASP: MBL-associated serine protease; MBL: mannose-binding lectin; other AD: autoimmune disease (almost all possible diagnoses have been reported); other pyogenic: serious deep or systemic infection due to, or typically caused by, a pyogenic bacterium (abscess, osteomyelitis, pneumonia, bacteraemia other than pneumococcal, meningitis other than meningococcal or pneumococcal, cellulitis, myopericarditis, and peritonitis); SLE: typical systemic lupus erythematosus or an SLE-like syndrome without characteristic serologic findings].

TABLE 21.6: Diseases showing positive HLA antigen association.

System	Disease	HLA antigen	Relative risk
Rheumatologic	• Ankylosing spondylitis	B27	90.0
	• Reiter syndrome	B27	37.0
	• Acute anterior uveitis	B27	8.2
	• Reactive arthritis	B27	18.0
	• Psoriatic arthritis	B27	10.7
		B38	9.1
	• Juvenile rheumatoid arthritis	B27	3.9
	• Juvenile rheumatoid arthritis (pauciarticular)	DR5	3.3
	• Rheumatoid arthritis	DR4/Dw4	6.0
	• Sjögren syndrome	Dw3	10.0
	• Systemic lupus erythematosus	DR3	2.6
Gastrointestinal	• Gluten-sensitive enteropathy	DR3	12.0
	• Chronic active hepatitis	DR3	6.8
	• Ulcerative colitis	B5	3.8
	• IgA deficiency	DR3	13.0

Continued

Continued

System	Disease	HLA antigen	Relative risk
Haematologic	• Idiopathic haemochromatosis	A3	6.7
		B14	2.7
	• Pernicious anaemia	A3, B14	90.0
	• Hodgkin disease	DR5	5.0
		DP3	2.0
Dermatologic	• Dermatitis herpetiformis	DR3	17.3
	• Psoriasis vulgaris	Cw3	7.5
	• Psoriasis vulgaris (Japanese)	Cw6	8.5
	• Pemphigus vulgaris (Jewish)	DR4	24.0
	• Behçet disease (white)	A26	4.8
	• Behçet disease (Japanese)	B5	3.8
		B51	12.4
Endocrine	• Diabetes mellitus, type 1	DR4	6/7
		DR3	5.0
	• Graves' disease	DR2	0.25
		BfF1+	15.0
		B8	2.5
		DR3	3.7
	• Graves' disease (Japanese)	B35	4.4
		DR3	3.7
	• Addison disease	Dw3	10.5
	• Subacute thyroiditis	B35	13.7
	• Hashimoto thyroiditis	DR5	3.0
	• Congenital adrenal hyperplasia	B47	15.4
Neurologic	• Myasthenia gravis	B8	3.0
	• Multiple sclerosis	DR2/Dw2	6.0
	• Narcolepsy	DR2, DQ6	130.0
Psychiatric	• Bipolar disorder	B16	2.3
	• Schizophrenia	A28	2.3
Renal	• Idiopathic membranous nephropathy	DR3	5.7
	• Goodpasture syndrome	DR2	16.0
	• Minimal change disease	DR7	4.2
	• IgA nephropathy (French, Japanese)	DR4	3.1
	• Gold/penicillamine nephropathy	DR3	14.0
	• Polycystic kidney disease	B5	2.6
Infectious	• Tuberculoid leprosy (Asians)	B8	6.8
	• Paralytic polio	B16	4.3
	• Low vs. high response vaccinia	Cw3	12.7
	• Falciparum malaria, severe	B53	0.4/0.5
	• Progression to AIDS	B35	2–3
Others	• Birdshot retinochoroidopathy (BSRC)	HLA-A29	80–98
	• Cervical cancer	DR11-DQ3	2–3

(AIDS: acquired immunodeficiency syndrome; HLA: human leucocyte antigen)

Box 21.3: Classification of primary immunodeficiency disorders.

T-cell disorders:
- Severe combined immunodeficiency
- Wiskott–Aldrich syndrome (Xp11)
- Ataxia telangiectasia (11q)
- Digeorge anomaly

Phagocyte disorders:
- Chronic granulomatous disease
- Leucocyte adhesion defect
- Chédiak–Higashi syndrome
- Myeloperoxidase deficiency
- Cyclic neutropaenia (elastase defect)

B-cell defects:
- XL agammaglobulinaemia
- Common variable immunodeficiency
- Selective IgA deficiency
- AR agammaglobulinaemia
- Hyper-IgM syndrome-XL

Complement disorders:
- C1q deficiency
- Factor I deficiency
- Factor H deficiency
- Factor D deficiency
- Properdin deficiency

TABLE 21.7: Adult immunisation schedule.

	AT	BE	BG	HR	FI	FR	DE	GR	IT	NL	PL	RO	SP	SE	CH	UK
UMV for pregnant women																
Diphtheria	×	√	×	×	×	×	×	√	√	×	√	√	√	×	√	√
Tetanus	×	√	×	×	×	×	×	√	√	×	√	√	√	×	√	√
Pertussis	√	√	×	×	×	×	×	√	√	×	√	√	√	√	√	√
Influenza	√	√	×	√	√	√	√	√	×	√	√	√	√	√	√	√
UMV for adults																
Diphtheria	√	√	√	×	√	√	√	√	√	×	√	×	√	√	√	×
Tetanus	√	√	√	×	√	√	√	√	√	×	√	×	√	√	√	×
Pertussis	√	√	√	×	√	√	√	√	√	×	√	×	√	√	√	×
Hepatitis B	×	×	×	×	×	×	×	×	×	√	×	×	×	×	×	×
UMV for older adults (≥ 60 or 65 years of age)																
Zoster	√	×	×	×	×	√	×	√	√	×	×	×	×	×	×	√
Pneumococcal	√	√	√	×	√	×	√	√	√	×	√	×	×	×	×	√
Diphtheria	√	√	√	×	√	√	√	√	√	×	√	×	√	√	√	×
Tetanus	√	√	√	×	√	√	√	√	√	×	√	×	√	√	√	×
Pertussis	√	√	√	×	√	×	√	√	×	×	√	×	×	×	√	×
Influenza	√	√	√	√	√	√	√	√	√	√	√	×	√	√	√	√
Legend	√ Recommended for UMV					× Non recommended for UMV										
	Funded/reimbursed					Out-of-pocket (OOP)					Co-payment					

[AT: Austria; BE: Belgium; BG: Bulgaria; HR: Croatia; FI: Finland; FR: France; DE: Germany; GR: Greece; IT: Italy; NL:Netherlands; PL: Poland; RO: Romania; SP: Spain; SE: Sweden; CH: Switzerland (from Confoederatio Helvetica); UK: United Kingdom; UMV: universal mass vaccination]

BEST OF FIVES

1. A 70-year-old man presents with pyrexia, fatigue, weight loss, hypertension and mononeuritis multiplex. What will be the immunological test result?
   A. Positive extractable nuclear antigen (ENA)
   B. Antineutrophil cytoplasmic antibodies (ANCA)-negative
   C. Positive cytoplasmic ANCA (c-ANCA)
   D. Positive anti-citrullinated protein antibody (ACPA)
   E. Positive perinuclear ANCA (p-ANCA)

2. Sezary syndrome is
   A. Disorder of red blood cells
   B. T-cell malignancy
   C. Associated with dry mouth
   D. B-cell malignancy
   E. Thrombocytopaenia

3. What therapy can be useful in severe oral and genital ulceration?
   A. Etanercept
   B. Thalidomide
   C. Methotrexate
   D. Infliximab
   E. Nil

4. How are the majority of hereditary complement deficiencies inherited?
   A. Mitochondrial
   B. X-linked recessive
   C. X-linked dominant
   D. Autosomal recessive
   E. Autosomal dominant

5. A child has recurrent pyogenic infection. What is the most likely diagnosis?
   A. Helper T-cell deficiency
   B. B-cell deficiency
   C. Mannose-binding lectin deficiency
   D. C2 deficiency
   E. Killer T-cell deficiency

6. Which of the following confirms anaphylaxis over angioedema if there is any doubt of the diagnosis?
   A. Facial oedema
   B. Elevated serum mast cell tryptase
   C. Neutrophilia
   D. Rash
   E. Hypereosinophilia

7. What immunoglobulin (Ig) if present in low levels can be associated with coeliac disease?
   A. IgG
   B. IgE
   C. IgA
   D. IgM
   E. IgD

8. What is true about monoclonal free light chains?
   A. They are commonly found in the urine of multiple myeloma.
   B. They do not lead to renal damage.
   C. They are pathognomonic of monoclonal gammopathy of undetermined significance (MGUS).
   D. They are pathognomonic of Waldenström's macroglobulinaemia.
   E. They are found in amyloidosis.

9. What is the main contributory factor to the immunodeficiency seen in chronic lymphocytic leukaemia?
   A. Hypogammaglobulinaemia
   B. Neutropaenia
   C. T-cell deficiency
   D. Interleukin 10 activity
   E. Lymphopaenia

10. A 22-year-old male presents with easy bruising. You note that he is very tall and his sclerae have a blue tinge. He has marked hypermobility of his joints and has moderate elasticity of his skin. Which of the following is the most likely cause?
    A. Classical form of Ehlers–Danlos syndrome
    B. Hypermobility syndrome
    C. Osteogenesis imperfecta
    D. Hypermobile form of Ehlers–Danlos syndrome
    E. Marfan syndrome

11. A 24-year-old man with history of latex allergy is brought to the accident and emergency (A+E) department with anaphylactic shock. Which fruit is associated with latex allergy?
    A. Apple
    B. Banana
    C. Pear
    D. Grapefruit
    E. Orange

12. A man has had a previous splenectomy for immune thrombocytopenic purpura. Since his splenectomy, he has had two episodes of pneumonia. Post splenectomy, what type of immunodeficiency occurs?
    A. Complement mediated
    B. Killer T cells
    C. Cell mediated
    D. Helper T cells
    E. Humoral

13. Positive anti-Ro antibodies with no other autoantibodies present are indicative of what condition?
    A. Dermatomyositis
    B. Systemic lupus erythematosus (SLE)
    C. Rheumatoid arthritis
    D. Sjögren's syndrome
    E. Polymyositis

14. A patient presents with acute hereditary angioedema. On examination, there is evidence of stridor. How do you manage this patient?
    A. Intravenous (IV) fluids
    B. Adrenaline
    C. Icatibant
    D. Chlorphenamine
    E. Hydrocortisone

15. What autoimmune disorder is related to C1q deficiency?
    A. Systemic lupus erythematosus (SLE)
    B. Systemic sclerosis
    C. Churg-Strauss syndrome
    D. Goodpasture's syndrome
    E. Autoimmune hepatitis

16. Which of the following is a human leucocyte antigen (HLA)-class II antigen?
    A. HLA-A
    B. HLA-G
    C. HLA-DR
    D. HLA-C
    E. HLA-B

17. What statement is true regarding the immune system?
    A. CD8 T cells are responsible for antibody production.
    B. CD4 T cells interact with B cells via major histocompatibility complex (MHC) class I.
    C. CD8 T cells interact with all cells via MHC class II.
    D. CD4 T cells interact with B cells via MHC class II.
    E. Only macrophages express MHC 1.

18. In what percentage of the normal population would you expect to find raised immunoglobulin E (IgE) levels?
    A. 15%
    B. 2.5%
    C. 1%
    D. 5%
    E. 10%

19. In what compartment is the Mantoux test administered?
    A. Topical
    B. Intradermal
    C. Intravenous
    D. Subcutaneous
    E. Intramuscular

20. What immune cells are affected by chronic lymphocytic leukaemia predominantly?
    A. B cells
    B. CD4 T cells
    C. Macrophages
    D. CD8 cells
    E. NK cells

21. If adenosine deaminase is absent from a cell, i.e. in severe combined immunodeficiency disease, what does this result in?
    A. Synthesis of deoxyadenosine
    B. Leads to degeneration of deoxyadenosine
    C. Upregulation of receptors
    D. Leads to accumulation of deoxyadenosine
    E. Down-regulation of receptors

22. A patient presents with hypocalcaemic tetany. He has abnormal ears, hypertelorism and an absent thymus. What is the likely diagnosis if a patient has an absent thymus, hypocalcaemia and abnormal ears?
    A. Down syndrome
    B. Tay syndrome
    C. DiGeorge syndrome
    D. Wiskott–Aldrich syndrome
    E. Severe combined immunodeficiency

23. In systemic lupus erythematosus (SLE), what abnormal immune response is seen?
    A. Type IV hypersensitivity reaction
    B. Type I hypersensitivity reaction
    C. Alternative complement pathway activation

D. C3 complement deficiency
E. Type III hypersensitivity

24. A patient with partial lipodystrophy develops nephrotic syndrome. What investigation will indicate the likely renal pathology?
    A. Human immunodeficiency virus (HIV) testing
    B. Antistreptolysin titre (ASOT)
    C. Serum immunoglobulins
    D. Antinuclear antibody (ANA)
    E. Complement studies

25. One principal function of the Class I and Class II major histocompatibility complex S proteins is to
    A. Transduce the signal to the T-cell interior following antigen binding
    B. Mediate immunoglobulin class switching
    C. Present antigen for recognition by the T-cell antigen receptor
    D. Stimulate production of interleukins
    E. Bind complement

Answers

1-E, 2-B, 3-B, 4-D, 5-C, 6-B, 7-C, 8-A, 9-A, 10-D, 11-B, 12-E, 13-B, 14-C, 15-A, 16-C, 17-D, 18-B, 19-B, 20-A, 21-D, 22-C, 23-E, 24-E, 25-C

■ SUGGESTED READING

1. Frey NV, Porter DL. Cytokine release syndrome with novel therapeutics for acute lymphoblastic leukemia. Hematology Am Soc Hematol Educ Program. 2016; 2016(1):567-72.
2. Frey N, Porter D. Cytokine release syndrome with chimeric antigen receptor T cell therapy. Biol Blood Marrow Transplant. 2019;25(4):e123-7.
3. Tangye SG, Al-Herz W, Bousfiha A, Chatila T, Cunningham-Rundles C, Etzioni A, et al. Human Inborn Errors of Immunity: 2019 Update on the Classification from the International Union of Immunological Societies Expert Committee. J Clin Immunol. 2020;40(1):24-64.
4. Botto M, Kirschfink M, Macor P, Pickering MC, Würzner R, Tedesco F. Complement in human diseases: Lessons from complement deficiencies. Mol Immunol. 2009;46(14):2774-83.
5. Johansson SG, Bieber T, Dahl R, Friedmann PS, Lanier BQ, Lockey RF, et al. Revised nomenclature for allergy for global use: Report of the Nomenclature Review Committee of the World Allergy Organization, October 2003. J Allergy Clin Immunol. 2004;113(5):832-6.
6. Kyle RA. Amyloidosis: a convoluted story. Br J Haematol. 2001;114(3):529-38.
7. Kim DK, Hunter P, Advisory Committee on Immunization Practices. Recommended Adult Immunization Schedule, United States, 2019. Ann Intern Med. 2019;170(3):182-92.
8. Centers for Disease Control and Prevention. General best practice guidelines for immunization. [online] Available from: https://www.cdc.gov/vaccines/hcp/acip-recs/general-recs/index.html [Last accessed June, 2020].
9. Davidson A, Diamond B. Autoimmune diseases. N Engl J Med. 2001;345(5):340-50.
10. Arbuckle MR, McClain MT, Rubertone MV, Scofield RH, Dennis GJ, James JA, et al. Development of autoantibodies before the clinical onset of systemic lupus erythematosus. N Engl J Med. 2003;349(16):1526-33.
11. Rose NR. Predictors of autoimmune disease: autoantibodies and beyond. Autoimmunity. 2008;41(6):419-28.
12. Cunningham-Rundles C. How I treat common variable immunodeficiency. Blood. 2010;116(1):7-15.

22 CHAPTER

Maternal Medicine

Mohammed Shaheen

■ PHYSIOLOGICAL CHANGES IN PREGNANCY

The physiological changes in pregnancy are shown in **Figure 22.1**.

■ ANAEMIA IN PREGNANCY

The criteria for anaemia in pregnancy as per the World Health Organization (WHO) and Centre for Disease Control and Prevention (CDC) are given in **Table 22.1**.
- Iron deficiency is the most common cause of anaemia, followed by folic acid deficiency.
- The risks of preterm delivery and post-partum maternal infections are increased by anaemia.
- If Hb is < 11.5 g/dL at the onset of pregnancy, treatment must be done.
- Iron and folate supplementation is recommended.

■ HYPERTENSION IN PREGNANCY

The definitions for hypertension are as follows:
- Normal: < 120/80 mmHg
- Elevated: 120–129/< 80 mmHg
- Stage 1 hypertension: 130–139/80–89 mmHg
- Stage 2 hypertension: ≥ 140/90 mmHg

The American College of Obstetricians and Gynecologists (ACOG) defines chronic hypertension as systolic blood pressure (BP) ≥ 140 mmHg or diastolic BP ≥ 90 mmHg on two occasions before 20 weeks' gestation.

Hypertension during pregnancy can be classified as one of the following:
- Chronic hypertension: BP is high before pregnancy or before 20 weeks' gestation. Chronic hypertension complicates about 1–5% of all pregnancies (**Table 22.2**).
- Gestational hypertension: Hypertension develops after 20 weeks' gestation (typically after 37 weeks) and remits by 6 weeks' postpartum; it occurs in about 5–10% of pregnancies, more commonly in multifoetal pregnancy (**Table 22.2**).

Antihypertensives of choice: Methyldopa, beta-blockers or calcium channel blockers tried first. Methyldopa, beta-blockers or calcium channel blockers.

Drugs to be avoided: Angiotensin-converting enzyme (ACE) inhibitors, angiotensin II receptor blockers (ARBs), aldosterone antagonists.

Consider hospitalisation or termination of pregnancy if BP is > 180/110 mmHg.

■ GESTATIONAL DIABETES

The risk factors have been most recently defined by the National Institute for Health and Care Excellence (NICE) guidelines:
- Previous macrosomic infant (4.5 kg or above)
- Previous gestational diabetes
- First-degree relative with diabetes
- Obesity [body mass index (BMI) > 30 kg/m^2]
- Specific ethnic family origin with a high prevalence of diabetes: South Asian
- Macrosomia in current pregnancy
- Glycosuria ≥ 1+ on more than one occasion or ≥ 2+ on one occasion
- Previous unexpected and unexplained perinatal death
- Polycystic ovary syndrome
- Polyhydramnios

Gestational diabetes mellitus (GDM) is diagnosed by the derangement of values in an oral glucose tolerance test using 100 g of glucose. This is given in **Table 22.3**.

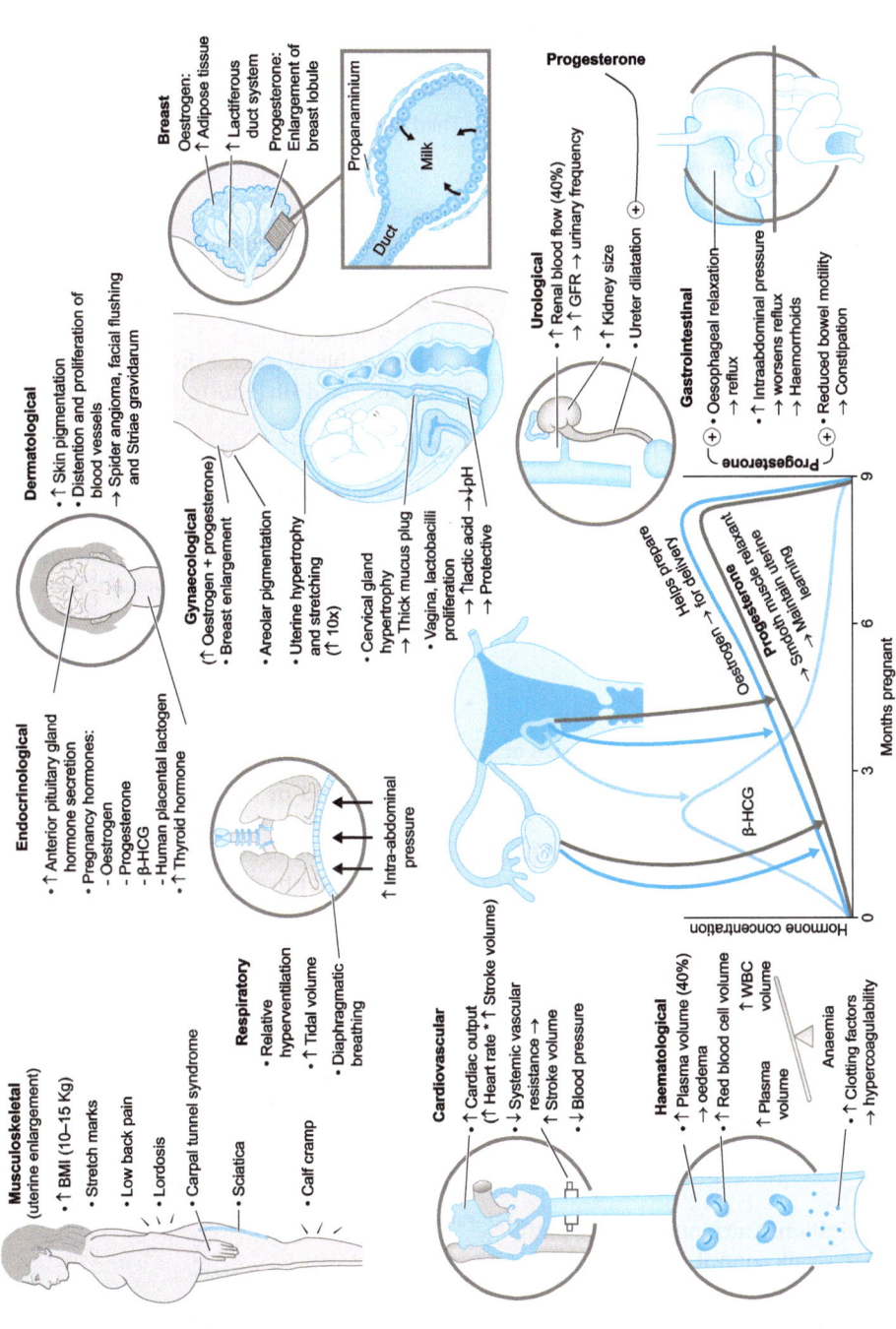

Fig. 22.1: Physiological changes in pregnancy.

TABLE 22.1: Criteria for anaemia in pregnancy as per World Health Organization (WHO) and Centres for Disease Control and Prevention (CDC).

Criteria given by	Mild	Moderate	Severe
WHO	8–11 g%	5–7 g%	< 5 g%
	First Trimester	Second Trimester	Third Trimester
CDC	< 11 g%	< 10.5 g%	< 11 g%

TABLE 22.2: Maternal and foetal risks in pregnancy.

Maternal risks	Foetal risks
• Pre-eclampsia and eclampsia • Hypertensive encephalopathy • Stroke • Renal failure • Left ventricular failure • HELLP syndrome (haemolysis, elevated liver enzymes and low platelet count) • Abruptio placentae	Decreased uteroplacental blood flow → growth restriction, hypoxia

TABLE 22.3: Commonly used criteria for diagnosis of GDM.

Timing of test	Carpenter and Coustan	NDDG
Fasting	95 mg/dL	105 mg/dL
1st hour	180 mg/dL	190 mg/dL
2nd hour	155 mg/dL	165 mg/dL
3rd hour	140 mg/dL	145 mg/dL

(NDDG: National Diabetes Data Group)

Foetal complications: Respiratory distress, hypoglycaemia, hypocalcaemia, hyperbilirubinaemia, hyperviscosity

Treatment

Lifestyle modification: Nutritional control, physical activity and weight control.

Insulin is the drug of choice.

The drugs recommended in pregnancy are metformin and glibenclamide, mainly because of their ease of administration and the reduced need for insulin.

TABLE 22.4: Normal physiological levels of thyroid-stimulating hormone by trimester.

Trimester	TSH reference value
First trimester	0.1–2.5 mIU/L
Second trimester	0.2–3.0 mIU/L
Third trimester	0.3–3.0 mIU/L

Goals of treatment are:
- Fasting blood glucose levels at < 95 mg/dL (< 5.3 mmol/L)
- 2-hour post-prandial levels at ≤ 120 mg/dL (≤ 6.6 mmol/L)
- No wide blood glucose fluctuations
- Glycosylated Hb (HbA1c) levels at < 6.5%

■ THYROID DISORDERS IN PREGNANCY

- Maternal hypothyroidism is an easily treatable condition that is associated with significant risk to the foetus: Low birth weight, foetal distress and impaired neuropsychological development. The most common causes of maternal hypothyroidism are Hashimoto thyroiditis and treatment of Graves' disease.
- Hyperthyroidism in pregnancy is rarer, as it usually poses a problem for conception.
- Post-partum maternal thyroid dysfunction: Hypothyroid or hyperthyroid dysfunction that occurs in 4–7% of women during the first 6 months after delivery
- The normal physiological levels of thyroid-stimulating hormone (TSH) by trimester is defined by the American Thyroid Association (**Table 22.4**).

Management/Treatment

For treatment of hypothyroidism for newly diagnosed cases, a replacement dose of 2–2.4 µg/kg/day of levothyroxine is recommended.

Hyperthyroidism: Propylthiouracil is recommended as the first-line anti-thyroid drug in pregnancy.

■ ASTHMA IN PREGNANCY

- Maternal bronchial asthma and its exacerbation is a major clinical problem that can lead to maternal and foetal morbidity and mortality.

- The short-acting beta-agonist of choice is Salbutamol. For patients who experience mild-to-severe asthma during pregnancy, inclusion of inhaled glucocorticoids reduces the risk of exacerbation.
- Peripartum usage of prostaglandin F2-alpha is contraindicated in asthmatics as it may cause sudden bronchoconstriction. Oxytocin, dinoprostone and misoprostol are recommended alternatives.

THROMBOEMBOLISM

- Pregnancy and post-pregnancy puerperium is known to be a prothrombotic state.
- Diagnose deep vein thrombosis using Doppler ultrasonography. Pelvic Venous Thrombosis must be ruled out. For the diagnosis of pulmonary embolism, a helical CT or a pulmonary angiography may be used.
- Low-molecular-weight heparin is the treatment of choice.
- Warfarin should be *avoided*.

HEPATIC DISORDERS OF PREGNANCY

- Hepatic disorders of pregnancy can be divided into three: Those that are induced by pregnancy (such as acute fatty liver of pregnancy or intrahepatic cholestasis), those that develop during pregnancy but are unrelated to it and pre-existing hepatobiliary disorders that complicate pregnancy.
- Acute viral hepatitis: Hepatitis E may be more fulminant during pregnancy.
- All pregnant women must be tested for hepatitis B surface antigen (HBsAg) to prevent perinatal transmission
- Intrahepatic cholestasis of pregnancy
  - Clinical features—intense pruritus and jaundice
  - Increased risk of foetal prematurity, stillbirth and respiratory distress syndrome
- Fatty liver of pregnancy
  - Occurs near term
  - Associated with preeclampsia
  - Needs prompt delivery or termination of pregnancy

INFECTIOUS DISEASES IN PREGNANCY

- The most common maternal infections [e.g. urinary tract infections (UTIs), skin and respiratory tract infections] are usually not serious problems during pregnancy.
- Maternal infections that can damage the foetus include cytomegalovirus infection, herpes simplex virus infection, rubella, toxoplasmosis, hepatitis B and syphilis.
- Safe anti-bacterials during pregnancy discussed later.

Human Immunodeficiency Virus (HIV)

- Vertical transmission usually occurs transplacentally during the pregnancy, at the time of delivery due to intermixing of blood and post-partum while breastfeeding.
- Withholding breastfeeding reduces the transmission rates by 20–25%.
- Women with viral loads high than 400 copies/mL are recommended to undergo a caesarean section.
- Neonatal screening for HIV is initiated at birth and continues till 3 months of age.
- Post-exposure prophylaxis for the child is recommended and women are advised to not breastfeed.

EPILEPSY AND SEIZURE DISORDERS IN PREGNANCY

- Seizure disorders may impair fertility. But certain anti-seizure drugs may make oral contraceptives less effective, resulting in unintentional pregnancy.
- Periconceptional management: Folic acid is supplemented for all women with epilepsy at a higher dose of 1 mg daily, initiated preconceptionally and continued throughout pregnancy.
- Management during pregnancy: Lamotrigine and levetiracetam are preferred as first-line therapy for pregnant women with seizure disorders. Risk of congenital malformations and haemorrhagic manifestations in the newborn in higher.

CARDIAC DISEASE IN PREGNANCY

The classification of cardiac disease in pregnancy as per the NYHA is given in **Box 22.1**.

DRUGS AND PREGNANCY

The drugs that are used in pregnancy and those that are contraindicated are given in **Tables 22.5** and **22.6**, respectively.

The common problems in pregnancy and the drugs that can be used to control them are given in **Table 22.7**.

TABLE 22.5: Current categories for drug use in pregnancy.

Category	Description
A	Adequate well-controlled studies in humans show no risk to the foetus (e.g. magnesium sulphate)
B	No well-controlled studies have been conducted in humans. Animal studies show no risk to the foetus (e.g. amoxicillin, amoxicillin + clavulanic acid, cefotaxime, methyldopa, metronidazole, erythromycin)
C	No well-controlled studies have been conducted in humans. Animal studies have shown an adverse effect on the foetus (e.g. diclofenac, rifampicin, fluoroquinolones, aminoglycosides, glyburide)
D	Human studies have demonstrated risk to the foetus. However, the benefits of therapy may outweigh the potential harm (e.g. tetracycline, phenytoin, valproic acid, carbamazepine, ACE inhibitors)
X	Controlled studies in animals or humans have demonstrated foetal abnormalities. The use of the product is contraindicated in women who are or may become pregnant (e.g. thalidomide, oral contraceptive pills, misoprostol)

Box 22.1: Cardiac disease in pregnancy.

Group 1: Mortality < 1%
- Atrial septal defect
- Ventricular septal defect
- Patent ductus arteriosus
- Pulmonary/tricuspid disease
- Corrected tetralogy of Fallot
- Bioprosthetic valve
- Mitral stenosis, NYHA class I and II

Group 2: Mortality 5–15%
- Group 2A
  - Mitral stenosis NYHA class III and IV
  - Aortic stenosis
  - Coarctation of aorta without valvular involvement
  - Uncorrected tetralogy of Fallot
  - Previous myocardial infarction
  - Marfan syndrome with normal aorta
- Group 2B
  - Mitral stenosis with atrial fibrillation
  - Artificial valve

Group 3: Mortality 25–50%
- Primary pulmonary hypertension
- Eisenmenger syndrome
- Coarctation of aorta with valvular involvement
- Marfan syndrome with aortic involvement

(NYHA: New York Heart Association)

TABLE 22.6: List of few drugs contraindicated during pregnancy and those which have teratogenic effects.

Drug	Side effects
Tetracycline	Yellow staining of the primary or deciduous teeth and diminished growth of the long bones
Phenytoin	Foetal hydantoin syndrome consisting of intrauterine, growth retardation, microcephaly, mental retardation, distal phalangeal hypoplasia
Retinoic acid	Craniofacial dysmorphism, cleft palate, thymic aplasia and neural tube defects
Thalidomide	Meromelia, absence of the limbs to rudimentary limbs to abnormally shortened limbs
Alcohol	Intrauterine growth retardation (IUGR), small head, small eyes or short eyes opening, or a poorly developed philtrum and congenital heart disease

Continued

Continued

Drug	Side effects
Nicotine	IUGR
Warfarin	Nasal hypoplasia, and a depressed nasal bridge, stippled epiphyses, termed foetal warfarin syndrome
Oestrogen and androgens	Genital tract malformations
Chloramphenicol	Gray baby syndrome

TABLE 22.7: **Common problems in pregnancy and drugs that can be safely used.**

Common problems in pregnancy	Drugs that can be safely used
Nausea and vomiting	Pyridoxine, meclizine diphenhydramine
Constipation	Mild purgative-like senna
Peptic ulcer	Sucralfate, H_2 blockers
Haematopoietic (iron and folic acid deficiency)	Iron and folic acid
Urinary tract infections	Ampicillin, amoxicillin, cefuroxime axetil
Other infections	β-lactam antibiotics, cephalosporins
Malaria	Chloroquine, quinine, proguanil
Amoebiasis	Metronidazole and diloxanide furoate
Worm infestation	Piperazine citrate, pyrantel pamoate
Fungal infection	Miconazole, clotrimazole, nystatin
HIV infection	None of the anti-HIV drugs are safe, except zidovudine and nevirapine
Tuberculosis	INH and ethambutol are safe. If third drug is needed, then rifampicin
Diabetes mellitus	Insulin
Hypothyroidism	Thyroxine
Thyrotoxicosis	Propylthiouracil
Hypertension	α-methyldopa, in emergency—hydralazine, β-blockers—labetalol, atenolol
Thromboembolic disease	Heparin
Headache and inflammatory condition	Paracetamol, avoid other NSAIDs
Epilepsy	Sodium valproate and phenytoin to be avoided, carbamazepine in lower dose can be used
Migraine	Paracetamol, propranolol, amitriptyline
Antidepressants	Amitriptyline and imipramine

(HIV: human immunodeficiency virus; INH: isoniazid; NSAIDs: non-steroidal anti-inflammatory drugs)

BEST OF FIVES

1. A 19-year-old female has a history of hypertension which is managed with a combination of ramipril and indapamide. Her past medical history includes 11-beta hydroxylase deficiency diagnosed shortly after birth along with cliteromegaly. Which of the following is likely to be markedly raised?
   A. 11-Deoxycortisol
   B. Oestradiol
   C. Oestrone
   D. 17-OH progesterone
   E. 17-OH pregnenolone

2. In which of the following heart diseases is maternal mortality found to be the highest?
   A. Eisenmenger's complex
   B. Coarctation of aorta
   C. Mitral stenosis
   D. Aortic stenosis
   E. Atrial septal defect (ASD)

3. A 29-year-old woman presents with amenorrhoea for the past 6 months. Her body mass index (BMI) is 23 kg/m². Investigations show follicle stimulating hormone (FSH) 40 U/L (< 15) and prolactin 200 mU/L (< 450). Which of the following is the most likely diagnosis?
   A. Androgen insensitivity syndrome
   B. Pituitary failure
   C. Polycystic ovarian syndrome
   D. Premature ovarian failure
   E. Prolactinoma

4. A 26-year-old female presents with a 1-year history of galactorrhoea and amenorrhoea. Magnetic resonance imaging (MRI) of the pituitary reveals a 1.5-cm tumour with some suprasellar extension. What is the most appropriate treatment for this woman?
   A. Cabergoline therapy
   B. Combined oral contraceptive
   C. Pituitary surgery
   D. Somatostatin analogue therapy
   E. Stereotactic pituitary irradiation

5. A 24-year-old woman presents with a 4-month history of amenorrhoea. Investigations show:

Serum oestradiol	97 pmol/L	(130–500)
Serum LH	2.0 mU/L	(3.0–6.6)
Serum FSH	1.2 mU/L	(3.3–10.1)
Serum prolactin	1,000 mU/L	(50–500)
Serum testosterone	2.1 pmol/L	(< 3.0)

   Which investigation is the most appropriate?
   A. 17 hydroxyprogesterone
   B. Insulin tolerance test
   C. Magnetic resonance imaging (MRI) of the pituitary
   D. Pregnancy test
   E. Urine free cortisol concentration

6. A 34-year-old female presents in the 30th week of pregnancy with profound tiredness and anxiety. Examination reveals a tremor, a pulse of 100 beats per minute and a soft bruit heard over the thyroid gland. Thyroid function tests show free T4 42.9 pmol/L (10–22) and thyroid-stimulating hormone (TSH) 0.02 mU/L(0.45). Which of the following treatments would you select for this patient?
   A. Carbimazole
   B. Lithium
   C. Potassium perchlorate
   D. Propranolol
   E. Radioactive iodine therapy

7. A 35-year-old woman had been diagnosed with microprolactinoma 5 years ago and was treated with cabergoline in the past, which she took for about 3 years. On examination, pulse was 78 beats per minute and blood pressure was 118/66 mmHg. There was no galactorrhoea to expression. Her visual acuity and papillary reflexes were normal.

   Investigations showed:

Plasma prolactin	3,980 mU/L	(< 360)
Plasma free T4	22.3 pmol/L	(10–22)
Plasma free T3	4.2 pmol/L	(5–10)
Plasma thyroid-stimulating hormone	0.22 mU/L	(0.4–5)

What is the next most appropriate management?
A. Complete pituitary hormonal profile
B. Computed tomography (CT) scan of pituitary
C. Magnetic resonance imaging (MRI) scan of pituitary
D. Reassurance
E. Repeat prolactin level

8. A 22-year-old woman presented with a 5-year history of hirsutism. Her periods are irregular with oligomenorrhoea. On examination, she had a body mass index of 26 kg/m². She had coarse, dark hair over her chin, lower back and inner thighs. Investigations during the follicular phase showed:

Serum androstenedione	12.1 nmol/L	(0.6–8.8)
Serum dehydroepiandrosterone sulphate	9.7 µmol/L	(2–10)
Serum 17-hydroxyprogesterone	5.8 nmol/L	(1–10)
Serum oestradiol	240 pmol/L	(200–400)
Serum testosterone	3.6 nmol/L	(0.5–3)
Serum sex hormone binding protein	32 nmol/L	(40–137)
Plasma luteinising hormone	4.8 U/L	(2.5–10)
Plasma follicle-stimulating hormone	2.5 U/L	(2.5–10)
Plasma prolactin	380 mU/L	(<360)

What is the most appropriate treatment for her hirsutism and her underlying condition?
A. Bromocriptine
B. Cabergoline
C. Clomiphene
D. Metformin
E. Oral contraceptive pill (OCP)

9. A 22-year-old woman with irregular periods presents with oligomenorrhoea. Investigations during the follicular phase show:

Serum androstenedione	10.1 nmol/L	(2–10)
Serum dehydroepiandrosterone sulphate	12.6 µmol/L	(2–10)
Serum 17-hydroxyprogesterone	5.6 nmol/L	(1–10)
Serum oestradiol	230 pmol/L	(200–400)
Serum testosterone	3.9 nmol/L	(<3)
Serum sex hormone binding protein	32 nmol/L	(19–80)
Plasma luteinising hormone	10.8 U/L	(2.5–10)
Plasma follicle-stimulating hormone	3.6 U/L	(2.5–10)
Plasma prolactin	980 mU/L	(<500)

What is the most likely diagnosis?
A. Adult-onset congenital adrenal hyperplasia
B. Drug-induced hyperprolactinaemia
C. Microprolactinoma
D. Polycystic ovarian syndrome (PCOS)
E. Testosterone-producing ovarian tumour

10. A 32-year-old pregnant woman is seen in the emergency department with right-sided facial weakness. She has no other focal neurology in the face, arms or legs and skin is intact with no lesions. Blood tests done on arrival are normal. Given the underlying diagnosis, what is the most appropriate management of this patient?
A. Computed tomography (CT) of head
B. Aspirin
C. Prednisolone
D. Aciclovir
E. Prednisolone + Aciclovir

11. A 28-year-old woman with bipolar disorder would like to get pregnant. She is taking lithium daily with active monitoring in the community. Her mood is currently stable. You counsel her about the risks associated with pregnancy and lithium. What foetal abnormality is associated with lithium?
A. Macrosomia
B. Ebstein's anomaly
C. Oligohydramnios
D. Transposition of great vessels
E. Ventricular septal defect

Answers
1-A, 2-A, 3-D, 4-A, 5-C, 6-A, 7-D, 8-E, 9-D, 10-C, 11-B

SUGGESTED READING

1. Ito S. Mother and child: Medication use in pregnancy and lactation. Clin Pharmacol Ther. 2016;100(1):8-11.
2. Society of Maternal-Fetal Medicine (SMFM) Publications Committee. SMFM Statement: Pharmacological treatment of gestational diabetes. Am J Obstet Gynecol. 2018;218(5):B2-4.
3. Hartling L, Dryden DM, Guthrie A, Muise M, Vandermeer B, Donovan L. Benefits and harms of treating gestational diabetes mellitus: a systematic review and meta-analysis for the U.S. Preventive Services Task Force and the National Institutes of Health Office of Medical Applications of Research. Ann Intern Med. 2013;159(2):123-9.
4. Poprzeczny AJ, Louise J, Deussen AR, Dodd JM. The mediating effects of gestational diabetes on fetal growth and adiposity in women who are overweight and obese: secondary analysis of the LIMIT randomised trial. BJOG. 2018;125(12):1558-66.
5. Gestational Hypertension and Preeclampsia: ACOG Practice Bulletin, Number 222. Obstet Gynecol. 2020;135(6):e237-60.
6. Heard AR, Dekker GA, Chan A, Jacobs DJ, Vreeburg SA, Priest KR. Hypertension during pregnancy in South Australia, part 1: pregnancy outcomes. Aust N Z J Obstet Gynaecol. 2004;44(5):404-9.
7. Hauth JC, Ewell MG, Levine RJ, J R Esterlitz, B Sibai, L B Curet, et al. Pregnancy outcomes in healthy nulliparas who developed hypertension. Calcium for Preeclampsia Prevention Study Group. Obstet Gynecol. 2000;95(1):24-8.
8. American College of Obstetricians and Gynecologists. ACOG Practice Bulletin No. 95: anemia in pregnancy. Obstet Gynecol. 2008;112(1):201-7.
9. World Health Organization. WHO recommendations on antenatal care for a positive pregnancy experience. Luxembourg: World Health Organization; 2016.
10. Pavord S, Myers B, Robinson S, Allard S, Strong J, Oppenheimer C. UK guidelines on the management of iron deficiency in pregnancy. Br J Haematol. 2012;156(5):588-600.
11. Pavord S, Daru J, Prasannan N, Robinson S, Stanworth S, Girling J, et al. UK guidelines on the management of iron deficiency in pregnancy. Br J Haematol. 2020;188(6):819-30.

CHAPTER 23

Environmental Medicine

■ HEAT-RELATED ILLNESSES

Heat Cramps
- Most benign heat disorder, generally associated with strenuous physical activity.
  - Loss of sodium in the sweat coupled with inadequate sodium replacement results in **hyponatraemia** that is thought to produce cramps through interference with calcium-dependent muscle relaxation.
  - Hyperventilation producing respiratory alkalosis and mild hypokalaemia may be a contributory factor.
- **Clinical features:**
  - Patients complain of painful spasm of skeletal muscles, both of extremities and abdomen.
  - Usually, the cramps occur in the muscles that have been subjected to excessive exercise. The body temperature does not rise and the sweating is normal or excessive.
- **Laboratory studies:**
  - Mild hyponatraemia, hypokalaemia and respiratory alkalosis
- **Treatment:**
  - Rest in a cool environment
  - Replacement of sodium, potassium and water
  - Avoid massage of the involved limbs as it generates heat.
- **Prevention:**
  - Liberal ingestion of sodium and water

Heat Oedema
- It manifests by ankle and wrist swelling occurring in the first few days of heat exposure. It may be pitting in a few patients.
- The oedema resolves within a few days of acclimatisation.

Heat Exhaustion
- Heat exhaustion is common in elderly patients and occurs due to fluid and electrolyte losses coupled with inadequate replacement.

Exertional Heat Injury
- It occurs in persons who exert in hot and humid environment. It is common in long-distance runners who run without adequate hydration and acclimatisation.
- **Clinical features:**
  - This disorder is characterised by headache, piloerection, chills, hyperventilation, nausea, vomiting, muscular incoordination and incoherent speech.
  - The patients sweat freely and the body temperature is elevated but usually not as high as that seen with heat stroke.
  - Some patients may develop loss of consciousness.
  - Examination shows a diaphoretic patient with tachycardia and hypotension.
  - Some patients also develop thrombocytopaenia, disseminated intravascular coagulation (DIC) and rhabdomyolysis.

Treatment

- The patient should be placed in a cool place covered with wet cold sheets so as to lower the temperature below 100.4°F (38°C).
- Massage of extremities is helpful in increasing flow of blood from the core to the periphery.
- Infuse 5% dextrose in N/2 saline.

Heat Stroke

- Heat stroke is of two types: Exertional (increased endogenous heat production) and classic (impairment of heat dissipation).
- **Exertional heat stroke:**
  - Occurs in healthy, young individuals, usually during the period of acclimatisation who exert in hot environment
  - The patient develops hyperthermia and loss of consciousness.
  - The patient sweats freely.
  - Complications include DIC, rhabdomyolysis, renal failure and lactic acidosis.
- **Classic heat stroke:**
  - It occurs more often in elderly persons with underlying predisposing conditions during hot weather.
  - Examination shows a temperature > 106°F (41.1°C).
  - Most of the patients do not sweat and the skin is dry.
  - Tachycardia, cardiac arrhythmias, low blood pressure, decreased deep tendon reflexes, lethargy, stupor or coma depending upon the severity
  - The pupils may be fixed and dilated.
  - Complications in the form of lactic acidosis, DIC, rhabdomyolysis and renal failure are uncommon as compared to exertional heat stroke.
- **Laboratory investigations:**
  - Leucocytosis
  - Proteinuria
  - Elevated blood urea
  - Respiratory alkalosis followed by metabolic acidosis (lactic acidosis)
  - Normo- or hypokalaemia
  - Hypocalcaemia
  - Hypophosphataemia
  - ST-T wave changes in the ECG
  - Thrombocytopaenia
  - Coagulopathy
  - DIC

Treatment

- Maintenance of airway, breathing and circulation
- IV line and oxygen administration
- Blood for various investigations
- The patient should be totally disrobed.
- Application of ice on lateral aspects of the trunk, axillae and groins
- Evaporative cooling involves the removal of clothing, spraying tepid water over the patient, and facilitating evaporation and convection with the use of a fan.
- Cold fluids intravenously
- Immersing the patient in ice-cold water is equally or possibly more effective.
- Other ice-water gastric lavage and enemas, and ice-water peritoneal dialysis

Malignant Hyperthermia

- It is characterised by a rapid increase in temperature in response to inhalational anaesthetics (halothane) or muscle relaxants (succinylcholine).

Clinical Features

- Reduced muscle relaxation, fasciculations and trismus during intubation
- Cardiac arrhythmia, muscle rigidity, hypotension and cyanosis
- **Complications:** Pulmonary oedema, DIC and acute renal failure

Laboratory Features

- Respiratory and metabolic acidosis, hyperkalaemia and hypermagnesaemia

Treatment

- Surgery should be stopped and inhalational anaesthetic is withdrawn.
- Oxygen is administered and external cooling is started.
- Dantrolene in a dose of 1 mg/kg

Neuroleptic Malignant Syndrome

- Neuroleptic malignant syndrome (NMS) is associated with therapeutic use of neuroleptic drugs such as phenothiazines, butyrophenones and thioxanthines.

Clinical Features

- NMS typically develops over a period of 24–72 hours and lasts for 5–10 days.
- The typical features are hyperthermia, hypertonia of muscles, fluctuating levels of consciousness and instability of autonomic nervous system.
- Autonomic features include pallor, sweating, fluctuating blood pressure, tachycardia, urinary incontinence and cardiac arrhythmias.
- Death usually occurs between 3 and 30 days and is due to respiratory failure, cardiovascular collapse, renal failure and cardiac arrhythmias.

Laboratory Features

- Leucocytosis with shift to the left is common.
- Elevated liver enzymes and creatine kinase
- Myoglobinuria and acute renal failure

Treatment

- Management focuses on the withdrawal of neuroleptic agent and meticulous supportive care that includes aggressive hydration and reduction of body temperature.
- Dantrolene and bromocriptine (2.5–10 mg TID) have produced variable results.

■ HYPOTHERMIA

- **Definition:** Hypothermia is defined as a core temperature below 35°C (95°F).
  - **Mild hypothermia:** Core temperature 32–35°C (90–95°F)
  - **Moderate hypothermia:** Core temperature 28–32°C (82–90°F)
  - **Severe hypothermia:** Core temperature below 28°C (82°F)
- **Primary hypothermia** happens because of overwhelming cold exposure. Heat production in itself is normal.
- **Secondary hypothermia:** Hypothyroidism, Addison's disease, malnutrition, burns, hypothalamic abnormalities, sepsis, thiamine deficiency, alcohol intoxication, hypoglycaemia, etc.

Clinical Symptoms of Hypothermia

Clinical symptoms of hypothermia are given in **Table 23.1**.

- **Electrocardiographic changes**—Prolongation of all the ECG intervals, including RR, PR, QRS and QT. Elevation of the J point (only if the ST segment is unaltered), producing a characteristic J or Osborn wave

TABLE 23.1: Clinical symptoms of hypothermia (HT).

Mild (HT I)	Moderate (HT II)	Severe (HT III)	Severe (HT IV)	Death (HT V)
• Estimated core temperature 32–35°C (90–95°F) • Normal mental status with shivering. • Increased metabolic rate • Maximum shivering thermogenesis, 'cold diuresis' • Amnesia/dysarthria/ataxia • Loss of coordination • Tachycardiac, tachypnoeic	• Estimated core temperature 28–32°C (82–90°F) • Altered mental status without shivering • Stupor • No shivering • Bradycardiac/atrial fibrillation • Decreased BP and RR • Pupils dilated (< 30°C)	• Estimated core temperature 24–28°C (75–82°F) • Unconscious.	• Core temperature 13.7–24°C (56.7–75°F) (resuscitation may be possible) • Apparent death • Coma • No corneal or oculocephalic reflexes • Decreased BP • Ventricular fibrillation (Maximum risk: 22°C) • Apnoea • Asystole • Areflexia/fixed pupils • Flat EEG (19°C)	• Core temperature < 9 to 13.7°C (48.2–56.7°F) (resuscitation not possible) • Due to irreversible hypothermia.

(BP: blood pressure; EEG: electroencephalogram)

Management

Methods of active external and internal rewarming are given in **Table 23.2**.

■ DROWNING (SUBMERSION INJURIES)

Drowning

Asphyxiation caused by submersion in a liquid that causes interruption of the body's oxygen absorption

Near-drowning

The term was formerly used to describe victim's survival at least 24 hours after submersion.

Wet Drowning

Aspiration of water into airways and lungs (85%)—1–3 cc of aspirated water will lead to destruction of surfactant, alveolar instability, non-cardiogenic pulmonary oedema and impaired gas exchange.

Dry Drowning

- Severe parasympathetically mediated laryngospasm (15%)
- **Signs and Symptoms:** About 70% develop signs within 7 hours.
  - **Pulmonary:** Fluid aspiration results in varying degrees of hypoxaemia, non-cardiogenic pulmonary oedema—acute respiratory distress syndrome (ARDS).
  - **Neurologic:** Hypoxaemia and ischaemia cause neuronal damage, which can produce cerebral oedema and elevations in intracranial pressure which can progress into hypoxic ischaemic encephalopathy.
  - **Cardiovascular:** Arrhythmias secondary to hypothermia and hypoxaemia such as sinus tachycardia, sinus bradycardia and atrial fibrillation.
  - **Acid-base and electrolytes:** A metabolic and/or respiratory acidosis is often observed.
  - **Renal:** Renal failure due to acute tubular necrosis resulting from hypoxaemia, shock, haemoglobinuria or myoglobinuria is rare.

Management

- Includes pre-hospital care, emergency department (ED) care and inpatient care
- Ventilation is the most important initial treatment of submersion injury.
- Standard cardiopulmonary resuscitation (CPR) protocol needs to be followed.
- Identify spine injuries and other major organ injuries and manage accordingly.
- Supportive care: Renal failure, shock, infections, etc.

■ RADIATION EXPOSURE

Classification and Types of Radiation Effects

The classification of radiation effects is given in **Figure 23.1** and the types of radiation effects are shown in **Figure 23.2**.

■ ILLNESSES AT HIGH ALTITUDE

Acute Mountain Sickness

- Acute mountain sickness (AMS) is a syndrome characterised by headache, fatigue, anorexia,

TABLE 23.2: Methods of active external rewarming and active internal (core) rewarming.

Active external rewarming	Active internal (core) rewarming
• Heat to body surfaces • Heating blankets (fluid-filled) • Air blankets • Radiant warmers • Immersion in hot bath • Water bottles/heating pads • Less effective than internal rewarming, if vasoconstricted. Concern about after drop • Rewarming rates: 1–2.5°C/h	• Warm IV fluids • Warm, humid oxygen • Peritoneal lavage • Gastric/oesophageal lavage • Bladder/rectal lavage • Pleural/mediastinal lavage • Microwaves (diathermy) • Extracorporeal circulatory rewarming

Classification of radiation effects

Effects on human body		Incubation period	Example	Mechanism of how radiation effects appear
Categories of effects	Physical effects	Within several weeks = Acute effects (early effects)	Acute radiation syndromes* / Acute skin disease	Deterministic effects caused by cell deaths or cell degeneration†
		After the lapse of several months = Late effects	Abnormal foetal development (malformation)	
			Opacity of the lens	
			Cancer and leukaemia	Stochastic effects due to mutation
	Hereditary effects		Hereditary disorders	

*: Major symptoms are vomiting within several hours after exposure, diarrhoea continuing for several days to several weeks, decrease of the number of blood cells, bleeding, hair loss, transient male sterility, etc.
†: Deterministic effects do not appear unless having been exposed to radiation exceeding a certain dose level.

Fig. 23.1: Classification of radiation effects.

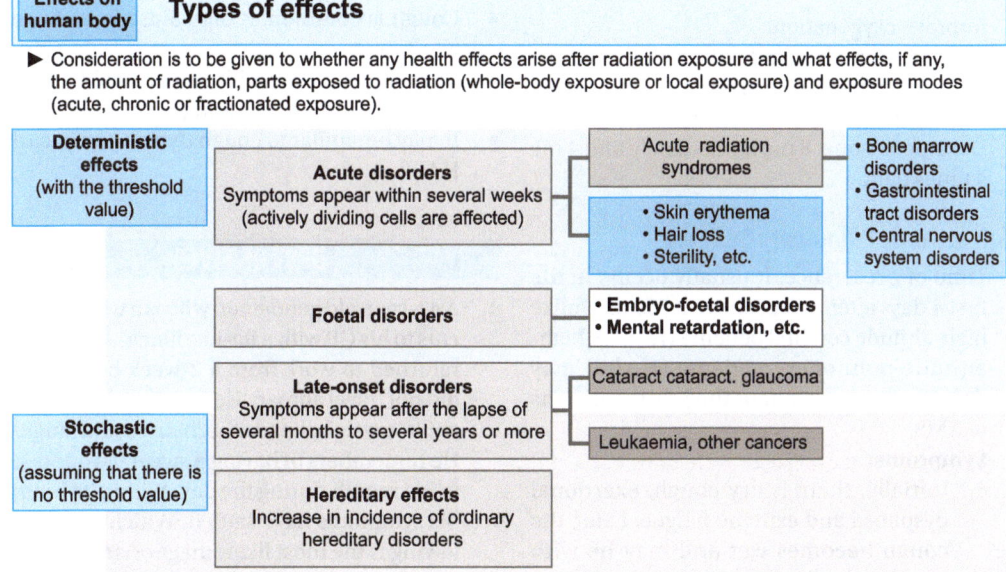

Fig. 23.2: Types of radiation effects.

nausea and vomiting, difficulty in sleeping or dizziness.
- Ataxia and peripheral oedema may be present.
- Symptoms develop within 6–12 hours of an ascent and vary in severity from trivial to completely incapacitating.

Treatment
- Mild cases require rest and simple analgesics.
- Acetazolamide (carbonic anhydrase inhibitor) that produces a metabolic acidosis and stimulates ventilation

Chronic Mountain Sickness (Monge's Disease)
- It occurs on long exposure to high altitude.
- **Symptoms:** Headache, poor concentration and signs of polycythaemia
- **Physical examination:** Cyanosis and clubbing of fingers

High-altitude Cerebral Oedema
- **Symptoms:** Ataxia and altered consciousness. In addition to features of AMS, the patient also develops confusion, disorientation, visual disturbance, lethargy and can lead to loss of consciousness.
- **Signs:** Papilloedema and retinal haemorrhages are common. Focal neurological signs may be detected.

Treatment
- Improve oxygenation.
- Descent is needed, and if descent is not possible, oxygen therapy in a portable pressurised bag is useful.
- Dexamethasone: 8 mg immediately and 4 mg 4 times daily

High-altitude Pulmonary Oedema
- Time of occurrence: It usually occurs in the first 4 days after ascent above 2,500 m. Unlike high-altitude cerebral oedema (HACE), high-altitude pulmonary oedema (HAPE) may develop de novo without the preceding signs of AMS.
- **Symptoms:**
  - Initially, there is dry cough, exertional dyspnoea and extreme fatigue. Later, the cough becomes wet and may be with blood-stained sputum.
  - Tachycardia and tachypnoea develop at rest. Crepitations may be heard in bilateral lung fields. Severe hypoxaemia and pulmonary hypertension may develop.

Treatment
- Reversal of hypoxia with immediate descent and oxygen administration.
- Nifedipine (20 mg 4 times daily) is given to reduce pulmonary arterial pressure.
- If there is a delay in descent, oxygen therapy in a portable pressurised bag should be given.

High-altitude Retinal Haemorrhage
- It may be found in about 30% of trekkers at 5,000 m and is usually asymptomatic and resolve spontaneously.
- Visual defects can develop when the haemorrhage involves the macula.
- There is no specific treatment.

Venous Thrombosis
- It can develop at altitudes over 6,000 m.
- Risk factors are dehydration, inactivity, cold and use of oral contraceptive pill at high altitude.

Refractory Cough
- Cough is common at high altitude and usually benign.
- Causes include breathing of dry, cold air and increased mouth breathing.
- It may be similar to cough that occurs in early HAPE.

BEST OF FIVES

1. A 42-year-old gentleman who is a welder presents to his GP with a flu-like illness. He has just returned to work from a 2-week holiday. He did not travel abroad. He presented with fever, chills, myalgia, headache, nausea and fatigue. He remembers of having a sweet flavour taste in his mouth during the day. Within 24 hours, his symptoms have settled. Which of the following is the most likely diagnosis?
   A. Common cold
   B. Extrinsic allergic alveolitis
   C. Influenzae A
   D. Influenzae B
   E. Metal fume fever

2. Which of the following food poisoning bacteria is transferred to food by coughing and sneezing?
   A. *Bacillus cereus*
   B. *Salmonella*
   C. *Staphylococcus aureus*
   D. *Clostridium perfringens*
   E. *Escherichia coli*

3. Stochastic effects of radiation exposure include:
   A. Carcinogenicity
   B. Anaemia
   C. Hypothyroidism
   D. Hair loss
   E. Pigmentation

4. The most sensitive indicator of radiation-induced haematopoietic toxicity is:
   A. Neutrophilia
   B. Neutropaenia
   C. Lymphopaenia
   D. Eosinophilia
   E. Anaemia

5. Above 2,500 m, high-altitude illnesses may develop in healthy individuals, and above 3,500 m symptoms commonly develop. Diseases commonly include all except:
   A. Retinal haemorrhage
   B. Pulmonary oedema
   C. Anaemia
   D. Venous thrombosis
   E. Cerebral oedema

6. Osborn J wave on electrocardiogram (ECG) is classically seen in cases of:
   A. Hyperkalaemia
   B. Hypocalcaemia
   C. Hypothermia
   D. Hyponatraemia
   E. Hypercalcaemia

7. Seawater can produce life-threatening electrolyte disturbances which include:
   A. Hypernatraemia, hypermagnesaemia and hypercalcaemia
   B. Hyponatraemia, hyperkalaemia and acidosis
   C. Hypocalcaemia, hypomagnesaemia and hyperphosphataemia
   D. Hyperuricaemia, hypokalaemia and hypocalcaemia
   E. Hypokalaemia, hypocalcaemia and alkalosis

8. Clinical features of heat stroke include all except:
   A. Hyperpyrexia (core temperature > 40°C)
   B. Hot dry skin
   C. Dilated pupils
   D. Tachycardia
   E. Delirium

9. Secondary hypothermia is seen in all the following conditions except:
   A. Hypothyroidism
   B. Addison's disease
   C. Sepsis
   D. Alcohol intoxication
   E. Hyperglycaemia

10. Poor prognostic signs in drowning include all except:
    A. Duration of submersion > 5 minutes
    B. Time to effective basic life support > 10 minutes
    C. Resuscitation duration > 25 minutes
    D. Glasgow coma scale < 5 (i.e. comatose)
    E. Arterial blood pH > 7.1 upon presentation

Answers

1-E, 2-C, 3-A, 4-C, 5-C, 6-C, 7-A, 8-C, 9-E, 10-E

SUGGESTED READING

1. Larach MG, Gronert GA, Allen GC, Brandom BW, Lehman EB. Clinical presentation, treatment, and complications of malignant hyperthermia in North America from 1987 to 2006. Anesth Analg. 2010;110(2):498-507.
2. Laskowski LK, Landry A, Vassallo SU, Hoffman RS. Ice water submersion for rapid cooling in severe drug-induced hyperthermia. Clin Toxicol (Phila). 2015;53(3):181-4.
3. Näyhä S. Environmental temperature and mortality. Int J Circumpolar Health. 2005;64(5):451-8.
4. Centers for Disease Control and Prevention (CDC). Hypothermia-related deaths--United States, 2003-2004. MMWR Morb Mortal Wkly Rep. 2005;54(7):173-5.
5. Headdon WG, Wilson PM, Dalton HR. The management of accidental hypothermia. BMJ. 2009;338:b2085.
6. Wolbarst AB, Wiley AL Jr, Nemhauser JB, Christensen DM, Hendee WR. Medical response to a major radiologic emergency: a primer for medical and public health practitioners. Radiology. 2010;254(3):660-77.
7. Bushberg JT, Kroger LA, Hartman MB, Leidholdt EM, Miller KL, Derlet R, et al. Nuclear/radiological terrorism: emergency department management of radiation casualties. J Emerg Med. 2007;32(1):71-85.
8. Roach RC, Lawley JS, Hackett PH. High-altitude physiology. In: Auerbach PS (Ed). Wilderness Medicine, 7th edition, Philadelphia: Elsevier; 2017. p. 2.

CHAPTER 24

Toxicology

■ TOXIDROMES

Various toxidromes and their related findings are given in **Table 24.1**.

■ TREATMENT OF A PATIENT WITH POISONING

Removing Unabsorbed Poison from Gut
- Syrup of Ipecac
- Gastric lavage
- Cathartics
- Activated charcoal
- Whole bowel irrigation: Isotonic solution of polyethylene glycol-electrolytes.

Enhancement of Excretion of Toxin
- Forced diuresis
- Multiple-dose activated charcoal
- Peritoneal and haemodialysis, haemoperfusion, haemofiltration

TABLE 24.1: Various toxidromes and related findings.

Toxidrome	Vital signs	Mental status	Pupils	Other findings	Examples
Anticholinergic	Hyperthermia, tachycardia, hypertensive, tachypnoea	Hyperthermia, agitated, hallucinating	Mydriasis	Dry flushed skin, urinary retention	Antihistamine, TCAs, atropine, scopolamine, antispasmodic
Cholinergic	Bradycardia (muscarinic), tachycardia and hypertension (nicotinic)	Confused, coma	Miosis	SLUDGE (Salivation, lacrimation, urination, diarrhoea, GI upset, emesis)	Organophosphate, pesticides, nerve agents, physostigmine
Hallucinogen	Hyperthermia, tachycardia, hypertension	Hallucination, synaesthesia, agitation	Mydriasis	Nystagmus	PCP (phencyclidine), LSD (lysergic and diethylamide), mescaline
Opioid	Hypothermia, bradycardia, hypotension, bradypnoea	CNS depression, coma	Miosis	Hyporeflexia, pulmonary oedema	Opioids (heroin, morphine, methadone, dilaudid, etc.)
Sedative-hypnotic	Hyperthermia, bradycardia, hypotension, bradypnoea	CNS depression, confusion, coma	Miosis	Hyporeflexia	Benzodiazepines, barbiturates, alcohols

Continued

Continued

Toxidrome	Vital signs	Mental status	Pupils	Other findings	Examples
Serotonin syndrome	Hyperthermia, tachycardia, hypertension, tachycardia	Confused, agitated coma	Mydriasis	Tremor, myoclonus, diaphoresis, hyperreflexia, trisum, rigidity	MAOIs, SSRIs, meperidine, dextromethorphan
Sympatho-mimetic	Hyperthermia, tachycardia, tachypnoea	Agitated hyperalert, paranoia	Mydriasis	Diaphoresis, tremors, hyperreflexia, seizures	Cocaine, amphetamine, pseudoephedrine

(MAOIs: monoamine oxidase inhibitors, SSRIs: selective serotonin reuptake inhibitors or serotonin specific reuptake inhibitors; TCAs: tricyclic antidepressants)

Specific Therapy
Antidotes
Different poisons and their antidotes are given in **Table 24.2**.

■ POISONOUS SNAKES
Clinical Manifestations
Bites by Elapidae (Cobras, Kraits)
- Neurotoxic effects
- Local pain and swelling are frequent in cobra bites. Krait bites are painless and without any local swelling.
- Paralysis—ptosis and external ophthalmoplegia. The palate, jaws, tongue, vocal cords, neck muscle and muscles of deglutition become paralysed.
- Respiratory failure due to paralysis of intercostal muscle and diaphragm

Bites by Viperidae (Vipers)
- In general, the Viperidae venoms are best known for their severe local manifestations and haemotoxic effects.
- There is local swelling, which spreads rapidly.
- Bruising, blistering and necrosis are very common. Necrosis, especially if it occurs in tight fascial compartments such as digits and anterior tibial compartment.
- Haemostatic abnormalities are characteristic resulting in bleeding.
- Acute renal failure

Bites by Hydrophidae (Sea Snakes)
- Sea snakes produce myotoxicity that produces muscle pains, muscle weakness and rhabdomyolysis producing myoglobinuria.

TABLE 24.2: Antidotes to different poisons.

Antidotes	Poison
Atropine	Cholinesterase inhibitors (organophosphates, carbamates)
2-PAM	Organophosphates
Naloxone	Opioids
Dextrose	Hypoglycaemic agents
Sodium bicarbonate	Tricyclic antidepressants
Methylene blue	Methaemoglobinaemia-producing agents
Ethanol	Methanol, ethylene glycol
Snake antivenom	Snake bites
Desferrioxamine	Iron
BAL (Dimercaprol)	Lead, arsenic, mercury
D-Penicillamine	Mercury, lead, arsenic
2,3-dimercaptosuccinic acid	Lead, mercury, arsenic
Fomepizole (4-MP)	Methanol, ethylene glycol
N-acetylcysteine	Paracetamol
Flumazenil	Benzodiazepines
Glucagon	β-blockers, calcium channel blockers

(2-PAM: 2-pyridine aldoxime methyl chloride; BAL: British anti-Lewisite)

- Cardiac involvement can occur due to release of potassium (hyperkalaemia) from necrosed muscles.

Investigations
- Total leucocyte count exceeding 20,000/mm^3 indicates severe envenomation.

- Anaemia results from bleeding, and rarely haemolysis.
- Thrombocytopaenia in viper bites
- Pink plasma and black urine indicate intravascular haemolysis.
- Urine shows red blood cells, red cell casts, protein and myoglobin.
- **20-minute whole blood clotting test** and clot quality test are useful. Incoagulable blood at 20 minutes indicates systemic envenomation.

Management

Hospital Treatment
- Maintain circulation, airway and breathing.
- Clean the site of bite and elevate it to reduce local oedema.
  Antivenom treatment
  Indications for antivenom

Signs of systemic envenomation as indicated by:
- Impaired consciousness
- Neurotoxicity
- Hypotension and shock, abnormal electrocardiogram (ECG)
- Haemostatic abnormalities: Spontaneous systemic bleeding/coagulopathy.
- Evidences of intravascular haemolysis
- Evidences of renal failure
  Polyspecific (polyvalent) antivenom available in India—against the four common varieties of snakes, i.e., cobra, krait, Russell's viper and saw-scaled viper.

There are two types of reactions: an early (anaphylactoid) reaction and a late (serum sickness type) reaction. These reactions are treated with adrenaline 0.5–1.0 mL subcutaneously (may be repeated). Chlorpheniramine maleate 10 mg intravenously and hydrocortisone 100 mg intravenously.

Cholinergics
- Cholinergic agents are useful in patients with neurotoxic features, particularly cobra bite.
- Neostigmine along with atropine.

Supportive Therapy
- Respiratory paralysis should be treated by artificial ventilation.
- Hypotension and shock should be treated with fresh whole blood or fresh frozen plasma, dopamine and hydrocortisone.
- Oliguria and renal failure should be treated conservatively, failing which dialysis should be done.
- Local infection should be prevented by antibiotics covering gram-negative organisms and anaerobes. All patients should receive anti-tetanus prophylaxis.
- At a later stage, some patients may require surgical debridement, skin grafting or fasciotomy.

■ TOXICITY CAUSED BY SCORPION STINGS

- The poisonous scorpions of India include the red scorpion (Mesobuthus) and the black scorpion (Palamnaeus).
- The glands in the terminal segment of the tail produce venom that is injected by a stinger.

Clinical Features

The clinical features of envenomation develop within 2–12 hours of sting by a poisonous scorpion.

Local Features
- Sting may be followed by the onset of intense pain at the site within several minutes.
- Often there is intense pain with mild palpation or tapping over the site (the 'tap test'). Pain or numbness may radiate up the extremity.

Systemic Features
- Initial features are due to **transient cholinergic hyperactivity** (restlessness, anxiety, vomiting, profuse sweating, salivation, sensation of tongue thickening, dysphagia, bradycardia, hypotension and priapism)→ followed by **sustained adrenergic hyperactivity** (resulting in hypertension, tachycardia, chest discomfort, cold extremities and myocardial failure).
- In late stages, hypotension and shock develop.
- Electrocardiographic features suggestive of myocarditis may be present.

Management
- Mild analgesics for relieving pain
- Correction of fluid deficit; avoid large amount of fluids without proper monitoring because of the risk of pulmonary oedema.
- Prazosin (0.25–0.5 mg every 4–6 h) to control hypertension. It is an antidote for scorpion stings. An alternative is to give nifedipine.

- Dopamine infusion for hypotension
- Glucose–insulin infusion may be beneficial in systemic envenomation.

■ ORGANOPHOSPHORUS AND CARBAMATE POISONING

Clinical Features
- Organophosphorus compounds produce muscarinic, nicotinic and central nervous system (CNS) effects.
- Carbamates produce a similar clinical picture but of shorter duration and lower order of toxicity.

Muscarinic Manifestations
- **D**iarrhoea, **U**rination, **M**iosis (small pupils), **B**radycardia, **E**mesis, **L**acrimation, **L**ethargy, and **S**alivation (DUMBELLS)
- Nausea, vomiting, abdominal pain and faecal incontinence
- Increased bronchial secretions, cough and occasionally pulmonary oedema
- Excessive sweating, salivation and lacrimation
- Blurring of vision and miosis
- Increased urinary frequency and incontinence
- Bradycardia, hypotension and conduction blocks

Nicotinic Manifestations
Twitching, fasciculations, weakness, diminished respiratory effort, hypertension and tachycardia

Central Nervous System Manifestations
Anxiety, restlessness, tremors, convulsions, confusion, weakness and coma

Intermediate Syndrome
- Syndrome of muscular paralysis, 24–96 hours after ingestion of an organophosphate and following treatment of acute cholinergic syndrome.
- Predominantly neck flexors, proximal limb muscles, those supplied by cranial nerves and respiratory muscles are involved.

Diagnosis
- Diagnosis of organophosphorus poisoning can be confirmed by demonstrating a reduction of cholinesterase activity in plasma or in red blood cells, to < 50% of normal.
- With carbamates reduction of cholinesterase level is rare because of the rapid reversibility of inhibition.

Management
General Measures
- Remove the patient from the site of exposure and wash the skin with soap and water.
- In the case of ingestion, gastric lavage should be done if the patient presents within the first 1 hour of ingestion.
- Activated charcoal is given orally.
- Meticulous care of the airway along with oxygenation is important. If there is respiratory insufficiency, the patient should be ventilated.
- Benzodiazepines for convulsions. They also reduce morbidity and mortality even in the absence of convulsions.

Specific Measures
- Atropine
- Pralidoxime (2-PAM)

■ ALUMINIUM PHOSPHIDE POISONING

Clinical Features
- Initial features include retrosternal burning, epigastric discomfort and recurrent vomiting and diarrhoea.
- Fishy smell from breath
- Next 6–8 hours—systemic features

Cardiovascular Features
- Important cardiovascular features are hypotension, shock, tachycardia or bradycardia and arrhythmias.
- Shock occurs because of cardiotoxicity, recurrent vomiting and widespread vascular injury.
- A few patients may develop congestive heart failure due to myocardial depression.

Respiratory Features

Cough, dyspnoea, cyanosis, pulmonary oedema and acute respiratory distress syndrome (ARDS)

Metabolic Features

Hypo- or hypermagnesaemia and metabolic acidosis are common.

Management

- Perform a gastric lavage using potassium permanganate.
- Activated charcoal also adsorbs phosphine.
- Adequate ventilation and urine output help to maintain adequate excretion of phosphine.
- Supportive care is the most important step in the management.

■ BARBITURATE POISONING

Clinical Features

- In large overdose, there is:
  o CNS depression ranging from lethargy to coma
  o Hypotension, pulmonary oedema and cardiac arrest
  o Hypothermia
  o Respiratory depression
  o Pupils are usually constricted but may dilate in terminal phases.
  o Bullous skin lesions may be seen with severe overdose.

Management

- Prompt gastrointestinal decontamination should be done by lavage. Repeated oral administration of activated charcoal 2–4 hourly is very effective.
- Alkalinisation of urine (without diuresis) is effective in Phenobarbital poisoning. It enhances renal excretion of Phenobarbital.
- Haemodialysis is effective in removing long-acting barbiturates.

■ METHANOL POISONING

Clinical Features

- Nausea, vomiting, abdominal pain, headache, vertigo, obtundation, convulsions and coma

- Late manifestations: Metabolic acidosis and retinal injury. The ophthalmologic manifestations include:
  o Clouding and diminished vision
  o Dancing and flashing spots
  o Hyperaemia of the optic disc
  o Retinal oedema and blindness

Management

- Gastrointestinal decontamination in early stages
- Correction of systemic acidosis with sodium bicarbonate
- Ethanol therapy is indicated in patients with visual symptoms or methanol level exceeding 20–30 mg/dL.
- Haemodialysis is indicated for:
  o Patients with methanol level exceeding 50 mg/dL
  o Patients with visual signs
  o Patients with metabolic acidosis unresponsive to bicarbonate
- Potent antidote of methanol poisoning is **4-methylpyrazole or fomepizole**.
- Folinic acid (leucovorin) is given in addition.

■ SALICYLATE POISONING

Children are more vulnerable in comparison to adults.

In adults, plasma salicylates level above 50 mg/dL indicate moderate-to-severe poisoning.

- The characteristic features are:
  o Tinnitus
  o Deafness
  o Blurring of vision
- Other features include:
  o Hyperventilation resulting in respiratory alkalosis, severe dehydration and hypokalaemia.
- The initial respiratory alkalosis is later followed by metabolic acidosis. Marked acidosis is regarded as a very serious feature as it may herald sudden respiratory or cardiac arrest.

Management

- General measures including gastric lavage and activated charcoal.

- Alkalinisation of urine in moderate or severe poisoning
- Peritoneal dialysis or haemodialysis may be required in severe cases.

PARACETAMOL (ACETAMINOPHEN) POISONING

- Toxicity unlikely to result from a single dose of < 150 mg/kg in a child or 7.5–10 g in an adult.
- Toxicity is likely with single ingestions > 250 mg/kg or those > 12 g over a 24-hour period.

Acetaminophen metabolism is shown in **Figure 24.1**.

Clinical Manifestations of Toxicity

- Stage I (0.5–24 h): No symptoms; nausea, vomiting and malaise.
- Stage II (24–72 h):
    - Subclinical elevations of hepatic aminotransferases [aspartate aminotransferase (AST), alanine aminotransferase (ALT)].
    - Right upper quadrant pain, with liver enlargement and tenderness. Elevations of prothrombin time (PT), total bilirubin, and oliguria and renal function abnormalities may become evident. Acute kidney injury is due primarily to acute tubular necrosis.
- Stage III (72–96 h): Fulminant hepatic failure; Jaundice, confusion (hepatic encephalopathy), a marked elevation in hepatic enzymes, hyperammonaemia, bleeding diathesis, hypoglycaemia, lactic acidosis, renal failure (25%) and death.
- Stage IV (4 days to 2 weeks): Recovery phase that usually begins by day 4 and is complete by 7 days after overdose.

Treatment

- Activated charcoal: Single oral dose of 1 g/kg.
- Gastric lavage: Only for massive ingestions (e.g., > 600 mg/kg).
- Antidote: **N-acetylcysteine (NAC)**
    - MOA: A glutathione precursor.
    - Limits the formation and accumulation of N-acetyl-p-benzoquinone imine (NAPQI).
    - Powerful anti-inflammatory and antioxidant effects:
        - IV infusion—150 mg/kg over 15 minutes; 50 mg/kg over the next 4 hours; 100 mg/kg over the next 16 hours up to 36 hours.
        - Oral NAC treatment regimen consists of a 72 hours oral course given as a 140 mg/kg loading dose followed by 17 doses of 70 mg/kg every 4 hours (total dose 1330 mg/kg).
- Alternate medication: Oral methionine.
- Liver transplantation: It is life-saving for fulminant hepatic necrosis.

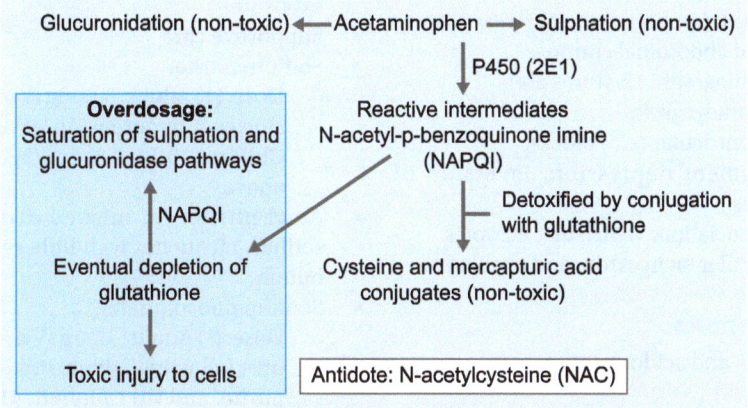

Fig. 24.1: Acetaminophen metabolism.

MUSHROOM POISONING

Ingestion of *Amanita phalloides* ('death cap'). It contains two types of toxins, both of which are heat stable and survive cooking.
1. 'Phallotoxins' causing severe gastroenteritis within 6–12 hours of ingestion
2. 'Amatoxins' causing delayed liver and renal tubular damage.

Management
- Gastric lavage
- Maintenance of fluid and electrolyte balance
- Penicillin and silymarin—inhibit uptake of amatoxin by hepatocytes.
- Otherwise, management is supportive and includes treatment of hepatic and renal failure.

OLEANDER POISONING

- Ingestion of yellow oleander (*Thevetia peruviana*) is toxic.
- Oleander plant contains glycosides that resemble digitoxin, a cardiac glycoside. These include thevetins A and B, and neriifolin.
- All parts contain the toxin, but the maximum amount is in the seeds.

Clinical Features
- It starts within 2–3 hours of ingestion.
- Gastrointestinal irritation produces nausea, vomiting, diarrhoea and abdominal pain.
- Other features include dizziness, papillary dilatation, tingling and numbness, restlessness, arrhythmias, hypotension, nervous system toxicity and abdominal cramps.
- Electrocardiographic features are:
  - Sinus bradycardia
  - Atrioventricular (AV) blocks
  - ST-segment depression, inversion of T waves
  - AV dissociation, ventricular ectopics
  - Ventricular tachycardia and fibrillation

Laboratory Features
Hyperkalaemia and acidosis.

Treatment
- Correction of fluid, electrolyte and acid-base disturbances
- Repeated dose of activated charcoal
- Atropine and pacing for bradycardia-related arrhythmias
- Lidocaine for ventricular tachyarrhythmias
- Digoxin-specific Fab antibody fragments may be tried.

CYANIDE POISONING

- Onset of cyanide poisoning—inhalation (rapid onset, seconds to minutes), ingestion and skin contact (delayed onset, 15–30 min)
- Death may occur within 6–8 minutes after inhalation of a high concentration. 2–5 mg/kg of it is lethal.
- Mechanism: Inhibits mitochondrial cytochrome oxidase and acts as 'asphyxiating' agent.

Clinical Features
- Metabolic acidosis: Non-specific symptoms.
- CNS: Dizziness, nausea, vomiting, drowsiness, tetanus, trismus, hallucinations.
- CVS: Dysrhythmia, hypotension. Tachycardia and hypertension may occur transiently in early stages.
- Respiratory: Dyspnoea, initial hyperventilation followed by hypoventilation and pulmonary oedema. Cyanosis not apparent, since blood is adequately oxygenated.

Treatment
- Activated charcoal: For alert, asymptomatic patients following ingestion.
- Supplemental oxygen: 100% for suspected exposure.
- Supportive care
- Sodium nitrite:
  - Dose: (1) Adults: 300 mg IV over 5 minutes; slower if hypotension develops and (2) Children: 0.12–0.33 mg/kg IV infused as above.
- Amyl nitrite: An inhaled drug, similar to sodium nitrite but with little systemic distribution.
- Sodium thiosulphate:
  - Dose: (i) Adults: 12.5 g IV over 10–20 minutes following administration of sodium nitrite, and (ii) Children: 412.5 mg/kg IV over 10–20 minutes.
- Hydroxocobalamin
  - Dose: 4–5 g IV

CARBON MONOXIDE POISONING

It produces toxicity by binding with haemoglobin and cytochrome oxidase, which decreases the delivery of oxygen to tissue and inhibits cellular respiration.

Clinical Features

Acute severe carbon monoxide poisoning produces non-specific symptoms such as headache, nausea, irritability, weakness and tachypnoea. Later, ataxia, nystagmus, drowsiness and hyperreflexia may develop leading to coma, respiratory depression, cardiovascular collapse and death. Myocardial ischaemia/infarction, cerebral oedema and rhabdomyolysis (with myoglobinuria and renal failure) may occur. Long-term exposure can lead to Parkinsonism.

Treatment

Administration of normobaric 100% oxygen/hyperbaric oxygen (severe cases).

BEST OF FIVES

1. A young woman who has acutely ingested immediate-release acetaminophen tablets 10 hours ago has a serum acetaminophen concentration of 100 µg/mL. She has vomited several times in the past 2 hours. Which of the following would be appropriate?
   A. Start vitamin K
   B. No active intervention is needed
   C. Start N-acetylcysteine
   D. Start on flumazenil
   E. Plan haemodialysis

2. A person is brought by police from the railway platform. He is talking irrelevant. He is having dry mouth with hot skin, dilated pupils, staggering gait and slurred speech. The most probable diagnosis is:
   A. Alcohol intoxication
   B. Carbamates poisoning
   C. Organophosphorous poisoning
   D. Datura poisoning
   E. Opioid poisoning

3. In methyl alcohol poisoning, there is central nervous system depression, cardiac depression and optic nerve atrophy. These effects are produced due to:
   A. Formaldehyde and formic acid
   B. Acetaldehyde
   C. Pyridine
   D. Acetic acid
   E. Cyanides

4. A farmer has taken arrack from the local shop. After about an hour, he develops confusion, vomiting and blurring of vision. He has been brought to the emergency department. He should be given:
   A. Naloxone
   B. Diazepam
   C. Atropine
   D. Flumazenil
   E. Ethyl alcohol

5. A housewife ingests a rodenticide white powder accidentally. She is brought to the hospital where the examination shows generalised, flaccid paralysis and an irregular pulse. Electrocardiogram shows multiple ventricular ectopics and generalised changes with ST-T. Serum potassium is 2.5 mEq/L. The most likely ingested poison is:
   A. Barium carbonate
   B. Superwarfarins
   C. Zinc phosphide
   D. Aluminium phosphide
   E. Paraquat

6. Hyperthermia in a patient of poisoning is a pointer to all except:
   A. Ecstasy
   B. Selective serotonin reuptake inhibitor
   C. Salicylates
   D. Chlorpromazine
   E. Barbiturates

7. Ophitoxaemia refers to:
   A. Organophosphorous poisoning
   B. Heavy metal poisoning
   C. Carbamate poisoning
   D. Scorpion venom poisoning
   E. Snake venom poisoning

8. A 30-year-old farmer had an alleged history of snakebite and presented to the hospital with inability to open eyes well and difficulty in breathing. He is very anxious and is having tachycardia and tachypnoea. On examination, the bite mark cannot be visualised and there is no swelling of the limb. He has bilateral ptosis. His 20-minute whole blood clotting test is of good quality. What is the next course of action?
   A. Do not give anti-snake venom (ASV), but observe the patient
   B. Give ASV and keep the patient in observation
   C. Give ASV and neostigmine and observe the patient
   D. Reassure the patient and send him home with anxiolytic
   E. Start plasmapheresis

9. Regarding Amanita phylloides mushroom toxicity, which is false?
   A. Large doses of penicillin IV may be useful
   B. Silibinin, a milk thistle extract, may inhibit hepatic uptake of Amatoxin
   C. Multiple dose charcoal is indicated
   D. Haemoperfusion may be useful if utilised within 48 hours of ingestion
   E. Symptoms typically occur within the first 4 hours of ingestion

10. With regard to organophosphates and carbamates, which is false?
    A. Both inactivate acetyl cholinesterase
    B. Both cause an acute cholinergic syndrome
    C. Both respond to treatment with atropine
    D. Both respond to treatment with pralidoxime
    E. If there are associated central nervous system (CNS) signs and muscle weakness, the cause is likely to be organophosphates

11. Digoxin toxicity is potentiated by all except:
    A. Hypokalaemia
    B. Hypomagnesaemia
    C. Hypermagnesaemia
    D. Hypocalcaemia
    E. Hypothyroidism

12. Which of the following toxins does NOT cause a syndrome comprising mydriasis, thirst, tachycardia and urinary retention?
    A. Tricyclic antidepressants
    B. Trumpet lily
    C. Scopolamine
    D. Organophosphates
    E. Antihistamines

13. Regarding acute theophylline toxicity, the true statement is:
    A. Theophylline has very poor oral bioavailability
    B. Metabolic complications include hyperkalaemia and hypophosphataemia
    C. Elimination is not increased by haemodialysis
    D. Signs of minor toxicity usually manifest at serum concentrations from 220 to 440 µmol/L (20–40 mg/L)
    E. Phenytoin is the anticonvulsant of choice in seizures resulting from toxicity

14. Haemodialysis would increase the excretion of which of these toxic drugs?
    A. Tricyclics
    B. Benzodiazepines
    C. Digoxin
    D. Lithium
    E. Calcium channel blockers

15. A patient who has been taking a monoamine oxidase (MAO) inhibitor for years presents to the emergency department with hyperthermia, confusion, hypertension and diaphoresis. He has no known allergies/adverse reactions. Which of the following agents should NOT be used in his management?
    A. Diazepam
    B. Pethidine
    C. Chlorpromazine
    D. Cyproheptadine
    E. Methysergide

16. The safest and most efficacious therapy for cyanide poisoning is:
    A. Sodium thiosulphate
    B. Amyl nitrite
    C. Sodium nitrite
    D. Cobalt ethylenediamine tetra-acetic acid (EDTA)
    E. Hydroxycobalamin

17. The best predictor of serious toxicity in tricyclic antidepressants (TCA) poisoning is:

A. Drug plasma levels
B. Glasgow Coma Score (GCS) < 8
C. Estimates of ingested drug dose
D. Rightward deviation of the QRS vector
E. QRS duration of > 100 msec

18. All of the following substances bind well to activated charcoal except:
    A. Thioridazine
    B. Atenolol
    C. Cyanide
    D. Benztropine
    E. Tetrahydrocannabinol (THC)

19. With regard to management of warfarin toxicity, which is false?
    A. Any major bleeding should be managed with 5–10 mg intravenous (IV) vitamin K and fresh frozen plasma (FFP)
    B. The onset of action of IV vitamin K is 1–3 hours
    C. With an international normalised ratio (INR) of 13, if a patient has minor or no bleeding then FFP is still warranted
    D. If a prothrombin time has an INR of 13 with minimal bleeding, an appropriate IV dose of vitamin K would be 1–2 mg IV
    E. If vitamin K is given for a toxic INR with no major bleeding, then the INR should be checked in 6–12 hours, and the warfarin withheld for 1–2 days

20. Regarding iron overdoses, which is true?
    A. 95% of ingested tablets are seen on plain X-ray
    B. Large overdose will produce a metabolic acidosis with a normal anion gap
    C. Charcoal is the recommended method of gastrointestinal tract (GIT) decontamination in the first hour
    D. Deferoxamine when given will produce rose-coloured urine
    E. They have no local GIT irritating effects

Answers

1-C, 2-D, 3-A, 4-E, 5-A, 6-B, 7-E, 8-C, 9-E, 10-D, 11-D, 12-D, 13-D, 14-D, 15-B, 16-E, 17-B, 18-C, 19-C, 20-E

SUGGESTED READING

1. Mowry JB, Spyker DA, Brooks DE, McMillan N, Schauben JL. 2014 Annual Report of the American Association of Poison Control Centers' National Poison Data System (NPDS): 32nd Annual Report. Clin Toxicol (Phila). 2015;53(10):962-1147.
2. Gjersing L, Jonassen KV, Biong S, Ravndal E, Waal H, Bramness JG, et al. Diversity in causes and characteristics of drug-induced deaths in an urban setting. Scand J Public Health. 2013;41(2):119-25.
3. Erickson TB, Thompson TM, Lu JJ. The approach to the patient with an unknown overdose. Emerg Med Clin North Am. 2007;25(2):249-81.
4. Yates C, Manini AF. Utility of the electrocardiogram in drug overdose and poisoning: theoretical considerations and clinical implications. Curr Cardiol Rev. 2012;8(2):137-51.
5. Hammett-Stabler CA, Pesce AJ, Cannon DJ. Urine drug screening in the medical setting. Clin Chim Acta. 2002;315(1-2):125-35.
6. Mowry JB, Spyker DA, Brooks DE, Zimmerman A, Schauben JL. 2015 Annual Report of the American Association of Poison Control Centers' National Poison Data System (NPDS): 33rd Annual Report. Clin Toxicol (Phila). 2016;54(10):924-1109.
7. Chadwick A, Ash A, Day J, Borthwick M. Accidental overdose in the deep shade of night: a warning on the assumed safety of 'natural substances'. BMJ Case Rep. 2015; 2015.
8. Dawson AH, Buckley NA. Pharmacological management of anticholinergic delirium - theory, evidence and practice. Br J Clin Pharmacol. 2016;81(3):516-24.
9. Warrell DA. Envenoming and injuries by venomous and nonvenomous reptiles worldwide. In: Auerbach PS (Ed). Wilderness Medicine, 6th edition. Philadelphia: Elsevier Mosby; 2012. p. 1040.
10. Maduwage K, Buckley NA, de Silva HJ, Lalloo DG, Isbister GK. Snake antivenom for snake venom induced consumption coagulopathy. Cochrane Database Syst Rev. 2015;(6):CD011428.
11. Chiew AL, Gluud C, Brok J, Buckley NA. Interventions for paracetamol (acetaminophen) overdose. Cochrane Database Syst Rev. 2018;2(2):CD003328.

CHAPTER 25

Oncology

■ ONCOGENES

Oncogenes can promote cell growth in the absence of normal growth, promoting mitogenic signals (**Tables 25.1** and **25.2**).

TABLE 25.1: Examples of oncogenes and associated tumours.

Classification of oncogenes	Examples of associated tumours
Growth factors	
Platelet-derived growth factor (PDGF)	Non-small cell cancer of lung
Transforming growth factor alpha (TGF-α)	Hepatocellular cancer
Growth factor receptors	
Epidermal growth factor receptor (EGFR)	Lung and gastrointestinal tumours
Human epidermal growth factor receptor 2 (HER2/neu)	Breast cancer
Signal transducing proteins	
KRAS	Adenocarcinoma of colon, lung and pancreas
NRAS	Haematopoietic tumours, melanomas
ABL	Chronic myeloid leukaemia, acute lymphoblastic leukaemia
Nuclear-regulatory proteins/transcription factors	
C-MYC	Burkitt lymphoma
N-MYC	Neuroblastoma
Cell cycle regulators	
Cyclin D	Breast, oesophageal and liver cancers

Tumour suppressor genes apply brakes to cell proliferation and prevent uncontrolled/abnormal cell proliferation and induce repair or self-death (apoptosis). Important tumour suppressor genes are *RB, p53, BRCA1, and BRCA2* genes (**Table 25.3**).

■ TUMOUR MARKERS

Common tumour markers are given in **Table 25.4**.

■ CHEMOTHERAPEUTIC AGENTS

Various chemotherapeutic drugs and their mechanism are shown in **Figure 25.1**.

Cyclophosphamide

Cyclophosphamide and its uses are given in **Box 25.1**.

TABLE 25.2: Structural abnormalities associated with oncogenes.

Oncogene	Aberration	Neoplasm
abl	t(9;22)	CML, AML, ALL
myc	t(8;14)	Burkitt lymphoma, B-ALL, T-ALL
bcl-1, bcl-2	t(11;14)	B-cell lymphoma
tcl-1, tcl-2	t(11;14)	T-cell lymphoma
p53, erb-A, erb-B	t(15;17)	APML
mos, ets-2	t(8;21)	AML-M2
ets-l, sis	t(11;22)	Ewing's sarcoma
myc	t(3;8)	Renal cell carcinoma
myb	t(6;14)	Ovarian carcinoma

(CML: chronic myeloid leukaemia; AML: acute myeloid leukaemia; ALL: acute lymphoid leukaemia; APML: acute promyelocytic leukaemia)

TABLE 25.3: Few examples of tumour suppressor genes and tumours in which it is affected.

Gene (locus)	Function	Tumours in which gene is affected	
		Familial	Sporadic
DCC (18q)	Cell surface interaction	Not known	Colorectal cancer
Rb1 (13q)	Transcription	Retinoblastoma	Small cell carcinoma of lung
p53 (17p)	Transcription	Li-Fraumeni syndrome	Cancer of breast, colon and lung
BRCA1(17q)	Transcription	Carcinoma of breast	Carcinoma breast/ovary
BRCA2 (13q)	Regulator/DNA repair		
WT1 (11p)	Transcription	Wilms' tumour	Lung cancer

TABLE 25.4: Common tumour markers.

Tumour marker	Associated tumours
Enzymes	
• Alkaline phosphatase (ALP)	Hepatoma, secondaries in liver, ovarian, lung, gastrointestinal cancers and Hodgkin's disease
• Placental alkaline phosphatase (PLAP)	Seminoma
• Prostatic acid phosphatase (PAP)	Prostate carcinoma
• Neuron-specific enolase (NSE)	Small-cell carcinoma of lung, neuroblastoma
• Tartrate-resistant acid phosphatase (TRAP)	Hairy cell leukaemia
Hormones	
• Human chorionic gonadotropin (hCG)	Trophoblastic tumours, non-seminomatous tumours of testis
• Calcitonin	Medullary carcinoma of thyroid
• Catecholamine	Phaeochromocytoma
• Ectopic hormones	Paraneoplastic syndromes
Oncofetal antigens	
• α-Foetoprotein	Cancer of liver, non-seminomatous germ cell tumours of testis
• Carcinoembryonic antigen (CEA)	Carcinomas of the colon, pancreas, lung, and stomach. May also be elevated in cigarette smoking, peptic ulcer disease, inflammatory bowel disease, pancreatitis, hypothyroidism, cirrhosis and biliary obstruction
Carbohydrate markers/mucins and other glycoproteins	
• CA-125	Ovarian cancer
• CA 15–3	Breast carcinoma, pancreatic, lung, ovarian, colorectal and liver cancer in some benign breast and liver diseases
• CA 19–9	Pancreatic and colorectal cancer
Specific proteins	
• Immunoglobulins	Multiple myeloma and other gammopathies
• Prostate-specific antigen (PSA)	Prostate carcinoma. Other conditions include prostatitis, benign prostatic hypertrophy, prostatic trauma and after ejaculation
• Ferritin	Non-specific, Hodgkin lymphoma, leukaemia, liver, lung and breast cancer

Continued

Continued

Tumour marker	Associated tumours
• Thyroglobulin	Differentiated thyroid cancer
• S-100	Melanoma
• İnhibin A and B	Granulosa cell tumour
• Catalase, profilin 1, CD59	Oral squamous cell carcinoma
Receptor markers	
• Oestrogen and progesterone receptors	Breast cancer as indicators for hormonal therapy
• C-erbB2 (HER2/neu)	Co-receptor in epidermal growth factor action, overexpression associated with cancer
Genetic changes	
• Bcr-Abl mutation	Chronic myeloid leukaemia
New molecular markers	
• p53, APC, RAS mutants in stool and serum	Carcinoma of colon
• p53 and RAS mutants in sputum and serum	Lung cancer
Mitochondrial markers (mtDNA)	Carcinoma of breast, prostate, lung, thyroid, colon

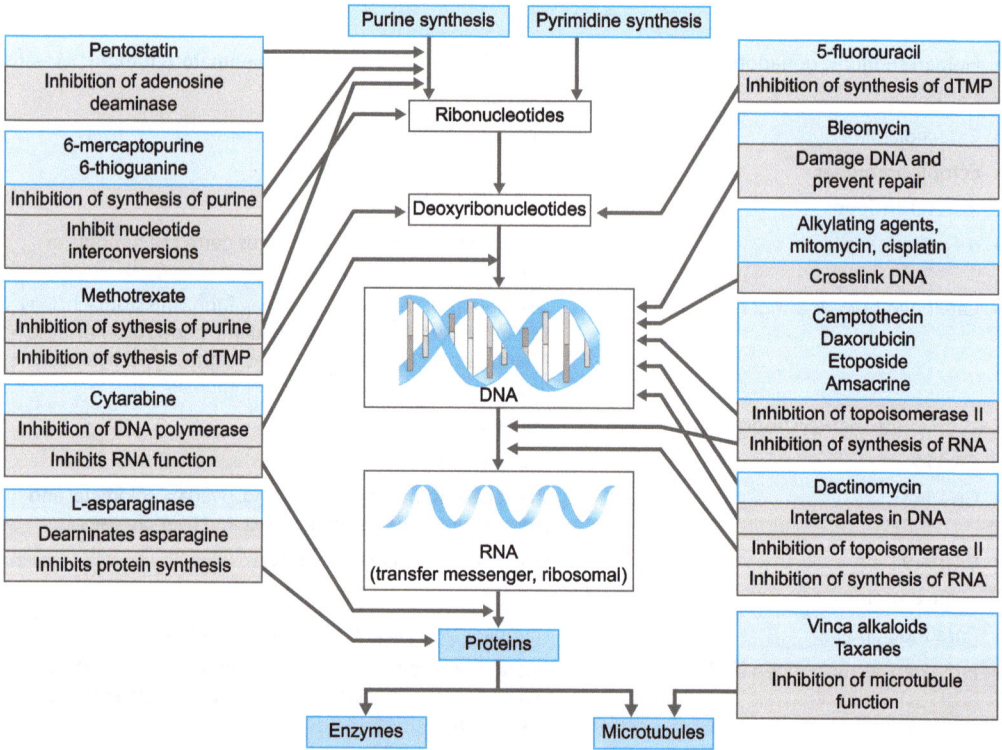

(dTMP: deoxythymidine monophosphate)

Fig. 25.1: Mechanism of action of various chemotherapeutic drugs.

Methotrexate

Methotrexate and its uses are given in **Box 25.2**.

Cisplatin

Cisplatin and its uses are given in **Box 25.3**.

TARGETED THERAPY IN CANCER PATIENTS

Common types of targeted therapies:
- Monoclonal antibodies (**Table 25.5**)
- Inhibitors of tyrosine kinases
- Inhibitors of proteasomes
- Immunotoxins
- Inhibitors of growth factor receptors

Box 25.2: Methotrexate and its uses.

- Uses
  - Choriocarcinoma
  - Leukaemias
  - Rheumatoid arthritis/connective tissue disorders
  - Psoriasis
- Toxicity
  - Hepatotoxicity
  - Bone marrow suppression
  - Megaloblastic anaemia
  - Ulcerative enteritis, ulcerative dermatitis
  - Pulmonary fibrosis
- Folinic acid (citrovorum factor) is used to antagonise the toxicity

---

Box 25.1: Cyclophosphamide and its uses.

- Uses
  - SLE, rheumatoid arthritis, Wegener's granulomatosis, PAN
  - Lymphomas
  - Leukaemias
- Toxicity
  - Alopecia
  - Bone marrow depression
  - Hepatotoxicity
  - Cystitis and bladder carcinoma
  - Severe cystitis can be treated by mercaptoethane sulphonate

(PAN: polyarteritis nodosa; SLE: systemic lupus erythematosus)

Box 25.3: Cisplatin and its uses.

- Uses
  - Sarcomas
  - Small cell cancer of lung
  - Ovarian carcinoma
  - Lymphoma
  - Germ cell tumours
  - Bladder carcinoma
  - Breast carcinoma
- Toxicity
  - Nausea and vomiting
  - Nephrotoxicity
  - Neurotoxicity
  - Ototoxicity
  - Alopecia

TABLE 25.5: Various monoclonal antibodies, their targets and cancers in which it is used.

Monoclonal antibodies	Target	Cancers
Alemtuzumab	CD52	CLL
Bevacizumab	VEGF	Colon, lung, breast, kidney, and brain
Cetuximab	EGFR1	Colon, H and N
Panitumumab	EGFR1	Colon
Rituximab	CD20	Lymphomas
Trastuzumab	HER2	Breast
Olaparib, rucaparib	PARP	Ovary
Onartuzumab, emibetuzumab	HGF/c-Met	Non-small cell lung cancer
Ipilimumab	CTLA4	Unresectable melanoma
Nivolumab, pembrolizumab	PD-1	Refractory non-small cell lung cancer

(EGFR: epidermal growth factor receptor ; VEGF: vascular endothelial growth factor; PARP: Poly ADP ribose polymerase; CTLA4: cytotoxic T-lymphocyte-associated protein 4; HER2: human epidermal growth factor receptor 2; CLL: chronic lymphocytic leukaemia; PD-1: programmed cell death protein 1; CD52: cluster of differentiation 52; HGF/c-Met: hepatocyte growth factor receptor/c-mesenchymal epithelial transition factor)

Conjugate of Monoclonal Antibody

- This involves conjugating chemotherapy molecules to monoclonal antibodies.
- Examples include gemtuzumab ozogamicin for acute myelogenous leukaemia.

Tyrosine Kinases and Their Inhibitors

Tyrosine kinases are activated by either growth factors or mutation of genes.

Non-receptor Tyrosine Kinase Inhibitors

Imatinib—chronic myeloid leukaemia.

Receptor Tyrosine Kinase Inhibitors

Gefitinib, erlotinib and lapatinib act in EGFR.

Proteasome Inhibitors

Bortezomib—treatment of relapsed/refractory multiple myeloma patients.

Different sites of targeted therapy are shown in **Figure 25.2**.

Immunotoxins

- Immunotoxin binds to the target cell, internalised and then the enzymatic fragment of the toxin kills the cell by inhibiting protein synthesis.
- Human interleukin-2 combined with truncated diphtheria toxin—for cutaneous T-cell lymphoma

Radioimmunotherapy

Prepared by combining the antibody with a radio conjugate, yttrium-90 or iodine-131 (e.g. tositumomab combined with iodine-131).

■ ONCOLOGIC EMERGENCIES

Oncologic emergencies are given in **Table 25.6**.

Febrile Neutropaenia

Defined as an oral temperature > 38.5°C and an absolute neutrophil count < 500/mm³ or expected to fall below 500/mm³.

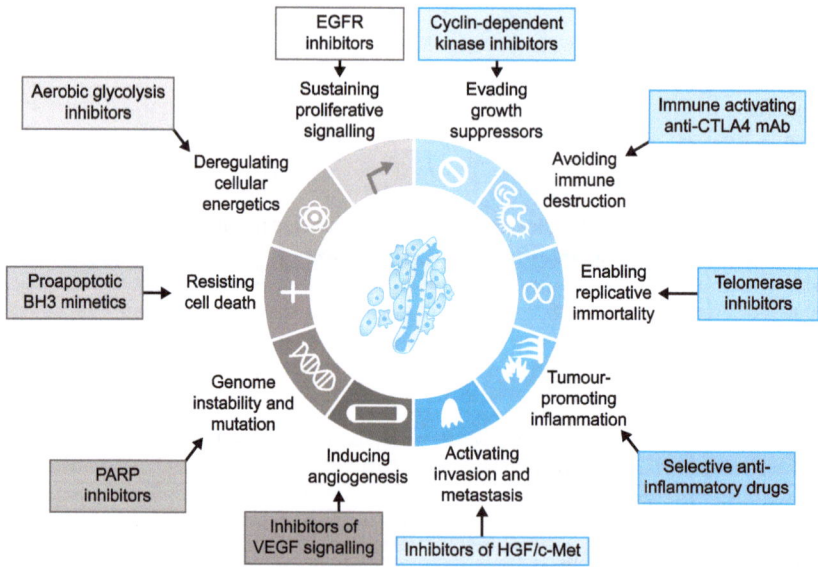

(EGFR: epidermal growth factor receptor; VEGF: vascular endothelial growth factor; PARP: poly ADP ribose polymerase; HGF/c-Met: hepatocyte growth factor receptor/c-mesenchymal epithelial transition factor; CTLA4: cytotoxic T-lymphocyte-associated protein 4)

Fig. 25.2: Sites of targeted therapy.

TABLE 25.6: Oncologic emergencies.

Metabolic or hormonal problems	Treatment related	Pressure or obstruction
• Hypercalcaemia • Syndrome of inappropriate antidiuretic hormone secretion (SIADH) • Lactic acidosis • Hypoglycaemia • Adrenal insufficiency	• Tumour lysis syndrome • Human antibody infusion reactions • Febrile neutropaenia • Thrombocytopaenia • Pulmonary infiltrates • Haemorrhagic cystitis • Hyperviscosity syndrome • Disseminated intravascular coagulation • Hypersensitivity reactions to antineoplastic drugs	• Superior vena cava syndrome • Epidural spinal cord compression • Pericardial effusion/cardiac tamponade • Intestinal obstruction • Urinary obstruction

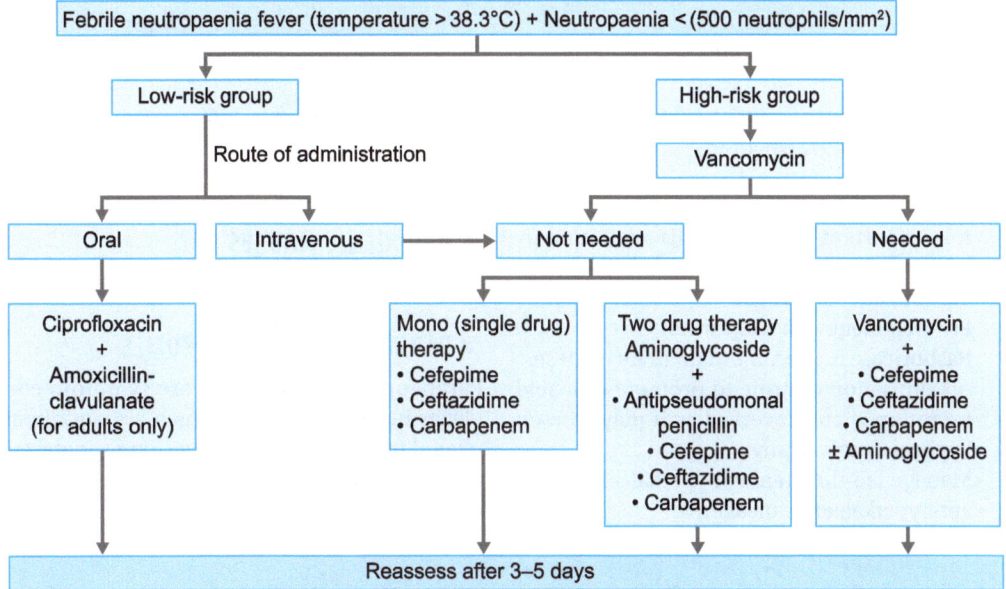

Flowchart 25.1: Algorithm for the antibiotic and their mode of administration in febrile neutropaenia.

Management

Management of febrile neutropaenia is shown in **Flowchart 25.1**.

Tumour Lysis Syndrome

- Occurs 1–5 days post-chemotherapy and is due to rapid release of intracellular contents and nucleic acids

- The syndrome is most common in lymphoma and leukaemia (**Fig. 25.3**).

Clinical Features

Lysis of malignant cells causes several metabolic disturbances. Hyperuricaemia produces acute renal failure; hyperkalaemia leads to cardiac arrhythmias; hyperphosphataemia produces acute renal failure and hyperkalaemia;

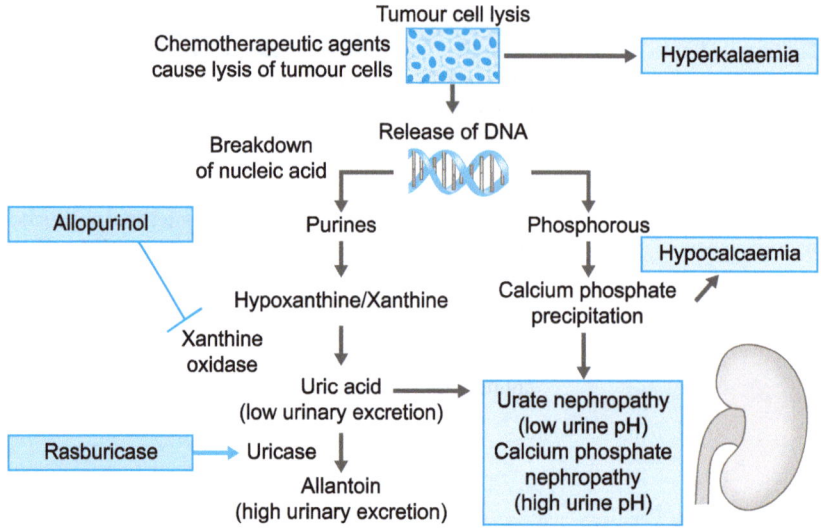

Fig. 25.3: Mechanism of tumour lysis.

and hypocalcaemia results in seizures, muscle cramps, tetany, and arrhythmia.

Treatment
- It is important to prevent this syndrome by adequate hydration and diuresis before, during, and after treatment.
- Pre-treatment with allopurinol
- Rasburicase is a recombinant urate oxidase.
- Alkalinisation of urine to promote uric acid excretion is controversial as it may worsen hypocalcaemic tetany.
- Manage life-threatening hyperkalaemia with antihyperkalaemic measures.
- For hypocalcaemia, infuse calcium gluconate under EGC monitoring.
- Early dialysis, if required.

ONCOGENIC VIRUSES

Oncogenic virus are given in **Table 25.7**.

PARANEOPLASTIC SYNDROMES

Paraneoplastic syndromes are symptom complexes in cancer patients which are not directly related to mass effects or invasion or metastasis or by the secretion of hormones indigenous to the tissue of origin (**Table 25.8**).

TABLE 25.7: Various viruses implicated in human tumours and associated lesions.

Type of virus	Lesions
Oncogenic RNA viruses	
Human T-cell lymphotropic virus type-1	Adult T-cell leukaemia/lymphoma
Oncogenic DNA viruses	
• Human papillomavirus (HPV)	
○ Low-oncogenic risk HPV—benign lesions of squamous epithelium	
– HPV types 1, 2, 4, and 7	Benign squamous papilloma (wart)
– HPV-6 and HPV-11	Condylomata acuminata (genital warts) of the vulva, penis, and perianal region
	Laryngeal papillomas

Continued

Continued

Type of virus	Lesions
○ High-oncogenic risk HPV—malignant tumours	
– HPV types 16 and 18	Squamous cell carcinoma of the cervix and anogenital region
	Oropharyngeal cancers (tonsil)
• Epstein–Barr virus	Burkitt lymphoma (requires cofactor-malaria)
	Nasopharyngeal cancer
• Hepatitis B and C viruses	Hepatocellular carcinoma
• Human herpes virus-8	Kaposi's sarcoma
	Pleural effusion lymphoma, multicentric Castleman disease
• Merkel cell polyomavirus	Merkel cell carcinoma

TABLE 25.8: Paraneoplastic syndromes.

Clinical syndromes	Cause/Mechanism	Associated cancer (example)
Endocrinopathies		
Cushing syndrome	ACTH or ACTH-like substance	Small-cell carcinoma of lung
Syndrome due to inappropriate antidiuretic hormone secretion	Antidiuretic hormone or atrial natriuretic hormones	Small-cell carcinoma of lung
Hypercalcaemia	PTHRP, TGF-α, TNF, IL-1	Squamous cell carcinoma of lung
		Renal carcinoma
Carcinoid syndrome	Serotonin, bradykinin	Bronchial carcinoid
Hypoglycaemia	Insulin or insulin-like substance	Fibrosarcoma
Polycythaemia	Erythropoietin	Renal carcinoma, hepatocellular carcinoma
Neurological (polyneuropathy, myelopathy, eaton–lambert syndrome, cerebellar degeneration, cortical degeneration, limbic encephalitis)		
Cutaneous syndromes		
Acanthosis nigricans	Immunological; secretion of epidermal growth factor	Carcinoma of stomach, lung and uterus
Paraneoplastic pemphigus	Immunological	B-cell lymphoproliferative disorders (80%), CLL, Castleman disease, thymoma
Dermatomyositis	Immunological	Bronchogenic, breast carcinoma
Sign of Leser-Trelat (rapid increase in number and size of seborrheic keratosis)	Immunological	Adenocarcinoma (stomach, rectum, breast, lungs, colon)
Exfoliative dermatitis	Immunological	Lymphoma
Acquired diffuse palmoplantar keratoderma	Immunological	Cancers of breast, lung, stomach and leukaemia

Continued

Continued

Clinical syndromes	Cause/Mechanism	Associated cancer (example)
Bazex syndrome (acrokeratosis paraneoplastica)	Immunological	Squamous cell carcinoma of the upper aerodigestive tract
Pityriasis rotunda	Immunological	Hepatocellular, gastric and prostate cancer, leukaemia, lymphoma
Paget's disease		Invasive breast carcinoma
Erythema gyratum repens	Immunological	Transitional carcinoma of the kidney and adenocarcinoma of lung, breast and oesophagus
Sweet's syndrome		Leukaemia
Pyoderma gangrenosum		AML, CML, myeloma
Necrolytic migratory erythema		Glucagonoma
Changes in osseous, articular, and soft tissue		
Hypertrophic osteoarthropathy and clubbing of the fingers	Not known	Bronchogenic carcinoma
Vascular and haematologic syndromes		
Venous thrombosis (Trousseau syndrome)	Tumour products like mucins which activate clotting	Pancreatic carcinoma
		Bronchogenic carcinoma
Disseminated intravascular coagulation	Procoagulant substance: Cytoplasmic granules (e.g. acute promyelocytic leukaemia cells), or mucus (adenocarcinomas)	Acute promyelocytic leukaemia, prostatic adenocarcinomas
Non-bacterial thrombotic endocarditis	Hypercoagulability	Advanced mucus-secreting adenocarcinomas
Renal syndromes		
Nephrotic syndrome	Tumour antigens, immune complexes	Various cancers
Amyloidosis		
Primary amyloidosis	Immunological amyloid light (AL) chain protein	Multiple myeloma
Secondary amyloidosis	Amyloid associated A protein	Renal cell carcinoma and other solid

(ACTH: adrenocorticotropic hormone; IL: interleukin; TGF: transforming growth factor; TNF: tumour necrosis factor; PTHRP: parathyroid hormone-related protein; AML: acute myeloid leukaemia; CML: chronic myeloid leukaemia; CLL: chronic lymphocytic leukaemia)

BEST OF FIVES

1. The DNA (deoxyribonucleic acid) damage checkpoints are located in which phase of the cell cycle?
   A. G1/S
   B. S/G2
   C. M
   D. M/G2
   E. G1/M

2. The presence of mutations in p53 has been associated with which of the following properties on cells?
   A. Loss of the G2 checkpoint following treatment with DNA (deoxyribonucleic acid)-damaging agents
   B. Enhanced capacity to undergo apoptosis following exposure to radiation
   C. Increased capacity for DNA amplification
   D. A and C
   E. All of the above

3. The correct order of mitosis is:
   A. Prometaphase, metaphase, anaphase, telophase, prophase
   B. Prometaphase, metaphase, prophase, anaphase, telophase
   C. Prophase, prometaphase, metaphase, anaphase, telophase
   D. Telophase, anaphase, prophase, metaphase, prometaphase
   E. Prophase, telophase, anaphase, metaphase, prometaphase

4. The Warburg effect describes:
   A. Exponential cell growth in response to an exogenous stimulant
   B. Inefficient energy production by most cancer cells, resulting in rapid adenosine triphosphate (ATP) depletion and necrotic cell death
   C. Initiation of neoplasia requires two somatic mutations for initiation of sporadic neoplasms and hereditary neoplasms require a genetic plus a somatic mutation
   D. Sculpting of normal human tissues as a result of cell death
   E. The susceptibility of a cancer cell depends on the mitotic activity in it

5. Metronomic low-dose chemotherapy describes:
   A. Continuous low-dose treatment with chemotherapeutics
   B. Pulse dosing with low doses of chemotherapeutics
   C. Continuous low-dose treatment with intermittent pulse dosings of chemotherapeutics
   D. Treatment of refractory tumours with continuous low doses of chemotherapeutics in conjunction with metronidazole
   E. Used in treatment of bladder carcinoma

6. The human papillomavirus (HPV) vaccine Gardasil
   A. Is a quadrivalent vaccine containing virus-like particles (VLPs) from four different types of HPV
   B. Protects from all HPV-causing cervical cancer
   C. Is recommended only for sexually active women
   D. Is recommended for treating cervical cancer
   E. All the above

7. *Helicobacter pylori* infection is associated with an increased risk of which of the following?
   A. Oesophageal adenocarcinoma
   B. Gastric cardia carcinoma
   C. Oesophageal squamous cell carcinoma
   D. Intestinal-type gastric adenocarcinoma
   E. Non-small-cell lung carcinoma

8. Which of the following malignancies is associated with germ line mutations in the *RET* proto-oncogene?
   A. Multiple endocrine neoplasia (MEN) 2A
   B. MEN 2B
   C. Sporadic medullary thyroid carcinoma
   D. All the above
   E. A and C

9. A 28-year-old woman with bilateral ductal cancer presents to the medical oncologist for assessment and treatment. Her medical history is notable for intussusception at 6 years of age. On her physical examination, the medicine resident notices small blue/black hyperpigmented macules on her lips, buccal mucosa and fingertips. What is her diagnosis?

A. Hereditary BRCA1 syndrome
B. Hereditary BRCA2 syndrome
C. Li–Fraumeni syndrome
D. Peutz–Jeghers syndrome
E. Cowden syndrome

10. The abscopal effect of radiation is
    A. Attributed to the activation of antigen and cytokine release
    B. Commonly seen because immune system evasion by cancer cells is rarely present
    C. Seen more frequently with lower doses and greater fractions
    D. Activation of the humoral immune response
    E. Double-stranded breaks in DNA in non-irradiated cells

11. Which of the following is a principle of epigenetic therapy?
    A. Epigenetic changes cause alterations in the sequencing of targeted genes.
    B. Epigenetic therapy is mostly utilised and has the greatest efficacy in solid tumours.
    C. The impact of epigenetic therapy is not seen immediately due to efficacy being based on cellular reprogramming.
    D. Combination therapy with histone deacetylase (HDAC) inhibitors and demethylating agents should not be pursued due to overlapping toxicities.
    E. It is best used in childhood cancer therapy.

12. Which of the following is an approach to cancer immunotherapy?
    A. Passive transfer of activated immune cells with anti-tumour activity
    B. Active immunisation to enhance anti-tumour reactions
    C. Non-specific stimulation of immune reactions
    D. All of the above
    E. A and B

13. What is the purpose of adoptive cell transfer therapies?
    A. Decreasing the number of reactive T cells ex vivo and transfer back to the patient
    B. Increasing the number of cytokines ex vivo and transfer back to the patient
    C. Activating and expanding tumour-reactive T cells and transfer back to the patient
    D. Modulating CD4+ tumour-specific T cells before transferring back to the patient
    E. Modulation of plasma cells to produce anti-tumour antibodies

14. A 35-year-old non-smoking female with a history of chronic oral lichen planus presented with a painful right oral tongue lesion measuring 2.5 cm. Biopsy revealed well-differentiated squamous cell carcinoma. Ultrasound revealed that the oral tongue lesion was 0.6 cm thick. Computed tomography (CT) showed no abnormal neck nodes. The lesion was widely excised and a right selective neck dissection (SND) was performed. Pathology revealed a 2.6-cm SCC, negative surgical margins, no perineural or lymphovascular invasion and all 15 lymph nodes without SCC. The pathologic stage was II (T2N0M0). The next most appropriate therapy is:
    A. Post-operative adjuvant radiation therapy
    B. Post-operative adjuvant concurrent chemotherapy and radiation therapy
    C. Close monitoring
    D. Left selective neck dissection
    E. Immunotherapy

15. A 45-year-old Asian woman, who is a non-smoker, presents to your office for consultation regarding systemic therapy for metastatic adenocarcinoma of the lung. Her tumour has an activating EGFR mutation. Which of the following is a valid first-line treatment option for this patient?
    A. Cetuximab
    B. Afatinib
    C. Necitumumab
    D. Crizotinib
    E. Rituximab

16. A 60-year-old man with a 45 pack-year history of smoking presents with chest pain. Chest X-ray reveals a right upper lobe mass. Computed tomography (CT) scan of the chest demonstrates a 4-cm right upper lobe lung mass, with right hilar and multiple ipsilateral enlarged mediastinal lymph nodes. Bronchoscopy and biopsy of the mass reveal non-squamous cell lung carcinoma (NSCLC). Positron emission tomography (PET) scan demonstrates increased fluorodeoxyglucose (FDG) uptake in the lung mass, right hilar and

mediastinal lymph brain nodes, but no other site of metastatic disease. CT of the abdomen and magnetic resonance imaging (MRI) of the brain are unremarkable. Mediastinoscopy and biopsy reveal NSCLC. His cancer is staged as T2aN2M0, stage IIIA NSCLC. His performance status is 1 and he is otherwise in good health. Which of the following is the best management for this patient?
   A. Definitive radiation to the chest
   B. Radiation to the chest, followed by platinum-based chemotherapy
   C. Concurrent radiation to the chest and platinum-based chemotherapy
   D. Platinum-based chemotherapy
   E. Surgery followed by radiation

17. Which of the following statements is TRUE regarding mediastinal germ cell tumours?
   A. The incidence of malignant mediastinal germ cell tumours is the same in men and women.
   B. Seminoma is the most common mediastinal germ cell tumour.
   C. An elevated serum alpha foetoprotein (AFP) in a patient with biopsy-proven seminoma indicates the presence of a non-seminomatous component.
   D. Mediastinal non-seminomatous germ cell tumours (NSGCTs) are associated with better overall survival than testicular NSGCTs.
   E. These tumours are common in men around 50 years of age.

18. Which of the following statements are TRUE? (Select two correct responses)
   A. Blood group B has been associated with gastric cancers.
   B. Most of the patients with *Helicobacter pylori* infection will develop gastric cancer.
   C. Epstein–Barr virus infection has been noted in a certain type of gastric carcinoma.
   D. WHO classifies *H. pylori* infection as class I carcinogen.
   E. Vegetarian diet is considered protective for gastric cancer.

19. Which of the following statements about staging systems for hepatocellular carcinoma is TRUE?
   A. The Okuda system takes into account several clinical features that include tumour size (> 50% of liver), ascites (positive or negative), hypoalbuminaemia (< 3 g/dL) and hyperbilirubinaemia (> 3 mg/dL).
   B. The Cancer of the Liver Italian Program system uses hepatic tumour morphology and extent of liver replacement, Child–Pugh score, portal vein thrombosis and serum alpha-foetoprotein (AFP) levels.
   C. The Barcelona Clinic Liver Cancer scoring system combines assessment of tumour stage, liver function and patient symptoms with a treatment algorithm and has been shown to correlate well with patient outcomes.
   D. All of the above
   E. None of the above

20. Which anti-emetic schedule is the most appropriate for a patient receiving 70 mg/m^2 cisplatin in combination with gemcitabine 1,250 mg/m^2 at day 1?
   A. Metoclopramide in combination with dexamethasone at day 1
   B. 5-HT3 receptor antagonist (e.g. ondansetron and ganister) and dexamethasone at day 1
   C. 5-HT3 receptor antagonist in combination with lorazepam at day 1
   D. 5-HT3 receptor antagonist, aprepitant or fosaprepitant, at day 1
   E. 5-HT3 receptor antagonist, aprepitant or fosaprepitant, and dexamethasone at day 1

Answers
1-A, 2-D, 3-C, 4-B, 5-A, 6-A, 7-D, 8-D, 9-D, 10-A, 11-C, 12-D, 13-C, 14-A, 15-B, 16-C, 17-C, 18-C & D, 19-D, 20-E

SUGGESTED READING
1. Siegel RL, Miller KD, Jemal A. Cancer statistics, 2019. CA Cancer J Clin. 2019;69(1):7-34.
2. Hanna NH, Schneider BJ, Temin S, Baker S, Brahmer J, Ellis PM, et al. Therapy for Stage IV Non-Small-Cell Lung

Cancer Without Driver Alterations: ASCO and OH (CCO) Joint Guideline Update. J Clin Oncol. 2020;38(14):1608-32.
3. Paik PK, Felip E, Veillon R, Sakai H, Cortot AB, Garassino MC, et al. Tepotinib in non-small-cell lung cancer with MET Exon 14 skipping mutations. N Engl J Med. 2020.
4. Yefimova M, Aslakson RA, Yang L, Garcia A, Boothroyd D, Gale RC, et al. Palliative care and end-of-life outcomes following high-risk surgery. JAMA Surg. 2020;155(2):138-46.
5. Dempke WCM, Fenchel K, Uciechowski P, Dale SP. Second- and third-generation drugs for immuno-oncology treatment- The more the better? Eur J Cancer. 2017;74:55-72.
6. Bhatt AN, Mathur R, Farooque A, Verma A, Dwarakanath BS. Cancer biomarkers – Current perspectives. Indian J Med Res. 2010;132:129-49.
7. Lenz HJ. Management and preparedness for infusion and hypersensitivity reactions. Oncologist. 2007;12(5):601-9.
8. Isabwe GAC, Garcia Neuer M, de Las Vecillas Sanchez L, Lynch DM, Marquis K, Castells M. Hypersensitivity reactions to therapeutic monoclonal antibodies: Phenotypes and endotypes. J Allergy Clin Immunol. 2018;142(1):159-70.
9. Sharma S. Tumor markers in clinical practice: General principles and guidelines. Indian J Med Paediatr Oncol. 2009;30(1):1-8.

CHAPTER 26

Geriatric Medicine

Sheetal Raj M

■ WHAT MAKES THE ASSESSMENT/ TREATMENT OF ELDERLY DIFFERENT? (TABLE 26.1)

- Individuals become more dissimilar as they grow.
- Abrupt decline in any system is always due to disease and not due to normal ageing.
- Multiple pathology

- **Missing symptoms**
  - Angina in an elderly patient with osteoarthritis—may not manifest
- **Masking symptoms**
  - History of fall and fracture neck of femur in an elderly female—masked a coexistent haemiparesis due to an internal capsule infarct

TABLE 26.1: Atypical disease presentations in older adults.

Diagnosis	Potential presenting symptoms and signs	Diagnosis	Potential presenting symptoms and signs
Myocardial infarction	• Altered mental status • Fatigue • Fever • Functional decline	Malignancy	• Altered mental status • Fever • Pathologic fracture
Infection	• Altered mental status • Functional decline • Hypothermia	Pulmonary embolus	• Altered mental status • Fatigue • Fever • Syncope
Hyperthyroidism	• Altered mental status • Anorexia • Atrial fibrillation • Chest pain • Constipation • Fatigue • Weight gain	Vitamin deficiency	• Altered mental status • Ataxia • Dementia • Fatigue
Depression	• Cognitive impairment • Failure to thrive • Functional decline	Faecal impaction	• Altered mental status • Chest pain • Diarrhoea • Urinary incontinence
Electrolyte disturbance	• Altered mental status • Falls • Fatigue • Personality changes	Aortic stenosis	• Altered mental status • Fatigue

GERIATRIC GIANTS

- Term coined by Sir Bernard Issacs
- He recognised that multiple illnesses of the senior years needed a broader perspective in socioeconomic and medical terms.
- 'Geriatric Giants' or the four I's:
  - Immobility
  - Instability
  - Incontinence
  - Impairment of intellect
    - Cognitive impairment
    - Delirium
    - Depression
- He asserted that if we look closely enough, all common problems of older adults lead to one of these four Giants.
- **Newer giants**
  - Frailty
  - Sarcopaenia
  - The 'anorexia of ageing'
  - Mild cognitive impairment

'The Modern Geriatric Giants'

The modern geriatric giants are shown in **Figure 26.1**.

DEMENTIA

- **Dementia** is a cluster of symptoms including: Forgetfulness, poor judgement, decline in intellectual functioning.
- **Mild cognitive impairment** demonstrates mild deficits (most commonly in short-term memory) on formal testing but does not meet criteria for dementia.
- Insidious Onset and Progressive
- Cognitive domains:
  - Complex attention
  - Executive function
  - Learning and memory
  - Language
  - Perceptual—motor
  - Social cognition

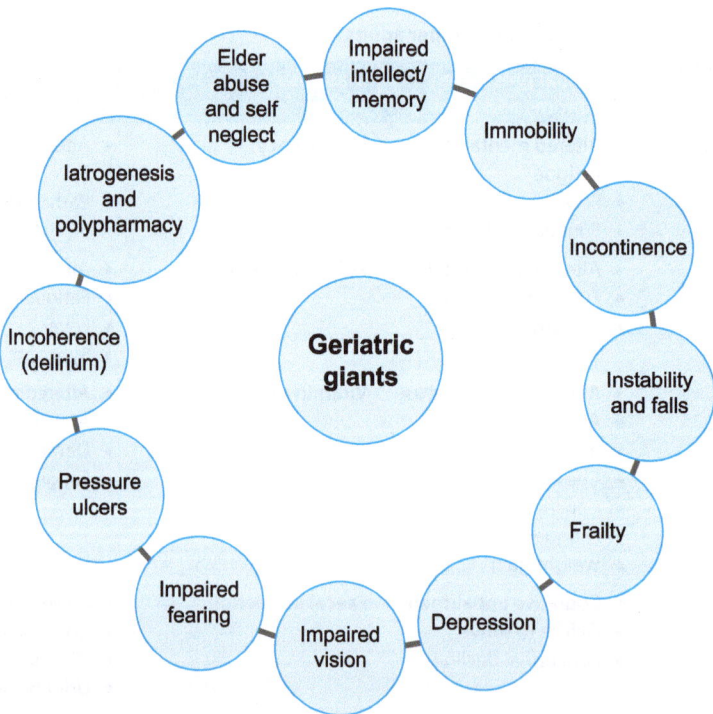

Fig. 26.1: Modern geriatric giants.

Geriatric Medicine

Major neurocognitive disorder (NCD): 2 or more cognitive domains impaired PLUS 1 or more impaired instrumental activities of daily living (IADLs)

Mild NCD: 1 or more cognitive domains impaired; Instrumental activities of daily living (IADLs) intact
   Not due to delirium or another mental disorder

Causes of Dementia

The causes of dementia are given in **Box 26.1**.

Alzheimer Disease
- Most common form of dementia in the elderly (60–80%)
- Magnetic resonance imaging (MRI)—bilateral hippocampal atrophy

Vascular Dementia
- Associated with a stroke. Abrupt onset of symptoms followed by stepwise deterioration

Frontotemporal Dementia
It presents with language abnormalities and behavioural disturbances

Normal-pressure Hydrocephalus
Triad of dementia, gait disturbance and urinary incontinence

Dementia with Lewy bodies
Hallucinations and delusions

'Modifiable' Causes of Dementia
Modifiable causes of dementia are given in **Box 26.2**.

Treatment
- Tacrine, donepezil
- Rivastigmine
- Galantamine
- Memantine
- Selegiline
- Vitamin E
- Ginkgo Biloba

Box 26.1: Causes of dementia.
- Alzheimer's disease
- Vascular dementia [Strokes and transient ischaemic attack (TIA)]
- Parkinson's disease
- Frontotemporal dementia (FTD)
- Normal-pressure hydrocephalus (NPH)
- Dementia with Lewy Bodies
- Delirium/Depression

Box 26.2: Modifiable causes of dementia.
- Depression
- Electrolyte disorders
- Hypothyroidism
- Vitamin deficiencies (B12, folate)
- Normal-pressure hydrocephalus
- Brain tumour
- Subdural haematoma (SDH)
- Subacute central nervous system (CNS) infections

■ DEPRESSION

- At least **FIVE** of the following, of which (1) or (2) must be present for 2 weeks or more:
  1. Depressed mood
  2. Anhedonia
  3. Weight loss/appetite loss
  4. Insomnia or hypersomnia
  5. Psychomotor agitation or retardation
  6. Fatigue or loss of energy
  7. Feelings of worthlessness/inappropriate guilt
  8. Decreased concentration/indecisiveness/inattention
  9. Recurrent thoughts of death, suicidal ideation or suicide plan or attempt
- The symptoms cause distress and/or impaired functioning.
- Symptoms not due to an underlying medical condition or better explained by another psychiatric condition (e.g. bipolar, schizoaffective)

Management of Depression in Older Adults
- Non-pharmacological therapy preferred
  - Cognitive behaviour therapy
- **Pharmacological therapy**
  - Selective serotonin reuptake inhibitors (SSRIs) preferred (risk of hyponatraemia +)
  - Mirtazapine, venlafaxine, duloxetine also useful
- Needs **referral to** a psychiatrist
  - If suicidal/homicidal OR refusing to eat/drink
  - If not responding to antidepressants (8–12-week trial at appropriate dose)
  - Uncertain diagnosis
  - Bipolar disorder present
- Electroconvulsive therapy safe in older adults—if indicated

DELIRIUM
- Rapid and abrupt onset of:
  - Impaired attention
  - Lack of awareness of environment
- Change in at least **ONE** cognitive domain:
  - Memory
  - Orientation
  - Language
  - Perception
- Associated with:
  - Change in sleep-wake cycle
  - Change in emotional states
  - Worsening behaviour in evenings

The characteristics of depression, delirium and dementia are given in **Table 26.2**.

FRAILTY SYNDROME
- Frailty is a term used to describe a subgroup of older adults who experience decreased functional reserve, functional decline and increased vulnerability for morbidity and mortality.
- Frailty is defined as the presence of three or more of these conditions:
  Fried Frailty score
  - Unintentional weight loss (at least 6 kg in 1 year)
  - Self-reported exhaustion
  - Reduced gait speed
  - Decreased physical activity
  - Reduced grip strength

Treatment
- Address the precipitating acute illness.
- Address the underlying loss of reserve.

TABLE 26.2: Characteristics of depression, delirium and dementia.

	Depression	Delirium	Dementia
Onset	Weeks to months	Hours to days	Months to years
Mood	Low/apathetic	Fluctuates	Fluctuates
Course	Chronic; responds to treatment	Acute; responds to treatment	Chronic, with deterioration over time
Self-awareness	Likely to be concerned about memory impairment	May be aware of changes in cognition; fluctuates	Likely to hide or be unaware of cognitive deficits
Activities of daily living (ADLs)	May neglect basic self-care	May be intact or impaired	May be intact early, impaired as disease progresses
Instrumental activities of daily living (IADLs)	May be intact or impaired	May be intact or impaired	May be intact early, impaired before ADLs as disease progresses

URINARY INCONTINENCE (UI)

- It is involuntary loss of urine in sufficient amount or frequency to constitute a social and/or health problem.
- It is a heterogeneous condition that ranges in severity from dribbling small amounts of urine to continuous urinary incontinence with concomitant faecal incontinence.
- The common reversible factors can be remembered by the mnemonic DRIP '**D**elirium; **R**estricted mobility, **R**etention; **I**nfection, **I**nflammation (atrophic vaginitis), **I**mpaction of stool; **P**olyuria, **P**harmaceuticals.'

Categories of Incontinence

Urge Incontinence (UI)
- Most common cause of UI
- Abrupt desire to void that cannot be suppressed
- Usually idiopathic
- **Causes:** Infection, tumour, stones, atrophic vaginitis or urethritis, stroke, Parkinson's disease, dementia

Stress Incontinence
- Occurs with increase in abdominal pressure, cough, sneeze, etc.
- **Causes:** Hypermotility of bladder neck and urethra; associated with ageing, hormonal changes, trauma of childbirth or pelvic surgery (85% of cases)
- **Other causes:** Intrinsic sphincter problems; due to pelvic/incontinence surgery, pelvic radiation, trauma, neurogenic causes (15% of cases)

Overflow Incontinence
- Overdistention of bladder produces incontinence.
- Bladder outlet obstruction: stricture, benign prostatic hyperplasia (BPH), cystocele, faecal impaction
- Non-contractile bladder (hypoactive detrusor or atonic bladder): Diabetes, multiple sclerosis (MS), spinal injury, medications

Functional Incontinence
- Does not involve lower urinary tract
- Result of psychological, cognitive or physical impairment

Treatment Options
- Reduce amount and timing of fluid intake.
- Avoid bladder stimulants (caffeine).

Pharmacological Interventions
- **Urge Incontinence:** Oxybutynin, propantheline, imipramine
- **Stress Incontinence:** Phenylpropanolamine, pseudoephedrine, oestrogen

Surgical Corrections
- **Urethral Hypermotility**
  - Marshall-Marchetti-Krantz procedure
  - Needle neck suspension
- **Intrinsic sphincter deficiency**
  - Sling procedure

FALLS IN THE ELDERLY

Common Causes Associated with Falls
The common causes that lead to falls are given in **Box 26.3**.

FAILURE TO THRIVE

- 'A syndrome of weight loss, decreased appetite, poor nutrition and inactivity, often accompanied by dehydration, depressive symptoms, impaired immune function and low cholesterol.'

Box 26.3: Common causes associated with falls.
- Ophthalmologic diseases
- Arthritis
- Foot problems
- Neurologic illness
  - Parkinson's and related disorders
  - Strokes
  - Peripheral neuropathy
  - Dizziness and disequilibrium

- Affects the following four main domains:
  i. **Functional:** Basic activity of daily living (BADL)/IADL
  ii. **Malnutrition:** Weight trend, body mass index (BMI), lymphocytes and albumin
  iii. **Depression:** +/− Geriatric Depression Scale (GDS)
  iv. **Cognition:** Confusion Assessment Method (CAM), Standardized Mini-Mental State Examination (SMMSE)

SARCOPAENIA

- Age-related loss of muscle mass
- Increases the risk for falls, fractures, dependency, use of hospital services, institutionalisation, poor quality of life and mortality

ANOREXIA OF AGEING

- Specific geriatric syndrome that can lead to malnutrition if not appropriately diagnosed and treated
- Features:
  - Body wasting (cachexia and sarcopaenia)
  - Poor endurance
  - Reduced physical performance
  - Slow gait speed
  - Impaired mobility

MULTIMORBIDITY AND POLYPHARMACY

Affects 55–98% of elderly

Multimorbidity

- The coexistence of ≥ 2 chronic conditions, where one is not necessarily more central than the others

Polypharmacy

- Administration of more medications than clinically indicated, representing unnecessary drug use
- ≥ 5 drugs during a 3-month period

ELDER ABUSE

Elder abuse is defined as any action or inaction that threatens the well-being of an older person.

Categories of Abuse

- **Physical and sexual abuse:**
  - Any act of violence or rough treatment, whether or not actual physical injury results from it
    - For example: slapping, punching, kicking, pinching, burning, restraints
- **Emotional and psychological abuse:**
  - Any act that diminishes dignity and self-worth
    - For example: confinement, isolation, verbal assault, humiliation and infantilisation
- **Financial abuse and material exploitation:**
  - Any improper conduct that results in monetary or personal loss for the older adult
- **Abandonment and neglect:**
  - *Active neglect:* Intentional (deliberate) withholding of basic necessities and/or care for physical or mental health
  - *Passive neglect:* Not providing basic necessities and care. There is no conscious attempt to inflict distress.
- **Medical abuse:**
  - Any medical procedure or treatment done without the permission of the older person or his/her 'Power of Attorney' or substitute decision maker.

COMPREHENSIVE GERIATRIC ASSESSMENT

- Comprehensive geriatric assessment (CGA) is a multi-dimensional, multi-disciplinary diagnostic and therapeutic process.
- It is conducted to determine the medical, mental and functional problems of older people with frailty so that a coordinated and integrated plan for treatment and follow-up can be developed **(Fig. 26.2)**.

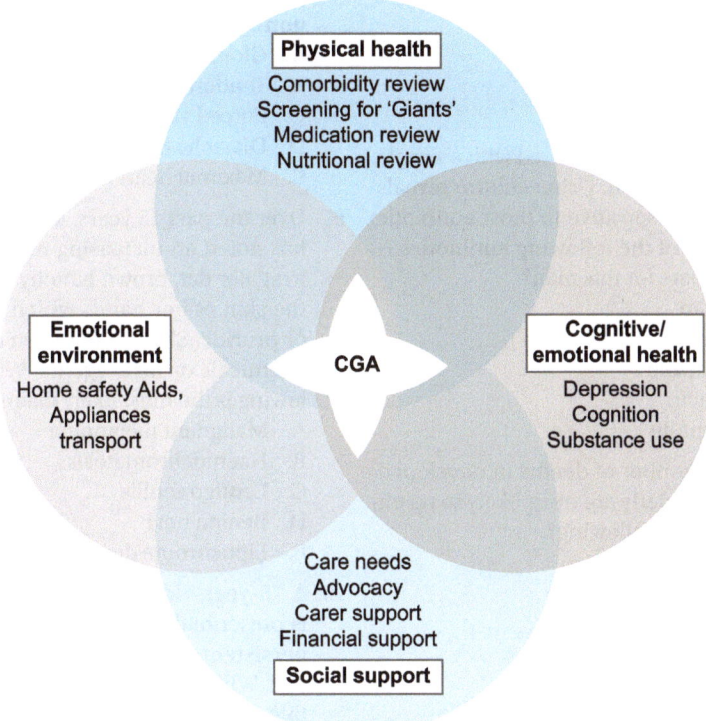

Fig. 26.2: Components of comprehensive geriatric assessment (CGA).

BEST OF FIVES

1. A 75-year-old woman has had decreasing visual acuity in both eyes for the past 5 years predominantly affecting the central visual fields. Funduscopic examination reveals discrete thickenings and atrophy of the retinal pigment epithelium. The intraocular pressure is normal. Which of the following conditions is he most likely to have?
   A. Macular degeneration
   B. Cataract formation
   C. Primary glaucoma
   D. Diabetic retinopathy
   E. Vitamin A deficiency

2. A 65-year-old man has difficulty hearing on the left, gradually worsening over the past 5 years. A lightly vibrating tuning fork is placed firmly on the midline of the patient's head, and sound lateralises to the bad ear. The base of a lightly vibrating tuning fork is then placed on the mastoid bone behind the bad ear and on level with the ear canal. Which of the following conditions is he most likely to have?
   A. Otosclerosis
   B. Otitis media
   C. Meniere disease
   D. Presbycusis
   E. Schwannoma

3. A 75-year-old man complains of increasing difficulty with joint pain in lower limbs over the past 10 years. The pain is worse with activity and as the day progresses. His knees are primarily affected, left worse than right. On physical examination, there is decreased range of motion of the knees, but no redness or swelling or joint deformity. Radiographs reveal joint space narrowing at the knees, with osteophyte formation involving the tibias. Which of the following conditions is he most likely to have?

A. Pseudogout
B. Osteoarthritis
C. Gouty arthritis
D. Lyme disease
E. Rheumatoid arthritis

4. A 68-year-old man is diagnosed with a simple urinary tract infection. Urine culture reveals a bacterial agent sensitive to most antibiotic classes. Which of the following antibiotics is most appropriate for this man?
   A. Amoxicillin
   B. Cephalexin
   C. Cotrimoxazole
   D. Levofloxacin
   E. Nitrofurantoin

5. The greatest number of deaths in developed nations in the elderly are most likely to result from which of the following?
   A. Traumatic injuries
   B. Cardiovascular diseases
   C. Neoplasia
   D. Infectious agents
   E. Immunologic diseases

6. An 80-year-old man has had no major medical illnesses during his life. He has decreased energy and fatigue for the past month. On physical examination, his skin shows wrinkling with loss of elasticity. He has visual acuity of 20/40 in both eyes. Pulmonary function studies show a decreased total lung capacity with normal FEV_1 and FEV_1/FVC ratio. Which of the following conditions is he most likely to have?
   A. Hypopituitarism
   B. Emphysema
   C. Skin cancer
   D. Macular degeneration
   E. Frailty

7. Which of the following conditions is most likely to be characteristic for elderly persons who have a history of diabetes mellitus?
   A. Bronchogenic carcinoma
   B. Presbyopia
   C. Hypertrophic cardiomyopathy
   D. Hepatic cirrhosis
   E. Renal failure

8. Which of the following physiologic parameters is most likely to be higher for the older population, compared to the younger population?
   A. Glomerular filtration rate
   B. Tendon tensile strength
   C. Forced vital capacity
   D. Diastolic blood pressure
   E. Maximal heart rate

9. Over the past 15 years, a 68-year-old woman has noted an increasing number and size of irregular flat, brown blotchy 1-2 cm areas on the skin of her hands which are not painful or pruritic. She has not been exposed to any chemicals or toxic agents. Which of the following is the most likely diagnosis?
   A. Malignant melanoma
   B. Haemochromatosis
   C. Lentigo senilis
   D. Benign nevi
   E. Lipochrome deposition

10. A 75-year-old man with Parkinson disease is prescribed an anticholinergic drug for the persistent tremor she experiences while at rest. Which of the following complications of this drug treatment is most likely to occur in this man?
    A. Urinary retention
    B. Bradycardia
    C. Diarrhoea
    D. Osteonecrosis
    E. Tardive dyskinesia

11. A 64-year-old woman has progressive memory loss and inability to carry out activities of daily living over the past 5 years. Which of the following conditions is she most likely to have?
    A. Progeria
    B. Vitamin B12 deficiency
    C. Dementia with Lewy bodies
    D. Alzheimer disease
    E. Diabetes mellitus

12. An 80-year-old woman is travelling to her native place on train. She takes an over-the-counter (OTC) medication to combat motion sickness. An hour later she becomes disoriented, anxious and confused. Which of the following drugs did she most likely ingest?
    A. Acetaminophen
    B. Caffeine

C. Diphenhydramine
D. Ephedrine
E. St John's wort

13. A 90-year-old woman is independently living in her own home. Her memory is good. She has no chronic medial ailments. She can perform all activities of daily living. Which of the following represents the greatest environmental risk hazard to this woman?
    A. Electric hair dryer
    B. Glass shower door
    C. Hot water heater set at 43°C
    D. Loose rug on the floor
    E. Natural gas appliance

14. Which of the following findings on blood gas analysis would be expected for an 80-year-old male?
    A. Carboxyhaemoglobin 5%
    B. O_2 saturation 60%
    C. PaO_2 90 mmHg
    D. $PaCO_2$ 50 mmHg
    E. pH 7.5

15. A 90-year old male presents with acute confusion. On physical examination, vital signs include temperature 38.2°C, pulse 100/min, respiratory rate 20/min and blood pressure 120/70 mmHg. He has photophobia and neck rigidity. Laboratory studies show a serum sodium of 140 mmol/L, potassium 4.7 mmol/L, chloride 100 mmol/L, CO_2 29 mmol/L, glucose 60 mg/dL and creatinine 1.2 mg/dL. Which of the following is he most likely to have?
    A. Meningitis
    B. Delirium
    C. Dementia
    D. Depression
    E. Diabetic coma

16. An elderly woman with a history of diabetes mellitus has experienced shortness of breath, nausea and lightheadedness for the past 2 hours. In the emergency department, her vital signs represent temperature 36.5°C, pulse 90/min, respiratory rate 22/min and blood pressure 110/75 mmHg. Her pulse has varying volumes and there are bibasal crackles. Which of the following laboratory tests is most useful for workup of this woman?
    A. Haematocrit
    B. Haemoglobin A1C
    C. Sputum eosinophil count
    D. Stool for ova and parasites
    E. Troponin

17. An elderly man has become bedridden following fracture of neck of femur worsened by osteoporosis. Which of the following complications is most serious to prevent through repositioning?
    A. Dependent oedema
    B. Fractures
    C. Muscle atrophy
    D. Pressure ulcers
    E. Venous thrombosis

18. An elderly man has a fall and fractured his left femoral neck. Surgical repair is performed. He develops altered sensorium post-operatively. Which of the following is the most probable cause in this patient?
    A. Antibiotic therapy
    B. Urinary infection
    C. Hyponatraemia
    D. Stroke
    E. Depression

19. A 76-year-old man is in the hospital for treatment of a stroke. On the second hospital day, he becomes agitated and confused. He is disoriented. He is fearful and thinks that the intravenous stand is a dangerous animal. What is the possible cause of this condition?
    A. Depression
    B. Delirium
    C. Dementia
    D. Meningitis
    E. Seizure

20. Age-related loss of muscle mass increases the risk for falls, fractures, dependency, use of hospital services, institutionalisation, poor quality of life and mortality. This is called:
    A. Failure to thrive
    B. Frailty
    C. Sacropaenia
    D. Anorexia of ageing
    E. Multimorbidity

Answers

1-A, 2-A, 3-B, 4-C, 5-B, 6-E, 7-E, 8-D, 9-C, 10-A, 11-D, 12-C, 13-D, 14-C, 15-A, 16-E, 17-D, 18-C, 19-B, 20-C

■ SUGGESTED READING

1. Blokzijl F, de Ligt J, Jager M, Sasselli V, Roerink S, Sasaki N, et al. Tissue-specific mutation accumulation in human adult stem cells during life. Nature. 2016; 538(5):260-4.
2. Slieker RC, Relton CL, Gaunt TR, Slagboom PE, Heijmans BT, et al. Age-related DNA methylation changes are tissue-specific with ELOVL2 promoter methylation as exception. Epigenetics Chromatin. 2018;11(1):25.
3. vB Hjelmborg J, Iachine I, Skytthe A, Vaupel JW, McGue M, Koskenvuo M, et al. Genetic influence on human lifespan and longevity. Hum Genet. 2006;119(3):312-21.
4. American Psychiatric Association. Diagnostic and Statistical Manual of Mental Disorders (DSM-5), 5th edition. Arlington: American Psychiatric Association; 2013.
5. Knopman DS, DeKosky ST, Cummings JL, Chui H, Corey-Bloom J, Relkin N, et al. Practice parameter: diagnosis of dementia (an evidence-based review). Report of the Quality Standards Subcommittee of the American Academy of Neurology. Neurology. 2001;56(9):1143-53.
6. Fried LP, Tangen CM, Walston J, Newman AB, Hirsch C, Gottdiener J, et al. Frailty in older adults: evidence for a phenotype. J Gerontol A Biol Sci Med Sci. 2001;56(3): M146-56.
7. Centers for Disease Control and Prevention and The Merck Company Foundation. The State of Aging and Health in America 2007. The Merck Company Foundation, Whitehouse Station, NJ 2007. [online] Available at: http://www.cdc.gov/aging/pdf/saha_2007.pdf. [Last accessed June, 2020].
8. United Nations, Department of Economic and Social Affairs, Population Division. World Population Ageing 2013. [online] Available from: http://www.un.org/en/development/desa/population/publications/pdf/ageing/WorldPopulationAgeing2013.pdf. [Last accessed June, 2020].

CHAPTER 27

Medical Genetics

■ HUMAN GENOME PROJECT
- The human genome is composed of 46 distinct chromosomes.
- Human Genome Project: Its main aim was to decode a total of approximately 3 billion DNA base pairs containing estimated 25,000–30,000 genes.

Potential Benefits of Human Genome Project
- Molecular medicine:
  - Earlier detection of genetic predispositions to disease
  - Gene therapy
  - Pharmacogenomics ('custom drugs' to target specific genetic composition so as to get best drug response with minimal side effects)
- Energy and environmental applications:
  - Use microbial genomics research to create new energy sources (biofuels) and to develop environmental monitoring techniques to detect pollutants.
- Risk assessment
- Assess health damage caused by radiation exposure and mutagenic chemicals
- DNA forensics (identification)

■ PHARMACOGENETICS
- Pharmacogenetics or pharmacogenomics is the study of interaction between genetics and therapeutic drugs.
- Pharmacogenetics is the study of unexpected drug response result and to look for a genetic cause.
- Pharmacogenomics is the study of identifying genetic differences within a population that explains certain observed responses to a drug or susceptibility to a health problem.
- Potential applications include:
  - Maximise therapeutic effects.
  - Decrease likelihood of adverse reactions.
  - Determine drug responses in the treatment of cardiac, respiratory and psychiatric conditions.
  - Develop targeted drugs.

■ EPIGENETICS
- Refers to variability in gene expression, heritable through mitosis and potentially meiosis, without any underlying modification in the actual genetic sequence.
- Potential clinical applications include:
  - Epigenetic tumour markers
  - Epigenetic therapeutic agents (e.g. azacitidine, decitabine, vorinostat) that are used in the treatment of myelodysplastic syndromes and progressive lymphoma

■ CHROMOSOMAL ABERRATIONS
- Chromosomal aberrations may be summarised as follows:
  - Autosomal abnormalities
  - Sex-linked abnormalities
- Both autosomal and sex-linked abnormalities may be due to:
  - Numerical abnormalities (number of chromosomes different from normal)

○ Structural abnormalities (change in structure of chromosomes due to addition or deletion of a part of it)

Numerical Abnormalities of Autosomal Chromosomes

- **Polyploidy:** One whole set of chromosomes (i.e. 23 chromosomes) is gained (3n, 4n: Normal pattern is 2n). This is not compatible with life.
- **Aneuploidy:** One or more chromosomes are either gained or lost.
  ○ Monosomy: Loss of one chromosome (instead of the typical two in humans) from a pair of autosomes (2n-1). This is lethal in males.
  ○ Trisomy: Addition of an extra autosome chromosome (2n+1), e.g.
    - Down syndrome (trisomy-21; 47 XY, +21).
    - Patau syndrome (trisomy-13; 47 XY, +13).
    - Edwards syndrome (trisomy-18; 47 XY,+18)

Numerical Abnormalities of Sex Chromosomes

- Monosomy is seen with Turner's syndrome (45 X or 45 X0).
- Presence of more than one X chromosome produces higher risk of mental retardation (e.g. Klinefelter syndrome—47 XXY).

Structural Abnormalities of Chromosome

Structural abnormalities of chromosome are discussed below and shown in **Figure 27.1**.
- **Deletion:** Loss of part of a chromosome (e.g. loss of short arm of chromosome number 5 produces Cri-du-chat syndrome 46 XY, 5 p-)
- **Inversion:** When a segment of chromosome is oriented in the reverse direction, such segment is said to be inverted and the phenomenon is termed as inversion.
- **Translocation:** Exchange of segments between two non-homologous chromosomes, i.e. recombination of two unrelated genes for new genetic information (e.g. Philadelphia chromosome)
  ○ **Robertsonian translocation/centric fusion:**
    - This results from the breakage of two acrocentric chromosomes (i.e. chromosome 13, 14, 15, 21 and 22) at or close to their centromeres and subsequent fusion of their long arms.
    - The short arms of each chromosome are lost, these being of no clinical

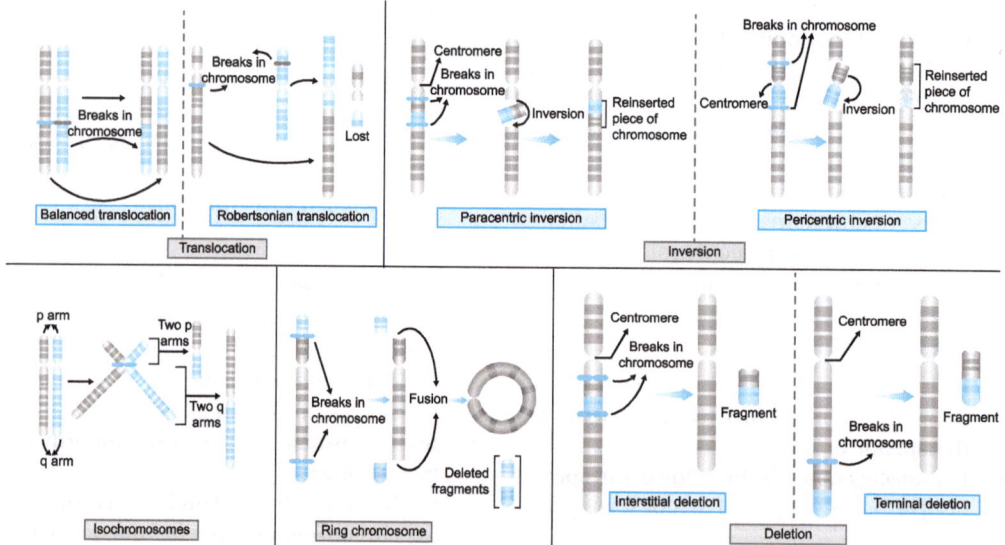

Fig. 27.1: Structural abnormalities of chromosome.

importance as they contain genes only for ribosomal RNA, for which there are multiple copies on various other chromosomes.
- The total chromosome number is reduced to 45. The major practical importance is that this can predispose to the birth of babies with Down syndrome.
- **Ring chromosomes**: Fusion of the two ends of the same chromosome; there is loss of genetic material at the ends of the chromosome prior to the fusion.
- **Isochromosomes**: A chromosome with two genetically identical arms, i.e. two 'p' or two 'q' arms (e.g. some cases of Turner's syndrome)

MIXOPLOIDY

- **Mosaicism:** Defined as the presence in an individual or in a tissue of two or more cell lines that differ in their genetic constitution but are derived from a single zygote, i.e. they have the same genetic origin. Seen in Down syndrome (1-2%) and Duchenne muscular dystrophy (DMD).
- **Chimerism:** Defined as the presence in an individual or in a tissue of two or more cell lines that are derived from more than one zygote, i.e. they have different genetic origins.

AUTOSOMAL DOMINANT DISEASES

- Characterised by (**Fig. 27.2**):
  ○ Vertical transmission to subsequent generations
  ○ One parent is affected in most cases
  ○ About 50% chances that the child of an affected parent will be affected
  ○ Males and females equally affected
- Some autosomal dominant diseases may show variable expression, i.e. variation in severity of the same disease (autosomal dominance with variable penetrance).
- Sometimes, the gene is not expressed at all (non-penetrance) which explains apparent skipping of generations.

Examples of autosomal dominant disorders are given in **Table 27.1**.

AUTOSOMAL RECESSIVE DISEASES

- Characterised by (**Fig. 27.3**):
  ○ Males and females are equally likely to be affected.

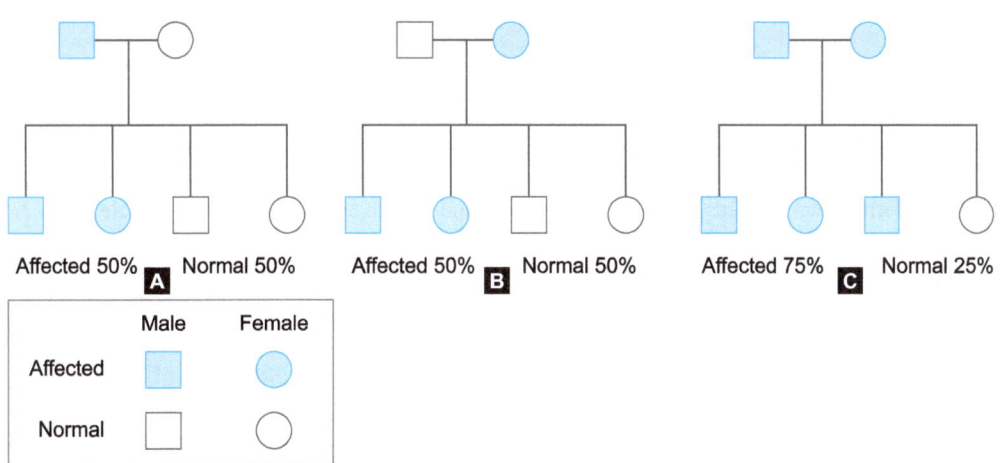

Fig. 27.2: Pedigree illustrating autosomal dominant transmission. (A and B) One parent is affected; (C) Both parents are affected. Note that both males and females are affected equally.

TABLE 27.1: Examples of autosomal dominant and autosomal recessive disorders.

System	Autosomal dominant disorder	Autosomal recessive disorder
Nervous	• Huntington disease • Neurofibromatosis • Tuberous sclerosis	• Neurogenic muscular atrophies • Friedreich's ataxia • Spinal muscular atrophy
Skeletal	• Marfan syndrome • Achondroplasia • Noonan syndrome	• Alkaptonuria • Ehlers–Danlos syndrome
Metabolic	• Familial hypercholesterolaemia • Intermittent porphyria	Cystic fibrosis, phenylketonuria, lysosomal storage diseases, galactosaemia, haemochromatosis, glycogen storage diseases
Haematopoietic	• Hereditary spherocytosis • von Willebrand disease	Sickle cell anaemia, thalassaemia
Renal	Polycystic kidney disease	Congenital adrenal hyperplasia
Gastrointestinal	Familial polyposis coli	Wilson's disease

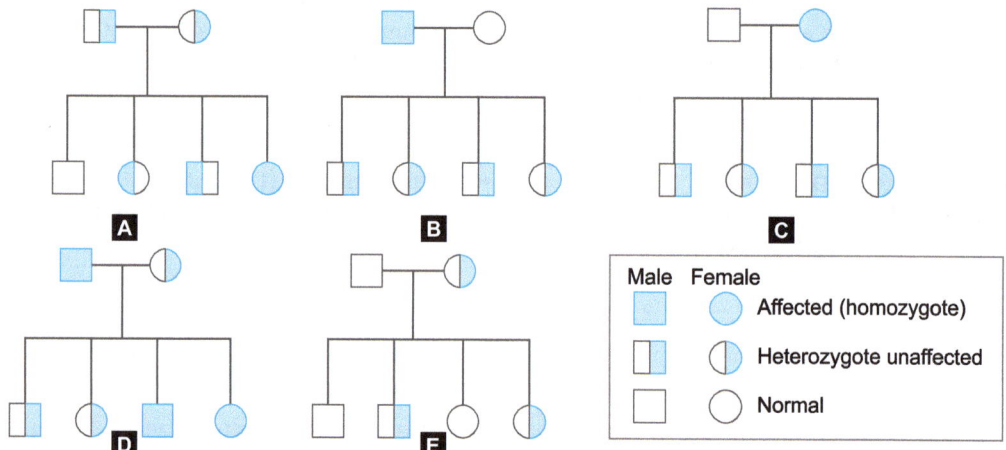

Fig. 27.3: Pedigree illustrating mechanism of autosomal recessive transmission. (A) Both parents are unaffected heterozygotes; (B and C) One parent is sufferer (homozygous) and other is normal; (D) One parent is sufferer and other is unaffected heterozygote; (E) One parent is normal and other is an unaffected heterozygote.

- o Disease not present in parents, offspring or other relatives of affected person (horizontal transmission)
- o Birth of an affected child establishes both parents as carriers of a single copy of the gene mutation.
- o Chance of a second affected child in the sibship is one in four or 25% in each pregnancy. About 50% are heterozygotes (clinically normal) and 25% are normal without any mutant gene.

Examples of autosomal recessive disorders are given in **Table 27.1**.

■ X-LINKED DOMINANT DISEASES

- Characterised by (**Fig. 27.4**):
  - o No carrier state as the disease will manifest even if single chromosome has abnormal gene.
  - o The trait is never passed from father to son, as the son's 'normal' X chromosome is from mother.

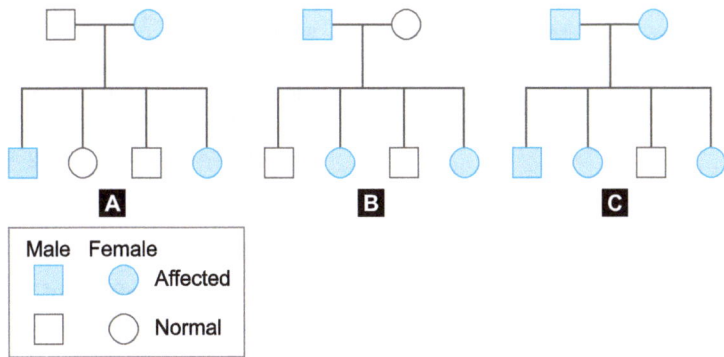

Figs. 27.4A to C: X-linked dominant transmission. Only females are affected. Usually males who inherit the mutant allele die in utero. (A) Normal male and female affected (sufferer); (B) Affected male and normal female; (C) Both male and female are affected.

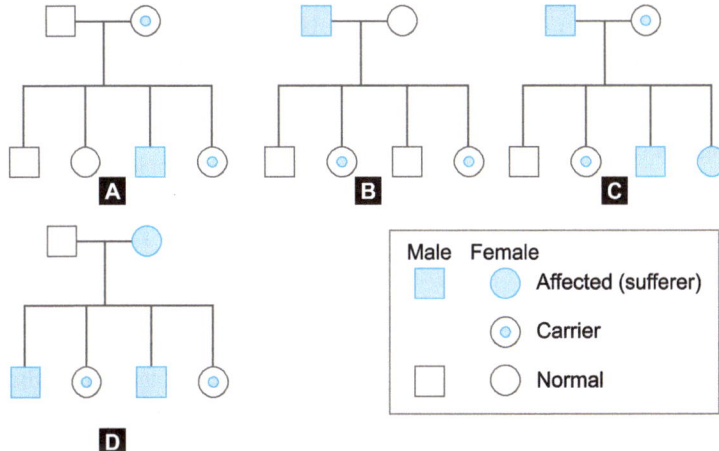

Figs. 27.5A to D: Mode of X-linked recessive transmission. Note the absence of male-to-male transmission. (A) Male is normal and female is a carrier; (B) Male is sufferer and female is normal; (C) Male is a sufferer and female is a carrier; (D) Male is normal and female is a sufferer.

- All daughters of an affected father are diseased as the daughter gets abnormal X from the father.
- If mother is affected and father is normal, 50% of both sons and daughters are affected.
- In general, males are more severely affected than females.
- For example, vitamin D resistance rickets, Alport syndrome

X-LINKED RECESSIVE DISEASES

- Characterised by (**Fig. 27.5**):
  o The disease is never passed from father to son.
  o Manifests only in males. In many diseases, males do not survive.
  o Mothers are always carriers and all their sons are affected.

Examples of X-linked recessive disorders are given in **Table 27.2**.

Y-LINKED DISEASES

- Characterised by:
  o Only men are affected.
  o Transmission of the gene occurs from an affected male to all his sons but never to the daughters.

TABLE 27.2: Examples of X-linked recessive disorders.

System	Related X-linked recessive disease
Musculoskeletal	Duchenne muscular dystrophy
Blood	Haemophilia A and B
	Glucose-6-phosphate dehydrogenase deficiency
Immune	Agammaglobulinaemia
Metabolic	Diabetes insipidus
Nervous	Fragile-X syndrome

■ DIGENIC INHERITANCE

- Digenic inheritance explicates how the retinitis pigmentosa (RP) manifests in those children whose parents carry a different RP-associated gene.
- Both parents have a normal vision, but the offsprings who were double heterozygotes developed RP.
- Digenic pedigrees exhibit characteristics of both autosomal dominant (vertical transmission) and autosomal recessive inheritance (1 in 4 recurrence risk).

■ MITOCHONDRIAL INHERITANCE

- An individual's mitochondrial genome is entirely derived from the mother.
- Examples include myopathy, encephalopathy, lactic acidosis, and stroke-like episodes (MELAS), myoclonic epilepsy associated with ragged red fibres (MERRF), and Kearns–Sayre syndrome (ophthalmoplegia, pigmentary retinopathy and cardiomyopathy)

■ GENETIC IMPRINTING

- The two copies of most genes are functionally equivalent. In a small number, only one of the pair is transcribed.
- The active gene will be that inherited from a specific parent, and the other copy is silenced associated with methylation of DNA (epigenetic modification of a gene not due to a DNA mutation).

Conditions associated with genetic imprinting:
- Prader–Willi syndrome with paternal chromosome deletion
- Angelman syndrome with maternal chromosome deletion
- Other conditions associated with imprinting are Beckwith–Wiedemann syndrome and Russell-Silver syndrome, DMD in females and epigenetic silencing in oncogenesis, e.g. colon cancer 3p21 MLH1.

■ PLEIOTROPY

- Genes that exert effects of the physiological and anatomical features are called pleiotropic.
- For example, Marfan syndrome (eyes, skeleton and the cardiovascular system are affected); cystic fibrosis (sweat glands, lungs, pancreas and genitourinary system are affected), osteogenesis imperfecta [(OI) bones, teeth and sclera are affected] and sickle cell anaemia (RBCs, bone and spleen are affected).

■ LOCUS HETEROGENEITY

- It is a disease which is caused due to mutations at different loci in different families and is said to exhibit locus heterogeneity.
- Osteogenesis imperfecta: Subunits of procollagen triple helix are encoded by two genes, one on chromosome 17 and the other on chromosome 7. Mutation in either of these genes can alter the structure of the collagen molecules and lead to OI; disease states are often indistinguishable.

■ POLYMORPHISMS

- A polymorphism is defined as one that exists with a population frequency of > 1%.
- Most common polymorphisms are neutral but may often cause small alterations in the protein structure and function of the gene. For example, cystic fibrosis, haemochromatosis, alpha 1 AT deficiency and spinomuscular dystrophy.

■ MONGOLISM (DOWN SYNDROME)

- Autosomal abnormality where the number of the autosomes are affected (autosomal imbalance)
  ○ Extra chromosome 21 (trisomy 21) due to non-disjunction during meiosis (95%)

- o 1% mosaicism
- o 4% due to translocation
- Significant relationship to increasing maternal age

Clinical Features
- Typical facies is characterised by flat nasal bridge, mouth hanging open, flat face, widely spaced eyes (hypertelorism) and upward, slanting eyes with epicanthic folds, malformed ears and protruding furrowed tongue (Mongoloid facies)
- Broad, short neck
- Brachycephaly
- Simian crease—single palmar flexion crease (50% cases)
- Mental deficiency
- An almond shape to the eyes caused by an epicanthic fold of the eyelid
- Brushfield spot on iris
- Short stature and hypotonia
- Fondness for music
- Congenital heart diseases, e.g. atrial septal defect (ASD), ventricular septal defect (VSD), tetralogy of Fallot and endocardial cushion defects
- Increased frequency of leukaemia
- Increased risk of sleep apnoea

The screens required to diagnose Down syndrome are given in **Box 27.1**.

> **Box 27.1: Down syndrome screens.**
> - **Triple screen (75% sensitive):** Maternal serum alpha-foetoprotein, estriol and human chorionic gonadotropin (hCG).
> - **Quad screen (79% sensitive):** Maternal serum alpha-foetoprotein, estriol, hCG and high inhibin-alpha (INHA).
> - **Nuchal translucency/free beta-hCG >/ pregnancy-associated plasma protein-A (PAPPA) screen (91% sensitive):** Ultrasound to measure nuchal translucency in addition to the free beta-hCG and PAPPA.
> - **The full integrated test** (first-trimester nuchal translucency, and PAPP-A plus second-trimester quadruple markers) detects 85% of Down syndrome foetuses.

■ KLINEFELTER SYNDROME
- Most common karyotype is XXX.
- Other karyotypes include XXXY/XXXXX/XXYY.

Clinical Features
- Sterility, small testes
- Gynaecomastia
- Eunuchoid body proportions
- Sparse facial, body and sexual hair
- Mental retardation

■ TURNER SYNDROME
Genetic constitution hence becomes 45 XO.

Clinical Features
- Short stature
- Webbed neck and low posterior hair line
- Broad chest → 'shield chest'
- Increased carrying angle at the elbows (cubitus valgus)
- Lymphoedema
- Mild mental retardation
- Infertility
- Primary amenorrhoea with elevated follicle-stimulating hormone (FSH)
- Coarctation of aorta or bicuspid aortic valve
- Lack of secondary sexual characteristics

■ GENE THERAPY
Gene therapy is a technique for correcting defective genes responsible for disease development by using genetic material.

Forms
- Germ-line gene therapy → modification of the germ-line cells. It is not accepted at present due to ethical reasons.
- Somatic germ therapy → modification of different somatic cells. This can be achieved by following ways:
  - o A normal gene is inserted in a non-specific location.
  - o Repair of defective gene through selective reverse mutation

o Alteration of the regulation of an abnormal gene

Approaches
- Two different approaches:
  o In 'ex vivo' gene therapy, genetic modifications are done on specific cells which are isolated and purified from patient and are re-infused.
  o In 'in vivo' gene therapy, which is also the most commonly used technique, a vector is used to directly transfer the genes into patient's tissue.
  o The disease-causing gene is replaced by a normal gene by inserting it in the genome.
  o Therapeutic gene is delivered by a carrier molecule, which is called a vector, into the patient's target cells. The commonly used vector is a virus. For instance, moloney murine leukaemia virus, adenoviruses, adeno-associated viruses and lentivirus.

Risks
- Potential for vectors producing disease
- May induce cancers
- Immune over-reactions

Therapeutic Applications
- Gene therapy has not been approved for clinical use.
- Trials are going in genetic disorders, cancers, infectious diseases and other diseases such as Alzheimer's disease and atherosclerosis.

A list of chromosomal disorders is given in **Table 27.3**.

TABLE 27.3: List of chromosomal disorders.

Chromosome	Abnormality	Disease association
X	XO	Turner's syndrome
Y	XXY	Klinefelter syndrome
Y	XYY	Double Y syndrome
Y	XXX	Trisomy X syndrome
Y	Xp21 deletion	Duchenne's/Becker syndrome congenital adrenal hypoplasia, chronic granulomatus disease
1	1p (somatic) monosomy trisomy	Neuroblastoma
2	Monosomy trisomy 2q	Growth retardation, developmental and mental delay, and minor physical abnormalities
3	Monosomy trisomy (somatic)	Non-Hodgkin's lymphoma
4	Monosomy trisomy (somatic)	Acute non-lymphocytic leukaemia (ANLL)
5	5p deletion	Cri-du-chat; Lejeune syndrome
5	5q (somatic) monosomy trisomy	Myelodysplastic syndrome (MDS)
6	Monosomy trisomy (somatic)	Clear-cell sarcoma
7	7q 11.23 deletion	William's syndrome
8	Monosomy trisomy	MDS; Warkany syndrome; chronic myelogenous leukaemia
9	Trisomy	Complete trisomy 9 syndrome: Mosaic trisomy 9 syndrome
10	Monosomy trisomy (somatic)	ALL or ANLL
11	11p-	Aniridia: Wilms tumor
11	Monosomy (somatic) trisomy	Myeloid lineages affected (ANLL, MDS)
12	Monosomy trisomy (somatic)	CLL, juvenile granulosa cell tumor (JGCT)
13	13q14 deletion	Retinoblastoma
13	Monosomy trisomy	Patau's syndrome

Continued

Continued

Chromosome	Abnormality	Disease association
14	Monosomy trisomy (somatic)	Myeloid disorders (MDS, ANLL, atypical CML)
15	15q11-q13 deletion monosomy	Prader-Wili, Angelman's syndrome
15	Trisomy (somatic)	Myeloid and lymphoid lineages affected, e.g. MDS, ANLL, ALL, CLL
16	16q13.3 deletion monosomy trisomy (somatic)	Rubinstein-Taybi, papillary renal cell carcinomas (malignant)
17	17p (somatic)	17p syndrome in myeloid malignancies
17	Monosomy trisomy (somatic)	Renal cortical adenomas
18	Monosomy trisomy	Edwards syndrome
19	Trisomy, deletion	
20	20p-	Trisomy 20p syndrome
20	20q-	MDS, ANLL, polycythaemia vera, chronic neutrophilic leukaemia
20	Monosomy trisomy (somatic)	Papillary renal cell carcinomas (malignant)
21	Monosomy trisomy	Down's syndrome
22	22q11.2 deletion	DiGeorge's syndrome, velocardiofacial syndrome, conotruncal anomaly face syndrome, CML-reciprocal translocation 9:22 Opitz G/BBB syndrome, Caylor cardiofacial syndrome
22	Monosomy trisomy	Complete trisomy 22 syndrome

(ALL: acute lymphoid leukaemia; CLL: . chronic lymphocytic leukaemia; CML: chronic myeloid leukaemia)

BEST OF FIVES

1. In sporadic Prader–Willi syndrome (PWS), there is a non-disjunction defect on chromosome 15, and both copies of the chromosomal region are derived from the mother. This is an example of:
   A. Isochromosomal disorder
   B. Chimerism
   C. Genomic imprinting
   D. Lyonisation
   E. Mosaicism

2. A 32-year-old primigravida with 11 weeks' gestation has been admitted with hyperemesis. She is worried about genetic defects in the foetus. The investigation panel done reveals moderately elevated human chorionic gonadotropin (hCG) and markedly elevated pregnancy-associated plasma protein-A (PAPP-A). These suggest the increased likelihood of:
   A. Huntington's disease
   B. Down syndrome
   C. Cri-du-chat syndrome
   D. Beckwith–Wiedemann syndrome
   E. Choriocarcinoma

3. A young male has a strong family history of cancers, i.e. mother and aunt had carcinoma of breast, maternal uncle had astrocytoma and elder sister had acute promyelocytic leukaemia. You suspect him to have Li-Fraumeni syndrome. On genetic analysis, you would expect:
   A. Loss-of-function mutations in the gene encoding p53
   B. Gain-of-function mutations in the gene encoding p53
   C. Inactivation mutations in the tumour suppressor gene on 5q
   D. Activation mutations in the tumour suppressor gene on 5q
   E. Activation of BCR-abl

4. A woman is at a risk of being a carrier of an X-linked recessive disease. Her grandfather and brother are affected, which make her

mother an obligate gene carrier. Her risk of being a carrier is therefore:
A. 50%
B. 25%
C. 75%
D. 100%
E. 0%

5. Telomeres are the protective end regions of chromosomes which shorten with each cell division because telomerase is absent in somatic cells. When telomeres are sufficiently eroded, cells stop dividing. Telomeres are particularly shortened and DNA is damaged due to lack of a helicase in patients resulting from premature ageing in:
A. Cockayne syndrome
B. Werner's syndrome
C. Rothmund–Thomson syndrome
D. Bloom syndrome
E. Pendred syndrome

6. Retinitis pigmentosa can occur as the result of mutations in more than 75 genes, each of which has a different chromosomal location. This phenomenon is called:
A. Polymorphic copy number variants
B. Gene polymorphism
C. Allelic heterogeneity
D. Chimerism
E. Locus heterogeneity

7. A 60-year-old patient presents with fatigue, weight loss, left upper quadrant fullness and heaviness from 6 months. The haematological tests revealed hemoglobin of 10 gm%, total count 500,000/mm and platelet count 4,00,000/mm. Differential count: Neutrophils 55, lymphocytes 4, monocytes 2, basophils 6, metamyelocytes 10, myelocytes 118, promyelocytes 2 and blasts 3. The most likely genetic abnormality in this case is:
A. t(9, 22)
B. t(8, 14)
C. t(4, 16)
D. Trisomy 12
E. Trisomy 18

8. A 22-year-old man presents to accident and emergency on a Saturday afternoon after collapsing while playing basketball. He has sharp central chest pain, a weak left radial pulse and a mild pectus excavatum. His grandfather died from a suspected heart attack while pushing his car in Africa last year. What is the inheritance of this condition?
A. Autosomal dominant
B. Autosomal recessive
C. Mitochondrial
D. X-linked dominant
E. Y-linked

9. A baby in the neonatal ward with a cleft palate has developed seizure. The calcium is noted to be low. There is a family history of schizophrenia. Chromosomal analysis is likely to reveal:
A. 22q11.2 microdeletions
B. Trisomy 18
C. 44 XXXX
D. 17 p deletion
E. 11p13 deletion

10. Regarding alpha 1 antitrypsin deficiency, all the following statements are TRUE except:
A. Homozygous mutation carriers are at a higher risk of neonatal jaundice and emphysema.
B. There is a possible increased risk of emphysema in heterozygous mutation carriers.
C. There is good evidence that ZZ homozygous alpha-1-antitrypsin mutation carriers have a far higher risk of emphysema if they smoke.
D. The ZZ phenotype is usually the most severe and leads to an inability to cope with airborne pathogens.
E. MZ carriers are at no increased risk if they smoke, so smoking can be continued.

11. A neonate with seizures on examination has macroglossia and asymmetry and weighs 4.5 kg. Bedside test reveals hypoglycaemia. The most likely syndromic diagnosis is:
A. Beckwith–Wiedemann syndrome
B. Russell–Silver syndrome
C. Neurofibromatosis type 1
D. Simpson–Golabi–Behmel syndrome
E. Klippel–Trenaunay–Weber syndrome

12. All are TRUE statements regarding Huntington's disease except:
A. Huntington's disease is caused by an autosomal dominant trinucleotide repeat.
B. Huntington's disease is associated with depression and motor disorders.

C. Huntington's disease has 100% penetrance so if an individual has the gene, he/she will develop the disease.
D. If an individual inherits the gene from his/her father, he/she is likely to have an earlier onset and a more severe form than if he/she had inherited the same gene from his/her mother.
E. Huntington's disease shows maternal anticipation.

13. In which of the following phenotypic females does a testis develop?
    A. 46, XY with an interstitial deletion of Yp involving the *SRY* gene
    B. 46, XY with a point mutation in the HMG domain of the *SRY* gene
    C. 46, XX
    D. 46, XY with X-linked androgen receptor deficiency
    E. 45, X

14. Which of the following will yield the highest recurrence risk for Down syndrome in a family?
    A. 35-year-old mother
    B. 65-year-old father
    C. 25-year-old mother with a previous child with trisomy 21
    D. 20-year-old mother who carries a 21/14 Robertsonian translocation and has had no previous children with Down syndrome
    E. 20-year-old father who carries a 21/14 Robertsonian translocation and has had no previous children with Down syndrome

15. What is the clinical diagnosis of a child with a karyotype 46,XY.del (15)(q11q12)pat?
    A. Angelman syndrome
    B. Edwards syndrome
    C. Prader–Willi syndrome
    D. Cri-du-chat syndrome
    E. William syndrome

Answers

1-C, 2-B, 3-A, 4-A, 5-B, 6-E, 7-A, 8-A, 9-A, 10-E, 11-A, 12-E, 13-D, 14-D, 15-C

SUGGESTED READING

1. Strachan T, Read A. Human Molecular Genetics, 4th edition. New York: Garland Science; 2010.
2. Murphy A, Chu JH, Xu M, Carey VJ, Lazarus R, Liu a, et al. Mapping of numerous disease-associated expression polymorphisms in primary peripheral blood CD4+ lymphocytes. Hum Mol Genet. 2010;19(23):4745-57.
3. Collins FS, Green ED, Guttmacher AE, Guyer MS, US National Human Genome Research Institute. A vision for the future of genomics research. Nature. 2003;422(6934):835-47.
4. Ranweiler R. Assessment and care of the newborn with Down syndrome. Adv Neonatal Care. 2009;9(1):17-24.
5. National Society of Genetic Counselors' Definition Task Force, Resta R, Biesecker BB, Bennett RL, Blum S, Hahn SE, et al. A new definition of Genetic Counseling: National Society of Genetic Counselors' Task Force report. J Genet Couns. 2006;15(2):77-83.
6. Richter M, Stone D, Miao C, Humbert O, Kiem HP, Papayannopoulou T, et al. In vivo hematopoietic stem cell transduction. Hematol Oncol Clin North Am. 2017;31(5): 771-85.
7. Reynolds PN, Zinn KR, Gavrilyuk VD, Balyasnikova IV, Rogers BE, Buchsbaum DJ, et al. A targetable, injectable adenoviral vector for selective gene delivery to pulmonary endothelium in vivo. Mol Ther. 2000;2(6):562-78.
8. Colella P, Ronzitti G, Mingozzi F. Emerging issues in AAV-mediated in vivo gene therapy. Mol Ther Methods Clin Dev. 2018;8:87-104.
9. Reddy UM, Page GP, Saade GR. The role of DNA microarrays in the evaluation of fetal death. Prenat Diagn. 2012;32(4):371-5.

CHAPTER 28

Epidemiology

INTRODUCTION

It is the study of *frequency, distribution and determinants of diseases and other health-related conditions* in a *human population* and the *application* of this study to the prevention of disease and promotion of health.

The components of the definition of epidemiology are given in **Box 28.1**.

Types of Epidemiology

There are two major categories of epidemiology, which are given in **Box 28.2**.

Box 28.1: Components of the definition of epidemiology.

Study:	Frequency:	Distribution:	Determinants:
• Systematic collection, analysis and interpretation of data • Epidemiology involves collection, analysis and interpretation of health-related data **Epidemiology is a science**	• The number of times an event occurs • Epidemiology studies the number of times a disease occurs • It answers the question 'How many?' **Epidemiology is a quantitative science**	• Distribution of an event by person, place and time • Epidemiology studies distribution of diseases • It answers the question 'who, where and when?' **Epidemiology describes health events**	• Factors the presence/absence of which affect the occurrence and level of an event • Epidemiology studies what determines health events • It answers the question 'how and why?' **Epidemiology analyses health events**
Diseases and other health-related events • Epidemiology is not only the study of diseases • The focus of epidemiology is not only patients • It studies all health-related conditions **Epidemiology is a broader science**	**Human population** • Epidemiology diagnoses and treats communities/populations • Clinical medicine diagnoses and treats patients **Epidemiology is a basic science of public health**		**Application** • Epidemiological studies have direct and practical applications for prevention of diseases and promotion of health • Epidemiology is a science and practice **Epidemiology is an applied science**

> **Box 28.2: Two major categories of epidemiology.**
>
> **Descriptive Epidemiology:**
> - Defines frequency and distribution of diseases and other health-related events
> - Answers the four major questions: How many, who, where and when?
>
> **Analytic Epidemiology:**
> - Analyses determinants of health problems
> - Answers two other major questions: How? and why?

MEASURES OF DISEASE OCCURRENCE

Four quantitative descriptors:
1. **Numbers**—use of the actual number of events
2. **Ratios**—quantify the magnitude of one occurrence X in relation to another event Y as X/Y
3. **Proportions**—a ratio in which the numerator is included in the denominator
4. **Rates**—a proportion with time element. It measures the occurrence of an event over time.

   Incidence describes the proportion of a population that develops a disease overtime.

   Prevalence is the measure of the proportion of a population to a particular disease during a specified point in time or period.

   Incidence versus prevalence
   Incidence rate takes into account only new cases of a disease; however, Prevalence rate considers both new and old cases of a given disease.

MEASURES OF ASSOCIATION

The measures of association are given in **Box 28.3**.

EVALUATION OF EVIDENCE (JUDGEMENT OF CAUSALITY)

Association and Causation

The existence of an association itself does not constitute a proof of causation. It could be a fact or an artefact. Therefore, an association is a necessary but not the only sufficient condition for causation.

Association could be due the following factors:
- Chance
- Bias
- Confounding
- Reverse causation

> **Box 28.3: Measures of association.**
>
> **Chi-square statistics**
> - Chi-square tests tell whether there is an association between two categorical variables.
> - If the calculated chi-square value is greater than the critical or $p < 0.05$, we say that there is association.
> - Chi-square statistics tells only whether there is association. It does not tell us how much strong an association is.
>
> **Relative risk (RR)**
> - RR = Incidence (risk) among exposed/Incidence (risk) among non-exposed
> - In general, strength of association can be considered as:
>   - High if RR > 3
>   - Moderate if RR is between 1.5 and 2.9
>   - Weak if RR is between 1.2 and 1.4
>
> **Odds ratio (OR)**
> - Odds ratio is the ratio of odds of exposure among diseased to odds of exposure among non-diseased.
> - OR = Odds of exposure among diseased/Odds of exposure among non-diseased
> - Interpretation of OR is the same as that of RR.
>
> **Attributable risk (AR)**
> - AR indicates how much of the risk is due to/attributable/to the exposure.
> - Quantifies the excess risk in the exposed that can be attributable to the exposure by removing the risk of the disease that occurred due to other causes.
> - AR = Risk (incidence) in exposed − Risk (incidence) in non-exposed
> - What does attributable risk of 10 mean?
>   - 10 of the exposed cases are attributable to the exposure.
>   - By removing the exposure, one can prevent 10 cases from getting the disease.
>
> **Possible outcomes in studying the relationship between exposure and disease**
> - No association
>   RR = 1
>   AR = 0
> - Positive association
>   RR > 1
>   AR > 0
> - Negative association
>   RR < 1 (fraction)
>   AR < 0 (negative)

- Reciprocal causation
- Cause–effect relationship

ROLE OF BIAS

Bias is any systematic error in the design, conduct or analysis of an epidemiologic study that results in an incorrect estimate of association between exposure and disease.

Unlike chance, bias cannot be statistically evaluated.

There are two major types of bias (**Box 28.4**):
1. Selection bias
2. Information bias

TYPES OF EPIDEMIOLOGIC STUDY DESIGNS

Epidemiologic study designs and their types are given in **Box 28.5**.

The various advantages and disadvantages of different types of epidemiologic study are given in **Table 28.1**.

LEVELS OF EVIDENCE

Levels of evidence are given in **Table 28.2**.

Box 28.4: Two major types of bias.

Selection bias:
- Is any systematic error that arises in the process of identifying the study population
- Affects the representativeness of the study
- Occurs when there is a difference between sample and population with respect to a variable

Examples:
- Diagnostic bias
- Volunteer bias
- Non-response bias
- Loss to follow-up bias

Information/Observation bias:
- Is any systematic error in the measurement of the information on exposure or disease

Examples:
- Interviewer bias/observer bias
- Recall bias/response bias
- Social desirability bias
- Placebo effect

Box 28.5: Types of epidemiologic study designs.

I. Based on objective/focus/research question
Descriptive studies
- Describe: Who, when, where and how many

Analytic studies
- Analyse: How and why

II. Based on the role of the investigator
Observational studies
- The investigator observes nature
- No intervention

Intervention/Experimental studies
- Investigator intervenes
- He has a control over the situation

III. Based on timing
One-time (one-spot) studies
- Conducted at a point in time
- An individual is observed at once

Longitudinal (follow-up) studies
- Conducted in a period of time
- Individuals are followed over a period of time

IV Based on the direction of follow-up/data collection
Prospective
- Conducted forwards in time

Retrospective
- Conducted backwards in time

V. Based on type of data they generate
Qualitative studies
- Generate contextual data
- Also called exploratory studies

Quantitative studies
- Generate numerical data
- It is also called explanatory studies

VI. Based on study setting
Community-based studies
- Conducted in communities

Institution-based studies
- Conducted in hospitals, colleges

Laboratory-based studies
- Conducted in major laboratories

VII. Standard classification
- Cross-sectional studies
- Case-control studies
- Cohort studies
- Experimental studies

TABLE 28.1: Types of study with its pros and cons.

Type of study	Description	Pros	Cons
RCT (Randomised controlled trial)	An experimental comparison study where participants are allocated to treatment/intervention or control/placebo groups using a random mechanism. Best for studying the effect of an intervention	• Unbiased distribution of confounders • Blinding more likely • Randomisation facilitates statistical analysis	• Expensive: Time and money • Volunteer bias • Ethically problematic at times
Crossover trial	A controlled trial where each participant has both therapies, i.e. randomised to treatment. A first then starts treatment B	• All participants serve as own controls and error variance is reduced, thus reducing sample size needed • All participants receive treatment (at least some of the time) • Statistical test assuming randomisation can be used • Blinding may be contained	• All participants receive placebo or alternative treatment at some point • Washout period lengthy or unknown • Cannot be used for treatments with permanent effects
Cohort study	Data obtained from groups who have already been exposed, or not exposed, to the factor of interest. No allocation of exposure is made by the researcher. Best for studying effects of risk factors on an outcome	• Ethically safe • Participants can be matched • Can establish timing and directionality of events • Eligibility criteria and outcome assessments can be standardised	• Controls may be difficult to identify • Exposure may be linked to a hidden confounder • Blinding is difficult for rare disease, large sample sizes or long follow-up necessary
Case-control study	Patients with a certain outcome or disease and an appropriate group of controls, without the outcome or disease, are selected (usually with some matching); then information is obtained on whether the subjects have been exposed to the factor under investigation	• Quick and cheap as fewer people needed than cross-sectional studies • Only feasible method for very rare disorders or those with long lag between exposure and outcome	• Reliance on recall or records to determine exposure status • Confounders • Selection of control groups is difficult • Potential bias: Recall, selection
Cross-sectional study	Examines the relationship between (1) diseases/other health-related characteristics and (2) other variables of interest as they exist in defined population at one time. Exposure and outcomes both measured at the same time. Quantifies prevalence, risk or diagnostic test accuracy	• Cheap and simple • Ethically safe	• Establishes association at most, not causality • Recall bias, social desirability bias • Researcher's (Neyman) bias • Group sizes may be unequal • Cofounders may be unequally distributed

TABLE 28.2: Levels of evidence.

Level of evidence (LOE)	Description
Level I	Evidence from a **systematic review or meta-analysis** of all revelant randomised controlled trial (RCTs) or evidence-based clinical practice guidelines based on systematic reviews of RCTs of good quality that have similar results
Level II	Evidence obtained from at least one well-designed **RCT** (e.g. large multisite RCT)
Level III	Evidence obtained from well-designed **controlled trials without randomisation** (i.e. quasi-experimental)
Level IV	Evidence from well-designed **case control or cohort studies**
Level V	Evidence from systematic reviews of descriptive and qualitative studies (metasynthesis)
Level VI	Evidence from a single descriptive or qualitative study
Level VII	Evidence from the opinion of authorities and/or reports of expert committees

TABLE 28.3: Types of blinding in clinical trials.

Type	Description
Unblinded or open label	All parties are aware of the treatment the participant receives
Single blind or single-masked	Only the participant is unaware of the treatment he/she receives
Double blind or double-masked	The participant and the clinicians/data collectors are unaware of the treatment the participant receives
Triple blind	Participant, clinicians/data collectors and outcome adjudicators/data analysts are all unaware of the treatment the participant receives

■ CONCEPT OF BLINDING IN CLINICAL TRIALS

Blinding is a procedure in which one or more parties in a trial are kept unaware of which treatment arms participants have been assigned to, in other words, which treatment was received. Blinding is an important aspect of any trial done in order to avoid and prevent conscious or unconscious bias in the design and execution of a clinical trial (**Table 28.3**).

BEST OF FIVES

1. Recall bias poses a substantial problem in which type of study?
   A. Crossover study
   B. Meta-analysis
   C. Retrospective case-controlled study
   D. Randomised double-blind control study
   E. Prospective cohort study

2. Regarding relative risk, which of the following is true?
   A. It can be positive or negative.
   B. It is calculated by the square root of the mean incidence in the exposed group divided by the mean incidence in the non-exposed group.
   C. It is the probability of an event occurring in an exposed group relative to a non-exposed group.
   D. When the risk is equal amongst the exposed and unexposed groups, the value is 0.
   E. It describes the chance of a patient's family developing a disease.

3. Data is said to be negatively skewed in distribution. What does it mean?
   A. Mode equals median
   B. Mean greater than median

C. Mean less than median
D. Normal distribution
E. Mean and median are the same

4. A study was conducted to compare calcium channel blocker (CCB), beta-blockers, angiotensin receptor blocker (ARB) and diuretics. One outcome of the study was to compare the blood pressure-lowering effect between the four medicines. Which of the following analysis would be most appropriate for the data?
   A. Correlation
   B. Student's t-test
   C. Cox regression
   D. ANOVA (analysis of variance)
   E. Regression

5. Which of the following statements is correct regarding random sampling?
   A. Increasing the sample size will not affect the standard error calculated from the sample.
   B. 95% of the sample means will lie within one standard error of the population mean.
   C. The distribution of the sample means is affected by the distribution of the variable in the population.
   D. The standard error of the mean is equivalent to the standard deviation of the sample means.
   E. Multiple samples are required to be taken in order to calculate the standard error of the mean.

6. With regards to a 95% confidence interval, which of the following is correct?
   A. 2.5% of measured values will lie below the lower limit of the interval.
   B. There is a 5% chance of the population mean lying above the upper limit of the interval.
   C. 5% of samples means will lie above the upper limit of the interval.
   D. 95% of the measured values will lie within the limits of the interval.
   E. The population mean lies within the limits of the interval with 95% confidence.

7. A multicentre double-blind randomised controlled trial (RCT) was conducted to compare the blood pressure (BP)-lowering effects of two antihypertensive drugs. Which of the following would be the most appropriate method for summarising the results?
   A. The mean and confidence interval for BP reduction for each antihypertensive drug
   B. The mean and confidence interval for final BP between the two antihypertensive drugs
   C. The mean and confidence interval for BP reduction between the two antihypertensive drugs
   D. The p-value for the difference in BP-lowering effects between the two antihypertensive drugs
   E. A box and whiskers plot displaying the minimum, maximum, median, lower quartile and upper quartile for the reduction in BP for each drug

8. Which is true of randomised parallel group studies?
   A. Randomisation ensures that variables between groups are balanced and do not affect outcomes.
   B. Randomisation minimises differences between the treatment groups at the onset.
   C. After a treatment has been run in one group, it is stopped and swapped with the treatment from another group.
   D. Differences in results between groups is due to the treatments.
   E. Group sizes should be equal.

9. A double-blinded randomised controlled trial was constructed and the two antiepileptic drugs were found to have major differences in the ratio of male to females. What should be done to improve the study?
   A. Restart the trial with only the sex being most affected by the condition.
   B. Restart the trial without randomisation
   C. No changes are needed.
   D. New participants should be brought in to equalise the ratio.
   E. The results should be analysed with this in mind to see if it affects the trial conclusions.

10. The end point for a double-blinded randomised controlled trial comparing treatments to prevent pulmonary embolism was death. Which of the following is true?
    A. Patients who do not survive a minimum time period should be excluded.
    B. If a severe side effect occurs frequently, then these patients should be excluded from the trial.
    C. Only the lead investigator should know details of the treatment groups during the trial.
    D. Only the participants should know details of which treatment they are on.
    E. A data monitoring committee should monitor patient safety and treatment data while the trial is running.

11. Power of a statistical test means:
    A. The strength of a relationship between two variables in a population
    B. The specificity of a test
    C. The power of a statistical test is the probability that the test will reject the null hypothesis when the null hypothesis is false
    D. The likelihood of a significant result occurring
    E. The estimate of a value or outcome based on a smaller sample

12. Which is true of confidence intervals?
    A. Confidence intervals describe the range of values around a median.
    B. They provide a measure of the statistical difference between two groups.
    C. A confidence interval describes the significance of the result.
    D. A 95% confidence interval means that there is a 95% chance that lies within the values shown.
    E. A 95% confidence interval means that the investigator is 95% sure that the outcome is correct.

13. Which of the statements is false?
    A. A high p value signifies a stronger result.
    B. Descriptive statistics summarise a data set to provide values such as the mean or the median.
    C. The null hypothesis declares that there is no link between two variables.
    D. The median is a value separating the higher and lower half of a sample.
    E. Correlation refers to a relationship between variables.

14. What is true regarding a studies sample?
    A. A random sample means that some members of a studies population have a 0% chance of being within the sample.
    B. A population sample must never have limiting criteria for selection.
    C. A population variable is an estimate of a sample statistic from a population sub-sample.
    D. A sample statistic is an estimate of a population variable from a population sub-sample.
    E. The mode is the middle value in an ordered sample.

15. Ivabradine was found safe in the initial test studies on healthy volunteers and a small trial of patients. What trial should be used next?
    A. Open label crossover study
    B. Double-blind parallel group randomised controlled trial
    C. Cross-sectional study
    D. Prospective cohort study
    E. Double-blind crossover randomised controlled trial

16. A study measuring the weights of 500 patients was performed. The mean weight was 198 lbs, the standard deviation was 50 lbs and the median weight was 155 lbs. Select the true statement.
    A. The largest patient weighs 249 lbs.
    B. The distribution is positively skewed.
    C. Half of all patients weigh 198 lbs or less.
    D. 95% of patients weigh between 97 and 299 lbs.
    E. The distribution is negatively skewed

17. The analysis of a study uses chi-squared test and the result is 2.668, $p = 0.04$. What does $p = 0.04$ signify?
    A. There is a 0.04 chance that the null hypothesis is true.
    B. The mean unnecessary investigation rate is 4%.
    C. The probability that the result is due to chance is 4%.

D. If there was no difference in unnecessary investigation rate, then the chance of this result occurring is 4%.
E. There is a fall of 4% in unnecessary investigations.

18. A study is done in patients with asthma to correlate the length of hospital stay with the respiratory rate on admission. The results show that the correlation coefficient is $R = 0.66$ with 95% confidence intervals of 0.60 and 0.73. Which of the following is true?
    A. A low respiratory rate at admission leads to a longer stay.
    B. We can be 95% certain that the respiratory rate affects stay length.
    C. Respiratory rate at admission is positively associated with the length of stay.
    D. The association is not significant.
    E. Respiratory rate at admission has very little effect on hospital stay.

19. Sodium-glucose cotransporter-2 (SGLT-2) inhibitor is compared with metformin on two patient samples. Which test would determine that the mean result is different in both groups?
    A. Unpaired t-test
    B. Spearman's rank correlation coefficient
    C. Mann–Whitney U test
    D. Paired t-test
    E. Pearson product moment correlation

20. A study is being planned to investigate any link between exposure to organophosphorus pesticides and new cases of neuropathy. Which would provide the best evidence?
    A. Retrospective case control study
    B. Randomised crossover trial
    C. Prospective cohort study
    D. Observational study
    E. Randomised controlled trial

Answers

1-C, 2-C, 3-C, 4-D, 5-D, 6-E, 7-C, 8-B, 9-E, 10-E, 11-C, 12-D, 13-A, 14-D, 15-E, 16-B, 17-D, 18-C, 19-A, 20-A

■ SUGGESTED READING

1. Coughlin SS, Beauchamp TL, Weed DL. Ethics and Epidemiology. London: Oxford University Press; 2009. p. 328.
2. Krieger N. Epidemiology and the People's Health: Theory and Context. 1st edition. Oxford: OUP USA; 2013. p. 400.
3. Wasserstein RL, Lazar NA. The ASA's Statement on p-Values: Context, Process, and Purpose. The American Statistician. 2016;70(2):129-33.
4. Bhopal R. Concepts of Epidemiology: Integrating the Ideas, Theories, Principles and Methods of Epidemiology, 2nd edition. Oxford; New York: Oxford University Press, USA; 2008. p. 456.
5. Rothman KJ. Epidemiology: An Introduction. Oxford: OUP USA; 2012. p. 281.
6. Wassertheil-Smoller S, Smoller JW. Biostatistics and epidemiology: a primer for health and biomedical professionals. 4th edition. New York: Springer; 2015.
7. Gerstman BB. Epidemiology Kept Simple: An Introduction to Classic and Modern Epidemiology, 2nd edition. Hoboken: Wiley-Liss; 2003.
8. Leening MJ, Vedder MM, Witteman JC, Pencina MJ, Steyerberg EW. Net reclassification improvement: computation, interpretation, and controversies: a literature review and clinician's guide. Ann Intern Med. 2014;160(2):122-31.
9. Pencina MJ, D'Agostino RB Sr, Demler OV. Novel metrics for evaluating improvement in discrimination: net reclassification and integrated discrimination improvement for normal variables and nested models. Stat Med. 2012;31(2):101-13.
10. Ioannidis JPA. The Proposal to Lower P Value Thresholds to .005. JAMA. 2018;319(14):1429-30.
11. Porta N, Bonet C, Cobo E. Discordance between reported intention-to-treat and per protocol analyses. J Clin Epidemiol. 2007;60(7):663-9.
12. Gravel J, Opatrny L, Shapiro S. The intention-to-treat approach in randomized controlled trials: are authors saying what they do and doing what they say? Clin Trials. 2007;4(4):350-6.

CHAPTER 29

Clinical Pharmacology

■ PHARMACODYNAMICS

It is the measurement of the effects of drugs on humans or an organ system.

It includes the mechanism of action and the end point.

Agonist
- Agonists are molecules that activate receptors.
- Agonists have both affinity and high intrinsic activity.
- For example, adrenergic (agonist: salbutamol), dopaminergic (agonist: dopamine), cholinergic (agonist: bethanechol)

Antagonist
- These drugs have affinity for a receptor but with no intrinsic activity.
- They prevent the activation of receptors by agonist.
- For example, atenolol, haloperidol, atropine

Partial agonist
Ligands with properties intermediate between agonist and antagonist.

Inverse agonist
Ligands that produce opposite effect to the full agonist when they bind to a receptor.

Therapeutic Index
- The ratio of the toxic dose to the therapeutic dose of a drug.
- The closer the ratio to 1, the more difficult the drug is to be used in clinical practice.
- For example, therapeutic index of digoxin—very low, amoxicillin—extremely high

Lethal dose, 50% (LD50): The single dose required to kill 50% of population. Not a helpful measure in clinical practice.

Median effective dose (ED50): Dose at which the response is 50% of the maximal effect. For example, increased intracellular calcium, reduced blood pressure or heart rate after giving drug.

■ PHARMACOKINETICS

It refers to the rate and manner in which drugs are absorbed, distributed, metabolised and eliminated within and from the body.

Volume of Distribution
- It describes how well a drug is removed from the plasma and distributed to the tissues.
- A large volume of distribution (Vd) means that the drug has a wide distribution or it is extensively bound to tissues or both.

Half-life
- Time required to clear 50% of drug
- Depends on Vd and clearance (CL)
- Multiphasic (if you can capture the distribution phase)
- Rule of thumb: Drug is cleared in five half-lives
- Half-life $(t_{1/2}) = 0.693 \times Vd/CL$

Bioavailability
It is defined as the fraction of unchanged drug reaching the systemic circulation following administration by any route (**Table 29.1**).

TABLE 29.1: Bio-availability of drugs based on various routes of administration.

Route	Bioavailability (%)	Characteristics
Intravenous (IV)	100 (by definition)	Most rapid onset
Intramuscular (IM)	75 to ≤ 100	Large volumes often feasible; may be painful
Subcutaneous (SC)	75 to ≤ 100	Smaller volumes than IM; may be painful
Oral (PO)	5 to < 100	Most convenient; first-pass effect may be significant
Rectal (PR)	30 to < 100	Less first-pass effect than oral
Inhalation	5 to < 100	Often very rapid onset
Transdermal	80 to ≤ 100	Usually very slow absorption; used for lack of first-pass effect; prolonged duration of action

TABLE 29.2: Types of conjugation.

Type of conjugation	Endogenous reactant	Examples
Glucuronidation	Uridine diphosphate (UDP) glucuronic acid	Nitrophenol, morphine, acetaminophen, diazepam, N-hydroxydapsone, sulphathiazole, meprobamate, digitoxin, digoxin
Acetylation	Acetyl-CoA	Sulphonamides, isoniazid, clonazepam, dapsone, mescaline
Glutathione conjugation	Glutathione (GSH)	Acetaminophen, ethacrynic acid, bromobenzene
Glycine conjugation	Glycine	Salicylic acid, benzoic acid, nicotinic acid, cinnamic acid, cholic acid, deoxycholic acid
Sulphation	Phosphoadenosyl phosphosulphate	Oestrone, aniline, phenol, 3-hydroxy coumarin, acetaminophen, methyldopa
Methylation	S-Adenosylmethionine	Dopamine, epinephrine, pyridine, histamine, thiouracil
Water conjugation	Water	Carbamazepine

First-pass Metabolism

Any drug is inactivated in the Gastrointestinal tract (GIT) or metabolised in the GIT wall or liver before it enters systemic circulation.

Bioavailability, defined as the ratio of the areas under the blood concentration-time curves, after extra- and intravascular drug administration (corrected for dosage if necessary), is often used as a measure of the extent of first-pass metabolism.

For example, drugs which undergo high first-pass metabolism are amitriptyline, lignocaine, morphine, neostigmine, nifedipine and propranolol.

■ DRUG METABOLISM

Phase I
Biotransformation:
- Attachment of new functional groups
- Transformation of the existing functional groups
- Activities of Phase I are increased by certain enzyme inducers. This is the basis for an important drug reaction.

For example, oxidation, reduction, hydroxylation and hydrolysis.

Phase II
Conjugation (**Table 29.2**):
- Masking of an existing functional group by for instance
- For example, acetylation, glycosylation, attachment of amino acid → More hydrophilic drug → Renal excretion

The phases of drug metabolism are shown in **Figure 29.1**.

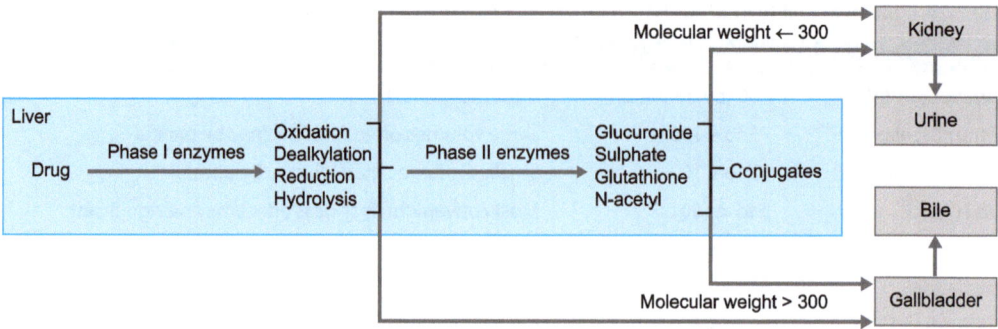

- Phase I enzymes catalyse the modification of existing functional groups in drug molecules (oxidation reactions).
- Conjugating enzymes (phase II) facilitate the addition of endogenous molecules such as sulphate, glucuronic acid and glutathione.

Fig. 29.1: Phases of drug metabolism.

TABLE 29.3: Genetic polymorphisms in drug metabolism.

Defect	Enzyme involved	Drug	Consequences
Oxidation	CYP2D6	Codeine	Reduced analgesia
Oxidation	Aldehyde dehydrogenase	Ethanol	Facial flushing, hypotension, tachycardia, nausea, vomiting
N-acetylation	N-acetyl transferase	Isoniazid	Peripheral neuropathy
Ester hydrolysis	Plasma cholinesterase	Succinylcholine	Prolonged apnoea
Oxidation	CYP2C9	Warfarin	Bleeding

■ PHARMACOGENETICS

Drug metabolism that varies on genetic basis is often called polymorphic drug metabolism (**Table 29.3**).

The commonest source is single nucleotide polymorphism.

■ DRUG INTERACTION

Definition

A measurable modification (in magnitude and/or duration) of the action of one drug by prior or concomitant administration of another substance, including prescription, non-prescription (including complementary medicines) drugs, food, alcohol, cigarette smoking or diagnostic tests.

Pharmacokinetic Interaction

Pharmacokinetic interaction of drugs is given in **Table 29.4**.

TABLE 29.4: Pharmacokinetic interaction.

Altered absorption	Tetracycline AND iron preparations → unabsorbable complexes
Displaced protein binding	Phenytoin and warfarin are highly bound to plasma protein and hence displace other drugs
Altered metabolism	• Carbamazepine increases its own metabolism • Phenytoin increases hepatic metabolism of theophylline
First-pass metabolism	Serum concentration of verapamil is reduced by rifampicin
Renal excretion	
Active tubular secretion: Probenecid → Decreases tubular secretion of methotrexate	Passive tubular reabsorption: Sodium bicarbonate increases lithium clearance and decreases action

Pharmacodynamic Interaction

It means alteration of the dug action without change in its serum concentration by pharmacokinetic factors.

Synergism means 1 + 1 = 3, Additive means 1 + 1 = 2, Potentiation means 1 + 0 = 2, Antagonism means 1 + 1 = 0 or 0.5.

■ ADVERSE DRUG REACTION

Definition

An unwanted or harmful reaction experienced following the administration of a drug or combination of drugs under normal conditions of use and suspected to be related to the drug.

Types of Adverse Drug Reaction

Types of adverse drug reaction (ADR) are given in **Box 29.1**.

Box 29.1: Classification of adverse drug reactions

Type A
- Response qualitatively normal but quantitatively abnormal
- Common, less serious, dose-related
- Corrected by dose adjustment
- Include side effect, toxic effect, and withdrawal

Type B
- Because of patient peculiarities such as allergy, idiosyncrasy, dose-related
- Uncommon
- Serious reactions need withdrawal of drug required
- Not always predictable OR preventable

Type C
- Associated with long-term drug therapy, e.g. benzodiazepine dependence and analgesic nephropathy
- They are well known and can be anticipated

Type D
- Refer to carcinogenic and teratogenic effects
- These reactions are delayed in onset

Type E
- End of dose effect
- For example, abrupt cessation of corticosteroids produces acute adrenal insufficiency and stoppage of propranolol can produce rebound effect

Type F
- Failure of therapy
- Oral contraceptive pill (OCP) failure when on antitubercular therapy

BEST OF FIVES

1. A 56-year-old man presented with an acute coronary syndrome. He was advised to take clopidogrel in addition to aspirin, atenolol, glyceryl trinitrate and low-molecular-weight heparin. What is the predominant mechanism through which clopidogrel inhibits platelet aggregation?
   A. It enhances the effect of circulating antithrombin.
   B. It inhibits binding of adenosine diphosphate.
   C. It inhibits cyclooxygenase 1.
   D. It irreversibly binds glycoprotein IIb/IIIa receptor sites.
   E. It prevents production of thromboxane A2.

2. A 30-year-old woman uses beclomethasone 800 µg/day and inhaled salbutamol as required via a metered-dose inhaler. She used the salbutamol two or three times a day and woke at night wheezing once or twice a week. What is the most appropriate management?
   A. Add montelukast.
   B. Add salmeterol.
   C. Change to a powder inhaler.
   D. Double the dose of beclomethasone.
   E. Maintain current treatment.

3. A 45-year-old man who had undergone a liver transplant developed hypertrichosis, hypertension and hyperplasia of gums. What medication is most likely to have been responsible?
   A. Aspirin
   B. Ciclosporin
   C. Mycophenolate mofetil
   D. Prednisolone
   E. Sodium valproate

4. In a clinical trial for heart failure, 34.8% of patients treated with digoxin and 35.1% of patients treated with placebo died (relative risk = 0.99; 95% confidence interval = 0.91–1.07; $p = 0.80$). Which is the most appropriate interpretation of these data?
   A. Digoxin has a small beneficial effect to reduce mortality in congestive heart failure (CHF).
   B. Digoxin has no effect on mortality in CHF.
   C. Digoxin is likely to reduce morbidity in CHF.

D. There is no clinically significant therapeutic effect of digoxin in patients with CHF.
E. There is no conclusive evidence of an effect of digoxin because of the limited power of the study.

5. A 62-year-old male presents with recurrent episodes of transient ischaemic attack (TIA). Examination reveals an obese subject with a body mass index (BMI) of 38 kg/m², a pulse of 76 beats per minute and regular and a pressure of 138/82 mmHg. Cardiovascular examination is normal. Which evidence-based intervention would be likely to prevent further episodes?
   A. Aspirin plus clopidogrel
   B. Aspirin plus dipyridamole
   C. Increase dose of aspirin 150 mg daily
   D. Switch clopidogrel alone
   E. Switch dipyridamole alone

6. Which of the following antihistamines likely causes sedation?
   A. Cetirizine
   B. Cyproheptadine
   C. Fexofenadine
   D. Loratadine
   E. Terfenadine

7. A lady with polymyalgia rheumatica was treated with prednisolone 15 mg daily along with calcium and vitamin D. Her symptoms have persistently relapsed when the dose of prednisolone was reduced below her current dose. How should her disease be managed?
   A. Continue the current dose of prednisolone.
   B. Continue the current dose of prednisolone and start methotrexate.
   C. Continue taper prednisolone. Treat any symptoms with non-steroidal anti-inflammatory drugs.
   D. Increase the dose of prednisolone and add a bisphosphonate.
   E. Stop both prednisolone and azathioprine.

8. A 65-year-old man with a long-standing history of bronchial asthma and on inhaled corticosteroids presents with fever and haemoptysis. Sputum sample proves to be positive with acid alcohol fast bacilli. Which of the following options would be an appropriate step in his management?
   A. Continue with antituberculous therapy and steroids at current dose.
   B. Continue with antituberculous therapy and reduce steroid dose.
   C. Continue with antituberculous therapy and increase steroid dose.
   D. Stop antituberculous therapy and continue with steroids at current dose.
   E. Stop antituberculous therapy and steroids and start broad-spectrum antibiotics.

9. A 45-year-old man presents with a 6-month history of weight loss of 10 kg and diarrhoea. Investigations revealed: 24-hour urine 5-hydroxyindoleacetic acid (5-HIAA) 100 mg/day (normal < 5 mg/day). Abdominal ultrasound scan showed numerous echo-dense deposits within the liver. What is the appropriate treatment for this patient's diarrhoea?
   A. Cyproheptadine
   B. Ketanserin
   C. Loperamide
   D. Methysergide
   E. Octreotide

10. A 27-year-old female presents with secondary amenorrhoea and galactorrhoea over the last 3 months.
Investigations show:
- Serum oestradiol 130 nmol/L (NR 130–600)
- Serum luteinising hormone (LH) 4.5 mU/L (NR 2–20)
- Serum follicle-stimulating hormone (FSH) 2.2 mU/L (NR 2–20)
- Serum prolactin 8,940 mU/L (NR 50–450)
- Free thyroxine (T4) 5.2 pmol/L (NR 9–22)
- Thyroid-stimulating hormone (TSH) 4.2 mU/L (NR 0.5–5.0)

What is the likely diagnosis?
   A. Drug induced
   B. Non-functional pituitary tumour
   C. Polycystic ovarian syndrome
   D. Pregnancy
   E. Prolactinoma

11. A chronic kidney disease patient develops haematuria post-dialysis. The activated partial thromboplastin time is mildly prolonged. What specific antidote should be administered?
   A. Fresh frozen plasma
   B. None—specific antidote exists

C. Platelet transfusion
D. Protamine sulphate
E. Vitamin K

12. A 50-year-old male with 7 year history of type II diabetes mellitus is currently on diet control. He takes other medications. Examination reveals that he is obese with a body mass index (BMI) of 34 kg/m². His pressure 180/90 mmHg and he has a pulse of 80 beats per minute and regular. He has mild non-proliferative diabetic retinopathy (NPDR). Investigations reveal urine albumin 220 µmol/day and HbA1c 7.4% (NR 5–6.8%). All of the following drugs have an evidence of a reduction of risk of developing a cardiac event in this man except:
    A. Angiotensin-converting enzyme (ACE) inhibitor
    B. Aspirin
    C. Insulin
    D. Metformin
    E. Statins

13. A 75-year-old man with atrial flutter was treated with amiodarone 200 mg daily. Examination of the patient reveals a fine tremor, a pulse of 56 beats per minute and a pressure of 146/88 mmHg. Investigations reveal: Serum free thyroxine (T4) 36.1 nmol/L (NR 9–22) and serum thyroid-stimulating hormone (TSH) <0.04 mU/L (NR 0.4–4). What is best management strategy for this patient?
    A. Continue amiodarone and start carbimazole.
    B. Stop amiodarone and start carbimazole.
    C. Stop amiodarone and start carbimazole flecainide.
    D. Stop amiodarone and start steroids.
    E. Stop amiodarone only.

14. A 74-year-old male presents with pins and needle sensation of legs, particularly at night, of 6 months' duration. He has a past history of hypertension for which he takes atenolol and ramipril. He stopped smoking 10 years ago and drinks little alcohol. On examination, he has a pressure of 148/88 mmHg. No abnormalities are found on neurological examination of legs. Both plantars are flexor and muscle power sensation is intact. Which of the following is an appropriate management plan for this patient?
    A. Start amitriptyline
    B. Start bromocriptine
    C. Start phenytoin
    D. Stop atenolol
    E. Stop ramipril

15. A 65-year-old man is brought to the casualty with a history of being stung by bees while working in his garden. He is arousable, without respiratory distress but has generalised rash. Systolic blood pressure (BP) was 75 mmHg and pulse rate was 102 bpm. What is the first drug that should be administered?
    A. Hydrocortisone
    B. Chlorpheniramine
    C. Adrenaline
    D. Montelukast
    E. Dopamine

16. A 24-year-old male with crush injury and acute kidney injury (AKI) has a serum potassium of 7 mmol/L. Which of the following is not used in the treatment of hyperkalaemia?
    A. Intravenous (IV) calcium gluconate
    B. IV furosemide
    C. IV hydrocortisone
    D. Beta-2 adrenergic agonists
    E. Haemodialysis

17. Which of the following drugs can cause lymphadenopathy?
    A. Phenytoin
    B. Acyclovir
    C. Zidovudine
    D. Ciprofloxacin
    E. Amoxicillin

18. A 64-year man was noted to have hypertension (180/100 mmHg). He has a history of a myocardial infarction 2 years ago and a background history of asthma. What is the choice of antihypertensive for this patient?
    A. Angiotensin-converting enzyme (ACE) inhibitor
    B. Alpha blocker
    C. Amlodipine
    D. Beta blocker
    E. Thiazide diuretic

19. A 55-year-old male diabetic for the past 12 years presented to his physician with erectile dysfunction. After evaluation, the

patient was started on sildenafil. The patient returned to his doctor after a month reporting good improvement of his earlier symptoms. However, he casually mentioned that he has been suffering from colour vision disturbances of late. This effect of the drug that occur at doses in the middle of the usual dose-response curve but in a tissue other than that in which the therapeutic action is sought is termed as:
A. Toxic effect
B. Hypersusceptible effect
C. Collateral effect
D. Cumulative effect
E. Hypersensitivity effect

20. What term is used to describe a decrease in responsiveness to a drug which develops in a few minutes?
A. Refractoriness
B. Cumulative effect
C. Tolerance
D. Tachyphylaxis
E. Collateral effect

Answers

1-D, 2-B, 3-B, 4-A, 5-A, 6-B, 7-B, 8-A, 9-E, 10-E, 11-D, 12-D, 13-D, 14-A, 15-C, 16-C, 17-A, 18-A, 19-C, 20-D

■ SUGGESTED READING

1. Aronson JK. Clinical pharmacology and therapeutics in the UK – a great instauration. Br J Clin Pharmacol. 2010;69(2):111-7.
2. Fitzgerald JD. An alternative view of the role of clinical pharmacology. Br J Clin Pharmacol. 2011;71(3):471-2.
3. Page C. A response to: 'A manifesto for clinical pharmacology from principles to practice' by Jeff Aronson. Br J Clin Pharmacol. 2010;70(6):912-3.
4. Waldman SA, Terzic A. Clinical pharmacology and therapeutics: the next five years. Clin Pharmacol Ther. 2015;97(1):2-6.
5. Pacanowski M, Huang SM. Precision Medicine. Clin Pharmacol Ther. 2016;99(2):124-9.
6. Honig PK, Hirsch G. Adaptive Biomedical Innovation. Clin Pharmacol Ther. 2016;100(6):574-8.
7. Blaschke TF. Global challenges for clinical pharmacology in the developing world. Clin Pharmacol Ther. 2009;85(6):579-81.
8. Suryawati S. Contribution of clinical pharmacology to improve the use of medicines in developing countries. Int J Risk Safety Med. 2005;17(1):57-64.

CHAPTER 30

ECG Interpretation

CONDUCTION SYSTEM OF THE HEART (FIG. 30.1)

The rate and rhythm of the heart are controlled by the sinoatrial node (SA node) situated at the junction of superior vena cava and right atrium.

- The impulse from the SA node spreads through the atrial musculature and down to the atrioventricular (AV) node that is situated above the tricuspid valve.
- Passage through the AV node is relatively slow, accounting for the normal physiological delay in ventricular depolarisation.
- The impulse then travels downwards to the bundle of His and through its branches (right bundle branch and left bundle branch) to the Purkinje network of fibres that convey the impulse to the ventricular endocardium and then epicardium.
- The SA node is the normal pacemaker of the heart as it has the fastest inherent discharge rate. However, potential pace-making properties also exist in the cells of the AV node, bundle of His and Purkinje fibres.
- SA node: Dominant pacemaker with an intrinsic rate of 60–100 beats per minute (bpm)
- AV node: Back-up pacemaker with an intrinsic rate of 40–60 bpm
- Ventricular cells: Back-up pacemaker with an intrinsic rate of 20–45 bpm

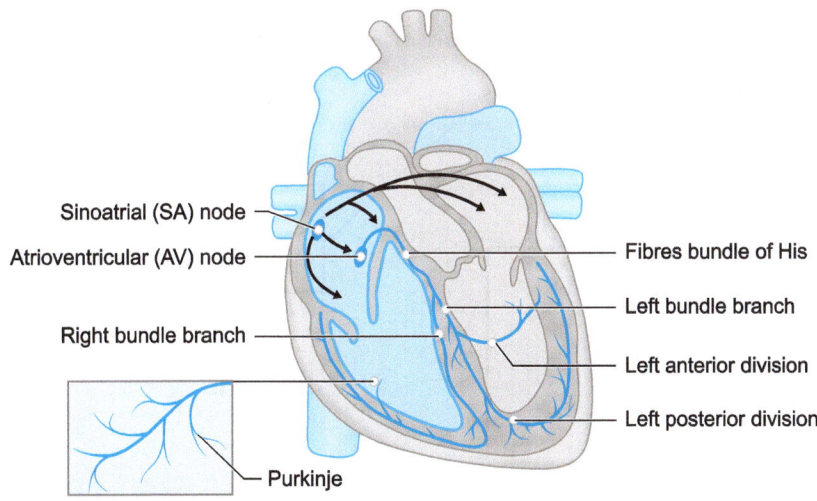

Fig. 30.1: Conduction system of the heart.

ECG Waveforms and Intervals

The electrocardiogram (ECG) ordinarily is recorded on special graph paper that is divided into 1 mm² grid-like boxes. Since the ECG paper speed is generally 2 mm/s, the smallest (1 mm) horizontal divisions correspond to 0.04 (40 ms), with heavier lines at intervals of 0.20 s (200 ms). Vertically, the ECG graph measures the amplitude of a specific wave or deflection (1 mV = 10 mm with standard calibration; the voltage criteria for hypertrophy are given in millimetres) (**Fig. 30.2**).

The ECG waveforms are labelled alphabetically (**Fig. 30.3**), beginning with the P wave, which represents atrial depolarisation. The QRS complex represents ventricular depolarisation, and the ST-T-U complex (ST segment, T wave, and U wave) represents ventricular repolarisation. The J point is the junction between the end of the QRS complex and the beginning of the ST segment. Atrial repolarisation is usually too low in amplitude to be detected, but it may become apparent in conditions such as acute pericarditis and atrial infarction.

There are four major ECG intervals: R-R, PR, QRS and QT. The heart rate (bpm) can be computed readily from the inter beat [R-number of small (0.04 s) units into 1,500]. The PR interval measures the time (normally 120–200 ms) between atrial and ventricular depolarisation, which includes the physiologic delay imposed by stimulation of cells in the AV junction area. The QRS interval (normally 100–110 ms or less) reflects the duration of ventricular depolarisation. The QT interval includes both ventricular depolarisation and repolarisation times and varies inversely with the heart rate. A rate-related ('corrected' Bazett's correction) QT interval, QTc, can be calculated as QT/Type equation here. R-R and normally is 0.44 s (some references give QTc upper normal limits as 0.43 s in men and 0.45 s in women. Also, a number of different formulas have been proposed, without consensus, for calculating the QTc). The QRS complex is subdivided into specific deflections or waves. If the initial QRS depletion in a particular lead is negative, it is termed a Q wave; the first positive deflection is termed an R wave. A negative deflection after an R wave is an S wave. Subsequent positive or negative waves are labelled 'R' and 'S', respectively. Lowercase letters (qrs) are used for waves of relatively small amplitude. An entirely negative QRS complex is termed a QS wave.

- U wave: Small, rounded, and upright wave following T wave. Most easily seen with a slow heart rate. Indicates repolarisation of Purkinje fibres

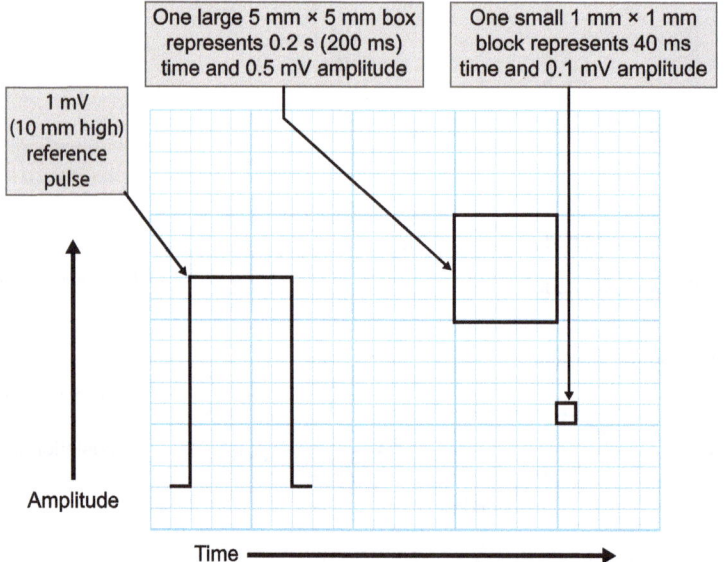

Fig. 30.2: Electrocardiogram (ECG) grid and standardisation.

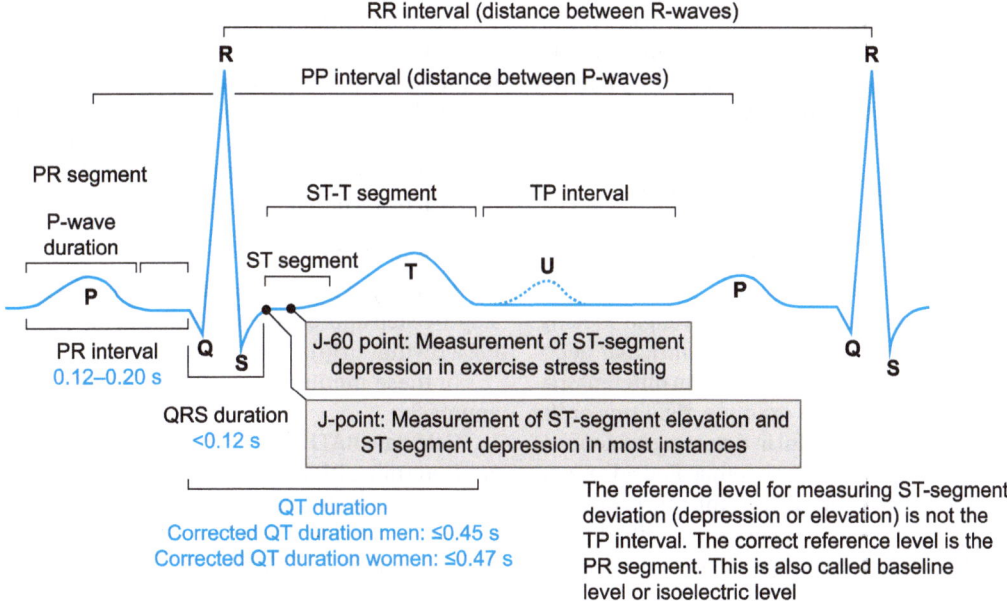

Fig. 30.3: Normal waves, segments and intervals.

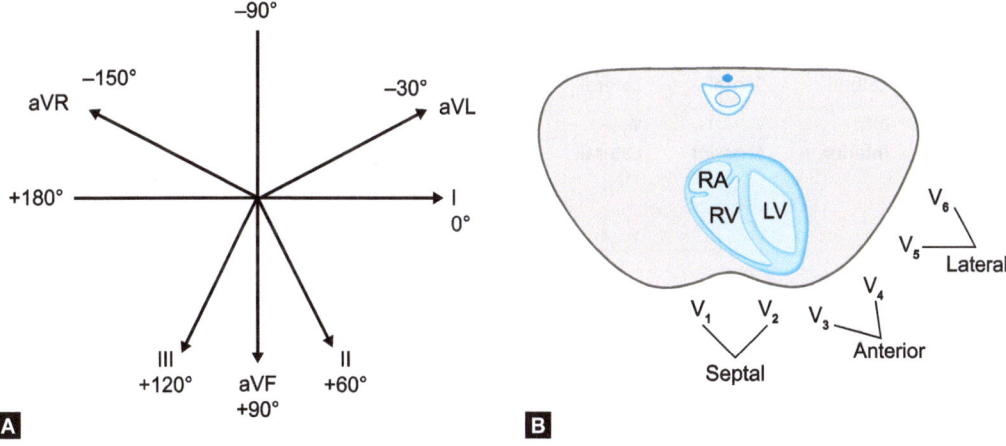

Figs. 30.4A and B: Anatomical relation of leads.

ECG Leads (Figs. 30.4A and B)

The 12 conventional ECG leads record the difference in potential between electrodes placed on the surface of the body. These leads are divided into two groups: Six limb (extremity) leads and six chest (precordial) leads. The limb leads record potentials transmitted onto the frontal plane, and the chest leads record potentials transmitted onto the horizontal plane.

The spatial orientation and polarity of the six frontal plane leads are represented on the hexaxial diagram. The six chest leads are unipolar recordings obtained by electrodes in the following positions; lead V_1, fourth intercostal space, just to the right of the sternum; lead V_2, fourth intercostal space, just to the left of the sternum; lead V_3, midway between V_2 and V_4; lead V_4, mid-clavicular line, fifth intercostal space; and lead V_5, anterior axillary line, same level as V4; and lead V_6, mid-axillary line, same level as V_4 and V_5.

Anatomic Groups of ECG Leads (Table 30.1)

Together, the frontal and horizontal plane electrodes provide a three-dimensional representation of cardiac electrical activity. Each lead can be likened to a different video camera angle 'looking' at the same events—atrial and ventricular depolarisation and repolarisation—from different spatial circumstances. For example, right precordial leads V_3R, V_4R, are useful in detecting evidence of acute right ventricular ischaemia. Bedside monitors and ambulatory ECG (Holter) recordings, usually employ only one or two modified leads. The ECG leads are configured so that a positive (upright) deflection is recorded in a lead, if a wave of depolarisation spreads towards the positive pole of the lead, and a negative deflection is recorded, if the wave spreads towards the negative pole. If the mean orientation of the depolarisation vector is at right angles to a particular lead axis, a biphasic (equally positive and negative) deflection will be recorded.

Reading 12-Lead ECGs

The best way to read 12-lead ECGs is to develop a step-by-step approach (just as we did for analysing a rhythm strip).

In these modules, we present a seven-step approach:
1. Calculate RATE
2. Determine RHYTHM
3. Determine QRS AXIS
4. Check individual WAVES
5. Calculate INTERVALS
6. Assess for HYPERTROPHY
7. Look for evidence of infarction/dyselectrolytemia

TABLE 30.1: Anatomic groups of electrocardiogram (ECG) Leads.

I Lateral	aVR None	V_1 Septal	V_4 Anterior
II Inferior	aVL Lateral	V_2 Septal	V_5 Lateral
III Inferior	aVL Inferior	V_3 Anterior	V_6 Lateral

Step 1: Determining the Heart Rate (Fig. 30.5A)

Rule of 300/1500

Heart rate can be calculated by dividing 1500 by the number of small squares between two R waves or by dividing 300 by the number of large squares between two R waves (R-R interval).

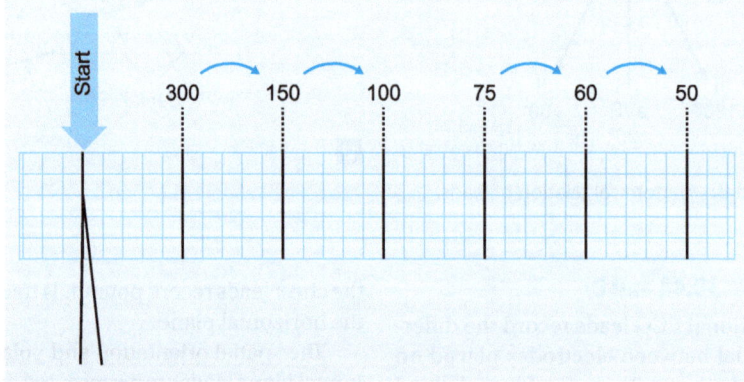

Fig. 30.5A: Calculation of heart rate.

6-second Rule

- Count the number of beats present on the ECG in 6 seconds.
- Multiply by 10.
- This is useful for irregular rhythms.

Common causes of tachycardia and bradycardia are listed in **Table 30.2**.

Step 2: Determine Regularity

- Look at the R-R distances (using a calliper or marking son a pen or paper)
- Regular (are they equidistant apart)? Occasionally irregular? Regularly irregular?
- Irregularly irregular?—atrial fibrillation (AF)

Common rhythm abnormalities described below

TABLE 30.2: Causes of tachycardia and bradycardia.

Interpretation	Beats per minute	Causes
Normal	60–99	–
Bradycardia	< 60	Hypothermia, increased vagal tone (due to vagal stimulation or drugs), athletes (fit people) hypothyroidism, beta blockade, marked intracranial hypertension, obstructive jaundice, uraemia, structural SA node disease, or ischaemia
Tachycardia	> 100	Any cause of adrenergic stimulation (including pain); thyrotoxicosis; hypovolaemia; vagolytic drugs (e.g. atropine) anaemia, pregnancy; vasodilator drugs, including many hypotensive agents; fever, myocarditis

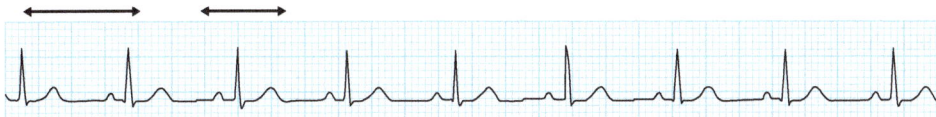

Sinus Rhythm

Cardiac impulse originates from the sinus node. Every QRS must be sinus node. Every QRS must be preceded by a P wave.

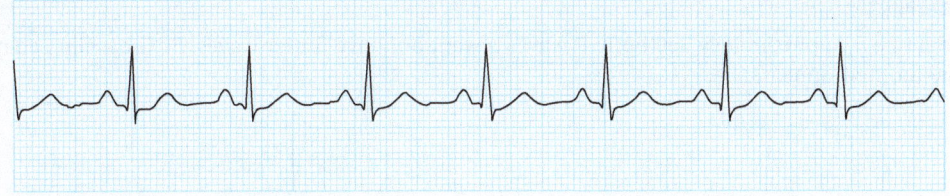

Sinus Bradycardia

Rhythm originates in the sinus node. Rate of < 60 bpm.

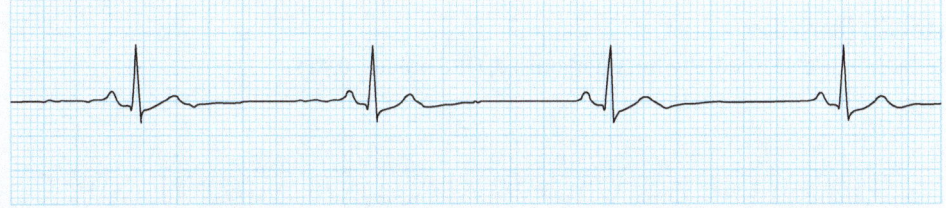

Sinus Tachycardia
Rate > 100 bpm, otherwise, normal.

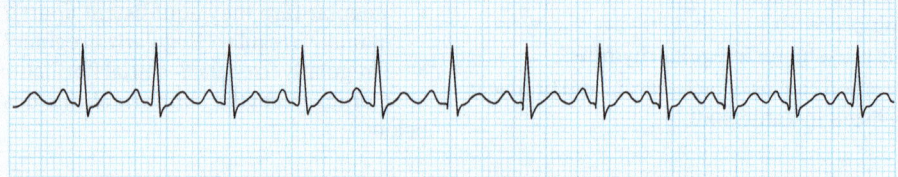

Sinus Pause
In disease (e.g. sick sinus syndrome), the SA node can fail in its pacing function. If failure is brief and recovery is prompt, the result is only a missed beat (sinus pause). If recovery is delayed and no other focus assumes pacing function, cardiac arrest follows.

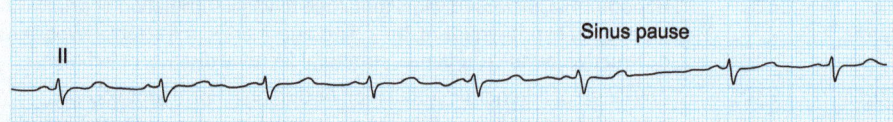

Atrial Fibrillation
Atrial rate approximately 400–600 bpm; ventricular rate approximately 150 bpm; irregularly irregular, baseline irregularity, no visible P waves, QRS occurs irregularly with its length usually < 0.12 s, fibrillary waves.

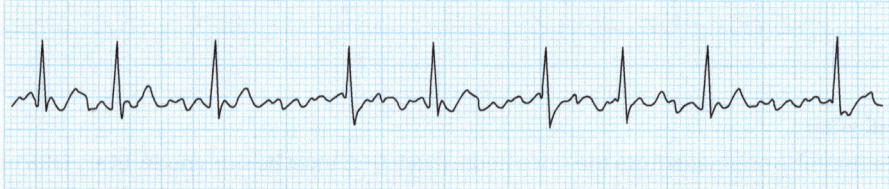

Atrial Flutter
Atrial rate = Approximately 300 bpm, P waves absent but have flutter waves, ECG baseline adapts 'saw-toothed' appearance.

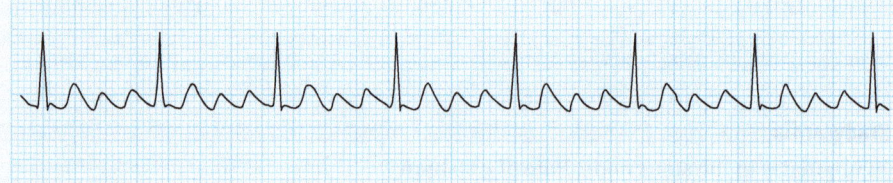

Ventricular Fibrillation
Rate cannot be discerned, rhythm unorganised, QRS broad > 0.12 s.

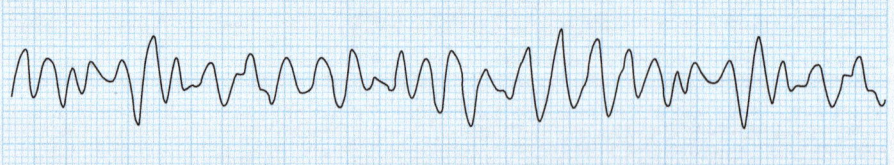

Ventricular Tachycardia

Rate = 100–250 bpm, broad QRS, regular

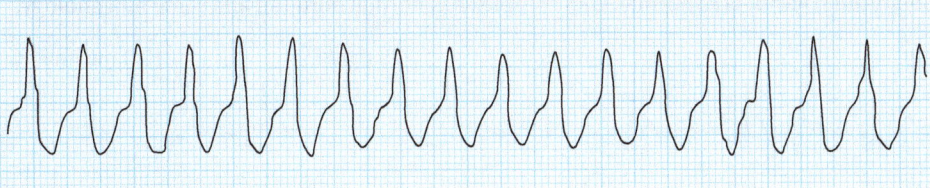

Torsades de Pointes

Literally meaning twisting of points is a distinctive form of polymorphic ventricular tachycardia characterised by a gradual change in the amplitude and twisting of the QRS complexes around the isoelectric line.

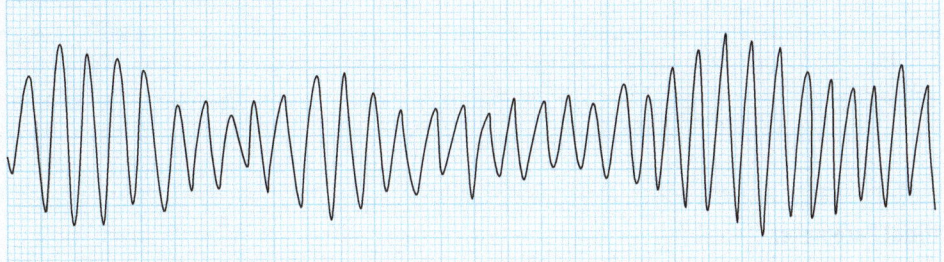

Supraventricular Tachycardia (SVT)

Tachycardic rhythm originating above the ventricular tissue. Atrial and ventricular rate = 150–250 bpm. Regular rhythm, P is usually not discernable.

Note:
Types of SVT:
- SA node re-entrant tachycardia (SANRT)
- Ectopic (unifocal) atrial tachycardia (EAT)
- Multifocal atrial tachycardia (MAT)
- A-fib or A flutter with rapid ventricular response. Without rapid ventricular response, both are usually not classified as SVT
- AV nodal re-entrant tachycardia (AVNRT— most common)
- Permanent (or persistent) junctional reciprocating tachycardia (PJRT)
- AV re-entrant tachycardia (AVRT)

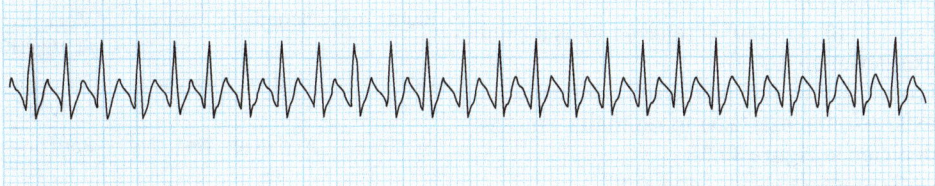

Atrial Premature Beat (aPB)

Arises from an irritable focus in one of the atria. aPB produces different looking P wave, because depolarisation vector is abnormal. QRS complex has normal duration and same morphology.

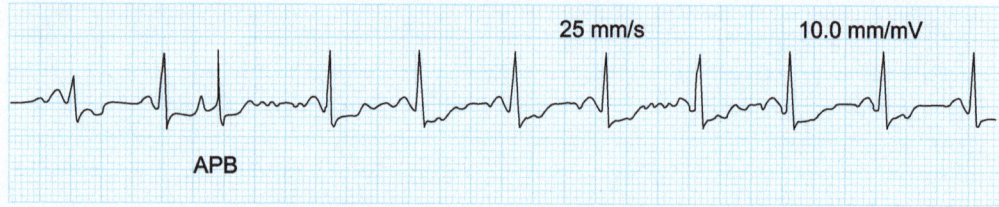

Premature Ventricular Complexes (PVCs)

- Occasionally irregular rhythm, broad QRS arising from ventricles
- No P-wave associated with PVCs. It can be monomorphic/polymorphic.

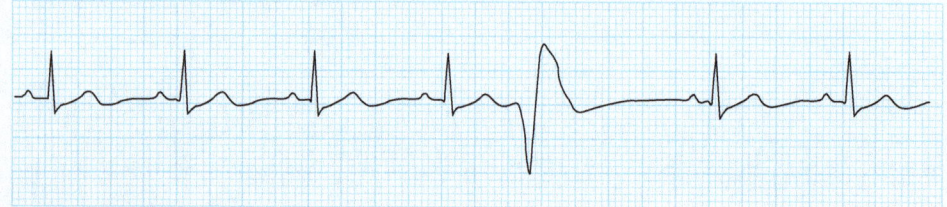

Artificial Pacemaker

Sharp, thin spike, before each complex, ventricular paced rhythm shows wide ventricular pacemaker spikes.

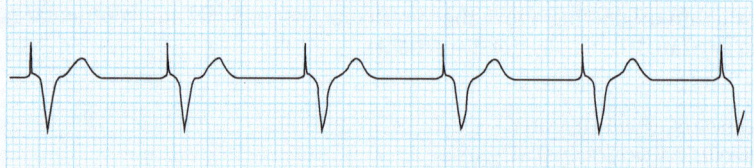

Step 3: Determining the Axis (Table 30.3)

- Normal QRS axis from −30° to +110°
- From −30° to −90° is referred to as a left axis deviation (LAD)
- From +110° to +180° is referred to as a right axis deviation (RAD)
- From −180° to −90° is referred as north-west axis/extreme axis/axis in no man's land as depicted in **Figure 30.5B**
- QRS complex in leads I and aVF
- Determine if they are predominantly positive or negative
- The combination should place the axis into one of the four quadrants above
  Causes of axis deviation listed in **Table 30.4**.

TABLE 30.3: Determining the axis.

Axis	LI	LIII or aVF	TIP (Fig. 30.5C)
Normal	Positive	Positive	Both up
Right	Negative	Positive	Meet-REACHING
Left	Positive	Negative	Separate-LEAVING
Northwest	Negative	Negative	Both down

Step 4: Check Individual Waves

Assess P Waves

- Always positive in leads I and II
- Always negative in lead aVR

ECG Interpretation

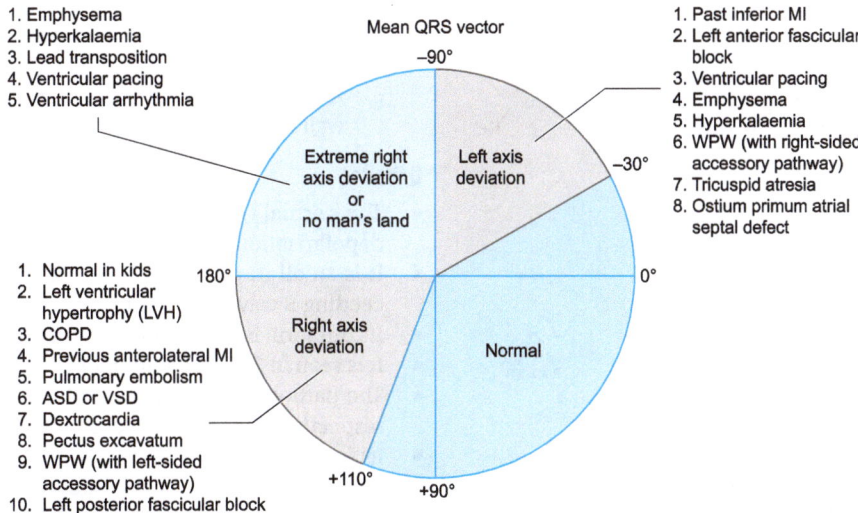

Fig. 30.5B: Pictorial representation of AXIS deviation with examples.

(ASD: atrial septal defects; COPD: chronic obstructive pulmonary disease; MI: myocardial infarction; VSD: ventricular septal defects; WPW: Wolff–Parkinson–White)

TABLE 30.4: Cardiac axis.

Cardiac axis	Causes
LAD	• Left anterior hemiblock, left ventricular hypertrophy (LVH), Wolff–Parkinson–White (WPW) syndrome, inferior myocardial infarction (MI), ostium primum atrial septal defect (ASD), and ventricular tachycardia • Normal variation in pregnancy, obesity, ascites
RAD	Normal finding in children and tall thin adults, right ventricular hypertrophy (RVH), chronic obstructive pulmonary disease (COPD), left posterior hemiblock, WPW syndrome, and anterolateral MI
North west	Dextrocardia, severe emphysema, hyperkalaemia, lead transposition, artificial cardiac pacing and ventricular tachycardia

- Less than 2.5 small squares in duration
- Less than 2.5 small squares in amplitude
- Commonly biphasic in lead V_1
- Best seen in leads II
- Tall (> 2.5 mm), pointed P waves (P pulmonale)—suggests right atrial enlargement (RAE)

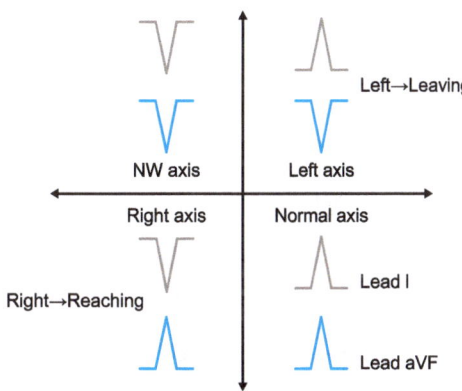

Fig. 30.5C: Axis determination based on direction of lead I and lead aVF.

  ○ Seen in COPD, ASD, TS, Ebstein anomaly (Himalayan P waves)
- Notched/bifid ('M' shaped) P wave (P 'mitrale') in limb leads—suggests left atrial enlargement (LAE)
  ○ Seen in mitral stenosis (MS), mitral regurgitation (MR), and systemic hypertension.
- Absent P waves—AF/flutter
- Inverted P waves in lead II—dextrocardia

P-wave abnormalities are depicted in **Figure 30.5D**.

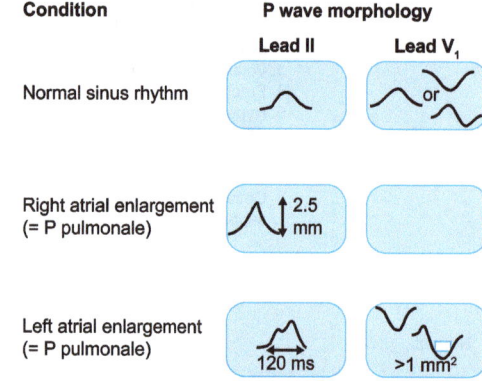

Fig. 30.5D: P-wave abnormality.

QRS Complex

Normal Characteristics

- *Duration:* 0.04–0.11 s
  - **Broad/wide QRS** (> 0.12 s)
    - Ventricular hypertrophy
    - Intra-ventricular conduction disturbance
    - Aberrant ventricular conduction
    - Ventricular pre-excitation
    - Ventricular ectopic or escape pacemaker
    - Ventricular pacing by cardiac pacemaker
- Q < 0.04 s, < 25% of R wave
- Height of QRS—**Sokolow index** (SV2 + RV5) < 35 mm (< 45 mm for young)
  - Increased in RV/LV hypertrophy
  - Decreased—**low voltage QRS** (< 5 mV in limbleads/< 10 mV in chest leads)
    - Obese patient
    - Restrictive cardiomyopathy
    - Pericardial effusion
    - Hypothyroidism
    - Hypothermia
    - Myocarditis
- Axis of ventricular depolarisation –30 to +110° (abnormalities already discussed)
- **Ventricular activation time (VAT)**—time from start of Q wave till top of R wave. Normal of LV < 0.04 s (V_5 and V_6 leads), RV < 0.03 s (V_1 Lead)
  - Prolonged in ischaemia, bundle branch block

- **Precordial R wave progression**, i.e. R wave amplitude progressively increases from V_1 to V_6
  - Absent R wave progression sign of anterior wall MI

Q Waves

- The normal Q wave in lead I is due to septal depolarisation.
- It is small in amplitude—< 25% of the succeeding R wave, or < 3 mm.
- Its duration is < 0.04 s or one small box.
- It is seen in L1 and sometimes in V_5 and V_6.
- The pathological Q wave of infarction in the respective leads is due to dead muscle.
- It is deep in amplitude—> 25% of the succeeding R wave, or > 4 mm. Its duration is > 0.04 s or > 1 small box.
- Pathological Q waves may be seen in cardiomyopathies—hypertrophic obstructive cardiomyopathy (HOCM) and infiltrative myocardial disease.
- Absent Q waves in V_5-V_6 is most commonly due to left bundle branch block (LBBB).

T Wave (Table 30.5)

- Normally repolarisation directs from epicardium to endocardium = T wave is concordant with QRS complex

TABLE 30.5: T wave.

Causes of T wave inversions	Tall T waves (more than two-thirds of neighbouring QRS)
• Coronary artery disease (CAD)/ischaemia • Cardiomyopathies—hypertrophic • Myocarditis and pericarditis • Wellens syndrome • Pulmonary embolism • Raised ICT—Central nervous system (CNS) bleed • Ventricular hypertrophy • Bundle branch block • Pacing • Persistent juvenile T wave pattern	• Hyperkalaemia—Steeple T waves • Hyperacute MI • Benign early repolarisation (BER)

- Ischaemic area: A repolarisation is delayed and an actionpotential is extended
- Vector of repolarisation is directed from ischemic area:
  - Sub-endocardial ischaemia—to epicardium—T wave elevation
  - Sub-epicardial ischaemia—to endocardium—T wave inversion
- Asymmetrical T wave inversion—the first half having more gradual slope than the second half
- Symmetrical→ T wave inversion seen in ischaemia
- Amplitude rarely exceeds 10 mm

U Waves

- The U wave is a wave on an ECG that is not always seen. It is typically small; and by definition, follows the T wave. U waves are thought to represent repolarisation of the papillary muscles or Purkinje fibres.
- Normal U waves are small, round and symmetrical and positive in lead II. It is the same direction as T wave in that lead.
- Prominent U waves are most often seen in hypokalaemia, but may be present in hypercalcaemia, thyrotoxicosis, or exposure to digitalis, epinephrine, and class 1A and 3 antiarrhythmics, as well as in congenital long QT syndrome, and in the setting of intracranial-haemorrhage.
- An inverted U wave may represent myocardial ischaemia or left ventricular volume overload.

The Osborn wave (J wave) is a positive deflection at the J point (negative in aVR and V_1), characteristically seen in hypothermia (typically temperature < 30°C), but also can be seen in raised intracranial tension, hypercalcaemia.

Epsilon wave is a small positive deflection buried in the end of the QRS complex. It is the characteristic of arrhythmogenic right ventricular dysplasia (ARVD).

Step 5: Calculate Intervals

PR Interval (Figs. 30.6A to C)

Normal: 0.12–0.20 seconds.

Long PR interval may indicate heart block.

First-degree Heart Block

P wave precedes QRS complex but PR intervals prolong (> 5 small squares) and remains constant from beat to beat.

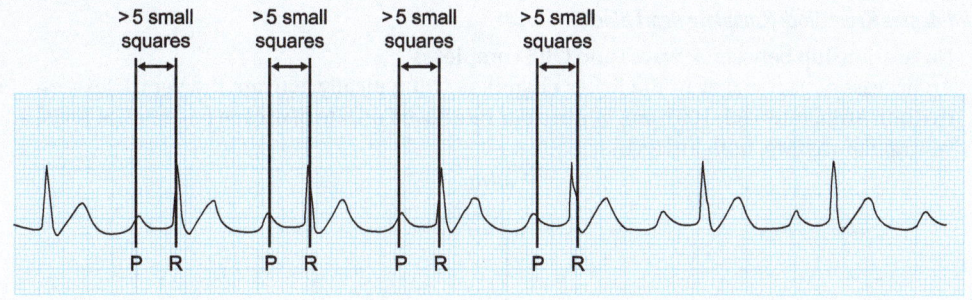

Second-degree Heart Block
- Mobitz Type I or Wenckebach
  - Runs in cycle, first PR interval is often normal. With successive beat, PR interval lengthens until there will be a P wave with no following QRS complex
  - The block is at AV node, often transient, may be asymptomatic

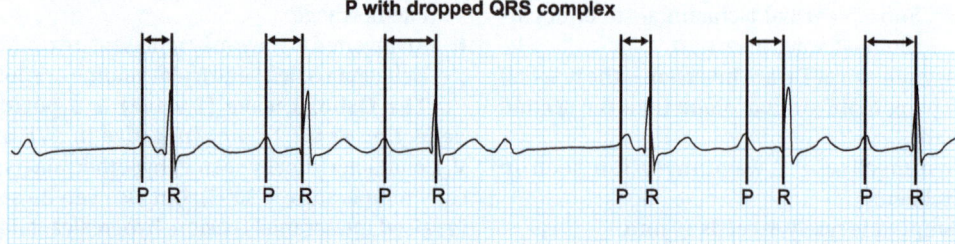

- Mobitz Type 2
  - PR interval is constant, duration is normal/prolonged. Periodically, no conduction between atria and ventricles—producing a P wave with no associated QRS complex (blocked P wave)
  - The block is most often below AV node, at bundle of His or BB
  - May progress to third-degree heart block

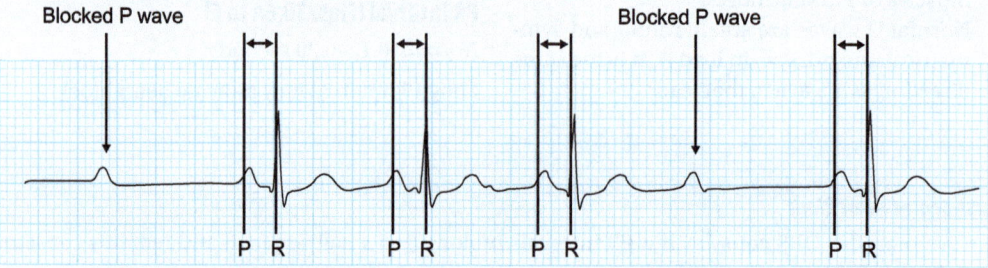

Third-degree Heart Block (Complete Heart Block)
- No relationship between P waves and QRS complexes
- An accessory pacemaker in the lower chambers will typically activate the ventricles—escape rhythm. Atrial rate = 60–100 bpm. Ventricular rate based on site of escape pacemaker. Atrial and ventricular rhythm, both are regular

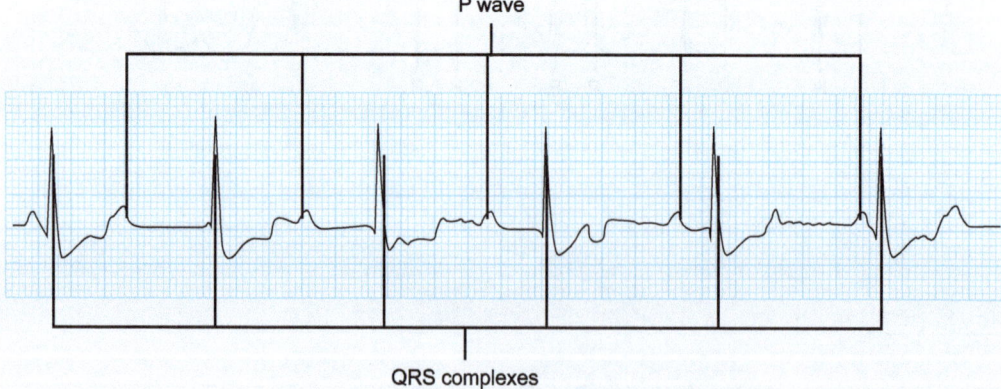

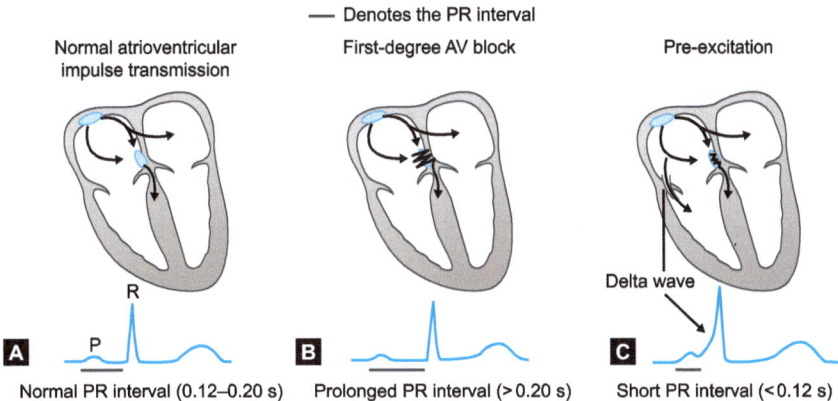

Figs. 30.6A to C: (A) Normal atrioventricular (AV) impulse transmissions; (B) First-degree AV block; (C) Pre-excitation.

Causes of Conduction Block
- CAD, acute MI, remote MI, pulmonary embolism
- Drugs
- Aortic stenosis, subacute bacterial endocarditis (SABE) + abscesses in conduction
- Cardiac trauma and hyperkalaemia
- Lenegre's disease (idiopathic fibrosis of conduction)
- Lev's disease (calcification of the cardiac skeleton)
- Cardiomyopathy—dilated and hypertrophic
- Infiltrative—Chagas disease
- Myxoedema, amyloidosis and ventricular hypertrophy
- Idiopathic

Short PR interval
- Tachycardia
- Pre-excitation syndromes
  - Lown-Ganong-Levine syndrome
  - Wolff-Parkinson-White syndrome
  - Mahaim pathway

The diagnostic triad of WPW consists of a wide QRS complex associated with a relatively short PR interval and slurring of the initial part of the QRS (delta wave), with the latter effect being due to aberrant activation of ventricular myocardium. The presence of a bypass tract predisposes to re-entrant supraventricular tachyarrhythmias.

QT Interval
It represents the time taken for ventricular depolarisation and repolarisation.

- The duration of the QT interval is proportionate to the heart rate. The faster the heart beats, the faster the ventricles repolarise so the shorter the QT interval. Therefore, what is a 'normal' QT varies with the heart rate
- QT interval should be 0.35–0.45 s
- For each heart rate you need to calculate an adjusted QT interval, called the 'corrected QT' (QTc): QTc = QT/square root of RR interval—**Bazett's formula**

Prolonged QTc (> 440 ms)—a prolonged QT can be very dangerous. It can predispose an individual to a type of ventricular tachycardia—Torsades de pointes.
- Hypokalaemia
- Hypomagnesaemia
- Hypocalcaemia
- Hypothermia
- Myocardial ischaemia
- Raised intracranial pressure
- Congenital long QT syndrome—Example: Jervell and Lange-Nielsen syndrome or Romano-Ward syndrome
- Drugs—chlorpromazine, haloperidol, quetiapine, quinidine, procainamide, disopyramide, flecainide, sotalol, amiodarone, amitriptyline, diphenhydramine, astemizole, loratadine, terfenadine, chloroquine, quinine, and macrolides.

Short QTc (< 350 ms)
- Hypercalcaemia
- Digoxin effect

Bundle branch blocks

Left bundle branch block (LBBB)—indirect activation causes left ventricle contracts later than the right ventricle

QS or rS complex in V_1—W-shaped

RsR' wave in V_6—M-shaped

Right bundle branch block (RBBB)—indirect activation causes right ventricle contracts later than the left ventricle

Terminal R wave (rSR') in V_1—M-shaped

Slurred S wave in V_6—W-shaped

Left bundle branch block

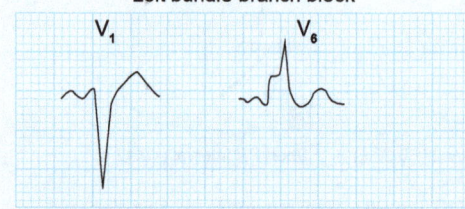

Right bundle branch block

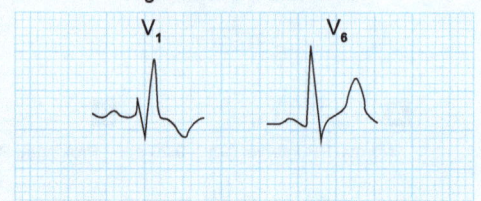

Mnemonic: WILLIAM

Mnemonic: MARROW

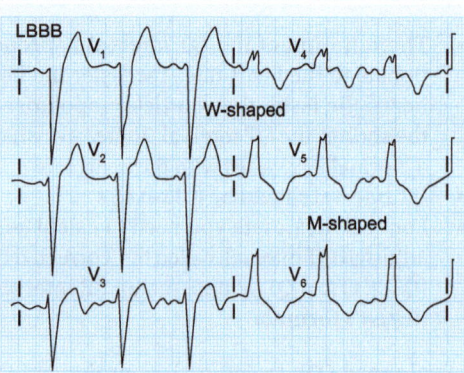

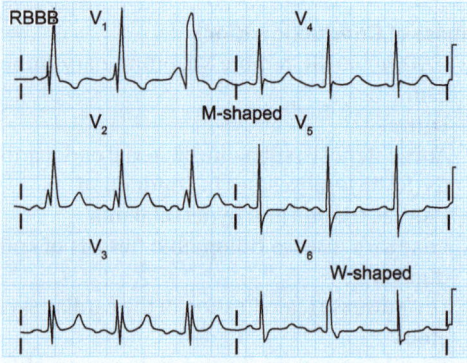

Step 6: Assess for Hypertrophy

Right Ventricular Hypertrophy

Criteria of Right Ventricular Hypertrophy

- Tall R in V_1 with R > S, or R/S ratio > 1
- Deep S waves in V_4, V_5, and V_6
- Associated RAD, RAE
- Deep T inversion in V_1, V_2, and V_3

Cause of Right Ventricular Hypertrophy

- Long-standing MS
- Pulmonary hypertension of any cause
- Ventricular septal defect (VSD) or ASD with initial L to R shunt
- Congenital heart with RV over load
- Tricuspid regurgitation, pulmonary stenosis

Left Ventricular Hypertrophy

Causes of Left Ventricular Hypertrophy

- Pressure overload—systemic hypertension and aortic stenosis
- Volume overload —AR or MR-dilated cardiomyopathy
- VSD—cause both right and left ventricular volume overload
- Hypertrophic cardiomyopathy

Criteria of Left Ventricular Hypertrophy

- High QRS voltages in limb leads:
  - Sokolow and Lyon criteria: S (V_1) + R (V_5 or V_6) > 35 mm
  - Cornell criteria: S (V_3) + R (aVL) > 28 mm (men) or > 20 mm (women)
  - Others: R (aVL) > 13 mm

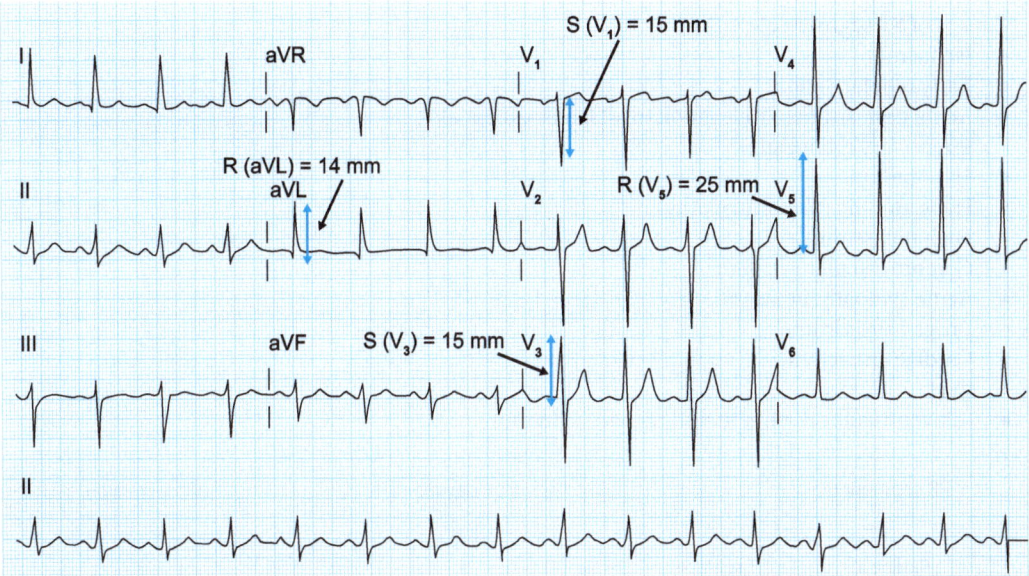

Fig. 30.7: Electrocardiogram (ECG) showing voltage criteria for left ventricular hypertrophy (LVH).

TABLE 30.6: Romhilt-Estes Score for LVH.

ECG criteria	Points
Voltage criteria (any of) (Fig. 30.7): • R or S in limb leads ≥ 20 mm • S in V_1 or V_2 ≥ 30 mm • R in V_5 or V_6 ≥ 30 mm	3
ST-T abnormalities: • ST-T vector opposite to QRS without digitalis	3
• ST-T vector opposite to QRS with digitalis	1
Negative terminal P mode in V_1, 1 mm in depth and 0.04 s in duration (indicates left atrial enlargement)	3
LAD (QRS of −30° or more)	2
QRS duration ≥ 0.09 s	1
Delayed intrinsicoid deflection in V_5 or V_6 (> 0.05 s)	1

- Deep symmetric T inversion in V_4, V_5, and V_6
- QRS duration > 0.09 sec, associated LAD, LAE.
- Romhilt-Estes Score: Score > 5—definite left ventricular hypertrophy (LVH), < 3 LVH unlikely (**Table 30.6**).

TABLE 30.7: Types of left ventricular hypertrophy (LVH).

Pressure overload	Volume overload
• Like in hypertension, ischaemic heart disease (IHD) • LV strain pattern—ST depression with T inversion in V_5, V_6, L1, and aVL leads	• Like in mitral or aortic regurgitation • Shows prominent Q waves, positive T waves in V_5, V_6, L1, and aVL

Types of Left Ventricular Hypertrophy
Types of LVH are given in **Table 30.7**.

ST segment
Abnormalities
ST Segment:
- ST segment is isoelectric and at the same level as subsequent PR interval
- The length between the end of the S wave (end of ventricular depolarisation) and the beginning of repolarisation
- From J point on the end of QRS complex, to inclination of T wave

Causes of ST segment elevation
- Ischaemia
- Early repolarisation
- Acute pericarditis: ST elevation in all leads, except aVR
- Pulmonary embolism
- Hypothermia
- Hypertrophic cardiomyopathy
- High potassium
- Cerebrovascular accident
- Acute sympathetic stress
- Brugada syndrome
- Cardiac aneurysm
- LVH
- Idioventricular rhythm including paced rhythm.

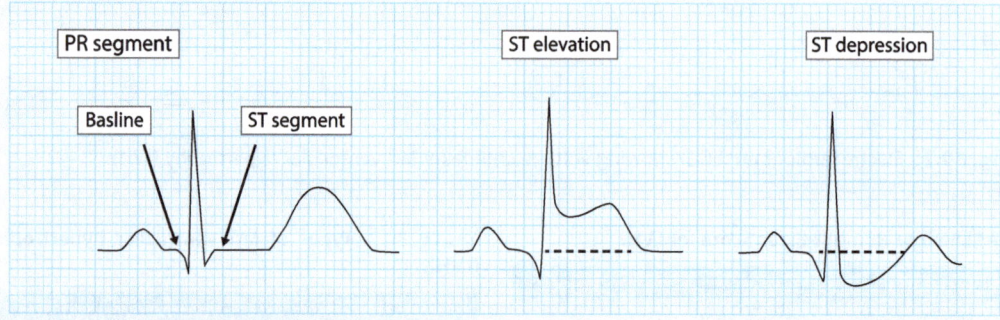

Causes of ST segment depression
- Myocardial ischaemia/non-ST-elevation myocardial infarction (NSTEMI)
- Reciprocal change in ST segment elevation myocardial infarction (STEMI)
- Posterior MI
- Digoxin effect (reverse tick mark/'sagging' morphology, resembling Salvador Dali's moustache)
- Hypokalaemia
- Bundle branch block
- Ventricular hypertrophy
- Ventricular pacing

Step 7: Look for any Evidence of Infarction

ECG Changes in Myocardial Infarction

There are two types of MI—STEMI and NSTEMI.

STEMI criteria
- ST elevation in > 2 chest leads > 2 mm elevation
- ST elevation in > 2 limb leads > 1 mm elevation
- Q wave > 0.04 s (1 small square)

Electrocardiogram localization of type of MI is listed in **Table 30.8**.

Electrocardiogram signs of ischemic heart disease are listed in **Table 30.9**.

Non-ST-Elevation MI

Non-ST-elevation MI is also known as sub-endocardial or non-Q-wave MI.

In a PT with acute coronary syndrome (ACS) in which the ECG does not show ST elevation, NSTEMI (sub-endocardia lMI) is suspected if
- ST depression (A)
- T wave inversion with or without ST depression (B)
- Q wave and ST elevation will never happen

TABLE 30.8: Electrocardiogram localization of type of myocardial infarction (MI).

Location of MI	Lead with ST changes	Affected coronary artery
Anterior	V_1, V_2, V_3, V_4	Left anterior descending (LADA) artery
Septum	V_1, V_2	LADA
Left lateral	I, aVL, V_5, V_6	Left circumflex
Inferior	II, III, aVF	Right coronary artery (RCA)
Right atrium	aVR, V1	RCA
Posterior	Posterior chest leads	RCA
Right ventricle	Right-sided leads	RCA

TABLE 30.9: Electrocardiogram signs of ischemic heart disease.

Ischaemia	Injury	Infarct
• T-wave inversion (flipped T) • ST segment depression • T wave flattening • Biphasic T waves	• ST segment elevation of > 1 mm in at least two contiguous leads • Heightened or peaked T waves • Directly related to portions of myocardium rendered electrically inactive	• Significant Q wave where none previously existed • Why? • Impulse travelling away from the positive lead • Necrotic tissue is electrically dead

Depressed ST segment

Peaked T waves

Inverted T waves

Elevated ST segment

Q wave

ELECTROLYTES AND ECG (Fig. 30.8)

Hypocalcaemia: Prolonged ST segment and QT intervals

Hypercalcaemia
- Shortened ST segment
- Widened T wave and short QT

Hypokalaemia
- ST depression
- Shallow, flat, and inverted T wave
- Prominent U wave and P waves

Hyperkalaemia
- Tall, peaked T waves
- Flat P waves
- Widened QRS complex
- Prolonged PR interval
- Sine wave

Hypomagnesaemia
- Tall T waves
- Depressed ST segment

Hypermagnesaemia
- Prolonged PR interval
- Widened QRS complexes

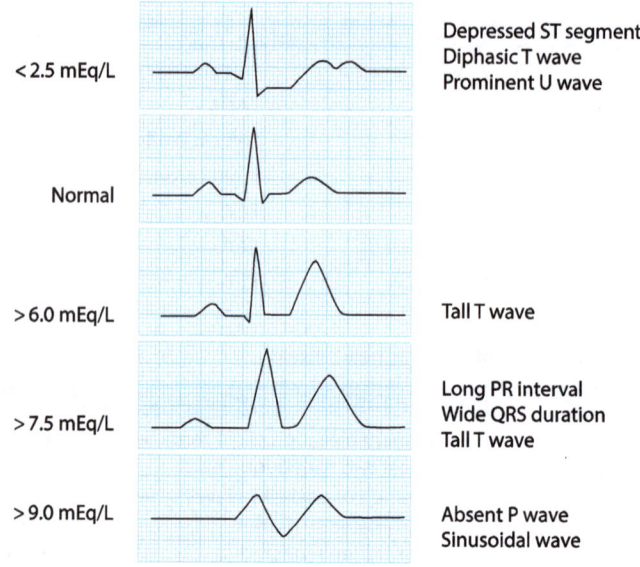

Fig. 30.8: Electrocardiogram (ECG) changes are seen with potassium.

EXAMPLES
Example 1

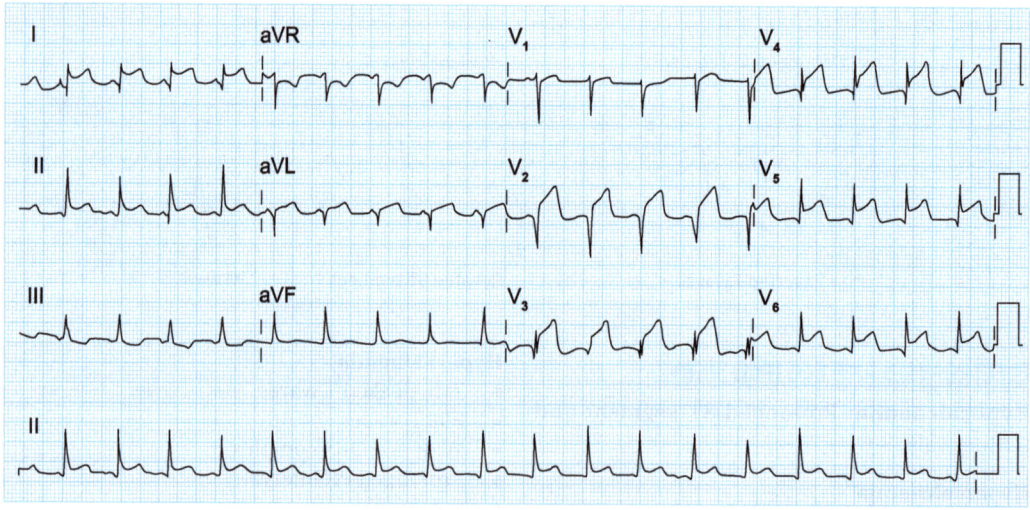

12-lead ECG Showing

Rate	110 bpm
Rhythm	Sinus rhythm
Axis	Normal
P wave	Duration 0.08 s and normal morphology
PR interval/segment	• 0.12 s • PR segment elevation in aVR
QRS	0.08 s
ST segment	• Elevation in V_2–V_6, I, aVL • Depression in aVR
T wave	Normal
QT interval	0.32 s
Final diagnosis	Acute pericarditis

Example 2

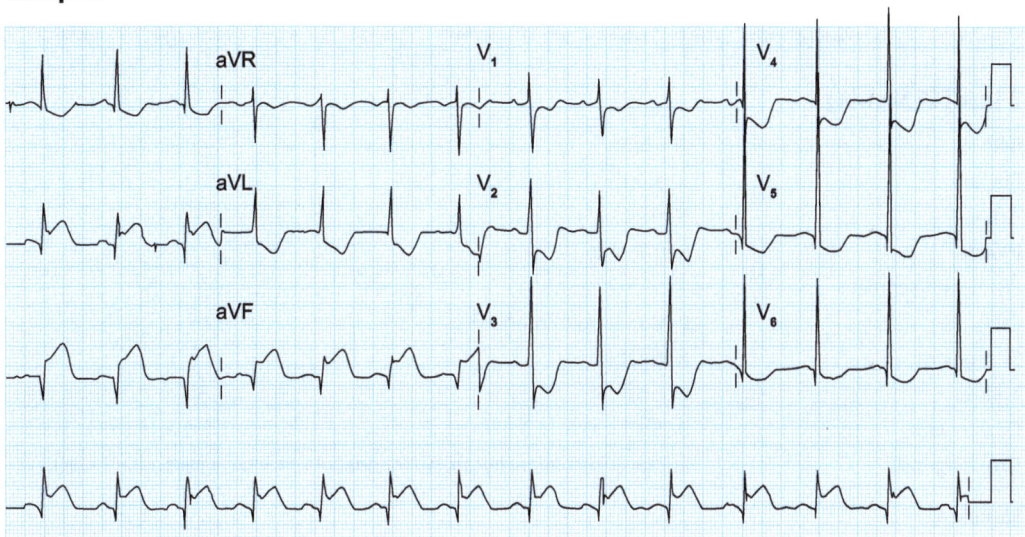

12-Lead ECG Showing

Rate	85 bpm
Rhythm	Sinus
Axis	Normal
P wave	Duration 0.12 s and normal morphology
PR interval/segment	0.16 s
QRS	0.08 s
ST segment	• Elevation in II, III, aVF (elevation in Lead III > II) • Depression in V_1-V_6, I, aVL
T wave	Corresponds to ST–T changes.
QT interval	0.36 s
Final diagnosis	Inferior wall MI with signs of RV infarction

Example 3

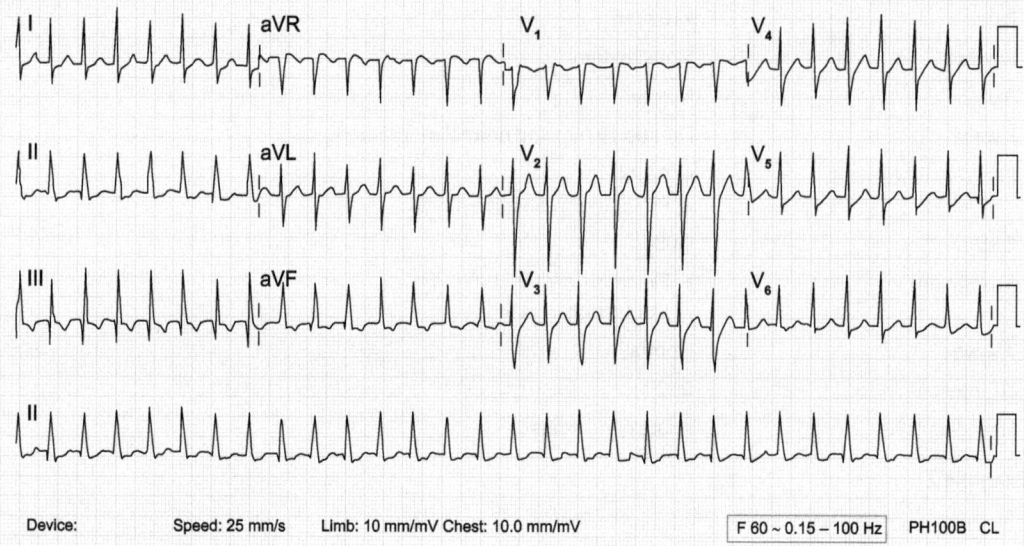

12-Lead ECG Showing

Rate	200 bpm
Rhythm	Regular
Axis	Normal
P wave	Retrograde
PR interval/segment	
QRS	0.08 s (narrow complex)
ST segment	Normal
T wave	Normal
QT interval	0.28 s
Final diagnosis	Supraventricular tachycardia-AV nodal re-entry tachycardia (SVT-AVNRT)

Example 4

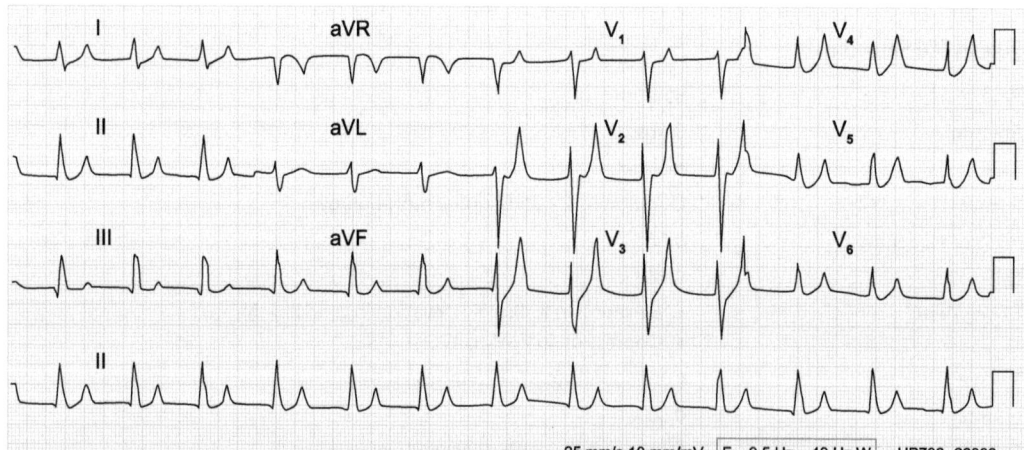

12-Lead ECG Showing

Rate	75 bpm
Rhythm	Junctional
Axis	Normal
P wave	Absent
PR interval/segment	–
QRS	0.14 s notching at J point (V$_2$)
ST segment	• Minimal elevation in V$_3$–V$_5$ • No reciprocal changes
T wave	Tall T steeple waves in precordial leads, concordant with QRS
QT interval	0.36 s
Final diagnosis	Hyperkalaemia

Example 5

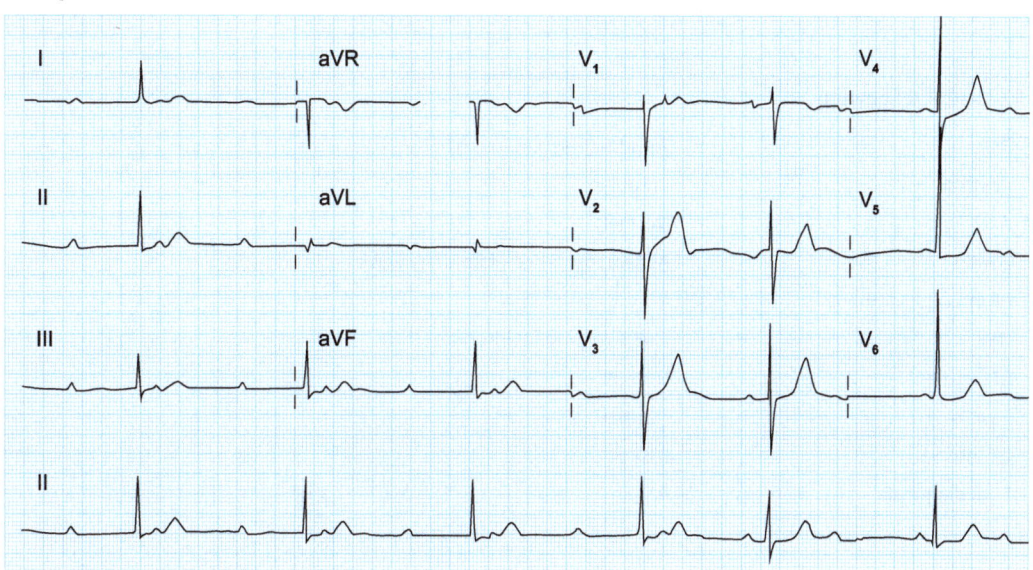

12-Lead ECG Showing

Rate	Atrial—80 bpm; Ventricular—50 bpm
Rhythm	Junctional escape
Axis	Normal
P wave	Present
PR interval/segment	–
QRS	0.08 s independent of P waves
ST segment	Normal
T wave	Normal
QT interval	0.36 s
Final diagnosis	Complete heart block

Example 6

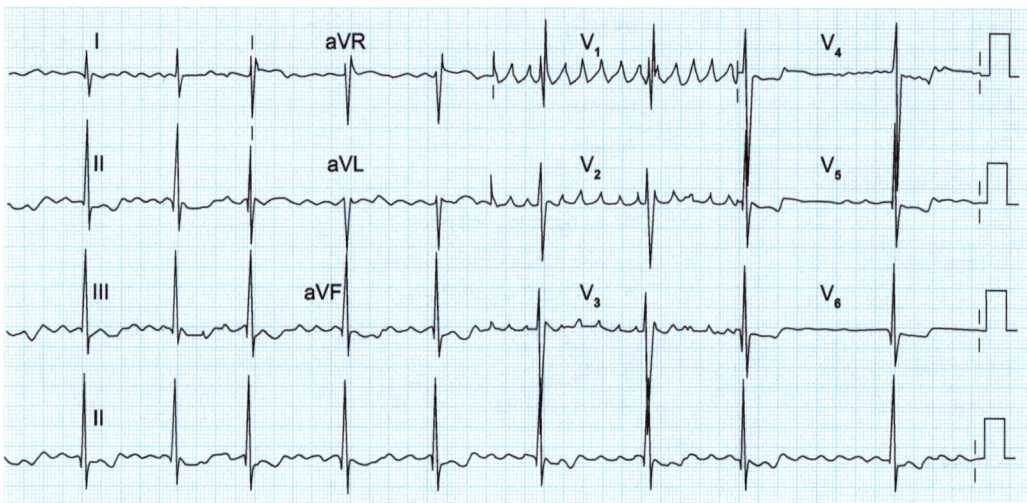

12-Lead ECG Showing

Rate	70 bpm (6-s rule)
Rhythm	Irregular
Axis	Normal
P wave	Absent, presence of fibrillary waves
PR interval/segment	–
QRS	0.08 s varying RR interval
ST segment	Normal
T wave	Normal
QT interval	0.32 s
Final diagnosis	AF

Example 7

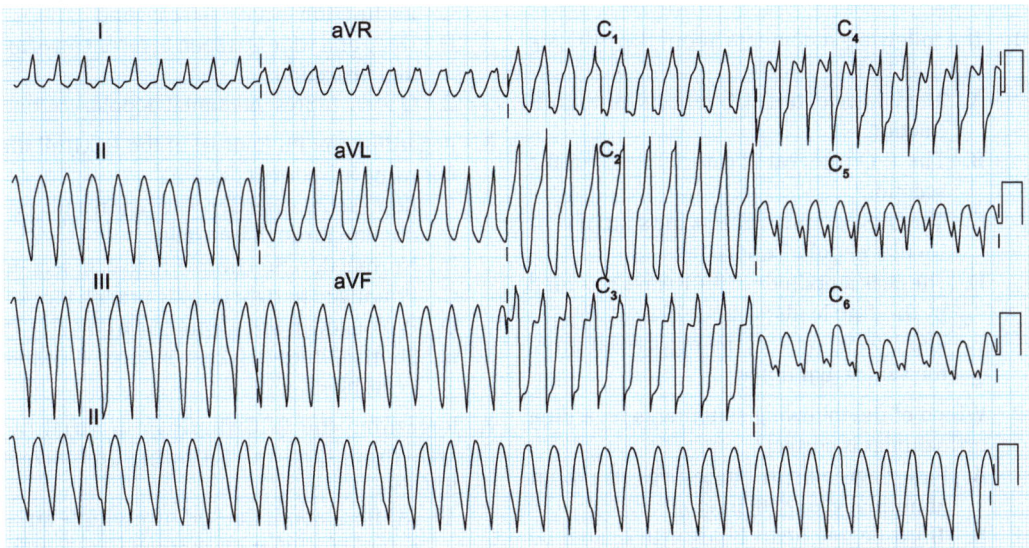

12-Lead ECG Showing

Rate	250 bpm
Rhythm	Regular
Axis	Left- northwest
P wave	AV dissociation
PR interval/segment	–
QRS	0.28 s (Broad complex) positive concordance
ST segment	–
T wave	–
QT interval	–
Final diagnosis	Monomorphic ventricular tachycardia (VT)

BEST OF FIVES

1. The following statements about the ECG are true EXCEPT
   A. The P wave of the ECG reflects atrial contraction.
   B. The P-Q interval is normally about 0.1 second.
   C. The QRS complex reflects the start of ventricular depolarisation.
   D. The peak amplitude of the R wave recorded by the limb leads is about 20 mV.
   E. The T-wave reflects the repolarisation of the ventricular fibres.

2. Which of the following statements regarding arrhythmias is correct?
   A. First-degree heart block gives rise to an abnormally long PR interval.
   B. Third-degree heart block is indicated by an abnormally long QRS complex following the P wave.
   C. An ECG with a sawtooth pattern on the baseline indicates atrial fibrillation
   D. In second-degree heart block, all P waves are not followed by a QRS complex.
   E. Ventricular premature beats are characterised by QRS width < 110 seconds.

3. The following statements about the ECG are true EXCEPT
   A. The Q-T interval varies with heart rate.
   B. In hyperkalaemia, the T wave is flattened.
   C. The U wave is more often seen when the heart rate is low.
   D. A long QT interval is characteristic of hypocalcaemia.
   E. Left-axis deviation occurs in left ventricular hypertrophy.

4. The P-wave of normal ECG:
   A. Has voltage and duration nearly equal to 2.5 × 2.5 mm
   B. Is upright in aVR
   C. Represents right atrial depolarisation in its second half
   D. Coincides with atrial systole
   E. Is biphasic in lead III

5. As regards Q wave, all the following are correct EXCEPT
   A. It represents septal depolarisation from left to right in V_5.
   B. Its depth is not > 1/4 its corresponding R.
   C. Its duration is not > 0.04 second.
   D. Deep and wide Q is seen in recent myocardial infarction.
   E. Q wave represents septal depolarisation.

6. Regarding the PR interval of the ECG, all the following are correct EXCEPT
   A. Represents atrial depolarisation and conduction through ventricle
   B. Normal duration from 0.12 to 0.30 second
   C. Prolonged in right bundle branch block
   D. Prolonged in first-degree heart block
   E. Short PR interval is seen in second-degree heart block

7. Regarding the ECG findings in atrial (A) arrhythmias, all the following are correct EXCEPT
   A. (A) fibrillation: Caused by multiple atrial ectopic foci that discharged very rapidly and irregularly
   B. (A) tachycardia: Paroxysmal rapid and irregular rate (150–200 bpm)
   C. (A) flutter: Sawtooth waves associated with partial atrioventricular (AV) block
   D. (A) fibrillation: Absence of P waves, very irregular rate and normal QRS
   E. Supraventricular tachycardia has regular narrow QRS morphology

8. Ventricular premature beat ("VPB") is
   A. Caused by an ectopic ventricular focus that discharges regularly
   B. Preceded by P wave and has bizarre prolonged QRS
   C. Followed by a compensatory pause
   D. Occurs in series without normal beats in between
   E. QRS complex is narrow

9. All of the following cause low-voltage ECG EXCEPT
   A. Hypothermia
   B. Body mass index (BMI) > 35 kg/m²
   C. Hypothyroidism
   D. Hypokalaemia
   E. Half-standardisation

10. Left-axis deviation of the ECG is described when:
    A. The axis of the heart is from –0 to +90°.
    B. The QRS complex is prominent positive in lead aVF.

C. The QRS is prominent positive in lead I and prominent negative in lead III.
D. Left posterior hemiblock causes left axis deviation (LAD).
E. Ostium secundum atrial septal defect (ASD) causes LAD.

11. Regarding the ECG findings in heart block (HB), all of the following are correct EXCEPT
    A. Complete (HB): Complete dissociation between P waves and QRS complexes
    B. First degree (HB): PR interval is abnormally long.
    C. Second degree (HB): A ventricular beat may follow every second or third atrial beat.
    D. First degree (HB): PR interval lengthens progressively until a ventricular beat is dropped.
    E. Mobitz type 1 (HB): PR interval lengthens progressively until a ventricular beat is dropped.

12. The ECG findings of bundle branch block (BBB):
    A. Associated with absence of P waves
    B. Heart rate is slowed to < 60 bpm.
    C. Double-hump QRS complex occurs in V_5 and V_6 in right BBB.
    D. QRS complexes are prolonged and deformed.
    E. QRS width < 10 seconds.

13. Regarding the ECG of ventricular hypertrophy (VH):
    A. Axis of the heart is from −30° to +90° in right VH.
    B. S wave in V_1 or V_2 plus R wave in V_5 or V_6 account > 35 mm in left VH in adults.
    C. S wave is deep in V_1 and V_2 and R wave is tall in V_5 and V_6 in right VH.
    D. Right VH may occur in systemic hypertension.
    E. Biventricular hypertrophy is seen in atrial septal defect (ASD).

14. Regarding the ECG findings of myocardial infarction (MI), all the following are correct EXCEPT
    A. Elevation of the ST segment in recent (acute) MI
    B. Deep and wide Q in old MI
    C. Low voltage in massive MI
    D. ST elevation in II, III and aVF suggests anterior wall MI
    E. Inferior wall MI is associated with right ventricular MI

15. Correct statement regarding ECG changes in electrolyte imbalance is:
    A. Tall and peaked T wave in hypokalaemia
    B. T wave inversion and prominent U wave in hyperkalaemia
    C. Prolonged QT interval in hypocalcaemia
    D. High voltage in hyponatraemia
    E. Absent p waves in hypokalaemia

16. Which electrical event of the heart is NOT recorded on the standard 12-lead ECG trace?
    A. Atrial depolarisation
    B. Atrial repolarisation
    C. Phase 2 of the ventricular action potential
    D. Ventricular repolarisation
    E. Phase 4 of the ventricular action potential

17. Wide QRS is seen in all EXCEPT
    A. Sinus rhythm with complete left bundle branch block
    B. Accelerated idioventricular rhythm
    C. Atrial fibrillation
    D. Atrial sensed and ventricular paced pattern
    E. Sinus rhythm with Wolff-Parkinson-White pre-excitation

18. Which of the following is associated with ST segment elevation in ECG?
    A. Left ventricular hypertrophy (LVH)
    B. Right VH (RVH)
    C. Digoxin effect
    D. Early repolarisation after an attack of angina
    E. Subendocardial infarction

19. The time necessary for ventricular depolarisation is represented by the:
    A. P-R interval
    B. QRS interval
    C. QT interval
    D. S-T segment
    E. QRS complex

20. The duration from the beginning of the P wave to the beginning of the QRS complex is the:
    A. P-R interval
    B. QRS duration
    C. Absolute refractory period
    D. Relative refractory period
    E. PR segment

Answers

1-D, 2-A, 3-B, 4-A, 5-D, 6-D, 7-B, 8-C, 9-D, 10-C, 11-D, 12-D, 13-B, 14-D, 15-C, 16-B, 17-C, 18-D, 19-B, 20-A

■ SUGGESTED READING

1. Goldberger AL, Goldberger ZE, Shvilkin AS. Goldberger's Clinical Electrocardiography: A Simplified Approach, 9th edition. Philadelphia: Elsevier; 2017.
2. Mirvis, DM, Goldberger, AL. Electrocardiography. In: Zipes DP, Libby P, Bonow RO, et al (Eds). Braunwald's Heart Disease: A Textbook of Cardiovascular Medicine, 11th edition. , Philadelphia: W.B. Saunders Company; 2018.
3. Kligfield P, Gettes LS, Bailey JJ, Childers R, Deal BJ, Hancock EW, et al. Recommendations for the standardization and interpretation of the electrocardiogram. Part I: The electrocardiogram and its technology. A scientific statement from the American Heart Association Electrocardiography and Arrhythmias Committee, Council on Clinical Cardiology; the American College of Cardiology Foundation; and the Heart Rhythm Society. Heart Rhythm. 2007; 4:394.
4. Surawicz B, Childers R, Deal BJ, Gettes LS, Bailey JJ, Gorgels A, et al. AHA/ACCF/HRS recommendations for the standardization and interpretation of the electrocardiogram: part III: intraventricular conduction disturbances: a scientific statement from the American Heart Association Electrocardiography and Arrhythmias Committee, Council on Clinical Cardiology; the American College of Cardiology Foundation; and the Heart Rhythm Society. Endorsed by the International Society for Computerized Electrocardiology. J Am Coll Cardiol. 2009;53(11):976-81.
5. Thygesen K, Alpert JS, Jaffe AS, Chaitman BR, Bax JJ, Morrow DA, et al. Fourth universal definition of myocardial infarction (2018). J Am Coll Cardiol. 2018;72(18):2231-64.
6. Rautaharju PM, Surawicz B, Gettes LS, Bailey JJ, Childers R, Deal BJ, et al. AHA/ACCF/HRS recommendations for the standardization and interpretation of the electrocardiogram: part IV: the ST segment, T and U waves, and the QT interval: a scientific statement from the American Heart Association Electrocardiography and Arrhythmias Committee, Council on Clinical Cardiology; the American College of Cardiology Foundation; and the Heart Rhythm Society. Endorsed by the International Society for Computerized Electrocardiology. J Am Coll Cardiol. 2009;53(11):982-91.
7. Fihn SD, Gardin JM, Abrams J, Berra K, Blankenship JC, Dallas AP, et al. 2012 ACCF/AHA/ACP/AATS/PCNA/SCAI/STS Guideline for the diagnosis and management of patients with stable ischemic heart disease: a report of the American College of Cardiology Foundation/American Heart Association Task Force on Practice Guidelines, and the American College of Physicians, American Association for Thoracic Surgery, Preventive Cardiovascular Nurses Association, Society for Cardiovascular Angiography and Interventions, and Society of Thoracic Surgeons. J Am Coll Cardiol. 2012;60(24):e44-164.
8. Myers J, Arena R, Franklin B, Pina I, Kraus WE, McInnis K, et al. Recommendations for clinical exercise laboratories: a scientific statement from the American Heart Association. Circulation. 2009;119(24):3144-61.
9. Gibbons RJ, Balady GJ, Bricker JT, Chaitman BR, Fletcher GF, Froelicher VF, et al. ACC/AHA 2002 guideline update for exercise testing: summary article: a report of the American College of Cardiology/American Heart Association Task Force on Practice Guidelines (Committee to Update the 1997 Exercise Testing Guidelines). Circulation. 2002;106(14):1883-92.

INDEX

Page numbers followed by *b* refer to box, *f* refer to figure, *fc* refer to flowchart, and *t* refer to table.

A

Abacavir 412
Abdomen
  CT scan of 150
  magnetic resonance imaging of 164
  ultrasound of 164
Abscess 501
  abdominal 371
  ultrasound-guided aspiration of 150
Absolute basophil count 293
Absolute polycythaemia 292
Acanthosis nigricans 522
Acetaminophen 563
  metabolism 563*f*
Acid-base
  and electrolytes 554
  imbalances 237
Acid-fast bacillus 334
Acidosis 241
Acid-pepsin versus mucosal resistance 82
Acne
  clinical variants of 515*b*
  conglobata 515
  excoriée 515
  fulminans 515
  venenata 515
  vulgaris 515
Acquired immunity 529
  types of 529
Acquired immunodeficiency syndrome 337, 373, 398, 402, 403, 405, 411, 501, 513, 537
  dementia complex 408
Acrokeratosis paraneoplastica 576
Acromegaly 171, 462
Activated partial thromboplastin time 272, 274, 277, 279
Active therapy 283
Acute adrenal crisis 180
Acute arthritis, causes of 208, 209*b*
Acute asthma 345*fc*
  treatment of severe 343
Acute attack, treatment of 219
Acute cardiogenic pulmonary oedema, treatment of 46

Acute circulatory failure 44
  causes of 44, 45*t*
  classification of 44, 45*t*
Acute coronary syndrome 55, 57*fc*, 183
  management of 59*fc*
Acute diarrhoea, causes of 78*b*, 364*t*
Acute endocarditis 52
  clinical features of 53
Acute hepatitis 117*f*, 144
  causes for 114, 118*b*
Acute hyperventilation syndrome 506
Acute idiopathic thrombocytopenic purpura 270*t*
Acute inflammatory demyelinating polyradiculoneuropathy 462
Acute kidney injury 237, 238, 242*fc*, 504
  clinical features of 239*t*
  type of 239
Acute leukaemias 248, 282, 310
  classification of 280
Acute liver failure 149
  complications of 125*t*
Acute lymphoblastic leukaemia 280, 286, 286*t*, 302
  precursor
    B-cell 281
    T-cell 281
Acute lymphocytic leukaemia 280, 284, 284*fc*
Acute lymphoid leukaemia 281, 568, 599
Acute mania, clinical features of 485*b*
Acute massive pulmonary embolism 66
Acute myeloblastic leukaemia 280
Acute myelocytic leukaemia 280
Acute myelogenous leukaemia 286, 286*t*
Acute myeloid leukaemia 281, 284, 568, 576
  therapy of 285*fc*
Acute myocardial infarction 55, 58, 58f, 58*t*
  emergency management of 24
  management of 58

Acute myocarditis 67
  aetiology of 67, 67*b*
Acute pancreatitis 163
  causes of 163, 163*b*
  complications of 165*b*
Acute promyelocytic leukaemia 285, 568
Acute pulmonary oedema
  clinical features of 45
  management of 11, 12*fc*
Acute renal failure 238*b*, 241*fc*
  causes of 239*fc*
  urinalysis in 240*fc*
Acute respiratory alkalosis 506
Acute respiratory distress syndrome 327, 327*t*, 356, 364, 554
Acute respiratory failure 324, 325
  causes of 325*b*
Acute rheumatic fever 48*b*
  diagnosis in 48
  management of 48
Acute stress ulcers, aetiology of 82
Acute tubular necrosis 240
Acute variceal bleeding, management of 132*b*
Acute variceal haemorrhage, treatment of 133*fc*
Acute viral hepatitis 111
  complications of 117*t*
Acyclovir 374
Adams–Stokes attacks 44
Addison's disease 179, 512, 517
Adefovir dipivoxil 122
Adeno respiratory syncytial virus 335
Adenoma 178
Adenosine 42
  deaminase levels 456
Adisintegrin 275
Adrenal tumours 178
Adrenocorticotropic hormone 178-180, 353, 576
Adriamycin 311
Adult immunisation schedule 538*t*
Adult T-cell
  leukaemia 311
  lymphoma 311
Adverse drug reaction 613
  classification of 613*b*
  types of 613

Aedes aegypti mosquitoes 374, 377
African trypanosomiasis 392
Agnosia 433, 435
Airborne allergens 511
Airflow limitation, reversibility of 322
Airway disease, chronic obstructive 337, 344
Akinesia 452
Alanine
   aminotransferase 105, 115, 117, 121, 376, 563
   transaminase 144
Albinism 476
Alcohol 60, 126, 128, 546
   consumption, amount of 158*t*
   dependence 487
      treatment 487
   intoxication, acute 488
   withdrawal syndrome, features of 488
Aldosterone
   antagonists 141
   receptor blockers 63
Alemtuzumab 57*t*
Alkaline phosphatase 103, 115, 310
Alkalosis 177
   correction of 178
Alkaptonuria 477
Allergens, common 533*b*
Allergic alveolitis, extrinsic 344
Allergic contact eczema 511
Allergy 532
Allodynia 439
Allogeneic bone marrow transplantation 296
Alopecia 524
   areata 517
   causes of 525*t*
   classification of 525*t*
Alpha-1-antitrypsin defeciency 154
Alpha-blockers 63
Alpha-foetoprotein 105, 148
   elevated levels of 105
Alpha-methyldopa 450
Alpha-thalassaemia syndromes 260
Alprazolam 486
Aluminium phosphide poisoning 561
Alzheimer's disease 436, 436*b*, 512, 583
   clinical features 436
   laboratory investigations 436
   management 436
Amanita phalloides 126, 564
American College of Rheumatism criteria 210, 213*t*
American Diabetes Association 193*t*

Amineptine 490
Amino acid metabolism 475
Aminoglycosides 371
Aminosalicylates 95
Aminotransferases 102
Amiodarone 41
Amitriptyline 439, 483
Amoebic liver abscess 151
Amoxicillin 381
Amprenavir 412
Amylase 139
Amyloidosis 350, 462, 576
   primary 298, 576
   secondary 576
Anacrotic pulse 37*b*
Anaemia 153, 248, 256, 259, 261, 282, 309, 313, 542
   acquired sideroblastic 264
   acute haemolytic 261
   autoimmune haemolytic 254
   classification of 248, 248*t*
   clinical features of 249*f*
   hypochromic microcytic 263, 264*t*
   immunohaemolytic 254
   inherited sideroblastic 264
   severe 260
   supportive therapy for 263
   treatment of 296
Anagrelide 295
Analgesics 210
Anaphylactic reactions 533
Anaphylactoid
   purpura 212
   reactions 533*b*
Anaphylaxis, management of 27, 27*fc*
Ancylostoma duodenale 390
Ancylostomiasis 390
   clinical features 390
   diagnosis 390
   treatment 390
Androgens 547
Aneuploidy 592
Aneurysm, dissecting 34
Angina
   management of 27
   pectoris 34, 55
   treatment of 28*fc*
   unstable 55, 59
Angioedema 533
Angiotensin converting enzyme 12, 59, 64, 393, 500, 533, 542
   inhibitors 63
Angiotensin receptor
   antagonists 63
   blockers 542
Anion gap 10, 498
Ankylosing spondylitis 211

Ann Arbor classification 313*t*
   Cotswold's modification of 309*t*
Anopheles mosquitoes 386
Anorexia 586
   nervosa 492, 493*t*
Antacids 83
Antibiotics 79, 117, 150, 277, 530, 533
   intravenous 366
   therapy, empiric 455*t*
Antibodies
   dependent cell-mediated cytotoxicity 531
   structure 530
Anticholinergic 512, 558
   drugs 512
Anticoagulants 25*fc*, 65, 448
Antidepressants 512
   atypical 490
   drugs 489
Antidiuretic hormone 501
Antidotes poisons 559*t*
Antiemetics 512
Anti-epileptic agents, newer 442
Antifibrinolytic drugs 280
Antigen 117, 530
   binding sites 530
   processing of 531
Antigenic determinant sites 530
Antihistamines 512
Antihypertensives 512
   drug 63*b*, 63*f*
Anti-inflammatory agents 520
Anti-inflammatory function 473
Antimicrobial therapy 334
Antimitochondrial antibody 144
Antimotility drugs 79
Anti-myeloperoxidase 232
Antineutrophil cytoplasmic antibody 217, 230, 232
Antinuclear antibody 213, 232, 302
Antiparkinsonian drugs 512
Antiphospholipid 213, 232
   antibody syndrome 65, 215
   clinical features of 215*t*
Antiplatelets 19
   antibodies 270
Antipsychotics 512
   atypical 490
   drugs 489
   classification of 490*b*
Antiretroviral drug 410, 412*b*
   common 412*t*
Antiretroviral regimens 410, 413*t*
Antiretroviral therapy 415
   indications for 410
Antisecretory agents 79
Antispasmodics 512
Antistreptococcal therapy 48

Antistreptolysin O 232
Antithrombin therapy 59
Antithrombotic, deficiency of 65
Antituberculous drugs 339, 340*t*
Antivenom
   indications for 560
   treatment 560
Antiviral agents 122
Anuria 226
Anxiety 560
   disorders 485
      generalised 486
   state 34, 485
Aorta, coarctation of 60, 70
Aortic component 38
Aortic regurgitation 39, 51
   acute 51
   aetiology of 51*b*
   chronic 51
   peripheral signs of 51*b*
Aortic stenosis 50, 581
   aetiology of 50, 51*b*
Apex beat, normal 36
Aphasia 408, 433
   type of 434, 434*t*
Apical impulse 36
Aplastic anaemia 248, 264, 266
   severe 266
Apnoea–hypopnoea index 326, 326*t*, 368
Apraxia 433, 435
Arboviral diseases 374
Arginine vasopressin 502
Aripiprazole 484
Arrhythmias 533
Arterial blood gas 9, 29, 30, 65, 321, 406
   levels, normal 321*t*
   studies 66
Arterial blood supply 150
Arterial oxygen saturation 293
Arterial thrombosis, prevention of 215
Arteriovenous fistula 40
Arthritis
   chronic 208, 209*b*
   inflammatory 208*t*
Artificial pacemaker 624
Artificially acquired
   active immunity 530
   passive immunity 530
Ascariasis 389
   clinical features 389
   treatment 390
Ascaris lumbricoides 389
Ascites 138
   pathogenesis of 139*t*

Ascitic fluid
   changes 139*t*
   examination of 141*t*, 146
   infection, classification of 138
   nature of 139, 140*b*, 141*b*
Ascorbic acid deficiency 470
Aseptic meningitis 455
Aspartate aminotransferase 105, 115, 117, 376, 563
Aspergilloma 350
Aspergillosis, allergic bronchopulmonary 341, 341*t*
Aspiration 327
   pneumonia 336
Aspirin 28
   low-dose 295
Assist control mode ventilation 328
Asteatotic eczema 512
Asthma
   chronic 342
   classification of 342*b*, 342*t*
   COPD overlap syndrome 348
   drugs useful in 343*t*
   episodic 342
   in pregnancy 544
   management of acute severe 28, 29*fc*
   severe acute 342
   stepwise management of 344*f*
Asymmetrical T wave inversion 627
Ataxia 443, 454
   acquired 454
   classification of 454, 454*t*
   hemiparesis syndrome 450
   hereditary 454
   telangiectasia 311, 524
Atazanavir 412, 413
Atherosclerosis 54
   risk factors of 55*b*
Atherosclerotic cardiovascular disease 183
Athetosis 453
Athlete's foot 521
Atomic bombing 281
Atopic dermatitis 513
   vascular stigmata of 512*t*
Atopic eczema 511, 512
Atria, disturbance of 40
Atrial fibrillation 41, 622
   aetiology of 41, 41*b*
Atrial flutter 42, 622
Atrial musculature 617
Atrial natriuretic peptide 502
Atrial premature beat 624
Atrial septal defect 39, 69, 625
Atrioventricular block 43
   complete 44

Atrioventricular node, disturbance of 40
Atropine 26
   dosage 26*t*
Atypical mycobacteria 336
   infections 407
Atypical pneumonias 335
   diagnosis of 335, 336*b*
Auscultatory signs 65
Auspitz sign 514
Autism 482
Autoantibodies 65, 119, 155
   against Smith antigen 213
Autoimmune disease 302, 474, 536
Autoimmune polyendocrinopathy syndrome 188
Autoimmunohaemolytic anaemia 265, 265*b*, 267*b*
Autologous stem-cell transplantation 300
Autonomic dysfunction 452
Autonomic neuropathy 199
   clinical features of 199*b*
Autosomal chromosomes, numerical abnormalities of 592
Autosomal dominant
   diseases 593
   polycystic kidney disease 242
Autosomal recessive
   diseases 593
   disorders 594*t*
Auxiliary orthotopic transplantation 149
Azathioprine 119
Azithromycin 380, 381, 388, 424
Azotaemia 226, 381

B

Bacillus cereus 382
Back pain, acute 1
Bacteraemia 536
Bacterial vaginosis-associated organisms 422
Bacteriuria
   asymptomatic 227
   types 227*t*
Balanced reciprocal translocation 288
Balloon tamponade 80, 134
Barbiturate poisoning 562
Bariatric surgery 475
Barlow's disease 470
Barlow's syndrome 50
Basal cell carcinoma 522
Basic life support 22
Basilar migraine 438

Basilar syndrome, top of 448
Bazett's formula 629
Bazex syndrome 576
B-cell
 function, abnormalities of 404
 origin 290
Becker muscular dystrophy 464
Behçet's disease 212
 criteria of 212, 212t
 minor criteria of 212t
Bell's palsy 437
 aetiology 437
 clinical features 437
 investigations 437
 treatment 437
Bence-Jones protein 300
Benedict's syndrome 447
Benzathine penicillin 428
Benzodiazepine 26
Beta-blockers 63
Beta-thalassaemia
 intermedia 260
 major 260
  pathogenesis of 262f
 minor 260
 syndromes 260, 260t
Bevacizumab 571
Bias
 role of 604
 types of 604, 604b
Bicarbonate 195
Bile acid sequestrants 192
Bile duct
 injury 144
 strictures 156
Biliary cirrhosis 128, 154
 clinical features of 155b
 primary 154
 secondary 154, 156
Biliary excretion 158
Biliary secretion 158
Bilirubin 105
 conjugation, impaired 107
 formation 157
 hepatic processing of 157
 increased production of 107
 metabolism 157
  intestinal phase of 158
 production 157
 renal excretion of 158
 unconjugated 158
Biliverdin 157
Binding 158
 protein 294
Binet staging 291, 291t
 clinical staging features of 291, 291t
Biopsy 309
Bisferiens pulse 37b

Bisphosphonates 12
Bite cells 263f
Bladder 226
 carcinoma 392
Blast crisis phase 288
Bleeding 279
 arteries, embolisation of 80
 distinguishing patterns of 267t
 into muscles 273
 manifestations 293
 tendency 299
 time 268, 270, 272, 274
Bleomycin 311
Bleuler's criteria 482b
Blinding, types of 606t
Blindness 408
Blood 66, 115
 ammonia estimation 129
 count 256, 282, 290, 313
  complete 240
 culture 53, 150
 investigations 164
 loss 248
 pressure 9, 193t, 334, 376, 553
  systolic 18, 44, 64, 392
 products, irradiated 304
 transfusion 256, 266, 303, 425
  complications of 304, 304t
 urea
  and creatinine 277
  nitrogen 237
Blunt chest trauma 327
Body
 iron stores, elevation of 152
 louse 519
 mass index 475
Bone 299
 marrow 250, 253, 255, 268, 270, 290, 294, 296, 298, 299
  aspirate 283
  aspirate and biopsy 302
  examination 300
  failure 282
  function 264t
  involvement 312
  iron 250, 253
  study 288
  transplantation 259, 261, 283, 304, 305
 metabolism 473t
 pain 288
 scan 300
Bortezomib 572
Botulism 379
 classification 379
 clinical features 379
 diagnosis 379
 treatment 379
Bourneville disease 524

Bowel movements 77
Bradycardia 36, 560, 561
 causes of 621t
Bradykinesia 452
Brain 405
 abscess 350
 involvement 153
Break-bone fever 375
Breakpoint cluster region 280
Breathing 22
Breathlessness 1
Bromosulphthalein clearance 105
Bronchial asthma 341
 classification 341
 clinical features 342
 management of 343
Bronchial disease 364
Bronchial obstruction 344
 causes of 344, 346t
Bronchiectasis 349, 358, 380
 causes of 349, 350b
 clinical features 349
 complications of 350, 350b
 management 350
Bronchitis, chronic 347, 348b, 349t
Bronchoalveolar lavage 334
Bronchodilator therapy 366
Bronchopneumonia 380, 452
Bronchopulmonary aspergillosis 341
 classification 341
Bronchoscopy 21, 363, 366
 indications of 365t
Brown-Séquard syndrome 458
 clinical manifestations of 459t
Brucella 515
 abortus 392
 canis 392
 suis 392
Brucellosis 392
Brudzinski's neck sign 455, 456
Brugada syndrome 43
Bubonic plague 378
Budd-Chiari syndrome 145
 causes of 145b
Bulbar palsy, progressive 459
Bulimia nervosa 493, 493t
Bulk laxatives 78
Bull-neck appearance 378
Bullous pemphigoid 520
Bundle branch block 40, 626, 630
Bundle of Kent 40
Bupropion 490
Burkitt leukaemia 281, 314
Burkitt lymphoma 314, 315b, 315t, 316f
Busulphan 289
Butyrophenones 450

C

Cachexia 347
Calcinosis 64
Calcitonin 12, 471
Calcium 471
  channel blocker 28, 63
  chloride 9
  gluconate 9
  homeostasis 473
  pyrophosphate dihydrate deposition disease 219
Calymmatobacterium granulomatis 422
Camel hump fever 388
Campylobacter 408
  jejuni 382
Candida 407, 411
  albicans 385, 422
  infection 385
Candidiasis 385, 405
  cutaneous 386
  treatment 386
Canines 389
Carbamate poisoning 561
Carbamazepine 437
Carbimazole 14
Carbohydrate 86
  markers 569
Carbon dioxide
  narcosis 347
  partial pressure of 505
Carbon monoxide 323
  poisoning 565
Carbon tetrachloride 462
Carcinoid syndrome 91
Carcinoid tumours 91
Cardiac arrest 43
  causes of 43, 43*b*
  management of 22, 22*fc*, 23*fc*
Cardiac arrhythmias 34, 40, 40*b*, 552
  classification 40
Cardiac disease 545, 546*b*
  classification of 545
Cardiac failure, congestive 9, 361
Cardiac function 283
Cardiac injury enzymes 57
Cardiogenic shock 45
  treatment of 45
Cardiology 34
Cardiomyopathy 67, 626
  congestive 67
  hypertrophic 67
Cardiopathy syndrome 524
Cardiorespiratory disease 65
Cardiovascular disease 183, 214, 364, 409, 489
Cardiovascular disorders 347
Cardiovascular function 473
Cardiovascular system 171, 237, 248, 299
Carditis 47
Carotid
  sinus syncope 35
  territory 443
Carpal spasm 177
Casal's necklace 471
Catamenial pneumothorax 363
Cataplexy 491
Catatonia 503
Cauda equina lesion 458*t*
Cavitation 501
Cefixime 381
Cefotaxime 381
Ceftriaxone 381
Cell
  count 138
  of origin 307
  tropism 400
Cellular bone marrow 296
Centers for Disease Control and Prevention 330, 402*t*
Central nervous system 53, 286, 299, 376, 391, 441, 444
  complications 61
  demyelinating diseases of 457
  manifestations 561
Central pontine myelinolysis 503
Central retinal artery occlusion 446
Central venous pressure 18, 392
Cephalosporins
  tetracyclines 533
  third-generation 142
Cerebellar diseases 454
  signs of 454*b*
Cerebral hemispheres 434*t*
Cerebral infarction 409
Cerebral ischaemia 446*t*
Cerebral oedema 124
  high-altitude 556
Cerebral salt wasting 502
Cerebral toxoplasmosis 409
Cerebral venous thrombosis 449
  causes of 450*b*
  clinical features 449
  treatment 449
Cerebrospinal fluid 461
  abnormalites 437
  examination 283
  findings 455, 456
Cerebrovascular accident 442
  risk factors of 444*t*
Cerebrum 253
Ceruloplasmin 104
Cetuximab 571
Chancroid 423, 423*b*
  diagnosis 423
Charcot's triad 111
Chelating drugs 154
Chelation therapy 153
Chemical 281
  aspiration pneumonia 336
Chemokine receptor 400
Chemotherapeutic drugs 570*f*
Chemotherapy 287, 289, 294, 301, 302, 308
  alternative 285
  induction 284
Chest
  pain 1, 34, 34*b*
  radiography 48, 57, 65, 150
  syndrome, acute 259
  X-ray 283
Chickenpox 373, 529
  clinical features 373
  complications 374
  management 374
Chikungunya 377
  clinical features 377
  diagnosis 377
  treatment 377
Child's-Pugh classification, modified 129*t*
Child-Turcotte-Pugh score 129*t*
Chimerism 593
Chi-square statistics 603
Chlamydia 515
  pneumonia 335
  strain of 424
  trachomatis 422-424
Chloramphenicol 381, 385, 547
Chloromas 282
Chloroquine 462
Cholangiopancreatography, endoscopic retrograde 105
Cholecystitis 34
Cholera 381
  clinical features 381
  diagnosis 382
  treatment 382
Cholestasis 143, 144
  chronic 144
  extrahepatic 109
  intrahepatic 109
  types of 109
Chorea 47, 452
Christmas disease 273
Chromosomal disorders, list of 598*t*
Chromosome
  analysis 315
  structural abnormalities of 592, 592*f*
Chronic alcohol misuse, consequences of 488*b*
Chronic disease, anaemia of 264, 266

Chronic dyspnoea 364
  causes of 364t
Chronic hepatitis
  causes of 118t
  grade of 114
Chronic kidney disease 183, 234, 235, 237, 472, 489
  causes of 234, 235b
  classification, revised 235f
  clinical features of 234
  clinical manifestations of 236f
  stages of 234, 234t
  treatment of 235, 238b
Chronic liver damage, hallmark of 118
Chronic lymphocytic leukaemia 280, 290, 302, 576, 599
Chronic myelogenous leukaemia 289, 302
Chronic myeloid leukaemia 287, 568, 576, 599
  chronic stable phase of 289f
Chronic obstructive pulmonary disease 65, 325, 330, 331, 344, 347b, 348f, 364, 625
  risk factors for 346b
  severity of 348f
Chronic respiratory failure 324, 325
  causes of 325b
Chronic stable phase 288, 289t
Chronic thromboembolic pulmonary hypertension 64
Churg–Strauss syndrome 218
Chvostek sign 177
Ciliary dyskinesia, primary 351
Ciprofloxacin 379, 381
Circadian rhythm sleep disorders 492
Circulation 22
Circulatory assist devices 45
Cirrhosis 122, 127, 129t, 131f, 139, 139t
  absence of 139
  alcoholic 127, 512
  cardiac 156
  causes of 149
  complications of 129b, 149
  drug-induced 128
  end stage of 128
  morphological classification of 127f, 127t
Cisplatin 571, 571b
Citalopram 436
Clarithromycin 380
Claude's syndrome 447
Clindamycin 388
Clonazepam 437, 486

Clostridium
  botulinum 379, 382
  difficile 92
  perfringens 382
Clotrimazole 521
Clotting orders 272
Clotting time 272
Clubbing 321
  causes of 321, 321b
  grade of 321, 321b
Cluster headache 439
  clinical features 439
  treatment 439
Coagulation disorders 267, 267t
Coagulopathy 16, 125, 282, 286
Cobalamin transport, abnormal 252
Coccidioides immitis 407
Coccidioidomycosis 405
Cockayne's syndrome 524
Cockcroft–Gault formula 226
Coeliac disease 87
Coffee worker's lung 346
Cognitive impairment, mild 435, 582
Cold haemolysin type 265
Colitis
  antibiotics-associated 92
  ischaemic 91
Collagen vascular disease 67
Collapsing pulse 37
Collar rash 471
Colloidal bismuth compounds 84
Colon, Crohn's disease of 97t
Colonic stasis 77
Coma 465
  causes of 465, 465b
  management of 16
  score 465
  severity of 465
Combination therapy 122
Common opportunistic infections, treatment of 411t
Community-acquired pneumonia 331, 331b, 332t, 333t
Comprehensive geriatric assessment 586
Compression 145, 308
Compressive myelopathy 457, 458t
Computed tomography 18, 179, 183, 334, 361
Condylomata lata 425
Confusion 1
Congenital heart disease 69
  classification of 69t
Congenital syphilis 425–427
  stigmata of 427b

Conjugation 158
  types of 611t
Conjunctiva 384
Conjunctival icterus 102
Conn's syndrome 178
Connective tissue disorder 208
Consciousness 136
Constipation 3, 77, 93
  causes 77
  investigations 78
  treatment 78
Contact dermatitis 513
Continuous ambulatory peritoneal dialysis 236
Continuous murmurs, causes of 40b
Continuous positive airway pressure 327, 329
Controlled mode ventilation 328
Conus medullaris lesion 458t
Conventional insulin therapy 193
Convulsions 380
Coombs' test 255, 290
Copper metabolism, normal 153
Cor pulmonale 347, 350
Coronary arteriography 55
Coronary artery
  bypass graft 25, 28, 56
  disease 171, 181, 626
Coronary sinus septal defect 69
Coronavirus
  disease 2019 392
  novel 331
Corticosteroids 48, 95, 210, 266, 276, 521
Corticotropin-releasing hormone 179
Corynebacterium diphtheriae 378
Costochondritis–Tietze syndrome 34
Cotrimoxazole 381
Cough 2, 389
Courvoisier's law 111
COVID-19 392
Coxiella burnettii 335
Coxiella endocarditis 385
Cradle cap 512
Cranial arteritis 217
C-reactive protein 48, 393
Creatine clearance 226
Crescentic glomerulonephritis 231
Creutzfeldt–Jakob disease 453
Crigler–Najjar syndrome 110
Crohn's disease 95, 97, 97t
Crusted scabies 518
Cryoglobulinaemia 298, 299, 462
Cryoprecipitate 280, 303

Cryptococcal meningitis 408, 415
Cryptococcosis 405
Cryptococcus neoformans 408
Cryptosporidium parvum 382
Crystalline penicillin 428
Curb 65 rule 334*b*
Cushing's disease 178
Cushing's syndrome 178, 179*fc*, 503
   causes of 178, 178*t*
   clinical features of 178, 178*t*
Cutaneous lupus erythematosus 214
Cyanide poisoning 564
Cyanosis 34
   central 35
   features 35*t*
   types of 35
Cyclophosphamide 311, 521, 568, 571*b*
Cycloserine 340
Cysticercosis 388
   clinical features 389
   diagnosis 389
   treatment 389
Cystinuria 477
Cytochemical staining 286
Cytology 139
Cytomegalovirus 405-407, 411, 415, 428, 456
   encephalitis 408
Cytoplasmic auer rods 286
Cytotoxic natural killer cells 531
Cytotoxic T-lymphocyte-associated protein 535, 571, 572

D

Dacarbazine 311
Dapsone 462, 521
Dark pigment 110
Dark stools 108
Darunavir 412, 413
D-dimer 66
   levels 66
   test 279
Deafness 524
Death, causes of 156
Deep tendon reflexes 459
Deep venous thrombosis 65, 392
   clinical features of 65
   treatment of 66
Dehydration 22*t*
   severe 21, 513
   severity of 79, 79*t*
Dejerine-Roussy syndrome 447, 448
Delavirdine 412

Delirium 1, 486, 487*t*, 488*t*, 583, 584, 584*t*
   causes of 487*b*
Delta hepatitis 113, 116
Delusions 481
Dementia 435, 487*t*, 488*t*, 582, 583, 584*t*
   causes of 435, 435*b*, 583, 583*b*
   clinical features 435
   frontotemporal 583
   modifiable causes of 583, 583*b*
Demyelination, causes of 456, 457*b*
Dendritic cells 400
Dengue 375, 376*f*
   fever 374, 376
      clinical features 375
   haemorrhagic fever 376
   severe 377
   shock syndrome 376
Deoxynucleotidyl transferase 286
Deoxyribonucleic acid 116, 117, 121
   double stranded 213, 232
Deoxythymidine monophosphate 570
Depression 483, 487, 581, 583, 584*t*
   management of 584
Depressive episode, major 484*b*
Dermal infiltrate 286
Dermal vasculitis 536
Dermatitis 511
   herpetiformis 513
Dermatomyositis 216, 216*t*
Dermatophytes 521
Devic's disease 460
Dexamethasone 393
Dextrose 559
   intravenous 196
Diabetes 190, 385
   cardiovascular complications of 196
   complications of 193, 195*t*
   insipidus 172, 181
      central 172
      types of 172
   mellitus 183, 187, 462, 512
      classification of 187, 187*t*
      diagnostic criteria of 190*t*
      general characteristics of 187, 187*t*
      gestational 199, 542
      permanent neonatal 188
      type 1 187, 189, 191*t*, 474
      type 2 187, 189, 189*f*, 191*t*, 194*fc*, 198*fc*, 474
      types of 188*fc*
   pharmacological treatment of 190

Diabetic ketoacidosis 193, 196, 197, 197*t*, 498
   management of 29, 30*fc*
Diabetic nephropathy 198
   stages of 198*f*
Diabetic neuropathy 198, 199
   classification of 199*b*
Diabetic retinopathy, features of 199*t*
Diagnostic spinal tap 314
Dialysis 13
   indication of 238*b*
Diarrhoea 2, 78, 93, 407, 415, 561
   causes of 407, 408*t*
   chronic 78
Dicrotic pulse 37
Didanosine 412
Dietary therapy 475
Dihydroergotamine 439
Dihydropyridine 28
Dilated cardiomyopathy 67
   causes of 67*b*
Dipeptidyl peptidase 4 194
Diphtheria 378, 462
   clinical features 378
   complications 378
   diagnosis 378
   management 378
   pertussis, tetanus 378
   tetanus 378
      acellular pertussis 378
Diplopia 6, 443
Direct lung injury 327
Discoid eczema 512
Discoid lupus erythematosus, typical 536
Disease-modifying antirheumatic drugs 210
Disseminated gonococcal infection 422, 536
Disseminated intravascular coagulation 278, 278*t*, 279*t*, 286, 551
   pathogenesis of 278, 278*f*
   signs of 279*t*
Diuretics 63
Dizziness 487
Dolutegravir 412
Donath-Landsteiner antibodies 265
Donepezil 583
Donovan bodies 424
Donovanosis 424
Doppler ultrasonography 66, 157
Down syndrome 596, 597*b*
Doxycycline 335, 424, 428
Drowning 554

Drugs 60, 126, 143, 172, 261, 281, 546
  interaction 612
  metabolism 611
    phases of 612f
  resistance 339
  therapy 348b
  treatment 55
Dry beriberi 471
Dry drowning 554
Dual-energy X-ray absorptiometry 176
Dubin–Johnson syndrome 110
Duchenne muscular dystrophy 464
Duct obstruction, large 108
Ductus arteriosus 69
Duloxetine 490
Duplex ultrasonography 66
Durie–Salmon staging 300t
Dysarthria 443, 503
  clumsy hand syndrome 450
Dysdiadochokinesia 454
Dyshidrotic eczema 512
Dyslipidaemias, management of 182t
Dysmetria 454
Dyspepsia 4, 85
  functional 85
Dysphagia 80, 435, 503, 560
  acquired 81t
Dyspnoea 389
  acute 364
  differential diagnosis of 363
Dyspraxia 436
Dystonia 453
Dysuria 4
Dysynergia 454

E

Early goal-directed therapy 392t
Eastern equine encephalitis 375
Eating disoders 492
Echinococcosis 389
  clinical features 389
  diagnosis 389
  treatment 389
Echinococcus granulosus 389
Echocardiography 12, 18, 48, 53, 55, 57, 65
Ectoparasites 422
Eculizumab 265
Eczema 511
  gravitational 512
Efalizumab 514
Efavirenz 412
Effusion, types of 358
Eisenmenger's syndrome 70
Ejection click 38

Ejection systolic murmurs 39
Elastography, hepatic 105
Electrocardiogram 40, 41, 42, 48, 57, 59, 65, 66, 505, 618
  leads, anatomic groups of 620t
Electrocardiography 55
Electroconvulsive therapy 489
Electroencephalogram 553
Electroencephalography 124
Electrolyte 237, 633
  alterations 171
  disturbance 581
  imbalance 453
Electrophoretic studies 300
Elevated immunoglobulin, types of 104t
Elevated mood, stages of 485t
Elevated serum aminotransferases, causes of 103
Emergency surgery 134
  indications of 95
Emesis 561
Emibetuzumab 571
Emollient laxatives 78
Emotional abuse 586
Emphysema 345, 349t
Empiric regimens 334
Empyema 350
  thoracis 358
    aetiology 358
    clinical features 360
    management of 360
Emtricitabine 412
Encephalitis 380, 409, 436, 453
Encephalopathy 124, 125
  acute hepatic 136
  chronic hepatic 136
  hypertensive 61
  treatment measures for 137b
Endemic typhus 385
Endocardial involvement, evidence of 53
Endocarditis 48
  clinical features of subacute 52
  post-operative 52
  right-sided 52
  subacute 52
Endocrine diseases 77
Endocrinology 171
Endocrinopathy 298
Endoscopic variceal band ligation 135
Endoscopy 130
Entamoeba histolytica 151, 422
Entecavir 122
Enteric fever 380
Enteric gram-negative bacilli 336
Enteropathy 188
  gluten-induced 87

Enteroviruses 456
Enzyme 103, 569
  immunoassay 427
  linked immunosorbent assay 302, 398
Eosinophilia 309
  pulmonary infiltrates with 336
Epidemic typhus 385
Epidemiologic study designs, types of 604, 604b
Epidemiology 602b
  types of 602
Epidermal growth factor receptor 571, 572
Epidermophyton 521
Epigenetics 591
Epilepsy 440, 545
  aetiology 440
  classification of 440, 440t
  clinical features 440
  diagnosis of 441
  treatment of 442f
  types of 442
Epitope 530
Epsilon wave 627
Epstein–Barr virus 307, 311, 373, 428, 456, 575
Ergotamine 439
Erythema
  gyratum repens 576
  marginatum 47
  multiforme 516, 516b
  nodosum 337, 514, 515b
Erythrocyte sedimentation rate 48, 115, 256, 279, 310
Erythrocytosis 292, 293
Erythromycin 380, 424
Erythropoietin levels 293
Escherichia coli 142, 276, 382, 408
Escitalopram 436
Esmolol 21
Ester hydrolysis 612
Esterase, non-specific 286
Estimated glomerular filtration rate 183
Ethambutol 340
Ethanol 559
Ethionamide 340
Ethylene glycol poisoning 498
Etoposide 311
Etravirine 413
Eukaryotic translation initiation factor 188
European Atherosclerosis Society guidelines 182t
European League Against Rheumatism 210
European Society of Cardiology 182t

Excessive fibrinolysis, causes of 274*b*
Expanded dengue syndrome 374
Expiratory reserve volume 323
Extracorpuscular defects 108
Extra-dural myelopathy 458
Extrahepatic biliary obstruction 128
Extralymphatic organs, involvement of 308
Extramedullary haematopoiesis 295
 treatment of 296
Extramedullary leukaemic infiltration 282
Extrathoracic metastasis, manifestations of 353*t*
Eye 357, 405
 involvement 286
  features of 153
 opening score 465
 signs 470
Eyebrows 512

F

Fabry's disease 524
Facial nerve palsy
 causes of 465, 465*t*
 differential diagnosis 465
Faecal impaction 581
Faecal-oral route 111
Falciparum malaria 386
 complications of 386
 neurological complications of 386
Falls 2, 474, 585
Famciclovir 437
Farmer's lung 346
Fat 86
Fatigue 401
Fatty liver 126, 143, 545
 alcoholic 158
 causes of 126*b*
Fava beans 261
Favipiravir 393
Febrile neutropaenia 572, 573*fc*
Felty's syndrome 209
Ferritin 393
Fever 2, 53, 401
Fibreoptic endoscopy 133
Fibrinogen concentration 276
Fibrosis 118
 hepatic 105, 143
Fine-needle aspiration cytology 302
First heart sound 38, 38*b*
Fits 2
Fitz-Hugh-Curtis syndrome 422
Flow cytometry 265
Flow volume curves 323
Fluconazole 521

Fluid
 analysis 358
 and electrolyte balance, maintenance of 283
 electrolytes and acid-base disorders 498
 replacement 22*t*
 therapy 377
Flu-like symptoms 282
Flunarizine 439
Fluorescent treponemal antibody absorption 427
Fluphenazine 453
Folate deficiency 254
Folic acid 252*t*
 deficiency 252, 253
 supplementation 259
Follicular lymphomas 312
Food borne botulism 379
Food poisoning 79, 381
 causes of 381*t*
 clinical features 381
 diagnosis 381
 management 381
Forced expiratory
 flow 324
 time 322
 volume 324, 343, 348, 474
Forced vital capacity 324, 343, 348
Formiminoglutamate 253
Fosamprenavir 412, 413
Fourth heart sound 38, 39*b*
Fragmentation syndromes 254
Frailty syndrome 584
Free fatty acid 197
Free thyroxine 173, 175
Free triiodothronine 173, 175
Fresh frozen plasma 24, 303
Froin's syndrome 437
Frozen red blood cells 304
Fulminant hepatic failure
 causes of 123*t*
 complications of 124*b*
Functional residual capacity 323
Fundoscopy 409
Fungal
 agents 422
 infections 405, 513
Furosemide 520

G

Gabapentin 437, 439
Gait ataxia 454
Galantamine 583
Gall stones 156
Gallium nitrate 13
Gamma-glutamyl transpeptidase 103, 144

Gas exchange, disorders of 506
Gastric
 hypersecretion 82
 lymphoma 311
 varices 130
Gastroenteritis 78
Gastroesophageal reflux disease 80, 489
Gastrointestinal disease 407
Gastrointestinal system 237
 diseases of 77
Gastrointestinal tract 302
Gene therapy 259, 597
Generalised lymphadenopathy 302
 causes of 302*t*
 diagnostic features of 302*t*
Genetic
 disorders 282
 imprinting 596
 testing 152
Genital discharge 4
Genital lesion, primary 424
Genital ulcer 427
 disease 427, 428
Genitalia, external 423, 424
Genitourinary system 409
Gentamicin 379
Geriatric medicine 581
German measles 372
Gestational diabetes mellitus 199, 542
 diagnosis of 199*t*
Ghon's complex 337
Ghon's lesion 337
Giant-cell arteritis 217
Giardia lamblia 90, 382, 422
Giardiasis 90
Gilbert's syndrome 110
Gingival hypertrophy 286
Ginkgo biloba 583
Glandular fever 373
Glasgow coma
 scale 9
 score 465
Glioblastoma multiforme 198
Globin synthesis 254
Glomerular basement membrane 217, 230-232
Glomerular disease
 primary 229
 spectrum of 229, 230*fc*
Glomerular filtration rate 198, 234, 235, 235*f*
Glomerulonephritis 53, 230, 536
 acute 232*fc*
 causes of 229, 229*b*
 rapidly progressive 231
Glomerulosclerosis, focal segmental 230

Glucagon 196
Glucagon-like peptide 1 192
　receptor agonist 194
Glucocorticoid 214
　deficiency 180
Glucokinase 188
Glucose
　6-phosphate dehydrogenase
　　deficiency 261, 263f
　tolerance, impaired 190
　transporter-2 194
Glucuronic acid 158
Glutamic acid decarboxylase
　antibodies 188
Glyceryl trinitrate 28
Glycine encephalopathy 477
Glycoprotein 59, 569
Gonadotropin-releasing hormone,
　deficiencies of 171
Gonorrhoea 422
　clinical features 422
　complications 422
　diagnosis 422
　treatment of 423, 423b
Gout 219
　aetiology of 219, 219b
Graft-versus-host disease 306
Gram stain 138, 422
Granulocyte 293
　concentrates 303
Granuloma 143
　hepatic 156
　inguinale 424, 424b
　　clinical features 424
　　diagnosis 424
　　treatment 424
Granulomatous interstitial
　inflammation 355
Ground itch dermatitis 390
Growth
　and development, retardation
　　of 260
　hormone-releasing hormone 171
Guillain–Barré syndrome 373, 436,
　437, 462, 501
Gummatous syphilis 426

H

H1N1 influenza 330, 330b
Haemarthroses 273
Haematemesis 2, 79
　aetiology of 80t
　management strategies of 80t
Haematocrit 252
　packed-cell volume 248
Haematologic system 237

Haematological disorders 254,
　364
Haematological tests 129
Haematology 248
Haematopoietic neoplasms,
　primary 248
Haematopoietic stem-cell
　transplantation
　complications of 304, 305, 306t
　indications for 305t
Haematuria 4, 53, 226
Haemochromatosis, hereditary 151
Haemodialysis 235
Haemoglobin 248, 252, 256, 282,
　288, 290, 293
　electrophoresis 256
　hlycosylated 190
　level 277, 296
　maintenance of 261
　quantitative defect in 256
　synthesis, defective 248
Haemoglobinopathies 254, 256,
　256b
　acquired 256
Haemolysis 108, 153
　causes of 255
　elevated liver enzymes, low
　　platelet count 123
　evidences of 256
　extravascular 255, 255t
　intravascular 255t, 261, 264
Haemolytic anaemias 249
　classification of 254t
　clinical features of 255t
　diagnosis of 255
　treatment of 256
Haemolytic disease 254
Haemolytic state, demonstration
　of 259
Haemolytic-uraemic syndrome
　274, 276
　aetiology of 277f
　pathogenesis of 277f
Haemophilia 272t, 273, 304
　A 272
　B 273
　clinical features of 273t
Haemophilus
　ducreyi 422, 423
　influenzae 259, 332
Haemoptysis 5, 350, 363
　causes of 363, 364t
　management of 20
Haemorrhage 278
　conjunctival 380
Haemorrhagic symptoms,
　management of 280

Haemorrhagic tendency 128
Haemosiderosis 260
Hair-on-end appearance 260
Hairy cell leukaemia 285
Hallucinations 481
　hypnagogic 491
Ham's acidified serum test 265
Hansen's disease 382
Hapten 530
Hartnup disease 477
Hashimoto's thyroiditis 174, 517
Head louse 519
Headache 2, 171, 386, 438
　classification of 439t
　primary 439
　red flags of 440b
　secondary 439
Heart 34, 357, 405
　block
　　complete 628
　　first-degree 43, 627
　　conduction system of 617, 617f
　disease, ischaemic 54, 633t
　failure 46, 258
　　acute 46
　　causes of 46, 46b
　　chronic 46
　　clinical manifestations of 46
　　congestive 192
　　diastolic 46
　　management of 47
　　signs of 47b
　　systolic 46
　　types of 46
　lung transplantation 70
　rate 18
　　calculation of 620
　　determining 620
Heat
　cramps 551
　exhaustion 551
　oedema 551
　stroke 552
　　classic 552
　　exertional 552
Heavy chain diseases 298
Heinz bodies 263f
Helicobacter pylori 82, 311
　infection
　　first-line treatment of 84t
　　natural history of 83f
　　persistent 84t
　　tests for 83t
Hemianopia 443
Hemiballismus 453
Hemimedullary syndrome 448
Hemiplegia 446f

Henoch–Schönlein purpura 212, 232
Heparin 280
Hepatic artery angiography 148
Hepatic complications 117, 150, 306
Hepatic encephalopathy 123, 134, 135*b*
  types of 136, 136*t*
Hepatic failure
  hyperacute 123
  subacute 123
Hepatic venous outflow tract obstruction 145
Hepatitis 111, 143, 144
  A 111, 116, 382
    virus 115, 116, 123
  alcoholic 159
  autoimmune 128
  B 112, 116, 123
    chronic 119
    core antigen 112, 116, 117
    surface antigen 116, 117
    treatment, chronic 121*fc*
    virus 115-117, 121, 123, 575
  B E antigen 112, 117
    antibodies against 116, 117
  C 113, 116
    chronic 122
    new drugs for 123*b*
  C virus 115-117, 118*t*, 123, 311, 416, 575
    infection, extrahepatic manifestations of 118*t*
    antibodies against 116
  cholestatic 144
  chronic
    hepatic 114, 117*f*, 120, 143, 144
    viral 128
  D 113, 116
    chronic 123
  D virus 115-117
    antibodies against 116
  E 113, 116
    antigen 117
    virus 115, 116
  granulomatous 144
  interface 118
  progressive 118
  stage of chronic 118
  type of 111
Hepatobiliary disorders 102
Hepatocellular carcinoma 147, 149
  risk factors for 147*b*
Hepatocyte
  growth factor receptor 572
  infection of 111
  nuclear factor 188

Hepatolenticular degeneration 153
Hepatopulmonary syndrome 149
Hepatorenal syndrome 137
  types of 138*b*
Hepatosplenomegaly 3, 108, 286
Hepatotoxic drugs 143*b*
Hepatotoxicity, dose-dependent 144
Hepatotropic viruses 115*t*
Hepcidin 250
Herpes simplex
  encephalitis 408
  virus 405, 407
Herpes zoster 408
Hess test 268, 274
High blood pressure, classification of 60*fc*
High serum ascites albumin gradient 141
High-resolution computed tomography 65
Histamine-2 receptor antagonists 83
Histocompatibility complex, major 534
Histoplasmosis 405, 407
Hoarseness 5
Hodgkin lymphoma 287, 307, 307*t*, 311*t*, 314
  characteristics of 314, 314*t*
  classification of 307, 308*f*
  staging of 309*t*, 310, 311
  treatment of 310*t*
Homocystinuria 477
Horizontal transmission 112
Hormones 569
Host cell
  chromosome of 398
  cytoplasm of 400
  membrane, penetration of 400
Human genome project 591
Human herpes virus 306, 311, 575
Human immunodeficiency virus 65, 233, 235, 304, 310, 331, 334, 339, 346, 355, 399, 399*f*, 400*f*, 402, 405, 406*f*, 408*t*, 423, 440, 441, 444, 536, 545, 547
  associated dementia 408
  classification 401
  clinical staging 401
  disease progression 403*f*
  genome 399
  infection 339, 371, 398, 462
    classification of 402*b*
    diagnosis of 398, 410
    management of 410
    natural history of 401
    of cells 399
    primary 402, 404

  life cycle 411*f*
  progression 404
  specific t-cell responses 404*f*
Human leucocyte antigen 306, 537
Human T-lymphotropic virus 311
Huntington's disease 450
Hutchinson's incisors 427
Hydralazine 21
Hydrocortisone 14, 15
Hydroxycarbamide 259, 289, 294
Hydroxychloroquine 214, 393
Hydroxytryptamine 490
Hydroxyurea 259, 289, 294
Hyperaldosteronism
  primary 178
  secondary 179
Hyperbilirubinaemia 110, 156
  congenital non-haemolytic 110
  fluctuating 102
  types of 102*t*
  unconjugated 108, 110
Hypercalcaemia 176, 300, 357, 633
  causes of 176, 176*b*
  management of severe 12
Hypercarbia 438
Hypercholesterolaemia 155
  familial 183
Hyperdynamic apex 36
Hyperglycaemic hyperosmolar state 196, 197, 197*t*
  management of 196, 196*b*
Hyperkalaemia 241, 504, 633
  management of severe 9
  treatment of 505*t*
Hyperkinetic pulse 36
  features of 36*b*
Hyperleucocytosis, treatment of 283
Hyperlipidaemia, causes of secondary 181*t*
Hypermagnesaemia 633
Hypermetabolic state 295
  symptoms of 288
Hypernatraemia 502, 502*t*
Hyperparathyroidism 175, 238, 473
  causes of 175, 175*t*
  classification of 175, 175*t*
Hyperphosphataemia 241
Hyperplasia 293
Hyperpyrexia 438
Hypersensitivity reactions 534*t*
  characteristic features of 534
Hypertension 9, 60, 63*f*, 241
  causes of 60, 60*b*
  classification 60*b*
  complications of 61
  control of 238
  essential 60
  gestational 542

in pregnancy 542
malignant 61
per se 60
primary 60
secondary 60, 62t
Hypertensive emergency 21, 62
Hyperthermia, malignant 552
Hyperthyroid crisis 174
Hyperthyroidism 172, 581
diagnosis in 173fc
primary 172
secondary 172
Hypertrophy 630
Hyperuricaemia 219, 293, 368
aetiology of 219, 219b
Hyperventilation 19
Hyperviscosity syndrome 299
Hypnozoites 386
Hypoalbuminaemia 139
Hypocalcaemia 177, 241, 633
Hypoglycaemia 11, 125, 196
Hypokalaemia 167, 503, 633
Hypokinesia 452
Hypokinetic apex 37
Hypokinetic pulse 36
features of 36b
Hypomagnesaemia 177, 633
Hypomelanosis of Ito 524
Hyponatraemia 195, 499, 500t, 551
causes of 499, 499t, 500fc
management of 503t
treatment of severe 501fc
Hypoparathyroidism 177
Hypopituarism 171
Hypoproteinaemia 350
Hypotension 125, 533, 560
Hypothermia 553
clinical symptoms of 553, 553t
mild 553
moderate 553
primary 553
secondary 553
severe 553
Hypothyroidism 174, 175fc
Hypotonia 454
Hypovolaemia 499
management of 17
Hypoxaemia 554
acute 324
chronic 324
correction of 328
Hypoxia 64, 438

I

Ibuprofen 520
Ichthyoses 513
Idiopathic pulmonary fibrosis 356

Idiopathic thrombocytopenic
purpura 271
chronic 270t
treatment of 271b
Idiosyncratic drug reactions 143
Imatinib mesylate 289
Imidazoles 521
Immune
disorders 311
acquired 311
chronic 266
dysfunction 385
dysregulation 188
reactions, types of 532, 532t
reconstitution inflammatory
syndrome 416
response 529
status 307
system 299, 530
thrombocytopenic purpura 269
characterisation of 269f
types of 270t
Immunisation, passive 112
Immunity 529
cell mediated 530
genetic 529
humoral 530
innate 529
Immunodeficiency disorders,
primary 535, 538b
Immunoglobulin 117, 290, 300,
304, 535
A 230, 231
nephropathy Berger's disease
231
classes 532t
determination 314
G 271
intravenous 266
Immunologic phenomena 53
Immunomodulatory monoclonal
antibodies, specific 271
Immunophenotype 290
Immunosuppressive
agents 95
therapy 266
Immunotherapy 302
Immunotoxins 572
Implantable cardioverter-
defibrillator 23, 43
Impulse
conduction, disturbances of 40
formation, disturbances of 40
Incontinence, categories of 585
Incontinentia pigmenti 524
Incubation period 111-114
Indian tick typhus 385
Indinavir 412, 413

Induction therapy, goal of 284
Industrial toxins 462
Infantile botulism 379
Infarction, evidence of 632
Infections 125, 261, 287
acute 159, 404
bacterial 405
chronic 159, 266
helminthic 405
intestinal 529
minor opportunistic 403
route of 142, 150
source of 111
Infectious diseases 229, 371
Infectious mononucleosis 373
aetiology 373
clinical features 373
complications 373
investigations 373
treatment 373
Infectious virus 401
Infective endocarditis 52, 52b, 53,
54t, 371
diagnosis of 54
predisposition to 53
types of 52
Inferior sinus venosus type defect
69
Inflammation 160
Inflammatory bowel disease 93
complications of 96, 97b
Inflammatory cells, spillover of 118
Influenza 329, 335, 405, 529
complications 329
management 330
pneumonia, primary 329
Injection sclerotherapy 133
Inotropic agents 45
Insect bites 513
Insomnia 487, 491
causes of 491b
Inspiratory reserve volume 323
Insulin 188, 195, 544
infusion, continuous
subcutaneous 193
preparations 192, 193t
regimens 192, 193b
therapy, general indications for
190
Integumentary system 237
Intensive care unit 334
Intention tremor 454
Intercostal space 13
Intermediate syndrome 561
International Staging System 300t
Interstitial lung disease 354, 489
causes of 355t
Intestinal mucosal cell 87

Intestine 93
  ulcers in 93b
Intoxication 382
Intra-aortic balloon pump 18
Intracorpuscular defects 108
Intracranial pressure, raised 438, 438b
Intra-dural extra-medullary myelopathy 458
Intra-dural intra-medullary myelopathy 458
Intraluminal digestion, disorders of 87
Intravascular volume 241
Intrinsic renal disorders 240
Invade portal vein 148
Invasive aspergillosis 407
Invasive ventilation 328
Inverted saucer' appearance 383
Ionising radiation 281
Ipilimumab 571
Iris lesion 517
Iron overload 151, 259, 261
  classification of 151, 151b
Iron-deficiency anaemia 249, 250, 251t, 264
  causes of 249, 250, 250t
Irritable bowel syndrome 77, 92
  treatment of 93t
Irritant contact eczema 511
Ischaemic lesions 462
Ischaemic strokes 18
  types of 442
Islet cell antigen 188
Isochromosomes 593
Isomorphic phenomenon 514
Isoniazid 340, 547
Isonicotinic acid hydrazide 339
Isospora belli 411
Itraconazole 521

J

Jacksonian seizures 441
Janus kinase 2 mutations 294
Japanese encephalitis 375, 377
  clinical features 378
  diagnosis 378
  treatment 378
Jaundice 2, 107, 111, 259, 415
  cholestatic 108
  classification of 107t, 108f
  haemolytic 107, 108
  hepatocellular 103, 108
  latent 107
  mild 108
  obstructive 108
  types of 109t
Joint swelling 5

Jones criteria, revised 48, 48b
Jugular veins 62
Jugular venous
  pressure 36
    causes of raised 36, 37b
  pulse 36
Juvenile myoclonic epilepsy 441

K

Kala-azar 387
  aetiology 387
  clinical features 388
  investigations 388
  treatment 388
Kallmann syndrome 171
Kaposi's sarcoma 311, 405
Katayama fever 391
Kayser–Fleischer ring 153
Kerion 521
Kernig's sign 455, 456
Ketoconazole 521
Kidney 53, 226, 357, 405
  disease 234, 408
  end-stage 238
  transplantation 235
Klebsiella granulomatis 424
Klinefelter syndrome 592, 597
Klippel–Trenaunay–Weber syndrome 524
Knob-like spikes 399
Koilonychia 249
Korsakoff's psychosis 471
Kussmaul's breathing 504
Kussmaul's sign 36

L

Labetalol 21
Lacrimation 561
Lactate dehydrogenase 140, 255, 277, 361
Lactic acidosis 498
Lactic dehydrogenase 104
Lactose intolerance 89
Lacunar infarction 449
Lacunar stroke
  signs of 450t
  symptoms of 450t
Laennec's cirrhosis 127
Lamivudine 122, 412
Lange-Nielsen syndrome 629
Language, defective 433
Lap score 296
Laryngeal injury 329
Late latent syphilis 426
Latent tuberculosis 417
  infection 339
  screening for 339

Lead intoxication 438
Lead poisoning 462
Left atrium to right atrium connection 40
Left bundle branch block 626, 630
Left ventricular failure 47
Left ventricular hypertrophy 630
  causes of 630
  criteria of 630
  types of 631, 631t
Legionella pneumophila 332, 335
Legs
  elephantiasis of 390
  lymphoedema of 390
Leigh syndrome 471
Leishmania donovani 387
Lentiginosis 524
Lentivirus family 398
Leonine facies 383
Lepromatous leprosy 383
  nasal symptoms 383
  skin involvement 383
Lepromin test 384
Leprosy 382, 462
  clinical features 383
  clinicopathological classification of 383, 383f
  diagnosis of 384
  treatment 384
Leptospira interrogans 384
Leptospirosis 384
  aetiology 384
  clinical features 384
  severe 384
Lesion
  in external genitalia 423
  location of 450t
Lethargy 401, 561
Leucocyte alkaline phosphatase 294
  score 289
Leucocytosis 296
  eosinophilic 389
Leucostasis 282
Leukaemia 280, 282
  aetiology of 281
  chronic 287
  traditional classification of 280t
Leukaemic blasts 286
Leukaemic meningitis 286
Levels of evidence 606t
Levothyroxine 14
Lewy bodies 583
  disease, diffuse 450
Lichen planus 513, 514
Lichen simplex chronicus 513
Lidocaine 41
Limb
  pain 2
  swelling 2

Linear naevus sebaceous syndrome 524
Lipid storage diseases 453
Lipoprotein
 cholesterol, low-density 183
 high-density 181, 188
Listeria 454
 monocytogenes 382
Liver 143, 357, 405
 abscess 371
 aspiration 148
 based metabolic conditions 149
 biochemistry 102
 biopsy 105, 110, 130, 146, 152, 153, 156, 157, 159, 309
  complications of 106*b*
  contraindications of 106*b*
  indications of 106*b*
 biosynthetic function of 104
 cancer, pathogenesis of 112
 direct invasion of 150
 disease
  alcoholic 158, 158*t*
  chronic 453
  chronic parenchymal 114
  drug-induced 144*t*
 failure, fulminant 149
 function
  biochemical tests for 152
  tests 105*t*
 involvement 153, 155
 miscellaneous 157
 transplantation 137, 148, 154
  complications of 150*b*
  contraindications of 150*b*
  indications of 149*b*
Lobes, functions of 433
Local ablation strategies 148
Local injection therapy 148
Locus heterogeneity 596
Loeffler's syndrome 336
Loop diuretics 63, 142
Lopinavir 331, 393, 412, 413
Lorazepam 486
Louis–Bar syndrome 524
Low serum ascites albumin gradient 141
Low-density lipoprotein 181
 goals, modify 181*t*
Lower gastrointestinal bleeding, causes of 92, 92*b*
Lower limb conditions 65
Lower motor neuron 448, 458, 459, 465
 lesion 433, 433*t*
Low-molecular-weight heparin 59
Lugol's iodine 14

Lumbar puncture 436
 contraindications 436
 indications 436
 indications of 436*b*
Lung 53
 abscess 350, 351, 358
  causes of 351*b*
 and pleura 34
 cancer 351, 353*t*
  clinical subgroups of 352*t*
  manifestations of 352*t*
 capacity of 323
 carcinoma of 354
 classification of tumours of 351*t*
 diffusing capacity of 323
 disease 64, 356*t*
  chronic obstructive 344, 348*f*
  diffuse parenchymal 354, 355*t*
 injury 306
  acute 327
  indirect 327
 parenchymal disease of 364
 perfusion scanning of 66
 secondary tuberculosis of 338*f*
 staging of carcinoma of 354*t*
 vascular diseases of 364
 volume measurements 323*f*
Lupus erythematosus 213
Lupus nephritis, classification of 212*b*
Lymph node 290, 357
 biopsy 309
Lymph, percolation of 139
Lymphadenopathy 5, 286, 401, 423
 generalised painless 426
 painless generalised 290
 persistent generalised 403
Lymphangioleiomyomatosis 363
Lymphatic filariasis 390
 clinical features 390
 investigations 390
 treatment 390
Lymphatic obstruction 139
Lymphocyte 409
Lymphocytic hypophysitis 171
Lymphocytosis 290
Lymphogranuloma venereum 424, 424*b*, 428, 429
 clinical features 424
 diagnosis 424
 treatment 424
Lymphoid neoplasm 312, 312*t*
Lymphoid tissue 403
Lymphoma 307
 malignant 307
Lymphopaenia 309
Lymphoplasmacytic lymphoma 311

M

Macronodular cirrhosis 127
Macrophages 400
Magnesium 41, 195
Magnetic resonance
 cholangiopancreatography 106
 elastography 105
 imaging 461
Malabsorption 155
Malabsorption syndrome 86
 aetiology of 87*t*
 classification of 87*t*
Malaria 249, 371, 386
 clinical features 386
 complicated 387*t*
 investigations 387
 management 387
  of uncomplicated 387
Malariae malaria 386
Malarial paroxysm, classic 386
Malassezia 512
 furfur 521
Malignant skin tumours, list of 522*b*
Mallorca acne 515
Malt worker's lung 346
Malta fever 392
Mania 484
Manic episode, diagnostic criteria for 485*b*
Mannose-binding lectin 536
Maple syrup urine disease 476
Marfan's syndrome 363
Marie–Foix syndrome 447
Marie–Strumpell disease 211
Marrow
 cytogenic study of 298
 infiltration 248
 replacement 248
Mask-like face 452
Massive splenomegaly 160, 287, 288
Massive transfusion 304
Maternal medicine 542
Maturity onset diabetes of young 188, 189
Mean arterial pressure 392
Mean corpuscular haemoglobin 250
 concentration 250
Mean corpuscular volume 250, 253
Measles 372
 clinical features 372
 complications 372
 treatment 372

Mechanical ventilation 328
  complications of 329
  indications of 328b
Medial medullary syndrome 448
Mediastinal masses 363
Mediastinum, localised disease
  of 307
Medical genetics 591
Medical nutrition therapy 190,
  190f, 192
Mediterranean fever 392
Megacolon 392
Megaloblastic anaemia 251, 252t
  diagnosis of 252t
  laboratory findings of 252t
Megaoesophagus 392
Melaena 2
Melanoma, malignant 523
Melphalan 289
Memantine 583
Membrane fusion 400
Membrane on tonsils 378
Membranoproliferative
  glomerulonephritis 230, 232
Membranous glomerulonephritis
  233, 234
Memory
  impairment of 435
  loss, progressive 5
Meningeal irritation, signs of 455
Meninges 405
Meningitis 409, 436, 536
  acute 408
    bacterial 454
  bacterial 455, 455t
Meningoencephalitis 373
Meningovascular disease, chronic
  426
Mental status 558
Merkel cell polyomavirus 575
Mesenchymal epithelial transition
  factor 572
Mesenchymal tumours 351
Mesobuthus 560
Metabolic abnormalities 282
Metabolic acidosis 10, 498, 504,
  505
  causes of 504, 505t
  management of 10fc
Metabolic causes 487
Metabolic defects 475
Metabolic diseases 77
Metabolic disturbances 237, 453
Metabolic encephalopathies 465
Metabolic liver disease, inherited
  128
Metabolic problems 573
Metabolic syndrome 200, 200b,
  476

Metalloproteinase 275
Metastatic neoplasms 248
Methaemogloinaemia 265
  causes of 265b
Methanol poisoning 498, 562
Methotrexate 143, 521, 571, 571b
Methyl prednisolone 393
Methylene blue 559
Methylenedioxyamphetamine 28
Methylmalonic acid 253
Methylprednisolone 331
Metoclopramide 439, 450
Metronidazole 151
Mianserine 490
Miconazole 521
Microalbuminuria 226
Microangiopathic haemolytic states
  274
Microcytic hypochromic anaemia
  250, 260
  differential diagnosis for 251t
Micronodular cirrhosis 127t
Microscopic polyangiitis 218
Microsporum 521
Microvascular angina 55
Microvascular thrombi 279
Migraine 438
  classical 438
  classification 438
  clinical features 438
  hemiplegic 438
  precipitating factors 438
  treatment of 439, 439b
Millard–Gubler syndrome 447
Miller's lung 346
Miller–Fisher syndrome 462
Mineralocorticoid deficiency 180
Minerals and electrolytes 87
Minimal change disease 233, 234
Mirtazapine 490
Mitochondrial inheritance 596
Mitral regurgitation 39, 49
  acute 50
  aetiology of 50b
  chronic 50
Mitral stenosis 49
  aetiology of 49, 49b
  complications of 49, 49b
  management of 49
Mitral valve prolapse 34, 39, 50
Mixed cirrhosis 127
Mixoploidy 593
Modafinil 491
Modern geriatric giants 582, 582f
Molecular genetics 272
Molecular medicine 591
Molluscum contagiosum 407
Monge's disease 556
Mongolism 596

Moniliasis 385
Monoamine oxidase 490
  inhibitor 483, 501, 559
Monoamine-depleting drug 453
Monoarthritis
  acute 209
  chronic 209
Monoclonal antibody 571, 571t
  conjugate of 572
Monoclonal gammopathies,
  malignant 298
Monoclonal protein 298, 301
Monocytes 400
Mononeuritis multiplex 462
Mononeuropathy 462
Monospot test 373
Mood disorder 473, 483
  classification of 484t
  spectrum of 484f
Moraxella catarrhalis 332
Morning stiffness 209
Mosaicism 593
Motor neuron disease 459
  classification 459
  treatment 460
Mountain sickness
  acute 554
  chronic 556
Mouth ulcers 6
Movement disorders 449, 451fc
Mucocutaneous diseases 407
Mucocutaneous lesions 425
Mucopurulent relapses 347
Mucosa-associated lymphoid tissue
  83
Mucosal cell 87
Mucosal lesions 425
Mucosal lymphoid tissue 400
Mucosal resistance 82
Mucous membranes 107, 112, 267,
  384, 385
Multibacillary leprosy 384
  treatment of 384
Multi-drug resistance protein 2,
  complete absence of 110
Multifocal leucoencephalopathy,
  progressive 405, 406, 408
Multilineage dysplasia 297
Multimorbidity 586
Multiorgan dysfunction syndrome
  279
Multiple myeloma 298, 299
  clinical features of 299t
  diagnosis of 299
Multiple sclerosis 460, 461, 501
  classification 460
  clinical features 460
  investigations 460
  treatment 460

Multiple subcutaneous injections 193
Multisystem diseases 229
Mumps 373, 529
  clinical features 373
  complications 373
Murine typhus 385
Murmurs 39
  diastolic 39b
  early
    diastolic 39
    systolic 39
  late systolic 39
  mid-diastolic 39
  systolic 39b
Muscarinic manifestations 561
Muscular dystrophies 464
Musculoskeletal system 237
  disorders of 506
Mushroom
  poisoning 564
  worker's lung 346
Mutations 110
Myalgias 401
Myasthenia gravis 463
Mycobacteria 336
  tuberculosis 403
Mycobacteriosis 405
Mycobacterium avium 407
  complex 406
  intracellulare complex 337
Mycobacterium leprae 336, 382
Mycobacterium tuberculosis 335, 339
  complex 336
Mycobacterium, atypical 337t
Mycophenolate mofetil 214, 521
Mycoplasma 335, 456, 515
  genitalium 423
  hominis 422
  pneumonia 332, 335
Mycosis fungoides 523
Myelodysplasia 264
Myelodysplastic syndrome 248, 264, 282, 296, 297, 297t
Myelofibrosis, primary 295
Myeloid neoplasms, classification of 292
Myeloma cells 300
Myeloperoxidase 286
Myelophthisic anaemia 248
Myeloproliferative diseases 291
Myeloproliferative neoplasm 287, 292t
  acquired 293
Myocardial infarction 12, 34, 581, 625, 632
  type of 633t
Myocarditis 48, 626

Myoclonic epilepsy 453
Myoclonus 453
Myopathic diseases 77
Myopathies, hereditary 464
Myositis, inclusion-body 216, 216t
Myotonic dystrophy 464
Myxoedema 462
  coma 13, 174
Myxoviruses, group of 329

N

N-acetylation 612
N-acetylcysteine 563
Nail 53
Nail polish 511
Naloxone 559
Narcolepsy 491
Nasal saline 18
Nasopharynx 384
Naturally acquired immunity 529
  active 529
  passive 529
Near-drowning 554
Necator americanus 390
Neck
  pain 5
  rigidity 455
  stiffness 455
Necrolytic migratory erythema 576
Needle aspiration 150
Neisseria gonorrhoeae 422
Nelfinavir 412, 413
Nelson's syndrome 178
Neonatal jaundice 261
  management of 263
Neoplasms, malignant 302
Nephritic syndrome 229, 232fc
Nephrology 226
Nephrotic syndrome 233, 308, 576
  causes of 233, 233t
Nerve involvement 383
Nervous dyspepsia 85
Nervous system 357
  diseases of 433
Neurocognitive disorder, major 583
Neurocutaneous melanosis 524
Neurocutaneous syndromes 523, 524b
Neurocysticercosis 389
Neurofibromatosis 524
  diagnostic criteria for 524b
Neurogenic
  shock 45
  syncope 35
Neuroichthyosis 524
Neuroleptic malignant syndrome 552
Neurologic system 237

Neurological disease 77
Neurological disorders, primary 465
Neurological manifestations 209, 299
Neurological symptoms 401
Neuromyelitis optica 460, 461t
  treatment 461
Neuropathy, focal 462
Neuropsychiatric symptoms 452
Neurosis 481t
Neurosyphilis 426
  asymptomatic 426
Neurotoxic snake bite 16, 17fc
Neutralisation 531
Neutropaenia 282
Neutrophil 531
  alkaline phosphatase 289
Nevirapine 413
Newer drugs 122
Nicardipine 21
Nicotine 547
  dependence 487
  withdrawal 487
Nightmare
  disorder 492
  flashbacks 486
Nikolsky's sign 520
Nitrates 135
Nitric oxide, inhaled 259
Nitroglycerin 12, 21
Nivolumab 571
Nocardiosis 405
Nocturnal angina 55
Non-alcoholic
  fatty liver disease 126, 128
  steatohepatitis 126
  steatosis 126
Non-cardiogenic pulmonary oedema 554
Non-cirrhotic portal fibrosis 157
Nondihydropyridine 28
Non-ejection click 39
Non-gonococcal urethritis 423
  causes of 423b
  treatment 423
Non-hepatic complications 150
Non-Hodgkin lymphoma 287, 310, 314
  characteristics of 314, 314t
  development of 311t
  grading of 312t
  high-grade 313t
  low-grade 313t
Noninflammatory arthritis 208t
Non-invasive ventilation 328
  contraindications for 328
  indications for 328

Non-malignant complications, late onset 306
Non-megaloblastic macrocytic anaemia, causes of 254, 254t
Non-nucleoside reverse transcriptase inhibitors 412
Nonorganic dyspepsia 85
Non-proliferative glomerulonephritis, causes of 230f
Non-receptor tyrosine kinase inhibitors 572
Non-selective beta blockers 135
Non-small cell
  carcinoma 354t
  lung
    cancer, treatment of 355b
    carcinoma 353
Non-ST elevation myocardial infarction 25, 55, 59
Non-steroidal anti-inflammatory drugs 60, 82, 214, 547
Non-surgical therapy 148
Non-thermal measures 80
Non-tranfusion therapy 273
Non-transforming human retrovirus 398
Nontropical sprue 87
Non-tuberculous mycobacteria 336, 337
Nonulcer dyspepsia 85, 86, 86t
Noradrenaline 490
Normal glutamic acid, replacement of 256
Normal-pressure hydrocephalus 583
Normochromic anaemia 263
Normochromic normocytic anaemia 150
Normocytic anaemia 263
Norwalk virus 382
Norwegian scabies 518
Nosocomial pneumonia 335
Nuclear antigens, antibodies against 155
Nuclear enzyme, terminal 286
Nucleated red cells 262f
Nucleic acid
  amplification tests 339, 456
  detection of 424
  sequence-based amplification 377
Numbness 3
Nummular eczema 512
Nutrition and metabolism 470
Nutritional deficiency 347, 462, 487
Nutritional therapy 238
Nystagmus 454

O

Obesity 474, 476t
  causes of 474, 475b
  classes of 475t
Obsessive-compulsive disorder 486
Obstructive sleep apnoea 60, 325, 326t
  clinical features of 326t
  degree of 326
  diagnosis 325
  risk factors for 326t
  treatment 325
  types of 326b
Obstructive ventilator defect 322
Occasional irregularity 36
Occupational lung diseases 356
Octreotide 80
Ocular diseases 409
Odynophagia 407
Oedema 249
  cardiogenic pulmonary 45
  high-altitude pulmonary 556
Oesophageal candidiasis 407
Oesophageal diseases 407
Oesophageal dysmotility 64
Oesophageal lumen 81
Oesophageal spasm, diffuse 34
Oesophageal wall 81
  causes in 81
Oesophagitis 407
Oestrogen 547
Ofloxacin 381
Olanzapine 484
Olaparib 571
Oleander poisoning 564
Oliguria 226
Onartuzumab 571
Oncofetal antigens 569
Oncogenes 568, 568t
  classification of 568
Oncogenic viruses 574
Oncologic emergencies 572, 573t
Oncology 568
Open pneumothorax 362
Ophthalmic complications 61
Ophthalmological manifestations 209
Opsonins 531
Optic neuritis 409
Oral acyclovir 437
Oral cavity 385, 520
Oral corticosteroids 271
Oral glucose tolerance test 190
Oral hypoglycaemic agent 11
Oral iron therapy 250
Oral levothyroxine 14
Oral rehydration solution 22

Oral therapy 122
Oral thrush 385
Organic psychiatry 486
Organophosphate poisoning 26
  treatment of 26t
Organophosphorus 561
Orthostatic syncope 35
Orthotopic liver transplantation 149
Osborn wave 627
Osler's nodes 53
Osler–Weber–Rendu syndrome 524
Osmotic demyelination syndrome 503
Osmotic fragility 259
Osmotic laxatives 78
Osteoarthritis 208, 473, 474
Osteoarthropathy, hypertrophic pulmonary 353
Osteomalacia 471, 473
Osteomyelitis 350
Osteopaenia 473
Osteoporosis 473
Osteosclerotic myeloma 299
Ostium
  primum 69
  secundum defects 69
Ovalocytes 256
Overflow incontinence 585
Oxidation 612
Oxygen therapy 327
  therapaeutic indications for 327t
Oxytetracycline 428

P

Packed red blood cell 392
Packed red cells 303
Packed-cell volume 50, 293
Paget's disease 473, 576
Pain 474
  abdominal 1
Painful crisis, acute 259
Palamnaeus 560
Palliative therapy 283
Pallor 108, 248, 288
Palpitations 2, 34
  causes of 34, 34b
Pancreas
  ductal adenocarcinoma of 167, 168b
  endocrine tumours of 166
  transcription factor 188
Pancreatic and duodenal homeobox 188
Pancreatic cancer 166
Pancreatic disorders 163
Pancreatic endocrine tumors 167t

Pancreatic tumours types 167*fc*
Pancreatitis 34, 125
　autoimmune 166
　　chronic 166
　chronic 164
Pancytopaenia 263, 264*t*, 287
Panic disorder 485
Panitumumab 571
Pansystolic murmurs 39
Paraaminosalicylic acid 340
Paracentesis, large-volume 142
Paracetamol 377
　poisoning 563
Paraesthesia 3
Paralysis 3
Paraneoplastic complications 313
Paraneoplastic syndromes 147, 352, 353*t*, 462, 574, 575*t*
Paranoid schizophrenia 483
Paraplegia, spinal causes of 456, 457*b*
Parasitic infestations 159
Parasomnias 492
　types of 492, 492*t*
Parathyroid hormone 176, 177, 471, 473
　related protein 576
Parenteral iron therapy 250
Parenteral route 113
Parietal cell antibody 251
Parinaud's syndrome 447
Parkinson's disease 583
Parkinsonism 449
　non-motor features of 452*t*
　plus 450
　primary 449
　secondary 450
Paroxysmal nocturnal haemoglobinuria 254, 263, 305
Paroxysmal supraventricular tachycardia 42
Partial agonist 610
Partial seizures 441
Partial thromboplastin time 276
Patent ductus arteriosus 39, 69
Patient's target cells 598
Patrick's test 211
Patterson-Kelly-brown dysphagia 249
Paucibacillary leprosy, treatment of 384
Paul–Bunnell test 373
Pautrier microabscess 523
Peak expiratory flow rate 322
Pediculosis 513, 519
Pediculus humanus
　capitis 519
　humanus 519

Pegvisomant 172
Pel-Ebstein fever, classical 308
Pellagra 471
Pelvic inflammatory disease 371, 422
Pembrolizumab 571
Pemphigus vulgaris 519
Pendular knee jerk 454
Penicillins 371, 533
Peptic ulcer disease 82
Peramivir 331
Percutaneous coronary intervention 25, 28, 56, 59
Percutaneous transhepatic cholangiography 106, 110
Pericardial effusion 68
Pericarditis 34, 48, 626
　acute 68
　chronic constrictive 68
Perihepatitis, acute 422
Perinephric abscesses 371
Periodic acid Schiff 90, 286
Peripheral arteries 53
Peripheral blood 157, 252, 299, 313
　film 259, 261
　investigations of 309*t*
　smear 262*f*, 263*f*, 277, 283, 290
Peripheral cyanosis 35
Peripheral destruction 264*t*
Peripheral nerves 253
Peripheral nervous system, demyelinating diseases of 457
Peripheral neuropathy 461
　types of 461, 462
Peripheral smear 252, 255, 260, 266, 279, 288, 296, 298
　examination 255
　sickle cell 256
Periportal fibrosis 392
Peritoneal dialysis 236
　continuous cycling 236
Peritoneum, inflammation of 139
Pernicious anaemia 251
Persistent ductus arteriosus 69
Persistent hypotension 44
Persistent juvenile 626*t*
Persistent vomiting 77
Pertussis 380
Phaeochromocytoma 180
Phagocyte disorders 538
Pharmacodynamic 610
　interaction 613
Pharmacogenetics 591, 612
Pharmacokinetic interaction 612, 612*t*
Pharmacotherapy 181
Phenothiazines 450
Phenylketonuria 475

Phenytoin 437, 462, 546
Philadelphia chromosome 280, 288, 296
Phlebotomus argentipes 388
Phobic disorders 485, 486
Phosphate binders 238
Phosphorus 195
Phthirus pubis 422
Physical abuse 586
Physiological levels, normal 544*t*
Pica 249
Pituitary gigantism 171
Pityriasis
　alba 518
　rotunda 576
　versicolor 521
Pityrosporum 512
　ovale 521
Pizotifen 439
Pizza pie 409
Plague 378
　clinical features 378
　diagnosis 379
　treatment 379
Plantar warts 519
Plasma 498, 498*t*
　biomarkers, characteristics of 58*t*
　cell
　　dyscrasias 298
　　proliferative disorders, classification of 298*t*
　enzymes 57
　exchange 276
　fibrinogen 279
　protease enzyme 275
　volume, expansion of 263
Plasmapheresis 271, 302
Plaster of Paris casts 513
Platelet 252, 288, 293
　concentrate 276, 303
　contraindication of 303*t*
　indications of 303*t*
　count 267, 268, 268*t*, 270, 272, 274, 276, 279, 282, 296
　disorders 267
　function disorders, classification of 269*t*
　transfusions 271
Pleiotropy 596
Pleural aspiration 358
Pleural effusion 357, 358
　causes of 358*t*
　classification of 358*t*
　diagnosis of 361*fc*
　management of 358
Pleural fluid parameters 359*t*
Pleural transudate, light's criteria for distinguishing 360*b*

Pleurisy 34
Pleuritic pain, treatment of 332
Pleuropulmonary manifestations 209
Plummer–Vinson syndrome 249
Pluripotent haematopoietic stem-cell 287
Pneumococcus 358
Pneumocystis Jirovecii infection 405
  management of 406, 407*t*
Pneumocystosis 405
Pneumonia 34, 331, 350, 501
  acute eosinophilic 336
  bacterial 358
  classification of 331*b*
  clinical features 332
  general complications of 332*b*
  hospital-acquired 335, 336*b*
  idiopathic interstitial 407
  investigations 332
  primary 332*t*
  secondary 379
  slow-resolving 335*t*
  treatment of 332, 335*t*
  unresolved 335
Pneumonic plague 379
Pneumonitis, hypersensitivity 344, 346*t*
Pneumothorax 34, 360
  aetiology 360
  classification of 361*fc*
  clinical features 360
  physical signs 360
  treatment 362
  types of 362
Podophyllin 519
POEMS syndrome 299
Poison 3
  from gut, removing unabsorbed 558
Poisoning, treatment of 558
Poisonous snakes 559
Poly ADP ribose polymerase 571, 572
Polyarteritis nodosa 217, 232, 462, 571
Polyarthritis 47
  acute 209
  chronic 209
Polycystic kidney disease 242
Polycystic ovary syndrome 474
Polycythaemia 292, 294*t*, 462
  classification of 292*b*
  primary 292
  secondary 292, 295, 295*t*, 347
  vera 293, 295
    features of 295*t*
Polydipsia 5
Polyendocrinopathy 188

Polymorphisms 596
Polymyalgia rheumatica 216
Polymyositis 216, 216*t*
Polyneuropathy 298
  causes of 461, 462*b*
  classification of 461, 462*b*
  generalised symmetrical 199
Polypharmacy 586
Polyploidy 592
Polyuria 5, 226
Pompholyx 512
Poorly absorbed antibiotics 137
Porphyria, acute intermittent 462
Portal hypertension 128, 130, 139
  classification of 130, 130*f*
  clinical consequences of 131*f*
  clinical features of 131*t*
  complications of 131*b*
  sequelae 128
  treatment of 132*b*
Portal systemic shunts, types of 135
Portal vein 150
Portal venous pressure 133
  measurement of 132
Portopulmonary hypertension 149
Portosystemic encephalopathy 135*b*, 136
Portosystemic shunts, complications of 135
Positive end-expiratory pressure 327, 329
Positive-pressure ventilation 501
Positron emission tomography 310
Post-exposure prophylaxis regimens 417*t*
Post-hypoxic brain injury 453
Postinfectious glomerulonephritis 229
Post-remission therapy 285
Post-streptococcal glomerulonephritis 229
Postural syncope 35
Postural tremor 454
Potassium 195
  chloride 503
  inwardly-rectifying channel 188
  sparing diuretics 63
Prader–Willi syndrome 596
Pralidoxime 26
Praziquantel 392
Prediabetes 190
Prednisolone 216
Prednisone 311
Predominant cells 288
Predominantly unconjugated hyperbilirubinaemia 107
Pre-eclamptic toxaemia 60
Pregnancy 545
  hepatic disorders of 545

Premature ventricular complexes 624
Priapism 288, 560
Prinzmetal's angina 55
Probenecid 428
Procaine penicillin 428
Procarbazine 311
Prochlorperazine 439
Prodromal symptoms 386
Profuse sweating 560
Progeria 524
Prognostic classifications 128
Prokinetic agents 78
Prolapsed rectum 380
Proliferative glomerulonephritis, causes of 230*f*
Prolonged fever, causes of 371
Prophylactic measures, primary 135
Prophylaxis 111
  pre-exposure 417
  secondary 135, 449
Propionibacterium acnes 515
Propranolol 14, 135, 439
Propylthiouracil 14
Prostaglandin analogues 83
Prostate 226
Prosthetic valve endocarditis 52
Protease inhibitors 412, 572
Protein 86, 138
  derivative, purified 366
  energy malnutrition 474
    complications of 474
  large precursor 399
  loss, consequences of 233
  mature 399
  specific 569
Proteinuria 226, 227*fc*
Prothrombin time 115, 272, 276, 279
Proton-pump inhibitor 80, 83, 84
Prototype disorder 534
Protozoal agents 422
Protozoal infections 405
Providing supportive care 266
Provirus 398
Pruritus 6, 513
  dermatological causes of 513*b*
  systemic causes of 513*b*
Pseudomembranous colitis 92
Pseudomonas aeruginosa 405
Psoriasis 513
  types of 514, 514*b*
Psoriatic arthritis 211
Psychiatric disease 409
Psychiatric manifestations 153
Psychiatric problems 491
Psychiatry 481
Psychological abuse 586

Psychological problems 491
Psychosis 481t, 487t
Pthirus pubis 519
Public louse 519
Pulmonary angiography 66
Pulmonary arterial hypertension 64
Pulmonary capillary pressure 45
Pulmonary component 38
Pulmonary embolism 34, 66, 626
  clinical features of 66
Pulmonary function tests 65, 321, 322b, 322t, 347
Pulmonary hypertension 62, 65, 347
  aetiology of 62, 64b
  classification of 62, 64b
  owing 64
  signs of 62
Pulmonary infarction 66, 327
  clinical features of 66
Pulmonary manifestations 356
Pulmonary oedema 45
  types of 45b
Pulmonary sarcoidosis, classic radiographic patterns of 357
Pulmonary stenosis 70
Pulmonary tuberculosis 337, 405
  complications of 337, 338t
  primary 336
Pulmonology 321
Pulse 50, 248
  character of 36, 37b
  clinical examination of 35, 36b
  Doppler sonography 146
  quality of 36, 37b
Pulsus alternans 37b
Pulsus bigeminus 37b
Pulsus paradoxus 37b
Pulsus parvus 37b
  et tardus 37b
Pulsus tardus 37b
Punch–Drunk syndrome 450
Pure motor syndrome 450
Pure red-cell aplasia 248
Pure sensory syndrome 450
Purkinje network 617
Pyelonephritis 243
  acute 228
  chronic 229
Pyoderma gangrenosum 576
Pyogenic meningitis 454, 455
Pyrazinamide 340
Pyrexia of unknown origin 371, 372t
  causes of 371t
Pyrophosphate arthropathy 219

Q

Q fever 385
Q waves 626
QRS complex 626
Quadruple therapy 84
Qualitative defects 274
Qualitative platelets defects 269
Quantitative deficiency 274
Quaternary syphilis 426
Quetiapine 484
Quinolones 340

R

Radiation effects
  classification of 554, 555f
  types of 554, 555f
Radiation exposure 554
Radiation injury 145
Radioactive 295
  iodine 174
    uptake 173
Radiofemoral delay 37
Radiofrequency ablation 42, 148
Radioimmunotherapy 572
Radiological examination 296, 300
Radiotherapy 301
Rai staging, clinical staging features of 291, 291t
Raltegravir 412
Ramsay Hunt syndrome 437
  aetiology 437
  clinical features 437
  treatment 437
Ranson criteria 164, 164b
Rapid eye movement 491, 492
Rapid plasma regain 427
Rapidly progressive glomerulonephritis, causes of 231, 231t
Rare sites 308
Rash 3
Raymond–Cestan syndrome 447
Raynaud phenomenon 64
Receptor tyrosine kinase inhibitors 572
Reciprocal translocation 287f
Recombinant tissue plasminogen activator 55, 59
Rectal stasis 77
Recurrent silent pulmonary embolism 66
Recurrent spontaneous pneumothorax 363

Recurrent variceal bleeding 135
Red blood cell 240, 248, 250, 252, 262, 277, 288, 392
  disorders 305
  saline-washed 304
Red cell 293
  concentrates 303
  count 293
  destruction 249
  distribution 250
    width 260
  enzyme deficiencies 254
  indices 252
  membrane, defects in 254
  production, impaired 248
  transfusion 251
Reduce proteinuria, measures to 233
Reed–Sternberg cell 307
Reflex epilepsy 441
Reflux nephropathy 229
Reflux oesophagitis 34, 80
Refractory anaemia 297
  with excess blasts 297
Refractory ascites, treatment of 142
Refractory cough 556
Refractory cytopaenia 297
Regional lymphadenopathy 424
Rehydration 15, 79
Reitan's number connection test 136
Reiter's syndrome 211
Relative polycythaemia 292
Remission induction 284
Remission maintenance 284
Renal biopsy 241
Renal complications 61
Renal cyst infection 243
Renal damage 299
Renal disease, end stage 198, 234
Renal failure 125
  chronic 238b, 453, 504
Renal function 300
  test 30
Renal imaging 241
Renal losses 499t
Renal manifestations 176
Renal replacement therapies 235, 241, 238t
  types of 235
Renal rickets 472
Renal syndromes 576
Renal transplantation 236
Renal tubular acidosis 241, 243fc
  types of 241, 241t

Renin inhibitors, direct 63
Repeated transfusions 258
Reperfusion therapy 45
Replacement therapy, indications of 273
Reproductive system 237
Reserpine 450
Residual volume 323, 324
Resistant rickets 472
Respiratory acidosis 506
　causes of 506*t*
Respiratory alkalosis 506
　causes of 506, 506*t*
Respiratory causes 321
Respiratory disease 489
Respiratory failure 125, 323, 325*t*, 347, 350, 453
　types of 324
Respiratory infections 407
Respiratory syndrome, severe acute 331
Respiratory system 237, 405, 473
Rest tremor 453
Restless leg syndrome 492
Restlessness 560
Restrictive ventilator defect 322
Resuscitation, cardiopulmonary 23
Reticulocyte count 250, 252
Reticuloendothelial system 531
Retinal haemorrhage, high-altitude 556
Retinal migraine 438
Retinal-neurocutaneous cavernous haemangioma syndrome 524
Retinoic acid 546
Retinopathy 409
　hypertensive 61
Retroviral genome 398
Reye's syndrome 126, 438
Reynolds pentad 111
Rheumatic fever 47
　prophylaxis 49
　prevention of 49
Rheumatoid arthritis 208, 209, 462
Rheumatoid vasculitis 209
Rhodococcus equi 407
Rhythm, types of 35, 36*b*
Rib fracture 34
Ribavirin 331
Ribonucleic acid 116
Rickets 471, 473
　drug-induced 472
　rosary 471
　secondary 472
　types of 471, 472*t*
Rickettsia 515
Rickettsial diseases 385, 385*t*
　treatment 385

Rickettsialpox 385
Rifampicin 340
Rifle criteria 238*t*
Right atrium 617
Right ventricular
　failure 47
　hypertrophy 70, 630
　causes of 630
Rilpivirine 413
Ring chromosomes 593
Ring sideroblasts 297
Risperidone 453, 484
Ritonavir 331, 393, 412, 413
Rituximab 266, 271, 276, 302, 571
Rivastigmine 583
Rizatriptan 439
Robertsonian translocation 592
Rocky mountain spotted fever 385
Romano-Ward syndrome 629
Romhilt-Estes score 631*t*
Rotavirus 382
Roth's spots 53
Rothmund-Thomson syndrome 524
Rotor syndrome 111
Rubella 372
　congenital 372
　syndrome 372
Rubeola 372
Rucaparib 571
Rye classification, histological type of 307*t*

S

Saber shin 427
Saddle nose deformity 426
Safety pin appearance 379
Saint vitus' dance 47
Salbutamol 322
Salicylate 48
　poisoning 498, 562
Saline, normal 30
Salivary glands 357
Salivation 560, 561
Salmonella 408, 515
　enterica serovar typhi 380
　enteritidis 382
　infections 405
　typhi 380
SAPHO syndrome 515
Saquinavir 412, 413
Sarcoidosis 356, 462
　clinical features 356
　extrapulmonary investigations of 357*t*
　radiological features of 357
Sarcopaenia 586

Sarcoptes scabiei 422
Scabies 513, 518
Scalp
　area 512
　dermatophytosis 521
Schistocytes 276
Schistosoma mansoni 391
Schistosomiasis 391
Schizophrenia 481-483
　acute 482
　catatonic 483
　clinical features 481
　diagnosis of 482*b*
　management 482
　symptoms of 482*t*
　types of 481, 482*b*
　undifferentiated type 483
Schizophrenic disorders, types of 483*b*
Schneider's 11 first rank symptoms of schizophrenia 482*b*
Sclera 107
Sclerodactyly 64
Sclerosing cholangitis 144, 156
Sclerosis, amyotrophic lateral 459, 501
Sclerotherapy, complications of 134*b*
Screening assays 279
Scrotal oedema 390
Scrub typhus 385
Scurvy 470
　types of 470, 470*t*
Sea snakes 559
Seborrhoeic eczema 512
Second heart sound 38, 38*b*
Second-degree heart block 44, 628
Secretory products 91
Seizure 2, 438
　causes of 441, 441*b*
　complex
　　absent 440
　　partial 441
　disorders 545
　focal 441
　secondary generalised 441
Selective serotonin reuptake inhibitor 483, 490, 501, 559
Selegiline 583
Sensorimotor syndrome 450
Sensory problems 452
Sepsis 390
　management of 391
　risk factors for 391*t*
　severity of 391*f*
Septic shock 45
　bundle 392
Septicaemia 350, 452

Septicaemic plague 379
Serologic tests 48
Serological markers 129
Serological tests 151, 424
   sensitivity of 427*t*
Serotonin specific reuptake
   inhibitors 559
Serotonin syndrome 559
Sertraline 436
Serum 498, 498*t*
   albumin 104
   alkaline phosphatase 300, 357
   ascites albumin gradient 138,
      140
   bilirubin 102, 150
      level, normal 107
   blood urea nitrogen 240
   ceruloplasmin levels 153
   copper 153
   creatinine concentration 240
   electrolytes 129
   enzymes 102
   ferritin 152
      raised 266
   globulins 104
   iron 152
      profile 152, 251*t*
      reduced 266
   markers 148
   methylmalonic acid 253*t*
   onstructural protein 377
   proteins 300
   sickness 534
   uric acid 294, 300
   vitamin B12 294, 296
   β2-microglobulin 300
Sex chromosomes, numerical
   abnormalities of 592
Sexual abuse 586
Sexually transmitted
   disease 422, 428
   infection 422*b*, 428
Sézary syndrome, diagnosis of 523
Sheehan's syndrome 171
Shigella 408
   species 422
Shock 44, 45*t*, 533
   anaphylactic 45
   cardinal features of 44
   hypovolaemic 45
   management of 17, 18*fc*, 44
   treatment of 18*fc*
   type of 45
Shunts 142
Sick sinus syndrome 43, 622
Sickle cell
   anaemia 256, 256*t*, 258*f*
      pathogenesis of 258*f*
   trait 256

Sickle solubility test 256
Sickling test 256
Sideroblastic anaemia 263, 264
   characteristics of 264*t*
Sideropenic dysphagia 249
Signal transducing proteins 568
Simple partial seizures 441
Sinoatrial blocks 40
Sinoatrial node 617
Sinus
   bradycardia 621
   mechanism, disturbances of 40
   pause 622
   rhythm 621
   tachycardia 622
   venosus defects 69
      superior 69
Sinusitis 329
Sjögren's syndrome 210, 462, 513
Sjögren–Larsson syndrome 524
Skeletal abnormalities 426
Skeletal manifestations 176
Skin 6, 267, 357, 405
   and mucous membranes, bluish
      discolouration of 34
   changes 298
   infection of 385
   involvement 383
   lesions 510*f*, 511*f*, 520
      primary 510
      secondary 510
   malignancies 522
   rashes 425
   yellowish pigmentation of 107
Sleep apnoea, types of 326
Sleep disorders 491
   primary 491
   secondary 491
Sleep paralysis 491
Sleep related xerostomia 513
Sleep studies 65
Sleeping sickness 392
Slit-lamp examination 153
Small cell carcinoma, treatment of
   354, 355*t*
Small duct obstruction 108
Small fibre polyneuropathy 461
Smoking cessation 489
Snake antivenom 559
Snakebite 16
   management of 16
Sodium
   bicarbonate 559
   fractional excretion of 240
   ipodate 14
   nitroprusside 21
   oxybate 492
Sore throat 47, 401
Speech disturbance 6

Spherocytes 259
Spherocytosis, hereditary 259
Spinal cord 253
   diseases 456
Spirochaete *Treponema pallidum*
   424
Spirometry interpretation 324*t*
Splanchnic vasodilation 139
Spleen 53, 269, 357, 405
Splenectomy 259, 261, 266, 271,
   276, 290
Splenic irradiation 296
Splenic marginal zone lymphoma
   311
Splenic vein occlusion 130
Splenomegaly
   causes of 159, 159*t*
   moderate 160
   treatment of 296
Splenoportovenography 157
Split livers 149
Spontaneous bacterial peritonitis
   142
Spontaneous bleeding 4
Sporadic ataxias 454
Spotted fever group 385
Sputum examination 337
Squamous cell carcinoma 522, 523
ST elevation myocardial infarction
   55, 59
St Louis encephalitis 375
ST segment
   depression, causes of 632
   elevation, causes of 632
Stable angina, management of 56*fc*
Staccato speech 454
Staphylococcus 358, 518
   aureus 52, 332, 366, 382, 405, 454
Starry sky appearance 315*f*
Static tremor 453
Statins 19
Status asthmaticus 342, 343
Status epilepticus 442
   management of 15
   treatment of 442, 443*b*
Stavudine 412
Steatohepatitis 144
   alcoholic 126
Steatorrhoea 156
Steatosis 126
   acute 144
   alcoholic 126
Stem cell
   differentiation of 248
   disorders, acquired 282
   disturbed proliferation of 248
   therapy 304
      clinical application of 305*t*
   transplantation 266, 290

Step-Ladder pattern 380
Sterile pyuria 422
  causes of 228b
Sternal tenderness 288
Steroids 156, 267
Stevens–Johnson syndrome 516, 517
Still's disease, adult-onset 210
Stimulant laxatives 78
Stokes–Adams–Morgagni attacks 44
Stool softeners 78
Streptococcal antibody tests 48
Streptococcus 358, 518
  pneumoniae 332
  pyogenes 366
Streptomycin 340, 379
Stress
  disorder, post-traumatic 486
  incontinence 585
  myocardial perfusion scanning 55
  ulcers, aetiology of 82
Stroke
  classification of 444fc, 445, 445t
  clinical features of 447t
  haemorrhagic 442
Structural disease 77
Sturge–Weber syndrome 524
Subacute combined degeneration 458
Subcutaneous nodules 47
Subfulminant hepatic failure 123
Subphrenic abscess, rupture of 358
Subtertian malaria 386
Subvalvular aortic stenosis 51
Sucralfate 84
Sucrose haemolysis test 265
Sudden cardiac death 43
  causes of 43b
Sulphonamides 371, 388
Sulphonylures 194
Sumatriptan 439
Sunburn 513
Supravalvular aortic stenosis 51
Supraventricular tachycardia 623
Surgical portosystemic shunting 135
Surgical therapy 20
Sweet's syndrome 576
Swimmer's itch 391
Swine flu 330
  diagnosis 330
  treatment 330
Sydenham's chorea 47, 452
Sympathomimetic amines 45
Symptomatic bacteriuria 227
Symptomatic disease 426
Symptomatic icteric phase 114
Synchronised cardioversion 42

Synchronised intermittent mandatory ventilation 329
Syncope 34
  cardiac 35
  drug-induced 35
  types of 34, 35b
Syndrome of inappropriate antidiuresis hormone 500, 502f
  secretion 501
Syphilis 409, 424
  acquired 425
  benign tertiary 426
  cardiovascular 426
  classification of 425, 425b
  early congenital 426
  latent 426
  management of 428t
  primary 425
  secondary 425
  untreated 427t
Syphilitic periostitis 426
Syringomyelia 457
Systemic diseases associated with malabsorption 86
Systemic disorders 327
Systemic inflammatory response syndrome 391
Systemic lupus erythematosus 88, 212, 213b, 214fc, 230, 232, 233, 274, 305, 327, 462, 474, 490, 535, 571
Systemic sclerosis 215
Systemic to pulmonary communication 40
Systemic to right heart connection 40

T

T cell
  depletion, mechanism of 403
  disorders 538
  origin 290
  significant depletion of 401
T wave 626, 626t
Tabes dorsalis 426
Tachycardia 36, 533, 552
  causes of 621, 621t
  wide-complex 40
Tachycardic rhythm 623
Tacrine 583
Tamponade, cardiac 68
Tapping apex 37
Target cells 256
Tear drop-shaped red cells 296
Telangiectasia 64
Telbivudine 122
Temporal arteritis 217, 462

Tender hepatomegaly, causes of 159, 159b
Tenofovir 122, 412
Tension pneumothorax 13, 362, 362t, 363
  management of 13f
Testicular involvement 286
Tetany 177
  causes of 177b
  control of 177
Tetracycline 424, 438, 521, 546
Tetralogy of Fallot 40, 70
Thalassaemia 260
  trait 264
Thalassaemic facies 260
Thalidomide 546
Therapeutic applications 598
Therapeutic index 610
Therapeutic procedure 106
Therapeutic radiation 281
Thermal measures 80
Thevetia peruviana 564
Thiacetazone 340
Thiamine 470
Thiazide diuretics 63
Thiazolidinedione 194
Third heart sound 38, 39b
Third-degree heart block 628
Third-line therapy 271
Thoracentesis 366
Thrombectomy, endovascular mechanical 19
Thrombin time 279
Thrombocytopaenia 267, 282
  autoimmune 266
  causes of 268t
Thrombocytosis 271, 309
  causes of 271t
Thromboembolism 545
Thrombolysis 20, 58
Thrombolytic agents 58
Thrombolytic therapy 58, 59, 67, 449
Thrombopoietin 271
Thrombosis 265, 278
Thrombotic episodes 293
Thrombotic thrombocytopaenia purpura 274, 275
  aetiology of 275f
  pathogenesis of 275f
Thyroid
  cancer 287
  disorders 172, 544
  function tests 172
  peroxidase antibodies 175
  stimulating hormone 172, 173, 175, 544t
  storm 14, 174
Thyrotoxic crisis 14, 174

Thyrotoxicosis 172, 172b
Thyrotropin-releasing hormone 171
Tianeptine 490
Tic 453
  douloureux 437
Tidal volume 323
Tinea
  barbae 521
  corporis 521
  cruris 521
  pedis 521
  unguium 521
  versicolor 521
Tipranavir 412, 413
Titubation 454
Tobacco use, complications of 487, 489b
Tocilizumab 393
Todd's palsy 441
Tongue thickening, sensation of 560
Tonic-clonic seizures 440
Topiramate 439
Torsades de pointes 41, 623
Total cholesterol 183
Total homocysteine 253
Total iron binding capacity 152
  reduced 266
Total leucocyte count 282, 286, 288, 296, 309
Total lung capacity 323, 324
Tourette syndrome 453
Tourniquet test 270, 274
Toxic 143
  epidermal necrolysis 516, 517
  gas, inhalation of 327
  hepatitis, direct 143
  substances 135b
Toxicity, clinical manifestations of 563
Toxicology 558
Toxidrome 558, 558t
Toxin 381, 462
  excretion of 558
  induced gastroenteritis 78
Toxoplasma 409, 411
  gondii 388, 409
Toxoplasmosis 388
  clinical manifestations 388
  diagnosis 388
  management 388
  transmission 388
Tracheal stenosis 329
Tracheomalacia 329
Traizoles 521
Trans arterial embolisation 148
Transaminases 102

Transarterial chemoembolisation 148
Transcriptase inhibitor, nucleotide reverse 412
Transforming growth factor 346, 576
Transient cholinergic hyperactivity 560
Transient ischaemic attack 183, 442, 583
  signs 442
  symptoms 442
Transient ST segment elevation 55
Transjugular intrahepatic portosystemic shunt 24, 133, 134
Transjugular portosystemic stent shunts 135
Transplacental transmission 425
Transverse myelitis 373, 456
  causes 456
Trastuzumab 571
Trauma 163, 462
  to liver 145
Traveller's diarrhoea 90
Trazodone 490
Treat underlying disease, measures to 234
Tremors 453
Trench fever 385
Treponema pallidum
  haemagglutination test 302
  particle agglutination 427
Triatomine bugs 392
Trichomonas vaginalis 422
Trichophyton 521
Tricuspid regurgitation 39
Tricyclic antidepressants 453, 490, 559
Trigeminal neuralgia 437
  clinical features 437
  treatment 437
Triggering agent, removal of 261
Triglycerides 188
Triiodothyronine 14
Trilineage 293
Trimethoprim 424
  sulphamethoxazole 533
Tropheryma whipplei 90
Tropical pancreatitis 166
Tropical pulmonary eosinophilia 336
Trousseau syndrome 576
Trousseau's sign 177, 279
Truncal neuropathy 34
Trypanosoma brucei gambiense 392

Trypanosoma cruzi 392
Trypanosomiasis 392
Tsetse fly 392
Tuberculin test 337
Tuberculoid leprosy 383
Tuberculosis 336, 339, 339b, 361, 371, 501, 535
  chemoprophylaxis 341
  extrapulmonary 339
  meningitis 409, 437, 456
  post-primary 337
Tuberous sclerosis 524
  complex 525t
Tumour 144
  benign epithelial 351
  induced rickets 472
  infiltration 301
  lysis
    mechanism of 574f
    syndrome 573
  malignant 266, 522
  markers 568
    common 569t
  necrosis factor 339, 535, 576
  primary 352t
  suppressor genes 568, 569t
  uncommon malignant 522
Turner syndrome 597
Typhoid 371, 380, 516
  clinical features 380
  complications of 380
  diagnosis 380
  fever 381t
  treatment 381
Typhus group 385
Typical antipsychotic 490
Tyrosine kinases 572

U

U wave 618, 627
  prominent 627
Ulcer 93
  dyspepsia 86, 86t
Ulceration 4
Ulcerative colitis 93, 97, 97t
Ultrasound elastography 105
Uncertain significance, monoclonal gammopathy of 301
Undulant fever 392
Unfractionated heparin 55, 59
Unilineage dysplasia 297
Upper gastrointestinal
  bleed 24
    management of 24fc
  scopy 131
Upper motor neuron 433t, 459, 465

Upper respiratory tract infection 230
Uraemia
  signs of 237t
  symptoms of 237t
Uraemic acidosis 498
Ureaplasma urealyticum 422
Ureter 226
Urethra 226
Urge incontinence 585
Urgent endoscopy 132
Uric acid levels, measurement of 314
Urinalysis 240
Urinary copper 153
Urinary incontinence 435, 585
Urinary sodium 500
Urinary system 237
Urinary tract infection 227, 371, 477
  clinical features of 228b
  complicated 228
  types of 228t
  uncomplicated 228
Urinary urobilinogen 108
Urine 115, 124, 276, 277, 300
  no bilirubin in 108
  osmolality 240
  sodium excretion 240
  tests 105
  turns dark yellow 108
  urobilinogen 105
Urobilinogen 105
  excretion of 158
  reabsorption of 158
Ursodeoxycholic acid 156
Urticaria 532
Uveitis 409

V

Vacuolar myelopathy 408
Vagal manoeuvres 42
Vagina 384, 385
Vaginal candidiasis 386
Valproate 439
  sodium 438
Valvular aortic stenosis 51
Van den Bergh reaction 158
Vanishing bile duct syndrome 144
Variceal banding 133
Variceal bleeding 132
  prevention of 134
Varicella 373
  zoster virus 405
Vascular dementia 583
Vascular disorders 144, 267
Vascular endothelial growth factor 571, 572

Vascular liver disease 145
Vascular obstruction, site of 130f
Vascular phenomena 53
Vasculitis 217, 462
  classification of 217f
  granulomatous 218
Vasoconstrictor therapy 132, 133
Vasopressin 80
Vasovagal syncope 35
Venereal disease research laboratory 302, 427
Venesection 294
Venezuelan encephalitis 375
Venlafaxine 486, 490
Venography, hepatic 146
Veno-occlusive disease 146
Venous obstruction 139
Venous thrombosis 145, 556, 576
  sites of 65
  treatment of 215
Ventilation-perfusion scanning 65
Ventilatory capacity 321
Ventricles, disturbance of 40
Ventricular activation time 626
Ventricular cells 617
Ventricular depolarisation 617
  axis of 626
Ventricular fibrillation 23, 622
  management of 22, 23fc
Ventricular hypertrophy 626
Ventricular septal defect 39, 69, 625
Ventricular tachycardia 23, 40, 41b, 623
Verner–Morrison syndrome 167
Verruca
  plana 519
  plantaris 519
  vulgaris 519
Vertebrobasilar territory 443
Vertigo 6
Vessels, invasion of 148
Vincristine 311, 462
Vipers 559
Viraemia 401, 403
Viral diseases 401
Viral enzymes, three 398
Viral genome 112, 400
Viral glycoproteins 399
Viral hepatitis 117t
  aetiology of 111t
  clinical features of 113, 114b
  investigations for 115t
  serological markers for 114, 116t
Viral infection 405
  direct detection of 410
Viral replication 401
  high levels of 112
Virus 282

particle 401
specific antibodies, detection of 410
type of 574
Visceral leishmaniasis 387
Viscus, rupture of 139
Visual impairment 171
Vital capacity 323, 324
Vital signs 558
Vitamin 3, 86
  A 470
  B12 294
    deficiency 251, 252, 252t, 253
  C 470
  D 176, 471
    deficiency 474b
    physiology of 471, 472f
    role of 473t
  deficiency 581
  E 583
  K deficiency 274
Vitiligo 517
Vomiting 560
von Hippel–Lindau disease 524
von Willebrand factor 274
  assay 274
von Willebrand's disease 273, 304

W

Waardenburg syndrome 524
Waldenström macroglobulinaemia 301
Warfarin 547
Warts 519
  common 519
  flat 519
Washer women's skin 381
Water-borne infection 113
Water-hammer pulse 37
Waterhouse–Friderichsen syndrome 180, 279
Water-soluble bilirubin diglucuronide 158
Watery diarrhoea 167
Weber's syndrome 447
Wegener's granulomatosis 218, 226
Weight loss 6
Weil syndrome 384
Wellcome classification 474
Wellens syndrome 626
Wells probability score 66
Wells scoring system 66
Werner syndrome 524
Wernicke's encephalopathy 471
Weskamp–Cotlier syndrome 524
West nile encephalitis 375
Western equine encephalitis 375
Wet drowning 554
Wheeze 389

Whipple's disease 90
White blood cell 240, 288, 311, 336, 522
 count 298
 disorders 305
Whooping cough 380
Wide fixed splitting 38
Wide mobile split 38
Willis-Ekbom disease 492
Wilson's disease 153, 450
Winterbottom sign 392
Wiskott-Aldrich syndrome 311
Wolff-Parkinson-White syndrome 42, 625
Woltman's sign 174
World Health Organisation 383
 classification 281*f*, 307*t*
Wound botulism 379
Wuchereria 336
 bancrofti 390
Wyburn-Mason syndrome 524

X

Xeroderma pigmentosum 524
Xerosis 513
Xerostomia 512
X-linked dominant diseases 594, 595
X-linked recessive disorders 596*t*

Y

Yellow fever 375
Yersinia 515
 pestis 378
Y-linked diseases 595

Z

Zalcitabine 412*b*
Zanamivir 331
Zidovudine 412*b*
Zollinger-Ellison syndrome 84, 87, 167
Zoonotic disease 113